# COMPLETE GUIDE TO PRESCRIPTION & NON-PRESCRIPTION

# DRUGS

By H. WINTER GRIFFITH, M.D.

Technical consultants:
John D. Palmer, M.D., Ph.D.
William N. Jones, B.S., M.S.

## NEW!

Revised for 1988
NOW INCLUDES
over 5000 Brand Names
over 550 Generic Names

## The Body Press

THE BODY PRESS
A division of Price Stern Sloan, Inc.
360 North La Cienega Boulevard
Los Angeles, California 90048


Library of Congress Cataloging-in-Publication Data

Griffith, H. Winter (Henry Winter), 1926-    )
  **Complete guide to prescription and non-prescription
drugs.**

  Includes index.
  1. Drugs—Popular works. 2. Drugs, Nonprescription—
Popular works. I. Title. II. Title: Complete guide
to prescription and non-prescription drugs. [DNLM:
1. Drugs—popular works. 2. Drugs, Non-Prescription—
popular works.   QV 55 G853c]
RM301.15.G75    1988    615'.1    87-25596
ISBN 0-89586-594-7
ISBN 0-89586-593-9 (pbk.)


©1983, 1985, 1987, 1988    HPBooks, Inc.
Printed in U.S.A.
Fifth Edition.

# CONTENTS

# ABOUT THE AUTHOR

H. Winter Griffith has authored several medical books, including the *Complete Guide to Symptoms, Illness & Surgery* and *Complete Guide to Sports Injuries,* both published by The Body Press. Others are *Instructions for Patients, Drug Information for Patients, Instructions for Dental Patients, Information and Instructions for Pediatric Patients* and *Pediatrics for Parents.* Dr. Griffith received his medical degree from Emory University in 1953. After 20 years in private practice, he established a basic medical-science program at Florida State University. He then became an associate professor of family and community medicine at the University of Arizona College of Medicine.

## Technical Consultants

**John D. Palmer, M.D., Ph.D.**
    Associate professor of pharmacology, University of Arizona College of Medicine
    Associate professor of medicine (clinical pharmacology), University of Arizona
      College of Medicine

**William N. Jones, Pharmacist, B.S., M.S.**
    Clinical pharmacy coordinator, Veterans Administration Medical Center, Tucson,
      Arizona
    Adjunct assistant professor, Department of Pharmacy Practice, College of
      Pharmacy, University of Arizona

# DRUGS AND YOU

My first day of pharmacology class in medical school started with a jolt. The professor began by writing on the blackboard, "Drugs are poisons."

I thought the statement was extreme. New drug discoveries promised to solve medical problems that had baffled men for centuries. The medical community was intrigued with new possibilities for drugs.

In the 30 years since then, many drug "miracles" have lived up to those early expectations. But the years have also shown the damage drugs can cause when they are misused or not fully understood.

As a family doctor and teacher, I have developed a healthy respect for what drugs can and can't do. I now appreciate my professor's warning.

A drug cannot "cure." It aids the body's natural defenses to promote recovery.

Likewise, a manufacturer or doctor cannot guarantee a drug will be useful for everyone. The complexity of the human body, individual responses in different people and in the same person under different circumstances, past and present health, age and sex influence how well a drug works.

All effective drugs produce desirable changes in the body, but a drug can also cause undesirable adverse reactions or side effects in some people.

Despite uncertainties, the drug discoveries of the last 40 years have given us tools to save lives and reduce discomfort.

Before you decide whether to take a drug, you or your doctor must ask, "Will the benefits outweigh the risks?"

The purpose of this book is to give you enough information about the most widely used drugs so you can make a wise decision. The information will alert you to potential or preventable problems. You can learn what to do if problems arise.

The information is derived from several expert sources. Every effort has been made to ensure accuracy and completeness. When information from different sources conflicts, I have used the majority's opinion, coupled with my clinical judgment and that of my technical consultants. Drug information changes with continuing observations by clinicians and users.

Information in this book applies to generic drugs in both the United States and Canada. Generic names do not vary in these countries, but brand names do.


# BE SAFE! TELL YOUR DOCTOR

Some suggestions for wise drug use apply to all drugs. Always give the following information to your physician, dentist or other health-care professional. They must have complete information to prescribe drugs safely for you. This information includes your medical history, your medical plans and progress while under medication.

## MEDICAL HISTORY

Tell the important facts of your medical history dealing with drugs. Include allergic or adverse reactions you have had to any medicine in the past. Name the allergic symptoms you have, such as hay fever, asthma, eye watering and itching, throat irritation and reactions to food. People who have allergies to common substances are more likely to develop drug allergies.

List all drugs you take. Don't forget vitamin and mineral supplements, skin, rectal or vaginal medicines, antacids, antihistamines, cold and cough remedies, aspirin and aspirin combinations, motion-sickness remedies, weight-loss aids, salt and sugar substitutes, caffeine, oral contraceptives, sleeping pills or "tonics."

## FUTURE MEDICAL PLANS

Discuss plans for elective surgery, pregnancy and breast-feeding.

## QUESTIONS

Don't hesitate to ask questions about a drug. Your doctor, nurse or pharmacist may be able to provide more information if they are familiar with you and your medical history.

# YOUR ROLE

Learn the generic names and brand names of all your medicines. Write them down to help you remember. If a drug is a mixture, learn the names of its generic ingredients.

## TAKING A DRUG

Never take medicine in the dark! Recheck the label before each use. You could be taking the *wrong* drug! Tell your doctor about any unexpected new symptoms you have while taking medicine. You may need to change medicines or have a dose adjustment.

## STORAGE

Keep all medicines out of children's reach. Store drugs in a cool, dry place, such as a kitchen cabinet or bedroom. Avoid medicine cabinets in bathrooms. They get too moist and warm at times.

Keep medicine in its original container, tightly closed. Don't remove the label! If directions call for refrigeration, don't freeze.

## DISCARDING

Don't save leftover medicine to use later. Discard it on the expiration date shown on the container. Dispose safely to protect children and pets.

## REFILLS

All refills must be ordered by your doctor or dentist, either in the first prescription or later. Only the pharmacy that originally filled the prescription can refill it without checking with your doctor or previous pharmacy. If you go to a *new* pharmacy, you must have a new prescription, or the new pharmacist must call your doctor or original pharmacy to see if a refill is authorized. Pharmacies don't usually transfer prescriptions.

If you need a refill, call your pharmacist and order your refill by number and name.

Use one pharmacy for the whole family if you can. The pharmacist then has a record of all of your drugs and can communicate effectively with your doctor.

## LEARN ABOUT DRUGS

Study the information in this book's charts regarding your medications. Read each chart completely. Because of space limitations, most information that fits more than one category appears only once.

Take care of yourself. You are the most important member of your health-care team.

# GUIDE TO DRUG CHARTS

The drug information in this book is organized in condensed, easy-to-read charts. Each drug is described in a two-page format, as shown in the sample chart below and opposite. Charts are arranged alphabetically by drug generic names, and in a few instances, such as *ADRENOCORTICOIDS, TOPICAL*, by drug class name.

A *generic name* is the official chemical name for a drug. A *brand name* is a drug manufacturer's registered trademark for a generic drug. Brand names listed on the charts

18   17   19

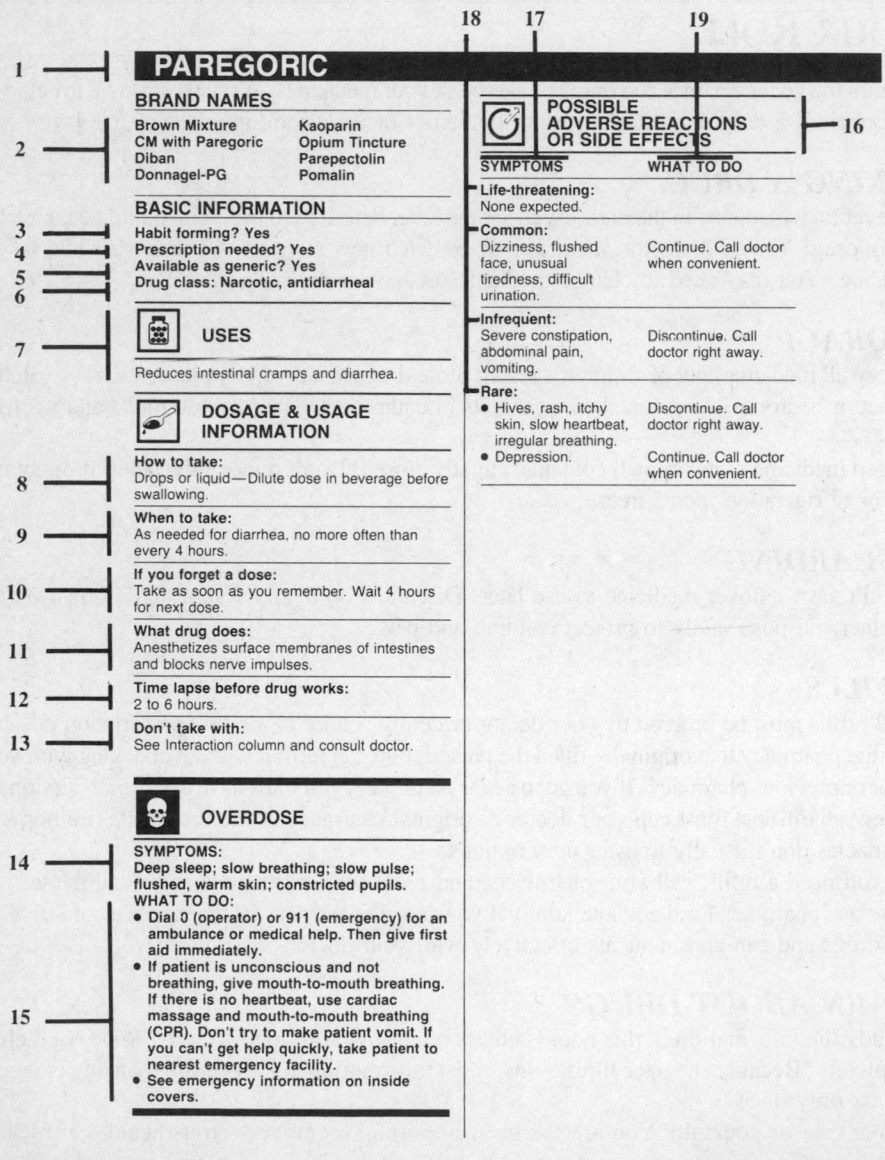

## PAREGORIC

### BRAND NAMES

| | |
|---|---|
| Brown Mixture | Kaoparin |
| CM with Paregoric | Opium Tincture |
| Diban | Parepectolin |
| Donnagel-PG | Pomalin |

### BASIC INFORMATION

Habit forming? Yes
Prescription needed? Yes
Available as generic? Yes
Drug class: Narcotic, antidiarrheal

### USES

Reduces intestinal cramps and diarrhea.

### DOSAGE & USAGE INFORMATION

How to take:
Drops or liquid—Dilute dose in beverage before swallowing.

When to take:
As needed for diarrhea, no more often than every 4 hours.

If you forget a dose:
Take as soon as you remember. Wait 4 hours for next dose.

What drug does:
Anesthetizes surface membranes of intestines and blocks nerve impulses.

Time lapse before drug works:
2 to 6 hours.

Don't take with:
See Interaction column and consult doctor.

### OVERDOSE

SYMPTOMS:
Deep sleep; slow breathing; slow pulse; flushed, warm skin; constricted pupils.
WHAT TO DO:
• Dial 0 (operator) or 911 (emergency) for an ambulance or medical help. Then give first aid immediately.
• If patient is unconscious and not breathing, give mouth-to-mouth breathing. If there is no heartbeat, use cardiac massage and mouth-to-mouth breathing (CPR). Don't try to make patient vomit. If you can't get help quickly, take patient to nearest emergency facility.
• See emergency information on inside covers.

### POSSIBLE ADVERSE REACTIONS OR SIDE EFFECTS

| SYMPTOMS | WHAT TO DO |
|---|---|
| **Life-threatening:** | |
| None expected. | |
| **Common:** | |
| Dizziness, flushed face, unusual tiredness, difficult urination. | Continue. Call doctor when convenient. |
| **Infrequent:** | |
| Severe constipation, abdominal pain, vomiting. | Discontinue. Call doctor right away. |
| **Rare:** | |
| • Hives, rash, itchy skin, slow heartbeat, irregular breathing. | Discontinue. Call doctor right away. |
| • Depression. | Continue. Call doctor when convenient. |

include those from the United States and Canada. A generic drug may have one or many brand names.

To find information about a generic drug, look it up in the alphabetical charts. To learn about a brand name, check the index first, where brand names are followed by their generic ingredients and chart page numbers.

The chart design is the same for every drug. When you are familiar with the chart, you can quickly find information you want to know about a drug.

On the next few pages, each of the numbered chart sections below is explained. This information will guide you in reading and understanding the charts that begin on page 2.

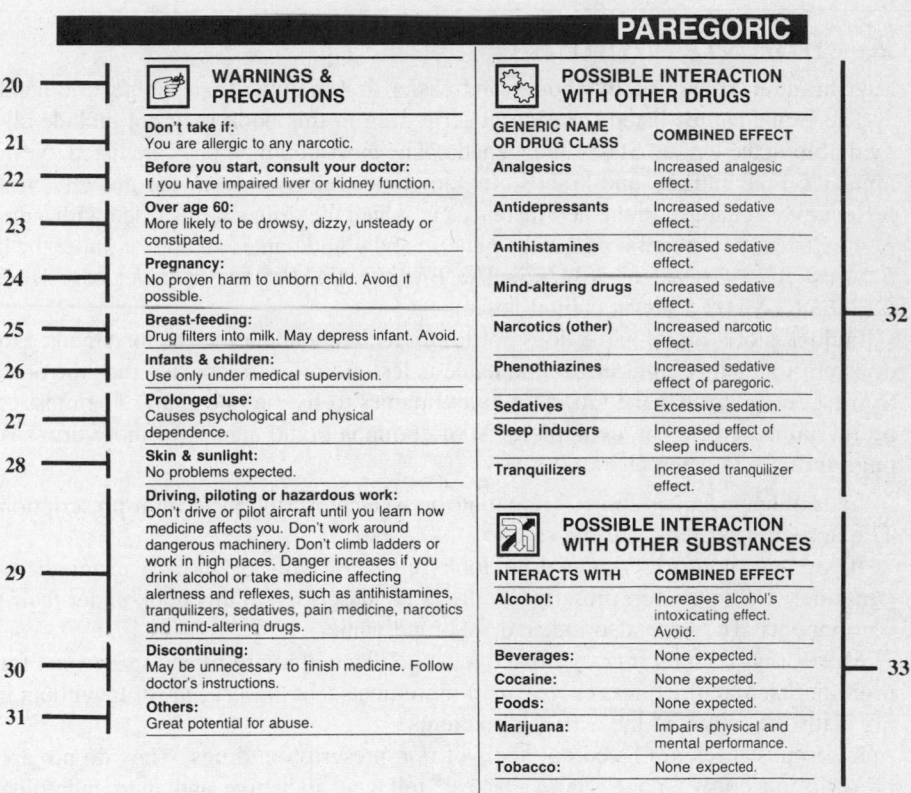

## PAREGORIC

**20** — WARNINGS & PRECAUTIONS

**21** — Don't take if:
You are allergic to any narcotic.

**22** — Before you start, consult your doctor:
If you have impaired liver or kidney function.

**23** — Over age 60:
More likely to be drowsy, dizzy, unsteady or constipated.

**24** — Pregnancy:
No proven harm to unborn child. Avoid if possible.

**25** — Breast-feeding:
Drug filters into milk. May depress infant. Avoid.

**26** — Infants & children:
Use only under medical supervision.

**27** — Prolonged use:
Causes psychological and physical dependence.

**28** — Skin & sunlight:
No problems expected.

**29** — Driving, piloting or hazardous work:
Don't drive or pilot aircraft until you learn how medicine affects you. Don't work around dangerous machinery. Don't climb ladders or work in high places. Danger increases if you drink alcohol or take medicine affecting alertness and reflexes, such as antihistamines, tranquilizers, sedatives, pain medicine, narcotics and mind-altering drugs.

**30** — Discontinuing:
May be unnecessary to finish medicine. Follow doctor's instructions.

**31** — Others:
Great potential for abuse.

### POSSIBLE INTERACTION WITH OTHER DRUGS

| GENERIC NAME OR DRUG CLASS | COMBINED EFFECT |
|---|---|
| Analgesics | Increased analgesic effect. |
| Antidepressants | Increased sedative effect. |
| Antihistamines | Increased sedative effect. |
| Mind-altering drugs | Increased sedative effect. |
| Narcotics (other) | Increased narcotic effect. |
| Phenothiazines | Increased sedative effect of paregoric. |
| Sedatives | Excessive sedation. |
| Sleep inducers | Increased effect of sleep inducers. |
| Tranquilizers | Increased tranquilizer effect. |

— **32**

### POSSIBLE INTERACTION WITH OTHER SUBSTANCES

| INTERACTS WITH | COMBINED EFFECT |
|---|---|
| Alcohol: | Increases alcohol's intoxicating effect. Avoid. |
| Beverages: | None expected. |
| Cocaine: | None expected. |
| Foods: | None expected. |
| Marijuana: | Impairs physical and mental performance. |
| Tobacco: | None expected. |

— **33**

# 1—GENERIC NAME

Each drug chart is titled by generic name, or in a few instances, by the name of the drug class, such as *DIGITALIS PREPARATIONS*.

Sometimes a drug is known by more than one generic name. The chart is titled by the most common one. Less-common generic names appear in parentheses following the first. For example, vitamin C is also known as ascorbic acid. Its chart title is *VITAMIN C (ASCORBIC ACID)*. The index will include a reference for each name.

Your drug container may show a generic name, a brand name or both. If you have only a brand name, use the index to find the drug's generic name and chart.

If your drug container shows no name, ask your doctor or pharmacist for the name.

# 2—BRAND NAMES

A brand name is usually shorter and easier to remember than the generic name.

The brand names listed for each generic drug in this book may not include all brands available in the United States and Canada. The most-common ones are listed. New brands appear on the market, and brands are sometimes removed from the market. No list can reflect every change. In the few instances in which the drug chart is titled with a drug class name instead of a generic name, the generic and brand names all appear under the heading *BRAND AND GENERIC NAMES*. The *BRAND NAMES* are in lower case letters, and *GENERIC NAMES* are in capital letters.

Inclusion of a brand name does not imply recommendation or endorsement. Exclusion does not imply that a missing brand name is less effective or less safe than the ones listed. Some generic drugs have too many brand names to list on one chart. The most common brand names appear, or a complete list of common brand names for those drugs is on the page indicated on the chart.

Lists of brand names don't differentiate between prescription and non-prescription drugs. The active ingredients are the same.

If you buy a non-prescription drug, look for generic names of the active ingredients on the container. Common non-prescription drugs are described in this book under their generic components. They are also indexed by brand name.

Most drugs contain *inert*, or inactive, ingredients that are *fillers* or *solvents* for active ingredients. Manufacturers choose inert ingredients that preserve the drug without interfering with the action of the active ingredients.

Inert substances are listed on labels of non-prescription drugs. They do not appear on prescription drugs. Your pharmacist can tell you all active and inert ingredients in a prescription drug.

Occasionally, a tablet, capsule or liquid may contain small amounts of sodium, sugar or potassium. If you are on a diet that severely restricts any of these, ask your pharmacist or doctor to suggest another form.

# BASIC INFORMATION

# 3—HABIT FORMING

A drug habit can be physical or psychological. A drug that produces physical dependence leads to addiction. It causes painful and sometimes dangerous effects when withdrawn.

Psychological dependence does not cause dangerous withdrawal effects. It may cause stress and unwanted behavior changes until the habit is broken.

# 4—PRESCRIPTION NEEDED?

"Yes" means a doctor must prescribe the drug for you. "No" means you can buy this drug without prescription. Sometimes low strengths of a drug are available without prescription, while high strengths require prescription.

The information about the generic drug applies whether it requires prescription or not. If the generic ingredients are the same, non-prescription drugs have the same dangers, warnings, precautions and interactions as prescribed drugs.

# 5—AVAILABLE AS GENERIC?

Some generic drugs have copyright restrictions that protect the manufacturer or distributor of that drug. These drugs may be purchased only by brand name.

In recent years, drug manufacturers have marketed more drugs under generic names. Drugs purchased by generic name sometimes are less expensive than brand names.

Some states allow pharmacists to fill prescriptions by brand names or generic names. This allows patients to buy the least-expensive form of a drug.

A doctor may specify a brand name because he or she trusts a known source more than an unknown manufacturer of generic drugs. You and your doctor should decide whether you should buy a medicine by generic or brand name.

Generic drugs manufactured in other countries are not subject to regulation by the U.S. Food and Drug Administration. Drugs manufactured in the United States are subject to regulation.

# 6—DRUG CLASS

Drugs that possess similar chemical structure and similar therapeutic effects are grouped into classes. Most drugs within a class produce similar benefits, side effects, adverse reactions and interactions with other drugs and substances. For example, there are 15 generic drugs in the narcotic drug class. All have similar effects on the body.

Some information on the charts applies to all drugs in a class. For example, a reference may be made to narcotics. The index lists the class—narcotics—and lists drugs in that class.

Drug classes are not standardized, so classes listed in other references may vary from the classes in this book.

# 7—USES

This section lists the disease or disorder for which a drug is prescribed.

Most uses listed are approved by the U.S. Food and Drug Administration. Some uses are listed if experiments and clinical trials indicate effectiveness and safety. Still, other uses are included that may not be officially sanctioned, but for which doctors commonly prescribe the drug.

The use for which your doctor prescribes the drug may not appear. You and your doctor should discuss the reason for any prescription medicine you take. You alone will probably decide whether to take a non-prescription drug. This section may help you make a decision.

# DOSAGE & USAGE INFORMATION

## 8—HOW TO TAKE

Drugs are available in tablets, capsules, liquids, suppositories, injections, aerosol inhalers and topical forms such as drops, sprays, creams, ointments and lotions. This section gives general instructions for taking each form.

This information supplements drug-label information. If your doctor's instructions differ from the suggestions, follow your *doctor's* instructions.

Instructions are left out for how *much* to take. Dose amounts can't be generalized. They must be individualized for you by your doctor, or you must read the drug label.

## 9—WHEN TO TAKE

Dose schedules vary for medicines and for patients.

Drugs prescribed on a schedule should usually be taken at approximately the same times each day. Some *must* be taken at regular intervals to maintain a steady level of the drug in the body. If the schedule interferes with your sleep, consult with your doctor.

Instructions to take on an empty stomach mean the drug is absorbed best in your body this way. Many drugs must be taken with liquid or food because they irritate the stomach.

Instructions for other dose schedules are usually on the label. Variations in standard dose schedules may apply because some medicines interact with others if you take them at the same time.

## 10—IF YOU FORGET A DOSE

Suggestions in this section vary from drug to drug. Most tell you when to resume taking the medicine if you forget a scheduled dose.

Establish habits so you won't forget doses. Forgotten doses decrease a drug's therapeutic effect.

## 11—WHAT DRUG DOES

This is a simple description of the drug's action in the body. The wording is generalized and may not be a complete explanation of the complex chemical process that takes place.

## 12—TIME LAPSE BEFORE DRUG WORKS

The times given are approximations. Times vary a great deal from person to person, and from time to time in the same person. The figures give you some idea of when to expect improvement.

## 13—DON'T TAKE WITH

Some drugs create problems when taken in combination with other substances. Most problems are detailed in the Interaction column of each chart. This section mentions substances that don't appear in the Interaction column.

Occasionally, an interaction is singled out if the combination is particularly harmful.

# OVERDOSE

## 14—SYMPTOMS

The symptoms listed are most likely to develop with accidental or purposeful overdose. An overdose patient may not show all symptoms listed. Sometimes symptoms are identical to ones listed as side effects. The difference is intensity and severity. You will have to judge. Consult a doctor or poison-control center if you have any doubt.

## 15—WHAT TO DO

If you suspect an overdose, whether symptoms are apparent or not, follow instructions in this section. Expanded instructions for emergency treatment for overdose are on the inside cover.

## 16—POSSIBLE ADVERSE REACTIONS OR SIDE EFFECTS

Adverse reactions or side effects are symptoms that may occur when you take a drug. They are effects on the body other than the desired therapeutic effect.

The term *side effect* implies expected and usually unavoidable effects of a drug. Side effects have nothing to do with the drug's intended use.

For example, the generic drug paregoric reduces intestinal cramps and vomiting. It also often causes a flushed face. The flushing is a side effect that is harmless and does not affect the drug's therapeutic potential.

The term *adverse reaction* is more significant. For example, paregoric can cause serious adverse allergic reaction in some people. This reaction can include hives, rash and severe itch.

Some adverse reactions can be prevented, which is one reason this information is included in the book. Most adverse reactions are minor and last only a short time. With many drugs, adverse reactions that might occur will frequently diminish in intensity as time passes.

The majority of drugs used properly for valid reasons offer benefits that outweigh potential hazards.

## 17—SYMPTOMS

Symptoms are grouped by various body systems. Symptoms that don't naturally apply to these body systems or which overlap systems are listed under "Others."

# 18—FREQUENCY

This is an estimation of how often symptoms occur in persons who take the drug. The four most common categories of frequency can be found under the **SYMPTOMS** heading and are as follows. **Life-threatening** means exactly what it says: Seek emergency treatment immediately. **Common** means these symptoms are expected and sometimes inevitable. **Infrequent** means the symptoms occur in approximately 1% to 10% of patients. **Rare** means symptoms occur in less than 1%.

# 19—WHAT TO DO

Carefully follow the instructions provided opposite the symptoms that apply to you.

# 20—WARNINGS AND PRECAUTIONS

Read these entries to determine special information that applies to you.

# 21—DON'T TAKE IF

This section lists circumstances that indicate the use of a drug may not be safe. On some drug labels and in formal medical literature, these circumstances are called *contraindications*.

# 22—BEFORE YOU START, CONSULT YOUR DOCTOR

This section lists conditions under which a drug should be used with caution.

# 23—OVER AGE 60

As a person ages, physical changes occur that require special consideration in drug use. Liver and kidney functions decrease, metabolism slows and the prostate gland enlarges in men.

Most drugs are metabolized or excreted at a rate dependent on kidney and liver functions. Small doses or longer intervals between doses may be necessary to prevent unhealthy concentration of a drug. Toxic effects and adverse reactions occur more frequently and cause more serious problems in this age group.

# 24—PREGNANCY

The best rule to follow during pregnancy is to avoid all drugs, including tobacco and alcohol. Any medicine—prescription or non-prescription—requires medical advice and supervision.

This section will alert you if there is evidence that a drug harms the unborn child. Lack of evidence does not guarantee a drug's safety. If safety is undetermined, and reasonable doubt exists, "No proven problems" is indicated.

## 25—BREAST-FEEDING

Many drugs filter into a mother's milk. Some drugs have dangerous or unwanted effects on the nursing infant. This section suggests ways to minimize harm to the child.

## 26—INFANTS & CHILDREN

Many drugs carry special warnings and precautions for children because of a child's size and immaturity. In medical terminology, *newborns* are babies up to 2 weeks old, *infants* are 2 weeks to 1 year, and *children* are 1 to 12 years.

## 27—PROLONGED USE

Most drugs produce no ill effects during short periods of treatment. However, relatively safe drugs taken for long periods may produce unwanted effects. These are listed. Drugs should be taken in the smallest dose and for the shortest time possible. Nevertheless, some diseases and conditions require an indefinite period of treatment. Your doctor may want to change drugs occasionally or alter your treatment regimen to minimize problems.

The words "functional dependence" sometimes appear in this section. This does not mean *physical* or *psychological addiction*. Sometimes a body function ceases to work naturally because it has been replaced or interfered with by the drug. The body then becomes dependent on the drug to continue the function.

## 28—SKIN & SUNLIGHT

Many drugs cause *photosensitivity*, which means increased skin sensitivity to ultraviolet rays from sunlight or artificial rays from a sunlamp. This section will alert you to this potential problem.

## 29—DRIVING, PILOTING OR HAZARDOUS WORK

Any drug that decreases alertness, muscular coordination or reflexes may make these activities hazardous. The effects may not appear in all people, or they may disappear after a short exposure to the drug. If this section contains a warning, use caution until you determine how a new drug affects you.

## 30—DISCONTINUING

Some patients stop taking a drug when symptoms begin to go away, although complete recovery may require longer treatment.

Other patients continue taking a drug when it is no longer needed. This section will tell you when you may safely discontinue a drug.

Some drugs cause symptoms days or weeks after discontinuing. This section warns you so the symptoms won't puzzle you if they occur.

# 31—OTHERS

Warnings and precautions appear here if they don't fit into the other categories. This section includes storage instructions, how to dispose of outdated drugs, weather influences on drug effect, changes in blood and urine tests, warnings to persons with chronic illness and other information.

# 32—POSSIBLE INTERACTION WITH OTHER DRUGS

Drugs interact in your body with other drugs, whether prescription or non-prescription. Interactions affect absorption, elimination or distribution of either drug. The chart lists interactions by generic name or drug class.

If a drug class appears, the generic drug interacts with any drug in that class. Drugs in each class that are included in the book are listed in the index.

Interactions are sometimes beneficial. You may not be able to determine from the chart which interactions are good and which are bad. Don't guess! Consult your doctor if you take drugs that interact. Some combinations are fatal!

Occasionally, drugs appear in the Interaction column that are not included in this book. These drugs are listed under Interactions for your safety.

Some drugs have too many interactions to list on one chart. The additional interactions appear on the page indicated at the bottom of the list.

# 33—POSSIBLE INTERACTION WITH OTHER SUBSTANCES

The substances listed here are repeated on every drug chart. All people eat food and drink beverages. Many adults consume alcohol. Many people use cocaine and smoke tobacco or marijuana. This section shows possible interactions between these substances and each drug.

# DRUGS OF ABUSE

Each of the drug charts beginning on page 2 contains a section listing the interactions of alcohol, marijuana and cocaine with the therapeutic drug in the bloodstream. These three drugs are singled out because of their widespread use and abuse. The information is factual, not judgmental.

The long-term effects of alcohol and tobacco abuse are numerous. They have been well-publicized and information is provided here as a reminder of the inherent dangers of these drugs.

Drugs of potential abuse include those that are addictive and harmful. They usually produce a temporary, false sense of well-being. The long-term effects, however, are harmful and can be devastating to the body and psyche of the addict.

Refresh your memory frequently about the potential harm from prolonged use of *any* drugs or substances you take. Avoid unwise use of habit-forming drugs.

These are the most common drugs of abuse:

# TOBACCO (NICOTINE)

**What it does:** Tobacco smoke contains noxious and cancer-producing ingredients. They include nicotine, carbon monoxide, ammonia, and a variety of harmful tars. Carcinogens in smoke probably come from the tars. Most are present in chewing tobacco and snuff as well as smoke from cigarettes, cigars, and pipes. Tobacco smoke interferes with the immune mechanisms of the body.

**Short-term effects of average amount:** Relaxation of mood if you are a steady smoker. Constriction of blood vessels.

**Short terms effects of large amount inhaled:** Headache, appetite loss, nausea.

**Long term effects:** Greatly enhanced chances of developing lung cancer. Impaired breathing and chronic lung disease (asthma, emphysema, bronchiectasis, lung abscess and others) much more likely. Heart and blood vessel disease more frequent and more severe when they happen. These include myocardial infarction (heart attack), coronary artery disease, heart beat irregularities, generalized atherosclerosis (hardening of the arteries making brain, heart, and kidney more vulnerable to disease), peripheral vascular disease such as intermittent claudication, Buerger's disease and others. Tobacco and nicotine lead to an increased incidence of abortion and significantly reduce the birth weight of children brought to term and delivered of women who smoke during pregnancy. Tobacco smoking causes higher frequency not only of lung cancer, but also increases the likelihood of developing cancer of the throat, larynx, mouth, esophagus, bladder, and pancreas.

Cigarette smoking has been linked to this many deaths per year in the U.S. alone:
80,000 lung cancer
22,000 other cancer
15,000 chronic lung disease
225,000 cardiovascular disease

346,000 TOTAL

# ALCOHOL

**What it does:**

● *Central Nervous System*

*Depresses,* does *not* stimulate, the action of all parts of the central nervous system, including the depression of normal mental activity and normal muscle function. Short term effects of an average amount: relaxation, breakdown of inhibitions, euphoria, decreased alertness. Short term effects of large amounts: nausea, stupor, hangover, unconsciousness, even death.

● *Gastrointestinal System*

Increases stomach acid, poisons liver function. Chronic alcoholism frequently leads to permanent damage to the liver.

● *Heart and Blood Vessels*

Decreased normal function, leading to heart diseases such as cardiomyopathy and disorders of the blood vessels and kidney such as high blood pressure. Bleeding from the esophagus and stomach frequently accompany chronic alcoholism.

● *Unborn Fetus (teratogenicity)*

Alcoholism in the mother carrying a fetus causes *fetal alcohol syndrome (FAS),* which includes the production of mental deficiency, facial abnormalities, slow growth and other major and minor malformations in the newborn.

**Signs of Use:**

*Early signs:* Prominent smell of alcohol on the breath, behavior changes (aggressive; passive; sexually uninhibited; poor judgment; outbursts of uncontrolled emotion, such as rage or tearfulness).

*Intoxication signs:* Unsteady gait, slurred speech, poor performance of any brain or muscle function, stupor or coma in *severe* alcoholic intoxication with slow, noisy breathing, cold and clammy skin, heartbeat faster than usual.

**Long term effects:**

*Addiction:* Compulsive use of alcohol. Persons addicted to alcohol have severe withdrawal symptoms when alcohol is unavailable. Even with successful treatment, addiction to alcohol (and other drugs that cause addiction) has a high tendency to relapse. (Memory of euphoric feelings plus family, social, emotional, psychological, and genetic factors probably are all important factors in producing the addiction.)

*Liver disease:* Usually cirrhosis; also, deleterious effects on the unborn child of an alcoholic mother.

*Loss of sexual function:* Impotence, erectile dysfunction, loss of libido.

*Increased incidence of cancer:* Mouth, pharynx, larynx, esophagus, liver, and lung.

*Changes in blood:* Makes it less likely for blood to clot efficiently.

*Heart disease:* Decreased normal function leading to possible damage and disease.

*Stomach and intestinal problems:* Increased production of stomach acid.

*Interference with expected or normal actions of many medications:* Detailed on every chart in this book, drugs such as sedatives, pain killers, narcotics, antihistamines, anticonvulsants, anticoagulants, and others.

# Marijuana (Cannabis, Hashish)

**What they do:** Heighten perception, cause mood swings, relax mind and body.
**Signs of use:** Red eyes, lethargy, uncoordinated body movements.
**Long-term effects:** Decreased motivation. Possible brain, heart, lung and reproductive system damage.

# Amphetamines

**What they do:** Speed up physical and mental processes to cause a false sense of energy and excitement. The moods are temporary and unreal.
**Signs of use:** Dilated pupils, insomnia, trembling.
**Long-term effects:** Violent behavior, paranoia, possible death from overdose.

# Barbiturates

**What they do:** Produce drowsiness and lethargy.
**Signs of use:** Confused speech, lack of coordination and balance.
**Long-term effects:** Disrupts normal sleep pattern. Possible death from overdose, especially in combination with alcohol.

# COCAINE

**What it does:** Stimulates the nervous system, heightens sensations and may produce hallucinations.
**Signs of use:** Trembling, intoxication, dilated pupils, constant sniffling.
**Long-term effects:** Ulceration of nasal passages where sniffed. Itching all over body, sometimes with open sores. Possible brain damage. Possible death from overdose.


# OPIATES (CODEINE, HEROIN, METHADONE, MORPHINE, OPIUM)

**What they do:** Relieve pain, create temporary and false sense of well-being.
**Signs of use:** Constricted pupils, mood swings, slurred speech, sore eyes, lethargy, weight loss, sweating.
**Long-term effects:** Malnutrition, extreme susceptibility to infection, the need to increase drug amount to produce the same effects. Possible death from overdose.


# PSYCHEDELIC DRUGS (LSD, MESCALINE)

**What they do:** Produce hallucinations, either pleasant or frightening.
**Signs of use:** Dilated pupils, sweating, trembling, fever, chills.
**Long-term effects:** Lack of motivation, unpredictable behavior, narcissism, recurrent hallucinations without drug use ("flashbacks"). Possible death from overdose.


# VOLATILE SUBSTANCES (GLUE, SOLVENTS)

**What they do:** Produce hallucinations, temporary, false sense of well-being and possible unconsciousness.
**Signs of use:** Dilated pupils, flushed face, confusion.
**Long-term effects:** Permanent brain, liver, kidney damage. Possible death from overdose.

# CHECKLIST FOR SAFER DRUG USE

- Tell your doctor about *any* drug you take (even aspirin, allergy pills, laxatives, vitamins, etc.) *before* you take *any* new drug.

- Learn all you can about drugs you may take *before* you take them. Information sources are your doctor, your nurse, your pharmacist, this book and other books in your public library.

- Don't take drugs prescribed for someone else—even if your symptoms are the same.

- Keep your prescription drugs to yourself. Your drugs may be harmful to someone else.

- Tell your doctor about any symptoms you believe are caused by a drug—prescription or non-prescription—that you take.

- Take only medicines that are *necessary*. Avoid taking non-prescription drugs while taking prescription drugs for a medical problem.

- Before your doctor prescribes for you, tell him about your previous experiences with any drug—beneficial results, adverse reactions or allergies.

- Take medicine in good light after you have identified it. If you wear glasses to read, put them on to check drug labels. It is easy to take the wrong drug at the wrong time.

- Don't keep any drugs that change mood, alertness or judgment—such as sedatives, narcotics or tranquilizers—by your bedside. These cause many accidental deaths by overdose. You may unknowingly repeat a dose when you are half asleep or confused.

- Know the names of your medicines. These include the generic name, the brand name and the generic names of all ingredients in a drug mixture. Your doctor, nurse or pharmacist can give you this information.

- Study the labels on all non-prescription drugs. If the information is incomplete or if you have questions, ask the pharmacist for more details.

- If you must deviate from your prescribed dose schedule, tell your doctor.

- Shake liquid medicines before taking.

- Store all medicines away from moisture and heat. Bathroom medicine cabinets are usually unsuitable.

- If a drug needs refrigeration, don't freeze.

- Obtain a standard measuring spoon from your pharmacy for liquid medicines. Kitchen teaspoons and tablespoons are not accurate enough.

- Follow diet instructions when you take medicines. Some work better on a full stomach, others on an empty stomach. Some drugs are more useful with special diets. For example, medicine for high blood pressure is more effective if accompanied by a sodium-restricted diet.

- Tell your doctor about any allergies you have. A previous allergy to a drug may make it dangerous to prescribe again. People with other allergies, such as eczema, hay fever, asthma, bronchitis and food allergies, are more likely to be allergic to drugs.

- Prior to surgery, tell your doctor, anesthesiologist or dentist about any drug you have taken in the past few weeks. Advise them of any cortisone drugs you have taken within two years.

- If you become pregnant while taking any medicine, including birth-control pills, tell your doctor immediately.

- Avoid *all* drugs while you are pregnant, if possible. If you must take drugs during pregnancy, record names, amounts, dates and reasons.

- If you see more than one doctor, tell each one about drugs others have prescribed.

- When you use non-prescription drugs, report it so the information is on your medical record.

- Store all drugs away from the reach of children.

- Note the expiration date on each drug label. Discard outdated ones safely.

- Pay attention to the information in the charts about safety while driving, piloting or working in dangerous places.

- Alcohol, cocaine, marijuana or other mood-altering drugs as well as tobacco—mixed with some drugs—can cause a life-threatening interaction, prevent your medicine from being effective or delay your return to health. Common sense dictates that you avoid them during illness.

# DRUG CHARTS

# ACEBUTOLOL

## BRAND NAMES

Sectral

## BASIC INFORMATION

**Habit forming? No**
**Prescription needed? Yes**
**Available as generic? No**
**Drug class: Beta-adrenergic blocker**

 ## USES

- Reduces frequency and severity of angina attacks.
- Stabilizes irregular heartbeat.
- Lowers blood pressure.
- Reduces frequency of migraine headaches. (Does not relieve headache pain.)

 ## DOSAGE & USAGE INFORMATION

**How to take:**
Tablet or capsule—Swallow with liquid. If you can't swallow whole, crumble tablet or open capsule and take with liquid or food.

**When to take:**
With meals or immediately after.

**If you forget a dose:**
Take as soon as you remember. Return to regular schedule, but allow 3 hours between doses.

**What drug does:**
- Blocks actions of sympathetic nervous system.
- Lowers heart's oxygen requirements.
- Slows nerve impulses through heart.
- Reduces blood-vessel contraction in several major organs and glands.

**Time lapse before drug works:**
1 to 4 hours.

*Continued next column*

 ## OVERDOSE

**SYMPTOMS:**
**Weakness, slow or weak pulse,**
**blood-pressure drop, fainting, convulsions,**
**cold and sweaty skin.**
**WHAT TO DO:**
- **Dial 0 (operator) or 911 (emergency) for an ambulance or medical help. Then give first aid immediately.**
- **See emergency information on inside covers.**

**Don't take with:**
Non-prescription drugs or drugs in interaction column without consulting doctor.

 ## POSSIBLE ADVERSE REACTIONS OR SIDE EFFECTS

| SYMPTOMS | WHAT TO DO |
|---|---|
| **Life-threatening:** | |
| None expected. | |
| **Common:** | |
| • Drowsiness, numbness or tingling in fingers and toes, dizziness, diarrhea, nausea, fatigue, weakness. | Continue. Call doctor when convenient. |
| • Pulse slower than 50 beats per minute. | Discontinue. Call doctor right away. |
| • Cold hands and feet; dry mouth, skin or eyes. | Continue. Tell doctor at next visit. |
| **Infrequent:** | |
| • Hallucinations, nightmares, insomnia, headache, difficulty breathing. | Discontinue. Call doctor right away. |
| • Confusion, depression, reduced alertness. | Continue. Call doctor when convenient. |
| • Constipation. | Continue. Tell doctor at next visit. |
| **Rare:** | |
| • Sore throat, fever, rash. | Discontinue. Call doctor right away. |
| • Unexplained bleeding and bruising. | Continue. Call doctor when convenient. |

 ## WARNINGS & PRECAUTIONS

**Don't take if:**
- You are allergic to any beta-adrenergic blocker.
- You have asthma.
- You have hay-fever symptoms.
- You have taken MAO inhibitors in past 2 weeks.

**Before you start, consult your doctor:**
- If you have heart disease or poor circulation to extremities.
- If you have hay fever, asthma, chronic bronchitis or emphysema.
- If you have overactive thyroid function.
- If you have impaired liver or kidney function.
- If you will have surgery within 2 months, including dental surgery, requiring general or spinal anesthesia.
- If you have diabetes or hypoglycemia.

**Over age 60:**
Adverse reactions and side effects may be more frequent and severe than in younger persons.

**Pregnancy:**
Risk to unborn child outweighs drug benefits. Don't use.

**Breast-feeding:**
Drug passes into milk. Avoid drug or discontinue nursing until you finish medicine. Consult doctor for advice on maintaining milk supply.

**Infants & children:**
Not recommended. Safety and dosage have not been established.

**Prolonged use:**
Weakens heart-muscle contractions.

**Skin & sunlight:**
No problems expected.

**Driving, piloting or hazardous work:**
Don't drive or pilot aircraft until you learn how medicine affects you. Don't work around dangerous machinery. Don't climb ladders or work in high places. Danger increases if you drink alcohol or take medicine affecting alertness and reflexes.

**Discontinuing:**
Don't discontinue without consulting doctor. Dose may require gradual reduction if you have taken drug for a long time. Doses of other drugs may also require adjustment.

**Others:**
May mask hypoglycemia.

## POSSIBLE INTERACTION WITH OTHER DRUGS

| GENERIC NAME OR DRUG CLASS | COMBINED EFFECT |
|---|---|
| Anesthetics used in surgery | Increased antihypertensive effect. |
| Antidiabetics | May make blood sugar more difficult to control. |
| Antihypertensives | Increased antihypertensive effect. |
| Anti-inflammatory drugs | Decreased antihypertensive effect. |
| Calcium-channel blockers | May worsen congestive heart failure. |
| Clonidine | Possible blood-pressure rise when clonidine is discontinued. |
| Digitalis preparations | Increased or decreased heart rate. Improves irregular heartbeat. |

| | |
|---|---|
| Diuretics | Increased antihypertensive effect. |
| Enalapril | Increased antihyperensive effect. Dosage of each may require adjustment. |
| Ketoprofen | Decreased antihypertensive effect of acebutolol. |
| Molindone | Increased tranquilizer effect. |
| MAO inhibitors | Possible excessive blood-pressure rise when MAO inhibitor is discontinued. |
| Pentoxifylline | Increased antihypertensive effect. |
| Reserpine | Possible excessively low blood pressure and slow heartbeat. |
| Suprofen | Decreased antihypertensive effect of acebutolol. |
| Sympathomimetics | Decreased effects of both drugs |
| Timolol eyedrops | Possible increased acebutolol effect. |
| Xanthine bronchodilators | Decreased effects of both drugs. |

## POSSIBLE INTERACTION WITH OTHER SUBSTANCES

| INTERACTS WITH | COMBINED EFFECT |
|---|---|
| Alcohol: | Excessive blood-pressure drop. Avoid. |
| Beverages: | None expected. |
| Cocaine: | Irregular heartbeat. Avoid. |
| Foods: | None expected. |
| Marijuana: | Daily use—Impaired circulation to hands and feet. |
| Tobacco: | Possible irregular heartbeat. |

# ACETAMINOPHEN

## BRAND NAMES

See complete list of brand names in the *Brand Name Directory,* page 940.

## BASIC INFORMATION

**Habit forming? No**
**Prescription needed? No**
**Available as generic? Yes**
**Drug class: Analgesic, fever-reducer**

## USES

Treatment of mild to moderate pain and fever. Acetaminophen does not relieve redness, stiffness or swelling of joints or tissue inflammation. Use aspirin or other drugs for inflammation.

## DOSAGE & USAGE INFORMATION

**How to take:**
- Tablet or capsule—Swallow with liquid.
- Effervescent granules—Dissolve granules in 4 oz. of cool water. Drink all the water.
- Suppositories—Remove wrapper and moisten suppository with water. Gently insert larger end into rectum. Push well into rectum with finger.

**When to take:**
As needed, no more often than every 3 hours.

**If you forget a dose:**
Take as soon as you remember. Wait 3 hours for next dose.

**What drug does:**
May affect hypothalamus—part of brain that helps regulate body heat and receives body's pain messages.

**Time lapse before drug works:**
15 to 30 minutes. May last 4 hours.

*Continued next column*

## OVERDOSE

**SYMPTOMS:**
**Stomach upset, irritability, convulsions, coma.**
**WHAT TO DO:**
- **Call your doctor or poison-control center for advice if you suspect overdose, even if not sure. Symptoms may not appear until damage has occurred.**
- **See emergency information on inside covers.**

**Don't take with:**
- Other drugs with acetaminophen. Too much acetaminophen can damage liver and kidneys.
- See Interaction column and consult doctor.

## POSSIBLE ADVERSE REACTIONS OR SIDE EFFECTS

| SYMPTOMS | WHAT TO DO |
|---|---|
| **Life-threatening:** None expected. | |
| **Common:** Lightheadedness. | Continue. Call doctor when convenient. |
| **Infrequent:** Trembling. | Continue. Call doctor when convenient. |
| **Rare:** • Extreme fatigue; rash, itch, hives; sore throat and fever after taking regularly a few days; unexplained bleeding or bruising; blood in urine; painful or frequent urination; jaundice; anemia. | Discontinue. Call doctor right away. |
| • Decreased volume of urine output. | Continue. Call doctor when convenient. |

## WARNINGS & PRECAUTIONS

**Don't take if:**
- You are allergic to acetaminophen.
- Your symptoms don't improve after 2 days use. Call your doctor.

**Before you start, consult your doctor:**
If you have bronchial asthma, kidney disease or liver damage.

**Over age 60:**
Don't exceed recommended dose. You can't eliminate drug as efficiently as younger persons.

**Pregnancy:**
No proven harm to unborn child. Avoid if possible.

**Breast-feeding:**
No proven harm to nursing infant.

**Infants & children:**
Use only under medical supervision.

**Prolonged use:**
May affect blood system and cause anemia. Limit use to 5 days for children 12 and under, and 10 days for adults.

**Skin & sunlight:**
No problems expected.

**Driving, piloting or hazardous work:**
Avoid if you feel drowsy. Otherwise, no restrictions.

**Discontinuing:**
Discontinue in 2 days if symptoms don't improve.

**Others:**
No problems expected.

## POSSIBLE INTERACTION WITH OTHER DRUGS

| GENERIC NAME OR DRUG CLASS | COMBINED EFFECT |
| --- | --- |
| Anticoagulants (oral) | May increase anticoagulant effect. If combined frequently, prothrombin time should be monitored. |
| Phenobarbital | Quicker elimination of and decreased effect of acetaminophen. |

## POSSIBLE INTERACTION WITH OTHER SUBSTANCES

| INTERACTS WITH | COMBINED EFFECT |
| --- | --- |
| Alcohol: | Drowsiness |
| Beverages: | None expected. |
| Cocaine: | None expected. However, cocaine may slow body's recovery. Avoid. |
| Foods: | None expected. |
| Marijuana: | Increased pain relief. However, marijuana may slow body's recovery. Avoid. |
| Tobacco: | None expected. |

# ACETAMINOPHEN & SALICYLATES

## BRAND NAMES

See complete list of brand names in the *Brand Name Directory*, page 940.

## BASIC INFORMATION

**Habit forming? No**
**Prescription needed?**
  **High strength: Yes**
  **Low strength: No**
**Yes, for some combinations**
**Available as generic? Yes**
**Drug class: Analgesic, fever-reducer
        (acetaminophen and salicylates),
        non-steroidal anti-inflammatory
        (salicylates)**

 ## USES

- Treatment of mild pain and fever.
- Salicylates are useful in the treatment of inflammatory conditions such as stiffness, swelling, joint pain of arthritis or rheumatism. For long term use for inflammatory problems, separate drugs instead of this combination may be safer and more effective.

 ## DOSAGE & USAGE INFORMATION

**How to take:**
- Tablet or capsule—swallow with liquid.
- Effervescent granules—dissolve granules in 4 oz. of cool water.

**When to take:**
As needed, no more often than every 3 hours or as prescribed by your doctor.

**If you forget a dose:**
Take as soon as you remember. Wait 3 hours for next dose.

**What drug does:**
- May affect hypothalamus, the part of the brain that helps regulate body heat and receives body's pain messages.

*Continued next column*

 ## OVERDOSE

**SYMPTOMS:**
**Ringing in ears; nausea; vomiting; dizziness; fever; deep, rapid breathing; hallucinations; coma; unusual sweating; blood in urine.**
**WHAT TO DO:**
- Dial 0 (operator) or 911 (emergency) for an ambulance or medical help. Then give first aid immediately.
- Emergency information on inside

6

- May affect production of prostaglandins to reduce inflammation.

**Time lapse before drug works:**
15 to 30 minutes. May last 4 hours.

**Don't take with:**
- Other drugs with acetaminophen or aspirin or other salicylates. Too much can cause damage to liver, kidneys and peripheral nerves.
- Any laxative containing cellulose.
- If medicine you take has a buffering agent added, don't take with tetracyclines.

 ## POSSIBLE ADVERSE REACTIONS OR SIDE EFFECTS

| SYMPTOMS | WHAT TO DO |
|---|---|
| **Life-threatening:** | |
| Wheezing and marked shortness of breath. | Seek emergency treatment immediately. |
| **Common:** | |
| • Jaundice, vomiting blood, black stools, cloudy urine, nausea and vomiting, discomfort on urinating, unexplained tiredness. | Discontinue. Call doctor right away. |
| • Indigestion or heartburn. | Continue. Call doctor when convenient. |
| **Infrequent:** | |
| Shortness of breath; wheezing (for medicines containing aspirin); urine volume decreased; feet swelling; black or tarry stools; pain on urinating; nausea and vomiting; skin rash, hives; sore throat, fever; easy bruising. | Discontinue. Call doctor right away. |
| **Rare:** | |
| • While taking medicine: Sudden decrease in urine volume. | Discontinue. Call doctor right away. |
| • After discontinuing medicine: Swelling of feet; rapid weight gain; bloating or puffiness; any urinary problems, such as painful, cloudy or bloody urine. | Check with doctor immediately. |

## WARNINGS & PRECAUTIONS

### Don't take if:
- You are allergic to acetaminophen or any salicylates (see Glossary).
- Your symptoms don't improve after 3 days use.
- You take a buffered form and need to restrict sodium in your diet.
- You have a peptic ulcer.
- You have a bleeding disorder.

### Before you start, consult your doctor:
- If you have ever had peptic ulcers.
- If you have had gout.
- If you have asthma or nasal polyps.
- If you have kidney disease or liver damage.

### Over age 60:
Don't exceed recommended dose. More likely to be harmful to kidney and liver or cause hidden bleeding in stomach or intestines. Watch for black stools or decreased urine output.

### Pregnancy:
Risk to unborn child outweighs drug benefits. Don't use.

### Breast-feeding:
Drug passes into milk. Avoid drug or discontinue nursing until you finish medicine. Consult doctor on maintaining milk supply.

### Infants & children:
Overdose frequent and severe. Keep bottles out of children's reach. Consult doctor before giving to persons under age 18 who have fever and discomfort of viral illness, especially chicken pox and influenza. Probably increases risk of Reye's syndrome (see Glossary).

### Prolonged use:
High doses for severe inflammatory conditions taken for long periods may increase likelihood of kidney damage.

### Skin & sunlight:
Aspirin combined with sunscreen may decrease sunburn.

### Driving, piloting or hazardous work:
No problems expected unless you feel drowsy.

### Discontinuing:
No problems expected.

### Others:
- Children up to 12 years—Don't take more than 5 doses per day for more than 5 consecutive days.
- Adults—Don't take for more than 10 consecutive days.
- Urine test for sugar may be inaccurate.
- Don't take if container has a strong vinegar-like odor.

## POSSIBLE INTERACTION WITH OTHER DRUGS

| GENERIC NAME OR DRUG CLASS | COMBINED EFFECT |
| --- | --- |
| Allupurinol | Decreased allopurinol effect. |
| Antacids | Decreased acetaminophen and salicylates effect. |
| Anticoagulants | Increased anticoagulant effect. Abnormal bleeding. |
| Antidiabetics (oral) | Low blood sugar. |
| Anti-inflammatory drugs (non-steroid) | Risk of stomach bleeding and ulcers. |
| Aspirin and other salicylates | Likely toxicity. |
| Cortisone drugs | Increased cortisone effect. Risk of ulcers and stomach bleeding. |
| Furosemide | Possible salicylate toxicity. |
| Indomethacin | Risk of stomach bleeding and ulcers. |
| Methotrexate | Increased methotrexate effect. |
| Para-aminosalicylic acid (PAS) | Possible salicylate toxicity. |
| Phenobarbital | Decreased effect of acetaminophen and salicylates because of quicker elimination. |

*Continued page 961*

## POSSIBLE INTERACTION WITH OTHER SUBSTANCES

| INTERACTS WITH | COMBINED EFFECT |
| --- | --- |
| Alcohol: | Increased chance of stomach irritation and bleeding. |
| Beverages: | None expected. |
| Cocaine: | None expected. However, cocaine may deter body's recovery. Avoid. |
| Foods: | None expected. |
| Marijuana: | Possible increased pain relief, but marijuana may deter body recovery. Avoid |
| Tobacco: | None expected |

8

# ACETOHEXAMIDE

## BRAND NAMES

Dimelor　　　　　　Dymelor

## BASIC INFORMATION

**Habit forming?** No
**Prescription needed?** Yes
**Available as generic?** No
**Drug class:** Antidiabetic (oral), sulfonurea

## USES

Treatment for diabetes in adults who can't control blood sugar by diet, weight loss and exercise.

## DOSAGE & USAGE INFORMATION

**How to take:**
Tablet—Swallow with liquid or food to lessen stomach irritation. If you can't swallow whole, crumble tablet and take with liquid or food.

**When to take:**
At the same times each day.

**If you forget a dose:**
Take as soon as you remember up to 2 hours late. If more than 2 hours, wait for next scheduled dose (don't double this dose).

**What drug does:**
Stimulates pancreas to produce more insulin. Insulin in blood forces cells to use sugar in blood.

**Time lapse before drug works:**
3 to 4 hours. May require 2 weeks for maximum benefit.

**Don't take with:**
See Interaction column and consult doctor.

## OVERDOSE

**SYMPTOMS:**
Excessive hunger, nausea, anxiety, cool skin, cold sweats, drowsiness, rapid heartbeat, weakness, unconsciousness, coma.
**WHAT TO DO:**
- Dial 0 (operator) or 911 (emergency) for an ambulance or medical help. Then give first aid immediately.
- See emergency information on inside covers.

## POSSIBLE ADVERSE REACTIONS OR SIDE EFFECTS

| SYMPTOMS | WHAT TO DO |
|---|---|
| **Life-threatening:** Low blood sugar (hunger, anxiety, cold sweats, rapid pulse). | Seek emergency treatment immediately. |
| **Common:** <br> • Dizziness. | Discontinue. Call doctor right away. |
| • Diarrhea, appetite loss, nausea, stomach pain, heartburn. | Continue. Call doctor when convenient. |
| **Infrequent:** Fatigue, itching or rash, ringing in ears. | Discontinue. Call doctor right away. |
| **Rare:** Sore throat, fever, unusual bleeding or bruising, jaundice. | Discontinue. Call doctor right away. |

## WARNINGS & PRECAUTIONS

**Don't take if:**
- You are allergic to any sulfonurea.
- You have impaired kidney or liver function.

**Before you start, consult your doctor:**
- If you have a severe infection.
- If you have thyroid disease.
- If you take insulin.
- If you have heart disease.

**Over age 60:**
Dose usually smaller than for younger adults. Avoid "low-blood-sugar" episodes because repeated ones can damage brain permanently.

**Pregnancy:**
No proven harm to unborn child. Avoid if possible.

**Breast-feeding:**
Drug filters into milk. May lower baby's blood sugar. Avoid.

**Infants & children:**
Don't give to infants or children.

**Prolonged use:**
None expected.

**Skin & sunlight:**
May cause rash or intensify sunburn in areas exposed to sun or sunlamp.

**Driving, piloting or hazardous work:**
No problems expected unless you develop hypoglycemia (low blood sugar). If so, avoid driving or hazardous activity.

**Discontinuing:**
Don't discontinue without consulting doctor. Dose may require gradual reduction if you have taken drug for a long time. Doses of other drugs may also require adjustment.

**Others:**
Don't exceed recommended dose. Hypoglycemia (low blood sugar) may occur, even with proper dose schedule. You must balance medicine, diet and exercise.

## POSSIBLE INTERACTION WITH OTHER DRUGS

| GENERIC NAME OR DRUG CLASS | COMBINED EFFECT |
|---|---|
| Anticoagulants (oral) | Unpredictable prothrombin times. |
| Anticonvulsants (hydantoin) | Decreased acetohexamide effect |
| Anti-inflammatory drugs (non-steroidal) | Increased acetohexamide effect. |
| Aspirin | Increased acetohexamide effect. |
| Beta-adrenergic blockers | Increased acetohexamide effect.May take blood sugar more difficult to control. |
| Chloramphenicol | Increased acetohexamide effect. |
| Clofibrate | Increased acetohexamide effect. |
| Contraceptives (oral) | Decreased acetohexamide effect. |
| Cortisone drugs | Decreased acetohexamide effect. |
| Diuretics (thiazide) | Decreased acetohexamide effect. |
| Epinephrine | Decreased acetohexamide effect. |
| Estrogens | Increased acetohexamide effect. |
| Guanethidine | Unpredictable acetohexamide effect. |
| Isoniazid | Decreased acetohexamide effect. |

| | |
|---|---|
| Labetolol | Increased antidiabetic effect, may mask hypoglycemia. |
| MAO inhibitors | Increased acetohexamide effect. |
| Oxyphenbutazone | Increased acetohexamide effect. |
| Phenylbutazone | Increased acetohexamide effect. |
| Phenyramidol | Increased acetohexamide effect. |
| Probenecid | Increased acetohexamide effect. |
| Pyrazinamide | Decreased acetohexamide effect. |
| Sulfa drugs | Increased acetohexamide effect. |
| Sulfaphenazole | Increased acetohexamide effect. |
| Thyroid hormones | Decreased acetohexamide effect. |

## POSSIBLE INTERACTION WITH OTHER SUBSTANCES

| INTERACTS WITH | COMBINED EFFECT |
|---|---|
| Alcohol: | Disulfiram reaction (see Glossary). Avoid. |
| Beverages: | None expected. |
| Cocaine: | No proven problems. |
| Foods: | None expected. |
| Marijuana: | Decreased acetohexamide effect. Avoid. |
| Tobacco: | None expected. |

# ACETOHYDROXAMIC ACID (AHA)

## BRAND NAMES

Lithostat

## BASIC INFORMATION

**Habit forming?** No
**Prescription needed?** Yes
**Available as generic?** No
**Drug class:** Antibacterial, antiurolithic

## USES

- Treatment for chronic urinary-tract infections.
- Prevents formation of urinary-tract stones. Will not dissolve stones already present.

## DOSAGE & USAGE INFORMATION

**How to take:**
Tablet or capsule—Swallow with liquid. If you can't swallow whole, crumble tablet or open capsule and take with liquid or food.

**When to take:**
At the same time each day, according to instructions on prescription label.

**If you forget a dose:**
Take as soon as you remember up to 2 hours late. If more than 2 hours, wait for next scheduled dose (don't double this dose).

**What drug does:**
Stops enzyme action that makes urine too alkaline. Alkaline urine favors bacterial growth and stone formation and growth.

**Time lapse before drug works:**
1 to 3 weeks.

**Don't take with:**
Alcohol or iron. See Interaction column and consult doctor.

## OVERDOSE

**SYMPTOMS:**
Loss of appetite, tremor, nausea, vomiting.
**WHAT TO DO:**
Overdose unlikely to threaten life. If person takes much larger amount than prescribed, call doctor, poison-control center or hospital emergency room for instructions.

## POSSIBLE ADVERSE REACTIONS OR SIDE EFFECTS

| SYMPTOMS | WHAT TO DO |
|---|---|
| **Life-threatening:** None expected. | |
| **Common:** | |
| • Appetite loss, nausea, vomiting. | Discontinue. Seek emergency treatment. |
| • Anxiety, depression, unusual tiredness. | Continue. Call doctor when convenient. |
| **Infrequent:** | |
| • Loss of coordination, slurred speech, severe headache, sudden change in vision, shortness of breath, clot or pain over a blood vessel, sudden chest pain, leg pain in calf (deep vein blood clot). | Discontinue. Seek emergency treatment. |
| • Rash on arms and face. | Discontinue. Call doctor right away. |
| **Rare:** Hair loss. | Continue. Call doctor when convenient. |

## WARNINGS & PRECAUTIONS

**Don't take if:**
You have severe chronic kidney disease.

**Before you start, consult your doctor:**
- If you are anemic.
- If you have or have had phlebitis or thrombophlebitis.

**Over age 60:**
Adverse reactions and side effects may be more frequent and severe than in younger persons.

**Pregnancy:**
Studies inconclusive on harm to unborn child. Animal studies show fetal abnormalities. Decide with your doctor whether drug benefits justify risk to unborn child.

**Breast-feeding:**
No proven problems. Avoid if possible.

**Infants & children:**
Not recommended. Safety and dosage have not been established.

**Prolonged use:**
No problems expected.

**Skin & sunlight:**
No problems expected.

**Driving, piloting or hazardous work:**
Don't drive or pilot aircraft until you learn how medicine affects you. Don't work around dangerous machinery. Don't climb ladders or work in high places. Danger increases if you drink alcohol or take medicine affecting alertness and reflexes, such as antihistamines, tranquilizers, sedatives, pain medicines, narcotics and mind-altering drugs.

**Discontinuing:**
Don't discontinue without consulting doctor. Dose may require gradual reduction if you have taken drug for a long time. Doses of other drugs may also require adjustment.

**Others:**
No problems expected.

## POSSIBLE INTERACTION WITH OTHER DRUGS

| GENERIC NAME OR DRUG CLASS | COMBINED EFFECT |
|---|---|
| Iron | Decreased effects of both drugs. |

## POSSIBLE INTERACTION WITH OTHER SUBSTANCES

| INTERACTS WITH | COMBINED EFFECT |
|---|---|
| Alcohol: | Severe skin rash common in many patients within 30 to 45 minutes after drinking alcohol. |
| Beverages: | None expected. |
| Cocaine: | None expected. |
| Foods: | None expected. |
| Marijuana: | None expected. |
| Tobacco: | None expected. |

# ACETOPHENAZINE

## BRAND NAMES

Tindal

## BASIC INFORMATION

**Habit forming? No**
**Prescription needed? Yes**
**Available as generic? Yes**
**Drug class: Tranquilizer, antiemetic**
**(phenothiazine)**

 ## USES

- Stops nausea, vomiting.
- Reduces anxiety, agitation.

 ## DOSAGE & USAGE INFORMATION

**How to take:**
- Tablet or capsule—Swallow with liquid or food to lessen stomach irritation.
- Suppositories—Remove wrapper and moisten suppository with water. Gently insert into rectum, large end first.
- Drops or liquid—Dilute dose in beverage.

**When to take:**
- Nervous and mental disorders—Take at the same times each day.
- Nausea and vomiting—Take as needed, no more often than every 4 hours.

**If you forget a dose:**
- Nervous and mental disorders—Take up to 2 hours late. If more than 2 hours, wait for next scheduled dose (don't double this).
- Nausea and vomiting—Take as soon as you remember. Wait 4 hours for next dose.

**What drug does:**
- Suppresses brain's vomiting center.
- Suppresses brain centers that control abnormal emotions and behavior.

*Continued next column*

 ## OVERDOSE

**SYMPTOMS:**
Stupor, convulsions, coma.
**WHAT TO DO:**
- **Dial 0 (operator) or 911 (emergency) for an ambulance or medical help. Then give first aid immediately.**
- **See emergency information on inside covers.**

**Time lapse before drug works:**
- Nausea and vomiting—1 hour or less.
- Nervous and mental disorders—4-6 weeks.

**Don't take with:**
- Antacid or medicine for diarrhea.
- Non-prescription drug for cough, cold or allergy.
- See Interaction column and consult doctor.

 ## POSSIBLE ADVERSE REACTIONS OR SIDE EFFECTS

| SYMPTOMS | WHAT TO DO |
|---|---|
| **Life-threatening:**<br>None expected. | |
| **Common:** | |
| • Muscle spasms of face and neck, unsteady gait. | Discontinue. Seek emergency treatment. |
| • Restlessness, tremor, drowsiness. | Discontinue. Call doctor right away. |
| • Decreased sweating, dry mouth. stuffy nose, constipation. | Continue. Call doctor when convenient. |
| **Infrequent:** | |
| • Fainting. | Discontinue. Seek emergency treatment. |
| • Rash. | Discontinue. Call doctor right away. |
| • Difficult or painful urination, diminished sex drive, swollen breasts, menstrual irregularities. | Continue. Call doctor when convenient. |
| **Rare:**<br>Change in vision, sore throat and fever, jaundice. | Discontinue. Call doctor right away. |

# ACETOPHENAZINE

 **WARNINGS & PRECAUTIONS**

**Don't take if:**
- You are allergic to any phenothiazine.
- You have a blood or bone-marrow disease.

**Before you start, consult your doctor:**
- If you will have surgery within 2 months, including dental surgery, requiring general or spinal anesthesia.
- If you have asthma, emphysema or other lung disorder.
- If you take non-prescription ulcer medicine, asthma medicine or amphetamines.

**Over age 60:**
Adverse reactions and side effects may be more frequent and severe than in younger persons. More likely to develop involuntary movement of jaws, lips, tongue, chewing. Report this to your doctor immediately. Early treatment can help.

**Pregnancy:**
Risk to unborn child outweighs drug benefits. Don't use.

**Breast-feeding:**
Drug passes into milk. Avoid drug or discontinue nursing until you finish medicine. Consult doctor for advice on maintaining milk supply.

**Infants & children:**
Don't give to children younger than 2.

**Prolonged use:**
May lead to tardive dyskinesia (involuntary movement of jaws, lips, tongue, chewing).

**Skin & sunlight:**
May cause rash or intensify sunburn in areas exposed to sun or sunlamp. Skin may remain sensitive for 3 months after discontinuing.

**Driving, piloting or hazardous work:**
Don't drive or pilot aircraft until you learn how medicine affects you. Don't work around dangerous machinery. Don't climb ladders or work in high places. Danger increases if you drink alcohol or take medicine affecting alertness and reflexes.

**Discontinuing:**
- Nervous and mental disorders—Don't discontinue without doctor's advice until you complete prescribed dose, even though symptoms diminish or disappear.
- Nausea and vomiting—May be unnecessary to finish medicine. Follow doctor's instructions.

 **POSSIBLE INTERACTION WITH OTHER DRUGS**

| GENERIC NAME OR DRUG CLASS | COMBINED EFFECT |
|---|---|
| Anticholinergics | Increased anticholinergic effect. |
| Antidepressants (tricyclic) | Increased acetophenazine effect. |
| Antihistamines | Increased antihistamine effect. Possible oversedation. |
| Appetite suppressants | Decreased suppressant effect. |
| Dronabinol | Increased effects of both drugs. Avoid. |
| Levodopa | Decreased levodopa effect. |
| Mind-altering drugs | Increased effect of mind-altering drugs. |
| Molindone | Increased tranquilizer effect. |
| Narcotics | Increased narcotic effect. |
| Phenytoin | Increased phenytoin effect. |
| Quinidine | Impaired heart function. Dangerous mixture. |
| Sedatives | Increased sedative effect. |
| Tranquilizers (other) | Increased tranquilizer effect. |

**POSSIBLE INTERACTION WITH OTHER SUBSTANCES**

| INTERACTS WITH | COMBINED EFFECT |
|---|---|
| Alcohol: | Dangerous oversedation. |
| Beverages: | None expected. |
| Cocaine: | Decreased acetophenazine effect. Avoid. |
| Foods: | None expected. |
| Marijuana: | Drowsiness. May increase antinausea effect. |
| Tobacco: | None expected. |

# ACYCLOVIR (ORAL & TOPICAL)

## BRAND NAMES

Zovirax          Zovirax Ointment

## BASIC INFORMATION

Habit forming? No
Prescription needed? Yes
Available as generic? No
Drug class: Antiviral

## USES

- Treatment of severe herpes infections of genitals occurring for first time in special cases.
- Treatment of severe herpes infections on mucous membrane of mouth and lips in special cases.
- Used (although not yet approved by FDA) for shingles (herpes zoster) and chicken pox (varicella) in special cases.

## DOSAGE & USAGE INFORMATION

How to take:
- Tablet or capsule—Swallow with liquid.
- Ointment—Apply to skin and mucous membranes every 3 hours (6 times a day) for 7 days. Use rubber glove when applying. Apply 1/2-inch strip to each sore or blister. Wash before using.

When to use:
As directed on label.

If you forget a dose:
Take as soon as you remember up to 2 hours late. If more than 2 hours, wait for next scheduled dose (don't double this dose).

What drug does:
- Inhibits reproduction of virus in cells without killing normal cells.
- Does not cure. Herpes may recur.

*Continued next column*

## OVERDOSE

SYMPTOMS:
Hallucinations, seizures, kidney shutdown.
WHAT TO DO:
- **Dial 0 (operator) or 911 (emergency) for an ambulance or medical help. Then give first aid immediately.**
- **See emergency information on inside covers.**

Time lapse before drug works:
2 hours.

Don't take with:
See Interaction column and consult doctor.

## POSSIBLE ADVERSE REACTIONS OR SIDE EFFECTS

| SYMPTOMS | WHAT TO DO |
|---|---|
| **Life-threatening:** None expected. | |
| **Common:** Rash, hives, itch, mild pain, burning or stinging of skin, lightheadedness, headache. | Continue. Call doctor when convenient. |
| **Infrequent:** Confusion, hallucinations, trembling. | Discontinue. Call doctor right away. |
| **Rare:** Abdominal pain, decreased appetite, nausea, vomiting, breathing difficulty, blood in urine, decreased urine volume. | Discontinue. Call doctor right away. |

## WARNINGS & PRECAUTIONS

**Don't take if:**
You are allergic to acyclovir.

**Before you start, consult your doctor:**
- If pregnant or plan pregnancy.
- If breast-feeding.
- If you have kidney disease.
- If you have any nerve disorder.

**Over age 60:**
Adverse reactions and side effects may be more frequent and severe than in younger persons.

**Pregnancy:**
Risk to unborn child outweighs drug benefits. Don't use.

**Breast-feeding:**
Drug passes into milk. Avoid drug or discontinue nursing until you finish medicine. Consult doctor for advice on maintaining milk supply.

**Infants & children:**
Use only under special medical supervision by experienced clinician.

**Prolonged use:**
Don't use longer than prescribed time.

**Skin & sunlight:**
No problems expected.

**Driving, piloting or hazardous work:**
No problems expected.

**Discontinuing:**
May be unnecessary to finish medicine. Follow doctor's instructions.

**Others:**
- Women: Get Pap smear every 6 months because those with herpes infections are more likely to develop cancer of cervix. Avoid sexual activity until all blisters or sores heal. Don't get medicine in eyes.
- Protect from freezing.
- Check with doctor if no improvement in 1 week.

## POSSIBLE INTERACTION WITH OTHER DRUGS

| GENERIC NAME OR DRUG CLASS | COMBINED EFFECT |
| --- | --- |
| Interferon | Neurological abnormalities. Avoid. |
| Methotrexate | Neurological abnormalities. Avoid. |
| Other medications that can cause toxic effects on kidneys: Amikacin Amphotericin B Capreomycin Colistimethate Colistin Gentamycin Kanamycin Neomycin Netilmicin Polymixin B Probenecid Streptomycin Tobramycin Vancomycin | Increase kidney toxicity. |

## POSSIBLE INTERACTION WITH OTHER SUBSTANCES

| INTERACTS WITH | COMBINED EFFECT |
| --- | --- |
| Alcohol: | Increased chance of brain and nervous system adverse reaction. Avoid. |
| Beverages: | No problems expected. |
| Cocaine: | Increased chance of brain and nervous system adverse reaction. Avoid. |
| Foods: | No problems expected. |
| Marijuana: | Increased chance of brain and nervous system adverse reaction. Avoid. |
| Tobacco: | No problems expected. |

# ADRENOCORTICOIDS (TOPICAL)

## BRAND NAMES

Some of these brand names are available as oral medicine. Look under specific generic name for each brand. See complete list of brand names in the *Brand Name Directory*, page 941.

## BASIC INFORMATION

**Habit forming? No**
**Prescription needed? Yes**
**Available as generic? Yes**
**Drug class: Adrenocorticoid (topical)**

 ## USES

Relieves redness, swelling, itching, skin discomfort of hemorrhoids, insect bites, poison ivy, oak, sumac, soaps, cosmetics and jewelry.

 ## DOSAGE & USAGE INFORMATION

**How to use:**
- Cream, lotion, ointment—Apply small amount and rub in gently.
- Topical aerosol—Follow directions on container. Don't breathe vapors.

**When to use:**
When needed or as directed. Don't use more often than directions allow.

**If you forget an application:**
Use as soon as you remember.

**What drug does:**
Reduces inflammation by affecting enzymes that produce inflammation.

**Time lapse before drug works:**
15 to 20 minutes.

**Don't use with:**
See Interaction column and consult doctor.

 ## OVERDOSE

**SYMPTOMS:**
**None expected.**
**WHAT TO DO:**
**If person swallows or inhales drug, call doctor, poison-control center or hospital emergency room for instructions.**

 ## POSSIBLE ADVERSE REACTIONS OR SIDE EFFECTS

| SYMPTOMS | WHAT TO DO |
|---|---|
| **Life-threatening:** None expected. | |
| **Common:** None expected. | |
| **Infrequent:** Infection on skin with pain, redness, blisters, pus; skin irritation with burning, itching, blistering or peeling; acne-like skin eruptions. | Continue. Call doctor when convenient. |
| **Rare:** None expected. | |

## WARNINGS & PRECAUTIONS

**Don't take if:**
You are allergic to any topical adrenocorticoid (cortisone) preparation.

**Before you start, consult your doctor:**
- If you plan pregnancy within medication period.
- If you have diabetes.
- If you have infection at treatment site.
- If you have stomach ulcer.
- If you have tuberculosis.

**Over age 60:**
Adverse reactions and side effects may be more frequent and severe than in younger persons, especially thinning of the skin.

**Pregnancy:**
Risk to unborn child outweighs drug benefits. Don't use.

**Breast-feeding:**
No problems expected.

**Infants & children:**
- Use only under medical supervision. Too much for too long can be absorbed into bloodstream through skin and retard growth.
- For infants in diapers, avoid plastic pants or tight diapers.

**Prolonged use:**
- Increases chance of absorption into bloodstream to cause side effects of oral cortisone drugs.
- May thin skin where used.

**Skin & sunlight:**
No problems expected.

**Driving, piloting or hazardous work:**
No problems expected.

**Discontinuing:**
May be unnecessary to finish medicine. Follow doctor's instructions.

**Others:**
- Don't use a plastic dressing longer than 2 weeks.
- Aerosol spray—Store in cool place. Don't use near heat or open flame or while smoking. Don't puncture, break or burn container.

## POSSIBLE INTERACTION WITH OTHER DRUGS

| GENERIC NAME OR DRUG CLASS | COMBINED EFFECT |
|---|---|
| Antibiotics (topical) | Decreased antibiotic effects. |
| Antifungals (topical) | Decreased antifungal effect. |

## POSSIBLE INTERACTION WITH OTHER SUBSTANCES

| INTERACTS WITH | COMBINED EFFECT |
|---|---|
| Alcohol: | None expected. |
| Beverages: | None expected. |
| Cocaine: | None expected. |
| Foods: | None expected. |
| Marijuana: | None expected. |
| Tobacco: | None expected. |

# ALBUTEROL

## BRAND AND GENERIC NAMES

ALBUTEROL          Salbutamol
Proventil          Ventolin

## BASIC INFORMATION

**Habit forming?** No
**Prescription needed?** Yes
**Available as generic?** Yes
**Drug class:** Bronchodilator,
                sympathomimetic

## USES

- Relieves wheezing and shortness of breath in bronchial asthma attacks, allergies, bronchitis, emphysema or other conditions that cause spasm of the bronchial tubes.
- Temporarily increases blood pressure.

## DOSAGE & USAGE INFORMATION

**How to take:**
- Oral liquid or tablet—Swallow with liquid or food to lessen stomach irritation.
- Inhaler—Follow instructions on package.

**When to take:**
When needed according to doctor's instructions. Don't take more than 2 doses 1 hour apart.

**If you forget a dose:**
Take when you remember. Wait 2 hours before next dose.

**What drug does:**
Relaxes smooth muscles to relieve constriction of bronchial tubes.

*Continued next column*

## OVERDOSE

**SYMPTOMS:**
Chest pain, irregular heartbeat, convulsions, coma.
**WHAT TO DO:**
- Dial 0 (operator) or 911 (emergency) for an ambulance or medical help. Then give first aid immediately.
- If patient is unconscious and not breathing, give mouth-to-mouth breathing.
- If there is no heartbeat, use cardiac massage and mouth-to-mouth breathing (CPR). Don't try to make patient vomit. If you can't get help quickly, take patient to nearest emergency facility.
- See emergency information on inside covers.

**Time lapse before drug works:**
5 to 30 minutes

**Don't take with:**
See Interaction column and consult doctor.

## POSSIBLE ADVERSE REACTIONS OR SIDE EFFECTS

| SYMPTOMS | WHAT TO DO |
| --- | --- |
| **Life-threatening:**<br>Severe chest pain, extremely rapid heart-beat (200/min or more). | Seek emergency treatment immediately. |
| **Common:**<br>Dizziness, lightheadedness, headache, nausea or vomiting, large pupils, blurred vision. | Discontinue. Call doctor right away. |
| **Infrequent:**<br>Difficult or painful urination, muscle cramps in legs, dry mouth. | Continue. Call doctor when convenient. |
| **Rare:**<br>Light chest pain, hallucinations, mood changes. | Discontinue. Call doctor right away. |

## WARNINGS & PRECAUTIONS

**Don't take if:**
You are allergic to any sympathomimetic.

**Before you start, consult your doctor:**
- If you have irregular or rapid heartbeat, congestive heart failure, coronary-artery disease or high blood pressure.
- If you have diabetes.
- If you have overactive thyroid.

**Over age 60:**
Adverse reactions and side affects may be more frequent and severe than in younger persons.

**Pregnancy:**
Risk to unborn child outweights drug benefits. Don't use.

**Breast-feeding:**
Drug passes into milk. Avoid drug or discontinue nursing until you finish medicine. Consult doctor for advice on maintaining milk supply.

**Infants & children:**
Use only under medical supervision.

**Prolonged use:**
No problems expected.

**Skin & sunlight:**
No problems expected.

**Driving, piloting or hazardous work:**
Don't drive or pilot aircraft until you learn how medicine affects you. Don't work around dangerous machinery. Don't climb ladders or work in high places. Danger increases if you drink alcohol or take medicine affecting alertness and reflexes, such as antihistamines, tranquilizers, sedatives, pain medicine, narcotics and mind-altering drugs.

**Discontinuing:**
No problems expected.

**Others:**
- May change blood glucose laboratory determinations (increased).
- May increase serum lactic acid concentrations.

## POSSIBLE INTERACTION WITH OTHER DRUGS

| GENERIC NAME OR DRUG CLASS | COMBINED EFFECT |
|---|---|
| Antidepressant (tricyclic) | Increased effect of both drugs. |
| Beta-adrenergic blockers | Decreased albuterol effect and beta-adrenergic blocker effect. |
| Digitalis | Increased risk of heartbeat irregularity. |
| Hydralazine | Decreased hydralazine effect. |
| Levodopa | Increased risk of heartbeat irregularity. |
| Sympathomimetics (others) | Increased effects of both drugs, especially harmful side effects. |

## POSSIBLE INTERACTION WITH OTHER SUBSTANCES

| INTERACTS WITH | COMBINED EFFECT |
|---|---|
| Alcohol: | Decreased albuterol effect. |
| Beverages: | None expected. |
| Cocaine: | Likely albuterol toxicity. |
| Foods: | None expected. |
| Marijuana: | Overstimulation. Avoid. |
| Tobacco: | No proven problems. |

# ALLOPURINOL

## BRAND NAMES

| | |
|---|---|
| Alloprin | Purinol |
| Aluline | Roucol |
| Apo-Allopurinol | Zurinol |
| Caplenal | Zyloprim |
| Lopurin | Zyloric |
| Novopurol | |

## BASIC INFORMATION

**Habit forming? No**
**Prescription needed? Yes**
**Available as generic? Yes**
**Drug class: Antigout**

 **USES**

- Treatment for chronic gout.
- Prevention of kidney stones caused by uric acid.

 **DOSAGE & USAGE INFORMATION**

**How to take:**
Tablet—Swallow with liquid or food to lessen stomach irritation.

**When to take:**
At the same times each day.

**If you forget a dose:**
- 1 dose per day—Take as soon as you remember up to 6 hours late. If more than 6 hours, wait for next scheduled dose (don't double this dose).
- More than 1 dose per day—Take as soon as you remember up to 3 hours late. If more than 3 hours, wait for next scheduled dose (don't double this dose).

**What drug does:**
Slows formation of uric acid by inhibiting enzyme (xanthine oxidase) activity.

**Time lapse before drug works:**
Reduces blood uric acid in 1 to 3 weeks. May require 6 months to prevent acute gout attacks.

*Continued next column*

 **OVERDOSE**

**SYMPTOMS:**
None expected.
**WHAT TO DO:**
Overdose unlikely to threaten life. If person takes much larger amount than prescribed, call doctor, poison-control center or hospital emergency room for instructions.

**Don't take with:**
See Interaction column and consult doctor.

 **POSSIBLE ADVERSE REACTIONS OR SIDE EFFECTS**

| SYMPTOMS | WHAT TO DO |
|---|---|
| **Life-threatening:** None expected. | |
| **Common:** Rash, hives, itch. | Discontinue. Call doctor right away. |
| **Infrequent:** | |
| • Jaundice. | Discontinue. Call doctor right away. |
| • Drowsiness, diarrhea, stomach pain, nausea, vomiting. | Continue. Call doctor when convenient. |
| **Rare:** | |
| • Sore throat, fever, unusual bleeding or bruising. | Discontinue. Call doctor right away. |
| • Numbness, tingling, pain in hands or feet. | Continue. Call doctor when convenient. |

 **WARNINGS & PRECAUTIONS**

**Don't take if:**
You are allergic to allopurinol.

**Before you start, consult your doctor:**
If you have had liver or kidney problems.

**Over age 60:**
Adverse reactions and side effects may be more frequent and severe than in younger persons.

**Pregnancy:**
Studies inconclusive on harm to unborn child. Animal studies show fetal abnormalities. Decide with your doctor whether drug benefits justify risk to unborn child.

**Breast-feeding:**
Drug passes into milk. Avoid drug or discontinue nursing.

**Infants & children:**
Not recommended.

**Prolonged use:**
No problems expected.

**Skin & sunlight:**
No problems expected.

**Driving, piloting or hazardous work:**
Avoid if you feel drowsy. Use may disqualify you for piloting aircraft.

# ALLOPURINOL

**Discontinuing:**
Don't discontinue without doctor's advice until you complete prescribed dose, even though symptoms diminish or disappear.

**Others:**
Acute gout attacks may increase during first weeks of use. If so, consult doctor about additional medicine.

 **POSSIBLE INTERACTION WITH OTHER DRUGS**

| GENERIC NAME OR DRUG CLASS | COMBINED EFFECT |
| --- | --- |
| Ampicillin | Likely skin rash. |
| Anticoagulants (oral) | Increased anticoagulant effect. |
| Antidiabetics (oral) | Increased uric-acid elimination. |
| Azathioprine | Increased azathioprine effect. |
| Chlorthalidone | Decreased allopurinol effect. |
| Cyclophosphamide | Increased cyclophosphamide toxicity. |
| Diuretics (thiazide) | Decreased allopurinol effect. |
| Ethacrynic acid | Decreased allopurinol effect. |
| Furosemide | Decreased allopurinol effect. |
| Indapamide | Decreased allopurinol effect. |
| Iron supplements | Excessive accumulation of iron in tissues. |
| Mercaptopurine | Increased mercaptopurine effect. |
| Metolazone | Decreased allopurinol effect. |
| Probenecid | Increased allopurinol effect. |

 **POSSIBLE INTERACTION WITH OTHER SUBSTANCES**

| INTERACTS WITH | COMBINED EFFECT |
| --- | --- |
| Alcohol: | None expected, but may impair management of gout. |
| Beverages: Caffeine drinks. | Decreased allopurinol effect. |
| Cocaine: | Decreased allopurinol effect. Avoid. |
| Foods: | None expected. Low-purine diet recommended (see Glossary). |
| Marijuana: | Occasional use—None expected. Daily use—Possible increase in uric-acid level. |
| Tobacco: | None expected. |

# ALPRAZOLAM

## BRAND NAMES

Xanax

## BASIC INFORMATION

Habit forming? Yes
Prescription needed? Yes
Available as generic? No
Drug class: Tranquilizer (benzodiazepine)

 **USES**

Treatment for nervousness or tension.

 **DOSAGE & USAGE INFORMATION**

**How to take:**
Tablet or capsule—Swallow with liquid. If you can't swallow whole, crumble tablet or open capsule and take with liquid or food.

**When to take:**
At the same time each day, according to instructions on prescription label.

**If you forget a dose:**
Take as soon as you remember up to 2 hours late. If more than 2 hours, wait for next scheduled dose (don't double this dose).

**What drug does:**
Affects limbic system of brain—part that controls emotions.

**Time lapse before drug works:**
2 hours. May take 6 weeks for full benefit.

**Don't take with:**
See Interaction column and consult doctor.

 **OVERDOSE**

**SYMPTOMS:**
Drowsiness, weakness, tremor, stupor, coma.
**WHAT TO DO:**
- Dial 0 (operator) or 911 (emergency) for an ambulance or medical help. Then give first aid immediately.
- If patient is unconscious and not breathing, give mouth-to-mouth breathing. If there is no heartbeat, use cardiac massage and mouth-to-mouth breathing (CPR). Don't try to make patient vomit. If you can't get help quickly, take patient to nearest emergency facility.
- See emergency information on inside covers.

 **POSSIBLE ADVERSE REACTIONS OR SIDE EFFECTS**

| SYMPTOMS | WHAT TO DO |
|---|---|
| **Life-threatening:** | |
| None expected. | |
| **Common:** | |
| Clumsiness, drowsiness, dizziness. | Continue. Call doctor when convenient. |
| **Infrequent:** | |
| • Hallucinations, confusion, depression, irritability, rash, itch, vision changes. | Discontinue. Call doctor right away. |
| • Constipation or diarrhea, nausea, vomiting, difficult or painful urination. | Continue. Call doctor when convenient. |
| **Rare:** | |
| • Slow heartbeat, breathing difficulty. | Discontinue. Seek emergency treatment. |
| • Mouth or throat ulcers, jaundice | Discontinue. Call doctor right away. |

## WARNINGS & PRECAUTIONS

**Don't take if:**
- You are allergic to any benzodiazepine.
- You have myasthenia gravis.
- You are active or recovering alcoholic.
- Patient is younger than 6 months.

**Before you start, consult your doctor:**
- If you have liver, kidney or lung disease.
- If you have diabetes, epilepsy or porphyria.

**Over age 60:**
Adverse reactions and side effects may be more frequent and severe than in younger persons. You need smaller doses for shorter periods of time. May develop agitation, rage or "hangover" effect.

**Pregnancy:**
Risk to unborn child outweighs drug benefits. Don't use.

**Breast-feeding:**
Drug passes into milk. Avoid drug or discontinue nursing until you finish medicine. Consult doctor for advice on maintaining milk supply.

**Infants & children:**
Use only under medical supervision for children older than 6 months.

**Prolonged use:**
May impair liver function.

**Skin & sunlight:**
No problems expected.

**Driving, piloting or hazardous work:**
Don't drive or pilot aircraft until you learn how medicine affects you. Don't work around dangerous machinery. Don't climb ladders or work in high places. Danger increases if you drink alcohol or take medicine affecting alertness and reflexes.

**Discontinuing:**
Don't discontinue without consulting doctor. Dose may require gradual reduction if you have taken drug for a long time. Doses of other drugs may also require adjustment.

**Others:**
- Hot weather, heavy exercise and profuse sweat may reduce excretion and cause overdose.
- Blood sugar may rise in diabetics, requiring insulin adjustment.

## POSSIBLE INTERACTION WITH OTHER DRUGS

| GENERIC NAME OR DRUG CLASS | COMBINED EFFECT |
|---|---|
| Anticonvulsants | Change in seizure frequency or severity. |
| Antidepressants | Increased sedative effect of both drugs. |
| Antihistamines | Increased sedative effect of both drugs. |
| Antihypertensives | Excessively low blood pressure. |
| Cimetidine | Excess sedation. |
| Disulfiram | Increased alprazolam effect. |
| Dronabinol | Increased effects of both drugs. Avoid. |
| MAO inhibitors | Convulsions, deep sedation, rage. |
| Molindone | Increased tranquilizer effect. |
| Narcotics | Increased sedative effect of both drugs. |
| Sedatives | Increased sedative effect of both drugs. |
| Sleep inducers | Increased sedative effect of both drugs. |
| Tranquilizers | Increased sedative effect of both drugs. |

## POSSIBLE INTERACTION WITH OTHER SUBSTANCES

| INTERACTS WITH | COMBINED EFFECT |
|---|---|
| Alcohol: | Heavy sedation. Avoid. |
| Beverages: | None expected. |
| Cocaine: | Decreased alprazolam effect. |
| Foods: | None expected. |
| Marijuana: | Heavy sedation. Avoid. |
| Tobacco: | Decreased alprazolam effect. |

# ALUMINUM, CALCIUM & MAGNESIUM ANTACIDS

## BRAND NAMES

**Camalox**

## BASIC INFORMATION

Habit forming? No
Prescription needed? No
Available as generic? No
Drug class: Antacids

 **USES**

- Binds excess phosphate in intestine.
- Treatment for hyperacidity in upper gastrointestinal tract, including stomach and esophagus. Symptoms may be heartburn or acid indigestion. Diseases include peptic ulcer, gastritis, esophagitis, hiatal hernia.
- Constipation relief.

 **DOSAGE & USAGE INFORMATION**

**How to take:**
- Tablet or capsule—Swallow with liquid.
- Chewable tablets or wafers—Chew well before swallowing.
- Liquid—Shake well and take undiluted.

**When to take:**
1 to 3 hours after meals unless directed otherwise by your doctor.

**If you forget a dose:**
Take as soon as you remember, but not simultaneously with any other medicine.

**What drug does:**
- Neutralizes some of the hydrochloric acid in the stomach.
- Reduces action of pepsin, a digestive enzyme.
- Stimulates muscles in lower bowel wall.

*Continued next column*

 **OVERDOSE**

**SYMPTOMS:**
Dry mouth, diarrhea, shallow breathing, weakness, fatigue, stupor.
**WHAT TO DO:**
- Dial 0 (operator) or 911 (emergency) for an ambulance or medical help. Then give first aid immediately.
- See emergency information on inside covers.

**Time lapse before drug works:**
15 minutes.

**Don't take with:**
Other medicines at the same time. Decreases absorption of other drugs. Wait 2 hours between doses.

 **POSSIBLE ADVERSE REACTIONS OR SIDE EFFECTS**

| SYMPTOMS | WHAT TO DO |
|---|---|
| **Life-threatening:** | |
| Heartbeat irregularity in patient with heart disease. | Discontinue. Seek emergency treatment. |
| **Common:** | |
| • Constipation, headache, appetite loss, distended stomach. | Discontinue. Call doctor right away. |
| • Unpleasant taste in mouth, abdominal pain, laxative effect, belching. | Continue. Call doctor when convenient. |
| **Infrequent:** | |
| Bone pain, frequent urination, dizziness, urgent urination, muscle weakness or pain, nausea. | Discontinue. Call doctor right away. |
| **Rare:** | |
| Mood changes, vomiting, nervousness, swollen feet and ankles. | Discontinue. Call doctor right away. |

 **WARNINGS & PRECAUTIONS**

**Don't take if:**
- You are allergic to any antacid.
- You have a high blood-calcium level.

**Before you start, consult your doctor:**
- If you have kidney disease.
- If you have chronic constipation, colitis or diarrhea.
- If you have symptoms of appendicitis.
- If you have stomach or intestinal bleeding.
- If you have irregular heartbeat.

**Over age 60:**
Adverse reactions and side effects may be more frequent and severe than in younger persons. Diarrhea or constipation particularly likely.

**Pregnancy:**
Risk to unborn child outweighs drug benefits. Don't use.

**Breast-feeding:**
Drug passes into milk. Avoid drug or discontinue nursing until you finish medicine. Consult doctor for advice on maintaining milk supply.

**Infants & children:**
Use only under medical supervision.

**Prolonged use:**
- Decreased phosphate level in blood weakens bones.
- High blood level of calcium which disturbs electrolyte balance.
- Kidney stones, impaired kidney function.

**Skin & sunlight:**
No problems expected.

**Driving, piloting or hazardous work:**
No problems expected.

**Discontinuing:**
May be unnecessary to finish medicine. Follow doctor's instructions.

**Others:**
Don't take longer than 2 weeks unless under medical supervision.

| Para-aminosalicylic acid (PAS) | Decreased PAS effect. |
|---|---|
| Penicillins | Decreased penicillin effect. |
| Pentobarbital | Decreased pentobarbital effect. |
| Phenylbutazone | Decreased phenylbutazone effect. |
| Pseudoephedrine | Increased pseudoephedrine effect. |
| Quinidine | Increased quinidine effect. |
| Salicylates | Increased salicylate effect. |
| Sulfa drugs | Decreased sulfa effect. |
| Tetracyclines | Decreased tetracycline effect. |
| Vitamins A and C | Decreased vitamin effect. |
| Vitamin D | Too much calcium in blood. |

## POSSIBLE INTERACTION WITH OTHER DRUGS

| GENERIC NAME OR DRUG CLASS | COMBINED EFFECT |
|---|---|
| Anticoagulants | Decreased anticoagulant effect. |
| Calcitonin | Decreased calcitonin effect. |
| Chlorpromazine | Decreased chlorpromazine effect. |
| Digitalis preparations | Decreased digitalis effect. |
| Diuretics | Increased calcium in blood. |
| Iron supplements | Decreased iron effect. |
| Isoniazid | Decreased isoniazid effect. |
| Levodopa | Increased levodopa effect. |
| Meperidine | Increased meperidine effect. |
| Nalidixic acid | Decreased effect of nalidixic acid |
| Oxyphenbutazone | Decreased oxyphenbutazone effect. |

## POSSIBLE INTERACTION WITH OTHER SUBSTANCES

| INTERACTS WITH | COMBINED EFFECT |
|---|---|
| Alcohol: | Decreased antacid effect. |
| Beverages: | No proven problems. |
| Cocaine: | No proven problems. |
| Foods: | Decreased antacid effect. Wait 1 hour after eating. |
| Marijuana: | No proven problems. |
| Tobacco: | Decreased antacid effect. |

# ALUMINUM HYDROXIDE

## BRAND NAMES

See complete list of brand names in the *Brand Name Directory,* page 941.

## BASIC INFORMATION

**Habit forming? No**
**Prescription needed? No**
**Available as generic? Yes**
**Drug class: Antacid, antidiarrheal**

 ## USES

- Binds excess phosphate in intestine.
- Treatment for hyperacidity in upper gastrointestinal tract, including stomach and esophagus. Symptoms may be heartburn or acid indigestion. Diseases include peptic ulcer, gastritis, esophagitis, hiatal hernia.
- Treatment for diarrhea.

 ## DOSAGE & USAGE INFORMATION

**How to take:**
- Tablet or capsule—Swallow with liquid.
- Chewable tablets or wafers—Chew well before swallowing.
- Liquid—Shake well and take undiluted.

**When to take:**
1 to 3 hours after meals unless directed otherwise by your doctor.

**If you forget a dose:**
Take as soon as you remember, but not simultaneously with any other medicine.

**What drug does:**
- Neutralizes some of the hydrochloric acid in the stomach.
- Reduces action of pepsin, a digestive enzyme.

**Time lapse before drug works:**
15 minutes.

*Continued next column*

 ## OVERDOSE

**SYMPTOMS:**
Weakness, fatigue, dizziness.
**WHAT TO DO:**
Overdose unlikely to threaten life. If person takes much larger amount than prescribed, call doctor, poison-control center or hospital emergency room for instructions.

**Don't take with:**
Other medicines at the same time. Decreases absorption of other drugs. Wait 2 hours between doses.

 ## POSSIBLE ADVERSE REACTIONS OR SIDE EFFECTS

| SYMPTOMS | WHAT TO DO |
|---|---|
| **Life-threatening:** None expected. | |
| **Common:** Constipation, appetite loss. | Continue. Call doctor when convenient. |
| **Infrequent:** | |
| • Lower abdominal pain and swelling, bone pain, muscle weakness, swollen wrists or ankles. | Discontinue. Call doctor right away. |
| • Mood changes, nausea, vomiting, weight loss. | Continue. Call doctor when convenient. |
| **Rare:** None expected. | |

 ## WARNINGS & PRECAUTIONS

**Don't take if:**
You are allergic to any antacid.

**Before you start, consult your doctor:**
- If you have kidney disease.
- If you have chronic constipation, colitis or diarrhea.
- If you have symptoms of appendicitis.
- If you have have stomach or intestinal bleeding.

**Over age 60:**
Adverse reactions and side effects may be more frequent and severe than in younger persons. Diarrhea or constipation particularly likely.

**Pregnancy:**
Risk to unborn child outweighs drug benefits. Don't use.

**Breast-feeding:**
Drug passes into milk. Avoid drug or discontinue nursing until you finish medicine. Consult doctor for advice on maintaining milk supply.

**Infants & children:**
Use only under medical supervision.

**Prolonged use:**
Decreased phosphate level in blood weakens bones.

**Skin & sunlight:**
No problems expected.

**Driving, piloting or hazardous work:**
No problems expected.

**Discontinuing:**
May be unnecessary to finish medicine. Follow doctor's instructions.

**Others:**
Don't take longer than 2 weeks unless under medical supervision.

## POSSIBLE INTERACTION WITH OTHER DRUGS

| GENERIC NAME OR DRUG CLASS | COMBINED EFFECT |
|---|---|
| Anticoagulants | Decreased anticoagulant effect. |
| Chlorpromazine | Decreased chlorpromazine effect. |
| Digitalis preparations | Decreased digitalis effect. |
| Iron supplements | Decreased iron effect. |
| Meperidine | Increased meperidine effect. |
| Nalidixic acid | Decreased effect of nalidixic acid. |
| Oxyphenbutazone | Decreased oxyphenbutazone effect. |
| Para-aminosalicylic acid (PAS) | Decreased PAS effect. |
| Penicillins | Decreased penicillin effect. |
| Pentobarbital | Decreased pentobarbital effect. |
| Phenylbutazone | Decreased phenylbutazone effect. |
| Pseudoephedrine | Increased pseudoephedrine effect. |
| Sulfa drugs | Decreased sulfa effect. |
| Tetracyclines | Decreased tetracycline effect. |
| Vitamins A and C | Decreased vitamin effect. |

## POSSIBLE INTERACTION WITH OTHER SUBSTANCES

| INTERACTS WITH | COMBINED EFFECT |
|---|---|
| Alcohol: | Decreased antacid effect. |
| Beverages: | No proven problems. |
| Cocaine: | No proven problems. |
| Foods: | Decreased antacid effect. Wait 1 hour after eating. |
| Marijuana: | No proven problems. |
| Tobacco: | Decreased antacid effect. |

# ALUMINUM & MAGNESIUM ANTACIDS

## BRAND NAMES

See complete list of brand names in the *Brand Name Directory,* page 942.

## BASIC INFORMATION

**Habit forming? No**
**Prescription needed? No**
**Available as generic? Yes**
**Drug class: Antacids**

## USES

- Binds excess phosphate in intestine.
- Treatment for hyperacidity in upper gastrointestinal tract, including stomach and esophagus. Symptoms may be heartburn or acid indigestion. Diseases include peptic ulcer, gastritis, esophagitis, hiatal hernia.
- Constipation relief.

## DOSAGE & USAGE INFORMATION

**How to take:**
- Tablet or capsule—Swallow with liquid.
- Chewable tablets or wafers—Chew well before swallowing.
- Liquid—Shake well and take undiluted.

**When to take:**
1 to 3 hours after meals unless directed otherwise by your doctor.

**If you forget a dose:**
Take as soon as you remember, but not simultaneously with any other medicine.

**What drug does:**
- Neutralizes some of the hydrochloric acid in the stomach.
- Reduces action of pepsin, a digestive enzyme.
- Stimulates muscles in lower bowel wall.

**Time lapse before drug works:**
15 minutes for acid relief.

*Continued next column*

## OVERDOSE

**SYMPTOMS:**
**Weakness, fatigue, dizziness, dry mouth, diarrhea, shallow breathing, stupor.**
**WHAT TO DO:**
- **Dial 0 (operator) or 911 (emergency) for an ambulance or medical help. Then give first aid immediately.**
- **See emergency information on inside covers.**

---

**Don't take with:**
Other medicines at the same time. Decreases absorption of other drugs. Wait 2 hours between doses.

## POSSIBLE ADVERSE REACTIONS OR SIDE EFFECTS

| SYMPTOMS | WHAT TO DO |
|---|---|
| **Life-threatening:** | |
| Heartbeat irregularity in patient with heart disease. | Discontinue. Seek emergency treatment. |
| **Common:** | |
| • Constipation, headache, appetite loss, distended stomach. | Discontinue. Call doctor right away. |
| • Unpleasant taste in mouth, abdominal pain, laxative effect, belching. | Continue. Call doctor when convenient. |
| **Infrequent:** | |
| Bone pain, frequent or urgent urination, dizziness, muscle weakness or pain, nausea. | Discontinue. Call doctor right away. |
| **Rare:** | |
| Mood changes, vomiting, nervousness, swollen feet and ankles. | Discontinue. Call doctor right away. |

## WARNINGS & PRECAUTIONS

**Don't take if:**
You are allergic to any antacid.

**Before you start, consult your doctor:**
If you have kidney disease, chronic constipation, colitis, diarrhea, symptoms of appendicitis, stomach or intestinal bleeding.

**Over age 60:**
Adverse reactions and side effects may be more frequent and severe than in younger persons. Diarrhea or constipation particularly likely.

**Pregnancy:**
Risk to unborn child outweighs drug benefits. Don't use.

**Breast-feeding:**
Drug passes into milk. Avoid drug or discontinue nursing until you finish medicine. Consult doctor for advice on maintaining milk supply.

**Infants & children:**
Use only under medical supervision.

**Prolonged use:**
Decreased phosphate level in blood weakens bones.

**Skin & sunlight:**
No problems expected.

**Driving, piloting or hazardous work:**
No problems expected.

**Discontinuing:**
May be unnecessary to finish medicine. Follow doctor's instructions.

**Others:**
Don't take longer than 2 weeks unless under medical supervision.

 ## POSSIBLE INTERACTION WITH OTHER DRUGS

| GENERIC NAME OR DRUG CLASS | COMBINED EFFECT |
|---|---|
| Anticoagulants (oral) | Decreased anticoagulant effect. |
| Chlorpromazine | Decreased chlorpromazine effect. |
| Digitalis preparations | Decreased digitalis effect. |
| Iron supplements | Decreased iron effect. |
| Isoniazid | Decreased isoniazid effect. |
| Levodopa | Increased levodopa effect. |
| Meperidine | Increased meperidine effect. |
| Nalidixic acid | Decreased effect of nalidixic acid. |
| Oxyphenbutazone | Decreased oxyphenbutazone effect. |
| Para-aminosalicylic acid (PAS) | Decreased PAS effect. |
| Penicillins | Decreased penicillin effect. |
| Pentobarbital | Decreased pentobarbital effect. |
| Phenylbutazone | Decreased phenylbutazone effect. |
| Pseudoephedrine | Increased pseudoephedrine effect. |
| Sulfa drugs | Decreased sulfa effect. |
| Tetracyclines | Decreased tetracycline effect. |
| Vitamin D | Too much calcium in blood. |

 ## POSSIBLE INTERACTION WITH OTHER SUBSTANCES

| INTERACTS WITH | COMBINED EFFECT |
|---|---|
| Alcohol: | Decreased antacid effect. |
| Beverages: | No proven problems. |
| Cocaine: | No proven problems. |
| Foods: | Decreased antacid effect. Wait 1 hour after eating. |
| Marijuana: | No proven problems. |
| Tobacco: | Decreased antacid effect. |

# ALUMINUM, MAGNESIUM, MAGALDRATE & SIMETHICONE ANTACIDS

## BRAND NAMES

See complete list of brand names in the *Brand Name Directory,* page 942.

## BASIC INFORMATION

**Habit forming?** No
**Prescription needed?** No
**Available as generic?** No
**Drug class:** Antacid, antiflatulent

## USES

- Treatment for hyperacidity in upper gastrointestinal tract, including stomach and esophagus. Symptoms may be heartburn or acid indigestion. Diseases include peptic ulcer, gastritis, esophagitis, hiatal hernia.
- Relief of constipation or diarrhea (sometimes).
- Treatment for retention of abdominal gas.
- Used prior to x-ray of abdomen to reduce gas shadows.

## DOSAGE & USAGE INFORMATION

**How to take:**
- Tablet or capsule—Swallow with liquid.
- Liquid—Dissolve in water. Drink complete dose.
- Chewable tablets—Chew completely. Don't swallow whole.

**When to take:**
1 to 3 hours after meals unless directed otherwise by your doctor.

**If you forget a dose:**
Take as soon as you remember, but not simultaneously with any other medicine.

*Continued next column*

## OVERDOSE

**SYMPTOMS:**
Dry mouth, shallow breathing, diarrhea, weakness, fatigue, dizziness, stupor.
**WHAT TO DO:**
- Dial 0 (operator) or 911 (emergency) for an ambulance or medical help. Then give first aid immediately.
- See emergency information on inside covers.

**What drug does:**
- Neutralizes some of the hydrochloric acid in the stomach.
- Reduces action of pepsin, a digestive enzyme.
- Stimulates muscles in lower bowel wall.

**Time lapse before drug works:**
15 minutes.

**Don't take with:**
Other medicines at the same time. Decreases absorption of other drugs. Wait 2 hours between doses.

## POSSIBLE ADVERSE REACTIONS OR SIDE EFFECTS

| SYMPTOMS | WHAT TO DO |
|---|---|
| **Life-threatening:** | |
| Heartbeat irregularity in patient with heart disease. | Discontinue. Seek emergency treatment. |
| **Common:** | |
| • Constipation, headache, appetite loss, distended stomach. | Discontinue. Call doctor right away. |
| • Unpleasant taste in mouth, abdominal pain, laxative effect, belching. | Continue. Call doctor when convenient. |
| **Infrequent:** | |
| Bone pain, frequent urination, dizziness, urgent urination, muscle weakness or pain, nausea. | Discontinue. Call doctor right away. |
| **Rare:** | |
| Mood changes, vomiting, nervousness, swollen feet and ankles. | Discontinue. Call doctor right away. |

## WARNINGS & PRECAUTIONS

**Don't take if:**
You are allergic to any antacid or simethicone.

**Before you start, consult your doctor:**
If you have kidney disease, chronic constipation, colitis, diarrhea, symptoms of appendicitis, stomach or intestinal bleeding.

**Over age 60:**
Adverse reactions and side effects may be more frequent and severe than in younger persons. Diarrhea or constipation particularly likely.

# ALUMINUM, MAGNESIUM, MAGALDRATE & SIMETHICONE ANTACIDS

**Pregnancy:**
Risk to unborn child outweighs drug benefits. Don't use.

**Breast-feeding:**
Drug passes into milk. Avoid drug or discontinue nursing until you finish medicine. Consult doctor for advice on maintaining milk supply.

**Infants & children:**
Use only under medical supervision.

**Prolonged use:**
Decreased phosphate level in blood weakens bones.

**Skin & sunlight:**
No problems expected.

**Driving, piloting or hazardous work:**
No problems expected.

**Discontinuing:**
May be unnecessary to finish medicine. Follow doctor's instructions.

**Others:**
Don't take longer than 2 weeks unless under medical supervision.

 **POSSIBLE INTERACTION WITH OTHER DRUGS**

| GENERIC NAME OR DRUG CLASS | COMBINED EFFECT |
|---|---|
| Anticoagulants (oral) | Decreased anticoagulant effect. |
| Chlorpromazine | Decreased chlorpromazine effect. |
| Digitalis preparations | Decreased digitalis effect. |
| Iron supplements | Decreased iron effect. |
| Isoniazid | Decreased isoniazid effect. |
| Levodopa | Increased levodopa effect. |
| Meperidine | Increased meperidine effect. |
| Nalidixic acid | Decreased effect of nalidixic acid. |
| Oxyphenbutazone | Decreased oxyphenbutazone effect. |
| Para-aminosalicylic acid (PAS) | Decreased PAS effect. |
| Penicillins | Decreased penicillin effect. |
| Pentobarbital | Decreased pentobarbital effect. |
| Phenylbutazone | Decreased phenylbutazone effect. |
| Pseudoephedrine | Increased pseudoephedrine effect. |
| Sulfa drugs | Decreased sulfa effect. |
| Tetracyclines | Decreased tetracycline effect. |
| Vitamins A and C | Decreased vitamin effect. |
| Vitamin D | Too much calcium in blood. |

 **POSSIBLE INTERACTION WITH OTHER SUBSTANCES**

| INTERACTS WITH | COMBINED EFFECT |
|---|---|
| Alcohol: | Decreased antacid effect. |
| Beverages: | No proven problems. |
| Cocaine: | No proven problems. |
| Foods: | Decreased antacid effect. Wait 1 hour after eating. |
| Marijuana: | No proven problems. |
| Tobacco: | Decreased antacid effect. |

# ALUMINUM, MAGNESIUM & SODIUM BICARBONATE ANTACIDS

## BRAND NAMES

Gas-Is-Gon                    Triconsil

## BASIC INFORMATION

**Habit forming? No**
**Prescription needed? No**
**Available as generic? No**
**Drug class: Antacid, antiflatulent**

## USES

- Binds excess phosphate in intestine.
- Treatment for hyperacidity in upper gastrointestinal tract, including stomach and esophagus. Symptoms may be heartburn or acid indigestion. Diseases include peptic ulcer, gastritis, esophagitis, hiatal hernia.
- Relief of constipation or diarrhea (sometimes).

## DOSAGE & USAGE INFORMATION

**How to take:**
- Liquid—Shake well and take undiluted.
- Powder—Dilute dose in beverage before swallowing.

**When to take:**
1 to 3 hours after meals unless directed otherwise by your doctor.

**If you forget a dose:**
Take as soon as you remember, but not simultaneously with any other medicine.

*Continued next column*

## OVERDOSE

**SYMPTOMS:**
**Dry mouth, shallow breathing, diarrhea, weakness, fatigue, dizziness, stupor.**
**WHAT TO DO:**
- **Overdose unlikely to threaten life. Depending on severity of symptoms and amount taken, call doctor, poison-control center or hospital emergency room for instructions.**
- **Dial 0 (operator) or 911 (emergency) for an ambulance or medical help. Then give first aid immediately.**
- **See emergency information on inside covers.**

**What drug does:**
- Neutralizes some of the hydrochloric acid in the stomach.
- Reduces action of pepsin, a digestive enzyme.
- Stimulates muscles in lower bowel wall.

**Time lapse before drug works:**
15 minutes.

**Don't take with:**
Other medicines at the same time. Decreases absorption of other drugs. Wait 2 hours between doses.

## POSSIBLE ADVERSE REACTIONS OR SIDE EFFECTS

| SYMPTOMS | WHAT TO DO |
|---|---|
| **Life-threatening:** | |
| Heartbeat irregularity in patient with heart disease. | Discontinue. Seek emergency treatment. |
| **Common:** | |
| • Constipation, headache, appetite loss, distended stomach. | Discontinue. Call doctor right away. |
| • Unpleasant taste in mouth, abdominal pain, laxative effect, belching. | Continue. Call doctor when convenient. |
| **Infrequent:** | |
| Bone pain, frequent or urgent urination, dizziness, muscle weakness or pain, nausea, weight gain. | Discontinue. Call doctor right away. |
| **Rare:** | |
| Mood changes, vomiting, nervousness, swollen feet and ankles. | Discontinue. Call doctor right away. |

## WARNINGS & PRECAUTIONS

**Don't take if:**
You are allergic to any antacid.

**Before you start, consult your doctor:**
If you have kidney or liver disease, high blood pressure, congestive heart failure, chronic constipation, colitis, diarrhea, symptoms of appendicitis, stomach or intestinal bleeding.

**Over age 60:**
Adverse reactions and side effects may be more frequent and severe than in younger persons. Diarrhea or constipation particularly likely.

**Pregnancy:**
Risk to unborn child outweighs drug benefits. Don't use.

**Breast-feeding:**
Drug passes into milk. Avoid drug or discontinue nursing until you finish medicine. Consult doctor for advice on maintaining milk supply.

**Infants & children:**
Use only under medical supervision.

**Prolonged use:**
- Decreased phosphate level in blood weakens bones.
- Prolonged use with calcium supplements or milk leads to too much calcium in blood.

**Skin & sunlight:**
No problems expected.

**Driving, piloting or hazardous work:**
No problems expected.

**Discontinuing:**
May be unnecessary to finish medicine. Follow doctor's instructions.

**Others:**
Don't take longer than 2 weeks unless under medical supervision.

## POSSIBLE INTERACTION WITH OTHER DRUGS

| GENERIC NAME OR DRUG CLASS | COMBINED EFFECT |
| --- | --- |
| Anticoagulants (oral) | Decreased anticoagulant effect. |
| Chlorpromazine | Decreased chlorpromazine effect. |
| Digitalis preparations | Decreased digitalis effect. |
| Iron supplements | Decreased iron effect. |

| | |
| --- | --- |
| Isoniazid | Decreased isoniazid effect. |
| Levodopa | Increased levodopa effect. |
| Meperidine | Increased meperidine effect. |
| Nalidixic acid | Decreased effect of nalidixic acid. |
| Oxyphenbutazone | Decreased oxyphenbutazone effect. |
| Para-aminosalicylic acid (PAS) | Decreased PAS effect. |
| Penicillins | Decreased penicillin effect. |
| Pentobarbital | Decreased pentobarbital effect. |
| Phenylbutazone | Decreased phenylbutazone effect. |
| Pseudoephedrine | Increased pseudoephedrine effect. |
| Sulfa drugs | Decreased sulfa effect. |
| Tetracyclines | Decreased tetrcycline effect. |
| Vitamina A and C | Decreased vitamin effect. |
| Vitamin D | Too much calcium in blood. |

## POSSIBLE INTERACTION WITH OTHER SUBSTANCES

| INTERACTS WITH | COMBINED EFFECT |
| --- | --- |
| Alcohol: | Decreased antacid effect. |
| Beverages: | No proven problems. |
| Cocaine: | No proven problems. |
| Foods: | Decreased antacid effect. Wait 1 hour after eating. |
| Marijuana: | Decreased antacid effect. |
| Tobacco: | No proven problems. |

# AMANTADINE

## BRAND NAMES

Symmetrel

## BASIC INFORMATION

Habit forming? No
Prescription needed? Yes
Available as generic? No
Drug class: Antiviral, antiparkinsonism

## USES

- Treatment for Type-A flu infections.
- Relief for symptoms of Parkinson's disease.

## DOSAGE & USAGE INFORMATION

**How to take:**
- Tablet or capsule—Swallow with liquid or food to lessen stomach irritation.
- Syrup—Dilute dose in beverage before swallowing.

**When to take:**
At the same times each day. For Type-A flu it is especially important to take regular doses as prescribed.

**If you forget a dose:**
Take as soon as you remember. Wait 4 hours for next dose. Return to schedule.

**What drug does:**
- Type-A flu—May block penetration of tissue cells by infectious material from virus cells.
- Parkinson's disease—Improves muscular condition and coordination.

**Time lapse before drug works:**
- Type-A flu—48 hours.
- Parkinson's disease—2 days to 2 weeks.

**Don't take with:**
- Alcohol
- See Interaction column and consult doctor.

## OVERDOSE

**SYMPTOMS:**
Heart-rhythm disturbances, blood-pressure drop, convulsions, toxic psychosis.
**WHAT TO DO:**
- Dial 0 (operator) or 911 (emergency) for an ambulance or medical help. Then give first aid immediately.
- See emergency information on inside covers.

## POSSIBLE ADVERSE REACTIONS OR SIDE EFFECTS

| SYMPTOMS | WHAT TO DO |
|---|---|
| **Life-threatening:** | |
| None expected. | |
| **Common:** | |
| • Hallucinations, confusion, lightheadedness. | Continue. Call doctor when convenient. |
| • Dizziness, headache, purple blotches, appetite loss, nausea. | Continue. Tell doctor at next visit. |
| • Dry mouth. | No action necessary. |
| **Infrequent:** | |
| • Fainting, slurred speech. | Discontinue. Call doctor right away. |
| • Difficult or painful urination. | Continue. Call doctor when convenient. |
| **Rare:** | |
| • Rash, uncontrollable rolling of eyes, blurred vision, sore throat, fever. | Discontinue. Call doctor right away. |
| • Vomiting. | Continue. Call doctor when convenient. |
| • Constipation. | Continue. Tell doctor at next visit. |

## WARNINGS & PRECAUTIONS

**Don't take if:**
You are allergic to amantadine.

**Before you start, consult your doctor:**
- If you have had epilepsy or other seizures.
- If you have had heart disease or heart failure.
- If you have had liver or kidney disease.
- If you have had peptic ulcers.
- If you have had eczema or skin rashes.
- If you have had emotional or mental disorders or taken drugs for them.

**Over age 60:**
Adverse reactions and side effects may be more frequent and severe than in younger persons.

**Pregnancy:**
Studies inconclusive on harm to unborn child. Animal studies show fetal abnormalities. Decide with your doctor whether benefits justify risk to unborn child.

**Breast-feeding:**
Drug passes into milk. Avoid drug or discontinue nursing until you finish medicine. Consult doctor for advice on maintaining milk supply.

**Infants & children:**
Use only under medical supervision.

**Prolonged use:**
Skin splotches, feet swelling, rapid weight gain, shortness of breath. Consult doctor.

**Skin & sunlight:**
No problems expected.

**Driving, piloting or hazardous work:**
Don't drive or pilot aircraft until you learn how medicine affects you. Don't work around dangerous machinery. Don't climb ladders or work in high places. Danger increases if you drink alcohol or take medicine affecting alertness and reflexes.

**Discontinuing:**
- Parkinson's disease—Don't discontinue without doctor's advice until you complete prescribed dose, even though symptoms diminish or disappear.
- Type-A flu—Discontinue 48 hours after symptoms disappear.

**Others:**
- Parkinson's disease—May lose effectiveness in 3 to 6 months. Consult doctor.
- Amantadine may increase susceptibility to German measles.

## POSSIBLE INTERACTION WITH OTHER DRUGS

| GENERIC NAME OR DRUG CLASS | COMBINED EFFECT |
|---|---|
| Amphetamines | Increased amantadine effect. Possible excessive stimulation and agitation. |
| Anticholinergics | Increased benefit, but excessive anticholinergic dose produces mental confusion, hallucinations, delirium. |
| Appetite suppressants | Increased amantadine effect. Possible excessive stimulation and agitation. |
| Levodopa | Increased benefit of levodopa. Can cause agitation. |
| Sympathomimetics | Increased amantadine effect. Possible excessive stimulation and agitation. |

## POSSIBLE INTERACTION WITH OTHER SUBSTANCES

| INTERACTS WITH | COMBINED EFFECT |
|---|---|
| Alcohol: | Increased alcohol effect. Possible fainting. |
| Beverages: | None expected. |
| Cocaine: | Dangerous overstimulation. |
| Foods: | None expected. |
| Marijuana: | None expected. |
| Tobacco: | None expected. |

# AMBENONIUM

## BRAND NAMES

Mytelase

## BASIC INFORMATION

Habit forming? No
Prescription needed? Yes
Available as generic? No
Drug class: Cholinergic (anticholinesterase)

 **USES**

- Treatment of myasthenia gravis.
- Treatment of urinary retention and abdominal distention.

 **DOSAGE & USAGE INFORMATION**

**How to take:**
Capsule—Swallow with liquid or food to lessen stomach irritation.

**When to take:**
As directed, usually 3 or 4 times a day.

**If you forget a dose:**
Take as soon as you remember up to 2 hours late. If more than 2 hours, wait for next scheduled dose (don't double this dose).

**What drug does:**
Inhibits the chemical activity of an enzyme (cholinesterase) so nerve impulses can cross the junction of nerves and muscles.

**Time lapse before drug works:**
3 hours.

**Don't take with:**
See Interaction column and consult doctor.

 **OVERDOSE**

**SYMPTOMS:**
**Muscle weakness, cramps, twitching or clumsiness; severe diarrhea, nausea, vomiting, stomach cramps or pain; breathing difficulty; confusion, irritability, nervousness, restlessness, fear; unusually slow heartbeat; seizures.**
**WHAT TO DO:**
- **Dial 0 (operator) or 911 (emergency) for an ambulance or medical help. Then give first aid immediately.**
- **See emergency information on inside covers.**

 **POSSIBLE ADVERSE REACTIONS OR SIDE EFFECTS**

| SYMPTOMS | WHAT TO DO |
|---|---|
| **Life-threatening:** None expected. | |
| **Common:** | |
| • Mild diarrhea, nausea, vomiting, stomach cramps or pain. | Discontinue. Call doctor right away. |
| • Excess saliva, unusual sweating. | Continue. Call doctor when convenient. |
| **Infrequent:** | |
| • Confusion, irritability. | Discontinue. Seek emergency treatment. |
| • Constricted pupils, watery eyes, lung congestion, urgent or frequent urination. | Continue. Call doctor when convenient. |
| **Rare:** None expected. | |

## WARNINGS & PRECAUTIONS

**Don't take if:**
- You are allergic to any cholinergic or bromide.
- You take mecamylamine.

**Before you start, consult your doctor:**
- If you plan to become pregnant within medication period.
- If you have bronchial asthma.
- If you have heartbeat irregularities.
- If you have urinary obstruction or urinary-tract infection.

**Over age 60:**
Adverse reactions and side effects may be more frequent and severe than in younger persons.

**Pregnancy:**
No proven harm to unborn child. Avoid if possible. May increase uterus contractions close to delivery.

**Breast-feeding:**
No problems expected, but consult doctor.

**Infants & children:**
Not recommended.

**Prolonged use:**
Medication may lose effectiveness. Discontinuing for a few days may restore effect.

**Skin & sunlight:**
No problems expected.

**Driving, piloting or hazardous work:**
Don't drive or pilot aircraft until you learn how medicine affects you. Don't work around dangerous machinery. Don't climb ladders or work in high places. Danger increases if you drink alcohol or take medicine affecting alertness and reflexes, such as antihistamines, tranquilizers, sedatives, pain medicine, narcotics and mind-altering drugs.

**Discontinuing:**
Don't discontinue without doctor's advice until you complete prescribed dose, even though symptoms diminish or disappear.

**Others:**
No problems expected.

## POSSIBLE INTERACTION WITH OTHER DRUGS

| GENERIC NAME OR DRUG CLASS | COMBINED EFFECT |
|---|---|
| Anesthetics (local or general) | Decreased ambenonium effect. |
| Antiarrhythmics | Decreased ambenonium effect. |
| Antibiotics | Decreased ambenonium effect. |
| Anticholinergics | Decreased ambenonium effect. May mask severe side effects. |
| Cholinergics (other) | Reduced intestinal-tract function. Possible brain and nervous-system toxicity. |
| Mecamylamine | Decreased ambenonium effect. |
| Nitrates | Decreased ambenonium effect. |
| Quinidine | Decreased ambenonium effect. |

## POSSIBLE INTERACTION WITH OTHER SUBSTANCES

| INTERACTS WITH | COMBINED EFFECT |
|---|---|
| Alcohol: | No proven problems with small doses. |
| Beverages: | None expected. |
| Cocaine: | Decreased ambenonium effect. Avoid. |
| Foods: | None expected. |
| Marijuana: | No proven problems. |
| Tobacco: | No proven problems. |

# AMILORIDE

## BRAND NAMES

Midamor

## BASIC INFORMATION

Habit forming? No
Prescription needed? Yes
Available as generic? Yes
Drug class: Diuretic

 ## USES

Treatment for high blood pressure and congestive heart failure. Decreases fluid retention and prevents potassium loss.

 ## DOSAGE & USAGE INFORMATION

How to take:
Tablet—Swallow with liquid.

When to take:
At the same time each day, preferably in the morning. May interfere with sleep if taken after 6 p.m.

If you forget a dose:
Take as soon as you remember up to 8 hours late. If more than 8 hours, wait for next scheduled dose (don't double this dose).

What drug does:
Blocks exchange of certain chemicals in the kidney so sodium is excreted. Conserves potassium.

*Continued next column*

 ## OVERDOSE

SYMPTOMS:
**Rapid, irregular heartbeat; confusion; shortness of breath; nervousness; extreme weakness.**
WHAT TO DO:
- **Dial 0 (operator) or 911 (emergency) for an ambulance or medical help. Then give first aid immediately.**
- **If patient is unconscious and not breathing, give mouth-to-mouth breathing. If there is no heartbeat, use cardiac massage and mouth-to-mouth breathing (CPR). Don't try to make patient vomit. If you can't get help quickly, take patient to nearest emergency facility.**
- **See emergency information on inside covers.**

Time lapse before drug works:
2 hours.

Don't take with:
See Interaction column and consult doctor.

 ## POSSIBLE ADVERSE REACTIONS OR SIDE EFFECTS

| SYMPTOMS | WHAT TO DO |
|---|---|
| **Life-threatening:**<br>None expected. | |
| **Common:**<br>Headache, nausea, appetite loss, vomiting, diarrhea. | Continue. Call doctor when convenient. |
| **Infrequent:**<br>• Cough, shortness of breath. | Discontinue. Call doctor right away. |
| • Dizziness, constipation, pain, bloating, muscle cramps. | Continue. Call doctor when convenient. |
| **Rare:**<br>None expected. | |

 ## WARNINGS & PRECAUTIONS

Don't take if:
- You are allergic to amiloride.
- Your serum potassium level is high.

Before you start, consult your doctor:
- If you plan to become pregnant within medication period.
- If you have diabetes.
- If you have heart disease.
- If you have kidney or liver disease.

Over age 60:
Adverse reactions and side effects may be more frequent and severe than in younger persons. More likely to exceed safe potassium blood levels.

Pregnancy:
No proven harm to unborn child. Avoid if possible.

Breast-feeding:
No problems expected, but consult doctor.

Infants & children:
Not recommended.

Prolonged use:
No problems expected.

Skin & sunlight:
No problems expected.

**Driving, piloting or hazardous work:**
Don't drive or pilot aircraft until you learn how medicine affects you. Don't work around dangerous machinery. Don't climb ladders or work in high places. Danger increases if you drink alcohol or take medicine affecting alertness and reflexes, such as antihistamines, tranquilizers, sedatives, pain medicine, narcotics and mind-altering drugs.

**Discontinuing:**
Don't discontinue without doctor's advice until you complete prescribed dose, even though symptoms diminish or disappear.

**Others:**
Periodic physical checkups and potassium-level tests recommended.

## POSSIBLE INTERACTION WITH OTHER DRUGS

| GENERIC NAME OR DRUG CLASS | COMBINED EFFECT |
|---|---|
| Acebutolol | Increased antihypertensive effect. Dosages may require adjustment. |
| Amiodarone | Increased risk of heartbeat irregularity due to low potassium. |
| Antihypertensives | Increased effect of both drugs. |
| Blood-bank blood | Increased potassium levels. |
| Calcium supplements | Increased calcium in blood. |
| Diuretics (other) | Increased effect of both drugs. |
| Enalapril | Possible excessive potassium in blood. |
| Labetolol | Increased antihypertensive effects. |
| Lithium | Possible lithium toxicity. |
| Nitrates | Excessive blood-pressure drop. |
| Oxprenolol | Increased antihypertensive effect. Dosages may require adjustment. |
| Pentoxifylline | Increased antihypertensive effect. |
| Potassium supplements | Increased potassium levels. |
| Sodium bicarbonate | Decreased potassium levels. |

## POSSIBLE INTERACTION WITH OTHER SUBSTANCES

| INTERACTS WITH | COMBINED EFFECT |
|---|---|
| Alcohol: | Increased blood-pressure drop. Avoid. |
| Beverages: Low-salt milk. | Possible excess potassium levels. Low-salt milk has extra potassium. |
| Cocaine: | Blood-pressure rise. Avoid. |
| Foods: Salt substitutes. | Possible excess potassium levels. |
| Marijuana: | None expected. |
| Tobacco: | None expected. |

# AMILORIDE & HYDROCHLOROTHIAZIDE

## BRAND NAMES

**Moduretic**

## BASIC INFORMATION

**Habit forming?** No
**Prescription needed?** Yes
**Available as generic?** No
**Drug class:** Diuretic (thiazide),
        antihypertensive

## USES

- Controls, but doesn't cure, high blood pressure.
- Reduces fluid retention (edema), decreasing likelihood of congestive heart failure.

## DOSAGE & USAGE INFORMATION

**How to take:**
Tablet or capsule—Swallow with liquid. If you can't swallow whole, crumble tablet or open capsule and take with liquid or food.

**When to take:**
At the same time each day, no later than 6 p.m.

**If you forget a dose:**
Take as soon as you remember up to 2 hours late. If more than 2 hours, wait for next scheduled dose (don't double this dose).

**What drug does:**
- Forces sodium and water excretion, conserves potassium, reducing body fluid.
- Relaxes muscle cells of small arteries.
- Reduced body fluid and relaxed arteries lower blood pressure.

**Time lapse before drug works:**
2-6 hours. May require several weeks to lower blood pressure.

*Continued next column*

## OVERDOSE

**SYMPTOMS:**
Cramps, weakness, drowsiness, weak pulse, coma, rapid, irregular heartbeat.
**WHAT TO DO:**
- **Dial 0 (operator) or 911 (emergency) for an ambulance or medical help. Then give first aid immediately.**
- **See emergency information on inside covers.**

**Don't take with:**
- See Interaction column and consult doctor.
- Non-prescription drugs without consulting doctor.

## POSSIBLE ADVERSE REACTIONS OR SIDE EFFECTS

| SYMPTOMS | WHAT TO DO |
|---|---|
| **Life-threatening:**<br>None expected. | |
| **Common:**<br>• Increased thirst, irregular heartbeat, cramps in muscles, numbness and tingling in hands and feet, thready pulse, shortness of breath. | Discontinue. Call doctor right away. |
| • Tiredness, weakness, dry mouth, diarrhea, headache, appetite loss, nausea. | Continue. Call doctor when convenient. |
| **Infrequent:**<br>Mood changes, constipation, decreased sex function, dizziness, lightheadedness. | Continue. Call doctor when convenient. |
| **Rare:**<br>Jaundice; unusual bleeding or bruising; abdominal pain with nausea and vomiting; sore throat, fever, sores in mouth; hives; skin rash; joint pain. | Discontinue. Seek emergency treatment. |

## WARNINGS & PRECAUTIONS

**Don't take if:**
You are allergic to amiloride or any thiazide diuretic drug.

**Before you start, consult your doctor:**
- If you are allergic to any sulfa drug.
- If you have gout, diabetes, heart disease.
- If you have liver, pancreas or kidney disorder.

**Over age 60:**
Adverse reactions and side effects may be more frequent and severe than in younger persons, especially dizziness and excessive potassium loss.

**Pregnancy:**
Risk to unborn child outweighs drug benefits. Don't use.

**Breast-feeding:**
Drug passes into milk. Avoid drug or discontinue nursing until you finish medicine.

**Infants & children:**
Not recommended unless closely supervised.

**Prolonged use:**
You may need medicine to treat high blood pressure for the rest of your life.

**Skin & sunlight:**
May cause rash or intensify sunburn in areas exposed to sun or sunlamp. Avoid overexposure.

**Driving, piloting or hazardous work:**
Don't drive or pilot aircraft until you learn how medicine affects you. Don't work around dangerous machinery. Don't climb ladders or work in high places. Danger increases if you drink alcohol or take medicine affecting alertness and reflexes, such as antihistamines, tranquilizers, sedatives, pain medicine, narcotics and mind-altering drugs.

**Discontinuing:**
Don't discontinue without medical advice.

**Others:**
- Hot weather and fever may cause dehydration and drop in blood pressure. Dose may require temporary adjustment. Weigh daily and report any unexpected weight decreases to your doctor.
- May cause rise in uric acid, leading to gout.
- May cause blood-sugar rise in diabetics.
- Get periodic check-ups and potassium-level laboratory tests.

## POSSIBLE INTERACTION WITH OTHER DRUGS

| GENERIC NAME OR DRUG CLASS | COMBINED EFFECT |
| --- | --- |
| Acebutolol | Increased antihypertensive effect. Dosages of both drugs may require adjustments. |
| Allopurinol | Decreased allopurinol effect. |
| Antidepressants (tricyclic) | Dangerous drop in blood pressure. Avoid combination unless under medical supervision. |
| Antihypertensives (other) | Increased effect of both drugs. |
| Barbiturates | Increased hydrochlorothiazide effect. |

| | |
| --- | --- |
| Blood-bank blood | Increased potassium levels. |
| Cortisone drugs | Excessive potassium loss that causes dangerous heart rhythms. |
| Digitalis preparations | Excessive potassium loss that causes dangerous heart rhythms. |
| Diuretics (thiazide) | Increased diuretic effect. |
| Diuretics (other) | Increased effect of both drugs. |
| Indapamide | Increased diuretic effect. |
| Lithium | Possible lithium toxicity. |
| MAO inhibitors | Increased hydrochlorothiazide effect. |
| Nitrates | Excessive blood-pressure drop. |
| Oxprenolol | Increased antihypertensive effect. Dosages may require adjustment. |
| Probenecid | Decreased probenecid effect. |
| Sodium bicarbonate | Decreased potassium levels. |

## POSSIBLE INTERACTION WITH OTHER SUBSTANCES

| INTERACTS WITH | COMBINED EFFECT |
| --- | --- |
| Alcohol: | Dangerous blood-pressure drop. |
| Beverages: Low-salt milk. | Possible excess potassium levels. Low-salt milk has extra potassium. |
| Cocaine: | None expected. |
| Foods: Salt substitutes. | Possible excess potassium levels. |
| Marijuana: | May increase blood pressure. |
| Tobacco: | None expected. |

# AMINOBENZOATE POTASSIUM

## BRAND NAMES

KPAB
Potaba
Potassium
  Aminobenzoate

Potassium
Para-
  aminobenzoate

## BASIC INFORMATION

**Habit forming? No**
**Prescription needed? Yes**
**Available as generic? Yes**
**Drug class: Antifibrosis**

## USES

Reduces inflammation and relieves contractions in tissues lying under the skin that have become tight from such disorders as dermatomyositis, Peyronie's disease, scleroderma, pemphigus, morphea.

## DOSAGE & USAGE INFORMATION

**How to take:**
- Tablets—Dissolve in liquid to prevent stomach upset.
- Capsules—Take with full glass of liquid.

**When to take:**
At the same times each day, according to instructions on prescription label. Usually taken with meals and at bedtime with a snack.

**If you forget a dose:**
Take as soon as you remember up to 2 hours late. If more than 2 hours, wait for next scheduled dose (don't double this dose).

**What drug does:**
May increase ability of diseased tissues to use oxygen.

**Time lapse before drug works:**
May require 3 to 10 months for improvement to begin.

**Don't take with:**
See Interaction column and consult doctor.

## OVERDOSE

**SYMPTOMS:**
Nausea, vomiting.
**WHAT TO DO:**
Overdose unlikely to threaten life. If person takes much larger amount than prescribed, call doctor, poison-control center or hospital emergency room for instructions.

## POSSIBLE ADVERSE REACTIONS OR SIDE EFFECTS

| SYMPTOMS | WHAT TO DO |
|---|---|
| **Life-threatening:**<br>None expected. | |
| **Common:**<br>Appetite loss, nausea. | Continue. Call doctor when convenient. |
| **Infrequent:**<br>• Low blood sugar (hunger, anxiety, cold sweats, rapid pulse). | Discontinue. Seek emergency treatment. (Note: Take sugar or honey on the way to emergency room.) |
| • Sore throat. | Discontinue. Call doctor right away. |
| **Rare:**<br>None expected. | |

## WARNINGS & PRECAUTION

**Don't take if:**
You are allergic to aminobenzoate potassium or aminobenzoic acid (PABA).

**Before you start, consult your doctor:**
- If you have low blood sugar.
- If you have diabetes mellitus.
- If you have kidney disease.

**Over age 60:**
Adverse reactions and side effects may be more frequent and severe than in younger persons, particularly low blood sugar.

**Pregnancy:**
No proven problems.

**Breast-feeding:**
Drug passes into milk. Avoid drug or discontinue nursing.

**Infants & children:**
Not recommended. Safety and dosage have not been established.

**Prolonged use:**
No problems expected.

**Skin & sunlight:**
No problems expected.

**Driving, piloting or hazardous work:**
No problems expected.

**Discontinuing:**
No problems expected.

**Others:**
If you become acutely ill and cannot eat well for even a short while, tell your doctor. These circumstances can lead to low blood sugar, and dosage may need adjustment.

 ## POSSIBLE INTERACTION WITH OTHER DRUGS

| GENERIC NAME OR DRUG CLASS | COMBINED EFFECT |
|---|---|
| Sulfa drugs (sulfonamides) | Decreased sulfa effect. |

 ## POSSIBLE INTERACTION WITH OTHER SUBSTANCES

| INTERACTS WITH | COMBINED EFFECT |
|---|---|
| Alcohol: | None expected. |
| Beverages: | None expected. |
| Cocaine: | None expected. |
| Foods: | None expected. |
| Marijuana: | None expected. |
| Tobacco: | None expected. |

# AMIODARONE

## BRAND NAMES

Cordarone

## BASIC INFORMATION

**Habit forming? No**
**Prescription needed? Yes**
**Available as generic? No**
**Drug class: Antiarrhythmic**

 ## USES

Prevents and treats life-threatening heartbeat irregularities involving both the large chambers of the heart (auricles and ventricles).

 ## DOSAGE & USAGE INFORMATION

**How to take:**
Tablets—Swallow whole with liquid or food to lessen stomach irritation. If you can't swallow whole, crumble tablet and take with liquid or food.

**When to take:**
According to prescription instructions.

**If you forget a dose:**
Skip this dose and resume regular schedule. Do not double the next dose. If you forget 2 doses or more, consult your doctor.

**What drug does:**
- Slows nerve impulses in the heart.
- Makes heart muscle fibers less responsive to abnormal electrical impulses arising in the electrical regulatory system of the heart.

*Continued next column*

 ## OVERDOSE

**SYMPTOMS:**
**Irregular heartbeat, loss of consciousness, seizures.**
**WHAT TO DO:**
- **Dial 0 (operator) or 911 (emergency) for an ambulance or medical help. Then give first aid immediately.**
- **If patient is unconscious and not breathing, give mouth-to-mouth breathing. If there is no heartbeat, use cardiac massage and mouth-to-mouth breathing (CPR). Don't try to make patient vomit. If you can't get help quickly, take patient to nearest emergency facility.**
- **See emergency information on inside covers.**

**Time lapse before drug works:**
2 to 3 days to 2 to 3 months.

**Don't take with:**
See Interaction column and consult doctor.

 ## POSSIBLE ADVERSE REACTIONS OR SIDE EFFECTS

| SYMPTOMS | WHAT TO DO |
|---|---|
| **Life-threatening:**<br>Shortness of breath, difficulty breathing, cough. (Not uncommon) | Discontinue. Seek emergency treatment. |
| **Common:**<br>• Walking difficulty, fever, numbness or tingling in hands or feet, shakiness, weakness in arms and legs. | Discontinue. Call doctor right away. |
| • Constipation, headache, appetite loss, nausea, vomiting. | Continue. Call doctor when convenient. |
| **Infrequent:**<br>• Skin color change to blue-gray, blurred vision, cold feeling, dry eyes, nervousness, scrotum swelling or pain, insomnia, swollen feet and ankles, fast or slow heartbeat, eyes hurt in light, weight gain or loss. | Discontinue. Call doctor right away. |
| • Bitter or metallic taste, diminished sex drive, dizziness, flushed face. | Continue. Call doctor when convenient. |
| **Rare:**<br>Jaundice, skin rash. | Discontinue. Call doctor right away. |

## WARNINGS & PRECAUTIONS

**Don't take if:**
You are allergic to amiodarone.

**Before you start, consult your doctor:**
- If you have liver or kidney disease.
- If you have high blood pressure.
- If you have heart disease other than coronary artery disease.

**Over age 60:**
- Adverse reactions and side effects may be more frequent and severe than in younger persons. Ask about smaller doses.
- Pain in legs (while walking) considerably more likely.

**Pregnancy:**
Safety to unborn child unestablished. Avoid if possible.

**Breast-feeding:**
Drug passes into milk. Avoid drug or discontinue nursing until you finish medicine. Consult doctor for advice on maintaining milk supply.

**Infants & children:**
Use only under close medical supervision.

**Prolonged use:**
- Blue-gray discoloration of skin may appear.
- Don't discontinue without consulting doctor. Dose may require gradual reduction if you have taken drug for a long time. Doses of other drugs may also require adjustment.

**Skin & sunlight:**
May cause rash or intensify sunburn in areas exposed to sun or sunlamp. Avoid undue exposure.

**Driving, piloting or hazardous work:**
Avoid if you feel dizzy or lightheaded. Otherwise, no problems expected.

**Discontinuing:**
- Don't discontinue without consulting doctor. Dose may require gradual reduction if you have taken drug for a long time. Doses of other drugs may also require adjustment.
- Notify doctor if cough, fever, breathing difficulty or shortness of breath occur after discontinuing medicine.

**Others:**
Learn to check your own pulse. If it drops to lower than 50 or rises to higher than 100 beats per minute, don't take amiodarone until you consult your doctor.

## POSSIBLE INTERACTION WITH OTHER DRUGS

| GENERIC NAME OR DRUG CLASS | COMBINED EFFECT |
|---|---|
| Anticoagulants | Increased anticoagulant effect. |
| Antiarrhythmics (other) | Increased likelihood of heartbeat irregularity. |
| Beta-blockers (acebutolol, atenolol, labetolol, metaprolol, nadolol, oxprenol, pindolol, propranolol, sotalol, timolol) | Increased likelihood of slow heartbeat. |
| Digitalis | Increased digitalis effect. |
| Diltiazam | Increased likelihood of slow heartbeat. |
| Diuretics | Increased risk of heartbeat irregularity due to low potassium level. |
| Nifedipine | Increased likelihood of slow heartbeat. |
| Phenytoin | Increased effect of phenytoin. |
| Verapamil | Increased likelihood of slow heartbeat. |

## POSSIBLE INTERACTION WITH OTHER SUBSTANCES

| INTERACTS WITH | COMBINED EFFECT |
|---|---|
| Alcohol: | Increased risk of heartbeat irregularity. Avoid. |
| Beverages: | None expected. |
| Cocaine: | Increased risk of heartbeat irregularity. Avoid. |
| Foods: | None expected. |
| Marijuana: | Possible irregular heartbeat. Avoid. |
| Tobacco: | Possible irregular heartbeat. Avoid. |

# AMOBARBITAL

## BRAND NAMES

Amytal      Novamobarb
Dexamyl    Tuinal
Isobec

## BASIC INFORMATION

**Habit forming? Yes**
**Prescription needed? Yes**
**Available as generic? Yes**
**Drug class: Sedative, hypnotic (barbiturate)**

## USES

- Reduces anxiety or nervous tension (low dose).
- Relieves insomnia (higher bedtime dose).

## DOSAGE & USAGE INFORMATION

**How to take:**
Tablet, capsule or liquid—Swallow with food or liquid to lessen stomach irritation. If you can't swallow whole, crumble tablet or open capsule and take with liquid or food.

**When to take:**
At the same times each day.

**If you forget a dose:**
Take as soon as you remember up to 2 hours late. If more than 2 hours, wait for next scheduled dose (don't double this dose).

**What drug does:**
May partially block nerve impulses at nerve-cell connections.

*Continued next column*

## OVERDOSE

**SYMPTOMS:**
**Deep sleep, weak pulse, coma.**
**WHAT TO DO:**
- **Dial 0 (operator) or 911 (emergency) for an ambulance or medical help. Then give first aid immediately.**
- **If patient is unconscious and not breathing, give mouth-to-mouth breathing. If there is no heartbeat use cardiac massage and mouth-to-mouth breathing (CPR). Don't try to make patient vomit. If you can't help quickly, take patient to nearest emergency facility.**
- **See emergency information on inside covers.**

**Time lapse before drug works:**
60 minutes.

**Don't take with:**
- Non-prescription drugs without consulting doctor.
- See Interaction column and consult doctor.

## POSSIBLE ADVERSE REACTIONS OR SIDE EFFECTS

| SYMPTOMS | WHAT TO DO |
|---|---|
| **Life-threatening:**<br>None expected. | |
| **Common:**<br>Dizziness, drowsiness, "hangover" effect. | Continue. Call doctor when convenient. |
| **Infrequent:**<br>• Rash or hives; swollen face, lips, eyelids; sore throat, fever. | Discontinue. Call doctor right away. |
| • Depression, confusion, slurred speech, nausea, vomiting, joint or muscle pain. | Continue. Call doctor when convenient. |
| **Rare:**<br>• Agitation, slow heartbeat, breathing difficulty, jaundice. | Discontinue. Call doctor right away. |
| • Unexplained bleeding or bruising. | Continue. Call doctor when convenient. |

## WARNINGS & PRECAUTIONS

**Don't take if:**
- You are allergic to any barbiturate.
- You have porphyria.

**Before you start, consult your doctor:**
- If you have epilepsy.
- If you have kidney or liver damage.
- If you have asthma.
- If you have anemia.
- If you have chronic pain.
- If you will have surgery within 2 months, including dental surgery, requiring general or spinal anesthesia.

**Over age 60:**
Adverse reactions and side effects may be more frequent and severe than in younger persons. Use small doses.

**Pregnancy:**
Risk to unborn child outweighs drug benefits. Don't use.

**Breast-feeding:**
Drug passes into milk. Avoid drug or discontinue nursing until you finish medicine. Consult doctor for advice on maintaining milk supply.

**Infants & children:**
Use only under doctor's supervision.

**Prolonged use:**
- May cause addiction, anemia, chronic intoxication.
- May lower body temperature, making exposure to cold temperatures hazardous.

**Skin & sunlight:**
May cause rash or intensify sunburn in areas exposed to sun or sunlamp.

**Driving, piloting or hazardous work:**
Don't drive or pilot aircraft until you learn how medicine affects you. Don't work around dangerous machinery. Don't climb ladders or work in high places. Danger increases if you drink alcohol or take medicine affecting alertness and reflexes.

**Discontinuing:**
May be unnecessary to finish medicine. Follow doctor's instructions. If you develop withdrawal symptoms of hallucinations, agitation or sleeplessness after discontinuing, call doctor right away.

**Others:**
Great potential for abuse.

 **POSSIBLE INTERACTION WITH OTHER DRUGS**

| GENERIC NAME OR DRUG CLASS | COMBINED EFFECT |
|---|---|
| Anticoagulants (oral) | Decreased anticoagulant effect. |
| Anticonvulsants | Changed seizure patterns. |
| Antidepressants (tricyclics) | Decreased antidepressant effect. Possible dangerous oversedation. |
| Antidiabetics (oral) | Increased amobarbital effect. |
| Antihistamines | Dangerous sedation. Avoid. |
| Anti-inflammatory drugs (non-steroidal) | Decreased anti-inflammatory effect. |
| Aspirin | Decreased aspirin effect. |
| Beta-adrenergic blockers | Decreased effect of beta-adrenergic blocker. |

| | |
|---|---|
| Contraceptives (oral) | Decreased contraceptive effect. |
| Cortisone drugs | Decreased cortisone effect. |
| Digitoxin | Decreased digitoxin effect. |
| Doxycycline | Decreased doxycycline effect. |
| Dronabinol | Increased effects of both drugs. Avoid. |
| Griseofulvin | Decreased griseofulvin effect. |
| Indapamide | Increased indapamide effect. |
| MAO inhibitors | Increased amobarbital effect. |
| Mind-altering drugs | Dangerous sedation. Avoid. |
| Narcotics | Dangerous sedation. Avoid. |
| Pain relievers | Dangerous sedation. Avoid. |
| Sedatives | Dangerous sedation. Avoid. |
| Sleep inducers | Dangerous sedation. Avoid. |
| Tranquilizers | Dangerous sedation. Avoid. |
| Valproic acid | Increased amobarbital effect. |

 **POSSIBLE INTERACTION WITH OTHER SUBSTANCES**

| INTERACTS WITH | COMBINED EFFECT |
|---|---|
| Alcohol: | Possible fatal oversedation. Avoid. |
| Beverages: | None expected. |
| Cocaine: | Decreased amobarbital effect. |
| Foods: | None expected. |
| Marijuana: | Excessive sedation. Avoid. |
| Tobacco: | None expected. |

# AMOXICILLIN

## BRAND NAMES

| | |
|---|---|
| Amoxil | Polymox |
| Augmentin | Robamox |
| Larotid | Sumox |
| Moxilean | Trimox |
| Novamoxin | Utimox |
| Penamox | Wymox |

## BASIC INFORMATION

**Habit forming? No**
**Prescription needed? Yes**
**Available as generic? Yes**
**Drug class: Antibiotic (penicillin)**

## USES

Treatment of bacterial infections that are susceptible to amoxicillin.

## DOSAGE & USAGE INFORMATION

**How to take:**
- Tablet or capsule—Swallow with liquid on an empty stomach 1 hour before or 2 hours after eating.
- Liquid—Take with cold beverage. Liquid form is perishable and effective for only 7 days at room temperature. Effective for 14 days if stored in refrigerator. Don't freeze.

**When to take:**
Follow instructions on prescription label or side of package. Doses should be evenly spaced. For example, 4 times a day means every 6 hours.

**If you forget a dose:**
Take as soon as you remember. Continue regular schedule.

**What drug does:**
Destroys susceptible bacteria. Does not kill viruses.

*Continued next column*

## OVERDOSE

**SYMPTOMS:**
**Severe diarrhea, nausea or vomiting.**
**WHAT TO DO:**
**Overdose unlikely to threaten life. If person takes much larger amount than prescribed, call doctor, poison-control center or hospital emergency room for instructions.**

**Time lapse before drug works:**
May be several days before medicine affects infection.

**Don't take with:**
See Interaction column and consult doctor.

## POSSIBLE ADVERSE REACTIONS OR SIDE EFFECTS

| SYMPTOMS | WHAT TO DO |
|---|---|
| **Life-threatening:**<br>Hives, rash, intense itching, faintness soon after a dose (anaphylaxis). | Seek emergency treatment immediately. |
| **Common:**<br>Dark or discolored tongue. | Continue. Tell doctor at next visit. |
| **Infrequent:**<br>Mild nausea, vomiting, diarrhea. | Continue. Call doctor when convenient. |
| **Rare:**<br>Unexplained bleeding. | Discontinue. Call doctor right away. |

## WARNINGS & PRECAUTIONS

**Don't take if:**
You are allergic to amoxicillin, cephalosporin antibiotics, other penicillins or penicillamine. Life-threatening reaction may occur.

**Before you start, consult your doctor:**
If you are allergic to any substance or drug.

**Over age 60:**
You may have skin reactions, particularly around genitals and anus.

**Pregnancy:**
Studies inconclusive on harm to unborn child. Animal studies show fetal abnormalities. Decide with your doctor whether drug benefits justify risk to unborn child.

**Breast-feeding:**
Drug passes into milk. Child may become sensitive to penicillins and have allergic reactions to penicillin drugs. Avoid amoxicillin or discontinue nursing until you finish medicine. Consult doctor for advice on maintaining milk supply.

**Infants & children:**
No problems expected.

**Prolonged use:**
You may become more susceptible to infections caused by germs not responsive to amoxicillin.

**Skin & sunlight:**
No problems expected.

**Driving, piloting or hazardous work:**
Usually not dangerous. Most hazardous reactions likely to occur a few minutes after taking amoxicillin.

**Discontinuing:**
Don't discontinue without doctor's advice until you complete prescribed dose, even though symptoms diminish or disappear.

**Others:**
No problems expected.

## POSSIBLE INTERACTION WITH OTHER DRUGS

| GENERIC NAME OR DRUG CLASS | COMBINED EFFECT |
|---|---|
| Beta-adrenergic blockers | Increased chance of anaphylaxis (see emergency information on inside front cover). |
| Chloramphenicol | Decreased effect of both drugs. |
| Erythromycins | Decreased effect of both drugs. |
| Loperamide | Decreased amoxicillin effect. |
| Paromomycin | Decreased effect of both drugs. |
| Tetracyclines | Decreased effect of both drugs. |
| Troleandomycin | Decreased effect of both drugs. |

## POSSIBLE INTERACTION WITH OTHER SUBSTANCES

| INTERACTS WITH | COMBINED EFFECT |
|---|---|
| Alcohol: | Occasional stomach irritation. |
| Beverages: | None expected. |
| Cocaine: | No proven problems. |
| Foods: | None expected. |
| Marijuana: | No proven problems. |
| Tobacco: | None expected. |

# AMPHETAMINE

## BRAND NAMES

| | |
|---|---|
| Amphaplex 10 & 20 | Biphetamine |
| Benzedrine | Declobese |
| Bexedrine | Obetrol 10 & 20 |

## BASIC INFORMATION

**Habit forming? Yes**
**Prescription needed? Yes**
**Available as generic? Yes**
**Drug class: Central-nervous-system**
  **stimulant (amphetamine)**

 ## USES

- Prevents narcolepsy (attacks of uncontrollable sleepiness).
- Controls hyperactivity in children.

 ## DOSAGE & USAGE INFORMATION

**How to take:**
- Tablet—Swallow with liquid.
- Extended-release capsules—Swallow each dose whole with liquid.

**When to take:**
- At the same times each day.
- Short-acting form—Don't take later than 6 hours before bedtime.
- Long-acting form—Take on awakening.

**If you forget a dose:**
- Short-acting form—Take up to 2 hours late. If more than 2 hours, wait for next dose (don't double this dose).
- Long-acting form—Take as soon as you remember. Wait 20 hours for next dose.

*Continued next column*

 ## OVERDOSE

**SYMPTOMS:**
**Rapid heartbeat, hyperactivity, high fever, hallucinations, suicidal or homicidal feelings, convulsions, coma.**
**WHAT TO DO:**
- **Dial 0 (operator) or 911 (emergency) for an ambulance or medical help. Then give first aid immediately.**
- **See emergency information on inside covers.**

**What drug does:**
- Narcolepsy—Apparently affects brain centers to decrease fatigue or sleepiness and increase alertness and motor activity.
- Hyperactive children—Calms children, opposite to effect on narcoleptic adults.

**Time lapse before drug works:**
15 to 30 minutes.

**Don't take with:**
See Interaction column and consult doctor.

 ## POSSIBLE ADVERSE REACTIONS OR SIDE EFFECTS

| SYMPTOMS | WHAT TO DO |
|---|---|
| **Life-threatening:** None expected. | |
| **Common:** | |
| • Irritability, nervousness, insomnia. | Continue. Call doctor when convenient. |
| • Dry mouth. | Continue. Tell doctor at next visit. |
| **Infrequent:** | |
| • Dizziness; reduced alertness; blurred vision; fast, pounding heartbeat; unusual sweating. | Discontinue. Call doctor right away. |
| • Headache. | Continue. Call doctor when convenient. |
| • Diarrhea or constipation, appetite loss, stomach pain, nausea, vomiting, weight loss, diminished sex drive, impotence. | Continue. Tell doctor at next visit. |
| **Rare:** | |
| • Rash, hives; chest pain or irregular heartbeat; uncontrollable movements of head, neck, arms, legs. | Discontinue. Call doctor right away. |
| • Mood changes, swollen breasts. | Continue. Call doctor when convenient. |

**WARNINGS & PRECAUTIONS**

**Don't take if:**
- You are allergic to any amphetamine.
- You will have surgery within 2 months, including dental surgery, requiring general or spinal anesthesia.

**Before you start, consult your doctor:**
- If you plan to become pregnant within medication period.
- If you have glaucoma.
- If you have heart or blood-vessel disease, or high blood pressure.
- If you have overactive thyroid, anxiety or tension.
- If you have a severe mental illness (especially children).

**Over age 60:**
Adverse reactions and side effects may be more frequent and severe than in younger persons.

**Pregnancy:**
Risk to unborn child outweighs drug benefits. Don't use.

**Breast-feeding:**
Drug passes into milk. Avoid drug or discontinue nursing.

**Infants & children:**
Not recommended for children under 12.

**Prolonged use:**
Habit forming.

**Skin & sunlight:**
No problems expected.

**Driving, piloting or hazardous work:**
Don't drive or pilot aircraft until you learn how medicine affects you. Don't work around dangerous machinery. Don't climb ladders or work in high places. Danger increases if you drink alcohol or take medicine affecting alertness and reflexes.

**Discontinuing:**
May be unnecessary to finish medicine. Follow doctor's instructions.

**Others:**
- This is a dangerous drug and must be closely supervised. Don't use for appetite control or depression. Potential for damage and abuse.
- During withdrawal phase, may cause prolonged sleep of several days.

 **POSSIBLE INTERACTION WITH OTHER DRUGS**

| GENERIC NAME OR DRUG CLASS | COMBINED EFFECT |
|---|---|
| Anesthesias (general) | Irregular heartbeat. |
| Antidepressants (tricyclic) | Decreased amphetamine effect. |
| Antihypertensives | Decreased antihypertensive effect. |
| Carbonic anhydrase inhibitors | Increased amphetamine effect. |
| Guanethidine | Decreased guanethidine effect. |
| Haloperidol | Decreased amphetamine effect. |
| MAO inhibitors | May severely increase blood pressure. |
| Phenothiazines | Decreased amphetamine effect. |
| Sodium bicarbonate | Increased amphetamine effect. |

 **POSSIBLE INTERACTION WITH OTHER SUBSTANCES**

| INTERACTS WITH | COMBINED EFFECT |
|---|---|
| Alcohol: | Decreased amphetamine effect. Avoid. |
| Beverages: Caffeine drinks. | Overstimulation. Avoid. |
| Cocaine: | Dangerous stimulation of nervous system. Avoid. |
| Foods: | None expected. |
| Marijuana: | Frequent use—Severely impaired mental function. |
| Tobacco: | None expected. |

# AMPICILLIN

## BRAND NAMES

| | |
|---|---|
| Alpen | Penbritin |
| Amcill | Polycillin |
| Ampicin | Prinicipen |
| Ampilean | SK-Ampicillin |
| Novo-Ampicillin | Supen |
| Omnipen | Totacillin |

## BASIC INFORMATION

**Habit forming? No**
**Prescription needed? Yes**
**Available as generic? Yes**
**Drug class: Antibiotic (penicillin)**

 ## USES

Treatment of bacterial infections that are susceptible to ampicillin.

 ## DOSAGE & USAGE INFORMATION

**How to take:**
- Tablets or capsules—Swallow with liquid on an empty stomach 1 hour before or 2 hours after eating.
- Liquid—Take with cold beverage. Liquid form is perishable and effective for only 7 days at room temperature. Effective for 14 days if stored in refrigerator. Don't freeze.

**When to take:**
Follow instructions on prescription label or side of package. Doses should be evenly spaced. For example, 4 times a day means every 6 hours.

**If you forget a dose:**
Take as soon as you remember. Continue regular schedule.

**What drug does:**
Destroys susceptible bacteria. Does not kill viruses.

**Time lapse before drug works:**
May be several days before medicine affects infection.

*Continued next column*

 ## OVERDOSE

**SYMPTOMS:**
**Severe diarrhea, nausea or vomiting.**
**WHAT TO DO:**
**Overdose unlikely to threaten life. If person takes much larger amount than prescribed, call doctor, poison-control center or hospital emergency room for instructions.**

**Don't take with:**
See Interaction column and consult doctor.

 ## POSSIBLE ADVERSE REACTIONS OR SIDE EFFECTS

| SYMPTOMS | WHAT TO DO |
|---|---|
| **Life-threatening:** | |
| Hives, rash, intense itching, faintness soon after a dose (anaphylaxis). | Seek emergency treatment immediately. |
| **Common:** | |
| Dark or discolored tongue. | Continue. Tell doctor at next visit. |
| **Infrequent:** | |
| Mild nausea, vomiting, diarrhea. | Continue. Call doctor when convenient. |
| **Rare:** | |
| Unexplained bleeding. | Discontinue. Call doctor right away. |

## WARNINGS & PRECAUTIONS

**Don't take if:**
You are allergic to ampicillin, cephalosporin antibiotics, other penicillins or penicillamine. Life-threatening reaction may occur.

**Before you start, consult your doctor:**
If you are allergic to any substance or drug.

**Over age 60:**
You may have skin reactions, particularly around genitals and anus.

**Pregnancy:**
Studies inconclusive on harm to unborn child. Animal studies show fetal abnormalities. Decide with your doctor whether drug benefits justify risk to unborn child.

**Breast-feeding:**
Drug passes into milk. Child may become sensitive to penicillins and have allergic reactions to penicillin drugs. Avoid ampicillin or discontinue nursing until you finish medicine. Consult doctor for advice on maintaining milk supply.

**Infants & children:**
No problems expected.

**Prolonged use:**
You may become more susceptible to infections caused by germs not responsive to ampicillin.

**Skin & sunlight:**
No problems expected.

**Driving, piloting or hazardous work:**
Usually not dangerous. Most hazardous reactions likely to occur a few minutes after taking ampicillin.

**Discontinuing:**
Don't discontinue without doctor's advice until you complete prescribed dose, even though symptoms diminish or disappear.

**Others:**
Urine sugar test for diabetes may show false positive result.

## POSSIBLE INTERACTION WITH OTHER DRUGS

| GENERIC NAME OR DRUG CLASS | COMBINED EFFECT |
|---|---|
| Beta-adrenergic blockers | Increased chance of anaphylaxis (see emergency information on inside front cover). |
| Chloramphenicol | Decreased effect of both drugs. |
| Erythromycins | Decreased effect of both drugs. |
| Loperamide | Decreased ampicillin effect. |
| Oral contraceptives | Occasionally impairs contraceptive efficiency. |
| Paromomycin | Decreased effect of both drugs. |
| Tetracyclines | Decreased effect of both drugs. |
| Troleandomycin | Decreased effect of both drugs. |

## POSSIBLE INTERACTION WITH OTHER SUBSTANCES

| INTERACTS WITH | COMBINED EFFECT |
|---|---|
| Alcohol: | Occasional stomach irritation. |
| Beverages: | None expected. |
| Cocaine: | No proven problems. |
| Foods: | None expected. |
| Marijuana: | No proven problems. |
| Tobacco: | None expected. |

# ANDROGENS

## BRAND AND GENERIC NAMES

See complete list of brand names in the *Brand Name Directory,* page 942.

## BASIC INFORMATION

**Habit forming? No**
**Available as generic? Yes**
**Prescription needed? Yes**
**Drug class: Androgens**

 ## USES

- Corrects male hormone deficiency.
- Reduces "male menopause" symptoms (loss of sex drive, depression, anxiety).
- Decreases calcium loss of osteoporosis (softened bones).
- Blocks growth of breast-cancer cells in females.
- Corrects undescended testicles in male children.
- Reduces breast pain and fullness following childbirth.
- Augments treatment of aplastic anemia.
- Stimulates weight gain after illness, injury or for chronically underweight persons.
- Stimulates growth in treatment of dwarfism.

 ## DOSAGE & USAGE INFORMATION

**How to take:**
- Tablets—With food to lessen stomach irritation.
- Injection—Once or twice a month.

**When to take:**
At the same time each day.

**If you forget a dose:**
Take as soon as you remember up to 2 hours late. If more than 2 hours, wait for next scheduled dose (don't double this dose).

*Continued next column*

 ## OVERDOSE

**SYMPTOMS:**
**None expected.**
**WHAT TO DO:**
**Overdose unlikely to threaten life. If person takes much larger amount than prescribed, call doctor, poison-control center or hospital emergency room for instructions.**

**What drug does:**
- Stimulates cells that produce male sex characteristics.
- Replaces hormone deficiencies.
- Stimulates red-blood-cell production.
- Suppresses production of estrogen (female sex hormone).

**Time lapse before drug works:**
Varies with problems treated. May require 2 or 3 months of regular use for desired effects.

**Don't take with:**
See Interaction column and consult doctor.

 ## POSSIBLE ADVERSE REACTIONS OR SIDE EFFECTS

| SYMPTOMS | WHAT TO DO |
|---|---|
| **Life-threatening:** | |
| Intense itching, weakness, loss of consciousness. | Seek emergency treatment immediately. |
| **Common:** | |
| • Acne or oily skin in females, deep voice, enlarged clitoris, frequent erections, swollen breasts in men. | Continue. Call doctor when convenient. |
| • Sore mouth, higher sex drive. | Continue. Tell doctor at next visit. |
| **Infrequent:** | |
| • Jaundice. | Discontinue. Seek emergency treatment. |
| • Depression or confusion, flushed face, rash or itch, nausea, vomiting, diarrhea, swollen feet or legs, vaginal bleeding. | Discontinue. Call doctor right away. |
| **Rare:** | |
| • Hives, black stool. | Discontinue. Seek emergency treatment. |
| • Sore throat, fever, abdominal pain. | Discontinue. Call doctor right away. |

## WARNINGS & PRECAUTIONS

**Don't take if:**
You are allergic to any male hormone.

**Before you start, consult your doctor:**
- If you might be pregnant.
- If you have cancer of prostate.
- If you have heart disease or arteriosclerosis.
- If you have kidney or liver disease.
- If you have breast cancer (males).
- If you have high blood pressure.
- If you have migraine attacks.
- If you have high level of blood calcium.
- If you have epilepsy.

**Over age 60:**
- May stimulate sexual activity.
- Can make high blood pressure or heart disease worse.
- Can enlarge prostate and cause urinary retention.

**Pregnancy:**
Risk to unborn child outweighs drug benefits. Don't use.

**Breast-feeding:**
Drug passes into milk. Avoid drug or discontinue nursing until you finish medicine. Consult doctor for advice on maintaining milk supply.

**Infants & children:**
Don't give to children younger than 2. Use with older children only under medical supervision.

**Prolonged use:**
- Reduces sperm count and volume of semen.
- Possible kidney stones.
- Unnatural hair growth and deep voice in women.

**Skin & sunlight:**
No problems expected.

**Driving, piloting or hazardous work:**
No problems expected.

**Discontinuing:**
No problems expected.

**Others:**
- May cause atrophy of testicles.
- Will not increase strength in athletes.

## POSSIBLE INTERACTION WITH OTHER DRUGS

| GENERIC NAME OR DRUG CLASS | COMBINED EFFECT |
| --- | --- |
| Anticoagulants | Increased anticoagulant effect. |
| Antidiabetics (oral) | Increased antidiabetic effect. |
| Chlorzoxazone | Decreased androgen effect. |
| Oxyphenbutazone | Decreased androgen effect. |
| Phenobarbital | Decreased androgen effect. |
| Phenylbutazone | Decreased androgen effect. |

## POSSIBLE INTERACTION WITH OTHER SUBSTANCES

| INTERACTS WITH | COMBINED EFFECT |
| --- | --- |
| Alcohol: | None expected. |
| Beverages: | None expected. |
| Cocaine: | No proven problems. |
| Foods: Salt. | Excessive fluid retention (edema). Decrease salt intake while taking male hormones. |
| Marijuana: | Decreased blood levels of androgens. |
| Tobacco: | No proven problems. |

# ANESTHETICS (TOPICAL)

## BRAND AND GENERIC NAMES

See complete list of brand names in the *Brand Name Directory,* page 942.

## BASIC INFORMATION

**Habit forming? No**
**Prescription needed?**
  **High strength: Yes**
  **Low strength: No**
**Available as generic? Yes**
**Drug class: Anesthetic (topical)**

 ## USES

- Relieves pain and itch of sunburn, insect bites, scratches and other minor skin irritations.
- Relieves discomfort and itch of hemorrhoids and other disorders of anus and rectum.

 ## DOSAGE & USAGE INFORMATION

**How to use:**
- Suppositories—Remove wrapper and moisten suppository with water. Gently insert larger end into rectum. Push well into rectum with finger.
- All other forms—Use only enough to cover irritated area. Follow instructions on label.

**When to use:**
When needed for discomfort, no more often than every hour.

**If you forget an application:**
Use as needed.

**What drug does:**
Blocks pain impulses from skin to brain.

**Time lapse before drug works:**
3 to 15 minutes.

**Don't take with:**
See Interaction column and consult doctor.

 ## OVERDOSE

**SYMPTOMS:**
**If swallowed or inhaled—Dizziness, nervousness, trembling, seizures.**
**WHAT TO DO:**
- **Dial 0 (operator) or 911 (emergency) for an ambulance or medical help. Then give first aid immediately.**
- **See emergency information on inside covers.**

 ## POSSIBLE ADVERSE REACTIONS OR SIDE EFFECTS

| SYMPTOMS | WHAT TO DO |
|---|---|
| **Life-threatening:** None expected. | |
| **Common:** None expected. | |
| **Infrequent:** | |
| • Nervousness; trembling; hives, rash, itch; inflammation or tenderness not present before application; slow heartbeat. | Discontinue. Call doctor right away. |
| • Dizziness, blurred vision, swollen feet. | Continue. Call doctor when convenient. |
| **Rare:** | |
| • Blood in urine. | Discontinue. Call doctor right away. |
| • Increased or painful urination. | Continue. Call doctor when convenient. |

# ANESTHETICS (TOPICAL)

## WARNINGS & PRECAUTIONS

**Don't use if:**
You are allergic to any topical anesthetic.

**Before you start, consult your doctor:**
- If you have skin infection at site of treatment.
- If you have had severe or extensive skin disorders such as eczema or psoriasis.
- If you have bleeding hemorrhoids.

**Over age 60:**
Adverse reactions and side effects may be more frequent and severe than in younger persons.

**Pregnancy:**
No proven harm to unborn child. Avoid if possible.

**Breast-feeding:**
No problems expected.

**Infants & children:**
Use caution. More likely to be absorbed through skin and cause adverse reactions.

**Prolonged use:**
Possible excess absorption. Don't use longer than 3 days for any one problem.

**Skin & sunlight:**
No problems expected.

**Driving, piloting or hazardous work:**
No problems expected.

**Discontinuing:**
May be unnecessary to finish medicine. Follow doctor's instructions.

**Others:**
No problems expected.

## POSSIBLE INTERACTION WITH OTHER DRUGS

| GENERIC NAME OR DRUG CLASS | COMBINED EFFECT |
|---|---|
| Sulfa drugs | Decreased effect of sulfa drugs for infection. |

## POSSIBLE INTERACTION WITH OTHER SUBSTANCES

| INTERACTS WITH | COMBINED EFFECT |
|---|---|
| Alcohol: | None expected. |
| Beverages: | None expected. |
| Cocaine: | Possible nervous-system toxicity. Avoid. |
| Foods: | None expected. |
| Marijuana: | None expected. |
| Tobacco: | None expected. |

# ANTICOAGULANTS (ORAL)

## BRAND AND GENERIC NAMES

ANISINDIONE
Anthrombin-K
Coumadin
Danilone
DICUMAROL
Dufalone
Hedulin
Liquamar
Marcumar
Marevan

Melitoxin
Miradon
Panwarfin
PHENINDIONE
PHENPROCOUMON
WARFARIN
 POTASSIUM
WARFARIN SODIUM
Warfilone
Warnerin

## BASIC INFORMATION

**Habit forming? No**
**Prescription needed? Yes**
**Available as generic? Yes**
**Drug class: Anticoagulant**

 ## USES

Reduces blood clots. Used for abnormal clotting inside blood vessels.

 ## DOSAGE & USAGE INFORMATION

**How to take:**
Tablet—Swallow with liquid. If you can't swallow whole, crumble tablet and take with liquid or food.

**When to take:**
At the same time each day.

**If you forget a dose:**
Take as soon as you remember up to 12 hours late. If more than 12 hours, wait for next scheduled dose (don't double this dose). Inform your doctor of any missed doses.

**What drug does:**
Blocks action of vitamin K necessary for blood clotting.

**Time lapse before drug works:**
36 to 48 hours.

*Continued next column*

 ## OVERDOSE

**SYMPTOMS:**
**Bloody vomit and bloody or black stools, red urine.**
**WHAT TO DO:**
- **Dial 0 (operator) or 911 (emergency) for an ambulance or medical help. Then give first aid immediately.**
- **See emergency information on inside covers.**

**Don't take with:**
See Interaction column and consult doctor.

 ## POSSIBLE ADVERSE REACTIONS OR SIDE EFFECTS

| SYMPTOMS | WHAT TO DO |
|---|---|
| **Life-threatening:** None expected. | |
| **Common:** Bloating, gas. | Continue. Tell doctor at next visit. |
| **Infrequent:** | |
| • Black stools or bloody vomit, coughing up blood. | Discontinue. Seek emergency treatment. |
| • Rash, hives, itch, blurred vision, sore throat, easy bruising, bleeding, cloudy or red urine, back pain, jaundice, fever, chills, fatigue, weakness. | Discontinue. Call doctor right away. |
| • Diarrhea, cramps, nausea, vomiting, swollen feet or legs, hair loss. | Continue. Call doctor when convenient. |
| **Rare:** Dizziness, headache, mouth sores. | Discontinue. Call doctor right away. |

 ## WARNINGS & PRECAUTIONS

**Don't take if:**
- You have been allergic to any oral anticoagulant.
- You have a bleeding disorder.
- You have an active peptic ulcer.
- You have ulcerative colitis.

**Before you start, consult your doctor:**
- If you take any other drugs, including non-prescription drugs.
- If you have high blood pressure.
- If you have heavy or prolonged menstrual periods.
- If you have diabetes.
- If you have a bladder catheter.
- If you have serious liver or kidney disease.
- If you will have surgery within 2 months, including dental surgery, requiring general or spinal anesthesia.

**Over age 60:**
Adverse reactions and side effects may be more frequent and severe than in younger persons.

**Pregnancy:**
Risk to unborn child outweighs drug benefits. Don't use.

**Breast-feeding:**
Drug filters into milk. May harm child. Avoid.

**Infants & children:**
Use only under doctor's supervision.

**Prolonged use:**
No problems expected.

**Skin & sunlight:**
No problems expected.

**Driving, piloting or hazardous work:**
- Avoid hazardous activities that could cause injury.
- Don't drive if you feel dizzy or have blurred vision.

**Discontinuing:**
Don't discontinue without consulting doctor. Dose may require gradual reduction if you have taken drug for a long time. Doses of other drugs may also require adjustment.

**Others:**
Carry identification to state you take anticoagulants.

## POSSIBLE INTERACTION WITH OTHER DRUGS

| GENERIC NAME OR DRUG CLASS | COMBINED EFFECT |
|---|---|
| Acetaminophen | Increased effect of anticoagulant. |
| Allopurinol | Increased effect of anticoagulant. |
| Amiodarone | Increased effect of anticoagulant. |
| Androgens | Increased effect of anticoagulant. |
| Antacids (large doses) | Decreased effect of anticoagulant. |
| Antibiotics | Increased effect of anticoagulant. |
| Anticonvulsants (hydantoin) | Increased effect of both drugs. |
| Antidepressants (tricyclic) | Increased effect of anticoagulant. |
| Antidiabetics (oral) | Increased effect of anticoagulant. |
| Antihistamines | Unpredictable increased or decreased effect of anticoagulant. |
| Aspirin | Possible spontaneous bleeding. |

| | |
|---|---|
| Barbiturates | Decreased effect of anticoagulant. |
| Benzodiazepines | Unpredictable increased or decreased anticoagulant effect. |
| Calcium supplements | Decreased anticoagulant effect. |
| Carbamazepine | Decreased effect of anticoagulant. |
| Ketoprofen | Increased risk of bleeding. |
| Suprofen | Increased risk of bleeding. |

## POSSIBLE INTERACTION WITH OTHER SUBSTANCES

| INTERACTS WITH | COMBINED EFFECT |
|---|---|
| Alcohol: | Can increase or decrease effect of anticoagulant. Use with caution. |
| Beverages: | None expected. |
| Cocaine: | None expected. |
| Foods: High in vitamin K such as fish, liver, spinach, cabbage. | May decrease anticoagulant effect. |
| Marijuana: | None expected. |
| Tobacco: | None expected. |

# ANTICONVULSANTS (DIONE-TYPE)

## BRAND AND GENERIC NAMES

**PARAMETHADIONE**    **TRIMETHADIONE**
Paradione                Tridione

## BASIC INFORMATION

**Habit forming? No**
**Prescription needed? Yes**
**Available as generic? No**
**Drug class: Anticonvulsant (Dione-type)**

 ## USES

Controls but does not cure petit mal seizures
(absence seizures).

 ## DOSAGE & USAGE INFORMATION

**How to take:**
Tablets, capsules or liquid: Take with food or
milk to lessen stomach irritation.

**When to take:**
At the same time each day.

**If you forget a dose:**
Take as soon as you remember up to 2 hours
late. If more than 2 hours, wait for next
scheduled dose (don't double this dose).

**What drug does:**
Raises threshold of seizures in cerebral cortex.
Does not alter seizure pattern.

**Time lapse before drug works:**
1 to 3 hours.

**Don't take with:**
See Interaction column and consult doctor.

 ## OVERDOSE

**SYMPTOMS:**
Bleeding, coma.
**WHAT TO DO:**

- Dial 0 (operator) or 911 (emergency) for an
  ambulance or medical help. Then give first
  aid immediately.
- If patient is unconscious and not
  breathing, give mouth-to-mouth breathing.
  If there is no heartbeat, use cardiac
  massage and mouth-to-mouth breathing
  (CPR). Don't try to make patient vomit. If
  you can't get help quickly, take patient to
  nearest emergency facility.
- See emergency information on inside
  covers.

 ## POSSIBLE ADVERSE REACTIONS OR SIDE EFFECTS

| SYMPTOMS | WHAT TO DO |
|---|---|
| **Life-threatening:** None expected. | |
| **Common:** Dizziness, drowsiness, headache, rash. | Continue. Call doctor when convenient. |
| **Infrequent:** Itching, nausea, vomiting. | Continue. Call doctor when convenient. |
| **Rare:** • Changes in vision; sore throat with fever and mouth sores; bleeding gums; easy bleeding or bruising; smoky or bloody urine; jaundice; puffed hands, face, feet or legs; swollen lymph glands; unusual weakness and fatigue. | Discontinue. Call doctor right away. |
| • Sensitivity to light. | Continue. Call doctor when convenient. |

## WARNINGS & PRECAUTIONS

**Don't take if:**
You are allergic to this drug or any anticonvulsant.

**Before you start, consult your doctor:**
- If you are pregnant or plan pregnancy.
- If you have blood disease.
- If you have liver or kidney disease.
- If you have disease of optic nerve or eye.
- If you will have surgery within 2 months, including dental surgery, requiring general or spinal anesthesia.

**Over age 60:**
Adverse reactions and side effects may be more frequent and severe than in younger persons.

**Pregnancy:**
Risk to unborn child outweighs drug benefits. Don't use.

**Breast-feeding:**
No problems proven. Avoid if possible. Consult doctor.

**Infants & children:**
Use only under close medical supervision of clinician experienced in convulsive disorders.

**Prolonged use:**
Have regular checkups, especially during early months of treatment.

**Skin & sunlight:**
Increased sensitivity to sunlight or sun lamp. Avoid overexposure.

**Driving, piloting or hazardous work:**
Don't drive or pilot aircraft until you learn how medicine affects you. Don't work around dangerous machinery. Don't climb ladders or work in high places. Danger increases if you drink alcohol or take medicine affecting alertness and reflexes, such as antihistamines, tranquilizers, sedatives, pain medicine, narcotics and mind-altering drugs. Be especially careful driving at night because medicine can affect vision.

**Discontinuing:**
Don't discontinue without consulting doctor. Dose may require gradual reduction if you have taken drug for a long time. Doses of other drugs may also require adjustment.

**Others:**
Arrange for eye exams every 6 months as well as blood counts and kidney-function studies.

## POSSIBLE INTERACTION WITH OTHER DRUGS

| GENERIC NAME OR DRUG CLASS | COMBINED EFFECT |
|---|---|
| Antidepressants (tricyclic) | Greater likelihood of seizures. |
| Antipsychotic medicines | Greater likelihood of seizures. |
| Anticonvulsants | Increased chance of blood toxicity. |
| Sedatives, sleeping pills, antihistamines, pain medicine, alchohol, tranquilizers, narcotics, mind-altering drugs. | Extreme drowsiness. Avoid. |

## POSSIBLE INTERACTION WITH OTHER SUBSTANCES

| INTERACTS WITH | COMBINED EFFECT |
|---|---|
| Alcohol: | Increased chance of seizures and liver damage. Avoid. |
| Beverages: Caffeine drinks. | May decrease anticonvulsant effect. |
| Cocaine: | Increased chance of seizures. Avoid. |
| Foods: | No problems expected. |
| Marijuana: | Increased chance of seizures. Avoid. |
| Tobacco: | Decreased absorption of medicine leading to uneven control of disease. |

# ANTITHYROID MEDICINES

## BRAND AND GENERIC NAMES

METHIMAZOLE     Tapazole
PROPYLTHIOURACIL    Thiamazole
Propyl-Thyracil

## BASIC INFORMATION

**Habit forming? No**
**Prescription needed? Yes**
**Available as generic? Yes**
**Drug class: Antihyperthyroid**

 **USES**

- Treatment of overactive thyroid (hyperthyroidism).
- Treatment of angina in patients who have overactive thyroid.

 **DOSAGE & USAGE INFORMATION**

**How to take:**
Tablet or capsule—Swallow with liquid or food to lessen stomach irritation. If you can't swallow whole, crumble tablet or open capsule and take with liquid or food.

**When to take:**
At the same times each day.

**If you forget a dose:**
Take as soon as you remember up to 2 hours late. If more than 2 hours, wait for next scheduled dose (don't double this dose).

**What drug does:**
Prevents thyroid gland from producing excess thyroid hormone.

**Time lapse before drug works:**
10 to 20 days.

**Don't take with:**
- Anticoagulants
- See Interaction column and consult doctor.

 **OVERDOSE**

**SYMPTOMS:**
Bleeding, spots on skin, jaundice (yellow eyes and skin), loss of consciousness.
**WHAT TO DO:**
Overdose unlikely to threaten life. If person takes much larger amount than prescribed, call doctor, poison-control center or hospital emergency room for instructions.

 **POSSIBLE ADVERSE REACTIONS OR SIDE EFFECTS**

| SYMPTOMS | WHAT TO DO |
|---|---|
| **Life-threatening:**<br>None expected. | |
| **Common:**<br>Skin rash, itching, dryness. | Discontinue. Call doctor right away. |
| **Infrequent:**<br>Dizziness, taste loss, sore throat with chills and fever, abdominal pain, constipation, diarrhea. | Discontinue. Call doctor right away. |
| **Rare:**<br>Headache; enlarged lymph glands; irregular or rapid heartbeat; unusual bruising or bleeding; backache; numbness or tingling in toes, fingers or face; joint pain; muscle aches; menstrual irregularities; jaundice; tired, weak, sleepy, listless; swollen eyes or feet. | Discontinue. Call doctor right away. |

## WARNINGS & PRECAUTIONS

**Don't take if:**
You are allergic to antithyroid medicines.

**Before you start, consult your doctor:**
- If you have liver disease.
- If you have blood disease.
- If you have an infection.
- If you take anticoagulants.

**Over age 60:**
Adverse reactions and side effects may be more frequent and severe than in younger persons.

**Pregnancy:**
Risk to unborn child outweighs drug benefits. Don't use.

**Breast-feeding:**
Drug filters into milk. May harm child. Avoid.

**Infants & children:**
Use only under special medical supervision by experienced clinician.

**Prolonged use:**
Adverse reactions and side effects more common.

**Skin & sunlight:**
No problems expected.

**Driving, piloting or hazardous work:**
Don't drive or pilot aircraft until you learn how medicine affects you. Don't work around dangerous machinery. Don't climb ladders or work in high places. Danger increases if you drink alcohol or take medicine affecting alertness and reflexes, such as antihistamines, tranquilizers, sedatives, pain medicine, narcotics and mind-altering drugs.

**Discontinuing:**
Don't discontinue without consulting doctor. Dose may require gradual reduction if you have taken drug for a long time. Doses of other drugs may also require adjustment.

**Others:**
No problems expected.

## POSSIBLE INTERACTION WITH OTHER DRUGS

| GENERIC NAME OR DRUG CLASS | COMBINED EFFECT |
|---|---|
| Anticoagulants | Increased effect of anticoagulants. |
| Antineoplastic drugs | Increased chance to suppress bone marrow. |
| Chloramphenicol | Increased chance to suppress bone marrow. |

## POSSIBLE INTERACTION WITH OTHER SUBSTANCES

| INTERACTS WITH | COMBINED EFFECT |
|---|---|
| Alcohol: | Increased possibility of liver toxicity. Avoid. |
| Beverages: | No problems expected. |
| Cocaine: | Increased toxicity potential of medicines. Avoid. |
| Foods: | No problems expected. |
| Marijuana: | Increased rapid or irregular heartbeat. Avoid. |
| Tobacco: | Increased chance of rapid heartbeat. Avoid. |

# APPETITE SUPPRESSANTS

## BRAND AND GENERIC NAMES

See complete list of brand names in the *Brand Name Directory*, page 943.

## BASIC INFORMATION

**Habit forming? Yes**
**Prescription needed? Yes**
**Available as generic? Yes**
**Drug class: Appetite suppressant**

## USES

Suppresses appetite.

## DOSAGE & USAGE INFORMATION

**How to take:**
- Tablet or capsule—Swallow with liquid. You may chew or crush tablet.
- Extended-release tablets or capsules—Swallow each dose whole with liquid.

**When to take:**
- Long-acting forms—10 to 14 hours before bedtime.
- Short-acting forms—1 hour before meals. Last dose no later than 4 to 6 hours before bedtime.

**If you forget a dose:**
- Long-acting form—Take as soon as you remember up to 2 hours late. If more than 2 hours, wait for next scheduled dose (don't double this dose).
- Short-acting form—Wait for next scheduled dose. Don't double this dose.

**What drug does:**
Apparently stimulates brain's appetite-control center.

*Continued next column*

## OVERDOSE

**SYMPTOMS:**
Irritability, overactivity, trembling, insomnia, mood changes, rapid heartbeat, confusion, disorientation, hallucinations, convulsions, coma.
**WHAT TO DO:**
- Dial 0 (operator) or 911 (emergency) for an ambulance or medical help. Then give first aid immediately.
- See emergency information on inside covers.

---

**Time lapse before drug works:**
Begins in 1 hour. Short-acting form lasts 4 hours. Long-acting form lasts 14 hours.

**Don't take with:**
- Non-prescription drugs without consulting doctor.
- See Interaction column and consult doctor.

## POSSIBLE ADVERSE REACTIONS OR SIDE EFFECTS

| SYMPTOMS | WHAT TO DO |
|---|---|
| **Life-threatening:**<br>None expected. | |
| **Common:**<br>Irritability, nervousness, insomnia, false sense of well-being. | Continue. Call doctor when convenient. |
| **Infrequent:**<br>• Irregular or pounding heartbeat, urgent or difficult urination. | Discontinue. Call doctor right away. |
| • Blurred vision, unpleasant taste or dry mouth, constipation or diarrhea, nausea, vomiting, cramps, changes in sex drive, increased sweating. | Continue. Call doctor when convenient. |
| **Rare:**<br>• Mood changes, rash or hives, breathing difficulty. | Discontinue. Call doctor right away. |
| • Hair loss. | Continue. Call doctor when convenient. |

## WARNINGS & PRECAUTIONS

**Don't take if:**
- You are allergic to any sympathomimetic or phenylpropanolamine.
- You have glaucoma.
- You have taken MAO inhibitors within 2 weeks.
- You plan to become pregnant within medication period.
- You have a history of drug abuse.
- You have irregular or rapid heartbeat.

**Before you start, consult your doctor:**
- If you have high blood pressure or heart disease.
- If you have an overactive thyroid, nervous tension or "anxiety."
- If you have epilepsy.
- If you will have surgery within 2 months, including dental surgery, requiring general or spinal anesthesia.

**Over age 60:**
Adverse reactions and side effects may be more frequent and severe than in younger persons.

**Pregnancy:**
Safety not established. Avoid.

**Breast-feeding:**
No proven problems. Consult doctor.

**Infants & children:**
Don't give to children younger than 12.

**Prolonged use:**
Loses effectiveness. Avoid.

**Skin & sunlight:**
No problems expected.

**Driving, piloting or hazardous work:**
Don't drive or pilot aircraft until you learn how medicine affects you. Don't work around dangerous machinery. Don't climb ladders or work in high places. Danger increases if you drink alcohol or take medicine affecting alertness and reflexes, such as antihistamines, tranquilizers, sedatives, pain medicine, narcotics and mind-altering drugs.

**Discontinuing:**
Don't discontinue without consulting doctor. Dose may require gradual reduction if you have taken drug for a long time. Doses of other drugs may also require adjustment.

**Others:**
Don't increase dose.

## POSSIBLE INTERACTION WITH OTHER DRUGS

| GENERIC NAME OR DRUG CLASS | COMBINED EFFECT |
| --- | --- |
| Appetite suppressants (other) | Dangerous overstimulation. |
| Caffeine | Increased stimulant effect of phentermine. |
| Guanethidine | Decreased guanethidine effect. |
| Hydralazine | Decreased hydralazine effect. |
| MAO inhibitors | Dangerous blood-pressure rise. |
| Methyldopa | Decreased methyldopa effect. |
| Molindone | Decreased suppressant effect. |
| Phenothiazines | Decreased appetite suppressant effect. |
| Rauwolfia alkaloids | Decreased effect of rauwolfia alkaloids. |

## POSSIBLE INTERACTION WITH OTHER SUBSTANCES

| INTERACTS WITH | COMBINED EFFECT |
| --- | --- |
| **Alcohol:** Beer, chianti wines, vermouth. | Dangerous blood-pressure rise. |
| **Beverages:** <br>• Caffeine drinks. <br>• Drinks containing tyramine (see Glossary). | Excessive stimulation. <br>Blood-pressure rise. |
| **Cocaine:** | Excessive stimulation. |
| **Foods:** Foods containing tyramine (see Glossary). | Blood-pressure rise. |
| **Marijuana:** | Frequent use—Irregular heartbeat. |
| **Tobacco:** | None expected. |

# ASPIRIN

## BRAND NAMES

See complete list of brand names in the *Brand Name Directory,* page 943.

## BASIC INFORMATION

**Habit forming? No**
**Prescription needed? No**
**Available as generic? Yes**
**Drug class: Analgesic, anti-inflammatory (salicylate)**

 ## USES

- Reduces pain, fever, inflammation.
- Relieves swelling, stiffness, joint pain of arthritis or rheumatism.

 ## DOSAGE & USAGE INFORMATION

**How to take:**
- Tablet or capsule—Swallow with liquid.
- Extended-release tablets or capsules—Swallow each dose whole.
- Suppositories—Remove wrapper and moisten suppository with water. Gently insert into rectum, large end first.

**When to take:**
Pain, fever, inflammation—As needed, no more often than every 4 hours.

**If you forget a dose:**
- Pain, fever—Take as soon as you remember. Wait 4 hours for next dose.
- Arthritis—Take as soon as you remember up to 2 hours late. Return to regular schedule.

**What drug does:**
- Affects hypothalamus, the part of the brain which regulates temperature by dilating small blood vessels in skin.

*Continued next column*

 ## OVERDOSE

**SYMPTOMS:**
**Ringing in ears; nausea; vomiting; dizziness; fever; deep, rapid breathing; hallucinations; convulsions; coma.**
**WHAT TO DO:**
- **Dial 0 (operator) or 911 (emergency) for an ambulance or medical help. Then give first aid immediately.**
- **See emergency information on inside covers.**

- Prevents clumping of platelets (small blood cells) so blood vessels remain open.
- Decreases prostaglandin effect.
- Suppresses body's pain messages.

**Time lapse before drug works:**
30 minutes for pain, fever, arthritis.

**Don't take with:**
- Tetracyclines. Space doses 1 hour apart.
- See Interaction column and consult doctor.

 ## POSSIBLE ADVERSE REACTIONS OR SIDE EFFECTS

| SYMPTOMS | WHAT TO DO |
|---|---|
| **Life-threatening:** | |
| Black or bloody vomit, blood in urine. Hives, rash, intense itching, faintness soon after a dose (anaphylaxis). | Seek emergency treatment immediately. |
| **Common:** | |
| ● Nausea, vomiting. | Discontinue. Seek emergency treatment. |
| ● Heartburn, indigestion. | Continue. Call doctor when convenient. |
| ● Ringing in ears. | Continue. Tell doctor at next visit. |
| **Infrequent:** | |
| None expected. | |
| **Rare:** | |
| ● Black stools, unexplained fever. | Discontinue. Seek emergency treatment. |
| ● Rash, hives, itch, diminished vision, shortness of breath, wheezing, jaundice. | Discontinue. Call doctor right away. |
| ● Drowsiness. | Continue. Call doctor when convenient. |

 ## WARNINGS & PRECAUTIONS

**Don't take if:**
- You need to restrict sodium in your diet. Buffered effervescent tablets and sodium salicylate are high in sodium.
- Aspirin has a strong vinegar-like odor, which means it has decomposed.
- You have a peptic ulcer of stomach or duodenum.
- You have a bleeding disorder.

**Before you start, consult your doctor:**
- If you have had stomach or duodenal ulcers.
- If you have had gout.
- If you have asthma or nasal polyps.

**Over age 60:**
More likely to cause hidden bleeding in stomach or intestines. Watch for dark stools.

**Pregnancy:**
Risk to unborn child outweighs drug benefits. Don't use.

**Breast-feeding:**
Drug passes into milk. Avoid drug or discontinue nursing until you finish medicine. Consult doctor for advice on maintaining milk supply.

**Infants & children:**
- Overdose frequent and severe. Keep bottles out of children's reach.
- Consult doctor before giving to persons under age 18 who have fever and discomfort of viral illness, especially chicken pox and influenza. Probably increases risk of Reye's syndrome.

**Prolonged use:**
Kidney damage. Periodic kidney-function test recommended.

**Skin & sunlight:**
Aspirin combined with sunscreen may decrease sunburn.

**Driving, piloting or hazardous work:**
No restrictions unless you feel drowsy.

**Discontinuing:**
For chronic illness—Don't discontinue without doctor's advice until you complete prescribed dose, even though symptoms diminish or disappear.

**Others:**
- Aspirin can complicate surgery, pregnancy, labor and delivery, and illness.
- For arthritis—Don't change dose without consulting doctor.
- Urine tests for blood sugar may be inaccurate.

## POSSIBLE INTERACTION WITH OTHER DRUGS

| GENERIC NAME OR DRUG CLASS | COMBINED EFFECT |
|---|---|
| Acebutolol | Decreased antihypertensive effect of acebutolol. |
| Allopurinol | Decreased allopurinol effect. |
| Antacids | Decreased aspirin effect. |
| Anticoagulants | Increased anticoagulant effect. Abnormal bleeding. |
| Antidiabetics (oral) | Low blood sugar. |
| Anti-inflammatory drugs (non-steroid) | Risk of stomach bleeding and ulcers. |

| | |
|---|---|
| Aspirin (other) | Likely aspirin toxicity. |
| Cortisone drugs | Increased cortisone effect. Risk of ulcers and stomach bleeding. |
| Furosemide | Possible aspirin toxicity. |
| Gold compounds | Increased likelihood of kidney damage. |
| Indomethacin | Risk of stomach bleeding and ulcers. |
| Ketoprofen | Increased risk of stomach ulcer. |
| Methotrexate | Increased methotrexate effect. |
| Minoxidil | Decreased minoxidil effect. |
| Oxprenolol | Decreased antihypertensive effect of oxprenolol. |
| Para-aminosalicylic acid (PAS) | Possible aspirin toxicity. |
| Penicillins | Increased effect of both drugs. |
| Phenobarbital | Decreased aspirin effect. |
| Phenytoin | Increased phenytoin effect. |
| Probenecid | Decreased probenecid effect. |
| Propranolol | Decreased aspirin effect. |
| Rauwolfia alkaloids | Decreased aspirin effect. |
| Salicylates (other) | Likely aspirin toxicity. |

*Continued page 961*

## POSSIBLE INTERACTION WITH OTHER SUBSTANCES

| INTERACTS WITH | COMBINED EFFECT |
|---|---|
| Alcohol: | Possible stomach irritation and bleeding. Avoid. |
| Beverages: | None expected. |
| Cocaine: | None expected. |
| Foods: | None expected. |
| Marijuana: | Possible increased pain relief, but marijuana may slow body's recovery. Avoid. |
| Tobacco: | None expected. |

# ATENOLOL

## BRAND NAMES

Tenormin

## BASIC INFORMATION

**Habit forming? No**
**Prescription needed? Yes**
**Available as generic? No**
**Drug class: Beta-adrenergic blocker**

## USES

- Reduces angina attacks.
- Stabilizes irregular heartbeat.
- Lowers blood pressure.
- Reduces frequency of migraine headaches. (Does not relieve headache pain.)
- Other uses prescribed by your doctor.

## DOSAGE & USAGE INFORMATION

**How to take:**
Tablet or capsule—Swallow with liquid. If you can't swallow whole, crumble tablet or open capsule and take with liquid or food.

**When to take:**
With meals or immediately after.

**If you forget a dose:**
Take as soon as you remember. Return to regular schedule, but allow 3 hours between doses.

**What drug does:**
- Blocks certain actions of sympathetic nervous system.
- Lowers heart's oxygen requirements.
- Slows nerve impulses through heart.
- Reduces blood vessel contraction in heart, scalp and other body parts.

**Time lapse before drug works:**
1 to 4 hours.

*Continued next column*

## OVERDOSE

**SYMPTOMS:**
**Weakness, slow or weak pulse, blood pressure drop, fainting, convulsions, cold and sweaty skin.**
**WHAT TO DO:**
- **Dial 0 (operator) or 911 (emergency) for an ambulance or medical help. Then give first aid immediately.**
- **See emergency information on inside covers.**

**Don't take with:**
Non-prescription drugs or drugs in Interaction column without consulting doctor.

## POSSIBLE ADVERSE REACTIONS OR SIDE EFFECTS

| SYMPTOMS | WHAT TO DO |
|---|---|
| **Life-threatening:**<br>None expected. | |
| **Common:** | |
| • Pulse slower than 50 beats per minute. | Discontinue. Call doctor right away. |
| • Drowsiness, numbness or tingling in fingers or toes, dizziness, diarrhea, nausea, fatigue, weakness. | Continue. Call doctor when convenient. |
| • Cold hands or feet; dry mouth, eyes, skin. | Continue. Tell doctor at next visit. |
| **Infrequent:** | |
| • Hallucinations, nightmares, insomnia, headache, breathing difficulty, joint pain. | Discontinue. Call doctor right away. |
| • Confusion, depression, reduced alertness. | Continue. Call doctor when convenient. |
| • Constipation. | Continue. Tell doctor at next visit. |
| **Rare:** | |
| • Rash, sore throat, fever. | Discontinue. Call doctor right away. |
| • Unusual bleeding or bruising. | Continue. Call doctor when convenient. |

## WARNINGS & PRECAUTIONS

**Don't take if:**
- You are allergic to any beta-adrenergic blocker.
- You have asthma.
- You have hay fever symptoms.
- You have taken MAO inhibitors in past 2 weeks.

**Before you start, consult your doctor:**
- If you have heart disease or poor circulation to the extremities.
- If you have hay fever, asthma, chronic bronchitis, emphysema.
- If you have overactive thyroid function.
- If you have impaired liver or kidney function.
- If you will have surgery within 2 months, including dental surgery, requiring general or spinal anesthesia.
- If you have diabetes or hypoglycemia.

**Over age 60:**
Adverse reactions and side effects may be more frequent and severe than in younger persons.

**Pregnancy:**
Risk to unborn child outweighs drug benefits. Don't use.

**Breast-feeding:**
Drug passes into milk. Avoid drug or discontinue nursing until you finish medicine. Consult doctor for advice on maintaining milk supply.

**Infants & children:**
Not recommended.

**Prolonged use:**
Weakens heart muscle contractions.

**Skin & sunlight:**
No problems expected.

**Driving, piloting or hazardous work:**
Don't drive or pilot aircraft until you learn how medicine affects you. Don't work around dangerous machinery. Don't climb ladders or work in high places. Danger increases if you drink alcohol or take medicine affecting alertness and reflexes.

**Discontinuing:**
Don't discontinue without consulting doctor. Dose may require gradual reduction if you have taken drug for a long time. Doses of other drugs may also require adjustment.

**Others:**
May mask hypoglycemia.

## POSSIBLE INTERACTION WITH OTHER DRUGS

| GENERIC NAME OR DRUG CLASS | COMBINED EFFECT |
|---|---|
| Acebutolol | Increased antihypertensive effects of both drugs. |
| Albuterol | Decreased albuterol effect and Beta-adronergic blocking effect. |
| Antidiabetics | Increased antidiabetic effect. |
| Antihistamines | Decreased antihistamine effect. |
| Antihypertensives | Increased effect of antihypertensive. |
| Anti-inflammatory drugs | Decreased effect of anti-inflammatory. |
| Barbiturates | Increased barbiturate effect. Oversedation. |

| | |
|---|---|
| Digitalis preparations | Increased or decreased heart rate. Improves irregular heartbeat. |
| Enalapril | Possible excessive potassium in blood. |
| Narcotics | Increased narcotic effect. Oversedation. |
| Nitrates | Possible excessive blood-pressure drop. |
| Pentoxifylline | Increased antihypertensive effect. |
| Phenytoin | Increased atenolol effect. |
| Quinidine | Slows heart excessively. |
| Reserpine | Increased reserpine effect. Excessive sedation and depression. |
| Tocainide | May worsen congestive heart failure. |

## POSSIBLE INTERACTION WITH OTHER SUBSTANCES

| INTERACTS WITH | COMBINED EFFECT |
|---|---|
| Alcohol: | Excessive blood pressure drop. Avoid. |
| Beverages: | None expected. |
| Cocaine: | Irregular heartbeat. |
| Foods: | None expected. |
| Marijuana: | Daily use—Impaired circulation to hands and feet. |
| Tobacco: | Possible irregular heartbeat. |

# ATROPINE

## BRAND NAMES

See complete list of brand names in the *Brand Name Directory,* page 944.

## BASIC INFORMATION

**Habit forming? No**
**Prescription needed?**
  **Low strength: No**
  **High strength: Yes**
**Available as generic? Yes**
**Drug class: Antispasmodic, anticholinergic**

## USES

Reduces spasms of digestive system, bladder and urethra.

## DOSAGE & USAGE INFORMATION

**How to take:**
Tablet—Swallow with liquid or food to lessen stomach irritation.

**When to take:**
30 minutes before meals (unless directed otherwise by doctor).

**If you forget a dose:**
Take as soon as you remember up to 2 hours late. If more than 2 hours, wait for next scheduled dose (don't double this dose).

**What drug does:**
Blocks nerve impulses at parasympathetic nerve endings, preventing muscle contractions and gland secretions of organs involved.

**Time lapse before drug works:**
15 to 30 minutes.

**Don't take with:**
See Interaction column and consult doctor.

## OVERDOSE

**SYMPTOMS:**
**Dilated pupils, rapid pulse and breathing, dizziness, fever, hallucinations, confusion, slurred speech, agitation, flushed face, convulsions, coma.**
**WHAT TO DO:**
- **Dial 0 (operator) or 911 (emergency) for an ambulance or medical help. Then give first aid immediately.**
- **See emergency information on inside covers.**

## POSSIBLE ADVERSE REACTIONS OR SIDE EFFECTS

| SYMPTOMS | WHAT TO DO |
|---|---|
| **Life-threatening:** | |
| None expected. | |
| **Common:** | |
| • Confusion, delirium, rapid heartbeat. | Discontinue. Call doctor right away. |
| • Nausea, vomiting, decreased sweating, | Continue. Call doctor when convenient. |
| • Constipation. | Continue. Tell doctor at next visit. |
| • Dryness in ears, nose, throat. | No action necessary. |
| **Infrequent:** | |
| Headache, difficult or painful urination. | Continue. Call doctor when convenient. |
| **Rare:** | |
| Rash or hives, pain, blurred vision. | Discontinue. Call doctor right away. |

## WARNINGS & PRECAUTIONS

**Don't take if:**
- You are allergic to any anticholinergic.
- You have trouble with stomach bloating.
- You have difficulty emptying your bladder completely.
- You have narrow-angle glaucoma.
- You have severe ulcerative colitis.

**Before you start, consult your doctor:**
- If you have open-angle glaucoma.
- If you have angina.
- If you have chronic bronchitis or asthma.
- If you have liver disease.
- If you have hiatal hernia.
- If you have enlarged prostate.
- If you have myasthenia gravis.
- If you have peptic ulcer.
- If you will have surgery within 2 months, including dental surgery, requiring general or spinal anesthesia.

**Over age 60:**
Adverse reactions and side effects may be more frequent and severe than in younger persons.

**Pregnancy:**
Studies inconclusive on harm to unborn child. Animal studies show fetal abnormalities. Decide with your doctor whether drug benefits justify risk to unborn child.

**Breast-feeding:**
Drug passes into milk and decreases milk flow. Avoid drug or discontinue nursing until you finish medicine. Consult doctor for advice on maintaining milk supply.

**Infants & children:**
Use only under medical supervision.

**Prolonged use:**
Chronic constipation, possible fecal impaction. Consult doctor immediately.

**Skin & sunlight:**
No problems expected.

**Driving, piloting or hazardous work:**
Use disqualifies you for piloting aircraft. Otherwise, no problems expected.

**Discontinuing:**
May be unnecessary to finish medicine. Follow doctor's instructions.

**Others:**
No problems expected.

## POSSIBLE INTERACTION WITH OTHER DRUGS

| GENERIC NAME OR DRUG CLASS | COMBINED EFFECT |
| --- | --- |
| **Amantadine** | Increased atropine effect. |
| **Anticholinergics (other)** | Increased atropine effect. |
| **Antidepressants (tricyclic)** | Increased atropine effect. Increased sedation. |
| **Antihistamines** | Increased atropine effect. |
| **Cortisone drugs** | Increased internal-eye pressure. |
| **Haloperidol** | Increased internal-eye pressure. |
| **MAO inhibitors** | Increased atropine effect. |
| **Meperidine** | Increased atropine effect. |
| **Methylphenidate** | Increased atropine effect. |
| **Molindone** | Increased anticholinergic effect. |
| **Nitrates** | Increased internal-eye pressure. |
| **Orphenadrine** | Increased atropine effect. |

| | |
| --- | --- |
| **Phenothiazines** | Increased atropine effect. |
| **Pilocarpine** | Loss of pilocarpine effect in glaucoma treatment. |
| **Potassium supplements** | Possible intestinal ulcers with oral potassium tablets. |
| **Vitamin C** | Decreased atropine effect. Avoid large doses of vitamin C. |

## POSSIBLE INTERACTION WITH OTHER SUBSTANCES

| INTERACTS WITH | COMBINED EFFECT |
| --- | --- |
| **Alcohol:** | None expected. |
| **Beverages:** | None expected. |
| **Cocaine:** | Excessively rapid heartbeat. Avoid. |
| **Foods:** | None expected. |
| **Marijuana:** | Drowsiness and dry mouth. |
| **Tobacco:** | None expected. |

# ATROPINE, HYOSCYAMINE, METHENAMINE, METHYLENE BLUE, PHENYLSALICYLATE & BENZOIC ACID

## BRAND NAMES

| | |
|---|---|
| Dolsed | Urinary Antiseptic |
| Hexalol | No. 2 |
| Prosed | Urised |
| Trac Tabs | Urisep |
| U-Tract | Uritab |
| UAA | Urithol |
| Uramine | Uritin |
| Uridon Modified | Uroblue |
| Urimed | Uro-Ves |

## BASIC INFORMATION

**Habit forming?** No
**Prescription needed?** Yes
**Available as generic?** No
**Drug class:** Urinary tract analgesic, antispasmodic, anti-infective

## USES

A combination medicine to control infection, spasms and pain caused by urinary tract infections.

## DOSAGE & USAGE INFORMATION

**How to take:**
Tablet—Swallow with liquid or food to lessen stomach irritation.

**When to take:**
30 minutes before meals (unless directed otherwise by doctor).

**If you forget a dose:**
Take as soon as you remember up to 2 hours late. If more than 2 hours, wait for next scheduled dose (don't double this dose).

*Continued next column*

## OVERDOSE

**SYMPTOMS:**
**Dilated pupils, rapid pulse and breathing, dizziness, fever, hallucinations, confusion, slurred speech, agitation, flushed face, convulsions, coma.**
**WHAT TO DO:**
- **Dial 0 (operator) or 911 (emergency) for an ambulance or medical help. Then give first aid immediately.**
- **See emergency information on inside covers.**

**What drug does:**
Makes urine acid. Blocks nerve impulses at parasympathetic nerve endings, preventing muscle contractions and gland secretions of organs involved. Methenamine destroys some germs.

**Time lapse before drug works:**
15 to 30 minutes.

**Don't take with:**
See Interaction column and consult doctor.

## POSSIBLE ADVERSE REACTIONS OR SIDE EFFECTS

| SYMPTOMS | WHAT TO DO |
|---|---|
| **Life-threatening:** | |
| Heartbeat irregularity, shortness of breath or difficulty breathing. | Seek emergency treatment immediately. |
| **Common:** | |
| Dry mouth, throat. | Continue. Call doctor when convenient. |
| **Infrequent:** | |
| Flushed, red face; drowsiness; difficult urination; nausea and vomiting; abdominal pain; ringing or buzzing in ears; severe drowsiness; back pain. | Discontinue. Call doctor right away. |
| **Rare:** | |
| Blurred vision; pain in eyes; skin rash, hives. | Discontinue. Seek emergency treatment. |

## WARNINGS & PRECAUTIONS

**Don't take if:**
- You are allergic to any of the ingredients or aspirin.
- Brain damage in child.
- You have glaucoma.

**Before you start, consult your doctor:**
- If you are on any special diet such as low-sodium.
- If you have had a hiatal hernia, bronchitis, asthma, liver disease, stomach or duodenal ulcers.
- If you have asthma, nasal polyps, bleeding disorder or enlarged prostate.
- If you will have any surgery within 2 months.

# ATROPINE, HYOSCYAMINE, METHENAMINE, METHYLENE BLUE, PHENYLSALICYLATE & BENZOIC ACID

**Over age 60:**
- Adverse reactions and side effects may be more frequent and severe than in younger persons.
- More likely to cause hidden bleeding in stomach or intestines. Watch for dark stools.

**Pregnancy:**
Risk to unborn child outweighs benefits. Don't use.

**Breast-feeding:**
Drug passes into milk. Avoid or discontinue nursing until you finish medicine.

**Infants & children:**
Side effects more likely. Not recommended in children under 12.

**Prolonged use:**
May lead to constipation or kidney damage. Request lab studies to monitor effects of prolonged use.

**Skin & sunlight:**
No problems expected.

**Driving, piloting or hazardous work:**
May disqualify for piloting aircraft during time you take medicine.

**Discontinuing:**
May be unnecessary to finish medicine. Follow your symptoms and doctor's advice.

**Others:**
- Salicylates can complicate surgery, pregnancy, labor and delivery, and illness.
- Urine tests for blood sugar may be inaccurate.
- Drink cranberry juice or eat prunes or plums to help make urine more acid.

## POSSIBLE INTERACTION WITH OTHER DRUGS

| GENERIC NAME OR DRUG CLASS | COMBINED EFFECT |
|---|---|
| Acebutolol | Decreased antihypertensive effect of acebutolol. |
| Allopurinol | Decreased allopurinol effect. |
| Amantadine | Increased atropine and belladonna effect. |
| Antacids | Decreased salicylate and methenamine effect. |
| Anticoagulants | Increased anticoagulant effect. Abnormal bleeding. |

| | |
|---|---|
| Anticholinergics (other) | Increased atropine and belladonna effect. |
| Antidepressants (other) | Increased hyoscyamine and belladonna effect. Increased sedation. |
| Antidiabetics (oral) | Low blood sugar. |
| Anti-inflammatory drugs (non-steroid) | Risk of stomach bleeding and ulcers. |
| Antihistamines | Increased atropine and hyoscyamine effect. |
| Aspirin | Likely salicylate toxicity. |
| Carbonic anhydrase inhibitors | Decreased methenamine effect. |
| Cortisone drugs | Increased internal-eye pressure, increased cortisone effect. Risk of ulcers and stomach bleeding. |
| Diuretics (thiazide) | Decreased urine acidity. |
| Furosemide | Possible salicylate toxicity. |
| Gold compounds | Increased likelihood of kidney damage. |
| Haloperidol | Increased internal-eye pressure. |
| Indomethacin | Risk of stomach bleeding and ulcers. |
| MAO inhibitors | Increased belladonna and atropine effect. |

*Continued page 961*

## POSSIBLE INTERACTION WITH OTHER SUBSTANCES

| INTERACTS WITH | COMBINED EFFECT |
|---|---|
| Alcohol: | Excessive sedation. Possible stomach irritation and bleeding. Avoid. |
| Beverages: | None expected. |
| Cocaine: | Excessively rapid heartbeat. Avoid. |
| Foods: | None expected. |
| Marijuana: | Drowsiness and dry mouth. May slow body's recovery. |
| Tobacco: | Dry mouth. |

# AZATADINE

## BRAND NAMES

Optimine                 Trinalin Repetabs

## BASIC INFORMATION

**Habit forming? No**
**Prescription needed? Yes**
**Available as generic? No**
**Drug class: Antihistamine**

 ## USES

- Reduces allergic symptoms such as hay fever, hives, rash or itching.
- Induces sleep.

 ## DOSAGE & USAGE INFORMATION

**How to take:**
Tablet—Swallow with liquid or food to lessen stomach irritation.

**When to take:**
Varies with form. Follow label directions.

**If you forget a dose:**
Take as soon as you remember up to 2 hours late. If more than 2 hours, wait for next scheduled dose (don't double this dose).

**What drug does:**
Blocks action of histamine after an allergic response triggers histamine release in sensitive cells.

**Time lapse before drug works:**
30 minutes.

**Don't take with:**
See Interaction column and consult doctor.

 ## OVERDOSE

**SYMPTOMS:**
Convulsions, red face, hallucinations, coma.
**WHAT TO DO:**
- **Dial 0 (operator) or 911 (emergency) for an ambulance or medical help. Then give first aid immediately.**
- **If patient is unconscious and not breathing, give mouth-to-mouth breathing. If there is no heartbeat, use cardiac massage and mouth-to-mouth breathing (CPR). Don't try to make patient vomit. If you can't get help quickly, take patient to nearest emergency facility.**
- **See emergency information on inside covers.**

 ## POSSIBLE ADVERSE REACTIONS OR SIDE EFFECTS

| SYMPTOMS | WHAT TO DO |
|---|---|
| **Life-threatening:** None expected. | |
| **Common:** Drowsiness; dizziness; dry mouth, nose, throat; nausea. | Continue. Tell doctor at next visit. |
| **Infrequent:** | |
| • Changes in vision. | Discontinue. Call doctor right away. |
| • Less tolerance for contact lenses, difficult urination. | Continue. Call doctor when convenient. |
| • Appetite loss. | Continue. Tell doctor at next visit. |
| **Rare:** Nightmares, agitation, irritability, sore throat, fever, rapid heartbeat, unusual bleeding or bruising, fatigue, weakness. | Discontinue. Call doctor right away. |

## WARNINGS & PRECAUTIONS

**Don't take if:**
You are allergic to any antihistamine.

**Before you start, consult your doctor:**
- If you have glaucoma.
- If you have enlarged prostate.
- If you have asthma.
- If you have kidney disease.
- If you have peptic ulcer.
- If you will have surgery within 2 months, including dental surgery, requiring general or spinal anesthesia.

**Over age 60:**
Don't exceed recommended dose. Adverse reactions and side effects may be more frequent and severe than in younger persons, especially urination difficulty, diminished alertness and other brain and nervous-system symptoms.

**Pregnancy:**
No proven harm to unborn child. Avoid if possible.

**Breast-feeding:**
Drug passes into milk. Avoid drug or discontinue nursing until you finish medicine. Consult doctor for advice on maintaining milk supply.

**Infants & children:**
Not recommended for premature or newborn infants. Otherwise, no problems expected.

**Prolonged use:**
Avoid. May damage bone-marrow and nerve cells.

**Skin & sunlight:**
May cause rash or intensify sunburn in areas exposed to sun or sunlamp.

**Driving, piloting or hazardous work:**
Don't drive or pilot aircraft until you learn how medicine affects you. Don't work around dangerous machinery. Don't climb ladders or work in high places. Danger increases if you drink alcohol or take medicine affecting alertness and reflexes, such as antihistamines, tranquilizers, sedatives, pain medicine, narcotics and mind-altering drugs.

**Discontinuing:**
No problems expected.

**Others:**
May mask symptoms of hearing damage from aspirin, other salicylates, cisplatin, paromomycin, vancomycin or anticonvulsants. Consult doctor if you use these.

## POSSIBLE INTERACTION WITH OTHER DRUGS

| GENERIC NAME OR DRUG CLASS | COMBINED EFFECT |
|---|---|
| Anticholinergics | Increased anticholinergic effect. |
| Antidepressants | Excess sedation. Avoid. |
| Antihistamines (other) | Excess sedation. Avoid. |
| Dronabinol | Increased effects of both drugs. Avoid. |
| Hypnotics | Excess sedation. Avoid. |
| MAO inhibitors | Increased azatadine effect. |
| Mind-altering drugs | Excess sedation. Avoid. |
| Molindone | Increased antihistamine effect. |
| Narcotics | Excess sedation. Avoid. |
| Sedatives | Excess sedation. Avoid. |
| Sleep inducers | Excess sedation. Avoid. |
| Tranquilizers | Excess sedation. Avoid. |

## POSSIBLE INTERACTION WITH OTHER SUBSTANCES

| INTERACTS WITH | COMBINED EFFECT |
|---|---|
| Alcohol: | Excess sedation. Avoid. |
| Beverages: Caffeine drinks. | Less azatadine sedation. |
| Cocaine: | Decreased azatadine effect. Avoid. |
| Foods: | None expected. |
| Marijuana: | Excess sedation. Avoid. |
| Tobacco: | None expected. |

# AZT (AZIDOTHYMIDINE), Also Called ZIDOVUDINE

## BRAND NAMES

**Retrovir**

## BASIC INFORMATION

**Habit forming? No**
**Prescription needed? Yes**
**Available as generic? No**
**Drug class: Antiviral**

## USES

Treatment of selected adult patients with AIDS (Acquired Immune Deficiency Syndrome) and advanced ARC (AIDS Related Complex) who have a history of pneumonia caused by *Pneumocystis carinii*.

## DOSAGE & USAGE INFORMATION

**How to take:**
Tablet or capsule—Swallow with liquid.

**When to take:**
Every 4 hours around the clock unless instructed otherwise.

**If you forget a dose:**
Take as soon as you remember.

**What drug does:**
Inhibits reproduction of some viruses, including HIV virus (the virus that causes AIDS).

**Time lapse before drug works:**
May require several weeks of treatment for full effect.

**Don't take with:**
See Interaction column and consult doctor.

## OVERDOSE

**SYMPTOMS:**
No cases reported. However, if overdose occurs, follow instructions below.
**WHAT TO DO:**
- **Dial 0 (operator) or 911 (emergency) for an ambulance or medical help. Then give first aid immediately.**
- **See emergency information on inside covers.**

## POSSIBLE ADVERSE REACTIONS OR SIDE EFFECTS

| SYMPTOMS | WHAT TO DO |
|---|---|
| **Life-threatening:** None expected. | |
| **Common:** | |
| • Anemia, low white-blood-cell count. | Discontinue. Call doctor right away. |
| • Severe headache, nausea, insomnia. | Continue. Call doctor when convenient. |
| **Infrequent:** Severe headache, sweating, fever, appetite loss, abdominal pain, vomiting, aching muscles, dizziness, numbness in hands and feet, shortness of breath, skin rash, strange taste. | Continue. Call doctor when convenient. |
| **Rare:** None expected. | |

## WARNINGS & PRECAUTIONS

**Don't take if:**
You are allergic to any component of this capsule.

**Before you start, consult your doctor:**
- If you know you have a low white-blood-cell count or severe anemia.
- If you have severe kidney or liver disease.

**Over age 60:**
Adverse reactions and side effects may be more frequent and severe than in younger persons. Ask doctor about smaller doses.

**Pregnancy:**
Effect unknown at present.

**Breast-feeding:**
Drug passes into milk. If possible, avoid drug or discontinue until you finish medicine. Consult your doctor for advice on maintaining milk supply.

**Infants & children:**
Not recommended.

**Prolonged use:**
Not recommended.

**Skin & sunlight:**
No problems expected.

**Driving, piloting, or hazardous work:**
Don't drive or pilot aircraft until you learn how medicine affects you. Don't work around dangerous machinery. Don't climb ladders or work in high places. Danger increases if you drink alcohol or take medicine affecting alertness and reflexes, such as antihistamines, tranquilizers, sedatives, pain medicine, narcotics and mind-altering drugs.

**Discontinuing:**
Don't discontinue without consulting your doctor. Dose may require gradual reduction if you have taken drug for a long time. Doses of other drugs may also require adjustment.

**Others:**
- Drug is still considered experimental so full safety and effectiveness are unknown.
- AZT does *not cure* HIV virus infections. Transfusions or dose modification may be necessary if toxicity develops.
- Have blood counts followed closely during treatment to detect anemia or lowered white-blood-cell count.
- AZT does not reduce risk of transmitting disease to others.

## POSSIBLE INTERACTION WITH OTHER DRUGS

| GENERIC NAME OR DRUG CLASS | COMBINED EFFECT |
|---|---|
| Acetaminophen | May increase toxic effects of AZT. |
| Acyclovir | Lethargy, convulsions. |
| Aspirin | May increase toxic effects of AZT. |
| Indomethacin | May increase toxic effects of AZT. |
| Probenecid | May increase toxic effects of AZT. |

## POSSIBLE INTERACTION WITH OTHER SUBSTANCES

| INTERACTS WITH | COMBINED EFFECT |
|---|---|
| Alcohol: | Unknown. Best avoid. |
| Beverages: | None expected. |
| Cocaine: | Unknown. Best avoid. |
| Foods: | None expected. |
| Marijuana: | Unknown. Best avoid. |
| Tobacco: | None expected. |

# BACAMPICILLIN

## BRAND NAMES

**Spectrobid**

## BASIC INFORMATION

**Habit forming? No**
**Prescription needed? Yes**
**Available as generic? No**
**Drug class: Antibiotic (penicillin)**

 **USES**

Treatment of bacterial infections that are
susceptible to bacampicillin.

 **DOSAGE & USAGE INFORMATION**

**How to take:**
- Tablets or capsules—Swallow with liquid on
  an empty stomach 1 hour before meals or 2
  hours after eating.
- Liquid—Take with cold beverage. Liquid form
  is perishable and effective for only 7 days at
  room temperature. Effective for 14 days if
  stored in refrigerator. Don't freeze.

**When to take:**
Follow instructions on prescription label or side
of package. Doses should be evenly spaced.
For example, 4 times a day means every 6
hours.

**If you forget a dose:**
Take as soon as you remember. Continue
regular schedule.

**What drug does:**
Destroys susceptible bacteria. Does not kill
viruses.

**Time lapse before drug works:**
May be several days before medicine affects
infection.

**Don't take with:**
See Interaction column and consult doctor.

 **OVERDOSE**

**SYMPTOMS:**
**Severe diarrhea, nausea or vomiting.**
**WHAT TO DO:**
**Overdose unlikely to threaten life. If person
takes much larger amount than prescribed,
call doctor, poison-control center or hospital
emergency room for specific instructions.**

 **POSSIBLE ADVERSE REACTIONS OR SIDE EFFECTS**

| SYMPTOMS | WHAT TO DO |
|---|---|
| **Life-threatening:** | |
| Hives, rash, intense itching, faintness soon after a dose (anaphylaxis). | Seek emergency treatment immediately. |
| **Common:** | |
| Dark or discolored tongue. | Continue. Tell doctor at next visit. |
| **Infrequent:** | |
| Mild nausea, vomiting, diarrhea. | Continue. Call doctor when convenient. |
| **Rare:** | |
| Unexplained bleeding. | Discontinue. Call doctor right away. |

## WARNINGS & PRECAUTIONS

**Don't take if:**
You are allergic to bacampicillin, cephalosporin antibiotics, other penicillins or penicillamine. Life-threatening reaction may occur.

**Before you start, consult your doctor:**
If you are allergic to any substance or drug.

**Over age 60:**
You may have skin reactions, particularly around genitals and anus.

**Pregnancy:**
Studies inconclusive on harm to unborn child. Animal studies show fetal abnormalities. Decide with your doctor whether drug benefits justify risk to unborn child.

**Breast-feeding:**
Drug passes into milk. Child may become sensitive to this and all penicillins. Avoid bacampicillin or discontinue nursing until you finish medicine. Consult doctor for advice on maintaining milk supply.

**Infants & children:**
No problems expected.

**Prolonged use:**
You may become more susceptible to infections caused by germs not responsive to bacampicillin.

**Skin & sunlight:**
No problems expected.

**Driving, piloting, or hazardous work:**
Usually not dangerous. Most hazardous reactions likely to occur a few minutes after taking bacampicillin.

**Discontinuing:**
Don't discontinue without doctor's advice until you complete prescribed dose, even though symptoms diminish or disappear.

**Others:**
Urine sugar test for diabetes may show false positive result.

## POSSIBLE INTERACTION WITH OTHER DRUGS

| GENERIC NAME OR DRUG CLASS | COMBINED EFFECT |
|---|---|
| Beta-adrenergic blockers | Increased chance of anaphylaxis (see emergency information on inside front cover). |
| Chloramphenicol | Decreased effect of both drugs. |
| Erythromycins | Decreased effect of both drugs. |
| Loperamide | Decreased bacampicillin effect. |
| Paromomycin | Decreased effect of both drugs. |
| Tetracyclines | Decreased effect of both drugs. |
| Troleandomycin | Decreased effect of both drugs. |

## POSSIBLE INTERACTION WITH OTHER SUBSTANCES

| INTERACTS WITH | COMBINED EFFECT |
|---|---|
| Alcohol: | Occasional stomach irritation. |
| Beverages: | None expected. |
| Cocaine: | No proven problems. |
| Foods: | None expected. |
| Marijuana: | No proven problems. |
| Tobacco: | None expected. |

# BACLOFEN

## BRAND NAMES

Lioresal

## BASIC INFORMATION

Habit forming? No
Prescription needed? Yes
Available as generic? No
Drug class: Muscle relaxant (analgesic)

 **USES**

- Relieves spasms, cramps and spasticity of muscles caused by medical problems, including multiple sclerosis and spine injuries.
- Reduces number and severity of trigeminal neuralgia attacks.

 **DOSAGE & USAGE INFORMATION**

**How to take:**
Tablet or capsule—Swallow with liquid or food to lessen stomach irritation.

**When to take:**
3 or 4 times daily as directed.

**If you forget a dose:**
Take as soon as you remember up to 2 hours late. If more than 2 hours, wait for next scheduled dose (don't double this dose).

**What drug does:**
Blocks body's pain and reflex messages to brain.

**Time lapse before drug works:**
Variable. Few hours to weeks.

*Continued next column*

 **OVERDOSE**

**SYMPTOMS:**
**Blurred vision, blindness, difficult breathing, muscle weakness, convulsive seizures.**
**WHAT TO DO:**
- **Dial 0 (operator) or 911 (emergency) for an ambulance or medical help. Then give first aid immediately.**
- **If patient is unconscious and not breathing, give mouth-to-mouth breathing. If there is no heartbeat, use cardiac massage and mouth-to-mouth breathing (CPR). Don't try to make patient vomit. If you can't get help quickly, take patient to nearest emergency facility.**
- **See emergency information on inside covers.**

**Don't take with:**
See Interaction column and consult doctor.

 **POSSIBLE ADVERSE REACTIONS OR SIDE EFFECTS**

| SYMPTOMS | WHAT TO DO |
|---|---|
| **Life-threatening:**<br>None expected. | |
| **Common:**<br>Dizziness, lightheadedness, confusion, drowsiness, nausea. | Continue. Call doctor when convenient. |
| **Infrequent:** | |
| • Rash with itching, numbness or tingling in hands or feet. | Discontinue. Call doctor right away. |
| • Headache, abdominal pain, diarrhea or constipation, appetite loss, muscle weakness, difficult or painful urination, male sex problems. | Continue. Call doctor when convenient. |
| **Rare:** | |
| • Fainting, hallucinations, depression, weakness, chest pain. | Discontinue. Call doctor right away. |
| • Ringing in ears, lowered blood pressure, pounding heartbeat. | Continue. Call doctor when convenient. |

## WARNINGS & PRECAUTIONS

**Don't take if:**
You are allergic to any muscle relaxant.

**Before you start, consult your doctor:**
- If you have Parkinson's disease.
- If you have cerebral palsy.
- If you have had a recent stroke.
- If you have had a recent head injury.
- If you have arthritis.
- If you have diabetes.
- If you have epilepsy.
- If you have psychosis.
- If you have kidney disease.
- If you will have surgery within 2 months, including dental surgery, requiring general or spinal anesthesia.

**Over age 60:**
Adverse reactions and side effects may be more frequent and severe than in younger persons.

**Pregnancy:**
Risk to unborn child outweighs drug benefits. Don't use.

**Breast-feeding:**
Avoid nursing or discontinue until you finish medicine.

**Infants & children:**
Not recommended.

**Prolonged use:**
Epileptic patients should be monitored with EEGs. Diabetics should more closely monitor blood sugar levels. Obtain periodic liver function tests.

**Skin & sunlight:**
No problems expected.

**Driving, piloting or hazardous work:**
Don't drive or pilot aircraft until you learn how medicine affects you. Don't work around dangerous machinery. Don't climb ladders or work in high places. Danger increases if you drink alcohol or take medicine affecting alertness and reflexes, such as antihistamines, tranquilizers, sedatives, pain medicine, narcotics and mind-altering drugs.

**Discontinuing:**
Don't discontinue without consulting doctor. Dose may require gradual reduction if you have taken drug for a long time. Doses of other drugs may also require adjustment.

**Others:**
No problems expected.

## POSSIBLE INTERACTION WITH OTHER DRUGS

| GENERIC NAME OR DRUG CLASS | COMBINED EFFECT |
| --- | --- |
| CNS depressants: antidepressants, antihistamines, muscle relaxants (other), narcotics, sedatives, sleeping pills, tranquilizers. | Increased sedation. Low blood pressure. Avoid. |
| General anesthetics | Increased sedation. Low blood pressure. Avoid. |
| Insulin and oral medications for diabetes | Need to adjust diabetes medicine dosage. |

## POSSIBLE INTERACTION WITH OTHER SUBSTANCES

| INTERACTS WITH | COMBINED EFFECT |
| --- | --- |
| Alcohol: | Increased sedation. Low blood pressure. Avoid. |
| Beverages: | No problems expected. |
| Cocaine: | Increased spasticity. Avoid. |
| Foods: | No problems expected. |
| Marijuana: | Increased spasticity. Avoid. |
| Tobacco: | May interfere with absorption of medicine. |

# BECLOMETHASONE

## BRAND NAMES

Beclovent Inhaler      Vancenase Inhaler
Beconase Inhaler      Vanceril Inhaler
Propaderm

## BASIC INFORMATION

Habit forming? No
Prescription needed? Yes
Available as generic? No
Drug class: Cortisone drug (adrenal
           corticosteroid), antiasthmatic

 ## USES

Prevents attacks of bronchial asthma and
allergic hay fever. Does not stop an active
asthma attack.

 ## DOSAGE & USAGE INFORMATION

**How to take:**
Follow package instructions. Don't inhale more
than twice per dose. Rinse mouth after use to
prevent hoarseness, throat irritation and mouth
infection.

**When to take:**
Regularly at the same times each day.

**If you forget a dose:**
Take as soon as you remember up to 2 hours
late. If more than 2 hours, wait for next
scheduled dose (don't double this dose).

**What drug does:**
Reduces inflammation in bronchial tubes.

**Time lapse before drug works:**
1 to 4 weeks.

**Don't take with:**
See Interaction column and consult doctor.

 ## OVERDOSE

**SYMPTOMS:**
Fluid retention, flushed face, nervousness,
stomach irritation.
**WHAT TO DO:**
Overdose unlikely to threaten life. If person
inhales much larger amount than prescribed,
call doctor, poison-control center or hospital
emergency room for instructions.

 ## POSSIBLE ADVERSE REACTIONS OR SIDE EFFECTS

| SYMPTOMS | WHAT TO DO |
|---|---|
| **Life-threatening:**<br>None expected. | |
| **Common:**<br>Fungus infection with white patches in mouth, dryness, sore throat. | Continue. Call doctor when convenient. |
| **Infrequent:**<br>• Rash. | Discontinue. Call doctor right away. |
| • Lung inflammation, spasm of bronchial tubes. | Continue. Call doctor when convenient. |
| **Rare:**<br>None expected. | |

## WARNINGS & PRECAUTIONS

**Don't take if:**
- You are allergic to beclomethasone.
- You have had tuberculosis.
- You are having an asthma attack.

**Before you start, consult your doctor:**
- If you take other cortisone drugs.
- If you have an infection.

**Over age 60:**
More likely to develop lung infections.

**Pregnancy:**
Risk to unborn child outweighs drug benefits. Don't use.

**Breast-feeding:**
Drug passes into milk. Avoid drug or discontinue nursing.

**Infants & children:**
Use only under medical supervision.

**Prolonged use:**
No problems expected.

**Skin & sunlight:**
No problems expected.

**Driving, piloting or hazardous work:**
No problems expected.

**Discontinuing:**
Don't discontinue without doctor's advice until you complete prescribed dose, even though symptoms diminish or disappear.

**Others:**
- Unrelated illness or injury may require cortisone drugs by mouth or injection. Notify your doctor.
- Consult doctor as soon as possible if your asthma returns while using beclamethasone as a preventive.
- Drug can reactivate tuberculosis.

## POSSIBLE INTERACTION WITH OTHER DRUGS

| GENERIC NAME OR DRUG CLASS | COMBINED EFFECT |
|---|---|
| Antiasthmatics (other) | Increased antiasthmatic effect. |
| Ephedrine | Increased beclomethasone effect. |
| Epinephrine | Increased beclomethasone effect. |
| Indapamide | Possible excessive potassium loss, causing dangerous heartbeat irregularity. |
| Isoetharine | Increased beclomethasone effect. |
| Isoproterenol | Increased beclomethasone effect. |
| Potassium supplements | Decreased potassium effect |
| Terbutaline | Increased beclomethasone effect. |
| Theophylline | Increased beclomethasone effect. |

## POSSIBLE INTERACTION WITH OTHER SUBSTANCES

| INTERACTS WITH | COMBINED EFFECT |
|---|---|
| Alcohol: | None expected. |
| Beverages: | None expected. |
| Cocaine: | None expected. |
| Foods: | None expected. |
| Marijuana: | Decreased beclomethasone effect. |
| Tobacco: | Decreased beclomethasone effect. |

# BELLADONNA

## BRAND NAMES

See complete list of brand names in the *Brand Name Directory,* page 944.

## BASIC INFORMATION

Habit forming? No
Prescription needed?
  Low strength: No
  High strength: Yes
Available as generic? Yes
Drug class: Antispasmodic, anticholinergic

 **USES**

Reduces spasms of digestive system, bladder and urethra.

 **DOSAGE & USAGE INFORMATION**

**How to take:**
- Tablet, elixir or capsule—Swallow with liquid or food to lessen stomach irritation.
- Drops—Dilute dose in beverage before swallowing.

**When to take:**
30 minutes before meals (unless directed otherwise by doctor).

**If you forget a dose:**
Take as soon as you remember up to 2 hours late. If more than 2 hours, wait for next scheduled dose (don't double this dose).

**What drug does:**
Blocks nerve impulses at parasympathetic nerve endings, preventing muscle contractions and gland secretions of organs involved.

**Time lapse before drug works:**
15 to 30 minutes.

**Don't take with:**
See Interaction column and consult doctor.

 **OVERDOSE**

**SYMPTOMS:**
**Dilated pupils, rapid pulse and breathing, dizziness, fever, hallucinations, confusion, slurred speech, agitation, flushed face, convulsions, coma.**
**WHAT TO DO:**
- **Dial 0 (operator) or 911 (emergency) for an ambulance or medical help. Then give first aid immediately.**
- **See emergency information on inside covers.**

 **POSSIBLE ADVERSE REACTIONS OR SIDE EFFECTS**

| SYMPTOMS | WHAT TO DO |
|---|---|
| **Life-threatening:** None expected. | |
| **Common:** | |
| • Confusion, delirium, rapid heartbeat. | Discontinue. Call doctor right away. |
| • Nausea, vomiting, decreased sweating, | Continue. Call doctor when convenient. |
| • Constipation. | Continue. Tell doctor at next visit. |
| • Dryness in ears, nose, throat. | No action necessary. |
| **Infrequent:** Headache, difficult urination. | Continue. Call doctor when convenient. |
| **Rare:** Rash or hives, pain, blurred vision. | Discontinue. Call doctor right away. |

 **WARNINGS & PRECAUTIONS**

**Don't take if:**
- You are allergic to any anticholinergic.
- You have trouble with stomach bloating.
- You have difficulty emptying your bladder completely.
- You have narrow-angle glaucoma.
- You have severe ulcerative colitis.

**Before you start, consult your doctor:**
- If you have open-angle glaucoma.
- If you have angina.
- If you have chronic bronchitis or asthma.
- If you have hiatal hernia.
- If you have liver disease.
- If you have enlarged prostate.
- If you have myasthenia gravis.
- If you have peptic ulcer.
- If you will have surgery within 2 months, including dental surgery, requiring general or spinal anesthesia.

**Over age 60:**
Adverse reactions and side effects may be more frequent and severe than in younger persons.

**Pregnancy:**
Studies inconclusive on harm to unborn child. Animal studies show fetal abnormalities. Decide with your doctor whether drug benefits justify risk to unborn child.

**Breast-feeding:**
Drug passes into milk and decreases milk flow. Avoid drug or discontinue nursing until you finish medicine. Consult doctor for advice on maintaining milk supply.

**Infants & children:**
Use only under medical supervision.

**Prolonged use:**
Chronic constipation, possible fecal impaction. Consult doctor immediately.

**Skin & sunlight:**
No problems expected.

**Driving, piloting or hazardous work:**
Use disqualifies you for piloting aircraft. Otherwise, no problems expected.

**Discontinuing:**
May be unnecessary to finish medicine. Follow doctor's instructions.

**Others:**
No problems expected.

## POSSIBLE INTERACTION WITH OTHER DRUGS

| GENERIC NAME OR DRUG CLASS | COMBINED EFFECT |
|---|---|
| Amantadine | Increased belladonna effect. |
| Anticholinergics (other) | Increased belladonna effect. |
| Antidepressants (tricyclic) | Increased belladonna effect. Increased sedation. |
| Antihistamines | Increased belladonna effect. |
| Cortisone drugs | Increased internal-eye pressure. |
| Haloperidol | Increased internal-eye pressure. |
| MAO inhibitors | Increased belladonna effect. |
| Meperidine | Increased belladonna effect. |
| Methylphenidate | Increased belladonna effect. |
| Molindone | Increased anticholinergic effect. |
| Nitrates | Increased internal-eye pressure. |
| Orphenadrine | Increased belladonna effect. |
| Phenothiazines | Increased belladonna effect. |

| | |
|---|---|
| Pilocarpine | Loss of pilocarpine effect in glaucoma treatment. |
| Potassium supplements | Possible intestinal ulcers with oral potassium tablets. |
| Vitamin C | Decreased belladonna effect. Avoid large doses of vitamin C. |

## POSSIBLE INTERACTION WITH OTHER SUBSTANCES

| INTERACTS WITH | COMBINED EFFECT |
|---|---|
| Alcohol: | None expected. |
| Beverages: | None expected. |
| Cocaine: | Excessively rapid heartbeat. Avoid. |
| Foods: | None expected. |
| Marijuana: | Drowsiness and dry mouth. |
| Tobacco: | None expected. |

# BELLADONNA ALKALOIDS & BARBITURATES

## BRAND NAMES

See complete list of brand names in the *Brand Name Directory,* page 945.

## BASIC INFORMATION

**Habit forming? Yes**
**Prescription needed? Yes**
**Available as generic? Some yes, some no**
**Drug class: Antispasmodic, anticholinergic, sedative**

 ## USES

- Reduces spasms of digestive system, bladder and urethra.
- Reduces anxiety or nervous tension (low dose).
- Relieves insomnia (higher bedtime dose).

 ## DOSAGE & USAGE INFORMATION

**How to take:**

- Tablet, liquid or capsule—Swallow with liquid or food to lessen stomach irritation. If you can't swallow whole, crumble tablet or open capsule and take with liquid or food.
- Extended-release tablets or capsules—Swallow each dose whole.
- Drops—Dilute dose in beverage before swallowing.

**When to take:**
At the same times each day.

**If you forget a dose:**
Take as soon as you remember up to 2 hours late. If more than 2 hours, wait for next scheduled dose (don't double this dose).

**What drug does:**

- May partially block nerve impulses at nerve-cell connections.

*Continued next column*

 ## OVERDOSE

**SYMPTOMS:**
**Blurred vision, confusion, convulsions, irregular heartbeat, hallucinations, coma.**
**WHAT TO DO:**

- **Dial 0 (operator) or 911 (emergency) for an ambulance or medical help. Then give first aid immediately.**
- **See emergency information on inside covers.**

- Blocks nerve impulses at parasympathetic nerve endings, preventing muscle contractions and gland secretions of organs involved.

**Time lapse before drug works:**
15 to 30 minutes.

**Don't take with:**
See Interaction column and consult doctor.

 ## POSSIBLE ADVERSE REACTIONS OR SIDE EFFECTS

| SYMPTOMS | WHAT TO DO |
|---|---|
| **Life-threatening:** | |
| Unusual excitement, restlessness, fast heartbeat, breathing difficulty. | Seek emergency treatment immediately. |
| **Common:** | |
| • Dry mouth, throat, nose; drowsiness; constipation; dizziness; nausea; vomiting; "hangover" effect; depression; confusion. | Discontinue. Call doctor right away. |
| • Reduced sweating, slurred speech, agitation. | Continue. Call doctor when convenient. |
| **Infrequent:** | |
| Difficult urination; difficult swallowing; rash or hives; face, lip or eyelid swelling; joint or muscle pain. | Discontinue. Call doctor right away. |
| **Rare:** | |
| Jaundice; unusual bruising or bleeding; hives, skin rash; pain in eyes; blurred vision; sore throat, fever, mouth sores; unexplained bleeding or bruising. | Discontinue. Call doctor right away. |

 ## WARNINGS & PRECAUTIONS

**Don't take if:**

- You are allergic to any barbiturate or any anticholinergic.
- You have porphyria, trouble with stomach bloating, difficulty emptying your bladder completely, narrow-angle glaucoma, severe ulcerative colitis.

## Before you start, consult your doctor:
- If you have open-angle glaucoma, angina, chronic bronchitis or asthma, hiatal hernia, liver disease, enlarged prostate, myasthenia gravis, peptic ulcer, epilepsy, kidney or liver damage, anemia, chronic pain.
- If you will have surgery within 2 months, including dental surgery, requiring general or spinal anesthesia.

## Over age 60:
Adverse reactions and side effects may be more frequent and severe than in younger persons. Ask your doctor about small doses.

## Pregnancy:
Risk to unborn child outweighs drug benefits. Don't use.

## Breast-feeding:
Drug passes into milk. Avoid drug or discontinue nursing until you finish medicine.

## Infants & children:
Use only under doctor's supervision.

## Prolonged use:
- May cause addiction, anemia, chronic intoxication.
- May lower body temperature, making exposure to cold temperatures hazardous.

## Skin & sunlight:
May cause rash or intensify sunburn in areas exposed to sun or sunlamp.

## Driving, piloting or hazardous work:
Don't drive or pilot aircraft until you learn how medicine affects you. Don't work around dangerous machinery. Don't climb ladders or work in high places. Danger increases if you drink alcohol or take medicine affecting alertness and reflexes.

## Discontinuing:
May be unnecessary to finish medicine. Follow doctor's instructions. If you develop withdrawal symptoms of hallucinations, agitation or sleeplessness after discontinuing, call doctor right away.

## Others:
Great potential for abuse.

## POSSIBLE INTERACTION WITH OTHER DRUGS

| GENERIC NAME OR DRUG CLASS | COMBINED EFFECT |
|---|---|
| Amantadine | Increased belladonna effect. |
| Anticoagulants (oral) | Decreased anticoagulant effect. |
| Anticholinergics (other) | Increased belladonna effect. |
| Anticonvulsants | Changed seizure patterns. |
| Antidepressants (tricyclics) | Possible dangerous oversedation. Avoid. |
| Antidiabetics (oral) | Increased barbiturate effect. |
| Antihistamines | Dangerous sedation. Avoid. |
| Anti-inflammatory drugs (non-steroidal) | Decreased anti-inflammatory effect. |
| Aspirin | Decreased aspirin effect. |
| Beta-adrenergic | Decreased effects of beta-adrenergic blocker. |
| Contraceptives (oral) | Decreased contraceptive effect. |
| Cortisone drugs | Increased internal-eye pressure. Decreased cortisone effect. |
| Digitoxin | Decreased digitoxin effect. |
| Doxycycline | Decreased doxycycline effect. |
| Dronabinol | Increased effects of both drugs. Avoid. |
| Griseofulvin | Decreased griseofulvin effect. |
| Haloperidol | Increased internal-eye pressure. |
| Indapamide | Increased indapamide effect. |
| MAO inhibitors | Increased belladonna and barbiturate effect. |

*Continued page 962*

## POSSIBLE INTERACTION WITH OTHER SUBSTANCES

| INTERACTS WITH | COMBINED EFFECT |
|---|---|
| Alcohol: | Possible fatal oversedation. Avoid. |
| Beverages: | None expected. |
| Cocaine: | Excessively rapid heartbeat. Avoid. |
| Foods: | None expected. |
| Marijuana: | Drowsiness and dry mouth. Avoid. |
| Tobacco: | Decreased effectiveness of acid reduction in stomach. |

# BENDROFLUMETHIAZIDE

## BRAND NAMES

Corzide         Rauzide
Naturetin

## BASIC INFORMATION

Habit forming? No
Prescription needed? Yes
Available as generic? Yes
Drug class: Antihypertensive, diuretic
(thiazide)

## USES

- Controls, but doesn't cure, high blood
pressure.
- Reduces fluid retention (edema) caused by
conditions such as heart disorders and liver
disease.

## DOSAGE & USAGE INFORMATION

How to take:
Tablet or capsule—Swallow with liquid. If you
can't swallow whole, crumble tablet or open
capsule and take with liquid or food. Don't
exceed dose.

When to take:
At the same time each day.

If you forget a dose:
Take as soon as you remember up to 2 hours
late. If more than 2 hours, wait for next
scheduled dose (don't double this dose).

What drug does:
- Forces sodium and water excretion, reducing
body fluid.
- Relaxes muscle cells of small arteries.
- Reduced body fluid and relaxed arteries lower
blood pressure.

Time lapse before drug works:
4 to 6 hours. May require several weeks to
lower blood pressure.

*Continued next column*

## OVERDOSE

SYMPTOMS:
Cramps, weakness, drowsiness, weak pulse,
coma.
WHAT TO DO:
- **Dial 0 (operator) or 911 (emergency) for an
ambulance or medical help. Then give first
aid immediately.**
- **See emergency information on inside
covers.**

Don't take with:
- See Interaction column and consult doctor.
- Non-prescription drugs without consulting
doctor.

## POSSIBLE ADVERSE REACTIONS OR SIDE EFFECTS

| SYMPTOMS | WHAT TO DO |
|---|---|
| **Life-threatening:**<br>None expected. | |
| **Common:**<br>None expected. | |
| **Infrequent:** | |
| • Blurred vision, severe abdominal pain, nausea, vomiting, irregular heartbeat, weak pulse. | Discontinue. Call doctor right away. |
| • Dizziness, mood changes, headaches, weakness, tiredness, weight changes. | Continue. Call doctor when convenient. |
| • Dry mouth, thirst. | Continue. Tell doctor at next visit. |
| **Rare:** | |
| • Rash or hives. | Discontinue. Seek emergency treatment. |
| • Sore throat, fever, jaundice. | Discontinue. Call doctor right away. |

## WARNINGS & PRECAUTIONS

Don't take if:
You are allergic to any thiazide diuretic drug.

Before you start, consult your doctor:
- If you are allergic to any sulfa drug.
- If you have gout.
- If you have liver, pancreas or kidney disorder.

Over age 60:
Adverse reactions and side effects may be
more frequent and severe than in younger
persons, especially dizziness and excessive
potassium loss.

Pregnancy:
Risk to unborn child outweighs drug benefits.
Don't use.

Breast-feeding:
Drug passes into milk. Avoid this medicine or
discontinue nursing.

Infants & children:
No problems expected.

Prolonged use:
You may need medicine to treat high blood
pressure for the rest of your life.

**Skin & sunlight:**
May cause rash or intensify sunburn in areas exposed to sun or sunlamp.

**Driving, piloting or hazardous work:**
Don't drive or pilot aircraft until you learn how medicine affects you. Don't work around dangerous machinery. Don't climb ladders or work in high places. Danger increases if you drink alcohol or take medicine affecting alertness and reflexes, such as antihistamines, tranquilizers, sedatives, pain medicine, narcotics and mind-altering drugs.

**Discontinuing:**
Don't discontinue without medical advice.

**Others:**
- Hot weather and fever may cause dehydration and drop in blood pressure. Dose may require temporary adjustment. Weigh daily and report any unexpected weight decreases to your doctor.
- May cause rise in uric acid, leading to gout.
- May cause blood-sugar rise in diabetics.

## POSSIBLE INTERACTION WITH OTHER DRUGS

| GENERIC NAME OR DRUG CLASS | COMBINED EFFECT |
|---|---|
| Acebutolol | Increased antihypertensive effect. Dosages of both drugs may require adjustments. |
| Allopurinol | Decreased allopurinol effect. |
| Amiodarone | Increased risk of heartbeat irregularity due to low potassium. |
| Antidepressants (tricyclic) | Dangerous drop in blood pressure. Avoid combination unless under medical supervision. |
| Barbiturates | Increased bendroflumethiazide effect. |
| Calcium supplements | Decreased calcium in blood. |
| Cholestyramine | Decreased bendroflumethiazide effect. |
| Cortisone drugs | Excessive potassium loss that causes dangerous heart rhythms. |

| | |
|---|---|
| Digitalis preparations | Excessive potassium loss that causes dangerous heart rhythms. |
| Diuretics (thiazide) | Increased effect of other thiazide diuretics. |
| Indapamide | Increased diuretic effect. |
| Labetolol | Increased antihypertensive effects. |
| Lithium | Increased effect of lithium. |
| MAO inhibitors | Increased bendroflumethiazide effect. |
| Nitrates | Excessive blood-pressure drop. |
| Oxprenolol | Increased antihypertensive effect. Dosages of both drugs may require adjustments. |
| Potassium supplements | Decreased potassium effect. |
| Probenecid | Decreased probenecid effect. |

## POSSIBLE INTERACTION WITH OTHER SUBSTANCES

| INTERACTS WITH | COMBINED EFFECT |
|---|---|
| Alcohol: | Dangerous blood-pressure drop. |
| Beverages: | None expected. |
| Cocaine: | None expected. |
| Foods: Licorice. | Excessive potassium loss that causes dangerous heart rhythms. |
| Marijuana: | May increase blood pressure. |
| Tobacco: | None expected. |

## BRAND NAMES

See complete list of brand names in the *Brand Name Directory,* page 945.

## BASIC INFORMATION

**Habit forming? No**
**Prescription needed? No**
**Available as generic? Yes**
**Drug class: Antiacne (topical)**

 ## USES

- Treatment for acne.
- Decreases wrinkles in face.

 ## DOSAGE & USAGE INFORMATION

**How to use:**
Cream, gel, pads, sticks or lotion—Wash affected area with plain soap and water. Dry gently with towel. Rub medicine into affected areas. Keep away from eyes, nose, mouth.

**When to use:**
Apply 1 or more times daily. If you have a fair complexion, start with single application at bedtime.

**If you forget an application:**
Use as soon as you remember.

**What drug does:**
Slowly releases oxygen from skin, which controls some skin bacteria. Also causes peeling and drying, helping control blackheads and whiteheads.

**Time lapse before drug works:**
1 to 2 weeks.

**Don't use with:**
See Interaction column and consult doctor.

 ## OVERDOSE

**SYMPTOMS:**
**None expected.**
**WHAT TO DO:**
- **If person swallows drug, call doctor, poison-control center or hospital emergency room for instructions.**
- **See emergency information on inside covers.**

 ## POSSIBLE ADVERSE REACTIONS OR SIDE EFFECTS

| SYMPTOMS | WHAT TO DO |
|---|---|
| **Life-threatening:** | |
| None expected. | |
| **Common:** | |
| None expected. | |
| **Infrequent:** | |
| • Rash, excessive dryness. | Discontinue. Call doctor right away. |
| • Painful skin irritation. | Continue. Call doctor when convenient. |
| **Rare:** | |
| None expected. | |

## WARNINGS & PRECAUTIONS

**Don't take if:**
You are allergic to benzoyl peroxide.

**Before you start, consult your doctor:**
- If you plan to become pregnant within medication period.
- If you take oral contraceptives.

**Over age 60:**
No problems expected.

**Pregnancy:**
No proven problems. Consult doctor.

**Breast-feeding:**
No proven problems. Consult doctor.

**Infants & children:**
Not recommended.

**Prolonged use:**
Permanent rash or scarring.

**Skin & sunlight:**
No problems expected.

**Driving, piloting or hazardous work:**
No problems expected.

**Discontinuing:**
- May be unnecessary to finish medicine. Discontinue when acne improves.
- If acne doesn't improve in 2 weeks, call doctor.

**Others:**
- Keep away from hair and clothing. May bleach.
- Store away from heat in cool, dry place.
- Avoid contact with eyes, lips, nose and sensitive areas of the neck.

## POSSIBLE INTERACTION WITH OTHER DRUGS

| GENERIC NAME OR DRUG CLASS | COMBINED EFFECT |
|---|---|
| Antiacne topical preparations (other) | Excessive skin irritation. |
| Skin-peeling agents (salicylic acid, sulfur, resorcinol, tretinoin) | Excessive skin irritation. |

## POSSIBLE INTERACTION WITH OTHER SUBSTANCES

| INTERACTS WITH | COMBINED EFFECT |
|---|---|
| Alcohol: | None expected. |
| Beverages: | None expected. |
| Cocaine: | None expected. |
| Foods: Cinnamon, foods with benzoic acid. | Skin rash. |
| Marijuana: | None expected. |
| Tobacco: | None expected. |

# BENZTHIAZIDE

## BRAND NAMES

Aquastat          Exna
Aquatag          Hydrex

## BASIC INFORMATION

**Habit forming?** No
**Prescription needed?** Yes
**Available as generic?** Yes
**Drug class:** Antihypertensive, diuretic
(thiazide)

 **USES**

- Controls, but doesn't cure, high blood pressure.
- Reduces fluid retention (edema) caused by conditions such as heart disorders and liver disease.

 **DOSAGE & USAGE INFORMATION**

**How to take:**
Tablet or capsule—Swallow with liquid. If you can't swallow whole, crumble tablet or open capsule and take with liquid or food. Don't exceed dose.

**When to take:**
At the same time each day.

**If you forget a dose:**
Take as soon as you remember up to 2 hours late. If more than 2 hours, wait for next scheduled dose (don't double this dose).

**What drug does:**
- Forces sodium and water excretion, reducing body fluid.
- Relaxes muscle cells of small arteries.
- Reduced body fluid and relaxed arteries lower blood pressure.

**Time lapse before drug works:**
4 to 6 hours. May require several weeks to lower blood pressure.

*Continued next column*

 **OVERDOSE**

**SYMPTOMS:**
Cramps, weakness, drowsiness, weak pulse, coma.
**WHAT TO DO:**
- Dial 0 (operator) or 911 (emergency) for an ambulance or medical help. Then give first aid immediately.
- See emergency information on inside covers.

---

**Don't take with:**
- See Interaction column and consult doctor.
- Non-prescription drugs without consulting doctor.

 **POSSIBLE ADVERSE REACTIONS OR SIDE EFFECTS**

| SYMPTOMS | WHAT TO DO |
|---|---|
| **Life-threatening:** None expected. | |
| **Common:** None expected. | |
| **Infrequent:** | |
| • Blurred vision, severe abdominal pain, nausea, vomiting, irregular heartbeat, weak pulse. | Discontinue. Call doctor right away. |
| • Dizziness, mood changes, headaches, weakness, tiredness, weight changes. | Continue. Call doctor when convenient. |
| • Dry mouth, thirst. | Continue. Tell doctor at next visit. |
| **Rare:** | |
| • Rash or hives. | Discontinue. Seek emergency treatment. |
| • Sore throat, fever, jaundice. | Discontinue. Call doctor right away. |

 **WARNINGS & PRECAUTIONS**

**Don't take if:**
You are allergic to any thiazide diuretic drug.

**Before you start, consult your doctor:**
- If you are allergic to any sulfa drug.
- If you have gout.
- If you have liver, pancreas or kidney disorder.

**Over age 60:**
Adverse reactions and side effects may be more frequent and severe than in younger persons, especially dizziness and excessive potassium loss.

**Pregnancy:**
Risk to unborn child outweighs drug benefits. Don't use.

**Breast-feeding:**
Drug passes into milk. Avoid drug or discontinue nursing.

**Infants & children:**
No problems expected.

**Prolonged use:**
You may need medicine to treat high blood pressure for the rest of your life.

**Skin & sunlight:**
May cause rash or intensify sunburn in areas exposed to sun or sunlamp.

**Driving, piloting or hazardous work:**
Don't drive or pilot aircraft until you learn how medicine affects you. Don't work around dangerous machinery. Don't climb ladders or work in high places. Danger increases if you drink alcohol or take medicine affecting alertness and reflexes, such as antihistamines, tranquilizers, sedatives, pain medicine, narcotics and mind-altering drugs.

**Discontinuing:**
Don't discontinue without medical advice.

**Others:**
- Hot weather and fever may cause dehydration and drop in blood pressure. Dose may require temporary adjustment. Weigh daily and report any unexpected weight decreases to your doctor.
- May cause rise in uric acid, leading to gout.
- May cause blood-sugar rise in diabetics.

## POSSIBLE INTERACTION WITH OTHER DRUGS

| GENERIC NAME OR DRUG CLASS | COMBINED EFFECT |
| --- | --- |
| Acebutolol | Increased antihypertensive effect. Dosages of both drugs may require adjustments. |
| Allopurinol | Decreased allopurinol effect. |
| Amiodarone | Increased risk of heartbeat irregularity due to low potassium. |
| Antidepressants (tricyclic) | Dangerous drop in blood pressure. Avoid combination unless under medical supervision. |
| Barbiturates | Increased benzthiazide effect. |
| Calcium supplements | Increased calcium in blood. |
| Cholestyramine | Decreased benzthiazide effect. |
| Cortisone drugs | Excessive potassium loss that causes dangerous heart rhythms. |
| Digitalis preparations | Excessive potassium loss that causes dangerous heart rhythms. |

| Diuretics (thiazide) | Increased effect of other thiazide diuretics. |
| --- | --- |
| Indapamide | Increased diuretic effect. |
| Labetolol | Increased antihypertensive effects. |
| Lithium | Increased effect of lithium. |
| MAO inhibitors | Increased benzthiazide effect. |
| Nitrates | Excessive blood-pressure drop. |
| Oxprenolol | Increased antihypertensive effect. Dosages of both drugs may require adjustments. |
| Potassium supplements | Decreased potassium effect. |
| Probenecid | Decreased probenecid effect. |

## POSSIBLE INTERACTION WITH OTHER SUBSTANCES

| INTERACTS WITH | COMBINED EFFECT |
| --- | --- |
| Alcohol: | Dangerous blood-pressure drop. |
| Beverages: | None expected. |
| Cocaine: | None expected. |
| Foods: Licorice. | Excessive potassium loss that causes dangerous heart rhythms. |
| Marijuana: | May increase blood pressure. |
| Tobacco: | None expected. |

# BENZTROPINE

## BRAND NAMES

Apo-Benztropine    Cogentin
Bensylate    PMS-Benztropine

## BASIC INFORMATION

Habit forming? No
Prescription needed? Yes
Available as generic? Yes
Drug class: Antidyskinetic, antiparkinsonism

## USES

- Treatment of Parkinson's disease.
- Treatment of adverse effects of phenothiazines.

## DOSAGE & USAGE INFORMATION

**How to take:**
Tablets or capsules—Take with food to lessen stomach irritation.

**When to take:**
At the same times each day.

**If you forget a dose:**
Take as soon as you remember up to 2 hours late. If more than 2 hours, wait for next scheduled dose (don't double this dose).

**What drug does:**
- Balances chemical reactions necessary to send nerve impulses within base of brain.
- Improves muscle control and reduces stiffness.

**Time lapse before drug works:**
1 to 2 hours.

*Continued next column*

## OVERDOSE

**SYMPTOMS:**
Agitation, dilated pupils, hallucinations, dry mouth, rapid heartbeat, sleepiness.
**WHAT TO DO:**
- Dial 0 (operator) or 911 (emergency) for an ambulance or medical help. Then give first aid immediately.
- If patient is unconscious and not breathing, give mouth-to-mouth breathing. If there is no heartbeat, use cardiac massage and mouth-to-mouth breathing (CPR). Don't try to make patient vomit. If you can't get help quickly, take patient to nearest emergency facility.
- See emergency information on inside covers.

**Don't take with:**
- Non-prescription drugs for colds, cough or allergy.
- See Interaction column and consult doctor.

## POSSIBLE ADVERSE REACTIONS OR SIDE EFFECTS

| SYMPTOMS | WHAT TO DO |
|---|---|
| **Life-threatening:** None expected. | |
| **Common:** | |
| • Blurred vision, light sensitivity, constipation, nausea, vomiting. | Continue. Call doctor when convenient. |
| • Difficult or painful urination. | Continue. Tell doctor at next visit. |
| **Infrequent:** None expected. | |
| **Rare:** | |
| • Rash, pain in eyes. | Discontinue. Call doctor right away. |
| • Confusion, dizziness, sore mouth or tongue, muscle cramps, numbness or weakness in hands or feet. | Continue. Call doctor when convenient. |

## WARNINGS & PRECAUTIONS

**Don't take if:**
You are allergic to any antidyskinetic.

**Before you start, consult your doctor:**
- If you have had glaucoma.
- If you have had high blood pressure or heart disease.
- If you have had impaired liver function.
- If you have had kidney disease or urination difficulty.

**Over age 60:**
More sensitive to drug. Aggravates symptoms of enlarged prostate. Causes impaired thinking, hallucinations, nightmares. Consult doctor about any of these.

**Pregnancy:**
Studies inconclusive on harm to unborn child. Animal studies show fetal abnormalities. Decide with your doctor whether drug benefits justify risk to unborn child.

**Breast-feeding:**
No problems expected.

**Infants & children:**
Not recommended for children 3 and younger. Use for older children only under doctor's supervision.

**Prolonged use:**
Possible glaucoma.

**Skin & sunlight:**
No problems expected.

**Driving, piloting or hazardous work:**
Don't drive or pilot aircraft until you learn how medicine affects you. Don't work around dangerous machinery. Don't climb ladders or work in high places. Danger increases if you drink alcohol or take medicine affecting alertness and reflexes, such as antihistamines, tranquilizers, sedatives, pain medicine, narcotics and mind-altering drugs.

**Discontinuing:**
Don't discontinue without consulting doctor. Dose may require gradual reduction if you have taken drug for a long time. Doses of other drugs may also require adjustment.

**Others:**
- Internal eye pressure should be measured regularly.
- Avoid becoming overheated.

## POSSIBLE INTERACTION WITH OTHER DRUGS

| GENERIC NAME OR DRUG CLASS | COMBINED EFFECT |
| --- | --- |
| Amantadine | Increased amantadine effect. |
| Antidepressants (tricyclic) | Increased benztropine effect. May cause glaucoma. |
| Antihistamines | Increased benztropine effect. |
| Levodopa | Increased levodopa effect. Improved results in treating Parkinson's disease. |
| Meperidine | Increased benztropine effect. |
| MAO inhibitors | Increased benztropine effect. |
| Orphenadrine | Increased benztropine effect. |
| Phenothiazines | Behavior changes. |
| Primidone | Excessive sedation. |
| Procainamide | Increased procainamide effect. |
| Quinidine | Increased benztropine effect. |
| Tranquilizers | Excessive sedation. |

## POSSIBLE INTERACTION WITH OTHER SUBSTANCES

| INTERACTS WITH | COMBINED EFFECT |
| --- | --- |
| Alcohol: | None expected. |
| Beverages: | None expected. |
| Cocaine: | Decreased benztropine effect. Avoid. |
| Foods: | None expected. |
| Marijuana: | None expected. |
| Tobacco: | None expected. |

# BETA-ADRENERGIC BLOCKING AGENTS & THIAZIDE DIURETICS

## BRAND AND GENERIC NAMES

ATENOLOL &
  CHLORTHALIDONE
Corzide
Inderide
Lopressor HCT
METOPROLOL &
  HYDROCHLORO-
  THIAZIDE
NADOLOL &
  BENDROFLUME-
  THIAZIDE

PINDOLOL &
  HYDROCHLORO-
  THIAZIDE
PROPRANOLOL &
  HYDROCHLORO-
  THIAZIDE
Tenoretic
Timolide
TIMOLOL & HYDRO-
  CHLOROTHIAZIDE
Viskazide

## BASIC INFORMATION

**Habit forming? No**
**Prescription needed? Yes**
**Available as generic? No**
**Drug class: Beta-adrenergic blocker, thiazide**
    **diuretic**

 ## USES

- Controls, but doesn't cure, high blood pressure.
- Reduces fluid retention (edema).
- Reduces angina attacks.
- Stabilizes irregular heartbeat.
- Lowers blood pressure.
- Reduces frequency of migraine headaches. (Does not relieve headache pain.)
- Other uses prescribed by your doctor.

 ## DOSAGE & USAGE INFORMATION

**How to take:**
Tablet or capsule—Swallow with liquid. If you can't swallow whole, crumble tablet or open capsule and take with liquid or food.

*Continued next column*

 ## OVERDOSE

**SYMPTOMS:**
**Irregular heartbeat (usually too slow), fainting, convulsions, coma.**
**WHAT TO DO:**
- **Dial 0 (operator) or 911 (emergency) for an ambulance or medical help. Then give first aid immediately.**
- **See emergency information on inside covers.**

**When to take:**
At the same time each day.

**If you forget a dose:**
Take as soon as you remember up to 4 hours late. If more than 4 hours, wait for next scheduled dose (don't double this dose).

**What drug does:**
- Forces sodium and water excretion, reducing body fluid.
- Relaxes muscle cells of small arteries.
- Reduced body fluid and relaxed arteries lower blood pressure.
- Blocks some of the actions of sympathetic nervous system.
- Lowers heart's oxygen requirements.
- Slows nerve impulses through heart.
- Reduces blood vessel contraction in heart, scalp and other body parts.

**Time lapse before drug works:**
- 1 to 4 hours for beta-blocker effect.
- May require several weeks to lower blood pressure.

**Don't take with:**
Any other medicines, even OTC drugs such as cough/cold medicines, diet pills, nose drops, caffeine, without consulting your doctor.

 ## POSSIBLE ADVERSE REACTIONS OR SIDE EFFECTS

| SYMPTOMS | WHAT TO DO |
|---|---|
| **Life-threatening:**<br>Wheezing, chest pain, irregular heartbeat. | Seek emergency treatment immediately. |
| **Common:**<br>• Dry mouth, weak pulse, vomiting, muscle cramps, increased thirst, mood changes. | Discontinue. Call doctor right away. |
| • Weakness, tiredness, dizziness, mental depression, diminished sex drive, constipation, nightmares, insomnia. | Continue. Call doctor when convenient. |
| **Infrequent:**<br>Cold feet and hands, chest pain, breathing difficulty, anxiety, nervousness, headache, appetite loss, numbness and tingling in fingers and toes. | Discontinue. Call doctor right away. |

# BETA-ADRENERGIC BLOCKING AGENTS & THIAZIDE DIURETICS

**Rare:**
Hives, skin rash; joint pain; jaundice; fever, sore throat, mouth ulcers.

Discontinue. Call doctor right away.

 ## WARNINGS & PRECAUTIONS

**Don't take if:**
- You are allergic to any beta-adrenergic blocker or any thiazide diuretic drug.
- You have asthma or hay fever symptoms.
- You have taken MAO inhibitors in past two weeks.

**Before you start, consult your doctor:**
- If you have heart disease or poor circulation to the extremities.
- If you have hay fever, asthma, chronic bronchitis, emphysema, overactive thyroid function, impaired liver or kidney function, gout, diabetes, hypoglycemia, liver, pancreas or kidney disorder.
- If you are allergic to any sulfa drug.
- If you will have surgery within 2 months, including dental surgery, requiring general or spinal anesthesia.

**Over age 60:**
Adverse reactions and side effects may be more frequent and severe than in younger persons, especially dizziness and excessive potassium loss.

**Pregnancy:**
Risk to unborn child outweighs drug benefits. Don't use.

**Breast-feeding:**
Drug passes into milk. Avoid drug or discontinue nursing until you finish medicine. Consult doctor for advice on maintaining milk supply.

**Infants & children:**
Not recommended.

**Prolonged use:**
- Weakens heart muscle contractions.
- You may need medicine to treat high blood pressure for the rest of your life.

**Skin & sunlight:**
May cause rash or intensify sunburn in areas exposed to sun or sunlamp.

**Driving, piloting or hazardous work:**
Don't drive or pilot aircraft until you learn how medicine affects you. Don't work around dangerous machinery. Don't climb ladders or work in high places. Danger increases if you drink alcohol or take medicine affecting alertness and reflexes, such as antihistamines, tranquilizers, sedatives, pain medicine, narcotics and mind-altering drugs.

**Discontinuing:**
Don't discontinue without consulting doctor. Dose may require gradual reduction if you have taken drug for a long time. Doses of other drugs may also require adjustment.

**Others:**
- May mask hypoglycemia.
- Hot weather and fever may cause dehydration and drop in blood pressure. Dose may require temporary adjustment. Weigh daily and report any unexpected weight decreases to your doctor.
- May cause rise in uric acid, leading to gout.
- May cause blood-sugar rise in diabetics.

 ## POSSIBLE INTERACTION WITH OTHER DRUGS

| GENERIC NAME OR DRUG CLASS | COMBINED EFFECT |
|---|---|
| Acebutolol | Increased antihypertensive effect of acebutolol. Dosage of both drugs may require adjustment. |
| Allopurinol | Decreased allopurinol effect. |
| Antidepressants (tricyclic) | Dangerous drop in blood pressure. Avoid combination unless under medical supervision. |

*Continued page 962*

 ## POSSIBLE INTERACTION WITH OTHER SUBSTANCES

| INTERACTS WITH | COMBINED EFFECT |
|---|---|
| Alcohol: | Dangerous blood-pressure drop. Avoid. |
| Beverages: | None expected. |
| Cocaine: | Irregular heartbeat. Avoid. |
| Foods: Licorice. | Excessive potassium loss that causes dangerous heart rhythms. |
| Marijuana: | May increase blood pressure. |
| Tobacco: | May increase blood pressure and make heart work harder. Avoid. |

# BETAMETHASONE

## BRAND NAMES

See complete list of brand names in the *Brand Name Directory*, page 945.

## BASIC INFORMATION

**Habit forming? No**
**Prescription needed? Yes**
**Available as generic? Yes**
**Drug class: Cortisone drug (adrenal corticosteroid)**

## USES

- Reduces inflammation caused by many different medical problems.
- Treatment for some allergic diseases, blood disorders, kidney diseases, asthma and emphysema.
- Replaces corticosteroid deficiencies.

## DOSAGE & USAGE INFORMATION

**How to take:**
- Tablet or liquid—Swallow with liquid or food to lessen stomach irritation. If you can't swallow whole, crumble tablet and take with liquid or food.
- Inhaler—Follow label instructions.

**When to take:**
At the same times each day. Take once-a-day or once-every-other-day doses in mornings.

**If you forget a dose:**
- Several-doses-per-day prescription—Take as soon as you remember up to 2 hours late. If more than 2 hours, wait for next scheduled dose (don't double this dose).
- Once-a-day dose or less—Wait for next dose. Double this dose.

**What drug does:**
Decreases inflammatory responses.

**Time lapse before drug works:**
2 to 4 days.

*Continued next column*

## OVERDOSE

**SYMPTOMS:**
**Headache, convulsions, heart failure.**
**WHAT TO DO:**
- **Dial 0 (operator) or 911 (emergency) for an ambulance or medical help. Then give first aid immediately.**
- **See emergency information on inside covers.**

**Don't take with:**
See Interaction column and consult doctor.

## POSSIBLE ADVERSE REACTIONS OR SIDE EFFECTS

| SYMPTOMS | WHAT TO DO |
|---|---|
| **Life-threatening:**<br>None expected. | |
| **Common:**<br>Acne, poor wound healing, thirst, indigestion, nausea, vomiting. | Continue. Call doctor when convenient. |
| **Infrequent:** | |
| • Bloody or black, tarry stool. | Discontinue. Seek emergency treatment. |
| • Blurred vision, halos around lights, sore throat, fever. | Discontinue. Call doctor right away. |
| • Mood changes, insomnia, restlessness, frequent urination, weight gain, round face, fatigue, weakness, TB recurrence, menstrual irregularities. | Continue. Call doctor when convenient. |
| **Rare:** | |
| • Irregular heartbeat. | Discontinue. Seek emergency treatment. |
| • Rash. | Discontinue. Call doctor right away. |

## WARNINGS & PRECAUTIONS

**Don't take if:**
- You are allergic to any cortisone drug.
- You have tuberculosis or fungus infection.
- You have herpes infection of eyes, lips or genitals.

**Before you start, consult your doctor:**
- If you have had tuberculosis.
- If you have congestive heart failure.
- If you have diabetes.
- If you have peptic ulcer.
- If you have glaucoma.
- If you have underactive thyroid.
- If you have high blood pressure.
- If you have myasthenia gravis.
- If you have blood clots in legs or lungs.

**Over age 60:**
Adverse reactions and side effects may be more frequent and severe than in younger persons. Likely to aggravate edema, diabetes or ulcers. Likely to cause cataracts and osteoporosis (softening of the bones).

**Pregnancy:**
Risk to unborn child outweighs drug benefits. Don't use.

**Breast-feeding:**
Drug passes into milk. Avoid drug or discontinue nursing until you finish medicine. Consult doctor for advice on maintaining milk supply.

**Infants & children:**
Use only under medical supervision.

**Prolonged use:**
- Retards growth in children.
- Possible glaucoma, cataracts, diabetes, fragile bones and thin skin.
- Functional dependence.

**Skin & sunlight:**
No problems expected.

**Driving, piloting or hazardous work:**
No problems expected.

**Discontinuing:**
- Don't discontinue without doctor's advice until you complete prescribed dose, even though symptoms diminish or disappear.
- Drug affects your response to surgery, illness, injury or stress for up to 2 years after discontinuing. Inform doctor.

**Others:**
Avoid immunizations if possible.

## POSSIBLE INTERACTION WITH OTHER DRUGS

| GENERIC NAME OR DRUG CLASS | COMBINED EFFECT |
|---|---|
| Amphoterecin B | Potassium depletion. |
| Anticholinergics | Possible glaucoma. |
| Anticoagulants (oral) | Decreased anticoagulant effect. |
| Anticonvulsants (hydantoin) | Decreased betamethasone effect. |
| Antidiabetics (oral) | Decreased antidiabetic effect. |
| Antihistamines | Decreased betamethasone effect. |
| Aspirin | Increased betamethasone effect. |
| Barbiturates | Decreased betamethasone effect. Oversedation. |
| Beta-adrenergic blockers | Decreased betamethasone effect. |
| Chloral hydrate | Decreased betamethasone effect. |
| Chlorthalidone | Potassium depletion. |
| Cholinergics | Decreased cholinergic effect. |
| Contraceptives (oral) | Increased betamethasone effect. |
| Digitalis preparations | Dangerous potassium depletion. Possible digitalis toxicity. |
| Diuretics (thiazide) | Potassium depletion. |
| Ephedrine | Decreased betamethasone effect. |
| Estrogens | Increased betamethasone effect. |
| Ethacrynic acid | Potassium depletion. |
| Furosemide | Potassium depletion. |
| Glutethimide | Decreased betamethasone effect. |
| Indapamide | Possible excessive potassium loss, causing dangerous heartbeat irregularity. |
| Indomethacin | Increased betamethasone effect. |
| Insulin | Decreased insulin effect. |
| Isoniazid | Decreased isoniazid effect. |
| Oxyphenbutazone | Possible ulcers. |
| Phenylbutazone | Possible ulcers. |
| Potassium supplements | Decreased potassium effect. |
| Rifampin | Decreased betamethasone effect. |
| Sympathomimetics | Possible glaucoma. |

## POSSIBLE INTERACTION WITH OTHER SUBSTANCES

| INTERACTS WITH | COMBINED EFFECT |
|---|---|
| Alcohol: | Risk of stomach ulcers. |
| Beverages: | No proven problems. |
| Cocaine: | Overstimulation. Avoid. |
| Foods: | No proven problems. |
| Marijuana: | Decreased immunity. |
| Tobacco: | Increased betamethasone effect. Possible toxicity. |

# BETHANECHOL

## BRAND NAMES

Duvoid                    Urecholine
Myotonachol

## BASIC INFORMATION

Habit forming? No
Prescription needed? Yes
Available as generic? Yes
Drug class: Cholinergic

## USES

Helps initiate urination following surgery, or for persons with urinary infections or enlarged prostate.

## DOSAGE & USAGE INFORMATION

**How to take:**
Tablet or capsule—Swallow with liquid, 1 hour before or 2 hours after eating.

**When to take:**
At the same times each day.

**If you forget a dose:**
Take as soon as you remember up to 2 hours late. If more than 2 hours, wait for next scheduled dose (don't double this dose).

**What drug does:**
Affects chemical reactions in the body that strengthen bladder muscles.

**Time lapse before drug works:**
30 to 90 minutes.

*Continued next column*

## OVERDOSE

**SYMPTOMS:**
Shortness of breath, wheezing or chest tightness, unconsciousness, coma.
**WHAT TO DO:**
- Dial 0 (operator) or 911 (emergency) for an ambulance or medical help. Then give first aid immediately.
- If patient is unconscious and not breathing, give mouth-to-mouth breathing. If there is no heartbeat, use cardiac massage and mouth-to-mouth breathing (CPR). Don't try to make patient vomit. If you can't get help quickly, take patient to nearest emergency facility.
- See emergency information on inside covers.

**Don't take with:**
See Interaction column and consult doctor.

## POSSIBLE ADVERSE REACTIONS OR SIDE EFFECTS

| SYMPTOMS | WHAT TO DO |
|---|---|
| **Life-threatening:** None expected. | |
| **Common:** None expected. | |
| **Infrequent:** Dizziness, headache, faintness, blurred or changed vision, diarrhea, nausea, vomiting, stomach discomfort, belching, excessive urge to urinate. | Continue. Call doctor when convenient. |
| **Rare:** Shortness of breath, wheezing, tightness in chest. | Discontinue. Call doctor right away. |

## WARNINGS & PRECAUTIONS

**Don't take if:**
You are allergic to any cholinergic.

**Before you start, consult your doctor:**
- If you plan to become pregnant within medication period.
- If you have asthma.
- If you have epilepsy.
- If you have heart or blood-vessel disease.
- If you have high or low blood pressure.
- If you have overactive thyroid.
- If you have intestinal blockage.
- If you have Parkinson's disease.
- If you have stomach problems (including ulcer).
- If you have had bladder or intestinal surgery within 1 month.

**Over age 60:**
Adverse reactions and side effects may be more frequent and severe than in younger persons.

**Pregnancy:**
Risk to unborn child outweighs drug benefits. Don't use.

**Breast-feeding:**
Drug filters into milk. May harm child. Avoid.

**Infants & children:**
Use only under medical supervision.

**Prolonged use:**
No problems expected.

**Skin & sunlight:**
No problems expected.

**Driving, piloting or hazardous work:**
Don't drive or pilot aircraft until you learn how medicine affects you. Don't work around dangerous machinery. Don't climb ladders or work in high places. Danger increases if you drink alcohol or take medicine affecting alertness and reflexes, such as antihistamines, tranquilizers, sedatives, pain medicine, narcotics and mind-altering drugs.

**Discontinuing:**
May be unnecessary to finish medicine. Follow doctor's instructions.

**Others:**
- Be cautious about standing up suddenly.
- Interferes with laboratory studies of liver and pancreas function.
- Side effects more likely with injections.

## POSSIBLE INTERACTION WITH OTHER DRUGS

| GENERIC NAME OR DRUG CLASS | COMBINED EFFECT |
| --- | --- |
| Cholinergics (other) | Increased effect of both drugs. Possible toxicity. |
| Nitrates | Decreased bethanechol effect. |
| Procainamide | Decreased bethanechol effect. |
| Quinidine | Decreased bethanechol effect. |

## POSSIBLE INTERACTION WITH OTHER SUBSTANCES

| INTERACTS WITH | COMBINED EFFECT |
| --- | --- |
| Alcohol: | None expected. |
| Beverages: | None expected. |
| Cocaine: | None expected. |
| Foods: | None expected. |
| Marijuana: | None expected. |
| Tobacco: | None expected. |

# BIPERIDEN

## BRAND NAMES

Akineton

## BASIC INFORMATION

**Habit forming? No**
**Prescription needed? Yes**
**Available as generic? No**
**Drug class: Antidyskinetic, antiparkinsonism**

 USES

- Treatment of Parkinson's disease.
- Treatment of adverse effects of phenothiazines.

 DOSAGE & USAGE INFORMATION

**How to take:**
Tablets or capsules—Take with food to lessen stomach irritation.

**When to take:**
At the same times each day.

**If you forget a dose:**
Take as soon as you remember up to 2 hours late. If more than 2 hours, wait for next scheduled dose (don't double this dose).

**What drug does:**
- Balances chemical reactions necessary to send nerve impulses within base of brain.
- Improves muscle control and reduces stiffness.

**Time lapse before drug works:**
1 to 2 hours.

*Continued next column*

 OVERDOSE

**SYMPTOMS:**
**Agitation, dilated pupils, hallucinations, dry mouth, rapid heartbeat, sleepiness.**
**WHAT TO DO:**
- **Dial 0 (operator) or 911 (emergency) for an ambulance or medical help. Then give first aid immediately.**
- **If patient is unconscious and not breathing, give mouth-to-mouth breathing. If there is no heartbeat, use cardiac massage and mouth-to-mouth breathing (CPR). Don't try to make patient vomit. If you can't get help quickly, take patient to nearest emergency facility.**
- **See emergency information on inside covers.**

**Don't take with:**
- Non-prescription drugs for colds, cough or allergy.
- See Interaction column and consult doctor.

 POSSIBLE ADVERSE REACTIONS OR SIDE EFFECTS

| SYMPTOMS | WHAT TO DO |
|---|---|
| **Life-threatening:**<br>None expected. | |
| **Common:** | |
| • Blurred vision, light sensitivity, constipation, nausea, vomiting. | Continue. Call doctor when convenient. |
| • Difficult or painful urination. | Continue. Tell doctor at next visit. |
| **Infrequent:**<br>None expected. | |
| **Rare:** | |
| • Rash, pain in eyes. | Discontinue. Call doctor right away. |
| • Confusion, dizziness, sore mouth or tongue, muscle cramps, numbness or weakness in hands or feet. | Continue. Call doctor when convenient. |

# BIPERIDEN

## WARNINGS & PRECAUTIONS

**Don't take if:**
You are allergic to any antidyskinetic.

**Before you start, consult your doctor:**
- If you have had glaucoma.
- If you have had high blood pressure or heart disease.
- If you have had impaired liver function.
- If you have had kidney disease or urination difficulty.

**Over age 60:**
More sensitive to drug. Aggravates symptoms of enlarged prostate. Causes impaired thinking, hallucinations, nightmares. Consult doctor about any of these.

**Pregnancy:**
Studies inconclusive on harm to unborn child. Animal studies show fetal abnormalities. Decide with your doctor whether drug benefits justify risk to unborn child.

**Breast-feeding:**
May inhibit milk secretion. Consult doctor.

**Infants & children:**
Not recommended for children 3 and younger. Use for older children only under doctor's supervision.

**Prolonged use:**
Possible glaucoma.

**Skin & sunlight:**
No problems expected.

**Driving, piloting or hazardous work:**
Don't drive or pilot aircraft until you learn how medicine affects you. Don't work around dangerous machinery. Don't climb ladders or work in high places. Danger increases if you drink alcohol or take medicine affecting alertness and reflexes, such as antihistamines, tranquilizers, sedatives, pain medicine, narcotics and mind-altering drugs.

**Discontinuing:**
Don't discontinue without consulting doctor. Dose may require gradual reduction if you have taken drug for a long time. Doses of other drugs may also require adjustment.

**Others:**
- Internal eye pressure should be measured regularly.
- Avoid becoming overheated.

## POSSIBLE INTERACTION WITH OTHER DRUGS

| GENERIC NAME OR DRUG CLASS | COMBINED EFFECT |
|---|---|
| Amantadine | Increased amantadine effect. |
| Antidepressants (tricyclic) | Increased biperiden effect. May cause glaucoma. |
| Antihistamines | Increased biperiden effect. |
| Levodopa | Increased levodopa effect. Improved results in treating Parkinson's disease. |
| Meperidine | Increased biperiden effect. |
| MAO inhibitors | Increased biperiden effect. |
| Orphenadrine | Increased biperiden effect. |
| Phenothiazines | Behavior changes. |
| Primidone | Excessive sedation. |
| Procainamide | Increased procainamide effect. |
| Quinidine | Increased biperiden effect. |
| Tranquilizers | Excessive sedation. |

## POSSIBLE INTERACTION WITH OTHER SUBSTANCES

| INTERACTS WITH | COMBINED EFFECT |
|---|---|
| Alcohol: | None expected. |
| Beverages: | None expected. |
| Cocaine: | Decreased biperiden effect. Avoid. |
| Foods: | None expected. |
| Marijuana: | None expected. |
| Tobacco: | None expected. |

# BISACODYL

## BRAND NAMES

| | |
|---|---|
| Apo-Bisacodyl | Dulcolax |
| Bisco-Lax | Evac-Q-Kwik |
| Cenalax | Fleet Bisacodyl |
| Clysodrast | Fleet Enema |
| Codylax | Nulac |
| Dacodyl | Theralax |
| Deficol | |

## BASIC INFORMATION

**Habit forming? No**
**Prescription needed? No**
**Available as generic? Yes**
**Drug class: Laxative (stimulant)**

## USES

Constipation relief.

## DOSAGE & USAGE INFORMATION

**How to take:**
- Tablet—Swallow with liquid.
- Suppository—Remove wrapper and moisten suppository with water. Gently insert larger end into rectum. Push well into rectum with finger.

**When to take:**
Usually at bedtime with a snack, unless directed otherwise.

**If you forget a dose:**
Take as soon as you remember.

**What drug does:**
Acts on smooth muscles of intestine wall to cause vigorous bowel movement.

**Time lapse before drug works:**
6 to 10 hours.

**Don't take with:**
- See Interaction column and consult doctor.
- Don't take within 2 hours of taking another medicine. Laxative interferes with medicine absorption.

## OVERDOSE

**SYMPTOMS:**
**Vomiting, electrolyte depletion.**
**WHAT TO DO:**
**Overdose unlikely to threaten life. If person takes much larger amount than prescribed, call doctor, poison-control center or hospital emergency room for instructions.**

## POSSIBLE ADVERSE REACTIONS OR SIDE EFFECTS

| SYMPTOMS | WHAT TO DO |
|---|---|
| **Life-threatening:**<br>None expected. | |
| **Common:**<br>Rectal irritation. | Continue. Call doctor when convenient. |
| **Infrequent:**<br>• Dangerous potassium loss. | Discontinue. Call doctor right away. |
| • Belching, cramps, nausea. | Continue. Call doctor when convenient. |
| **Rare:**<br>• Irritability, confusion, headache, rash, breathing difficulty, irregular heartbeat, muscle cramps, unusual tiredness or weakness. | Discontinue. Call doctor right away. |
| • Burning on urination. | Continue. Call doctor when convenient. |

# BISACODYL

## WARNINGS & PRECAUTIONS

**Don't take if:**
- You have symptoms of appendicitis, inflamed bowel or intestinal blockage.
- You are allergic to a stimulant laxative.
- You have missed a bowel movement for only 1 or 2 days.

**Before you start, consult your doctor:**
- If you have a colostomy or ileostomy.
- If you have congestive heart disease.
- If you have diabetes.
- If you have high blood pressure.
- If you have a laxative habit.
- If you have rectal bleeding.
- If you take other laxatives.

**Over age 60:**
Adverse reactions and side effects may be more frequent and severe than in younger persons.

**Pregnancy:**
Risk to mother and unborn child outweighs drug benefits. Don't use.

**Breast-feeding:**
Drug passes into milk. Avoid drug or discontinue nursing until you finish medicine. Consult doctor for advice on maintaining milk supply.

**Infants & children:**
Use only under medical supervision.

**Prolonged use:**
Don't take for more than 1 week unless under doctor's supervision. May cause laxative dependence.

**Skin & sunlight:**
No problems expected.

**Driving, piloting or hazardous work:**
No problems expected.

**Discontinuing:**
May be unnecessary to finish medicine. Follow doctor's instructions.

**Others:**
Don't take to "flush out" your system or as a "tonic."

## POSSIBLE INTERACTION WITH OTHER DRUGS

| GENERIC NAME OR DRUG CLASS | COMBINED EFFECT |
|---|---|
| Antacids | Tablet coating may dissolve too rapidly, irritating stomach or bowel. |
| Antihypertensives | May cause dangerous low potassium level. |
| Cimetidine | Stomach or bowel irritation. |
| Diuretics | May cause dangerous low potassium level. |
| Ranitidine | Stomach or bowel irritation. |

## POSSIBLE INTERACTION WITH OTHER SUBSTANCES

| INTERACTS WITH | COMBINED EFFECT |
|---|---|
| Alcohol: | None expected. |
| Beverages: | None expected. |
| Cocaine: | None expected. |
| Foods: | None expected. |
| Marijuana: | None expected. |
| Tobacco: | None expected. |

# BROMOCRIPTINE

## BRAND NAMES

**Parlodel**

## BASIC INFORMATION

**Habit forming? No**
**Prescription needed? Yes**
**Available as generic? Yes**
**Drug class: Antiparkinsonism**

## USES

- Controls Parkinson's disease symptoms such as rigidity, tremors and unsteady gait.
- Treats female infertility.
- Prevents lactation.

## DOSAGE & USAGE INFORMATION

**How to take:**
Tablet or capsule—Swallow with liquid or food to lessen stomach irritation. If you can't swallow whole, crumble tablet or open capsule and take with liquid or food.

**When to take:**
At the same times each day.

**If you forget a dose:**
Take as soon as you remember up to 2 hours late. If more than 2 hours, wait for next scheduled dose (don't double this dose).

**What drug does:**
Restores chemical balance necessary for normal nerve impulses.

*Continued next column*

## OVERDOSE

**SYMPTOMS:**
**Muscle twitch, spastic eyelid closure, nausea, vomiting, diarrhea, irregular and rapid pulse, weakness, fainting, confusion, agitation, hallucination, coma.**
**WHAT TO DO:**
- **Dial 0 (operator) or 911 (emergency) for an ambulance or medical help. Then give first aid immediately.**
- **If patient is unconscious and not breathing, give mouth-to-mouth breathing. If there is no heartbeat, use cardiac massage and mouth-to-mouth breathing (CPR). Don't try to make patient vomit. If you can't get help quickly, take patient to nearest emergency facility.**
- **See emergency information on inside covers.**

**Time lapse before drug works:**
2 to 3 weeks to improve; 6 weeks or longer for maximum benefit.

**Don't take with:**
See Interaction column and consult doctor.

## POSSIBLE ADVERSE REACTIONS OR SIDE EFFECTS

| SYMPTOMS | WHAT TO DO |
|---|---|
| **Life-threatening:** | |
| None expected. | |
| **Common:** | |
| • Mood changes, uncontrollable body movements, diarrhea. | Continue. Call doctor when convenient. |
| • Dry mouth, body odor. | No action necessary. |
| **Infrequent:** | |
| • Fainting, severe dizziness, headache, insomnia, nightmares, rash, itch, nausea, vomiting, irregular heartbeat. | Discontinue. Call doctor right away. |
| • Flushed face, blurred vision, muscle twitching, discolored or dark urine, difficult urination. | Continue. Call doctor when convenient. |
| • Constipation, tiredness. | Continue. Tell doctor at next visit. |
| **Rare:** | |
| • High blood pressure. | Discontinue. Call doctor right away. |
| • Anemia, duodenal ucler. | Continue. Call doctor when convenient. |

## WARNINGS & PRECAUTIONS

**Don't take if:**
- You are allergic to bromocriptine.
- You have taken MAO inhibitors in past 2 weeks.
- You have glaucoma (narrow-angle type).

**Before you start, consult your doctor:**
- If you have diabetes or epilepsy.
- If you have had high blood pressure, heart or lung disease.
- If you have had liver or kidney disease.
- If you have a peptic ulcer.
- If you have malignant melanoma.
- If you will have surgery within 2 months, including dental surgery, requiring general or spinal anesthesia.

**Over age 60:**
Adverse reactions and side effects may be more frequent and severe than in younger persons.

**Pregnancy:**
Risk to unborn child outweighs drug benefits. Don't use.

**Breast-feeding:**
Drug filters into milk. May harm child. Avoid.

**Infants & children:**
Not recommended.

**Prolonged use:**
May lead to uncontrolled movements of head, face, mouth, tongue, arms or legs.

**Skin & sunlight:**
No problems expected.

**Driving, piloting or hazardous work:**
Don't drive or pilot aircraft until you learn how medicine affects you. Don't work around dangerous machinery. Don't climb ladders or work in high places. Danger increases if you drink alcohol or take medicine affecting alertness and reflexes, such as antihistamines, tranquilizers, sedatives, pain medicine, narcotics and mind-altering drugs.

**Discontinuing:**
Don't discontinue without doctor's advice until you complete prescribed dose, even though symptoms diminish or disappear.

**Others:**
Expect to start with small doses and increase gradually to lessen frequency and severity of adverse reactions.

## POSSIBLE INTERACTION WITH OTHER DRUGS

| GENERIC NAME OR DRUG CLASS | COMBINED EFFECT |
|---|---|
| Antiparkinsonism drugs (other) | Increased bromocriptine effect. |
| Haloperidol | Decreased bromocriptine effect. |
| MAO inhibitors | Dangerous rise in blood pressure. |
| Methyldopa | Decreased bromocriptine effect. |
| Papaverine | Decreased bromocriptine effect. |
| Phenothiazines | Decreased bromocriptine effect. |
| Pyridoxine (Vitamin B-6) | Decreased bromocriptine effect. |
| Rauwolfia alkaloids | Decreased bromocriptine effect. |

## POSSIBLE INTERACTION WITH OTHER SUBSTANCES

| INTERACTS WITH | COMBINED EFFECT |
|---|---|
| Alcohol: | None expected. |
| Beverages: | None expected. |
| Cocaine: | Decreased bromocriptine effect. Avoid. |
| Foods: | None expected. |
| Marijuana: | Increased fatigue, lethargy, fainting. Avoid. |
| Tobacco: | Interferes with absorption. Avoid. |

# BROMODIPHENHYDRAMINE

## BRAND NAMES

Ambenyl Expectorant          Ambodryl

## BASIC INFORMATION

Habit forming? No
Prescription needed? Yes
Available as generic? No
Drug class: Antihistamine

 USES

- Reduces allergic symptoms such as hay fever, hives, rash or itching.
- Induces sleep.

 DOSAGE & USAGE INFORMATION

**How to take:**
Capsule or liquid—Swallow with liquid or food to lessen stomach irritation.

**When to take:**
Varies with form. Follow label directions.

**If you forget a dose:**
Take as soon as you remember up to 2 hours late. If more than 2 hours, wait for next scheduled dose (don't double this dose).

**What drug does:**
Blocks action of histamine after an allergic response triggers histamine release in sensitive cells.

**Time lapse before drug works:**
30 minutes.

**Don't take with:**
See Interaction column and consult doctor.

 OVERDOSE

**SYMPTOMS:**
Convulsions, red face, hallucinations, coma.
**WHAT TO DO:**
- **Dial 0 (operator) or 911 (emergency) for an ambulance or medical help. Then give first aid immediately.**
- **If patient is unconscious and not breathing, give mouth-to-mouth breathing. If there is no heartbeat, use cardiac massage and mouth-to-mouth breathing (CPR). Don't try to make patient vomit. If you can't get help quickly, take patient to nearest emergency facility.**
- **See emergency information on inside covers.**

 POSSIBLE ADVERSE REACTIONS OR SIDE EFFECTS

| SYMPTOMS | WHAT TO DO |
|---|---|
| **Life-threatening:** None expected. | |
| **Common:** Drowsiness, dizziness, dry mouth or throat, nausea. | Continue. Tell doctor at next visit. |
| **Infrequent:** | |
| • Vision changes. | Discontinue. Call doctor right away. |
| • Less tolerance for contact lenses, difficult or painful urination. | Continue. Call doctor when convenient. |
| • Appetite loss. | Continue. Tell doctor at next visit. |
| **Rare:** Nightmares, agitation, irritability, sore throat, fever, rapid heartbeat, unusual bleeding or bruising, fatigue, weakness. | Discontinue. Call doctor right away. |

# BROMODIPHENHYDRAMINE

## WARNINGS & PRECAUTIONS

**Don't take if:**
You are allergic to any antihistamine.

**Before you start, consult your doctor:**
- If you have glaucoma.
- If you have enlarged prostate.
- If you have asthma.
- If you have kidney disease.
- If you have peptic ulcer.
- If you will have surgery within 2 months, including dental surgery, requiring general or spinal anesthesia.

**Over age 60:**
Don't exceed recommended dose. Adverse reactions and side effects may be more frequent and severe than in younger persons, especially urination difficulty, diminished alertness and other brain and nervous-system symptoms.

**Pregnancy:**
No proven harm to unborn child. Avoid if possible.

**Breast-feeding:**
Drug passes into milk. Avoid drug or discontinue nursing until you finish medicine. Consult doctor for advice on maintaining milk supply.

**Infants & children:**
Not recommended for premature or newborn infants. Otherwise, no problems expected.

**Prolonged use:**
Avoid. May damage bone-marrow and nerve cells.

**Skin & sunlight:**
May cause rash or intensify sunburn in areas exposed to sun or sunlamp.

**Driving, piloting or hazardous work:**
Don't drive or pilot aircraft until you learn how medicine affects you. Don't work around dangerous machinery. Don't climb ladders or work in high places. Danger increases if you drink alcohol or take medicine affecting alertness and reflexes, such as antihistamines, tranquilizers, sedatives, pain medicine, narcotics and mind-altering drugs.

**Discontinuing:**
No problems expected.

**Others:**
May mask symptoms of hearing damage from aspirin, other salicylates, cisplatin, paromomycin, vancomycin or anticonvulsants. Consult doctor if you use these.

## POSSIBLE INTERACTION WITH OTHER DRUGS

| GENERIC NAME OR DRUG CLASS | COMBINED EFFECT |
|---|---|
| Anticholinergics | Increased anticholinergic effect. |
| Antidepressants | Excess sedation. Avoid. |
| Antihistamines (other) | Excess sedation. Avoid. |
| Dronabinol | Increased effects of both drugs. Avoid. |
| Hypnotics | Excess sedation. Avoid. |
| MAO inhibitors | Increased bromodiphenhydramine effect. |
| Mind-altering drugs | Excess sedation. Avoid. |
| Narcotics | Excess sedation. Avoid. |
| Sedatives | Excess sedation. Avoid. |
| Sleep inducers | Excess sedation. Avoid. |
| Tranquilizers | Excess sedation. Avoid. |

## POSSIBLE INTERACTION WITH OTHER SUBSTANCES

| INTERACTS WITH | COMBINED EFFECT |
|---|---|
| Alcohol: | Excess sedation. Avoid. |
| Beverages: Caffeine drinks. | Less bromodiphenhydramine sedation. |
| Cocaine: | Decreased bromodiphenhydramine effect. Avoid. |
| Foods: | None expected. |
| Marijuana: | Excess sedation. Avoid. |
| Tobacco: | None expected. |

# BROMPHENIRAMINE

## BRAND NAMES

See complete list of brand names in the *Brand Name Directory,* page 945.

## BASIC INFORMATION

**Habit forming? No**
**Prescription needed? Yes**
**Available as generic? Yes**
**Drug class: Antihistamine**

 **USES**

- Reduces allergic symptoms such as hay fever, hives, rash or itching.
- Induces sleep.

 **DOSAGE & USAGE INFORMATION**

**How to take:**
- Tablet, capsule or syrup—Swallow with liquid or food to lessen stomach irritation.
- Extended-release tablets or capsules—Swallow each dose whole.

**When to take:**
Varies with form. Follow label directions.

**If you forget a dose:**
Take as soon as you remember up to 2 hours late. If more than 2 hours, wait for next scheduled dose (don't double this dose).

**What drug does:**
Blocks action of histamine after an allergic response triggers histamine release in sensitive cells.

**Time lapse before drug works:**
30 minutes.

**Don't take with:**
See Interaction column and consult doctor.

 **OVERDOSE**

**SYMPTOMS:**
**Convulsions, red face, hallucinations, coma.**
**WHAT TO DO:**
- **Dial 0 (operator) or 911 (emergency) for an ambulance or medical help. Then give first aid immediately.**
- **See emergency information on inside covers.**

 **POSSIBLE ADVERSE REACTIONS OR SIDE EFFECTS**

| SYMPTOMS | WHAT TO DO |
|---|---|
| **Life-threatening:** None expected. | |
| **Common:** Drowsiness; dizziness; dry mouth, nose or throat; nausea. | Continue. Tell doctor at next visit. |
| **Infrequent:** | |
| ● Vision changes. | Discontinue. Call doctor right away. |
| ● Less tolerance for contact lenses, difficult or painful urination. | Continue. Call doctor when convenient. |
| ● Appetite loss. | Continue. Tell doctor at next visit. |
| **Rare:** Nightmares, agitation, irritability, sore throat, fever, rapid heartbeat, unusual bleeding or bruising, fatigue, weakness. | Discontinue. Call doctor right away. |

## WARNINGS & PRECAUTIONS

**Don't take if:**
You are allergic to any antihistamine.

**Before you start, consult your doctor:**
- If you have glaucoma.
- If you have enlarged prostate.
- If you have asthma.
- If you have kidney disease.
- If you have peptic ulcer.
- If you will have surgery within 2 months, including dental surgery, requiring general or spinal anesthesia.

**Over age 60:**
Don't exceed recommended dose. Adverse reactions and side effects may be more frequent and severe than in younger persons, especially urination difficulty, diminished alertness and other brain and nervous-system symptoms.

**Pregnancy:**
No proven harm to unborn child. Avoid if possible.

**Breast-feeding:**
Drug passes into milk. Avoid drug or discontinue nursing until you finish medicine. Consult doctor for advice on maintaining milk supply.

**Infants & children:**
Not recommended for premature or newborn infants. Otherwise, no problems expected.

**Prolonged use:**
Avoid. May damage bone marrow and nerve cells.

**Skin & sunlight:**
May cause rash or intensify sunburn in areas exposed to sun or sunlamp.

**Driving, piloting or hazardous work:**
Don't drive or pilot aircraft until you learn how medicine affects you. Don't work around dangerous machinery. Don't climb ladders or work in high places. Danger increases if you drink alcohol or take medicine affecting alertness and reflexes, such as antihistamines, tranquilizers, sedatives, pain medicine, narcotics and mind-altering drugs.

**Discontinuing:**
No problems expected.

**Others:**
May mask symptoms of hearing damage from aspirin, other salicylates, cisplatin, paromomycin, vancomycin or anticonvulsants. Consult doctor if you use these.

## POSSIBLE INTERACTION WITH OTHER DRUGS

| GENERIC NAME OR DRUG CLASS | COMBINED EFFECT |
| --- | --- |
| Anticholinergics | Increased anticholinergic effect. |
| Antidepressants | Excess sedation. Avoid. |
| Antihistamines (other) | Excess sedation. Avoid. |
| Dronabinol | Increased effects of both drugs. Avoid. |
| Hypnotics | Excess sedation. Avoid. |
| MAO inhibitors | Increased brompheniramine effect. |
| Mind-altering drugs | Excess sedation. Avoid. |
| Molindone | Increased antihistamine effect. |
| Narcotics | Excess sedation. Avoid. |
| Sedatives | Excess sedation. Avoid. |
| Sleep inducers | Excess sedation. Avoid. |
| Tranquilizers | Excess sedation. Avoid. |

## POSSIBLE INTERACTION WITH OTHER SUBSTANCES

| INTERACTS WITH | COMBINED EFFECT |
| --- | --- |
| Alcohol: | Excess sedation. Avoid. |
| Beverages: Caffeine drinks. | Less brompheniramine sedation. |
| Cocaine: | Decreased brompheniramine effect. Avoid. |
| Foods: | None expected. |
| Marijuana: | Excess sedation. Avoid. |
| Tobacco: | None expected. |

# BUCLIZINE

## BRAND NAMES

Bucladin-S

## BASIC INFORMATION

**Habit forming? No**
**Prescription needed?**
  **U.S.: No**
  **Canada: Yes**
**Available as generic? No**
**Drug class: Antihistamine, antiemetic**

 USES

Prevents motion sickness.

 DOSAGE & USAGE INFORMATION

**How to take:**
Tablet—Swallow with liquid or food to lessen stomach irritation. If you can't swallow whole, crumble tablet and chew or take with liquid or food.

**When to take:**
30 minutes to 1 hour before traveling.

**If you forget a dose:**
Take as soon as you remember. Wait 4 hours for next dose.

**What drug does:**
Reduces sensitivity of nerve endings in inner ear, blocking messages to brain's vomiting center.

**Time lapse before drug works:**
30 to 60 minutes.

**Don't take with:**
See Interaction column and consult doctor.

 OVERDOSE

**SYMPTOMS:**
**Drowsiness, confusion, incoordination, stupor, coma, weak pulse, shallow breathing.**
**WHAT TO DO:**
● **Dial 0 (operator) or 911 (emergency) for an ambulance or medical help. Then give first aid immediately.**
● **See emergency information on inside covers.**

 POSSIBLE ADVERSE REACTIONS OR SIDE EFFECTS

| SYMPTOMS | WHAT TO DO |
|---|---|
| **Life-threatening:**<br>None expected. | |
| **Common:**<br>Drowsiness. | Continue. Tell doctor at next visit. |
| **Infrequent:**<br>● Headache, diarrhea or constipation, fast heartbeat. | Continue. Call doctor when convenient. |
| ● Dry mouth, nose, throat. | Continue. Tell doctor at next visit. |
| **Rare:**<br>● Rash or hives. | Discontinue. Call doctor right away. |
| ● Restlessness, excitement, insomnia, blurred vision, frequent urination, difficult urination. | Continue. Call doctor when convenient. |
| ● Appetite loss, nausea. | Continue. Tell doctor at next visit. |

## WARNINGS & PRECAUTIONS

**Don't take if:**
- You are allergic to meclizine, buclizine or cyclizine.
- You have taken MAO inhibitors in the past 2 weeks.

**Before you start, consult your doctor:**
- If you have glaucoma.
- If you have prostate enlargement.
- If you have reacted badly to any antihistamine.

**Over age 60:**
Adverse reactions and side effects may be more frequent and severe than in younger persons, especially impaired urination from enlarged prostate gland.

**Pregnancy:**
Studies inconclusive on harm to unborn child. Animal studies show fetal abnormalities. Decide with your doctor whether drug benefits justify risk to unborn child.

**Breast-feeding:**
Drug passes into milk. Avoid drug or discontinue nursing until you finish medicine. Consult doctor for advice on maintaining milk supply.

**Infants & children:**
No problems expected.

**Prolonged use:**
No problems expected.

**Skin & sunlight:**
No problems expected.

**Driving, piloting or hazardous work:**
Don't fly aircraft. Don't drive until you learn how medicine affects you. Don't work around dangerous machinery. Don't climb ladders or work in high places. Danger increases if you drink alcohol or take medicine affecting alertness and reflexes, such as antihistamines, tranquilizers, sedatives, pain medicine, narcotics and mind-altering drugs.

**Discontinuing:**
No problems expected.

**Others:**
No problems expected.

 ## POSSIBLE INTERACTION WITH OTHER DRUGS

| GENERIC NAME OR DRUG CLASS | COMBINED EFFECT |
| --- | --- |
| Amphetamines | May decrease drowsiness caused by buclizine. |
| Anticholinergics | Increased effect of both drugs. |
| Antidepressants (tricyclic) | Increased effect of both drugs. |
| MAO inhibitors | Increased buclizine effect. |
| Narcotics | Increased effect of both drugs. |
| Pain relievers | Increased effect of both drugs. |
| Sedatives | Increased effect of both drugs. |
| Sleep inducers | Increased effect of both drugs. |
| Tranquilizers | Increased effect of both drugs. |

 ## POSSIBLE INTERACTION WITH OTHER SUBSTANCES

| INTERACTS WITH | COMBINED EFFECT |
| --- | --- |
| Alcohol: | Increased sedation. Avoid. |
| Beverages: Caffeine drinks. | May decrease drowsiness. |
| Cocaine: | None expected. |
| Foods: | None expected. |
| Marijuana: | Increased drowsiness, dry mouth. |
| Tobacco: | None expected. |

# BUMETANIDE

## BRAND NAMES

**Bumex**

## BASIC INFORMATION

**Habit forming? No**
**Prescription needed? Yes**
**Available as generic? No**
**Drug class: Diuretic**

 **USES**

Decreases fluid retention.

 **DOSAGE & USAGE INFORMATION**

**How to take:**
Tablet or capsule—Swallow with liquid or food to lessen stomach irritation. If you can't swallow whole, crumble tablet or open capsule and take with liquid or food.

**When to take:**
- 1 dose a day—Take after breakfast.
- More than 1 dose a day—Take last dose no later than 6 p.m. unless otherwise directed.

**If you forget a dose:**
- 1 dose a day—Take as soon as you remember up to 12 hours late. If more than 12 hours, wait for next scheduled dose (don't double this dose).
- More than 1 dose a day—Take as soon as you remember up to 2 hours late. If more than 2 hours, wait for next scheduled dose (don't double this dose).

**What drug does:**
Increases elimination of sodium and water from body. Decreased body fluid reduces blood pressure.

**Time lapse before drug works:**
1 hour to increase water loss.

*Continued next column*

 **OVERDOSE**

**SYMPTOMS:**
**Weakness, lethargy, dizziness, confusion, nausea, vomiting, leg-muscle cramps, thirst, stupor, deep sleep, weak and rapid pulse, cardiac arrest.**
**WHAT TO DO:**
- **Dial 0 (operator) or 911 (emergency) for an ambulance or medical help. Then give first aid immediately.**
- **See emergency information on inside covers.**

**Don't take with:**
See Interaction column and consult doctor.

 **POSSIBLE ADVERSE REACTIONS OR SIDE EFFECTS**

| SYMPTOMS | WHAT TO DO |
|---|---|
| **Life-threatening:**<br>None expected. | |
| **Common:**<br>Dizziness. | Continue. Call doctor when convenient. |
| **Infrequent:**<br>Mood changes, appetite loss, diarrhea, irregular heartbeat, muscle cramps, fatigue, weakness. | Discontinue. Call doctor right away. |
| **Rare:**<br>Rash or hives; yellow vision; ringing in ears; hearing loss; sore throat, fever; dry mouth; thirst; side or stomach pain; nausea; vomiting; unusual bleeding or bruising; joint pain; jaundice. | Discontinue. Call doctor right away. |

 **WARNINGS & PRECAUTIONS**

**Don't take if:**
You are allergic to bumetanide.

**Before you start, consult your doctor:**
- If you have liver or kidney disease.
- If you have gout.
- If you have diabetes.
- If you have impaired hearing.
- If you will have surgery within 2 months, including dental surgery, requiring general or spinal anesthesia.

**Over age 60:**
Adverse reactions and side effects may be more frequent and severe than in younger persons.

**Pregnancy:**
Risk to unborn child outweighs drug benefits. Don't use.

**Breast-feeding:**
Drug filters into milk. May harm child. Avoid.

**Infants & children:**
Use only under medical supervision.

**Prolonged use:**
- Impaired balance of water, salt and potassium in blood and body tissues. Request periodic laboratory studies of electrolytes in blood.
- Possible diabetes.

**Skin & sunlight:**
May cause rash or intensify sunburn in areas exposed to sun or sunlamp.

**Driving, piloting or hazardous work:**
No problems expected.

**Discontinuing:**
Don't discontinue without doctor's advice until you complete prescribed dose, even though symptoms diminish or disappear.

**Others:**
Frequent laboratory studies to monitor potassium level in blood recommended. Eat foods rich in potassium or take potassium supplements. Consult doctor.

## POSSIBLE INTERACTION WITH OTHER DRUGS

| GENERIC NAME OR DRUG CLASS | COMBINED EFFECT |
|---|---|
| Acebutolol | Increased antihypertensive effect. Dosages may require adjustment. |
| Amiodarone | Increased risk of heartbeat irregularity due to low potassium. |
| Amitracin, gentamycin, kanamycin, streptomycin, tobramycin, cisplatin, ethacrynic acid, furosemide, mercaptopurine, polymixins. | Increased possibility of hearing loss. |
| Amitriptyline | Increased amitriptyline effect. |
| Antihypertensives | Increased blood-pressure drop. |
| Calcium supplements | Increased calcium in blood. |
| Cephalosporin antibiotics | Increased possibility of hearing loss. |
| Enalapril | Possible excessive potassium in blood. |
| Indapamide | Increased diuretic effect. |
| Indomethicin | Decreased effect of bumetanide. |

| | |
|---|---|
| Labetolol | Increased antihypertensive effects. |
| Lithium | Increased possibility of lithium toxicity. |
| Nitrates | Excessive blood-pressure drop. |
| Oxprenolol | Increased antihypertensive effect. Dosages may require adjustment. |
| Pentoxifylline | Increased antihypertensive effect. |
| Potassium supplements | Decreased potassium effect. |
| Probenecid | Decreased effect of bumetanide. |

## POSSIBLE INTERACTION WITH OTHER SUBSTANCES

| INTERACTS WITH | COMBINED EFFECT |
|---|---|
| Alcohol: | Blood-pressure drop. Avoid. |
| Beverages: Caffeine. | Decreased bumetanide effect. |
| Cocaine: | Dangerous blood-pressure drop. Avoid. |
| Foods: | None expected. |
| Marijuana: | Increased thirst and urinary frequency, fainting. |
| Tobacco: | Decreased bumetanide effect. |

# BUSPIRONE

## BRAND NAMES

BuSpar

## BASIC INFORMATION

**Habit forming? Unknown**
**Prescription needed? Yes**
**Available as generic? No**
**Drug class: Antianxiety (tranquilizer)**

 USES

Treats anxiety disorders with nervousness or tension. Not intended for treatment of ordinary stress of daily living. Causes less sedation than some antianxiety drugs.

 DOSAGE & USAGE INFORMATION

**How to take:**
Tablets—Take with a glass of liquid.

**When to take:**
As directed. Usually 3 times daily. Food does not interfere with absorption.

**If you forget a dose:**
Take as soon as you remember, but skip this dose and don't double the next dose if it is almost time for the next dose.

**What drug does:**
Chemical family azaspirodecanedione; *not* a benzodiazepine. Probably has an effect on neurotransmitter systems.

**Time lapse before drug works:**
1 or 2 weeks before beneficial effects may be observed.

**Don't take with:**
Alcohol, other tranquilizers, antihistamines, muscle relaxants, sedatives or narcotics.

 OVERDOSE

**SYMPTOMS:**
**Severe drowsiness or nausea, vomiting, small pupils, unconsciousness.**
**WHAT TO DO:**
- **Dial 0 (operator) or 911 (emergency) for an ambulance or medical help. Then give first aid immediately.**
- **See emergency information on inside covers.**

 POSSIBLE ADVERSE REACTIONS OR SIDE EFFECTS

| SYMPTOMS | WHAT TO DO |
| --- | --- |
| **Life-threatening:**<br>Chest pain; pounding, fast heartbeat (rare). | Discontinue. Seek emergency treatment. |
| **Common:**<br>Lightheadedness, headache, nausea, restlessness. | Discontinue. Call doctor right away. |
| **Infrequent:**<br>Drowsiness, dry mouth, ringing in ears, nightmares or vivid dreams, unusual fatigue. | Continue. Call doctor when convenient. |
| **Rare:**<br>Numbness or tingling in feet or hands; sore throat; fever; depression or confusion; uncontrollable movements of tongue, lips, arms and legs. | Discontinue. Call doctor right away. |

 WARNINGS & PRECAUTIONS

**Don't take if:**
If you are allergic to buspirone.

**Before you start, consult your doctor:**
- If you have ever been addicted to any substance.
- If you have chronic kidney or liver disease.
- If you are already taking *any* medicine.

**Over age 60:**
Adverse reactions and side effects may be more frequent and severe than in younger persons.

**Pregnancy:**
No problems expected, but better to avoid if possible.

**Breast-feeding:**
Buspirone passes into milk of lactating experimental animals. Avoid if possible.

**Infants & children:**
Use only under close medical supervision.

**Prolonged use:**
Not recommended for prolonged use. Adverse side effects more likely.

**Skin & sunlight:**
No problems expected.

**Driving, piloting or hazardous work:**
Don't drive or pilot aircraft until you learn how medicine affects you. Don't work around dangerous machinery. Don't climb ladders or work in high places. Danger increases if you drink alcohol or take medicine affecting alertness and reflexes, such as antihistamines, tranquilizers, sedatives, pain medicine, narcotics and mind-altering drugs.

**Discontinuing:**
No problems expected.

**Others:**
Before elective surgery requiring local or general anesthesia, tell your dentist, surgeon or anesthesiologist that you take buspirone.

## POSSIBLE INTERACTION WITH OTHER DRUGS

| GENERIC NAME OR DRUG CLASS | COMBINED EFFECT |
|---|---|
| Antihistamines | Excessive sedation. Sedative effect of both drugs may be increased. |
| Barbiturates | Excessive sedation. Sedative effect of both drugs may be increased. |
| Muscle relaxants | Excessive sedation. Sedative effect of both drugs may be increased. |
| Narcotics | Excessive sedation. Sedative effect of both drugs may be increased. |
| Other tranquilizers | Excessive sedation. Sedative effect of both drugs may be increased. |
| Sedatives | Excessive sedation. Sedative effect of both drugs may be increased. |

## POSSIBLE INTERACTION WITH OTHER SUBSTANCES

| INTERACTS WITH | COMBINED EFFECT |
|---|---|
| Alcohol: | Excess sedation. Avoid. |
| Beverages: Caffeine-containing drinks. | Avoid. Decreased antianxiety effect of busiprone. |
| Cocaine: | Avoid. Decreased antianxiety effect of busiprone. |
| Foods: | None expected. |
| Marijuana: | Avoid. Decreased antianxiety effect of busiprone. |
| Tobacco: | Avoid. Decreased antianxiety effect of busiprone. |

# BUSULFAN

## BRAND NAMES

**Myleran**

## BASIC INFORMATION

**Habit forming? No**
**Prescription needed? Yes**
**Available as generic? No**
**Drug class: Antineoplastic,**
**immunosuppressant**

 **USES**

- Treatment for some kinds of cancer.
- Suppresses immune response after transplant and in immune disorders.

 **DOSAGE & USAGE INFORMATION**

**How to take:**
Tablet or capsule—Swallow with liquid after light meal. Don't drink fluids with meals. Drink extra fluids between meals. Avoid sweet or fatty foods.

**When to take:**
At the same time each day.

**If you forget a dose:**
Take as soon as you remember. Don't ever double dose.

**What drug does:**
Inhibits abnormal cell reproduction. May suppress immune system.

**Time lapse before drug works:**
Up to 6 weeks for full effect.

*Continued next column*

 **OVERDOSE**

**SYMPTOMS:**
**Bleeding, chills, fever, collapse, stupor, seizure.**
**WHAT TO DO:**
- **Dial 0 (operator) or 911 (emergency) for an ambulance or medical help. Then give first aid immediately.**
- **If patient is unconscious and not breathing, give mouth-to-mouth breathing. If there is no heartbeat, use cardiac massage and mouth-to-mouth breathing (CPR). Don't try to make patient vomit. If you can't get help quickly, take patient to nearest emergency facility.**
- **See emergency information on inside covers.**

**Don't take with:**
See Interaction column and consult doctor.

 **POSSIBLE ADVERSE REACTIONS OR SIDE EFFECTS**

| SYMPTOMS | WHAT TO DO |
|---|---|
| **Life-threatening:** None expected. | |
| **Common:** | |
| • Unusual bleeding or bruising, mouth sores with sore throat, chills and fever, black stools, lip sores, menstrual irregularities. | Discontinue. Call doctor right away. |
| • Hair loss, joint pain. | Continue. Call doctor when convenient. |
| • Nausea, vomiting, diarrhea (unavoidable), tiredness, weakness. | Continue. Tell doctor at next visit. |
| **Infrequent:** | |
| • Mental confusion, shortness of breath, may increase chance of developing leukemia. | Continue. Call doctor when convenient. |
| • Cough. | Continue. Tell doctor at next visit. |
| **Rare:** Jaundice. | Discontinue. Call doctor right away. |

## WARNINGS & PRECAUTIONS

**Don't take if:**
- You have had hypersensitivity to alkylating antineoplastic drugs.
- Your physician has not explained the serious nature of your medical problem and risks of taking this medicine.

**Before you start, consult your doctor:**
- If you have gout.
- If you have had kidney stones.
- If you have active infection.
- If you have impaired kidney or liver function.
- If you have taken other antineoplastic drugs or had radiation treatment in last 3 weeks.

**Over age 60:**
Adverse reactions and side effects may be more frequent and severe than in younger persons.

**Pregnancy:**
Consult doctor. Risk to child is significant.

**Breast-feeding:**
Drug passes into milk. Don't nurse.

**Infants & children:**
Use only under care of medical supervisors who are experienced in anticancer drugs.

**Prolonged use:**
Adverse reactions more likely the longer drug is required.

**Skin & sunlight:**
No problems expected.

**Driving, piloting or hazardous work:**
No problems expected.

**Discontinuing:**
Don't discontinue without doctor's advice until you complete prescribed dose, even though symptoms diminish or disappear. Some side effects may follow discontinuing. Report to doctor blurred vision, convulsions, confusion, persistent headache.

**Others:**
May cause sterility.

## POSSIBLE INTERACTION WITH OTHER DRUGS

| GENERIC NAME OR DRUG CLASS | COMBINED EFFECT |
|---|---|
| Antigout drugs | Decreased antigout effect. |
| Antineoplastic drugs (other) | Increased effect of all drugs (may be beneficial). |
| Chloramphenicol | Increased likelihood of toxic effects of both drugs. |

## POSSIBLE INTERACTION WITH OTHER SUBSTANCES

| INTERACTS WITH | COMBINED EFFECT |
|---|---|
| Alcohol: | May increase chance of intestinal bleeding. |
| Beverages: | No problems expected. |
| Cocaine: | Increases chance of toxicity. |
| Foods: | Reduces irritation in stomach. |
| Marijuana: | No problems expected. |
| Tobacco: | Increases lung toxicity. |

# BUTABARBITAL

## BRAND NAMES

See complete list of brand names in the *Brand Name Directory*, page 945.

## BASIC INFORMATION

**Habit forming? Yes**
**Prescription needed? Yes**
**Available as generic? Yes**
**Drug class: Sedative, hypnotic (barbiturate)**

 ## USES

- Reduces anxiety or nervous tension (low dose).
- Relieves insomnia (higher bedtime dose).

 ## DOSAGE & USAGE INFORMATION

**How to take:**
Tablet, capsule or liquid—Swallow with food or liquid to lessen stomach irritation. If you can't swallow whole, crumble tablet or open capsule and take with liquid or food.

**When to take:**
At the same times each day.

**If you forget a dose:**
Take as soon as you remember up to 2 hours late. If more than 2 hours, wait for next scheduled dose (don't double this dose).

**What drug does:**
May partially block nerve impulses at nerve-cell connections.

**Time lapse before drug works:**
60 minutes.

**Don't take with:**
- Non-prescription drugs without consulting doctor.
- See Interaction column and consult doctor.

 ## OVERDOSE

**SYMPTOMS:**
Deep sleep, weak pulse, coma.
**WHAT TO DO:**
- **Dial 0 (operator) or 911 (emergency) for an ambulance or medical help. Then give first aid immediately.**
- **See emergency information on inside covers.**

 ## POSSIBLE ADVERSE REACTIONS OR SIDE EFFECTS

| SYMPTOMS | WHAT TO DO |
|---|---|
| **Life-threatening:**<br>None expected. | |
| **Common:**<br>Dizziness, drowsiness, "hangover" effect. | Continue. Call doctor when convenient. |
| **Infrequent:**<br>• Rash or hives; swollen lips, face or eyelids; sore throat, fever. | Discontinue. Call doctor right away. |
| • Depression, confusion, slurred speech, diarrhea, nausea, vomiting, joint or muscle pain. | Continue. Call doctor when convenient. |
| **Rare:**<br>• Agitation, slow heartbeat, breathing difficulty, jaundice. | Discontinue. Call doctor right away. |
| • Unexplained bleeding or bruising. | Continue. Call doctor when convenient. |

 ## WARNINGS & PRECAUTIONS

**Don't take if:**
- You are allergic to any barbiturate.
- You have porphyria.

**Before you start, consult your doctor:**
- If you have epilepsy.
- If you have kidney or liver damage.
- If you have asthma.
- If you have anemia.
- If you have chronic pain.
- If you will have surgery within 2 months, including dental surgery, requiring general or spinal anesthesia.

**Over age 60:**
Adverse reactions and side effects may be more frequent and severe than in younger persons. Use small doses.

**Pregnancy:**
Risk to unborn child outweighs drug benefits. Don't use.

**Breast-feeding:**
Drug passes into milk. Avoid drug or discontinue nursing until you finish medicine. Consult doctor for advice on maintaining milk supply.

**Infants & children:**
Use only under doctor's supervision.

**Prolonged use:**
- May cause addiction, anemia, chronic intoxication.
- May lower body temperature, making exposure to cold temperatures hazardous.

**Skin & sunlight:**
May cause rash or intensify sunburn in areas exposed to sun or sunlamp.

**Driving, piloting or hazardous work:**
Don't drive or pilot aircraft until you learn how medicine affects you. Don't work around dangerous machinery. Don't climb ladders or work in high places. Danger increases if you drink alcohol or take medicine affecting alertness and reflexes.

**Discontinuing:**
May be unnecessary to finish medicine. Follow doctor's instructions. If you develop withdrawal symptoms of hallucinations, agitation or sleeplessness after discontinuing, call doctor right away.

**Others:**
High potential for abuse.

 ## POSSIBLE INTERACTION WITH OTHER DRUGS

| GENERIC NAME OR DRUG CLASS | COMBINED EFFECT |
| --- | --- |
| Anticoagulants (oral) | Decreased anticoagulant effect. |
| Anticonvulsants | Changed seizure patterns. |
| Antidepressants (tricyclics) | Decreased antidepressant effect. Possible dangerous oversedation. |
| Antidiabetics (oral) | Increased butabarbital effect. |
| Antihistamines | Dangerous sedation. Avoid. |
| Anti-inflammatory drugs (non-steroidal) | Decreased anti-inflammatory effect. |
| Aspirin | Decreased aspirin effect. |
| Beta-adrenergic blockers | Decreased effect of beta-adrenergic blocker. |
| Contraceptives (oral) | Decreased contraceptive effect. |
| Cortisone drugs | Decreased cortisone effect. |
| Digitoxin | Decreased digitoxin effect. |

| | |
| --- | --- |
| Doxycycline | Decreased doxycycline effect. |
| Dronabinol | Increased effects of both drugs. Avoid. |
| Griseofulvin | Decreased griseofulvin effect. |
| Indapamide | Increased indapamide effect. |
| MAO inhibitors | Increased butabarbital effect. |
| Mind-altering drugs | Dangerous sedation. Avoid. |
| Molindone | Increased sedative effect. |
| Narcotics | Dangerous sedation. Avoid. |
| Pain relievers | Dangerous sedation. Avoid. |
| Sedatives | Dangerous sedation. Avoid. |
| Sleep inducers | Dangerous sedation. Avoid. |
| Tranquilizers | Dangerous sedation. Avoid. |
| Valproic acid | Increased butabarbital effect. |

 ## POSSIBLE INTERACTION WITH OTHER SUBSTANCES

| INTERACTS WITH | COMBINED EFFECT |
| --- | --- |
| Alcohol: | Possible fatal oversedation. Avoid. |
| Beverages: | None expected. |
| Cocaine: | Decreased butabarbital effect. |
| Foods: | None expected. |
| Marijuana: | Excessive sedation. Avoid. |
| Tobacco: | None expected. |

# BUTALBITAL & ASPIRIN
## (Also contains caffeine)

## BRAND AND GENERIC NAMES

Buff-A-Comp
BUTALBITAL,
  ASPIRIN &
  CAFFEINE
Butal Compound
Fiorinal

Isollyl (Improved)
Lanorinal
Marnal
Protension
Tenstan

## BASIC INFORMATION

Habit forming? Yes
Prescription needed? Yes
Available as generic? Yes
Drug class: Analgesic, anti-inflammatory,
    sedative

 ## USES

- Reduces anxiety or nervous tension (low dose).
- Reduces pain, fever, inflammation.

 ## DOSAGE & USAGE INFORMATION

How to take:
- Tablet, liquid or capsule—Swallow with liquid or food to lessen stomach irritation. If you can't swallow whole, crumble tablet or open capsule and take with liquid or food.
- Extended-release tablets or capsules—Swallow each dose whole.
- Suppositories—Remove wrapper and moisten suppository with water. Gently insert into rectum, large end first.

When to take:
At the same times each day. No more often than every 4 hours.

*Continued next column*

 ## OVERDOSE

SYMPTOMS:
**Deep sleep, weak pulse, ringing in ears, nausea, vomiting, dizziness, fever, deep and rapid breathing, hallucinations, convulsions, coma.**
WHAT TO DO:
- **Dial 0 (operator) or 911 (emergency) for an ambulance or medical help. Then give first aid immediately.**
- **See emergency information on inside covers.**

### If you forget a dose:
Take as soon as you remember up to 2 hours late. If more than 2 hours, wait for next scheduled dose (don't double this dose).

### What drug does:
- May partially block nerve impulses at nerve-cell connections.
- Affects hypothalamus, the part of the brain which regulates temperature by dilating small blood vessels in skin.
- Prevents clumping of platelets (small blood cells) so blood vessels remain open.
- Decreases prostaglandin effect.
- Suppresses body's pain messages.

### Time lapse before drug works:
30 minutes.

### Don't take with:
- Non-prescription drugs without consulting doctor.
- See Interaction column and consult doctor.

 ## POSSIBLE ADVERSE REACTIONS OR SIDE EFFECTS

| SYMPTOMS | WHAT TO DO |
|---|---|
| **Life-threatening:** | |
| Hives, rash, intense itching, faintness soon after a dose (anaphylaxis); wheezing; tightness in chest; black or bloody vomit; black stools; shortness of breath. | Seek emergency treatment immediately. |
| **Common:** | |
| Dizziness, drowsiness, heartburn. | Continue. Call doctor when convenient. |
| **Infrequent:** | |
| Jaundice; vomiting blood; easy bruising; skin rash, hives; confusion; depression; sore throat, fever, mouth sores; hearing loss; slurred speech; decreased vision. | Discontinue. Call doctor right away. |
| **Rare:** | |
| • Diminished vision, blood in urine, unexplained fever. | Discontinue. Call doctor right away. |
| • Insomnia, nightmares, constipation, headache, nervousness, jaundice. | Continue. Call doctor when convenient. |

## WARNINGS & PRECAUTIONS

**Don't take if:**
- You are allergic to any barbiturate.
- You have a peptic ulcer of stomach or duodenum, bleeding disorder, porphyria.

**Before you start, consult your doctor:**
- If you have had stomach or duodenal ulcers.
- If you have asthma, nasal polyps, epilepsy, kidney or liver damage, anemia, chronic pain.
- If you will have surgery within 2 months, including dental surgery, requiring general or spinal anesthesia.

**Over age 60:**
- Adverse reactions and side effects may be more frequent and severe than in younger persons.
- More likely to cause hidden bleeding in stomach or intestines. Watch for dark stools.

**Pregnancy:**
Risk to unborn child outweighs drug benefits. Don't use.

**Breast-feeding:**
Drug passes into milk. Avoid drug or discontinue nursing until you finish medicine. Consult doctor for advice on maintaining milk supply.

**Infants & children:**
- Overdose frequent and severe. Keep bottles out of children's reach.
- Use only under doctor's supervision.

**Prolonged use:**
- Kidney damage. Periodic kidney-function test recommended.
- May cause addiction, anemia, chronic intoxication.
- May lower body temperature, making exposure to cold temperatures hazardous.

**Skin & sunlight:**
May cause rash or intensify sunburn in areas exposed to sun or sunlamp.

**Driving, piloting or hazardous work:**
Don't drive or pilot aircraft until you learn how medicine affects you. Don't work around dangerous machinery. Don't climb ladders or work in high places. Danger increases if you drink alcohol or take medicine affecting alertness and reflexes, such as antihistamines, tranquilizers, sedatives, pain medicine, narcotics and mind-altering drugs.

**Discontinuing:**
May be unnecessary to finish medicine. Follow doctor's instructions. If you develop withdrawal symptoms of hallucinations, agitation or sleeplessness after discontinuing, call doctor right away.

**Others:**
- Aspirin can complicate surgery, pregnancy, labor and delivery, and illness.
- For arthritis—Don't change dose without consulting doctor.
- Urine tests for blood sugar may be inaccurate.
- Great potential for abuse.

## POSSIBLE INTERACTION WITH OTHER DRUGS

| GENERIC NAME OR DRUG CLASS | COMBINED EFFECT |
|---|---|
| Acebutolol | Decreased antihypertensive effect of acebutolol. |
| Allopurinol | Decreased allopurinol effect. |
| Antacids | Decreased aspirin effect. |
| Anticoagulants (oral) | Increased anticoagulant effect. Abnormal bleeding. |
| Anticonvulsants | Changed seizure patterns. |
| Antidepressants | Decreased antidepressant effect. Possible dangerous oversedation. |
| Antidiabetics (oral) | Increased butalbital effect. Low blood sugar. |
| Antihistamines | Dangerous sedation. Avoid. |

*Continued page 963*

## POSSIBLE INTERACTION WITH OTHER SUBSTANCES

| INTERACTS WITH | COMBINED EFFECT |
|---|---|
| Alcohol: | Possible stomach irritation and bleeding, possible fatal oversedation. Avoid. |
| Beverages: | None expected. |
| Cocaine: | Decreased butalbital effect. |
| Foods: | None expected. |
| Marijuana: | Possible increased pain relief, but marijuana may slow body's recovery. Avoid. |
| Tobacco: | None expected. |

# BUTALBITAL, ASPIRIN & CODEINE
## (Also contains caffeine)

## BRAND NAMES

**Buff-A-Comp 3**     **Isollyl with Codeine**
**Fiorinal with Codeine**

## BASIC INFORMATION

**Habit forming? Yes**
**Prescription needed? Yes**
**Available as generic? No**
**Drug class: Narcotic, analgesic**

## USES

- Reduces anxiety or nervous tension (low dose).
- Reduces pain, fever, inflammation.

## DOSAGE & USAGE INFORMATION

**How to take:**
- Tablet, liquid or capsule—Swallow with liquid or food to lessen stomach irritation. If you can't swallow whole, crumble tablet or open capsule and take with liquid or food.
- Extended-release tablets or capsules—Swallow each dose whole.

**When to take:**
When needed. No more often than every 4 hours.

*Continued next column*

## OVERDOSE

**SYMPTOMS:**
**Deep sleep, slow and weak pulse, ringing in ears, nausea, vomiting, dizziness, fever, deep and rapid breathing, hallucinations, convulsions, coma.**
**WHAT TO DO:**
- **Dial 0 (operator) or 911 (emergency) for an ambulance or medical help. Then give first aid immediately.**
- **If patient is unconscious and not breathing, give mouth-to-mouth breathing. If there is no heartbeat, use cardiac massage and mouth-to-mouth breathing (CPR). Don't try to make patient vomit. If you can't get help quickly, take patient to nearest emergency facility.**
- **See emergency information on inside covers.**

**If you forget a dose:**
Take as soon as you remember. Wait 4 hours for next dose.

**What drug does:**
- May partially block nerve impulses at nerve-cell connections.
- Affects hypothalamus, the part of the brain which regulates temperature by dilating small blood vessels in skin.
- Prevents clumping of platelets (small blood cells) so blood vessels remain open.
- Decreases prostaglandin effect.
- Blocks pain messages to brain and spinal cord.
- Reduces sensitivity of brain's cough-control center.

**Time lapse before drug works:**
30 minutes.

**Don't take with:**
- Non-prescription drugs without consulting doctor.
- See Interaction column and consult doctor.

## POSSIBLE ADVERSE REACTIONS OR SIDE EFFECTS

| SYMPTOMS | WHAT TO DO |
|---|---|
| **Life-threatening:** | |
| Wheezing, tightness in chest, pinpoint pupils. | Seek emergency treatment immediately. |
| **Common:** | |
| Dizziness, drowsiness, heartburn, flushed face, depression, false sense of well-being, increased urination. | Continue. Call doctor when convenient. |
| **Infrequent:** | |
| Jaundice; vomiting blood; easy bruising; skin rash, hives; confusion; depression; sore throat, fever, mouth sores; difficult urination; hearing loss; slurred speech; blood in urine; decreased vision. | Discontinue. Call doctor right away. |
| **Rare:** | |
| Insomnia, nightmares, constipation, headache, nervousness, flushed face, increased sweating, unusual tiredness. | Continue. Call doctor when convenient. |

# BUTALBITAL, ASPIRIN & CODEINE
## (Also contains caffeine)

 **WARNINGS & PRECAUTIONS**

**Don't take if:**
- You are allergic to any barbiturate or narcotic.
- You have a peptic ulcer of stomach or duodenum, bleeding disorder, porphyria.

**Before you start, consult your doctor:**
- If you have had stomach or duodenal ulcers.
- If you have asthma, epilepsy, kidney or liver damage, anemia, chronic pain, gout.
- If you will have surgery within 2 months, including dental surgery, requiring general or spinal anesthesia.

**Over age 60:**
- Adverse reactions and side effects may be more frequent and severe than in younger persons.
- More likely to cause hidden bleeding in stomach or intestines. Watch for dark stools.
- More likely to be drowsy, dizzy, unsteady or constipated. Use only if absolutely necessary.

**Pregnancy:**
Risk to unborn child outweighs drug benefits. Don't use.

**Breast-feeding:**
Drug passes into milk. Avoid drug or discontinue nursing until you finish medicine. Consult doctor for advice on maintaining milk supply.

**Infants & children:**
- Overdose frequent and severe. Keep bottles out of children's reach.
- Use only under doctor's supervision.
- Consult doctor before giving to persons under age 18 who have fever and discomfort of viral illness, especially chicken pox and influenza. Probably increases risk of Reye's syndrome.

**Prolonged use:**
- Kidney damage. Periodic kidney-function test recommended.
- May cause addiction, anemia, chronic intoxication.
- May lower body temperature, making exposure to cold temperatures hazardous.

**Skin & sunlight:**
May cause rash or intensify sunburn in areas exposed to sun or sunlamp.

**Driving, piloting or hazardous work:**
Don't drive or pilot aircraft until you learn how medicine affects you. Don't work around dangerous machinery. Don't climb ladders or work in high places. Danger increases if you drink alcohol or take medicine affecting alertness and reflexes, such as antihistamines, tranquilizers, sedatives, pain medicine, narcotics and mind-altering drugs.

**Discontinuing:**
May be unnecessary to finish medicine. Follow doctor's instructions. If you develop withdrawal symptoms of hallucinations, agitation or sleeplessness after discontinuing, call doctor right away.

**Others:**
- Aspirin can complicate surgery, pregnancy, labor and delivery, and illness.
- For arthritis—Don't change dose without consulting doctor.
- Urine tests for blood sugar may be inaccurate.
- Great potential for abuse.

 **POSSIBLE INTERACTION WITH OTHER DRUGS**

| GENERIC NAME OR DRUG CLASS | COMBINED EFFECT |
|---|---|
| Acebutolol | Decreased antihypertensive effect of acebutolol. |
| Allopurinol | Decreased allopurinol effect. |
| Analgesics (other) | Increased analgesic effect. |
| Antacids | Decreased aspirin effect. |
| Anticoagulants (oral) | Increased anticoagulant effect. Abnormal bleeding. |
| Anticonvulsants | Changed seizure patterns. |

*Continued page 963*

 **POSSIBLE INTERACTION WITH OTHER SUBSTANCES**

| INTERACTS WITH | COMBINED EFFECT |
|---|---|
| Alcohol: | Possible stomach irritation and bleeding, possible fatal oversedation. Avoid. |
| Beverages: | None expected. |
| Cocaine: | Increased cocaine toxic effects. Avoid. |
| Foods: | None expected. |
| Marijuana: | Possible increased pain relief, but marijuana may slow body's recovery. Impairs physical and mental performance. Avoid. |
| Tobacco: | None expected. |

# BUTAPERAZINE

## BRAND NAMES

Repoise

## BASIC INFORMATION

Habit forming? No
Prescription needed? Yes
Available as generic? Yes
Drug class: Tranquilizer, antiemetic
           (phenothiazine)

## USES

- Stops nausea, vomiting.
- Reduces anxiety, agitation.

## DOSAGE & USAGE INFORMATION

**How to take:**
- Tablet or capsule—Swallow with liquid or food to lessen stomach irritation.
- Suppositories—Remove wrapper and moisten suppository with water. Gently insert into rectum, large end first.
- Drops or liquid—Dilute dose in beverage.

**When to take:**
- Nervous and mental disorders—Take at the same times each day.
- Nausea and vomiting—Take as needed, no more often than every 4 hours.

**If you forget a dose:**
- Nervous and mental disorders—Take up to 2 hours late. If more than 2 hours, wait for next scheduled dose (don't double this).
- Nausea and vomiting—Take as soon as you remember. Wait 4 hours for next dose.

**What drug does:**
- Suppresses brain's vomiting center.
- Suppresses brain centers that control abnormal emotions and behavior.

**Time lapse before drug works:**
- Nausea and vomiting—1 hour or less.
- Nervous and mental disorders—4-6 weeks.

*Continued next column*

## OVERDOSE

**SYMPTOMS:**
Stupor, convulsions, coma.
**WHAT TO DO:**
- Dial 0 (operator) or 911 (emergency) for an ambulance or medical help. Then give first aid immediately.
- See emergency information on inside covers.

**Don't take with:**
- Antacid or medicine for diarrhea.
- Non-prescription drug for cough, cold or allergy.
- See Interaction column and consult doctor.

## POSSIBLE ADVERSE REACTIONS OR SIDE EFFECTS

| SYMPTOMS | WHAT TO DO |
|---|---|
| **Life-threatening:** | |
| None expected. | |
| **Common:** | |
| • Muscle spasms of face and neck, unsteady gait. | Discontinue. Seek emergency treatment. |
| • Restlessness, tremor, drowsiness. | Discontinue. Call doctor right away. |
| • Decreased sweating, dry mouth, stuffy nose, constipation. | Continue. Call doctor when convenient. |
| **Infrequent:** | |
| • Fainting. | Discontinue. Seek emergency treatment. |
| • Rash. | Discontinue. Call doctor right away. |
| • Difficult urination, diminished sex drive, swollen breasts, menstrual irregularities. | Continue. Call doctor when convenient. |
| **Rare:** | |
| Changes in vision, sore throat, fever, jaundice. | Discontinue. Call doctor right away. |

## WARNINGS & PRECAUTIONS

### Don't take if:
- You are allergic to any phenothiazine.
- You have a blood or bone-marrow disease.

### Before you start, consult your doctor:
- If you will have surgery within 2 months, including dental surgery, requiring general or spinal anesthesia.
- If you have asthma, emphysema or other lung disorder.
- If you take non-prescription ulcer medicine, asthma medicine or amphetamines.

### Over age 60:
Adverse reactions and side effects may be more frequent and severe than in younger persons. More likely to develop involuntary movement of jaws, lips, tongue, chewing. Report this to your doctor immediately. Early treatment can help.

### Pregnancy:
Risk to unborn child outweighs drug benefits. Don't use.

### Breast-feeding:
Drug passes into milk. Avoid drug or discontinue nursing until you finish medicine. Consult doctor for advice on maintaining milk supply.

### Infants & children:
Don't give to children younger than 2.

### Prolonged use:
May lead to tardive dyskinesia (involuntary movement of jaws, lips, tongue, chewing).

### Skin & sunlight: .
May cause rash or intensify sunburn in areas exposed to sun or sunlamp. Skin may remain sensitive for 3 months after discontinuing.

### Driving, piloting or hazardous work:
Don't drive or pilot aircraft until you learn how medicine affects you. Don't work around dangerous machinery. Don't climb ladders or work in high places. Danger increases if you drink alcohol or take medicine affecting alertness and reflexes.

### Discontinuing:
- Nervous and mental disorders—Don't discontinue without doctor's advice until you complete prescribed dose, even though symptoms diminish or disappear.
- Nausea and vomiting—May be unnecessary to finish medicine. Follow doctor's instructions.

### Others:
No problems expected.

## POSSIBLE INTERACTION WITH OTHER DRUGS

| GENERIC NAME OR DRUG CLASS | COMBINED EFFECT |
| --- | --- |
| Anticholinergics | Increased anticholinergic effect. |
| Antidepressants (tricyclic) | Increased butaperazine effect. |
| Antihistamines | Increased antihistamine effect. |
| Appetite suppressants | Decreased suppressant effect. |
| Dronabinol | Increased effects of both drugs. Avoid. |
| Levodopa | Decreased levodopa effect. |
| Mind-altering drugs | Increased effect of mind-altering drugs. |
| Narcotics | Increased narcotic effect. |
| Phenytoin | Increased phenytoin effect. |
| Quinidine | Impaired heart function. Dangerous mixture. |
| Sedatives | Increased sedative effect. |
| Tranquilizers (other) | Increased tranquilizer effect. |

## POSSIBLE INTERACTION WITH OTHER SUBSTANCES

| INTERACTS WITH | COMBINED EFFECT |
| --- | --- |
| Alcohol: | Dangerous oversedation. |
| Beverages: | None expected. |
| Cocaine: | Decreased butaperazine effect. Avoid. |
| Foods: | None expected. |
| Marijuana: | Drowsiness. May increase antinausea effect. |
| Tobacco: | None expected. |

# CAFFEINE

## BRAND NAMES

See complete list of brand names in the *Brand Name Directory,* page 945.

## BASIC INFORMATION

**Habit forming? Yes**
**Prescription needed? No**
**Available as generic? Yes**
**Drug class: Stimulant (xanthine),**
          **vasoconstrictor**

## USES

- Treatment for drowsiness and fatigue.
- Treatment for migraine and other vascular headaches in combination with ergot.

## DOSAGE & USAGE INFORMATION

**How to take:**
- Tablet—Swallow with liquid or food to lessen stomach irritation. If you can't swallow whole, crumble tablet or open capsule and take with liquid or food.
- Extended-release capsules—Swallow whole with liquid.

**When to take:**
At the same times each day.

**If you forget a dose:**
Take as soon as you remember up to 2 hours late. If more than 2 hours, wait for next scheduled dose (don't double this dose).

**What drug does:**
- Constricts blood-vessel walls.
- Stimulates central nervous system.

**Time lapse before drug works:**
30 minutes.

*Continued next column*

## OVERDOSE

**SYMPTOMS:**
**Excitement, rapid heartbeat, hallucinations, convulsions, coma.**
**WHAT TO DO:**
- **Dial 0 (operator) or 911 (emergency) for an ambulance or medical help. Then give first aid immediately.**
- **See emergency information on inside covers.**

---

**Don't take with:**
- Non-prescription drugs without consulting doctor.
- See Interaction column and consult doctor.

## POSSIBLE ADVERSE REACTIONS OR SIDE EFFECTS

| SYMPTOMS | WHAT TO DO |
|---|---|
| **Life-threatening:** None expected. | |
| **Common:** | |
| • Rapid heartbeat, low blood sugar (hunger, anxiety, cold sweats, rapid pulse) with tremor, irritability. | Continue. Call doctor when convenient. |
| • Nervousness, insomnia. | Continue. Tell doctor at next visit. |
| • Increased urination. | No action necessary. |
| **Infrequent:** | |
| • Confusion, irritability. | Discontinue. Call doctor right away. |
| • Nausea, indigestion, burning feeling, in stomach. | Continue. Call doctor when convenient. |
| **Rare:** None expected. | |

## WARNINGS & PRECAUTIONS

**Don't take if:**
- You are allergic to any stimulant.
- You have heart disease.
- You have active peptic ulcer of stomach or duodenum.

**Before you start, consult your doctor:**
- If you have irregular heartbeat.
- If you have hypoglycemia (low blood sugar).
- If you have epilepsy.

**Over age 60:**
Adverse reactions and side effects may be more frequent and severe than in younger persons.

**Pregnancy:**
Risk to unborn child outweighs drug benefits. Don't use.

**Breast-feeding:**
Drug passes into milk. Avoid drug or discontinue nursing until you finish medicine. Consult doctor for advice on maintaining milk supply.

**Infants & children:**
Not recommended.

**Prolonged use:**
Stomach ulcers.

**Skin & sunlight:**
No problems expected.

**Driving, piloting or hazardous work:**
No problems expected.

**Discontinuing:**
Will cause withdrawal symptoms of headache, irritability, drowsiness. Discontinue gradually if you use caffeine for a month or more.

**Others:**
May produce or aggravate fibrocystic disease of the breast in women.

## POSSIBLE INTERACTION WITH OTHER DRUGS

| GENERIC NAME OR DRUG CLASS | COMBINED EFFECT |
|---|---|
| Contraceptives (oral) | Increased caffeine effect. |
| Isoniazid | Increased caffeine effect. |
| MAO inhibitors | Dangerous blood-pressure rise. |
| Sedatives | Decreased sedative effect. |
| Sleep inducers | Decreased sedative effect. |
| Sympathomimetics | Overstimulation. |
| Thyroid hormones | Increased thyroid effect. |
| Tranquilizers | Decreased tranquilizer effect. |

## POSSIBLE INTERACTION WITH OTHER SUBSTANCES

| INTERACTS WITH | COMBINED EFFECT |
|---|---|
| Alcohol: | Decreased alcohol effect. |
| Beverages: Caffeine drinks. | Increased caffeine effect. |
| Cocaine: | Overstimulation. Avoid. |
| Foods: | No proven problems. |
| Marijuana: | Increased effect of both drugs. May lead to dangerous, rapid heartbeat. Avoid. |
| Tobacco: | Increased heartbeat. Avoid. |

# CALCIUM CARBONATE

## BRAND NAMES

See complete list of brand names in the *Brand Name Directory,* page 946.

## BASIC INFORMATION

**Habit forming? No**
**Prescription needed? No**
**Available as generic? Yes**
**Drug class: Antacid**

 **USES**

Treatment for hyperacidity in upper gastrointestinal tract, including stomach and esophagus. Symptoms may be heartburn or acid indigestion. Diseases include peptic ulcer, gastritis, esophagitis, hiatal hernia.

 **DOSAGE & USAGE INFORMATION**

**How to take:**
- Tablet—Swallow with liquid.
- Chewable tablets or wafers—Chew well before swallowing.

**When to take:**
1 to 3 hours after meals unless directed otherwise by your doctor.

**If you forget a dose:**
Take as soon as you remember.

**What drug does:**
- Neutralizes some of the hydrochloric acid in the stomach.
- Reduces action of pepsin, a digestive enzyme.

**Time lapse before drug works:**
15 minutes.

**Don't take with:**
Other medicines at the same time. Decreases absorption of other drugs.

 **OVERDOSE**

**SYMPTOMS:**
**Weakness, fatigue, dizziness.**
**WHAT TO DO:**
**Overdose unlikely to threaten life. If person takes much larger amount than prescribed, call doctor, poison-control center or hospital emergency room for instructions.**

 **POSSIBLE ADVERSE REACTIONS OR SIDE EFFECTS**

| SYMPTOMS | WHAT TO DO |
|---|---|
| **Life-threatening:**<br>None expected. | |
| **Common:**<br>Constipation, appetite loss. | Continue. Call doctor when convenient. |
| **Infrequent:**<br>• Lower abdominal pain and swelling, bone pain, muscle weakness, swollen wrists or ankles. | Discontinue. Call doctor right away. |
| • Mood changes, nausea, vomiting, weight loss. | Continue. Call doctor when convenient. |
| **Rare:**<br>Difficult or painful urination, unusual tiredness or weakness. | Discontinue. Call doctor right away. |

**WARNINGS & PRECAUTIONS**

**Don't take if:**
- You are allergic to any antacid.
- You have a high blood-calcium level.

**Before you start, consult your doctor:**
- If you have kidney disease.
- If you have chronic constipation, colitis or diarrhea.
- If you have symptoms of appendicitis.
- If you have stomach or intestinal bleeding.
- If you have irregular heartbeat.

**Over age 60:**
Adverse reactions and side effects may be more frequent and severe than in younger persons. Diarrhea or constipation particularly likely.

**Pregnancy:**
Risk to unborn child outweighs drug benefits. Don't use.

**Breast-feeding:**
Drug passes into milk. Avoid drug or discontinue nursing until you finish medicine. Consult doctor for advice on maintaining milk supply.

**Infants & children:**
Use only under medical supervision.

**Prolonged use:**
- High blood level of calcium which disturbs electrolyte balance.
- Kidney stones, impaired kidney function.

**Skin & sunlight:**
No problems expected.

**Driving, piloting or hazardous work:**
No problems expected.

**Discontinuing:**
May be unnecessary to finish medicine. Follow doctor's instructions.

**Others:**
Don't take longer than 2 weeks unless under medical supervision.

## POSSIBLE INTERACTION WITH OTHER DRUGS

| GENERIC NAME OR DRUG CLASS | COMBINED EFFECT |
|---|---|
| Anticoagulants | Decreased anticoagulant effect. |
| Calcitonin | Decreased calcitonin effect. |
| Chlorpromazine | Decreased chlorpromazine effect. |
| Digitalis preparations | Decreased digitalis effect. |
| Diuretics | Increased calcium in blood. |
| Iron supplements | Decreased iron effect. |
| Meperidine | Increased meperidine effect. |
| Mexiletine | May slow elimination of mexiletine and cause need to adjust dosage. |
| Nalidixic acid | Decreased effect of nalidixic acid. |
| Oxyphenbutazone | Decreased oxyphenbutazone effect. |
| Para-aminosalicylic acid (PAS) | Decreased PAS effect. |
| Penicillins | Decreased penicillin effect. |
| Pentobarbital | Decreased pentobarbital effect. |
| Phenylbutazone | Decreased phenylbutazone effect. |
| Pseudoephedrine | Increased pseudoephedrine effect. |
| Quinidine | Increased quinidine effect. |
| Salicylates | Increased salicylate effect. |
| Sulfa drugs | Decreased sulfa effect. |

| | |
|---|---|
| Tetracyclines | Decreased tetracycline effect. |
| Vitamin A | Decreased vitamin effect. |
| Vitamin D (large doses) | Excessive absorption of vitamin D. |

## POSSIBLE INTERACTION WITH OTHER SUBSTANCES

| INTERACTS WITH | COMBINED EFFECT |
|---|---|
| Alcohol: | Decreased antacid effect. |
| Beverages: | No proven problems. |
| Cocaine: | No proven problems. |
| Foods: | Decreased antacid effect if taken with food. Wait 1 hour after eating. |
| Marijuana: | No proven problems. |
| Tobacco: | Decreased antacid effect. |

# CALCIUM & MAGNESIUM ANTACIDS

## BRAND AND GENERIC NAMES

Alkets
Bisodol
CALCIUM &
  MAGNESIUM
  CARBONATES
CALCIUM &
  MAGNESIUM
  CARBONATES &
  MAGNESIUM
  OXIDE

CALCIUM
  CARBONATE &
  MAGNESIA
Marblen
Ratio
Spastosed

## BASIC INFORMATION

**Habit forming? No**
**Prescription needed? No**
**Available as generic? Yes**
**Drug class: Antacid**

## USES

- Treatment for hyperacidity in upper gastrointestinal tract, including stomach and esophagus. Symptoms may be heartburn or acid indigestion. Diseases include peptic ulcer, gastritis, esophagitis, hiatal hernia.
- Constipation relief.

## DOSAGE & USAGE INFORMATION

**How to take:**
- Tablet or capsule—Swallow with liquid.
- Chewable tablets or wafers—Chew well before swallowing.
- Liquid—Shake well and take undiluted.

*Continued next column*

## OVERDOSE

**SYMPTOMS:**
**Dry mouth, shallow breathing, diarrhea, weakness, fatigue, stupor.**
**WHAT TO DO:**
- **Overdose unlikely to threaten life. Depending on severity of symptoms and amount taken, call doctor, poison-control center or hospital emergency room for instructions.**
- **Dial 0 (operator) or 911 (emergency) for an ambulance or medical help. Then give first aid immediately.**
- **See emergency information on inside covers.**

**When to take:**
1 to 3 hours after meals unless directed otherwise by your doctor.

**If you forget a dose:**
Take as soon as you remember, but not simultaneously with any other medicine.

**What drug does:**
- Neutralizes some of the hydrochloric acid in the stomach.
- Reduces action of pepsin, a digestive enzyme.
- Stimulates muscles in lower bowel wall.

**Time lapse before drug works:**
15 minutes for antacid effect.

**Don't take with:**
Other medicines at the same time. Decreases absorption of other drugs. Wait 2 hours between doses.

## POSSIBLE ADVERSE REACTIONS OR SIDE EFFECTS

| SYMPTOMS | WHAT TO DO |
|---|---|
| **Life-threatening:** | |
| Heartbeat irregularity in patient with heart disease. | Discontinue. Seek emergency treatment. |
| **Common:** | |
| • Constipation, headache, appetite loss, distended stomach. | Discontinue. Call doctor right away. |
| • Unpleasant taste in mouth, abdominal pain, laxative effect, belching. | Continue. Call doctor when convenient. |
| **Infrequent:** | |
| Bone pain, frequent urination, dizziness, urgent urination, muscle weakness or pain, nausea, weight gain. | Discontinue. Call doctor right away. |
| **Rare:** | |
| Mood changes, vomiting, nervousness, swollen feet and ankles. | Discontinue. Call doctor right away. |

# CALCIUM & MAGNESIUM ANTACIDS

## WARNINGS & PRECAUTIONS

**Don't take if:**
- You are allergic to any antacid.
- You have a high blood-calcium level.

**Before you start, consult your doctor:**
If you have kidney disease, chronic constipation, colitis, diarrhea, symptoms of appendicitis, stomach or intestinal bleeding, irregular heartbeat.

**Over age 60:**
Adverse reactions and side effects may be more frequent and severe than in younger persons. Diarrhea or constipation particularly likely.

**Pregnancy:**
Risk to unborn child outweighs drug benefits. Don't use.

**Breast-feeding:**
Drug passes into milk. Avoid drug or discontinue nursing until you finish medicine. Consult doctor for advice on maintaining milk supply.

**Infants & children:**
Use only under medical supervision.

**Prolonged use:**
- High blood level of calcium which disturbs electrolyte balance.
- Kidney stones, impaired kidney function.

**Skin & sunlight:**
No problems expected.

**Driving, piloting or hazardous work:**
No problems expected.

**Discontinuing:**
May be unnecessary to finish medicine. Follow doctor's instructions.

**Others:**
Don't take longer than 2 weeks unless under medical supervision.

## POSSIBLE INTERACTION WITH OTHER DRUGS

| GENERIC NAME OR DRUG CLASS | COMBINED EFFECT |
|---|---|
| Anticoagulants (oral) | Decreased anticoagulant effect. |
| Calcitonin | Decreased calcitonin effect. |
| Chlorpromazine | Decreased chlorpromazine effect. |
| Digitalis preparations | Decreased digitalis effect. |
| Iron supplements | Decreased iron effect. |
| Isoniazid | Decreased isoniazid effect. |
| Levodopa | Increased levodopa effect. |
| Meperidine | Increased meperidine effect. |
| Nalidixic acid | Decreased nalidixic acid effect. |
| Oxyphenbutazone | Decreased oxyphenbutazone effect. |
| Para-aminosalicylic acid (PAS) | Decreased PAS effect. |
| Penicillins | Decreased penicillin effect. |
| Pentobarbital | Decreased pentobarbital effect. |
| Phenylbutazone | Decreased phenylbutazone effect. |
| Pseudoephedrine | Increased pseudoephedrine effect. |
| Quinidine | Increased quinidine effect. |
| Salicylates | Increased salicylate effect. |
| Sulfa drugs | Decreased sulfa effect. |

## POSSIBLE INTERACTION WITH OTHER SUBSTANCES

| INTERACTS WITH | COMBINED EFFECT |
|---|---|
| Alcohol: | Decreased antacid effect. |
| Beverages: | No proven problems. |
| Cocaine: | No proven problems. |
| Foods: | Decreased antacid effect. Wait 1 hour after eating. |
| Marijuana: | Decreased antacid effect. |
| Tobacco: | Decreased antacid effect. |

# CALCIUM SUPPLEMENTS

## BRAND NAMES

See complete list of brand names in the *Brand Name Directory,* page 946.

## BASIC INFORMATION

**Habit forming? No**
**Prescription needed? For some**
**Available as generic? Yes**
**Drug class: Antihypocalcemic**

 ## USES

- Treats or prevents osteoporosis (thin, porous, easily fractured bones). Frequently prescribed with estrogen beginning at menopause.
- Helps heart, muscle and nervous system to work properly.

 ## DOSAGE & USAGE INFORMATION

**How to take:**
- Take in addition to foods high in calcium (milk, yogurt, sardines, cheese, canned salmon, turnip greens, broccoli, shrimp, tofu).
- Swallow with liquid or food to lessen stomach irritation. If you can't swallow whole, crumble tablet and take with food or liquid.
- Syrup—Take before meals.

**When to take:**
As directed. Don't take within 2 hours of any other medicine you take by mouth.

**If you forget a dose:**
Use as soon as you remember.

**What drug does:**
Participates in metabolism of all activities essential for normal life and function of cells.

**Time lapse before drug works:**
15 to 30 minutes.

*Continued next column*

 ## OVERDOSE

**SYMPTOMS:**
Confusion, irregular heartbeat, depression, bone pain, coma.
**WHAT TO DO:**
- Dial 0 (operator) or 911 (emergency) for an ambulance or medical help. Then give first aid immediately.
- See emergency information on inside covers.

**Don't take with:**
- Any other medicine until 2 hours have passed since taking calcium.
- See Interaction column and consult doctor.

 ## POSSIBLE ADVERSE REACTIONS OR SIDE EFFECTS

| SYMPTOMS | WHAT TO DO |
|---|---|
| **Life-threatening:** | |
| Irregular or very slow heart rate. | Discontinue. Seek emergency treatment. |
| **Common:** | |
| None expected. | |
| **Infrequent:** | |
| Constipation, diarrhea, drowsiness, headache, appetite loss, dry mouth, weakness. | Discontinue. Call doctor right away. |
| **Rare:** | |
| Frequent, painful or difficult urination; increased thirst; nausea, vomiting; rash; urine frequency increased and volume larger; confusion; high blood pressure; eyes sensitive to light. | Discontinue. Call doctor right away. |

## WARNINGS & PRECAUTIONS

**Don't take if:**
- You are allergic to calcium.
- You have a high blood-calcium level.

**Before you start, consult your doctor:**
If you have diarrhea, heart disease, kidney stones, kidney disease, sarcoidosis, malabsorption.

**Over age 60:**
No problems expected.

**Pregnancy:**
No problems expected, but ask your doctor.

**Breast-feeding:**
No problems expected.

**Infants & children:**
Use only under close medical supervision.

**Prolonged use:**
Side effects more likely.

**Skin & sunlight:**
No problems expected.

**Driving, piloting or hazardous work:**
No problems expected.

**Discontinuing:**
No problems expected.

**Others:**
- Exercise, along with vitamin D from sunshine and calcium, helps prevent osteoporosis.
- Don't use bone meal or dolomite as a source for calcium supplement (they may contain lead).

## POSSIBLE INTERACTION WITH OTHER DRUGS

| GENERIC NAME OR DRUG CLASS | COMBINED EFFECT |
|---|---|
| Anticoagulants | Decreased anticoagulant effect. |
| Calcitonin | Decreased calcitonin effect. |
| Chlorpromazine | Decreased chlorpromazine effect. |
| Digitalis preparations | Decreased digitalis effect. |
| Diuretics | Increased calcium in blood. |
| Estrogens and birth control pills | May increase absorption of calcium— frequently a desirable combined effect. |
| Iron supplements | Decreased iron effect. |

| | |
|---|---|
| Meperidine | Increased meperidine effect. |
| Mexiletine | May slow elimination of mexiletine and cause need to adjust dosage. |
| Nalidixic acid | Decreased effect of nalidixic acid. |
| Oxyphenbutazone | Decreased oxyphenbutazone effect. |
| Para-aminosalicylic acid (PAS) | Decreased PAS effect. |
| Penicillins | Decreased penicillin effect. |
| Pentobarbital | Decreased pentobarbital effect. |
| Phenylbutazone | Decreased phenylbutazone effect. |
| Pseudoephedrine | Increased pseudoephedrine effect. |
| Quinidine | Increased quinidine effect. |
| Salicylates | Increased salicylate effect. |
| Sulfa drugs | Decreased sulfa effect. |
| Tetracyclines | Decreased tetracycline effect. |
| Vitamins A and C | Decreased vitamin effect. |

## POSSIBLE INTERACTION WITH OTHER SUBSTANCES

| INTERACTS WITH | COMBINED EFFECT |
|---|---|
| Alcohol: | Decreased absorption of calcium. |
| Beverages: | No problems expected. |
| Cocaine: | No proven problems. |
| Foods: Don't take within 1 or 2 hours of food. | Decreased absorption of calcium. |
| Marijuana: | Decreased absorption of calcium. |
| Tobacco: | Decreased absorption of calcium. |

# CAPTOPRIL

## BRAND NAMES

Capoten

## BASIC INFORMATION

**Habit forming? No**
**Prescription needed? Yes**
**Available as generic? No**
**Drug class: Antihypertensive, A.C.E.**
**inhibitor (See Glossary)**

 ## USES

Treatment for high blood pressure and congestive heart failure.

 ## DOSAGE & USAGE INFORMATION

**How to take:**
Tablets—Swallow with liquid. Instructions to take on empty stomach mean 1 hour before or 2 hours after eating.

**When to take:**
At the same times each day, usually 3 times daily. Take first dose at bedtime and lie down immediately.

**If you forget a dose:**
Take as soon as you remember up to 2 hours late. If more than 2 hours, wait for next scheduled dose (don't double this dose).

**What drug does:**
- Reduces resistance in arteries.
- Strengthens heartbeat.

**Time lapse before drug works:**
60 to 90 minutes.

**Don't take with:**
See Interaction column and consult doctor.

 ## OVERDOSE

**SYMPTOMS:**
**Fever, chills, sore throat, fainting, convulsions, coma.**
**WHAT TO DO:**
- **Dial 0 (operator) or 911 (emergency) for an ambulance or medical help. Then give first aid immediately.**
- **See emergency information on inside covers.**

 ## POSSIBLE ADVERSE REACTIONS OR SIDE EFFECTS

| SYMPTOMS | WHAT TO DO |
|---|---|
| **Life-threatening:**<br>None expected. | |
| **Common:**<br>Rash, loss of taste. | Discontinue. Call doctor right away. |
| **Infrequent:**<br>• Swelling of mouth, face, hands or feet. | Discontinue. Seek emergency treatment. |
| • Dizziness, fainting, chest pain, fast or irregular heartbeat. | Discontinue. Call doctor right away. |
| **Rare:**<br>• Sore throat, cloudy urine, fever, chills. | Discontinue. Call doctor right away. |
| • Nausea, vomiting, indigestion, abdominal pain. | Continue. Call doctor when convenient. |

 ## WARNINGS & PRECAUTIONS

**Don't take if:**
- You are allergic to captopril.
- You have any autoimmune disease, including AIDS or lupus.
- You are receiving blood from a blood bank.
- You take drugs for cancer.
- You will have surgery within 2 months, including dental surgery, requiring general or spinal anesthesia.

**Before you start, consult your doctor:**
- If you have had a stroke.
- If you have angina or heart or blood-vessel disease.
- If you have high level of potassium in blood.
- If you have kidney disease.
- If you are on severe salt-restricted diet.
- If you have lupus.

**Over age 60:**
Adverse reactions and side effects may be more frequent and severe than in younger persons.

**Pregnancy:**
Risk to unborn child outweighs drug benefits. Don't use.

**Breast-feeding:**
Drug passes into milk. Avoid drug or discontinue nursing.

**Infants & children:**
Not recommended.

**Prolonged use:**
May decrease white cells in blood or cause protein loss in urine. Request periodic laboratory blood counts and urine tests.

**Skin & sunlight:**
No problems expected.

**Driving, piloting or hazardous work:**
Avoid if you become dizzy or faint. Otherwise, no problems expected.

**Discontinuing:**
Don't discontinue without consulting doctor. Dose may require gradual reduction if you have taken drug for a long time. Doses of other drugs may also require adjustment.

**Others:**
- Stop taking diuretics or increase salt intake 1 week before starting captopril.
- Avoid exercising in hot weather.

## POSSIBLE INTERACTION WITH OTHER DRUGS

| GENERIC NAME OR DRUG CLASS | COMBINED EFFECT |
|---|---|
| Acebutolol | Increased antihypertensive effect. Dosage of each may require adjustment. |
| Amiloride | Possible excessive potassium in blood. |
| Antihypertensives (other) | Possible excessive blood-pressure drop. |
| Enalapril | Possible excessive potassium in blood. |
| Chloramphenicol | Possible blood disorders. |
| Diuretics | Possible severe blood-pressure drop with first dose. |
| Nitrates | Possible excessive blood-pressure drop. |
| Oxprenolol | Increased antihypertensive effect. Dosage of each may require adjustment. |
| Pentoxifylline | Increased antihypertensive effect. |
| Potassium supplements | Excessive potassium in blood. |
| Spironolactone | Possible excessive potassium in blood. |
| Triamterene | Possible excessive potassium in blood. |

## POSSIBLE INTERACTION WITH OTHER SUBSTANCES

| INTERACTS WITH | COMBINED EFFECT |
|---|---|
| Alcohol: | Possible excessive blood-pressure drop. |
| Beverages: Low-salt milk. | Possible excessive potassium in blood. |
| Cocaine: | Increased dizziness and chest pain. |
| Foods: Salt substitutes. | Possible excessive potassium. |
| Marijuana: | Increased dizziness. |
| Tobacco: | May decrease captopril effect. |

# CAPTOPRIL & HYDROCHLOROTHIAZIDE

## BRAND NAMES

Capozide

## BASIC INFORMATION

**Habit forming?** No
**Prescription needed?** Yes
**Available as generic?** No
**Drug class:** Antihypertensive, diuretic (thiazide), A.C.E. inhibitor (See Glossary)

 **USES**

- Treatment for high blood pressure and congestive heart failure.
- Reduces fluid retention.

 **DOSAGE & USAGE INFORMATION**

**How to take:**
Tablets—Swallow with liquid. Instructions to take on empty stomach mean 1 hour before or 2 hours after eating.

**When to take:**
At the same times each day, usually 3 times daily. Take first dose at bedtime and lie down immediately.

**If you forget a dose:**
Take as soon as you remember up to 2 hours late. If more than 2 hours, wait for next scheduled dose (don't double this dose).

**What drug does:**
- Forces sodium and water excretion, reducing body fluid.
- Relaxes muscle cells of small arteries.
- Reduced body fluid and relaxed arteries lower blood pressure.
- Reduces resistance in arteries.
- Strengthens heartbeat.

*Continued next column*

 **OVERDOSE**

**SYMPTOMS:**
**Cramps, weakness, drowsiness, weak pulse, fever, chills, sore throat, fainting, convulsions, coma.**
**WHAT TO DO:**
- **Dial 0 (operator) or 911 (emergency) for an ambulance or medical help. Then give first aid immediately.**
- **See emergency information on inside covers.**

**Time lapse before drug works:**
4 to 6 hours. May require several weeks to lower blood pressure.

**Don't take with:**
- Non-prescription drugs without consulting doctor.
- See Interaction column and consult doctor.

 **POSSIBLE ADVERSE REACTIONS OR SIDE EFFECTS**

| SYMPTOMS | WHAT TO DO |
|---|---|
| **Life-threatening:** | |
| Irregular heartbeat (fast or uneven). | Discontinue. Seek emergency treatment. |
| **Common:** | |
| • Dry mouth, thirst, tiredness, weakness, muscle cramps, vomiting, chest pain, skin rash. | Discontinue. Call doctor right away. |
| • Taste loss, dizziness. | Continue. Call doctor when convenient. |
| **Infrequent:** | |
| • Face, mouth, hands swell. | Discontinue. Call doctor right away. |
| • Nausea, diarrhea. | Continue. Call doctor when convenient. |
| **Rare:** | |
| None expected. | |

 **WARNINGS & PRECAUTIONS**

**Don't take if:**
- You are allergic to captopril, or any thiazide diuretic drug.
- You have any autoimmune disease, including AIDS or lupus.
- You are receiving blood from a blood bank.
- You take drugs for cancer.
- If you will have surgery within 2 months, including dental surgery, requiring general or spinal anesthesia.

**Before you start, consult your doctor:**
- If you have had a stroke.
- If you have angina, heart or blood-vessel disease, a high level of potassium in blood, lupus, gout, liver, pancreas or kidney disorder.
- If you are on severe salt-restricted diet.
- If you are allergic to any sulfa drug.

**Over age 60:**
Adverse reactions and side effects may be more frequent and severe than in younger persons, especially dizziness and excessive potassium loss.

**Pregnancy:**
Risk to unborn child outweighs drug benefits. Don't use.

**Breast-feeding:**
Drug passes into milk. Avoid drug or discontinue nursing until you finish medicine. Consult doctor for advice on maintaining milk supply.

**Infants & children:**
Not recommended.

**Prolonged use:**
May decrease white cells in blood or cause protein loss in urine. Request periodic laboratory blood counts and urine tests.

**Skin & sunlight:**
May cause rash or intensify sunburn in areas exposed to sun or sunlamp.

**Driving, piloting or hazardous work:**
Don't drive or pilot aircraft until you learn how medicine affects you. Don't work around dangerous machinery. Don't climb ladders or work in high places. Danger increases if you drink alcohol or take medicine affecting alertness and reflexes, such as antihistamines, tranquilizers, sedatives, pain medicine, narcotics and mind-altering drugs.

**Discontinuing:**
Don't discontinue without consulting doctor. Dose may require gradual reduction if you have taken drug for a long time. Doses of other drugs may also require adjustment.

**Others:**
- Hot weather and fever may cause dehydration and drop in blood pressure. Dose may require temporary adjustment. Weigh daily and report any unexpected weight decreases to your doctor.
- May cause rise in uric acid, leading to gout.
- May cause blood-sugar rise in diabetics.

 ## POSSIBLE INTERACTION WITH OTHER DRUGS

| GENERIC NAME OR DRUG CLASS | COMBINED EFFECT |
|---|---|
| Acebutolol | Increased antihypertensive effect. Dosages of both drugs may require adjustments. |
| Allopurinol | Decreased allopurinol effect. |
| Amiloride | Possible excessive potassium in blood. |

| | |
|---|---|
| Antidepressants (tricyclic) | Dangerous drop in blood pressure. Avoid combination unless under medical supervision. |
| Antihypertensives (other) | Possible excessive blood-pressure drop. |
| Barbiturates | Increased hydrochlorothiazide effect. |
| Chloramphenicol | Possible blood disorders. |
| Cholestyramine | Decreased hydrochlorothiazide effect. |
| Cortisone drugs | Excessive potassium loss that causes dangerous heart rhythms. |
| Digitalis preparations | Excessive potassium loss that causes dangerous heart rhythms. |
| Diuretics (thiazide) | Increased effect of other thiazide diuretics. |
| Indapamide | Increased diuretic effect. |
| Lithium | Increased effect of lithium. |
| MAO inhibitors | Increased hydrochlorothiazide effect. |

*Continued page 964*

 ## POSSIBLE INTERACTION WITH OTHER SUBSTANCES

| INTERACTS WITH | COMBINED EFFECT |
|---|---|
| Alcohol: | Dangerous blood-pressure drop. Avoid. |
| Beverages: Low-salt milk. | Possible excessive potassium in blood. |
| Cocaine: | Increased dizziness, chest pain. |
| Foods: Salt substitutes. | Possible excessive potassium. |
| Marijuana: | Increased dizziness, may increase blood pressure. |
| Tobacco: | May decrease captopril effect. |

# CARBAMAZEPINE

## BRAND NAMES

Apo-Carbamazepine     Tegretol
Mazepine

## BASIC INFORMATION

**Habit forming? No**
**Prescription needed? Yes**
**Available as generic? Yes**
**Drug class: Analgesic, anticonvulsant**

 ## USES

- Decreased frequency, severity and duration of attacks of tic douloureaux (See Glossary).
- Prevents seizures.

 ## DOSAGE & USAGE INFORMATION

**How to take:**
Regular or chewable tablet—Swallow with liquid or food to lessen stomach irritation.

**When to take:**
At the same times each day.

**If you forget a dose:**
Take as soon as you remember up to 2 hours late. If more than 2 hours, wait for next scheduled dose (don't double this dose).

**What drug does:**
- Reduces transmission of pain messages at certain nerve terminals.
- Reduces excitability of nerve fibers in brain, thus inhibiting repetitive spread of nerve impulses.

*Continued next column*

 ## OVERDOSE

**SYMPTOMS:**
Involuntary movements, dilated pupils, flushed skin, stupor, coma.
**WHAT TO DO:**
- **Dial 0 (operator) or 911 (emergency) for an ambulance or medical help. Then give first aid immediately.**
- **If patient is unconscious and not breathing, give mouth-to-mouth breathing. If there is no heartbeat, use cardiac massage and mouth-to-mouth breathing (CPR). Don't try to make patient vomit. If you can't get help quickly, take patient to nearest emergency facility.**
- **See emergency information on inside covers.**

**Time lapse before drug works:**
- Tic douloureaux—24 to 72 hours.
- Seizures—1 to 2 weeks.

**Don't take with:**
See Interaction column and consult doctor.

 ## POSSIBLE ADVERSE REACTIONS OR SIDE EFFECTS

| SYMPTOMS | WHAT TO DO |
|---|---|
| **Life-threatening:** None expected. | |
| **Common:** Blurred vision. | Continue. Call doctor when convenient. |
| **Infrequent:** | |
| • Confusion, slurred speech, fainting, depression, headache, hallucinations, hives, rash, mouth sores, sore throat, fever, unusual bleeding or bruising, unusual fatigue. | Discontinue. Call doctor right away. |
| • Diarrhea. | Continue. Call doctor when convenient. |
| **Rare:** | |
| • Back-and-forth eye movements; breathing difficulty; irregular, pounding or slow heartbeat; chest pain; uncontrollable body jerks; numbness, weakness or tingling in hands and feet; tender, bluish legs or feet; less urine; swollen lymph glands. | Discontinue. Call doctor right away. |
| • Frequent urination. | Continue. Call doctor when convenient. |

## WARNINGS & PRECAUTIONS

**Don't take if:**
- You are allergic to carbamazepine.
- You have had liver or bone-marrow disease.
- You have taken MAO inhibitors in the past 2 weeks.

**Before you start, consult your doctor:**
- If you have high blood pressure, thrombophlebitis or heart disease.
- If you have glaucoma.
- If you have emotional or mental problems.
- If you have liver or kidney disease.
- If you drink more than 2 alcoholic drinks per day.

**Over age 60:**
Adverse reactions and side effects may be more frequent and severe than in younger persons.

**Pregnancy:**
Studies inconclusive on harm to unborn child. Animal studies show fetal abnormalities. Decide with your doctor whether drug benefits justify risk to unborn child.

**Breast-feeding:**
Drug passes into milk. Avoid drug or discontinue nursing until you finish medicine. Consult doctor for advice on maintaining milk supply.

**Infants & children:**
Not recommended.

**Prolonged use:**
- Jaundice and liver damage.
- Hair loss.
- Ringing in ears.
- Lower sex drive.

**Skin & sunlight:**
May cause rash or intensify sunburn in areas exposed to sun or sunlamp.

**Driving, piloting or hazardous work:**
Don't drive or pilot aircraft until you learn how medicine affects you. Don't work around dangerous machinery. Don't climb ladders or work in high places. Danger increases if you drink alcohol or take medicine affecting alertness and reflexes.

**Discontinuing:**
Don't discontinue without doctor's advice until you complete prescribed dose, even though symptoms diminish or disappear.

**Others:**
Use only if less-hazardous drugs are not effective. Stay under medical supervision.

## POSSIBLE INTERACTION WITH OTHER DRUGS

| GENERIC NAME OR DRUG CLASS | COMBINED EFFECT |
|---|---|
| Anticoagulants (oral) | Decreased anticoagulant effect. |
| Anticonvulsants (hydantoin) | Decreased effect of both drugs. |
| Antidepressants (tricyclic) | Confusion. Possible psychosis. |
| Contraceptives (oral) | Reduced contraceptive protection. Use another birth-control method. |
| Digitalis preparations | Excess slowing of heart. |
| Doxycycline | Decreased doxycycline effect. |
| MAO inhibitors | Dangerous overstimulation. Avoid. |
| Tranquilizers (benzodiazepine) | Increased carbamazepine effect. |

## POSSIBLE INTERACTION WITH OTHER SUBSTANCES

| INTERACTS WITH | COMBINED EFFECT |
|---|---|
| Alcohol: | Increased sedative effect of alcohol. Avoid. |
| Beverages: | None expected. |
| Cocaine: | Increased adverse effects of carbamazepine. Avoid. |
| Foods: | None expected. |
| Marijuana: | Increased adverse effects of carbamazepine. Avoid. |
| Tobacco: | None expected. |

# CARBENICILLIN

## BRAND NAMES

**Geocillin**          **Pyopen**
**Geopen**

## BASIC INFORMATION

**Habit forming? No**
**Prescription needed? Yes**
**Available as generic? Yes**
**Drug class: Antibiotic (penicillin)**

 ## USES

Treatment of bacterial infections that are susceptible to carbenicillin.

 ## DOSAGE & USAGE INFORMATION

**How to take:**
Tablets or capsules—Swallow with liquid on an empty stomach 1 hour before or 2 hours after eating.

**When to take:**
Follow instructions on prescription label or side of package. Doses should be evenly spaced. For example, 4 times a day means every 6 hours.

**If you forget a dose:**
Take as soon as you remember. Continue regular schedule.

**What drug does:**
Destroys susceptible bacteria. Does not kill viruses.

**Time lapse before drug works:**
May be several days before medicine affects infection.

**Don't take with:**
See Interaction column and consult doctor.

 ## OVERDOSE

**SYMPTOMS:**
**Severe diarrhea, nausea or vomiting.**
**WHAT TO DO:**
**Overdose unlikely to threaten life. If person takes much larger amount than prescribed, call doctor, poison-control center or hospital emergency room for instructions.**

 ## POSSIBLE ADVERSE REACTIONS OR SIDE EFFECTS

| SYMPTOMS | WHAT TO DO |
|---|---|
| **Life-threatening:** | |
| Hives, rash, intense itching, faintness soon after a dose (anaphylaxis). | Seek emergency treatment immediately. |
| **Common:** | |
| Dark or discolored tongue. | Continue. Tell doctor at next visit. |
| **Infrequent:** | |
| Mild nausea, vomiting, diarrhea. | Continue. Call doctor when convenient. |
| **Rare:** | |
| Unexplained bleeding. | Discontinue. Call doctor right away. |

## WARNINGS & PRECAUTIONS

**Don't take if:**
You are allergic to carbenicillin, cephalosporin antibiotics, other penicillins or penicillamine. Life-threatening reaction may occur.

**Before you start, consult your doctor:**
If you are allergic to any substance or drug.

**Over age 60:**
You may have skin reactions, particularly around genitals and anus.

**Pregnancy:**
Studies inconclusive on harm to unborn child. Animal studies show fetal abnormalities. Decide with your doctor whether drug benefits justify risk to unborn child.

**Breast-feeding:**
Drug passes into milk. Child may become sensitive to penicillins and have allergic reactions to penicillin drugs. Avoid carbenicillin or discontinue nursing until you finish medicine. Consult doctor for advice on maintaining milk supply.

**Infants & children:**
No problems expected.

**Prolonged use:**
You may become more susceptible to infections caused by germs not responsive to carbenicillin.

**Skin & sunlight:**
No problems expected.

**Driving, piloting or hazardous work:**
Usually not dangerous. Most hazardous reactions likely to occur a few minutes after taking carbenicillin.

**Discontinuing:**
Don't discontinue without doctor's advice until you complete prescribed dose, even though symptoms diminish or disappear.

**Others:**
Injection forms may cause fluid retention (edema) with weakness and low potassium in the blood.

## POSSIBLE INTERACTION WITH OTHER DRUGS

| GENERIC NAME OR DRUG CLASS | COMBINED EFFECT |
|---|---|
| Beta-adrenergic blockers | Increased chance of anaphylaxis (see emergency information on inside front cover). |
| Chloramphenicol | Decreased effect of both drugs. |
| Erythromycins | Decreased effect of both drugs. |
| Loperamide | Decreased carbenicillin effect. |
| Paromomycin | Decreased effect of both drugs. |
| Tetracyclines | Decreased effect of both drugs. |
| Troleandomycin | Decreased effect of both drugs. |

## POSSIBLE INTERACTION WITH OTHER SUBSTANCES

| INTERACTS WITH | COMBINED EFFECT |
|---|---|
| Alcohol: | Occasional stomach irritation. |
| Beverages: | None expected. |
| Cocaine: | No proven problems. |
| Foods: | Decreased effect of oral carbenicillin. |
| Marijuana: | No proven problems. |
| Tobacco: | None expected. |

# CARBIDOPA & LEVODOPA

## BRAND NAMES

Dopar            Sinemet
Larodopa

## BASIC INFORMATION

Habit forming? No
Prescription needed? Yes
Available as generic? Yes
Drug class: Antiparkinsonism

## USES

Controls Parkinson's disease symptoms such as rigidity, tremor and unsteady gait.

## DOSAGE & USAGE INFORMATION

**How to take:**
Tablet or capsule—Swallow with liquid or food to lessen stomach irritation. If you can't swallow whole, crumble tablet or open capsule and take with liquid or food.

**When to take:**
At the same times each day.

**If you forget a dose:**
Take as soon as you remember up to 2 hours late. If more than 2 hours, wait for next scheduled dose (don't double this dose).

**What drug does:**
Restores chemical balance necessary for normal nerve impulses.

*Continued next column*

## OVERDOSE

**SYMPTOMS:**
Muscle twitch, spastic eyelid closure, nausea, vomiting, diarrhea, irregular and rapid pulse, weakness, fainting, confusion, agitation, hallucination, coma.
**WHAT TO DO:**
- Dial 0 (operator) or 911 (emergency) for an ambulance or medical help. Then give first aid immediately.
- If patient is unconscious and not breathing, give mouth-to-mouth breathing. If there is no heartbeat, use cardiac massage and mouth-to-mouth breathing (CPR). Don't try to make patient vomit. If you can't get help quickly, take patient to nearest emergency facility.
- See emergency information on inside covers.

**Time lapse before drug works:**
2 to 3 weeks to improve; 6 weeks or longer for maximum benefit.

**Don't take with:**
See Interaction column and consult doctor.

## POSSIBLE ADVERSE REACTIONS OR SIDE EFFECTS

| SYMPTOMS | WHAT TO DO |
|---|---|
| **Life-threatening:**<br>None expected. | |
| **Common:** | |
| ● Mood changes, uncontrollable body movements, diarrhea. | Continue. Call doctor when convenient. |
| ● Dry mouth, body odor. | No action necessary. |
| **Infrequent:** | |
| ● Fainting, severe dizziness, headache, insomnia, nightmares, rash, itch, nausea, vomiting, irregular heartbeat. | Discontinue. Call doctor right away. |
| ● Flushed face, blurred vision, muscle twitching, discolored or dark urine, difficult urination. | Continue. Call doctor when convenient. |
| ● Constipation, tiredness. | Continue. Tell doctor at next visit. |
| **Rare:** | |
| ● High blood pressure. | Discontinue. Call doctor right away. |
| ● Duodenal ulcer, anemia. | Continue. Call doctor when convenient. |

## WARNINGS & PRECAUTIONS

**Don't take if:**
- You are allergic to levodopa or carbidopa.
- You have taken MAO inhibitors in past 2 weeks.
- You have glaucoma (narrow-angle type).

**Before you start, consult your doctor:**
- You have diabetes or epilepsy.
- If you have had high blood pressure, heart or lung disease.
- If you have had liver or kidney disease.
- If you have a peptic ulcer.
- If you have malignant melanoma.
- If you will have surgery within 2 months, including dental surgery, requiring general or spinal anesthesia.

**Over age 60:**
Adverse reactions and side effects may be more frequent and severe than in younger persons.

**Pregnancy:**
Risk to unborn child outweighs drug benefits. Don't use.

**Breast-feeding:**
Drug filters into milk. May harm child. Avoid.

**Infants & children:**
Not recommended.

**Prolonged use:**
May lead to uncontrolled movements of head, face, mouth, tongue, arms or legs.

**Skin & sunlight:**
No problems expected.

**Driving, piloting or hazardous work:**
Don't drive or pilot aircraft until you learn how medicine affects you. Don't work around dangerous machinery. Don't climb ladders or work in high places. Danger increases if you drink alcohol or take medicine affecting alertness and reflexes, such as antihistamines, tranquilizers, sedatives, pain medicine, narcotics and mind-altering drugs.

**Discontinuing:**
Don't discontinue without doctor's advice until you complete prescribed dose, even though symptoms diminish or disappear.

**Others:**
Expect to start with small dose and increase gradually to lessen frequency and severity of adverse reactions.

## POSSIBLE INTERACTION WITH OTHER DRUGS

| GENERIC NAME OR DRUG CLASS | COMBINED EFFECT |
|---|---|
| Antiparkinsonism drugs (other) | Increased effect of carbidopa and levodopa. |
| Haloperidol | Decreased effect of carbidopa and levodopa. |
| MAO inhibitors | Dangerous rise in blood pressure. |
| Methyldopa | Decreased effect of carbidopa and levodopa. |
| Papaverine | Decreased effect of carbidopa and levodopa. |
| Phenothiazines | Decreased effect of carbidopa and levodopa. |
| Pyridoxine (Vitamin B-6) | Decreased effect carbidopa and levodopa. |
| Rauwolfia alkaloids | Decreased effect carbidopa and levodopa. |

## POSSIBLE INTERACTION WITH OTHER SUBSTANCES

| INTERACTS WITH | COMBINED EFFECT |
|---|---|
| Alcohol: | None expected. |
| Beverages: | None expected. |
| Cocaine: | Decreased carbidopa and levodopa effect. |
| Foods: | None expected. |
| Marijuana: | Increased fatigue, lethargy, fainting. |
| Tobacco: | None expected. |

# CARBINOXAMINE

## BRAND NAMES

Clistin         Clistin R-A

## BASIC INFORMATION

**Habit forming? No**
**Prescription needed? Yes**
**Available as generic? No**
**Drug class: Antihistamine**

 **USES**

Reduces allergic symptoms such as hay fever, hives, rash or itching.

 **DOSAGE & USAGE INFORMATION**

**How to take:**
- Tablet—Swallow with liquid or food to lessen stomach irritation.
- Extended-release tablets—Swallow each dose whole. If you take regular tablets, you may chew or crush them.

**When to take:**
Varies with form. Follow label directions.

**If you forget a dose:**
Take as soon as you remember up to 2 hours late. If more than 2 hours, wait for next scheduled dose (don't double this dose).

**What drug does:**
Blocks action of histamine after an allergic response triggers histamine release in sensitive cells.

**Time lapse before drug works:**
30 minutes.

*Continued next column*

 **OVERDOSE**

**SYMPTOMS:**
**Convulsions, red face, hallucinations, coma.**
**WHAT TO DO:**
- **Dial 0 (operator) or 911 (emergency) for an ambulance or medical help. Then give first aid immediately.**
- **If patient is unconscious and not breathing, give mouth-to-mouth breathing. If there is no heartbeat, use cardiac massage and mouth-to-mouth breathing (CPR). Don't try to make patient vomit. If you can't get help quickly, take patient to nearest emergency facility.**
- **See emergency information on inside covers.**

**Don't take with:**
See Interaction column and consult doctor.

 **POSSIBLE ADVERSE REACTIONS OR SIDE EFFECTS**

| SYMPTOMS | WHAT TO DO |
|---|---|
| **Life-threatening:**<br>None expected. | |
| **Common:**<br>Drowsiness; dizziness; nausea; dry mouth, nose, throat. | Continue. Tell doctor at next visit. |
| **Infrequent:**<br>• Changes in vision. | Discontinue. Call doctor right away. |
| • Less tolerance for contact lenses, urination difficulty. | Continue. Call doctor when convenient. |
| • Appetite loss. | Continue. Tell doctor at next visit. |
| **Rare:**<br>Nightmares, agitation, irritability, sore throat, fever, rapid heartbeat, unusual bleeding or bruising, fatigue, weakness. | Discontinue. Call doctor right away. |

146

## WARNINGS & PRECAUTIONS

**Don't take if:**
You are allergic to any antihistamine.

**Before you start, consult your doctor:**
- If you have glaucoma.
- If you have enlarged prostate.
- If you have asthma.
- If you have kidney disease.
- If you have peptic ulcer.
- If you will have surgery within 2 months, including dental surgery, requiring general or spinal anesthesia.

**Over age 60:**
Don't exceed recommended dose. Adverse reactions and side effects may be more frequent and severe than in younger persons, especially urination difficulty, diminished alertness and other brain and nervous-system symptoms.

**Pregnancy:**
No proven harm to unborn child. Avoid if possible.

**Breast-feeding:**
Drug passes into milk. Avoid drug or discontinue nursing until you finish medicine. Consult doctor for advice on maintaining milk supply.

**Infants & children:**
Not recommended for premature or newborn infants. Otherwise, no problems expected.

**Prolonged use:**
Avoid. May damage bone marrow and nerve cells.

**Skin & sunlight:**
May cause rash or intensify sunburn in areas exposed to sun or sunlamp.

**Driving, piloting or hazardous work:**
Don't drive or pilot aircraft until you learn how medicine affects you. Don't work around dangerous machinery. Don't climb ladders or work in high places. Danger increases if you drink alcohol or take medicine affecting alertness and reflexes, such as antihistamines, tranquilizers, sedatives, pain medicine, narcotics and mind-altering drugs.

**Discontinuing:**
No problems expected.

**Others:**
May mask symptoms of hearing damage from aspirin, other salicylates, cisplatin, paromomycin, vancomycin or anticonvulsants. Consult doctor if you use these.

## POSSIBLE INTERACTION WITH OTHER DRUGS

| GENERIC NAME OR DRUG CLASS | COMBINED EFFECT |
|---|---|
| Anticholinergics | Increased anticholinergic effect. |
| Antidepressants | Increased carbinoxamine effect. Excess sedation. Avoid. |
| Antihistamines (other) | Excess sedation. Avoid. |
| Dronabinol | Increased effects of both drugs. Avoid. |
| Hypnotics | Excess sedation. Avoid. |
| MAO inhibitors | Increased carbinoxamine effect. |
| Mind-altering drugs | Excess sedation. Avoid. |
| Molindone | Increased antihistamine effect. |
| Narcotics | Excess sedation. Avoid. |
| Sedatives | Excess sedation. Avoid. |
| Sleep inducers | Excess sedation. Avoid. |
| Tranquilizers | Excess sedation. Avoid. |

## POSSIBLE INTERACTION WITH OTHER SUBSTANCES

| INTERACTS WITH | COMBINED EFFECT |
|---|---|
| Alcohol: | Excess sedation. Avoid. |
| Beverages: Caffeine drinks. | Less carbinoxamine sedation. |
| Cocaine: | Decreased carbinoxamine effect. Avoid. |
| Foods: | None expected. |
| Marijuana: | Excess sedation. Avoid. |
| Tobacco: | None expected. |

# CARBONIC ANHYDRASE INHIBITORS

## BRAND AND GENERIC NAMES

Acetazolam
ACETAZOLAMIDE
Ak-Zol
Apo-Acetazolamide
Cetazol
Daranide
Dazamide

Diamox
Diamox Sequels
DICHLORPHENAMIDE
METHAZOLAMIDE
Neptazane
Oratrol

## BASIC INFORMATION

Habit forming? No
Prescription needed? Yes
Available as generic? Yes
Drug class: Carbonic anhydrase inhibitor
(See Glossary)

## USES

- Treatment of glaucoma.
- Treatment of epileptic seizures.
- Treatment of body-fluid retention.
- Treatment for shortness of breath, insomnia and fatigue in high altitudes.

## DOSAGE & USAGE INFORMATION

**How to take:**
Tablets—Swallow whole with liquid or food to lessen stomach irritation.

**When to take:**
- 1 dose per day—At the same time each morning.
- More than 1 dose per day—Take last dose several hours before bedtime.

**If you forget a dose:**
Take as soon as you remember. Continue regular schedule.

*Continued next column*

## OVERDOSE

**SYMPTOMS:**
Drowsiness, confusion, excitement, nausea, vomiting, numbness in hands and feet, coma.

**WHAT TO DO:**
- Call your doctor or poison-control center for advice if you suspect overdose, even if not sure. Symptoms may not appear until damage has occurred.
- See emergency information on inside covers.

---

**What drug does:**
- Inhibits action of carbonic anhydrase, an enzyme. This lowers the internal eye pressure by decreasing fluid formation in the eye.
- Forces sodium and water excretion, reducing body fluid.

**Time lapse before drug works:**
2 hours.

**Don't take with:**
- Non-prescription drugs without consulting doctor.
- See Interaction column and consult doctor.

## POSSIBLE ADVERSE REACTIONS OR SIDE EFFECTS

| SYMPTOMS | WHAT TO DO |
|---|---|
| **Life-threatening:** Convulsions. | Seek emergency treatment immediately. |
| **Common:** None expected. | |
| **Infrequent:** | |
| • Back pain. | Discontinue. Call doctor right away. |
| • Fatigue, weakness, tingling or burning in feet or hands. | Continue. Call doctor when convenient. |
| **Rare:** Headache; mood changes; nervousness; clumsiness; trembling; confusion; hives; itch, rash; sores; ringing in ears; hoarseness; dry mouth; thirst; sore throat; fever; appetite change; nausea; vomiting; black, tarry stool; breathing difficulty; irregular or weak heartbeat; easy bleeding or bruising; muscle cramps; painful or frequent urination; blood in urine. | Discontinue. Call doctor right away. |

## WARNINGS & PRECAUTIONS

**Don't take if:**
- You are allergic to any carbonic anhydrase inhibitor.
- You have liver or kidney disease.
- You have Addison's disease (adrenal gland failure).
- You have diabetes.

**Before you start, consult your doctor:**
- If you have gout or lupus.
- If you are allergic to any sulfa drug.
- If you will have surgery within 2 months, including dental surgery, requiring general or spinal anesthesia.

**Over age 60:**
- Don't exceed recommended dose.
- If you take a digitalis preparation, eat foods high in potassium content or take a potassium supplement.

**Pregnancy:**
No proven harm to unborn child. Avoid if possible, especially first 3 months.

**Breast-feeding:**
Avoid drug or don't nurse your infant.

**Infants & children:**
Not recommended for children younger than 12.

**Prolonged use:**
May cause kidney stones, vision change, loss of taste and smell, jaundice or weight loss.

**Skin & sunlight:**
No problems expected.

**Driving, piloting or hazardous work:**
Avoid if you feel drowsy or dizzy. Otherwise, no problems expected.

**Discontinuing:**
Don't discontinue without medical advice.

**Others:**
Medicine may increase sugar levels in blood and urine. Diabetics may need insulin adjustment.

## POSSIBLE INTERACTION WITH OTHER DRUGS

| GENERIC NAME OR DRUG CLASS | COMBINED EFFECT |
|---|---|
| Amphetamines | Increased amphetamine effect. |
| Anticonvulsants | Increased loss of bone minerals. |
| Antidepressants (tricyclic) | Increased antidepressant effect. |
| Antidiabetics (oral) | Increased potassium loss. |
| Aspirin | Decreased aspirin effect. |
| Cortisone drugs | Increased potassium loss. |
| Digitalis preparations | Possible digitalis toxicity. |
| Diuretics | Increased potassium loss. |
| Lithium | Decreased lithium effect. |
| Methenamine | Decreased methenamine effect. |
| Mexiletene | May slow elimination of mexilitene and cause need to adjust dosage. |
| Quinidine | Increased quinidine effect. |
| Salicylates | Salicylate toxicity. |
| Sympathomimetics | Increased sympathomimetic effect. |

## POSSIBLE INTERACTION WITH OTHER SUBSTANCES

| INTERACTS WITH | COMBINED EFFECT |
|---|---|
| Alcohol: | None expected. |
| Beverages: | None expected. |
| Cocaine: | Avoid. Decreased carbonic anhydrase inhibitor effect. |
| Foods: Potassium-rich foods (see Glossary). | Eat these to decrease potassium loss. |
| Marijuana: | Avoid. Increased carbonic anhydrase inhibitor effect. |
| Tobacco: | May decrease absorption of carbonic anhydrase inhibitors. |

# CARISOPRODOL

## BRAND NAMES

Rela          Soma Compound
Soma        Soprodol

## BASIC INFORMATION

**Habit forming? No**
**Prescription needed? Yes**
**Available as generic? Yes**
**Drug class: Muscle relaxant (skeletal)**

## USES

Treatment for sprains, strains and muscle spasms.

## DOSAGE & USAGE INFORMATION

**How to take:**
Tablet or capsule—Swallow with liquid.

**When to take:**
As needed, no more often than every 4 hours.

**If you forget a dose:**
Take as soon as you remember. Wait 4 hours for next dose.

**What drug does:**
Blocks body's pain messages to brain. May also sedate.

**Time lapse before drug works:**
60 minutes.

**Don't take with:**
See Interaction column and consult doctor.

## OVERDOSE

**SYMPTOMS:**
**Nausea, vomiting, diarrhea, headache. May progress to severe weakness, difficult breathing, sensation of paralysis, coma.**
**WHAT TO DO:**
- **Dial 0 (operator) or 911 (emergency) for an ambulance or medical help. Then give first aid immediately.**
- **See emergency information on inside covers.**

## POSSIBLE ADVERSE REACTIONS OR SIDE EFFECTS

| SYMPTOMS | WHAT TO DO |
|---|---|
| **Life-threatening:** | |
| None expected. | |
| **Common:** | |
| ● Drowsiness, fainting, dizziness. | Continue. Call doctor when convenient. |
| ● Orange or red-purple urine. | No action necessary. |
| **Infrequent:** | |
| Agitation, constipation or diarrhea; nausea; cramps; vomiting; wheezing; shortness of breath. | Discontinue. Call doctor right away. |
| **Rare:** | |
| ● Black, tarry or bloody stool. | Discontinue. Seek emergency treatment. |
| ● Rash, hives, or itch; sore throat; fever; jaundice; tiredness; weakness. | Discontinue. Call doctor right away. |

# CARISOPRODOL

## WARNINGS & PRECAUTIONS

**Don't take if:**
- You are allergic to any skeletal-muscle relaxant.
- You have porphyria.

**Before you start, consult your doctor:**
- If you have had liver or kidney disease.
- If you plan pregnancy within medication period.

**Over age 60:**
Adverse reactions and side effects may be more frequent and severe than in younger persons.

**Pregnancy:**
No proven harm to unborn child. Avoid if possible.

**Breast-feeding:**
Drug passes into milk. Avoid drug or discontinue nursing until you finish medicine. Consult doctor for advice on maintaining milk supply.

**Infants & children:**
Not recommended.

**Prolonged use:**
Periodic liver-function tests recommended if you use this drug for a long time.

**Skin & sunlight:**
No problems expected.

**Driving, piloting or hazardous work:**
Don't drive or pilot aircraft until you learn how medicine affects you. Don't work around dangerous machinery. Don't climb ladders or work in high places. Danger increases if you drink alcohol or take medicine affecting alertness and reflexes, such as antihistamines, tranquilizers, sedatives, pain medicine, narcotics and mind-altering drugs.

**Discontinuing:**
Don't discontinue without doctor's advice until you complete prescribed dose, even though symptoms diminish or disappear.

**Others:**
No problems expected.

## POSSIBLE INTERACTION WITH OTHER DRUGS

| GENERIC NAME OR DRUG CLASS | COMBINED EFFECT |
|---|---|
| Antidepressants | Increased sedation. |
| Antihistamines | Increased sedation. |
| Dronabinol | Increased effect of dronabinol on central nervous system. Avoid combination. |
| Mind-altering drugs | Increased sedation. |
| Muscle relaxants (others) | Increased sedation. |
| Narcotics | Increased sedation. |
| Sedatives | Increased sedation. |
| Sleep inducers | Increased sedation. |
| Testosterone | Decreased carisoprodol effect. |
| Tranquilizers | Increased sedation. |

## POSSIBLE INTERACTION WITH OTHER SUBSTANCES

| INTERACTS WITH | COMBINED EFFECT |
|---|---|
| Alcohol: | Increased sedation. |
| Beverages: | None expected. |
| Cocaine: | Lack of coordination, increased sedation. |
| Foods: | None expected. |
| Marijuana: | Lack of coordination, drowsiness, fainting. |
| Tobacco: | None expected. |

151

# CARPHENAZINE

## BRAND NAMES

Proketazine

## BASIC INFORMATION

**Habit forming? No**
**Prescription needed? Yes**
**Available as generic? Yes**
**Drug class: Tranquilizer, antiemetic**
**(phenothiazine)**

## USES

- Stops nausea, vomiting.
- Reduces anxiety, agitation.

## DOSAGE & USAGE INFORMATION

**How to take:**
- Tablet or capsule—Swallow with liquid or food to lessen stomach irritation.
- Suppositories—Remove wrapper and moisten suppository with water. Gently insert into rectum, large end first.
- Drops or liquid—Dilute dose in beverage.

**When to take:**
- Nervous and mental disorders—Take at the same times each day.
- Nausea and vomiting—Take as needed, no more often than every 4 hours.

**If you forget a dose:**
- Nervous and mental disorders—Take up to 2 hours late. If more than 2 hours, wait for next scheduled dose (don't double this dose).
- Nausea and vomiting—Take as soon as you remember. Wait 4 hours for next dose.

**What drug does:**
- Suppresses brain's vomiting center.
- Suppresses brain centers that control abnormal emotions and behavior.

**Time lapse before drug works:**
- Nausea and vomiting—1 hour or less.
- Nervous and mental disorders—4-6 weeks.

*Continued next column*

## OVERDOSE

**SYMPTOMS:**
**Stupor, convulsions, coma.**
**WHAT TO DO:**
- **Dial 0 (operator) or 911 (emergency) for an ambulance or medical help. Then give first aid immediately.**
- **See emergency information on inside covers.**

**Don't take with:**
- Antacid or medicine for diarrhea.
- Non-prescription drug for cough, cold or allergy.
- See Interaction column and consult doctor.

## POSSIBLE ADVERSE REACTIONS OR SIDE EFFECTS

| SYMPTOMS | WHAT TO DO |
|---|---|
| **Life-threatening:** | |
| None expected. | |
| **Common:** | |
| • Muscle spasms of face and neck, unsteady gait. | Discontinue. Seek emergency treatment. |
| • Restlessness, tremor, drowsiness. | Discontinue. Call doctor right away. |
| • Decreased sweating, dry mouth, stuffy nose, constipation. | Continue. Call doctor when convenient. |
| **Infrequent:** | |
| • Fainting. | Discontinue. Seek emergency treatment. |
| • Rash. | Discontinue. Call doctor right away. |
| • Difficult urination, diminished sex drive, swollen breasts, menstrual irregularities. | Continue. Call doctor when convenient. |
| **Rare:** | |
| Changes in vision, sore throat, fever, jaundice. | Discontinue. Call doctor right away. |

## WARNINGS & PRECAUTIONS

**Don't take if:**
- You are allergic to any phenothiazine.
- You have a blood or bone-marrow disease.

**Before you start, consult your doctor:**
- If you will have surgery within 2 months, including dental surgery, requiring general or spinal anesthesia.
- If you have asthma, emphysema or other lung disorder.
- If you take non-prescription ulcer medicine, asthma medicine or amphetamines.

**Over age 60:**
Adverse reactions and side effects may be more frequent and severe than in younger persons. More likely to develop involuntary movement of jaws, lips, tongue, chewing. Report this to your doctor immediately. Early treatment can help.

**Pregnancy:**
Risk to unborn child outweighs drug benefits. Don't use.

**Breast-feeding:**
Drug passes into milk. Avoid drug or discontinue nursing until you finish medicine. Consult doctor for advice on maintaining milk supply.

**Infants & children:**
Don't give to children younger than 2.

**Prolonged use:**
May lead to tardive dyskinesia (involuntary movement of jaws, lips, tongue, chewing).

**Skin & sunlight:**
May cause rash or intensify sunburn in areas exposed to sun or sunlamp. Skin may remain sensitive for 3 months after discontinuing.

**Driving, piloting or hazardous work:**
Don't drive or pilot aircraft until you learn how medicine affects you. Don't work around dangerous machinery. Don't climb ladders or work in high places. Danger increases if you drink alcohol or take medicine affecting alertness and reflexes.

**Discontinuing:**
- Nervous and mental disorders—Don't discontinue without doctor's advice until you complete prescribed dose, even though symptoms diminish or disappear.
- Nausea and vomiting—May be unnecessary to finish medicine. Follow doctor's instructions.

**Others:**
No problems expected.

## POSSIBLE INTERACTION WITH OTHER DRUGS

| GENERIC NAME OR DRUG CLASS | COMBINED EFFECT |
|---|---|
| Anticholinergics | Increased anticholinergic effect. |
| Antidepressants (tricyclic) | Increased carphenazine effect. |
| Antihistamines | Increased antihistamine effect. |
| Appetite suppressants | Decreased suppressant effect. |
| Dronabinol | Increased effects of both drugs. Avoid. |
| Levodopa | Decreased levodopa effect. |
| Mind-altering drugs | Increased effect of mind-altering drugs. |
| Narcotics | Increased narcotic effect. |
| Phenytoin | Increased phenytoin effect. |
| Quinidine | Impaired heart function. Dangerous mixture. |
| Sedatives | Increased sedative effect. |
| Tranquilizers (other) | Increased tranquilizer effect. |

## POSSIBLE INTERACTION WITH OTHER SUBSTANCES

| INTERACTS WITH | COMBINED EFFECT |
|---|---|
| Alcohol: | Dangerous oversedation. |
| Beverages: | None expected. |
| Cocaine: | Decreased carphenazine effect. Avoid. |
| Foods: | None expected. |
| Marijuana: | Drowsiness. May increase antinausea effect. |
| Tobacco: | None expected. |

# CASCARA

## BRAND NAMES

Aromatic Cascara
  Fluidextract
Cascara Sagrada
Cas-Evac

Milk of
  Magnesia-Cascara
Peri-Colace

## BASIC INFORMATION

**Habit forming? No**
**Prescription needed? No**
**Available as generic? Yes**
**Drug class: Laxative (stimulant)**

 ## USES

Constipation relief.

 ## DOSAGE & USAGE INFORMATION

**How to take:**
- Tablet—Swallow with liquid. If you can't swallow whole, chew or crumble tablet and take with liquid or food.
- Liquid—Drink 6 to 8 glasses of water each day, in addition to one taken with each dose.

**When to take:**
Usually at bedtime with a snack, unless directed otherwise.

**If you forget a dose:**
Take as soon as you remember.

**What drug does:**
Acts on smooth muscles of intestine wall to cause vigorous bowel movement.

**Time lapse before drug works:**
6 to 10 hours.

**Don't take with:**
- See Interaction column and consult doctor.
- Don't take within 2 hours of taking another medicine. Laxative interferes with medicine absorption.

 ## OVERDOSE

**SYMPTOMS:**
Vomiting, electrolyte depletion.
**WHAT TO DO:**
Overdose unlikely to threaten life. If person takes much larger amount than prescribed, call doctor, poison-control center or hospital emergency room for instructions.

 ## POSSIBLE ADVERSE REACTIONS OR SIDE EFFECTS

| SYMPTOMS | WHAT TO DO |
|---|---|
| **Life-threatening:** | |
| None expected. | |
| **Common:** | |
| Rectal irritation. | Continue. Call doctor when convenient. |
| **Infrequent:** | |
| • Dangerous potassium loss. | Discontinue. Call doctor right away. |
| • Belching, cramps, nausea. | Continue. Call doctor when convenient. |
| **Rare:** | |
| • Irritability, confusion, headache, rash, breathing difficulty, irregular heartbeat, muscle cramps, unusual tiredness or weakness. | Discontinue. Call doctor right away. |
| • Burning on urination. | Continue. Call doctor when convenient. |

## WARNINGS & PRECAUTIONS

**Don't take if:**
- You have symptoms of appendicitis, inflamed bowel or intestinal blockage.
- You are allergic to a stimulant laxative.
- You have missed a bowel movement for only 1 or 2 days.

**Before you start, consult your doctor:**
- If you have a colostomy or ileostomy.
- If you have congestive heart disease.
- If you have diabetes.
- If you have high blood pressure.
- If you have a laxative habit.
- If you have rectal bleeding.
- If you take other laxatives.

**Over age 60:**
Adverse reactions and side effects may be more frequent and severe than in younger persons.

**Pregnancy:**
Risk to mother and unborn child outweighs drug benefits. Don't use.

**Breast-feeding:**
Drug passes into milk. Avoid drug or discontinue nursing until you finish medicine. Consult doctor for advice on maintaining milk supply.

**Infants & children:**
Use only under medical supervision.

**Prolonged use:**
Don't take for more than 1 week unless under a doctor's supervision. May cause laxative dependence.

**Skin & sunlight:**
No problems expected.

**Driving, piloting or hazardous work:**
No problems expected.

**Discontinuing:**
May be unnecessary to finish medicine. Follow doctor's instructions.

**Others:**
Don't take to "flush out" your system or as a "tonic."

## POSSIBLE INTERACTION WITH OTHER DRUGS

| GENERIC NAME OR DRUG CLASS | COMBINED EFFECT |
|---|---|
| Antihypertensives | May cause dangerous low potassium level. |
| Diuretics | May cause dangerous low potassium level. |

## POSSIBLE INTERACTION WITH OTHER SUBSTANCES

| INTERACTS WITH | COMBINED EFFECT |
|---|---|
| Alcohol: | None expected. |
| Beverages: | None expected. |
| Cocaine: | None expected. |
| Foods: | None expected. |
| Marijuana: | None expected. |
| Tobacco: | None expected. |

# CASTOR OIL

## BRAND NAMES

Alphamul
Emulsoil
Fleet Prep Kit
Granulex
Hydrisinol

Kellogg's
Neoloid
Purge
Stimuzyme Plus
Unisoil

## BASIC INFORMATION

**Habit forming? No**
**Prescription needed? No**
**Available as generic? Yes**
**Drug class: Laxative (stimulant)**

 ## USES

Constipation relief.

 ## DOSAGE & USAGE INFORMATION

**How to take:**
Liquid—Drink 6 to 8 glasses of water each day, in addition to one taken with each dose.

**When to take:**
Usually at bedtime with a snack, unless directed otherwise.

**If you forget a dose:**
Take as soon as you remember.

**What drug does:**
Acts on smooth muscles of intestine wall to cause vigorous bowel movement.

**Time lapse before drug works:**
2 to 6 hours.

**Don't take with:**
- See Interaction column and consult doctor.
- Don't take within 2 hours of taking another medicine. Laxative interferes with medicine absorption.

 ## OVERDOSE

**SYMPTOMS:**
**Vomiting, electrolyte depletion.**
**WHAT TO DO:**
**Overdose unlikely to threaten life. If person takes much larger amount than prescribed, call doctor, poison-control center or hospital emergency room for instructions.**

 ## POSSIBLE ADVERSE REACTIONS OR SIDE EFFECTS

| SYMPTOMS | WHAT TO DO |
|---|---|
| **Life-threatening:** None expected. | |
| **Common:** Rectal irritation. | Continue. Call doctor when convenient. |
| **Infrequent:** | |
| • Dangerous potassium loss. | Discontinue. Call doctor right away. |
| • Belching, cramps, nausea. | Continue. Call doctor when convenient. |
| **Rare:** | |
| • Irritability, confusion, headache, rash, breathing difficulty, irregular heartbeat, muscle cramps, unusual tiredness or weakness. | Discontinue. Call doctor right away. |
| • Burning on urination. | Continue. Call doctor when convenient. |

## WARNINGS & PRECAUTIONS

**Don't take if:**
- You have symptoms of appendicitis, inflamed bowel or intestinal blockage.
- You are allergic to a stimulant laxative.
- You have missed a bowel movement for only 1 or 2 days.

**Before you start, consult your doctor:**
- If you have a colostomy or ileostomy.
- If you have congestive heart disease.
- If you have diabetes.
- If you have high blood pressure.
- If you have a laxative habit.
- If you have rectal bleeding.
- If you take other laxatives.

**Over age 60:**
Adverse reactions and side effects may be more frequent and severe than in younger persons.

**Pregnancy:**
Risk to mother and unborn child outweighs drug benefits. Don't use.

**Breast-feeding:**
Drug passes into milk. Avoid drug or discontinue nursing until you finish medicine. Consult doctor for advice on maintaining milk supply.

**Infants & children:**
Use only under medical supervision.

**Prolonged use:**
Don't take for more than 1 week unless under doctor's supervision. May cause laxative dependence.

**Skin & sunlight:**
No problems expected.

**Driving, piloting or hazardous work:**
No problems expected.

**Discontinuing:**
May be unnecessary to finish medicine. Follow doctor's instructions.

**Others:**
Don't take to "flush out" your system or as a "tonic."

 ## POSSIBLE INTERACTION WITH OTHER DRUGS

| GENERIC NAME OR DRUG CLASS | COMBINED EFFECT |
| --- | --- |
| Antihypertensives | May cause dangerous low potassium level. |
| Diuretics | May cause dangerous low potassium level. |

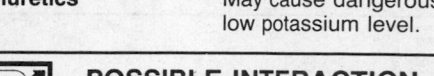 ## POSSIBLE INTERACTION WITH OTHER SUBSTANCES

| INTERACTS WITH | COMBINED EFFECT |
| --- | --- |
| Alcohol: | None expected. |
| Beverages: | None expected. |
| Cocaine: | None expected. |
| Foods: | None expected. |
| Marijuana: | None expected. |
| Tobacco: | None expected. |

# CEFACLOR

## BRAND NAMES

Ceclor

## BASIC INFORMATION

**Habit forming? No**
**Prescription needed? Yes**
**Available as generic? No**
**Drug class: Antibiotic (cephalosporin)**

 ## USES

Treatment of bacterial infections. Will not cure viral infections such as cold and flu.

 ## DOSAGE & USAGE INFORMATION

**How to take:**
- Tablet or capsule—Swallow with liquid. If you can't swallow whole, crumble tablet or open capsule and take with liquid or food.
- Liquid—Use measuring spoon.

**When to take:**
At same times each day, 1 hour before or 2 hours after eating.

**If you forget a dose:**
Take as soon as you remember or double next dose. Return to regular schedule.

**What drug does:**
Kills susceptible bacteria.

**Time lapse before drug works:**
May require several days to affect infection.

**Don't take with:**
See Interaction column and consult doctor.

 ## OVERDOSE

**SYMPTOMS:**
**Abdominal cramps, nausea, vomiting, severe diarrhea with mucus or blood in stool.**
**WHAT TO DO:**
**Overdose unlikely to threaten life. If person takes much larger amount than prescribed, call doctor, poison-control center or hospital emergency room for instructions.**

 ## POSSIBLE ADVERSE REACTIONS OR SIDE EFFECTS

| SYMPTOMS | WHAT TO DO |
|---|---|
| **Life-threatening:** | |
| Hives, rash, intense itching, faintness soon after a dose (anaphylaxis). | Seek emergency treatment immediately. |
| **Common:** | |
| Rash, redness, itching. | Discontinue. Call doctor right away. |
| **Infrequent:** | |
| Rectal itching. | Continue. Call doctor when convenient. |
| **Rare:** | |
| Mild nausea, vomiting, cramps, severe diarrhea with mucus or blood in stool, unusual weakness, tiredness, weight loss, fever. | Discontinue. Call doctor right away. |

## WARNINGS & PRECAUTIONS

**Don't take if:**
You are allergic to any cephalosporin antibiotic.

**Before you start, consult your doctor:**
- If you are allergic to any penicillin antibiotic.
- If you have a kidney disorder.
- If you have colitis or enteritis.

**Over age 60:**
Adverse reactions and side effects may be more frequent and severe than in younger persons. More likely to itch around rectum and genitals.

**Pregnancy:**
No proven harm to unborn child. Avoid if possible.

**Breast-feeding:**
Drug passes into milk. Avoid drug or discontinue nursing until you finish medicine. Consult doctor for advice on maintaining milk supply.

**Infants & children:**
No special warnings.

**Prolonged use:**
Kills beneficial bacteria that protect body against other germs. Unchecked germs may cause secondary infections.

**Skin & sunlight:**
No problems expected.

**Driving, piloting or hazardous work:**
No problems expected.

**Discontinuing:**
Don't discontinue without doctor's advice until you complete prescribed dose, even though symptoms diminish or disappear.

**Others:**
No problems expected.

 ## POSSIBLE INTERACTION WITH OTHER DRUGS

| GENERIC NAME OR DRUG CLASS | COMBINED EFFECT |
|---|---|
| Anticoagulants | Increased anticoagulant effect. |
| Loperamide | Reduced cefaclor effect. |
| Probenecid | Increased cefaclor effect. |

 ## POSSIBLE INTERACTION WITH OTHER SUBSTANCES

| INTERACTS WITH | COMBINED EFFECT |
|---|---|
| Alcohol: | None expected. |
| Beverages: | None expected. |
| Cocaine: | None expected, but cocaine may slow body's recovery. Avoid. |
| Foods: | Slow absorption. Take with liquid 1 hour before or 2 hours after eating. |
| Marijuana: | None expected, but marijuana may slow body's recovery. Avoid. |
| Tobacco: | None expected. |

# CEFADROXIL

## BRAND NAMES

Duricef                Ultracef

## BASIC INFORMATION

**Habit forming? No**
**Prescription needed? Yes**
**Available as generic? No**
**Drug class: Antibiotic (cephalosporin)**

 ## USES

Treatment of bacterial infections. Will not cure viral infections such as cold and flu.

 ## DOSAGE & USAGE INFORMATION

**How to take:**
- Tablet or capsule—Swallow with liquid. If you can't swallow whole, crumble tablet or open capsule and take with liquid or food.
- Liquid—Use measuring spoon.

**When to take:**
At same times each day, 1 hour before or 2 hours after eating.

**If you forget a dose:**
Take as soon as you remember or double next dose. Return to regular schedule.

**What drug does:**
Kills susceptible bacteria.

**Time lapse before drug works:**
May require several days to affect infection.

**Don't take with:**
See Interaction column and consult doctor.

 ## OVERDOSE

**SYMPTOMS:**
Abdominal cramps, nausea, vomiting, severe diarrhea with mucus or blood in stool.
**WHAT TO DO:**
Overdose unlikely to threaten life. If person takes much larger amount than prescribed, call doctor, poison-control center or hospital emergency room for instructions.

 ## POSSIBLE ADVERSE REACTIONS OR SIDE EFFECTS

| SYMPTOMS | WHAT TO DO |
|---|---|
| **Life-threatening:** | |
| Hives, rash, intense itching, faintness soon after a dose (anaphylaxis). | Seek emergency treatment immediately. |
| **Common:** | |
| Rash, redness, itching. | Discontinue. Call doctor right away. |
| **Infrequent:** | |
| Rectal itching. | Continue. Call doctor when convenient. |
| **Rare:** | |
| Mild nausea, vomiting, cramps, severe diarrhea with mucus or blood in stool, unusual weakness, tiredness, weight loss, fever. | Discontinue. Call doctor right away. |

## WARNINGS & PRECAUTIONS

**Don't take if:**
You are allergic to any cephalosporin antibiotic.

**Before you start, consult your doctor:**
• If you are allergic to any penicillin antibiotic.
• If you have a kidney disorder.
• If you have colitis or enteritis.

**Over age 60:**
Adverse reactions and side effects may be more frequent and severe than in younger persons. More likely to itch around rectum and genitals.

**Pregnancy:**
No proven harm to unborn child. Avoid if possible.

**Breast-feeding:**
Drug passes into milk. Avoid drug or discontinue nursing until you finish medicine. Consult doctor for advice on maintaining milk supply.

**Infants & children:**
No special warnings.

**Prolonged use:**
Kills beneficial bacteria that protect body against other germs. Unchecked germs may cause secondary infections.

**Skin & sunlight:**
No problems expected.

**Driving, piloting or hazardous work:**
No problems expected.

**Discontinuing:**
Don't discontinue without doctor's advice until you complete prescribed dose, even though symptoms diminish or disappear.

**Others:**
No problems expected.

 ## POSSIBLE INTERACTION WITH OTHER DRUGS

| GENERIC NAME OR DRUG CLASS | COMBINED EFFECT |
|---|---|
| Anticoagulants | Increased anticoagulant effect. |
| Loperamide | Reduced cefadroxil effect. |
| Probenecid | Increased cefadroxil effect. |

 ## POSSIBLE INTERACTION WITH OTHER SUBSTANCES

| INTERACTS WITH | COMBINED EFFECT |
|---|---|
| Alcohol: | None expected. |
| Beverages: | None expected. |
| Cocaine: | None expected, but cocaine may slow body's recovery. Avoid. |
| Foods: | Slow absorption. Take with liquid 1 hour before or 2 hours after eating. |
| Marijuana: | None expected, but marijuana may slow body's recovery. Avoid. |
| Tobacco: | None expected. |

161

# CEPHALEXIN

## BRAND NAMES

Ceporex               Novolexin
Keflex

## BASIC INFORMATION

**Habit forming? No**
**Prescription needed? Yes**
**Available as generic? No**
**Drug class: Antibiotic (cephalosporin)**

 **USES**

Treatment of bacterial infections. Will not cure viral infections such as cold and flu.

 **DOSAGE & USAGE INFORMATION**

**How to take:**
- Tablet or capsule—Swallow with liquid. If you can't swallow whole, crumble tablet or open capsule and take with liquid or food.
- Liquid—Use measuring spoon.

**When to take:**
At same times each day, 1 hour before or 2 hours after eating.

**If you forget a dose:**
Take as soon as you remember or double next dose. Return to regular schedule.

**What drug does:**
Kills susceptible bacteria.

**Time lapse before drug works:**
May require several days to affect infection.

**Don't take with:**
See Interaction column and consult doctor.

 **OVERDOSE**

**SYMPTOMS:**
**Abdominal cramps, nausea, vomiting, severe diarrhea with mucus or blood in stool.**
**WHAT TO DO:**
**Overdose unlikely to threaten life. If person takes much larger amount than prescribed, call doctor, poison-control center or hospital emergency room for instructions.**

 **POSSIBLE ADVERSE REACTIONS OR SIDE EFFECTS**

| SYMPTOMS | WHAT TO DO |
|---|---|
| **Life-threatening:** | |
| Hives, rash, intense itching, faintness soon after a dose (anaphylaxis). | Seek emergency treatment immediately. |
| **Common:** | |
| Rash, redness, itching. | Discontinue. Call doctor right away. |
| **Infrequent:** | |
| Rectal itching. | Continue. Call doctor when convenient. |
| **Rare:** | |
| Mild nausea, vomiting, cramps, severe diarrhea with mucus or blood in stool, unusual weakness, tiredness, weight loss, fever. | Discontinue. Call doctor right away. |

## WARNINGS & PRECAUTIONS

**Don't take if:**
You are allergic to any cephalosporin antibiotic.

**Before you start, consult your doctor:**
• If you are allergic to any penicillin antibiotic.
• If you have a kidney disorder.
• If you have colitis or enteritis.

**Over age 60:**
Adverse reactions and side effects may be more frequent and severe than in younger persons. More likely to itch around rectum and genitals.

**Pregnancy:**
No proven harm to unborn child. Avoid if possible.

**Breast-feeding:**
Drug passes into milk. Avoid drug or discontinue nursing until you finish medicine. Consult doctor for advice on maintaining milk supply.

**Infants & children:**
No special warnings.

**Prolonged use:**
Kills beneficial bacteria that protect body against other germs. Unchecked germs may cause secondary infections.

**Skin & sunlight:**
No problems expected.

**Driving, piloting or hazardous work:**
No problems expected.

**Discontinuing:**
Don't discontinue without doctor's advice until you complete prescribed dose, even though symptoms diminish or disappear.

**Others:**
No problems expected.

## POSSIBLE INTERACTION WITH OTHER DRUGS

| GENERIC NAME OR DRUG CLASS | COMBINED EFFECT |
|---|---|
| Anticoagulants | Increased anticoagulant effect. |
| Probenecid | Increased cephalexin effect. |

## POSSIBLE INTERACTION WITH OTHER SUBSTANCES

| INTERACTS WITH | COMBINED EFFECT |
|---|---|
| Alcohol: | None expected. |
| Beverages: | None expected. |
| Cocaine: | None expected, but cocaine may slow body's recovery. Avoid. |
| Foods: | Slow absorption. Take with liquid 1 hour before or 2 hours after eating. |
| Marijuana: | None expected, but marijuana may slow body's recovery. Avoid. |
| Tobacco: | None expected. |

# CEPHRADINE

## BRAND NAMES

Anspor                    Velosef

## BASIC INFORMATION

**Habit forming?** No
**Prescription needed?** Yes
**Available as generic?** No
**Drug class:** Antibiotic (cephalosporin)

 ## USES

Treatment of bacterial infections. Will not cure viral infections such as cold and flu.

 ## DOSAGE & USAGE INFORMATION

**How to take:**
- Tablet or capsule—Swallow with liquid. If you can't swallow whole, crumble tablet or open capsule and take with liquid or food.
- Liquid—Use measuring spoon.

**When to take:**
At same times each day, 1 hour before or 2 hours after eating.

**If you forget a dose:**
Take as soon as you remember or double next dose. Return to regular schedule.

**What drug does:**
Kills susceptible bacteria.

**Time lapse before drug works:**
May require several days to affect infection.

**Don't take with:**
See Interaction column and consult doctor.

 ## OVERDOSE

**SYMPTOMS:**
Abdominal cramps, nausea, vomiting, severe diarrhea with mucus or blood in stool.
**WHAT TO DO:**
Overdose unlikely to threaten life. If person takes much larger amount than prescribed, call doctor, poison-control center or hospital emergency room for instructions.

 ## POSSIBLE ADVERSE REACTIONS OR SIDE EFFECTS

| SYMPTOMS | WHAT TO DO |
|---|---|
| **Life-threatening:** | |
| Hives, rash, intense itching, faintness soon after a dose (anaphylaxis). | Seek emergency treatment immediately. |
| **Common:** | |
| Rash, redness, itching. | Discontinue. Call doctor right away. |
| **Infrequent:** | |
| Rectal itching. | Continue. Call doctor when convenient. |
| **Rare:** | |
| Mild nausea, vomiting, cramps, severe diarrhea with mucus or blood in stool, unusual weakness, tiredness, weight loss, fever. | Discontinue. Call doctor right away. |

## WARNINGS & PRECAUTIONS

**Don't take if:**
You are allergic to any cephalosporin antibiotic.

**Before you start, consult your doctor:**
- If you are allergic to any penicillin antibiotic.
- If you have a kidney disorder.
- If you have colitis or enteritis.

**Over age 60:**
Adverse reactions and side effects may be more frequent and severe than in younger persons. More likely to itch around rectum and genitals.

**Pregnancy:**
No proven harm to unborn child. Avoid if possible.

**Breast-feeding:**
Drug passes into milk. Avoid drug or discontinue nursing until you finish medicine. Consult doctor for advice on maintaining milk supply.

**Infants & children:**
No special warnings.

**Prolonged use:**
Kills beneficial bacteria that protect body against other germs. Unchecked germs may cause secondary infections.

**Skin & sunlight:**
No problems expected.

**Driving, piloting or hazardous work:**
No problems expected.

**Discontinuing:**
Don't discontinue without doctor's advice until you complete prescribed dose, even though symptoms diminish or disappear.

**Others:**
No problems expected.

## POSSIBLE INTERACTION WITH OTHER DRUGS

| GENERIC NAME OR DRUG CLASS | COMBINED EFFECT |
|---|---|
| Anticoagulants | Increased anticoagulant effect. |
| Probenecid | Increased cephradine effect. |

## POSSIBLE INTERACTION WITH OTHER SUBSTANCES

| INTERACTS WITH | COMBINED EFFECT |
|---|---|
| Alcohol: | None expected. |
| Beverages: | None expected. |
| Cocaine: | None expected, but cocaine may slow body's recovery. Avoid. |
| Foods: | Slow absorption. Take with liquid 1 hour before or 2 hours after eating. |
| Marijuana: | None expected, but marijuana may slow body's recovery. Avoid. |
| Tobacco: | None expected. |

# CHARCOAL, ACTIVATED

## BRAND NAMES

| | |
|---|---|
| Actidose-Aqua | Charcocaps |
| Arm-a-Char | Charcodote |
| Charcoaid | Insta-Char |
| Charcoalanti Dote | Liquid-Antidose |

## BASIC INFORMATION

**Habit forming? No**
**Prescription needed? No**
**Available as generic? Yes**
**Drug class: Antidote (adsorbent)**

## USES

- Treatment of poisonings from medication.
- Treatment (infrequent) for diarrhea or excessive gaseousness.

## DOSAGE & USAGE INFORMATION

**How to take:**
- Tablet or capsule—Swallow with liquid. If you can't swallow whole, crumble tablet or open capsule and take with liquid or food.
- Liquid—Take as directed on label.

**When to take:**
- For poisoning—Take immediately after poisoning. If your doctor or emergency poison control center has also recommended syrup of ipecac, don't take charcoal for 30 minutes or until vomiting from ipecac stops.
- For diarrhea or gas—Take at same times each day.

**If you forget a dose:**
- For poisonings—Not applicable.
- For diarrhea or gas—Take as soon as you remember up to 2 hours late. If more than 2 hours, wait for next scheduled dose (don't double this dose).

**What drug does:**
- Helps prevent poison from being absorbed from stomach and intestines.
- Helps absorb gas in intestinal tract.

*Continued next column*

## OVERDOSE

**SYMPTOMS:**
**None expected.**
**WHAT TO DO:**
**Overdose unlikely to threaten life. If person takes much larger amount than prescribed, call doctor, poison-control center or hospital emergency room for instructions.**

**Time lapse before drug works:**
Begins immediately.

**Don't take with:**
Ice cream or sherbet.

## POSSIBLE ADVERSE REACTIONS OR SIDE EFFECTS

| SYMPTOMS | WHAT TO DO |
|---|---|
| **Life-threatening:**<br>None expected. | |
| **Always:**<br>Black bowel movements. | No action necessary. |
| **Infrequent:**<br>None expected. | |
| **Rare:**<br>None expected. | |

## WARNINGS & PRECAUTIONS

**Don't take if:**
The poison was lye or other strong alkali, strong acids (such as sulfuric acid), cyanide, iron, ethyl alcohol or methyl alcohol. Charcoal will not prevent these poisons from causing ill effects.

**Before you start, consult your doctor:**
If you are taking it as an antidote for poison.

**Over age 60:**
No problems expected.

**Pregnancy:**
No problems expected.

**Breast-feeding:**
No problems expected.

**Infants & children:**
Don't give to children for more than 3 or 4 days for diarrhea. Continuing for longer periods can interfere with normal nutrition.

**Prolonged use:**
No problems expected.

**Skin & sunlight:**
No problems expected.

**Driving, piloting or hazardous work:**
No problems expected.

**Discontinuing:**
No problems expected.

**Others:**
No problems expected.

## POSSIBLE INTERACTION WITH OTHER DRUGS

| GENERIC NAME OR DRUG CLASS | COMBINED EFFECT |
|---|---|
| Any medicine taken at the same time | May decrease absorption of medicine. |

## POSSIBLE INTERACTION WITH OTHER SUBSTANCES

| INTERACTS WITH | COMBINED EFFECT |
|---|---|
| Alcohol: | None expected. |
| Beverages: | None expected. |
| Cocaine: | None expected. |
| Foods:<br>Ice cream or sherbet. | Decreased charcoal effect. |
| Marijuana: | None expected. |
| Tobacco: | None expected. |

# CHLOPHEDIANOL

## BRAND NAMES

Ulo                    Ulone

## BASIC INFORMATION

Habit forming? No
Prescription needed? Yes
Available as generic? No
Drug class: Cough suppressant

 ## USES

Reduces non-productive cough due to bronchial irritation.

 ## DOSAGE & USAGE INFORMATION

**How to take:**
Take syrup without diluting. Don't drink fluids immediately after medicine.

**When to take:**
3 or 4 times a day when needed. No more often than every 3 hours.

**If you forget a dose:**
Take as soon as you remember up to 2 hours late. If more than 2 hours, wait for next scheduled dose (don't double this dose).

**What drug does:**
Reduces cough reflex by direct effect on cough center in brain, and by local anesthetic action.

**Time lapse before drug works:**
30 minutes to 1 hour.

**Don't take with:**
- Alcohol or brain depressant or stimulant drugs.
- See Interaction column and consult doctor.

 ## OVERDOSE

**SYMPTOMS:**
Blurred vision, hallucinations, coma.
**WHAT TO DO:**
- Dial 0 (operator) or 911 (emergency) for an ambulance or medical help. Then give first aid immediately.
- If patient is unconscious and not breathing, give mouth-to-mouth breathing. If there is no heartbeat, use cardiac massage and mouth-to-mouth breathing (CPR). Don't try to make patient vomit. If you can't get help quickly, take patient to nearest emergency facility.
- See emergency information on inside covers.

 ## POSSIBLE ADVERSE REACTIONS OR SIDE EFFECTS

| SYMPTOMS | WHAT TO DO |
|---|---|
| **Life-threatening**<br>None expected. | |
| **Common:**<br>Difficult urination in older men with enlarged prostate. | Continue. Call doctor when convenient. |
| **Infrequent:**<br>None expected. | |
| **Rare:**<br>• Hallucinations, drowsiness, rash or hives, nausea, vomiting, irregular heartbeat. | Discontinue. Call doctor right away. |
| • Nightmares, excitement or irritability, blurred vision, dry mouth. | Continue. Call doctor when convenient. |

## WARNINGS & PRECAUTIONS

**Don't take if:**
You are allergic to chlophedianol.

**Before you start, consult your doctor:**
- If medicine is for hyperactive child who takes medicine for treatment.
- If your cough brings up sputum (phlegm).
- If you have heart disease.
- If you will have surgery within 2 months, including dental surgery, requiring general or spinal anesthesia.

**Over age 60:**
Adverse reactions and side effects may be more frequent and severe than in younger persons.

**Pregnancy:**
Risk to unborn child outweighs drug benefits. Don't use.

**Breast-feeding:**
Unknown whether medicine filters into milk. Consult doctor.

**Infants & children:**
Not recommended for children under age 2.

**Prolonged use:**
Not recommended. If cough persists despite medicine, consult doctor.

**Skin & sunlight:**
No problems expected.

**Driving, piloting or hazardous work:**
Don't drive or pilot aircraft until you learn how medicine affects you. Don't work around dangerous machinery. Don't climb ladders or work in high places. Danger increases if you drink alcohol or take medicine affecting alertness and reflexes, such as antihistamines, tranquilizers, sedatives, pain medicine, narcotics and mind-altering drugs.

**Discontinuing:**
May be unnecessary to finish medicine. Follow doctor's instructions.

**Others:**
Consult doctor if cough persists despite medication for 7 days or if fever, skin rash or headache accompany cough.

## POSSIBLE INTERACTION WITH OTHER DRUGS

| GENERIC NAME OR DRUG CLASS | COMBINED EFFECT |
|---|---|
| Anticonvulsants | Interferes with actions of both. |
| Antidepressants (tricyclic) | Excess sedation. |
| Appetite suppressants | Excess stimulation. |
| Central-nervous-system depressants: antidepressants, antihistamines, muscle relaxants, narcotics, pain pills, sedatives, sleeping pills, tranquilizers. | Excess sedation. |
| MAO inhibitors | Excess sedation. |
| Sympathomimetics | Excess stimulation. |

## POSSIBLE INTERACTION WITH OTHER SUBSTANCES

| INTERACTS WITH | COMBINED EFFECT |
|---|---|
| Alcohol: | Excess sedation. Avoid. |
| Beverages: Coffee, tea, cocoa, cola. | Excess stimulation. Avoid. |
| Cocaine: | Increased chance of toxic stimulation. Avoid. |
| Foods: | None expected. |
| Marijuana: | Increased chance of toxic stimulation. Avoid. |
| Tobacco: | Decreased effect of chlophedianol. |

# CHLORAL HYDRATE

## BRAND NAMES

Aquachloral
Aquachloral
  Supprettes
Colidrate
Noctec

Novochlorhydrate
Oradrate
SK-Chloral Hydrate

## BASIC INFORMATION

**Habit forming? Yes**
**Prescription needed? Yes**
**Available as generic? Yes**
**Drug class: Hypnotic**

## USES

- Reduces anxiety.
- Relieves insomnia.

## DOSAGE & USAGE INFORMATION

**How to take:**
- Tablet or capsule—Swallow with milk or food to lessen stomach irritation.
- Drops—Dilute dose in beverage before swallowing.
- Suppositories—Remove wrapper and moisten suppository with water. Gently insert larger end into rectum. Push well into rectum with finger.

**When to take:**
At the same time each day.

**If you forget a dose:**
Take as soon as you remember up to 2 hours late. If more than 2 hours, wait for next scheduled dose (don't double this dose).

*Continued next column*

## OVERDOSE

**SYMPTOMS:**
**Confusion, weakness, breathing difficulty, stagger, slow or irregular heartbeat.**
**WHAT TO DO:**
- **Dial 0 (operator) or 911 (emergency) for an ambulance or medical help. Then give first aid immediately.**
- **If patient is unconscious and not breathing, give mouth-to-mouth breathing. If there is no heartbeat, use cardiac massage and mouth-to-mouth breathing (CPR). Don't try to make patient vomit. If you can't get help quickly, take patient to nearest emergency facility.**
- **See emergency information on inside covers.**

**What drug does:**
Affects brain centers that control wakefulness and alertness.

**Time lapse before drug works:**
30 to 60 minutes.

**Don't take with:**
See Interaction column and consult doctor.

## POSSIBLE ADVERSE REACTIONS OR SIDE EFFECTS

| SYMPTOMS | WHAT TO DO |
|---|---|
| **Life-threatening:**<br>None expected. | |
| **Common:**<br>Nausea, stomach pain, vomiting. | Discontinue. Call doctor right away. |
| **Infrequent:**<br>"Hangover" effect, clumsiness or unsteadiness, drowsiness, dizziness, lightheadedness. | Continue. Call doctor when convenient. |
| **Rare:**<br>• Hallucinations, agitation, confusion. | Discontinue. Call doctor right away. |
| • Hives, rash. | Continue. Call doctor when convenient. |

## WARNINGS & PRECAUTIONS

**Don't take if:**
You are allergic to chloral hydrate.

**Before you start, consult your doctor:**
- If you have had liver, kidney or heart trouble.
- If you are prone to stomach upsets (if medicine is in oral form).
- If you have colitis or a rectal inflammation (if medicine is in suppository form).

**Over age 60:**
Adverse reactions and side effects may be more frequent and severe than in younger persons. More likely to have "hangover" effect.

**Pregnancy:**
Risk to unborn child outweighs drug benefits. Unborn child may become addicted to drug. Don't use.

**Breast-feeding:**
Drug filters into milk. May harm child. Avoid.

**Infants & children:**
Use only under medical supervision.

**Prolonged use:**
Addiction and possible kidney damage.

**Skin & sunlight:**
No problems expected.

**Driving, piloting or hazardous work:**
Don't drive or pilot aircraft until you learn how medicine affects you. Don't work around dangerous machinery. Don't climb ladders or work in high places. Danger increases if you drink alcohol or take medicine affecting alertness and reflexes, such as antihistamines, tranquilizers, sedatives, pain medicine, narcotics and mind-altering drugs.

**Discontinuing:**
Don't discontinue without consulting doctor. Dose may require gradual reduction if you have taken drug for a long time. Doses of other drugs may also require adjustment.

**Others:**
Frequent kidney-function tests recommended when drug is used for long time.

## POSSIBLE INTERACTION WITH OTHER DRUGS

| GENERIC NAME OR DRUG CLASS | COMBINED EFFECT |
| --- | --- |
| Anticoagulants | Possible hemorrhaging. |
| Antidepressants | Increased chloral hydrate effect. |
| Antihistamines | Increased chloral hydrate effect. |
| Cortisone drugs | Decreased cortisone effect. |
| MAO inhibitors | Increased chloral hydrate effect. |
| Mind-altering drugs | Increased chloral hydrate effect. |
| Molindone | Increased tranquilizer effect. |
| Narcotics | Increased chloral hydrate effect. |
| Pain relievers | Increased chloral hydrate effect. |
| Phenothiazines | Increased chloral hydrate effect. |
| Sedatives | Increased chloral hydrate effect. |
| Sleep inducers | Increased chloral hydrate effect. |
| Tranquilizers | Increased chloral hydrate effect. |

## POSSIBLE INTERACTION WITH OTHER SUBSTANCES

| INTERACTS WITH | COMBINED EFFECT |
| --- | --- |
| Alcohol: | Increased sedative effect of both. Avoid. |
| Beverages: | None expected. |
| Cocaine: | Decreased chloral hydrate effect. Avoid. |
| Foods: | None expected. |
| Marijuana: | May severely impair mental and physical functioning. Avoid. |
| Tobacco: | None expected. |

# CHLORAMBUCIL

## BRAND NAMES

Leukeran

## BASIC INFORMATION

Habit forming? No
Prescription needed? Yes
Available as generic? No
Drug class: Antineoplastic,
    immunosuppressant

 **USES**

- Treatment for some kinds of cancer.
- Suppresses immune response after transplant and in immune disorders.

 **DOSAGE & USAGE INFORMATION**

**How to take:**
Tablet or capsule—Swallow with liquid after light meal. Don't drink fluids with meals. Drink extra fluids between meals. Avoid sweet or fatty foods.

**When to take:**
At the same time each day.

**If you forget a dose:**
Take as soon as you remember. Don't ever double dose.

**What drug does:**
Inhibits abnormal cell reproduction. May suppress immune system.

**Time lapse before drug works:**
Up to 6 weeks for full effect.

*Continued next column*

 **OVERDOSE**

**SYMPTOMS:**
Bleeding, chills, fever, collapse, stupor, seizure.
**WHAT TO DO:**
- Dial 0 (operator) or 911 (emergency) for an ambulance or medical help. Then give first aid immediately.
- If patient is unconscious and not breathing, give mouth-to-mouth breathing. If there is no heartbeat, use cardiac massage and mouth-to-mouth breathing (CPR). Don't try to make patient vomit. If you can't get help quickly, take patient to nearest emergency facility.
- See emergency information on inside covers.

**Don't take with:**
See Interaction column and consult doctor.

 **POSSIBLE ADVERSE REACTIONS OR SIDE EFFECTS**

| SYMPTOMS | WHAT TO DO |
|---|---|
| **Life-threatening:**<br>None expected. | |
| **Common:** | |
| • Unusual bleeding or bruising, mouth sores with sore throat, chills and fever, black stools, mouth and lip sores, menstrual irregularities. | Discontinue. Call doctor right away. |
| • Hair loss, joint pain. | Continue. Call doctor when convenient. |
| • Nausea, vomiting, diarrhea (unavoidable), tiredness, weakness. | Continue. Tell doctor at next visit. |
| **Infrequent:** | |
| • Mental confusion, shortness of breath; may increase chance of developing leukemia. | Continue. Call doctor when convenient. |
| • Cough. | Continue. Tell doctor at next visit. |
| **Rare:**<br>Jaundice. | Discontinue. Call doctor right away. |

172

## WARNINGS & PRECAUTIONS

**Don't take if:**
- You have had hypersensitivity to alkylating antineoplastic drugs.
- Your physician has not explained serious nature of your medical problem and risks of taking this medicine.

**Before you start, consult your doctor:**
- If you have gout.
- If you have had kidney stones.
- If you have active infection.
- If you have impaired kidney or liver function.
- If you have taken other antineoplastic drugs or had radiation treatment in last 3 weeks.

**Over age 60:**
Adverse reactions and side effects may be more frequent and severe than in younger persons.

**Pregnancy:**
Consult doctor. Risk to child is significant.

**Breast-feeding:**
Drug passes into milk. Don't nurse.

**Infants & children:**
Use only under care of medical supervisors who are experienced in anticancer drugs.

**Prolonged use:**
Adverse reactions more likely the longer drug is required.

**Skin & sunlight:**
No problems expected.

**Driving, piloting or hazardous work:**
No problems expected.

**Discontinuing:**
Don't discontinue without doctor's advice until you complete prescribed dose, even though symptoms diminish or disappear. Some side effects may follow discontinuing. Report to doctor blurred vision, convulsions, confusion, persistent headache.

**Others:**
May cause sterility.

## POSSIBLE INTERACTION WITH OTHER DRUGS

| GENERIC NAME OR DRUG CLASS | COMBINED EFFECT |
|---|---|
| Antigout drugs | Decreased antigout effect. |
| Antineoplastic drugs (other) | Increased effect of all drugs, (may be beneficial). |
| Chloramphenicol | Increased likelihood of toxic effects of both drugs. |

## POSSIBLE INTERACTION WITH OTHER SUBSTANCES

| INTERACTS WITH | COMBINED EFFECT |
|---|---|
| Alcohol: | May increase chance of intestinal bleeding. |
| Beverages: | No problems expected. |
| Cocaine: | Increases chance of toxicity. |
| Foods: | Reduces irritation in stomach. |
| Marijuana: | No problems expected. |
| Tobacco: | Increases lung toxicity. |

# CHLORAMPHENICOL

## BRAND NAMES

| | |
|---|---|
| Amphicol | Mychel |
| Antibiopto | Mychel-S |
| Chloromycetin | Nova-Phenicol |
| Chloroptic | Novochlorocap |
| Econochlor | Ophthochlor |
| Fenicol | Ophthocort |
| Isopto Fenicol | Pentamycetin |
| Minims | Sopamycetin |

## BASIC INFORMATION

**Habit forming? No**
**Prescription needed? Yes**
**Available as generic? Yes**
**Drug class: Antibiotic**

## USES

Treatment of infections susceptible to chloramphenicol.

## DOSAGE & USAGE INFORMATION

**How to take:**
- Tablet or capsule—Swallow with liquid.
- Eye solution or ointment, ear solution or cream—Follow label instructions.

**When to take:**
Tablet or capsule—1 hour before or 2 hours after eating.

**If you forget a dose:**
Take as soon as you remember up to 2 hours late. If more than 2 hours, wait for next scheduled dose (don't double this dose).

**What drug does:**
Prevents bacteria from growing and reproducing. Will not kill viruses.

**Time lapse before drug works:**
2 to 5 days, depending on type and severity of infection.

**Don't take with:**
See Interaction column and consult doctor.

## OVERDOSE

**SYMPTOMS:**
**Nausea, vomiting, diarrhea.**
**WHAT TO DO:**
**Overdose unlikely to threaten life. If person takes much larger amount than prescribed, call doctor, poison-control center or hospital emergency room for instructions.**

## POSSIBLE ADVERSE REACTIONS OR SIDE EFFECTS

| SYMPTOMS | WHAT TO DO |
|---|---|
| **Life-threatening:** | |
| Hives, rash, intense itching, faintness soon after a dose (anaphylaxis). | Seek emergency treatment immediately. |
| **Common:** | |
| None expected. | |
| **Infrequent:** | |
| • Swollen face or extremities; diarrhea; nausea; vomiting; numbness, tingling, burning pain or weakness in hands and feet. | Discontinue. Call doctor right away. |
| • Headache, confusion. | Continue. Call doctor when convenient. |
| **Rare:** | |
| Pain, blurred vision, possible vision loss, sore throat, fever, jaundice, anemia. | Discontinue. Call doctor right away. |

## WARNINGS & PRECAUTIONS

**Don't take if:**
- You are allergic to chloramphenicol.
- It is prescribed for a minor disorder such as flu, cold or mild sore throat.

**Before you start, consult your doctor:**
- If you have had a blood disorder or bone-marrow disease.
- If you have had kidney or liver disease.
- If you have diabetes.

**Over age 60:**
Adverse reactions and side effects may be more frequent and severe than in younger persons, particularly skin irritation around rectum.

**Pregnancy:**
Risk to unborn child outweighs drug benefits. Don't use.

**Breast-feeding:**
Drug passes into milk. Avoid drug or discontinue nursing until you finish medicine. Consult doctor for advice on maintaining milk supply.

**Infants & children:**
Don't give to infants younger than 2.

**Prolonged use:**
You may become more susceptible to infections caused by germs not responsive to chloramphenicol.

**Skin & sunlight:**
No problems expected.

**Driving, piloting or hazardous work:**
Don't drive or pilot aircraft until you learn how medicine affects you. Don't work around dangerous machinery. Don't climb ladders or work in high places. Danger increases if you drink alcohol or take medicine affecting alertness and reflexes.

**Discontinuing:**
Don't discontinue without doctor's advice until you complete prescribed dose, even though symptoms diminish or disappear.

**Others:**
- Chloramphenicol can cause serious anemia. Frequent laboratory blood studies, liver and kidney tests recommended.
- Second medical opinion recommended before starting.

## POSSIBLE INTERACTION WITH OTHER DRUGS

| GENERIC NAME OR DRUG CLASS | COMBINED EFFECT |
|---|---|
| Anticoagulants | Increased anticoagulant effect. |
| Antidiabetics (oral) | Increased antidiabetic effect. |
| Cyclophosphamide | Decreased cyclophosphamide effect. |
| Flecainide | Possible decreased blood-cell production in bone marrow. |
| Penicillins | Decreased penicillin effect. |
| Phenytoin | Increased phenytoin effect. |
| Tocainide | Possible decreased blood-cell production in bone marrow. |

## POSSIBLE INTERACTION WITH OTHER SUBSTANCES

| INTERACTS WITH | COMBINED EFFECT |
|---|---|
| Alcohol: | Possible liver problems. May cause disulfiram reaction (see Glossary). |
| Beverages: | None expected. |
| Cocaine: | No proven problems. |
| Foods: | None expected. |
| Marijuana: | None expected. |
| Tobacco: | None expected. |

# CHLORDIAZEPOXIDE

## BRAND AND GENERIC NAMES

Apo-
  Chlordiazepoxide
CHLORDIAZEPOXIDE
Libritabs
Librium
Lipoxide
Medilium

Murcil
Novopoxide
Reposans
Sereen
SK-Lygen
Solium

## BASIC INFORMATION

**Habit forming? Yes**
**Prescription needed? Yes**
**Available as generic? Yes**
**Drug class: Tranquilizer (benzodiazepine)**

 ## USES

- Treatment for nervousness or tension.
- Treatment for muscle spasm.
- Treatment for convulsive disorders.

 ## DOSAGE & USAGE INFORMATION

**How to take:**
Tablet or capsule—Swallow with liquid. If you can't swallow whole, crumble tablet or open capsule and take with liquid or food.

**When to take:**
At the same time each day, according to instructions on prescription label.

**If you forget a dose:**
Take as soon as you remember up to 2 hours late. If more than 2 hours, wait for next scheduled dose (don't double this dose).

*Continued next column*

 ## OVERDOSE

**SYMPTOMS:**
**Drowsiness, weakness, tremor, stupor, coma.**
**WHAT TO DO:**
- **Dial 0 (operator) or 911 (emergency) for an ambulance or medical help. Then give first aid immediately.**
- **If patient is unconscious and not breathing, give mouth-to-mouth breathing. If there is no heartbeat, use cardiac massage and mouth-to-mouth breathing (CPR). Don't try to make patient vomit. If you can't get help quickly, take patient to nearest emergency facility.**
- **See emergency information on inside covers.**

**What drug does:**
Affects limbic system of brain—part that controls emotions.

**Time lapse before drug works:**
2 hours. May take 6 weeks for full benefit.

**Don't take with:**
See Interaction column and consult doctor.

 ## POSSIBLE ADVERSE REACTIONS OR SIDE EFFECTS

| SYMPTOMS | WHAT TO DO |
|---|---|
| **Life-threatening:** None expected. | |
| **Common:** Clumsiness, drowsiness, dizziness. | Continue. Call doctor when convenient. |
| **Infrequent:** | |
| • Hallucinations, confusion, depression, irritability, rash, itch, vision changes. | Discontinue. Call doctor right away. |
| • Constipation or diarrhea, nausea, vomiting, difficult urination. | Continue. Call doctor when convenient. |
| **Rare:** | |
| • Slow heartbeat, breathing difficulty. | Discontinue. Seek emergency treatment. |
| • Mouth, throat ulcers; jaundice. | Discontinue. Call doctor right away. |

## WARNINGS & PRECAUTIONS

**Don't take if:**
- You are allergic to any benzodiazepine.
- You have myasthenia gravis.
- You are active or recovering alcoholic.
- Patient is younger than 6 months.

**Before you start, consult your doctor:**
- If you have liver, kidney or lung disease.
- If you have diabetes, epilepsy or porphyria.

**Over age 60:**
Adverse reactions and side effects may be more frequent and severe than in younger persons. You need smaller doses for shorter periods of time. May develop agitation, rage or "hangover" effect.

**Pregnancy:**
Risk to unborn child outweighs drug benefits. Don't use.

**Breast-feeding:**
Drug passes into milk. Avoid drug or discontinue nursing until you finish medicine. Consult doctor for advice on maintaining milk supply.

**Infants & children:**
Use only under medical supervision for children older than 6 months.

**Prolonged use:**
May impair liver function.

**Skin & sunlight:**
No problems expected.

**Driving, piloting or hazardous work:**
Don't drive or pilot aircraft until you learn how medicine affects you. Don't work around dangerous machinery. Don't climb ladders or work in high places. Danger increases if you drink alcohol or take medicine affecting alertness and reflexes.

**Discontinuing:**
Don't discontinue without consulting doctor. Dose may require gradual reduction if you have taken drug for a long time. Doses of other drugs may also require adjustment.

**Others:**
- Hot weather, heavy exercise and profuse sweat may reduce excretion and cause overdose.
- Blood sugar may rise in diabetics, requiring insulin adjustment.

## POSSIBLE INTERACTION WITH OTHER DRUGS

| GENERIC NAME OR DRUG CLASS | COMBINED EFFECT |
|---|---|
| Anticonvulsants | Change in seizure frequency or severity. |
| Antidepressants | Increased sedative effect of both drugs. |
| Antihistamines | Increased sedative effect of both drugs. |
| Antihypertensives | Excessively low blood pressure. |
| Cimetidine | Excess sedation. |
| Disulfiram | Increased chlordiazepoxide effect. |
| Dronabinol | Increased effects of both drugs. Avoid. |
| MAO inhibitors | Convulsions, deep sedation, rage. |
| Molindone | Increased tranquilizer effect. |
| Narcotics | Increased sedative effect of both drugs. |
| Sedatives | Increased sedative effect of both drugs. |
| Sleep inducers | Increased sedative effect of both drugs. |
| Tranquilizers | Increased sedative effect of both drugs. |

## POSSIBLE INTERACTION WITH OTHER SUBSTANCES

| INTERACTS WITH | COMBINED EFFECT |
|---|---|
| Alcohol: | Heavy sedation. Avoid. |
| Beverages: | None expected. |
| Cocaine: | Decreased chlordiazepoxide effect. |
| Foods: | None expected. |
| Marijuana: | Heavy sedation. Avoid. |
| Tobacco: | Decreased chlordiazepoxide effect. |

# CHLORDIAZEPOXIDE & AMITRIPTYLINE

## BRAND NAMES

Limbitrol                    Limbitrol DS

## BASIC INFORMATION

Habit forming? Yes
Prescription needed? Yes
Available as generic? No
Drug class: Antidepressant, tranquilizer
            (benzodiazepine)

## USES

- Treatment for nervousness or tension.
- Gradually relieves, but doesn't cure, symptoms of depression.

## DOSAGE & USAGE INFORMATION

**How to take:**
Tablet or capsule—Swallow with liquid. If you can't swallow whole, crumble tablet or open capsule and take with liquid or food.

**When to take:**
At the same time each day, according to instructions on prescription label.

**If you forget a dose:**
Bedtime dose—If you forget your once-a-day bedtime dose, don't take it more than 3 hours late. If more than 3 hours, wait for next scheduled dose (don't double this dose).

**What drug does:**
Affects limbic system of brain—part that controls emotions.

*Continued next column*

## OVERDOSE

**SYMPTOMS:**
**Drowsiness, weakness, tremor, hallucinations, convulsions, stupor, coma.**
**WHAT TO DO:**
- **Dial 0 (operator) or 911 (emergency) for an ambulance or medical help. Then give first aid immediately.**
- **If patient is unconscious and not breathing, give mouth-to-mouth breathing. If there is no heartbeat, use cardiac massage and mouth-to-mouth breathing (CPR). Don't try to make patient vomit. If you can't get help quickly, take patient to nearest emergency facility.**
- **See emergency information on inside covers.**

**Time lapse before drug works:**
Begins in 1 to 2 weeks. May require 4 to 6 weeks for maximum benefit.

**Don't take with:**
- Non-prescription drugs without consulting doctor.
- See Interaction column and consult doctor.

## POSSIBLE ADVERSE REACTIONS OR SIDE EFFECTS

| SYMPTOMS | WHAT TO DO |
|---|---|
| **Life-threatening:** | |
| Slow heartbeat, irregular breathing. | Seek emergency treatment immediately. |
| **Common:** | |
| • Clumsiness, drowsiness, dizziness, headache, insomnia, dry mouth or unpleasant taste, constipation, fatigue, weakness. | Continue. Call doctor when convenient. |
| • "Sweet tooth." | Continue. Tell doctor at next visit. |
| **Infrequent:** | |
| • Hallucinations, confusion, depression, irritability, rash, itch, vision changes, jaundice, blurred vision, eye pain. | Discontinue. Call doctor right away. |
| • Constipation, diarrhea, nausea, vomiting, difficult urination, indigestion. | Continue. Call doctor when convenient. |
| **Rare:** | |
| Mouth or throat ulcers, fever. | Discontinue. Call doctor right away. |

## WARNINGS & PRECAUTIONS

**Don't take if:**
- You are allergic to any benzodiazepine or tricyclic antidepressant.
- You have myasthenia gravis, glaucoma, taken MAO inhibitors within 2 weeks, had a heart attack within 6 weeks.
- You are active or recovering alcoholic.
- Patient is younger than 12.

**Before you start, consult your doctor:**
- If you have liver, kidney or lung disease, diabetes, epilepsy, porphyria, enlarged prostate, heart disease, high blood pressure, stomach or intestinal problems, overactive thyroid, asthma.

# CHLORDIAZEPOXIDE & AMITRIPTYLINE

- If you will have surgery within 2 months, including dental surgery, requiring general or spinal anesthesia.

**Over age 60:**
More likely to develop urination difficulty and more side effects.

**Pregnancy:**
Risk to unborn child outweighs drug benefits. Don't use.

**Breast-feeding:**
Drug passes into milk. Avoid drug or discontinue nursing until you finish medicine. Consult doctor for advice on maintaining milk supply.

**Infants & children:**
Use only under medical supervision for children older than 6 months.

**Prolonged use:**
May impair liver function.

**Skin & sunlight:**
May cause rash or intensify sunburn in areas exposed to sun or sunlamp.

**Driving, piloting or hazardous work:**
Don't drive or pilot aircraft until you learn how medicine affects you. Don't work around dangerous machinery. Don't climb ladders or work in high places. Danger increases if you drink alcohol or take medicine affecting alertness and reflexes, such as antihistamines, tranquilizers, sedatives, pain medicine, narcotics and mind-altering drugs.

**Discontinuing:**
Don't discontinue without consulting doctor. Dose may require gradual reduction if you have taken drug for a long time. Doses of other drugs may also require adjustment.

**Others:**
- Hot weather, heavy exercise and profuse sweat may reduce excretion and cause overdose.
- Blood sugar may rise in diabetics, requiring insulin adjustment.

## POSSIBLE INTERACTION WITH OTHER DRUGS

| GENERIC NAME OR DRUG CLASS | COMBINED EFFECT |
|---|---|
| Anticoagulants (oral) | Increased anticoagulant effect. |
| Anticonvulsants | Change in seizure frequency or severity. |
| Anticholinergics | Increased anticholinergic effect. |
| Antidepressants | Increased sedative effect of both drugs. |

| | |
|---|---|
| Antihistamines | Increased sedative effect of both drugs. |
| Antihypertensives | Excessively low blood pressure. |
| Barbiturates | Decreased antidepressant effect. |
| Cimetidine | Excess sedation. |
| Clonidine | Decreased clonidine effect. |
| Disulfiram | Increased chlordiazepoxide effect. |
| Diuretics | Increased antidepressant effect. |
| Dronabinol | Increased effect of both drugs. |
| Ethchlorvynol | Delirium. |
| Guanethidine | Decreased guanethidine effect. |
| MAO inhibitors | Convulsions, deep sedation, rage. |
| Methyldopa | Decreased methyldopa effect. |
| Narcotics | Dangerous oversedation. |
| Phenytoin | Decreased phenytoin effect. |
| Quinidine | Irregular heartbeat. |
| Sedatives | Dangerous oversedation. |
| Sleep Inducers | Increased sedative effect of both drugs. |
| Sympathomimetics | Increased sympathomimetic effect. |

*Continued page 965*

## POSSIBLE INTERACTION WITH OTHER SUBSTANCES

| INTERACTS WITH | COMBINED EFFECT |
|---|---|
| **Alcohol:** Beverages or medicines with alcohol. | Excessive intoxication. Avoid. |
| **Beverages:** | None expected. |
| **Cocaine:** | Excessive intoxication. Avoid. |
| **Foods:** | None expected. |
| **Marijuana:** | Excessive drowsiness. Avoid. |
| **Tobacco:** | Decreased chlordiazepoxide effect. |

# CHLORDIAZEPOXIDE & CLIDINIUM

## BRAND NAMES

See complete list of brand names in the *Brand Name Directory,* page 946.

## BASIC INFORMATION

**Habit forming? Yes**
**Prescription needed? Yes**
**Available as generic? No**
**Drug class: Tranquilizer (benzodiazepine), antispasmodic, anticholinergic**

## USES

- Reduces spasms of digestive system, bladder and urethra.
- Treatment for nervousness or tension.
- Treatment for muscle spasm.

## DOSAGE & USAGE INFORMATION

**How to take:**
Tablet or capsule—Swallow with liquid. If you can't swallow whole, crumble tablet or open capsule and take with liquid or food.

**When to take:**
At the same time each day, according to instructions on prescription label.

**If you forget a dose:**
Take as soon as you remember up to 2 hours late. If more than 2 hours, wait for next scheduled dose (don't double this dose).

*Continued next column*

## OVERDOSE

**SYMPTOMS:**
**Dilated pupils, rapid pulse and breathing, dizziness, drowsiness, weakness, tremor, stupor, fever, hallucinations, confusion, slurred speech, agitation, flushed face, convulsions, coma.**
**WHAT TO DO:**
- **Dial 0 (operator) or 911 (emergency) for an ambulance or medical help. Then give first aid immediately.**
- **If patient is unconscious and not breathing, give mouth-to-mouth breathing. If there is no heartbeat, use cardiac massage and mouth-to-mouth breathing (CPR). Don't try to make patient vomit. If you can't get help quickly, take patient to nearest emergency facility.**
- **See emergency information on inside covers.**

**What drug does:**
- Blocks nerve impulses at parasympathetic nerve endings, preventing muscle contractions and gland secretions of organs involved.
- Affects limbic system of brain—part that controls emotions.

**Time lapse before drug works:**
15 to 30 minutes.

**Don't take with:**
See Interaction column and consult doctor.

## POSSIBLE ADVERSE REACTIONS OR SIDE EFFECTS

| SYMPTOMS | WHAT TO DO |
|---|---|
| **Life-threatening:** | |
| Slow or rapid heartbeat, breathing difficulty. | Discontinue. Seek emergency treatment. |
| **Common:** | |
| • Clumsiness, drowsiness, dizziness, delirium. | Discontinue. Call doctor right away. |
| • Dry mouth, throat, nose. | Continue. Tell doctor at next visit. |
| **Infrequent:** | |
| • Hallucinations, confusion, depression, irritability, rash, itch, vision changes, vomiting. | Discontinue. Call doctor right away. |
| • Constipation, diarrhea, nausea, urination difficulty. | Continue. Call doctor when convenient. |
| **Rare:** | |
| Jaundice, rash or hives, eye pain, blurred vision. | Discontinue. Call doctor right away. |

## WARNINGS & PRECAUTIONS

**Don't take if:**
- You are allergic to any anticholinergic or any benzodiazepine.
- You have trouble with stomach bloating, difficulty emptying your bladder completely, narrow-angle glaucoma, severe ulcerative colitis, myasthenia gravis.
- You are active or recovering alcoholic.
- Patient is younger than 6 months.

**Before you start, consult your doctor:**
- If you have open-angle glaucoma, angina, chronic bronchitis or asthma, hiatal hernia, enlarged prostate, myasthenia gravis, peptic ulcer, liver, kidney or lung disease, diabetes, epilepsy or porphyria.

- If you will have surgery within 2 months, including dental surgery, requiring general or spinal anesthesia.

**Over age 60:**
Adverse reactions and side effects may be more frequent and severe than in younger persons.

**Pregnancy:**
Risk to unborn child outweighs drug benefits. Don't use.

**Breast-feeding:**
Drug passes into milk. Avoid drug or discontinue nursing until you finish medicine. Consult doctor for advice on maintaining milk supply.

**Infants & children:**
Use only under medical supervision.

**Prolonged use:**
- Chronic constipation, possible fecal impaction.
- May impair liver function.

**Skin & sunlight:**
No problems expected.

**Driving, piloting or hazardous work:**
Don't drive or pilot aircraft until you learn how medicine affects you. Don't work around dangerous machinery. Don't climb ladders or work in high places. Danger increases if you drink alcohol or take medicine affecting alertness and reflexes, such as antihistamines, tranquilizers, sedatives, pain medicine, narcotics and mind-altering drugs.

**Discontinuing:**
Don't discontinue without consulting doctor. Dose may require gradual reduction if you have taken drug for a long time. Doses of other drugs may also require adjustment.

**Others:**
- Hot weather, heavy exercise and profuse sweat may reduce excretion and cause overdose.
- Blood sugar may rise in diabetics, requiring insulin adjustment.

## POSSIBLE INTERACTION WITH OTHER DRUGS

| GENERIC NAME OR DRUG CLASS | COMBINED EFFECT |
|---|---|
| Amantadine | Increased clidinium effect. |
| Antacids | Decreased clidinium effect. |
| Anticholinergics (other) | Increased clidinium effect. |
| Anticonvulsants | Change in seizure frequency or severity. |
| Antidepressants | Increased sedative effect of both drugs. |
| Antihistamines | Increased sedative effect of both drugs. |
| Antihypertensives | Excessively low blood pressure. |
| Cimetidine | Excess sedation. |
| Disulfiram | Increased chlordiazepoxide effect. |
| Dronabinol | Increased effects of both drugs. Avoid. |
| Haloperidol | Increased internal-eye pressure. |
| MAO inhibitors | Convulsions, deep sedation, rage. |
| Meperidine | Increased clidinium effect. |
| Methylphenidate | Increased clidinium effect. |
| Narcotics | Increased sedative effect of both drugs. |
| Nitrates | Increased internal-eye pressure. |
| Orphenadrine | Increased clidinium effect. |
| Phenothiazines | Increased clidinium effect. |
| Pilocarpine | Loss of pilocarpine effect in glaucoma treatment. |
| Potassium supplements | Possible intestinal ulcers with oral potassium tablets. |

*Continued page 965*

## POSSIBLE INTERACTION WITH OTHER SUBSTANCES

| INTERACTS WITH | COMBINED EFFECT |
|---|---|
| Alcohol: | Heavy sedation. Avoid. |
| Beverages: | None expected. |
| Cocaine: | Excessively rapid heartbeat. Avoid. |
| Foods: | None expected. |
| Marijuana: | Drowsiness and dry mouth, heavy sedation. Avoid. |
| Tobacco: | Decreased chlordiazepoxide effect. |

# CHLOROQUINE

## BRAND NAMES

**Aralen**

## BASIC INFORMATION

**Habit forming? No**
**Prescription needed? Yes**
**Available as generic? Yes**
**Drug class: Antiprotozoal, antirheumatic**

 ## USES

- Treatment for protozoal infections, such as malaria and amebiasis.
- Treatment for some forms of arthritis and lupus.

 ## DOSAGE & USAGE INFORMATION

**How to take:**
Tablet—Swallow with food or milk to lessen stomach irritation.

**When to take:**
- Depends on condition. Is adjusted during treatment.
- Malaria prevention—Begin taking medicine 2 weeks before entering areas with malaria.

**If you forget a dose:**
- 1 or more doses a day—Take as soon as you remember up to 2 hours late. If more than 2 hours, wait for next scheduled dose (don't double this dose).
- 1 dose weekly—Take as soon as possible, then return to regular dosing schedule.

**What drug does:**
- Inhibits parasite multiplication.
- Decreases inflammatory response in diseased joint.

**Time lapse before drug works:**
1 to 2 hours.

**Don't take with:**
See Interaction column and consult doctor.

 ## OVERDOSE

**SYMPTOMS:**
**Severe breathing difficulty, drowsiness, faintness.**
**WHAT TO DO:**
- **Dial 0 (operator) or 911 (emergency) for an ambulance or medical help. Then give first aid immediately.**
- **See emergency information on inside covers.**

 ## POSSIBLE ADVERSE REACTIONS OR SIDE EFFECTS

| SYMPTOMS | WHAT TO DO |
|---|---|
| **Life-threatening:** | |
| None expected. | |
| **Common:** | |
| Headache. | Continue. Tell doctor at next visit. |
| **Infrequent:** | |
| • Blurred or changed vision. | Discontinue. Call doctor right away. |
| • Rash or itch, diarrhea, nausea, vomiting. | Continue. Call doctor when convenient. |
| **Rare:** | |
| • Mood or mental changes, seizures, sore throat, fever, unusual bleeding or bruising, muscle weakness. | Discontinue. Call doctor right away. |
| • Ringing or buzzing in ears, hearing loss. | Continue. Call doctor when convenient. |

## WARNINGS & PRECAUTIONS

**Don't take if:**
You are allergic to chloroquine or hydroxychloroquine.

**Before you start, consult your doctor:**
- If you plan to become pregnant within the medication period.
- If you have blood disease.
- If you have eye or vision problems.
- If you have a G6PD deficiency.
- If you have liver disease.
- If you have nerve or brain disease (including seizure disorders).
- If you have porphyria.
- If you have psoriasis.
- If you have stomach or intestinal disease.
- If you drink more than 3 oz. of alcohol daily.

**Over age 60:**
Adverse reactions and side effects may be more frequent and severe than in younger persons.

**Pregnancy:**
Risk to unborn child outweighs drug benefits. Don't use.

**Breast-feeding:**
Drug passes into milk. Avoid drug or discontinue nursing.

**Infants & children:**
Not recommended. Dangerous.

**Prolonged use:**
Permanent damage to the retina (back part of the eye) or nerve deafness.

**Skin & sunlight:**
May cause rash or intensify sunburn in areas exposed to sun or sunlamp.

**Driving, piloting or hazardous work:**
Don't drive or pilot aircraft until you learn how medicine affects you. Don't work around dangerous machinery. Don't climb ladders or work in high places. Danger increases if you drink alcohol or take medicine affecting alertness and reflexes.

**Discontinuing:**
Don't discontinue without doctor's advice until you complete prescribed dose, even though symptoms diminish or disappear.

**Others:**
- Periodic physical and blood examinations recommended.
- If you are in a malaria area for a long time, you may need to change to another preventive drug every 2 years.

## POSSIBLE INTERACTION WITH OTHER DRUGS

| GENERIC NAME OR DRUG CLASS | COMBINED EFFECT |
| --- | --- |
| Estrogens | Possible liver toxicity. |
| Gold compounds | Risk of severe rash and itch. |
| Oxyphenbutazone | Risk of severe rash and itch. |
| Penicillamine | Possible blood or kidney toxicity. |
| Phenylbutazone | Risk of severe rash and itch. |
| Sulfa drugs | Possible liver toxicity. |

## POSSIBLE INTERACTION WITH OTHER SUBSTANCES

| INTERACTS WITH | COMBINED EFFECT |
| --- | --- |
| Alcohol: | Possible liver toxicity. Avoid. |
| Beverages: | None expected. |
| Cocaine: | None expected. |
| Foods: | None expected. |
| Marijuana: | None expected. |
| Tobacco: | None expected. |

# CHLOROTHIAZIDE

## BRAND NAMES

| | |
|---|---|
| Aldoclor | Diuril |
| Chloroserpine | SK-Chlorothiazide |
| Diupres | |

## BASIC INFORMATION

**Habit forming? No**
**Prescription needed? Yes**
**Available as generic? Yes**
**Drug class: Antihypertensive, diuretic
(thiazide)**

 **USES**

- Controls, but doesn't cure, high blood pressure.
- Reduces fluid retention (edema) caused by conditions such as heart disorders and liver disease.

 **DOSAGE & USAGE INFORMATION**

**How to take:**
Tablet or capsule—Swallow with liquid. If you can't swallow whole, crumble tablet or open capsule and take with liquid or food. Don't exceed dose.

**When to take:**
At the same time each day.

**If you forget a dose:**
Take as soon as you remember up to 2 hours late. If more than 2 hours, wait for next scheduled dose (don't double this dose).

**What drug does:**
- Forces sodium and water excretion, reducing body fluid.
- Relaxes muscle cells of small arteries.
- Reduced body fluid and relaxed arteries lower blood pressure.

*Continued next column*

 **OVERDOSE**

**SYMPTOMS:**
**Cramps, weakness, drowsiness, weak pulse, coma.**
**WHAT TO DO:**
- **Dial 0 (operator) or 911 (emergency) for an ambulance or medical help. Then give first aid immediately.**
- **See emergency information on inside covers.**

**Time lapse before drug works:**
4 to 6 hours. May require several weeks to lower blood pressure.

**Don't take with:**
- See Interaction column and consult doctor.
- Non-prescription drugs without consulting doctor.

 **POSSIBLE ADVERSE REACTIONS OR SIDE EFFECTS**

| SYMPTOMS | WHAT TO DO |
|---|---|
| **Life-threatening:**<br>None expected. | |
| **Common:**<br>None expected. | |
| **Infrequent:** | |
| • Blurred vision, severe abdominal pain, nausea, vomiting, irregular heartbeat, weak pulse. | Discontinue. Call doctor right away. |
| • Dizziness, mood changes, headaches, weakness, tiredness, weight changes. | Continue. Call doctor when convenient. |
| • Dry mouth, thirst. | Continue. Tell doctor at next visit. |
| **Rare:** | |
| • Rash or hives. | Discontinue. Seek emergency treatment. |
| • Jaundice. | Discontinue. Call doctor right away. |
| • Sore throat, fever. | Continue. Tell doctor at next visit. |

 **WARNINGS & PRECAUTIONS**

**Don't take if:**
You are allergic to any thiazide diuretic drug.

**Before you start, consult your doctor:**
- If you are allergic to any sulfa drug.
- If you have gout.
- If you have liver, pancreas or kidney disorder.

**Over age 60:**
Adverse reactions and side effects may be more frequent and severe than in younger persons, especially dizziness and excessive potassium loss.

**Pregnancy:**
Risk to unborn child outweighs drug benefits. Don't use.

**Breast-feeding:**
Drug passes into milk. Avoid drug or discontinue nursing.

**Infants & children:**
No problems expected.

**Prolonged use:**
You may need medicine to treat high blood pressure for the rest of your life.

**Skin & sunlight:**
May cause rash or intensify sunburn in areas exposed to sun or sunlamp.

**Driving, piloting or hazardous work:**
Don't drive or pilot aircraft until you learn how medicine affects you. Don't work around dangerous machinery. Don't climb ladders or work in high places. Danger increases if you drink alcohol or take medicine affecting alertness and reflexes, such as antihistamines, tranquilizers, sedatives, pain medicine, narcotics and mind-altering drugs.

**Discontinuing:**
Don't discontinue without medical advice.

**Others:**
- Hot weather and fever may cause dehydration and drop in blood pressure. Dose may require temporary adjustment. Weigh daily and report any unexpected weight decreases to your doctor.
- May cause rise in uric acid, leading to gout.
- May cause blood-sugar rise in diabetics.

 ## POSSIBLE INTERACTION WITH OTHER DRUGS

| GENERIC NAME OR DRUG CLASS | COMBINED EFFECT |
|---|---|
| Acebutolol | Increased antihypertensive effect. Dosages of both drugs may require adjustments. |
| Allopurinol | Decreased allopurinol effect. |
| Amiodarone | Increased risk of heartbeat irregularity due to low potassium. |
| Antidepressants (tricyclic) | Dangerous drop in blood pressure. Avoid combination unless under medical supervision. |
| Barbiturates | Increased chlorothiazide effect. |
| Calcium supplements | Increased calcium in blood. |
| Cholestyramine | Decreased chlorothiazide effect. |
| Cortisone drugs | Excessive potassium loss that causes dangerous heart rhythms. |
| Digitalis preparations | Excessive potassium loss that causes dangerous heart rhythms. |
| Diuretics (thiazide) | Increased effect of other thiazide diuretics. |
| Indapamide | Increased diuretic effect. |
| Labetolol | Increased antihypertensive effects. |
| Lithium | Increased effect of lithium. |
| MAO inhibitors | Increased chlorothiazide effect. |
| Nitrates | Excessive blood-pressure drop. |
| Oxprenolol | Increased antihypertensive effect. Dosages of both drugs may require adjustments. |
| Pentoxifylline | Increased antihypertensive effect. |
| Potassium supplements | Decreased potassium effect. |
| Probenecid | Decreased probenecid effect. |

 ## POSSIBLE INTERACTION WITH OTHER SUBSTANCES

| INTERACTS WITH | COMBINED EFFECT |
|---|---|
| Alcohol: | Dangerous blood-pressure drop. |
| Beverages: | None expected. |
| Cocaine: | None expected. |
| Foods: Licorice. | Excessive potassium loss that causes dangerous heart rhythms. |
| Marijuana: | May increase blood pressure. |
| Tobacco: | None expected. |

# CHLOROTRIANISENE

## BRAND NAMES

TACE

## BASIC INFORMATION

Habit forming? No
Prescription needed? Yes
Available as generic? Yes
Drug class: Female sex hormone (estrogen)

 USES

- Treatment for symptoms of menopause and menstrual-cycle irregularity.
- Replacement for female hormone deficiency.
- Treatment for cancer of prostate.

 DOSAGE & USAGE INFORMATION

**How to take:**
Capsule—Swallow with liquid. If you can't swallow whole, open capsule and take with liquid or food.

**When to take:**
At the same time each day.

**If you forget a dose:**
Take as soon as you remember up to 12 hours late. If more than 12 hours, wait for next scheduled dose (don't double this dose).

**What drug does:**
Restores normal estrogen level in tissues.

**Time lapse before drug works:**
10 to 20 days.

**Don't take with:**
See Interaction column and consult doctor.

 OVERDOSE

**SYMPTOMS:**
Nausea, vomiting, fluid retention, breast enlargement and discomfort, abnormal vaginal bleeding.
**WHAT TO DO:**
Overdose unlikely to threaten life. If person takes much larger amount than prescribed, call doctor, poison-control center or hospital emergency room for instructions.

 POSSIBLE ADVERSE REACTIONS OR SIDE EFFECTS

| SYMPTOMS | WHAT TO DO |
|---|---|
| **Life-threatening:** None expected. | |
| **Common:** | |
| • Stomach cramps. | Discontinue. Call doctor right away. |
| • Appetite loss. | Continue. Call doctor when convenient. |
| • Swollen ankles or feet; swollen, tender breasts; nausea; diarrhea. | Continue. Tell doctor at next visit. |
| **Infrequent:** | |
| • Rash, stomach or side pain. | Discontinue. Call doctor right away. |
| • Depression, dizziness, irritability, vomiting, breast lumps. | Continue. Call doctor when convenient. |
| • Brown blotches on skin, hair loss, vaginal discharge or bleeding, changes in sex drive. | Continue. Tell doctor at next visit. |
| **Rare:** Jaundice. | Discontinue. Call doctor right away. |

## WARNINGS & PRECAUTIONS

**Don't take if:**
- You are allergic to any estrogen-containing drugs.
- You have impaired liver function.
- You have had blood clots, stroke or heart attack.
- You have unexplained vaginal bleeding.

**Before you start, consult your doctor:**
- If you have had cancer of breast or reproductive organs, fibrocystic breast disease, fibroid tumors of the uterus or endometriosis.
- If you have had migraine headaches, epilepsy or porphyria.
- If you have diabetes, high blood pressure, asthma, congestive heart failure, kidney disease or gallstones.
- If you plan to become pregnant within 3 months.

**Over age 60:**
Controversial. You and your doctor must decide if drug risks outweigh benefits.

**Pregnancy:**
Risk to unborn child outweighs drug benefits. Don't use.

**Breast-feeding:**
Drug filters into milk. May harm child. Avoid.

**Infants & children:**
Not recommended.

**Prolonged use:**
Increased growth of fibroid tumors of uterus. Possible association with cancer of uterus.

**Skin & sunlight:**
May cause rash or intensify sunburn in areas exposed to sun or sunlamp.

**Driving, piloting or hazardous work:**
No problems expected.

**Discontinuing:**
You may need to discontinue chlorotrianisene periodically. Consult your doctor.

**Others:**
In rare instances, may cause blood clot in lung, brain or leg. Symptoms are *sudden* severe headache, coordination loss, vision change, chest pain, breathing difficulty, slurred speech, pain in legs or groin. Seek emergency treatment immediately.

## POSSIBLE INTERACTION WITH OTHER DRUGS

| GENERIC NAME OR DRUG CLASS | COMBINED EFFECT |
|---|---|
| Anticoagulants (oral) | Decreased anticoagulant effect. |
| Anticonvulsants (hydantoin) | Increased seizures. |
| Antidiabetics (oral) | Unpredictable increase or decrease in blood sugar. |
| Carbamazepine | Increased seizures. |
| Clofibrate | Decreased clofibrate effect. |
| Meprobamate | Increased chlorotrianisene effect. |
| Phenobarbital | Decreased chlorotrianisene effect. |
| Primidone | Decreased chlorotrianisene effect. |
| Rifampin | Decreased chlorotrianisene effect. |
| Thyroid hormones | Decreased thyroid effect. |

## POSSIBLE INTERACTION WITH OTHER SUBSTANCES

| INTERACTS WITH | COMBINED EFFECT |
|---|---|
| Alcohol: | None expected. |
| Beverages: | None expected. |
| Cocaine: | No proven problems. |
| Foods: | None expected. |
| Marijuana: | Possible menstrual irregularities and bleeding between periods. |
| Tobacco: | Increased risk of blood clots leading to stroke or heart attack. |

# CHLORPHENESIN

## BRAND NAMES

Maolate                    Mycil

## BASIC INFORMATION

Habit forming? No
Prescription needed? Yes
Available as generic? Yes
Drug class: Muscle relaxant (skeletal)

## USES

Treatment for sprains, strains and muscle spasms.

## DOSAGE & USAGE INFORMATION

**How to take:**
Tablet or capsule—Swallow with liquid.

**When to take:**
As needed, no more often than every 4 hours.

**If you forget a dose:**
Take as soon as you remember. Wait 4 hours for next dose.

**What drug does:**
Blocks body's pain messages to brain. May also sedate.

**Time lapse before drug works:**
60 minutes.

**Don't take with:**
See Interaction column and consult doctor.

## OVERDOSE

**SYMPTOMS:**
Nausea, vomiting, diarrhea, headache. May progress to severe weakness, difficult breathing, sensation of paralysis, coma.
**WHAT TO DO:**
- Dial 0 (operator) or 911 (emergency) for an ambulance or medical help. Then give first aid immediately.
- See emergency information on inside covers.

## POSSIBLE ADVERSE REACTIONS OR SIDE EFFECTS

| SYMPTOMS | WHAT TO DO |
|---|---|
| **Life-threatening:** | |
| None expected. | |
| **Common:** | |
| • Drowsiness, fainting, dizziness. | Continue. Call doctor when convenient. |
| • Orange or red-purple urine. | No action necessary. |
| **Infrequent:** | |
| Agitation, constipation or diarrhea, nausea, cramps, vomiting, wheezing, shortness of breath. | Discontinue. Call doctor right away. |
| **Rare:** | |
| • Bloody or tarry, black stool. | Discontinue. Seek emergency treatment. |
| • Rash, hives or itch; sore throat, fever; jaundice; tiredness; weakness. | Discontinue. Call doctor right away. |

# CHLORPHENESIN

## WARNINGS & PRECAUTIONS

**Don't take if:**
- You are allergic to any skeletal-muscle relaxant.
- You have porphyria.

**Before you start, consult your doctor:**
- If you have had liver or kidney disease.
- If you plan pregnancy within medication period.
- If you will have surgery within 2 months, including dental surgery, requiring general or spinal anesthesia.

**Over age 60:**
Adverse reactions and side effects may be more frequent and severe than in younger persons.

**Pregnancy:**
No proven harm to unborn child. Avoid if possible.

**Breast-feeding:**
Drug passes into milk. Avoid drug or discontinue nursing until you finish medicine. Consult doctor for advice on maintaining milk supply.

**Infants & children:**
Not recommended.

**Prolonged use:**
Periodic liver-function tests recommended if you use this drug for a long time.

**Skin & sunlight:**
No problems expected.

**Driving, piloting or hazardous work:**
Don't drive or pilot aircraft until you learn how medicine affects you. Don't work around dangerous machinery. Don't climb ladders or work in high places. Danger increases if you drink alcohol or take medicine affecting alertness and reflexes, such as antihistamines, tranquilizers, sedatives, pain medicine, narcotics and mind-altering drugs.

**Discontinuing:**
Don't discontinue without doctor's advice until you complete prescribed dose, even though symptoms diminish or disappear.

**Others:**
No problems expected.

## POSSIBLE INTERACTION WITH OTHER DRUGS

| GENERIC NAME OR DRUG CLASS | COMBINED EFFECT |
|---|---|
| Antidepressants | Increased sedation. |
| Antihistamines | Increased sedation. |
| Dronabinol | Increased effects of dronabinol on central nervous system. Avoid combination. |
| Mind-altering drugs | Increased sedation. |
| Muscle relaxants (other) | Increased sedation. |
| Narcotics | Increased sedation. |
| Sedatives | Increased sedation. |
| Sleep inducers | Increased sedation. |
| Testosterone | Decreased metaxalone effect. |
| Tranquilizers | Increased sedation. |

## POSSIBLE INTERACTION WITH OTHER SUBSTANCES

| INTERACTS WITH | COMBINED EFFECT |
|---|---|
| Alcohol: | Increased sedation. Avoid. |
| Beverages: | None expected. |
| Cocaine: | Lack of coordination, increased sedation. Avoid. |
| Foods: | None expected. |
| Marijuana: | Lack of coordination, drowsiness, fainting. Avoid. |
| Tobacco: | None expected. |

# CHLORPHENIRAMINE

## BRAND NAMES

See complete list of brand names in the *Brand Name Directory,* page 946.

## BASIC INFORMATION

**Habit forming? No**
**Prescription needed? No**
**Available as generic? Yes**
**Drug class: Antihistamine**

 ## USES

- Reduces allergic symptoms such as hay fever, hives, rash or itching.
- Prevents motion sickness, nausea, vomiting.
- Induces sleep.

 ## DOSAGE & USAGE INFORMATION

**How to take:**
- Tablet or syrup—Swallow with liquid or food to lessen stomach irritation.
- Extended-release tablets or capsules—Swallow each dose whole.

**When to take:**
Varies with form. Follow label directions.

**If you forget a dose:**
Take as soon as you remember up to 2 hours late. If more than 2 hours, wait for next scheduled dose (don't double this dose).

**What drug does:**
Blocks action of histamine after an allergic response triggers histamine release in sensitive cells.

**Time lapse before drug works:**
30 minutes.

**Don't take with:**
See Interaction column and consult doctor.

 ## OVERDOSE

**SYMPTOMS:**
**Convulsions, red face, hallucinations, coma.**
**WHAT TO DO:**
- **Dial 0 (operator) or 911 (emergency) for an ambulance or medical help. Then give first aid immediately.**
- **See emergency information on inside covers.**

 ## POSSIBLE ADVERSE REACTIONS OR SIDE EFFECTS

| SYMPTOMS | WHAT TO DO |
|---|---|
| **Life-threatening:** None expected. | |
| **Common:** Drowsiness; dizziness; dry mouth, nose, throat; nausea. | Continue. Tell doctor at next visit. |
| **Infrequent:** | |
| • Vision changes. | Discontinue. Call doctor right away. |
| • Less tolerance for contact lenses, difficult urination. | Continue. Call doctor when convenient. |
| • Appetite loss. | Continue. Tell doctor at next visit. |
| **Rare:** Nightmares, agitation, irritability, sore throat, fever, rapid heartbeat, unusual bleeding or bruising, fatigue, weakness. | Discontinue. Call doctor right away. |

## WARNINGS & PRECAUTIONS

**Don't take if:**
You are allergic to any antihistamine.

**Before you start, consult your doctor:**
- If you have glaucoma.
- If you have enlarged prostate.
- If you have asthma.
- If you have kidney disease.
- If you have peptic ulcer.
- If you will have surgery within 2 months, including dental surgery, requiring general or spinal anesthesia.

**Over age 60:**
Don't exceed recommended dose. Adverse reactions and side effects may be more frequent and severe than in younger persons, especially urination difficulty, diminished alertness and other brain and nervous-system symptoms.

**Pregnancy:**
No proven harm to unborn child. Avoid if possible.

**Breast-feeding:**
Drug passes into milk. Avoid drug or discontinue nursing until you finish medicine. Consult doctor for advice on maintaining milk supply.

**Infants & children:**
Not recommended for premature or newborn infants. Otherwise, no problems expected.

**Prolonged use:**
Avoid. May damage bone marrow and nerve cells.

**Skin & sunlight:**
May cause rash or intensify sunburn in areas exposed to sun or sunlamp.

**Driving, piloting or hazardous work:**
Don't drive or pilot aircraft until you learn how medicine affects you. Don't work around dangerous machinery. Don't climb ladders or work in high places. Danger increases if you drink alcohol or take medicine affecting alertness and reflexes, such as antihistamines, tranquilizers, sedatives, pain medicine, narcotics and mind-altering drugs.

**Discontinuing:**
No problems expected.

**Others:**
May mask symptoms of hearing damage from aspirin, other salicylates, cisplatin, paromomycin, vancomycin or anticonvulsants. Consult doctor if you use these.

## POSSIBLE INTERACTION WITH OTHER DRUGS

| GENERIC NAME OR DRUG CLASS | COMBINED EFFECT |
|---|---|
| Anticholinergics | Increased anticholinergic effect. |
| Antidepressants | Excess sedation. Avoid. |
| Antihistamines (other) | Excess sedation. Avoid. |
| Dronabinol | Increased effects of both drugs. Avoid. |
| Hypnotics | Excess sedation. Avoid. |
| MAO inhibitors | Increased chlorpheniramine effect. |
| Mind-altering drugs | Excess sedation. Avoid. |
| Molindone | Increased antihistamine effect. |
| Narcotics | Excess sedation. Avoid. |
| Sedatives | Excess sedation. Avoid. |
| Sleep inducers | Excess sedation. Avoid. |
| Tranquilizers | Excess sedation. Avoid. |

## POSSIBLE INTERACTION WITH OTHER SUBSTANCES

| INTERACTS WITH | COMBINED EFFECT |
|---|---|
| Alcohol: | Excess sedation. Avoid. |
| Beverages: Caffeine drinks. | Less chlorpheniramine sedation. |
| Cocaine: | Decreased chlorpheniramine effect. Avoid. |
| Foods: | None expected. |
| Marijuana: | Excess sedation. Avoid. |
| Tobacco: | None expected. |

# CHLORPROMAZINE

## BRAND NAMES

| | |
|---|---|
| Apo-Chlorpromazine | Ormazine |
| Chloramead | Promapar |
| Chlor-Promanyl | Promaz |
| Chlorprom | Promosol |
| Clorazine | Thorazine |
| Largactil | Thor-Prom |
| Novochlorpromazine | |

## BASIC INFORMATION

**Habit forming? No**
**Prescription needed? Yes**
**Available as generic? Yes**
**Drug class:** Tranquilizer, antiemetic
(phenothiazine)

## USES

- Stops nausea, vomiting.
- Reduces anxiety, agitation.

## DOSAGE & USAGE INFORMATION

**How to take:**
- Tablet or capsule—Swallow with liquid or food to lessen stomach irritation.
- Suppositories—Remove wrapper and moisten suppository with water. Gently insert into rectum, large end first.
- Drops or liquid—Dilute dose in beverage.

**When to take:**
- Nervous and mental disorders—Take at the same times each day.
- Nausea and vomiting—Take as needed, no more often than every 4 hours.

**If you forget a dose:**
- Nervous and mental disorders—Take up to 2 hours late. If more than 2 hours, wait for next scheduled dose (don't double this dose).
- Nausea and vomiting—Take as soon as you remember. Wait 4 hours for next dose.

*Continued next column*

## OVERDOSE

**SYMPTOMS:**
Stupor, convulsions, coma.
**WHAT TO DO:**
- **Dial 0 (operator) or 911 (emergency) for an ambulance or medical help. Then give first aid immediately.**
- **See emergency information on inside covers.**

**What drug does:**
- Suppresses brain's vomiting center.
- Suppresses brain centers that control abnormal emotions and behavior.

**Time lapse before drug works:**
- Nausea and vomiting—1 hour or less.
- Nervous and mental disorders—4-6 weeks.

**Don't take with:**
- Antacid or medicine for diarrhea.
- Non-prescription drug for cough, cold or allergy.
- See Interaction column and consult doctor.

## POSSIBLE ADVERSE REACTIONS OR SIDE EFFECTS

| SYMPTOMS | WHAT TO DO |
|---|---|
| **Life-threatening:** None expected. | |
| **Common:** | |
| • Muscle spasms of face and neck, unsteady gait. | Discontinue. Seek emergency treatment. |
| • Restlessness, tremor, drowsiness. | Discontinue. Call doctor right away. |
| • Decreased sweating, dry mouth, stuffy nose, constipation. | Continue. Call doctor when convenient. |
| **Infrequent:** | |
| • Fainting. | Discontinue. Seek emergency treatment. |
| • Rash. | Discontinue. Call doctor right away. |
| • Difficult urination, diminished sex drive, swollen breasts, menstrual irregularities. | Continue. Call doctor when convenient. |
| **Rare:** | |
| Vision changes, sore throat, fever, jaundice. | Discontinue. Call doctor right away. |

## WARNINGS & PRECAUTIONS

**Don't take if:**
- You are allergic to any phenothiazine.
- You have a blood or bone-marrow disease.

**Before you start, consult your doctor:**
- If you will have surgery within 2 months, including dental surgery, requiring general or spinal anesthesia.
- If you have asthma, emphysema or other lung disorder.
- If you take non-prescription ulcer medicine, asthma medicine or amphetamines.

**Over age 60:**
Adverse reactions and side effects may be more frequent and severe than in younger persons. More likely to develop involuntary movement of jaws, lips, tongue, chewing. Report this to your doctor immediately. Early treatment can help.

**Pregnancy:**
Risk to unborn child outweighs drug benefits. Don't use.

**Breast-feeding:**
Drug passes into milk. Avoid drug or discontinue nursing until you finish medicine. Consult doctor for advice on maintaining milk supply.

**Infants & children:**
Don't give to children younger than 2.

**Prolonged use:**
May lead to tardive dyskinesia (involuntary movement of jaws, lips, tongue, chewing).

**Skin & sunlight:**
May cause rash or intensify sunburn in areas exposed to sun or sunlamp. Skin may remain sensitive for 3 months after discontinuing.

**Driving, piloting or hazardous work:**
Don't drive or pilot aircraft until you learn how medicine affects you. Don't work around dangerous machinery. Don't climb ladders or work in high places. Danger increases if you drink alcohol or take medicine affecting alertness and reflexes.

**Discontinuing:**
- Nervous and mental disorders—Don't discontinue without doctor's advice until you complete prescribed dose, even though symptoms diminish or disappear.
- Nausea and vomiting—May be unnecessary to finish medicine. Follow doctor's instructions.

**Others:**
No problems expected.

## POSSIBLE INTERACTION WITH OTHER DRUGS

| GENERIC NAME OR DRUG CLASS | COMBINED EFFECT |
| --- | --- |
| Anticholinergics | Increased anticholinergic effect. |
| Antidepressants (tricyclic) | Increased chlorpromazine effect. |
| Antihistamines | Increased antihistamine effect. |
| Appetite suppressants | Decreased suppressant effect. |
| Calcium supplements | Decreased chlorpromazine effect. |
| Dronabinol | Increased effects of both drugs. Avoid. |
| Levodopa | Decreased levodopa effect. |
| Mind-altering drugs | Increased effect of mind-altering drugs. |
| Molindone | Increased tranquilizer effect. |
| Narcotics | Increased narcotic effect. |
| Phenytoin | Increased phenytoin effect. |
| Quinidine | Impaired heart function. Dangerous mixture. |
| Sedatives | Increased sedative effect. |
| Tranquilizers (other) | Increased tranquilizer effect. |

## POSSIBLE INTERACTION WITH OTHER SUBSTANCES

| INTERACTS WITH | COMBINED EFFECT |
| --- | --- |
| Alcohol: | Dangerous oversedation. |
| Beverages: | None expected. |
| Cocaine: | Decreased chlorpromazine effect. Avoid. |
| Foods: | None expected. |
| Marijuana: | Drowsiness. May increase antinausea effect. |
| Tobacco: | None expected. |

# CHLORPROPAMIDE

## BRAND NAMES

Apo-Chlorpropamide  Glucamide
Chloromide  Novopropamide
Chloronase  Stabinol
Diabinese

## BASIC INFORMATION

Habit forming? No
Prescription needed? Yes
Available as generic? Yes
Drug class: Antidiabetic (oral), sulfonurea

## USES

Treatment for diabetes in adults who can't control blood sugar by diet, weight loss and exercise.

## DOSAGE & USAGE INFORMATION

**How to take:**
Tablet—Swallow with liquid or food to lessen stomach irritation. If you can't swallow whole, crumble tablet and take with liquid or food.

**When to take:**
At the same times each day.

**If you forget a dose:**
Take as soon as you remember up to 2 hours late. If more than 2 hours, wait for next scheduled dose (don't double this dose).

**What drug does:**
Stimulates pancreas to produce more insulin. Insulin in blood forces cells to use sugar in blood.

**Time lapse before drug works:**
3 to 4 hours. May require 2 weeks for maximum benefit.

**Don't take with:**
See Interaction column and consult doctor.

## OVERDOSE

**SYMPTOMS:**
Excessive hunger, nausea, anxiety, cool skin, cold sweats, drowsiness, rapid heartbeat, weakness, unconsciousness, coma.
**WHAT TO DO:**
- Dial 0 (operator) or 911 (emergency) for an ambulance or medical help. Then give first aid immediately.
- See emergency information on inside covers.

## POSSIBLE ADVERSE REACTIONS OR SIDE EFFECTS

| SYMPTOMS | WHAT TO DO |
|---|---|
| **Life-threatening:** None expected. | |
| **Common:** | |
| ● Dizziness. | Discontinue. Call doctor right away. |
| ● Diarrhea, appetite loss, nausea, stomach pain, heartburn. | Continue. Call doctor when convenient. |
| **Infrequent:** Low blood sugar (hunger, anxiety, cold sweats, rapid pulse). | Discontinue. Seek emergency treatment. |
| **Rare:** Fatigue, itching or rash, sore throat, fever, ringing in ears, unusual bleeding or bruising, jaundice. | Discontinue. Call doctor right away. |

## WARNINGS & PRECAUTIONS

**Don't take if:**
- You are allergic to any sulfonurea.
- You have impaired kidney or liver function.

**Before you start, consult your doctor:**
- If you have a severe infection.
- If you have thyroid disease.
- If you take insulin.
- If you have heart disease.

**Over age 60:**
Dose usually smaller than for younger adults. Avoid "low-blood-sugar" episodes because repeated ones can damage brain permanently.

**Pregnancy:**
No proven harm to unborn child. Avoid if possible.

**Breast-feeding:**
Drug filters into milk. May lower baby's blood sugar. Avoid.

**Infants & children:**
Don't give to infants or children.

**Prolonged use:**
None expected.

**Skin & sunlight:**
May cause rash or intensify sunburn in areas exposed to sun or sunlamp.

**Driving, piloting or hazardous work:**
No problems expected unless you develop hypoglycemia (low blood sugar). If so, avoid driving or hazardous activity.

**Discontinuing:**
Don't discontinue without consulting doctor. Dose may require gradual reduction if you have taken drug for a long time. Doses of other drugs may also require adjustment.

**Others:**
Don't exceed recommended dose. Hypoglycemia (low blood sugar) may occur, even with proper dose schedule. You must balance medicine, diet and exercise.

## POSSIBLE INTERACTION WITH OTHER DRUGS

| GENERIC NAME OR DRUG CLASS | COMBINED EFFECT |
|---|---|
| Acebutolol | Possible increased difficulty in regulating blood-sugar levels. |
| Androgens | Increased chlorpropamide effect. |
| Anticoagulants (oral) | Unpredictable prothrombin times (see Glossary). |
| Anticonvulsants (hydantoin) | Decreased chlorpropamide effect. |
| Anti-inflammatory drugs (non-steroidal) | Increased chlorpropamide effect. |
| Aspirin | Increased chlorpropamide effect. |
| Beta-adrenergic blockers | Increased chlorpropamide effect. |
| Chloramphenicol | Increased chlorpropamide effect. |
| Clofibrate | Increased chlorpropamide effect. |
| Contraceptives (oral) | Decreased chlorpropamide effect. |
| Cortisone drugs | Decreased chlorpropamide effect. |
| Diuretics (thiazide) | Decreased chlorpropamide effect. |
| Epinephrine | Decreased chlorpropamide effect. |
| Estrogens | Increased chlorpropamide effect. |
| Guanethidine | Unpredictable chlorpropamide effect. |

| | |
|---|---|
| Isoniazid | Decreased chlorpropamide effect. |
| Labetolol | Increased antidiabetic effect, may mask hypoglycemia. |
| MAO inhibitors | Increased chlorpropamide effect. |
| Oxyphenbutazone | Increased chlorpropamide effect. |
| Phenylbutazone | Increased chlorpropamide effect. |
| Phenyramidol | Increased chlorpropamide effect. |
| Probenecid | Increased chlorpropamide effect. |
| Pyrazinamide | Decreased chlorpropamide effect. |
| Sulfa drugs | Increased chlorpropamide effect. |
| Sulfaphenazole | Increased chlorpropamide effect. |
| Thyroid hormones | Decreased chlorpropamide effect. |

## POSSIBLE INTERACTION WITH OTHER SUBSTANCES

| INTERACTS WITH | COMBINED EFFECT |
|---|---|
| Alcohol: | Disulfiram reaction (see Glossary). Avoid. |
| Beverages: | None expected. |
| Cocaine: | No proven problems. |
| Foods: | None expected. |
| Marijuana: | Decreased chlorpropamide effect. Avoid. |
| Tobacco: | None expected. |

# CHLORPROTHIXENE

## BRAND NAMES

Taractan          Tarasan

## BASIC INFORMATION

**Habit forming?** No
**Prescription needed?** Yes
**Available as generic?** No
**Drug class:** Tranquilizer (thioxanthine), antiemetic

 ## USES

- Reduces anxiety, agitation, psychosis.
- Stops vomiting.

 ## DOSAGE & USAGE INFORMATION

**How to take:**
- Tablet—Swallow with liquid. If you can't swallow whole, crumble tablet and take with liquid or food.
- Syrup—Dilute dose in beverage before swallowing.

**When to take:**
At the same time each day.

**If you forget a dose:**
Take as soon as you remember up to 2 hours late. If more than 2 hours, wait for next scheduled dose (don't double this dose).

**What drug does:**
Corrects imbalance of nerve impulses.

*Continued next column*

 ## OVERDOSE

**SYMPTOMS:**
**Drowsiness, dizziness, weakness, muscle rigidity, twitching, tremors, confusion, dry mouth, blurred vision, rapid pulse, shallow breathing, low blood pressure, convulsions, coma.**
**WHAT TO DO:**
- **Dial 0 (operator) or 911 (emergency) for an ambulance or medical help. Then give first aid immediately.**
- **If patient is unconscious and not breathing, give mouth-to-mouth breathing. If there is no heartbeat, use cardiac massage and mouth-to-mouth breathing (CPR). Don't try to make patient vomit. If you can't get help quickly, take patient to nearest emergency facility.**
- **See emergency information on inside covers.**

**Time lapse before drug works:**
3 weeks.

**Don't take with:**
See Interaction column and consult doctor.

 ## POSSIBLE ADVERSE REACTIONS OR SIDE EFFECTS

| SYMPTOMS | WHAT TO DO |
|---|---|
| **Life-threatening:**<br>None expected. | |
| **Common:** | |
| • Fainting; restlessness; jerky, involuntary, movements; blurred vision; rapid heartbeat. | Discontinue. Call doctor right away. |
| • Dizziness, drowsiness, constipation, muscle spasms, shuffling walk, decreased sweating. | Continue. Call doctor when convenient. |
| • Dry mouth, stuffy nose. | Continue. Tell doctor at next visit. |
| **Infrequent:** | |
| • Rash. | Discontinue. Call doctor right away. |
| • Less sexual ability, difficult urination. | Continue. Call doctor when convenient. |
| • Menstrual irregularities, swollen breasts. | Continue. Tell doctor at next visit. |
| **Rare:**<br>Sore throat, fever, jaundice. | Discontinue. Call doctor right away. |

 ## WARNINGS & PRECAUTIONS

**Don't take if:**
- You are allergic to any thioxanthine or phenothiazine tranquilizer.
- You have serious blood disorder.
- You have Parkinson's disease.
- Patient is younger than 12.

**Before you start, consult your doctor:**
- If you have had liver or kidney disease.
- If you have epilepsy or glaucoma.
- If you have high blood pressure or heart disease (especially angina).
- If you use alcohol daily.
- If you will have surgery within 2 months, including dental surgery, requiring general or spinal anesthesia.

**Over age 60:**
Adverse reactions and side effects may be more frequent and severe than in younger persons.

**Pregnancy:**
No proven harm to unborn child. Avoid if possible.

**Breast-feeding:**
Studies inconclusive. Consult your doctor.

**Infants & children:**
Not recommended.

**Prolonged use:**
- Pigment deposits in lens and retina of eye.
- Involuntary movements of jaws, lips, tongue (tardive dyskinesia).

**Skin & sunlight:**
May cause rash or intensify sunburn in areas exposed to sun or sunlamp.

**Driving, piloting or hazardous work:**
Don't drive or pilot aircraft until you learn how medicine affects you. Don't work around dangerous machinery. Don't climb ladders or work in high places. Danger increases if you drink alcohol or take medicine affecting alertness and reflexes.

**Discontinuing:**
Don't discontinue without consulting doctor. Dose may require gradual reduction if you have taken drug for a long time. Doses of other drugs may also require adjustment.

**Others:**
Hot temperatures increase chance of heat stroke.

## POSSIBLE INTERACTION WITH OTHER DRUGS

| GENERIC NAME OR DRUG CLASS | COMBINED EFFECT |
| --- | --- |
| Anticholinergics | Increased anticholinergic effect. |
| Anticonvulsants | Change in seizure pattern. |
| Antidepressants (tricyclic) | Increased chlorprothixene effect. Excessive sedation. |
| Antihistamines | Increased chlorprothixene effect. Excessive sedation. |
| Antihypertensives | Excessively low blood pressure. |
| Barbiturates | Increased chlorprothixene effect. Excessive sedation. |

| | |
| --- | --- |
| Bethanechol | Decreased bethanechol effect. |
| Dronabinol | Increased effects of both drugs. Avoid. |
| Guanethidine | Decreased guanethidine effect. |
| Levodopa | Decreased levodopa effect. |
| MAO inhibitors | Excessive sedation. |
| Mind-altering drugs | Increased chlorprothixene effect. Excessive sedation. |
| Narcotics | Increased chlorprothixene effect. Excessive sedation. |
| Sedatives | Increased chlorprothixene effect. Excessive sedation. |
| Sleep inducers | Increased chlorprothixene effect. Excessive sedation. |
| Tranquilizers | Increased chlorprothixene effect. Excessive sedation. |

## POSSIBLE INTERACTION WITH OTHER SUBSTANCES

| INTERACTS WITH | COMBINED EFFECT |
| --- | --- |
| Alcohol: | Excessive brain depression. Avoid. |
| Beverages: | None expected. |
| Cocaine: | Decreased chlorprothixene effect. Avoid. |
| Foods: | None expected. |
| Marijuana: | Daily use—Fainting likely, possible psychosis. |
| Tobacco: | None expected. |

# CHLORTHALIDONE

## BRAND NAMES

Apo-Chlorthalide
Combipres
Demi-Regroton
Hygroton
Novothalidone

Regroton
Tenoretic
Thalitone
Uridon

## BASIC INFORMATION

**Habit forming?** No
**Prescription needed?** Yes
**Available as generic?** Yes
**Drug class:** Antihypertensive, diuretic
(thiazide)

 **USES**

- Controls, but doesn't cure, high blood pressure.
- Reduces fluid retention (edema) caused by conditions such as heart disorders and liver disease.

 **DOSAGE & USAGE INFORMATION**

**How to take:**
Tablet or capsule—Swallow with liquid. If you can't swallow whole, crumble tablet or open capsule and take with liquid or food. Don't exceed dose.

**When to take:**
At the same time each day.

**If you forget a dose:**
Take as soon as you remember up to 2 hours late. If more than 2 hours, wait for next scheduled dose (don't double this dose).

**What drug does:**
- Forces sodium and water excretion, reducing body fluid.
- Relaxes muscle cells of small arteries.
- Reduced body fluid and relaxed arteries lower blood pressure.

*Continued next column*

 **OVERDOSE**

**SYMPTOMS:**
**Cramps, weakness, drowsiness, weak pulse, coma.**
**WHAT TO DO:**
- **Dial 0 (operator) or 911 (emergency) for an ambulance or medical help. Then give first aid immediately.**
- **See emergency information on inside covers.**

**Time lapse before drug works:**
4 to 6 hours. May require several weeks to lower blood pressure.

**Don't take with:**
- See Interaction column and consult doctor.
- Non-prescription drugs without consulting doctor.

 **POSSIBLE ADVERSE REACTIONS OR SIDE EFFECTS**

| SYMPTOMS | WHAT TO DO |
|---|---|
| **Life-threatening:**<br>None expected. | |
| **Common:**<br>None expected. | |
| **Infrequent:** | |
| • Blurred vision, severe abdominal pain, nausea, vomiting, irregular heartbeat, weak pulse. | Discontinue. Call doctor right away. |
| • Dizziness, mood changes, headaches, weakness, tiredness, weight changes. | Continue. Call doctor when convenient. |
| • Dry mouth, thirst. | Continue. Tell doctor at next visit. |
| **Rare:** | |
| • Rash or hives. | Discontinue. Seek emergency treatment. |
| • Jaundice, sore throat, fever. | Discontinue. Call doctor right away. |

 **WARNINGS & PRECAUTIONS**

**Don't take if:**
You are allergic to any thiazide diuretic drug.

**Before you start, consult your doctor:**
- If you are allergic to any sulfa drug.
- If you have gout.
- If you have liver, pancreas or kidney disorder.

**Over age 60:**
Adverse reactions and side effects may be more frequent and severe than in younger persons, especially dizziness and excessive potassium loss.

**Pregnancy:**
Risk to unborn child outweighs drug benefits. Don't use.

**Breast-feeding:**
Drug passes into milk. Avoid this medicine or discontinue nursing.

**Infants & children:**
No problems expected.

**Prolonged use:**
You may need medicine to treat high blood pressure for the rest of your life.

**Skin & sunlight:**
May cause rash or intensify sunburn in areas exposed to sun or sunlamp.

**Driving, piloting or hazardous work:**
Don't drive or pilot aircraft until you learn how medicine affects you. Don't work around dangerous machinery. Don't climb ladders or work in high places. Danger increases if you drink alcohol or take medicine affecting alertness and reflexes, such as antihistamines, tranquilizers, sedatives, pain medicine, narcotics and mind-altering drugs.

**Discontinuing:**
Don't discontinue without medical advice.

**Others:**
- Hot weather and fever may cause dehydration and drop in blood pressure. Dose may require temporary adjustment. Weigh daily and report any unexpected weight decreases to your doctor.
- May cause rise in uric acid, leading to gout.
- May cause blood-sugar rise in diabetics.

 ## POSSIBLE INTERACTION WITH OTHER DRUGS

| GENERIC NAME OR DRUG CLASS | COMBINED EFFECT |
|---|---|
| Acebutolol | Increased antihypertensive effect. Dosages of both drugs may require adjustments. |
| Allopurinol | Decreased allopurinol effect. |
| Amiodarone | Increased risk of heartbeat irregularity due to low potassium. |
| Antidepressants (tricyclic) | Dangerous drop in blood pressure. Avoid combination unless under medical supervision. |
| Barbiturates | Increased chlorthalidone effect. |
| Calcium supplements | Increased calcium in blood. |
| Cholestyramine | Decreased chlorthalidone effect. |
| Cortisone drugs | Excessive potassium loss that causes dangerous heart rhythms. |
| Digitalis preparations | Excessive potassium loss that causes dangerous heart rhythms. |
| Diuretics (thiazide) | Increased effect of other thiazide diuretics. |
| Enalapril | Possible excessive potassium in blood. |
| Indapamide | Increased diuretic effect. |
| Labetolol | Increased antihypertensive effects. |
| Lithium | Increased effect of lithium. |
| MAO inhibitors | Increased chlorthalidone effect. |
| Nitrates | Excessive blood-pressure drop. |
| Oxprenolol | Increased antihypertensive effect. Dosages of both drugs may require adjustments. |
| Pentoxifylline | Increased antihypertensive effect. |
| Potassium supplements | Decreased potassium effect. |
| Probenecid | Decreased probenecid effect. |

 ## POSSIBLE INTERACTION WITH OTHER SUBSTANCES

| INTERACTS WITH | COMBINED EFFECT |
|---|---|
| Alcohol: | Dangerous blood-pressure drop. |
| Beverages: | None expected. |
| Cocaine: | None expected. |
| Foods: Licorice. | Excessive potassium loss that causes dangerous heart rhythms. |
| Marijuana: | May increase blood pressure. |
| Tobacco: | None expected. |

# CHLORZOXAZONE

## BRAND NAMES

Algisin
Chlorzone Forte

Paraflex
Parafon Forte

## BASIC INFORMATION

**Habit forming? No**
**Prescription needed? Yes**
**Available as generic? Yes**
**Drug class: Muscle relaxant (skeletal)**

 ## USES

Treatment for sprains, strains and muscle spasms.

 ## DOSAGE & USAGE INFORMATION

**How to take:**
Tablet or capsule—Swallow with liquid.

**When to take:**
As needed, no more often than every 4 hours.

**If you forget a dose:**
Take as soon as you remember. Wait 4 hours for next dose.

**What drug does:**
Blocks body's pain messages to brain. May also sedate.

**Time lapse before drug works:**
60 minutes.

**Don't take with:**
See Interaction column and consult doctor.

 ## OVERDOSE

**SYMPTOMS:**
**Nausea, vomiting, diarrhea, headache, severe weakness, breathing difficulty, sensation of paralysis.**
**WHAT TO DO:**
**Overdose unlikely to threaten life. Depending on severity of symptoms and amount taken, call doctor, poison-control center or hospital emergency room for instructions.**

 ## POSSIBLE ADVERSE REACTIONS OR SIDE EFFECTS

| SYMPTOMS | WHAT TO DO |
|---|---|
| **Life-threatening:** None expected. | |
| **Common:** | |
| ● Drowsiness, dizziness. | Continue. Call doctor when convenient. |
| ● Orange or red-purple urine. | No action necessary. |
| **Infrequent:** Agitation, constipation or diarrhea, nausea, cramps, vomiting. | Discontinue. Call doctor right away. |
| **Rare:** | |
| ● Bloody or tarry, black stool. | Discontinue. Seek emergency treatment. |
| ● Rash or itch, sore throat, fever, jaundice, tiredness, weakness. | Discontinue. Call doctor right away. |

## WARNINGS & PRECAUTIONS

**Don't take if:**
You are allergic to any skeletal-muscle relaxant.

**Before you start, consult your doctor:**
- If you have had liver disease.
- If you plan pregnancy within medication period.

**Over age 60:**
Adverse reactions and side effects may be more frequent and severe than in younger persons.

**Pregnancy:**
No proven harm to unborn child. Avoid if possible.

**Breast-feeding:**
Drug passes into milk. Avoid drug or discontinue nursing until you finish medicine. Consult doctor for advice on maintaining milk supply.

**Infants & children:**
Not recommended.

**Prolonged use:**
No problems expected.

**Skin & sunlight:**
No problems expected.

**Driving, piloting or hazardous work:**
Don't drive or pilot aircraft until you learn how medicine affects you. Don't work around dangerous machinery. Don't climb ladders or work in high places. Danger increases if you drink alcohol or take medicine affecting alertness and reflexes, such as antihistamines, tranquilizers, sedatives, pain medicine, narcotics and mind-altering drugs.

**Discontinuing:**
Don't discontinue without doctor's advice until you complete prescribed dose, even though symptoms diminish or disappear.

**Others:**
Periodic liver-function tests recommended if you use this drug for a long time.

## POSSIBLE INTERACTION WITH OTHER DRUGS

| GENERIC NAME OR DRUG CLASS | COMBINED EFFECT |
|---|---|
| Antidepressants | Increased sedation. |
| Antihistamines | Increased sedation. |
| Dronabinol | Increased effect of dronabinol on central nervous system. Avoid combination. |
| MAO inhibitors | Increased effect of both drugs. |
| Mind-altering drugs | Increased sedation. |
| Muscle relaxants (others) | Increased sedation. |
| Narcotics | Increased sedation. |
| Sedatives | Increased sedation. |
| Sleep inducers | Increased sedation |
| Testosterone | Decreased chlorzoxazone effect. |
| Tranquilizers | Increased sedation. |

## POSSIBLE INTERACTION WITH OTHER SUBSTANCES

| INTERACTS WITH | COMBINED EFFECT |
|---|---|
| Alcohol: | Increased sedation. |
| Beverages: | No problems expected. |
| Cocaine: | Lack of coordination. |
| Foods: | No problems expected. |
| Marijuana: | Lack of coordination, drowsiness, fainting. |
| Tobacco: | No problems expected. |

# CHLORZOXAZONE & ACETAMINOPHEN

## BRAND NAMES

Blanex
Chlorofon-F
Chlorzone Forte
Flexaphen
Flexin
Lobac

Mus-Lax
Paracet Forte
Parafon Forte
Polyflex
Zoxaphen

## BASIC INFORMATION

Habit forming? No
Prescription needed? Yes
Available as generic? No
Drug class: Muscle relaxant (skeletal),
analgesic, fever-reducer

 ## USES

- Treatment for sprains, strains and muscle spasms.
- Treatment of mild to moderate pain and fever.

 ## DOSAGE & USAGE INFORMATION

How to take:
Tablet or capsule—Swallow with liquid.

When to take:
As needed, no more often than every 3 hours.

If you forget a dose:
Take as soon as you remember. Wait 3 hours for next dose.

*Continued next column*

 ## OVERDOSE

SYMPTOMS:
Nausea, vomiting, diarrhea, headache, severe weakness, unusual increase in sweating, fainting, breathing difficulty, irritability, convulsions, sensation of paralysis, coma.
WHAT TO DO:
- Overdose unlikely to threaten life. Depending on severity of symptoms and amount taken, call doctor, poison-control center or hospital emergency room for instructions.
- Dial 0 (operator) or 911 (emergency) for an ambulance or medical help. Then give first aid immediately.
- See emergency information on inside covers.

## What drug does:
- Blocks body's pain messages to brain. May also sedate.
- May affect hypothalamus, the part of the brain that helps regulate body heat and receives body's pain messages.

## Time lapse before drug works:
15 to 30 minutes. May last 4 hours.

## Don't take with:
- Other drugs with acetaminophen. Too much acetaminophen can damage liver and kidneys.
- See Interaction column and consult doctor.

 ## POSSIBLE ADVERSE REACTIONS OR SIDE EFFECTS

| SYMPTOMS | WHAT TO DO |
|---|---|
| **Life-threatening:** None expected. | |
| **Common:** Dizziness, lightheadedness, drowsiness. | Discontinue. Call doctor right away. |
| **Infrequent:** <br>• Difficult or frequent urination. | Discontinue. Call doctor right away. |
| • Nervousness, restlessness, irritability, constipation, headache, indigestion. | Continue. Call doctor when convenient. |
| **Rare:** <br>• Sudden decrease in urine output; swelling of lips, face or tongue. | Discontinue. Seek emergency treatment. |
| • Bloody or black stools, jaundice, unusual bleeding or bruising, sore mouth or throat, fever. | Discontinue. Call doctor right away. |

## WARNINGS & PRECAUTIONS

### Don't take if:
- You are allergic to any skeletal-muscle relaxant or acetaminophen.
- Your symptoms don't improve after 2 days use. Call your doctor.

### Before you start, consult your doctor:
- If you have had liver disease.
- If you have bronchial asthma, kidney disease or liver damage.
- If you plan pregnancy within medication period.

### Over age 60:
- Adverse reactions and side effects may be more frequent and severe than in younger persons.
- Don't exceed recommended dose. You can't eliminate drug as efficiently as younger persons.

### Pregnancy:
No proven harm to unborn child. Avoid if possible.

### Breast-feeding:
Drug passes into milk. Avoid drug or discontinue nursing until you finish medicine. Consult doctor for advice on maintaining milk supply.

### Infants & children:
Not recommended.

### Prolonged use:
May affect blood system and cause anemia. Limit use to 5 days for children 12 and under, and 10 days for adults.

### Skin & sunlight:
No problems expected.

### Driving, piloting or hazardous work:
Don't drive or pilot aircraft until you learn how medicine affects you. Don't work around dangerous machinery. Don't climb ladders or work in high places. Danger increases if you drink alcohol or take medicine affecting alertness and reflexes, such as antihistamines, tranquilizers, sedatives, pain medicine, narcotics and mind-altering drugs.

### Discontinuing:
Don't discontinue without consulting your doctor. Dose may require gradual reduction if you have taken drug for a long time. Doses of other drugs may also require adjustment.

### Others:
Periodic liver-function tests recommended if you use this drug for a long time.

## POSSIBLE INTERACTION WITH OTHER DRUGS

| GENERIC NAME OR DRUG CLASS | COMBINED EFFECT |
|---|---|
| Anticoagulants (oral) | May increase anticoagulant effect. If combined frequently, prothrombin time should be monitored. |
| Antidepressants | Increased sedation. |
| Antihistamines | Increased sedation. |
| Dronabinol | Increased effect of dronabinol on central nervous system. Avoid combination. |
| MAO inhibitors | Increased effect (but safety not established) of both drugs. |
| Mind-altering drugs | Increased sedation. |
| Muscle relaxants (others) | Increased sedation. |
| Narcotics | Increased sedation. |
| Phenobarbital | Quicker elimination and decreased effects of acetaminophen. |
| Sedatives | Increased sedation. |
| Sleep inducers | Increased sedation. |
| Testosterone | Decreased chlorzoxazone effect. |
| Tetracyclines (effervescent granules or tablets) | May slow tetracycline absorption. Space doses 2 hours apart. |
| Tranquilizers | Increased sedation. |

## POSSIBLE INTERACTION WITH OTHER SUBSTANCES

| INTERACTS WITH | COMBINED EFFECT |
|---|---|
| Alcohol: | Drowsiness, increased sedation. |
| Beverages: | No problems expected. |
| Cocaine: | Lack of coordination. May slow body's recovery. Avoid. |
| Foods: | No problems expected. |
| Marijuana: | Increased pain relief, lack of coordination, drowsiness, fainting. May slow body's recovery. Avoid. |
| Tobacco: | No problems expected. |

# CHOLESTYRAMINE

## BRAND NAMES

Questran

## BASIC INFORMATION

Habit forming? No
Prescription needed? Yes
Available as generic? No
Drug class: Antihyperlipidemic, antipruritic

 **USES**

- Removes excess bile acids that occur with some liver problems. Reduces persistent itch caused by bile acids.
- Lowers cholesterol level.

 **DOSAGE & USAGE INFORMATION**

**How to take:**
Powder, granules—Sprinkle into 8 oz. liquid. Let stand for 2 minutes, then mix with liquid before swallowing. Or mix with cereal, soup or pulpy fruit. Don't swallow dry.

**When to take:**
3 or 4 times a day on an empty stomach, 1 hour before or 2 hours after eating.

**If you forget a dose:**
Take as soon as you remember up to 2 hours late. If more than 2 hours, wait for next scheduled dose (don't double this dose).

**What drug does:**
Binds with bile acids to prevent their absorption.

**Time lapse before drug works:**
- Cholesterol reduction—1 day.
- Bile-acid reduction—3 to 4 weeks.

**Don't take with:**
- Any drug or vitamin simultaneously. Space doses 2 hours apart.
- See Interaction column and consult doctor.

 **OVERDOSE**

**SYMPTOMS:**
Increased side effects and adverse reactions.
**WHAT TO DO:**
Overdose unlikely to threaten life. Depending on severity of symptoms and amount taken, call doctor, poison-control center or hospital emergency room for instructions.

 **POSSIBLE ADVERSE REACTIONS OR SIDE EFFECTS**

| SYMPTOMS | WHAT TO DO |
|---|---|
| **Life-threatening:** None expected. | |
| **Common:** Constipation. | Continue. Call doctor when convenient. |
| **Infrequent:** Belching, bloating, diarrhea, mild nausea, vomiting, stomach pain. | Discontinue. Call doctor right away. |
| **Rare:** | |
| • Severe stomach pain; nausea; vomiting; black, tarry stool. | Discontinue. Seek emergency treatment. |
| • Rash. | Discontinue. Call doctor right away. |
| • Sore tongue. | Continue. Call doctor when convenient. |

## WARNINGS & PRECAUTIONS

**Don't take if:**
You are allergic to cholestyramine.

**Before you start, consult your doctor:**
- If you plan to become pregnant within medication period.
- If you have angina, heart or blood-vessel disease.
- If you have stomach problems (including ulcer).
- If you have constipation or hemorrhoids.
- If you have kidney disease.

**Over age 60:**
Adverse reactions and side effects may be more frequent and severe than in younger persons.

**Pregnancy:**
No proven harm to unborn child. Avoid if possible.

**Breast-feeding:**
No problems expected, but consult doctor.

**Infants & children:**
Not recommended.

**Prolonged use:**
No problems expected.

**Skin & sunlight:**
No problems expected.

**Driving, piloting or hazardous work:**
No problems expected.

**Discontinuing:**
Don't discontinue without doctor's advice until you complete prescribed dose, even though symptoms diminish or disappear.

**Others:**
No problems expected.

## POSSIBLE INTERACTION WITH OTHER DRUGS

| GENERIC NAME OR DRUG CLASS | COMBINED EFFECT |
|---|---|
| Anticoagulants | Increased anticoagulant effect. |
| Digitalis preparations | Decreased digitalis effect. |
| Indapamide | Decreased indapamide effect. |
| Thyroid hormones | Decreased thyroid effect. |
| All other medicines | Decreased absorption, so dosages or dosage intervals may require adjustment. |

## POSSIBLE INTERACTION WITH OTHER SUBSTANCES

| INTERACTS WITH | COMBINED EFFECT |
|---|---|
| Alcohol: | None expected. |
| Beverages: | None expected. |
| Cocaine: | None expected. |
| Foods: | Absorption of vitamins in foods decreased. Take vitamin supplements, particularly A, D, E & K. |
| Marijuana: | None expected. |
| Tobacco: | None expected. |

# CIMETIDINE

## BRAND NAMES

| | |
|---|---|
| Apo-Cimetidine | Peptol |
| Novo-Cimetine | Tagamet |

## BASIC INFORMATION

**Habit forming?** No
**Prescription needed?** Yes
**Available as generic?** No
**Drug class:** Histamine H-2 antagonist

## USES

Treatment for duodenal ulcers and other conditions in which stomach produces excess hydrochloric acid.

## DOSAGE & USAGE INFORMATION

**How to take:**
Tablet or capsule—Swallow with liquid.

**When to take:**
- 1 dose per day—Take at bedtime.
- 2 or more doses per day—Take at the same times each day.

**If you forget a dose:**
Take as soon as you remember up to 2 hours late. If more than 2 hours, wait for next scheduled dose (don't double this dose).

**What drug does:**
Blocks histamine release so stomach secretes less acid.

**Time lapse before drug works:**
Begins in 30 minutes. May require several days to relieve pain.

**Don't take with:**
See Interaction column and consult doctor.

## OVERDOSE

**SYMPTOMS:**
Confusion, slurred speech, breathing difficulty, rapid heartbeat, delirium.
**WHAT TO DO:**
Overdose unlikely to threaten life. If person takes much larger amount than prescribed, call doctor, poison-control center or hospital emergency room for instructions.

## POSSIBLE ADVERSE REACTIONS OR SIDE EFFECTS

| SYMPTOMS | WHAT TO DO |
|---|---|
| **Life-threatening:**<br>None expected. | |
| **Common:**<br>None expected. | |
| **Infrequent:** | |
| • Dizziness or headache, diarrhea, decreased sperm production. | Continue. Call doctor when convenient. |
| • Diminished sex drive, breast swelling and soreness in males, unusual milk flow in females, hair loss. | Continue. Tell doctor at next visit. |
| **Rare:**<br>Confusion; rash, hives; sore throat, fever; slow, fast or irregular heartbeat; unusual bleeding or bruising; muscle cramps or pain; fatigue; weakness. | Discontinue. Call doctor right away. |

## WARNINGS & PRECAUTIONS

**Don't take if:**
You are allergic to cimetidine or other histamine H-2 antagonist.

**Before you start, consult your doctor:**
- If you plan to become pregnant during medication period.
- If you take aspirin. Aspirin may irritate stomach.

**Over age 60:**
Adverse reactions and side effects may be more frequent and severe than in younger persons.

**Pregnancy:**
No proven harm to unborn child. Avoid if possible.

**Breast-feeding:**
No problems expected.

**Infants & children:**
Not recommended.

**Prolonged use:**
Possible liver damage.

**Skin & sunlight:**
No problems expected.

**Driving, piloting or hazardous work:**
Don't drive or pilot aircraft until you learn how medicine affects you. Don't work around dangerous machinery. Don't climb ladders or work in high places. Danger increases if you drink alcohol or take medicine affecting alertness and reflexes, such as antihistamines, tranquilizers, sedatives, pain medicine, narcotics and mind-altering drugs.

**Discontinuing:**
Don't discontinue without consulting doctor. Dose may require gradual reduction if you have taken drug for a long time. Doses of other drugs may also require adjustment.

**Others:**
Patients on kidney dialysis—Take at end of dialysis treatment.

## POSSIBLE INTERACTION WITH OTHER DRUGS

| GENERIC NAME OR DRUG CLASS | COMBINED EFFECT |
| --- | --- |
| Anticoagulants (oral) | Increased anticoagulant effect. |
| Anticholinergics | Decreased cimetidine effect. |
| Bethanechol | Increased cimetidine effect. |
| Carmustine (BCNU) | Severe impairment of red-blood-cell production; some interference with white-blood-cell formation. |
| Digitalis preparations | Increased digitalis effect. |
| Labetolol | Increased antihypertensive effects. |
| Penicillins | Increased penicillin effect. |
| Propranolol | May increase propranolol effect. |
| Quinidine | Increased quinidine effect. |
| Theophylline | Increased theophylline effect. |

## POSSIBLE INTERACTION WITH OTHER SUBSTANCES

| INTERACTS WITH | COMBINED EFFECT |
| --- | --- |
| Alcohol: | No interactions expected, but alcohol may slow body's recovery. Avoid. |
| Beverages: Milk. | Enhanced effectiveness. Small amounts useful for taking medication. |
| Caffeine drinks. | May increase acid secretion and delay healing. |
| Cocaine: | Decreased cimetidine effect. |
| Foods: | Enhanced effectiveness. Protein-rich foods should be eaten in moderation to minimize secretion of stomach acid. |
| Marijuana: | Increased chance of low sperm count. Marijuana may slow body's recovery. Avoid. |
| Tobacco: | No interactions expected, but tobacco may slow body's recovery. Avoid. |

# CINOXACIN

## BRAND NAMES

Azolinic Acid     Cinobactin
Cinobac

## BASIC INFORMATION

**Habit forming? No**
**Prescription needed? Yes**
**Available as generic? No**
**Drug class: Urinary anti-infective**

 ## USES

Treatment for urinary-tract infections.

 ## DOSAGE & USAGE INFORMATION

**How to take:**
- Tablet—Swallow with food or milk to lessen stomach irritation. If you can't swallow whole, crumble tablet and take with liquid or food.
- Liquid—Take with liquid or food.

**When to take:**
At the same times each day.

**If you forget a dose:**
Take as soon as you remember up to 2 hours late. If more than 2 hours, wait for next scheduled dose (don't double this dose).

**What drug does:**
Destroys bacteria susceptible to cinoxacin.

**Time lapse before drug works:**
1 to 2 weeks.

**Don't take with:**
See Interaction column and consult doctor.

 ## OVERDOSE

**SYMPTOMS:**
**Lethargy, stomach upset, behavioral changes, convulsions and stupor.**
**WHAT TO DO:**
- **Dial 0 (operator) or 911 (emergency) for an ambulance or medical help. Then give first aid immediately.**
- **If patient is unconscious and not breathing, give mouth-to-mouth breathing. If there is no heartbeat, use cardiac massage and mouth-to-mouth breathing (CPR). Don't try to make patient vomit. If you can't get help quickly, take patient to nearest emergency facility.**
- **See emergency information on inside covers.**

 ## POSSIBLE ADVERSE REACTIONS OR SIDE EFFECTS

| SYMPTOMS | WHAT TO DO |
|---|---|
| **Life-threatening:**<br>None expected. | |
| **Common:**<br>Rash, itch; decreased, blurred or double vision; halos around lights or excess brightness; changes in color vision; nausea, vomiting, diarrhea. | Discontinue. Call doctor right away. |
| **Infrequent:**<br>Dizziness, drowsiness, headache, ringing in ears, insomnia. | Continue. Call doctor when convenient. |
| **Rare:**<br>Severe stomach pain. | Discontinue. Call doctor right away. |

## WARNINGS & PRECAUTIONS

**Don't take if:**
- You are allergic to cinoxacin or nalidixic acid.
- You have a seizure disorder (epilepsy, convulsions).

**Before you start, consult your doctor:**
- If you plan to become pregnant during medication period.
- If you have or have had kidney or liver disease.
- If you have impaired circulation to the brain (hardened arteries).

**Over age 60:**
Adverse reactions and side effects may be more frequent and severe than in younger persons.

**Pregnancy:**
Risk to unborn child outweighs drug benefits. Don't use, especially during first 3 months.

**Breast-feeding:**
No problems expected, unless you have impaired kidney function. Consult doctor.

**Infants & children:**
Don't give to infants younger than 3 months.

**Prolonged use:**
No problems expected.

**Skin & sunlight:**
- May cause sunlight to hurt eyes.
- May cause rash or intensify sunburn in areas exposed to sun or sunlamp.

**Driving, piloting or hazardous work:**
Avoid if you feel drowsy, dizzy or have vision problems. Otherwise, no problems expected.

**Discontinuing:**
Don't discontinue without consulting doctor. Dose may require gradual reduction if you have taken drug for a long time. Doses of other drugs may also require adjustment.

**Others:**
Periodic blood counts, liver-function and kidney-function tests recommended.

 ## POSSIBLE INTERACTION WITH OTHER DRUGS

| GENERIC NAME OR DRUG CLASS | COMBINED EFFECT |
| --- | --- |
| None reported. | |

 ## POSSIBLE INTERACTION WITH OTHER SUBSTANCES

| INTERACTS WITH | COMBINED EFFECT |
| --- | --- |
| Alcohol: | Impaired alertness, judgment and coordination. |
| Beverages: | None expected. |
| Cocaine: | Impaired judgment and coordination. |
| Foods: | None expected. |
| Marijuana: | Impaired alertness, judgment and coordination. |
| Tobacco: | None expected. |

# CITRATES

## BRAND AND GENERIC NAMES

Albright's Solution
Bicitra
Citrolith
Modified Shohl's
  Solution
Oracit
Polycitra
Polycitra-K
POTASSIUM
  CITRATE

POTASSIUM
  CITRATE & CITRIC
  ACID
POTASSIUM
  CITRATE &
  SODIUM CITRATE
SODIUM CITRATE &
  CITRIC ACID
TRICITRATES
Urocit-K

## BASIC INFORMATION

**Habit forming?** No
**Prescription needed?** Yes
**Available as generic?** No
**Drug class:** Urinary alkalizer, antiurolithic
  (kidney stone)

 **USES**

- To make urine more alkaline (less acid).
- To treat or prevent recurrence of some types of kidney stones.

 **DOSAGE & USAGE INFORMATION**

**How to take:**
Tablets—Swallow whole with liquid. If tablets seem to stick in throat or esophagus, eat a banana to help ease it into the stomach.

**When to take:**
On full stomach, usually after meals or with food.

**If you forget a dose:**
Take as soon as you remember up to 2 hours late. If more than 2 hours, wait for next scheduled dose (don't double this dose).

*Continued next column*

 **OVERDOSE**

**SYMPTOMS:**
Convulsions, coma.
**WHAT TO DO:**
- Dial 0 (operator) or 911 (emergency) for an ambulance or medical help. Then give first aid immediately.
- See emergency information on inside covers.

**What drug does:**
Increases urinary alkalinity by excretion of bicarbonate ions.

**Time lapse before drug works:**
1 hour.

**Don't take with:**
- Any medicine that will decrease mental alertness or reflexes, such as alcohol, other mind-altering drugs, cough/cold medicines, antihistamines, allergy medicine, sedatives, tranquilizers (sleeping pills or "downers"), barbiturates, seizure medicine, narcotics, other prescription medicine for pain, muscle relaxants, anesthetics.
- See Interaction column and consult doctor.

 **POSSIBLE ADVERSE REACTIONS OR SIDE EFFECTS**

| SYMPTOMS | WHAT TO DO |
|---|---|
| **Life-threatening:** Black, tarry stools; vomiting blood; severe abdominal cramps; irregular heartbeat; shortness of breath. | Discontinue. Seek emergency treatment. |
| **Common:** Nausea or vomiting. | Continue. Call doctor when convenient. |
| **Infrequent:** Confusion, dizziness, swollen feet and ankles, irritability, depression, muscle pain, nervousness, numbness or tingling in hands or feet, unpleasant taste, weakness. | Discontinue. Call doctor right away. |
| **Rare:** None expected. | |

## WARNINGS & PRECAUTIONS

**Don't take if:**
You are allergic to any citrate.

**Before you start, consult your doctor:**
- If you have any disease involving the adrenal glands, diabetes, chronic diarrhea, heart problems, hypertension, kidney disease, stomach ulcer or gastritis, urinary tract infection, toxemia of pregnancy.
- If you plan strenuous exercise.

**Over age 60:**
Adverse reactions and side effects may be more frequent and severe than in younger persons. Ask doctor about smaller doses.

**Pregnancy:**
Safety to unborn child unestablished. Avoid if possible.

**Breast-feeding:**
Safety during lactation not established. Consult doctor.

**Infants & children:**
Use only under close medical supervision.

**Prolonged use:**
Adverse reactions more likely.

**Skin & sunlight:**
No problems expected.

**Driving, piloting or hazardous work:**
Don't drive or pilot aircraft until you learn how medicine affects you. Don't work around dangerous machinery. Don't climb ladders or work in high places. Danger increases if you drink alcohol or take medicine affecting alertness and reflexes, such as antihistamines, tranquilizers, sedatives, pain medicine, narcotics and mind-altering drugs.

**Discontinuing:**
Don't discontinue without consulting doctor. Dose may require gradual reduction if you have taken drug for a long time. Doses of other drugs may also require adjustment.

**Others:**
- Drink at least 8 ounces of water or other liquid (except milk) every hour while awake.
- Liquid may be chilled (don't freeze) to improve taste.

## POSSIBLE INTERACTION WITH OTHER DRUGS

| GENERIC NAME OR DRUG CLASS | COMBINED EFFECT |
|---|---|
| Antacids | Toxic effect of citrates (alkalosis). |
| Calcium supplements | Increases risk of kidney stones. |
| Methenamine | Decreases effects of methenamine. |
| Mexiletine | May slow elimination of mexiletine and cause need to adjust dosage. |
| Quinidine | Prolongs citrate effect. |

## POSSIBLE INTERACTION WITH OTHER SUBSTANCES

| INTERACTS WITH | COMBINED EFFECT |
|---|---|
| Alcohol: | Will decrease mental alertness. |
| Beverages: Salt-free milk. | May cause potassium toxicity. |
| Cocaine: | No proven problems. |
| Foods: Milk, cheese, ice cream, yogurt, buttermilk, salty foods, salt, salt substitutes. | May increase likelihood of kidney stones. |
| Marijuana: | No proven problems. |
| Tobacco: | Increases likelihood of stomach irritation. |

# CLEMASTINE

## BRAND NAMES

Tavist

## BASIC INFORMATION

Habit forming? No
Prescription needed? No
Available as generic? No
Drug class: Antihistamine

## USES

Reduces allergic symptoms such as hay fever, hives, rash or itching.

## DOSAGE & USAGE INFORMATION

**How to take:**
Tablet—Swallow with liquid or food to lessen stomach irritation.

**When to take:**
Varies with form. Follow label directions.

**If you forget a dose:**
Take as soon as you remember up to 2 hours late. If more than 2 hours, wait for next scheduled dose (don't double this dose).

**What drug does:**
Blocks action of histamine after an allergic response triggers histamine release in sensitive cells.

**Time lapse before drug works:**
30 minutes.

**Don't take with:**
See Interaction column and consult doctor.

## OVERDOSE

**SYMPTOMS:**
Convulsions, red face, hallucinations, coma.
**WHAT TO DO:**
- Dial 0 (operator) or 911 (emergency) for an ambulance or medical help. Then give first aid immediately.
- If patient is unconscious and not breathing, give mouth-to-mouth breathing. If there is no heartbeat, use cardiac massage and mouth-to-mouth breathing (CPR). Don't try to make patient vomit. If you can't get help quickly, take patient to nearest emergency facility.
- See emergency information on inside covers.

## POSSIBLE ADVERSE REACTIONS OR SIDE EFFECTS

| SYMPTOMS | WHAT TO DO |
|---|---|
| **Life-threatening:**<br>None expected. | |
| **Common:**<br>Drowsiness; dizziness; dry mouth, nose, throat; nausea. | Continue. Tell doctor at next visit. |
| **Infrequent:** | |
| • Vision changes. | Discontinue. Call doctor right away. |
| • Less tolerance for contact lenses; difficult urination. | Continue. Call doctor when convenient. |
| • Appetite loss. | Continue. Tell doctor at next visit. |
| **Rare:**<br>Nightmares, agitation, irritability; sore throat, fever; rapid heartbeat; unusual bleeding or bruising; fatigue, weakness. | Discontinue. Call doctor right away. |

## WARNINGS & PRECAUTIONS

**Don't take if:**
You are allergic to any antihistamine.

**Before you start, consult your doctor:**
- If you have glaucoma.
- If you have enlarged prostate.
- If you have asthma.
- If you have kidney disease.
- If you have peptic ulcer.
- If you will have surgery within 2 months, including dental surgery, requiring general or spinal anesthesia.

**Over age 60:**
Don't exceed recommended dose. Adverse reactions and side effects may be more frequent and severe than in younger persons, especially urination difficulty, diminished alertness and other brain and nervous-system symptoms.

**Pregnancy:**
No proven harm to unborn child. Avoid if possible.

**Breast-feeding:**
Drug passes into milk. Avoid drug or discontinue nursing until you finish medicine. Consult doctor for advice on maintaining milk supply.

**Infants & children:**
Not recommended for premature or newborn infants. Otherwise, no problems expected.

**Prolonged use:**
Avoid. May damage bone marrow and nerve cells.

**Skin & sunlight:**
May cause rash or intensify sunburn in areas exposed to sun or sunlamp.

**Driving, piloting or hazardous work:**
Don't drive or pilot aircraft until you learn how medicine affects you. Don't work around dangerous machinery. Don't climb ladders or work in high places. Danger increases if you drink alcohol or take medicine affecting alertness and reflexes, such as antihistamines, tranquilizers, sedatives, pain medicine, narcotics and mind-altering drugs.

**Discontinuing:**
No problems expected.

**Others:**
May mask symptoms of hearing damage from aspirin, other salicylates, cisplatin, paromomycin, vancomycin or anticonvulsants. Consult doctor if you use these.

 ## POSSIBLE INTERACTION WITH OTHER DRUGS

| GENERIC NAME OR DRUG CLASS | COMBINED EFFECT |
|---|---|
| Anticholinergics | Increased anticholinergic effect. |
| Antidepressants | Excess sedation. Avoid. |
| Antihistamines (other) | Excess sedation. Avoid. |
| Dronabinol | Increased effects of both drugs. Avoid. |
| Hypnotics | Excess sedation. Avoid. |
| MAO inhibitors | Increased clemastine effect. |
| Mind-altering drugs | Excess sedation. Avoid. |
| Molindone | Increased antihistamine effect. |
| Narcotics | Excess sedation. Avoid. |
| Sedatives | Excess sedation. Avoid. |
| Sleep inducers | Excess sedation. Avoid. |
| Tranquilizers | Excess sedation. Avoid. |

 ## POSSIBLE INTERACTION WITH OTHER SUBSTANCES

| INTERACTS WITH | COMBINED EFFECT |
|---|---|
| Alcohol: | Excess sedation. Avoid. |
| Beverages: Caffeine drinks. | Less clemastine sedation. |
| Cocaine: | Decreased clemastine effect. Avoid. |
| Foods: | None expected. |
| Marijuana: | Excess sedation. Avoid. |
| Tobacco: | None expected. |

# CLIDINIUM

## BRAND NAMES

Clipoxide          Quarzan
Librax

## BASIC INFORMATION

Habit forming? No
Prescription needed?
   Low strength: No
   High strength: Yes
Available as generic? Yes
Drug class: Antispasmodic, anticholinergic

 **USES**

Reduces spasms of digestive system, bladder and urethra.

 **DOSAGE & USAGE INFORMATION**

**How to take:**
Capsule—Swallow with liquid or food to lessen stomach irritation.

**When to take:**
30 minutes before meals (unless directed otherwise by doctor).

**If you forget a dose:**
Take as soon as you remember up to 2 hours late. If more than 2 hours, wait for next scheduled dose (don't double this dose).

**What drug does:**
Blocks nerve impulses at parasympathetic nerve endings, preventing muscle contractions and gland secretions of organs involved.

**Time lapse before drug works:**
15 to 30 minutes.

**Don't take with:**
See Interaction column and consult doctor.

 **OVERDOSE**

**SYMPTOMS:**
**Dilated pupils, rapid pulse and breathing, dizziness, fever, hallucinations, confusion, slurred speech, agitation, flushed face, convulsions, coma.**
**WHAT TO DO:**
- **Dial 0 (operator) or 911 (emergency) for an ambulance or medical help. Then give first aid immediately.**
- **See emergency information on inside covers.**

 **POSSIBLE ADVERSE REACTIONS OR SIDE EFFECTS**

| SYMPTOMS | WHAT TO DO |
|---|---|
| **Life-threatening:** None expected. | |
| **Common:** | |
| • Confusion, delirium, rapid heartbeat. | Discontinue. Call doctor right away. |
| • Nausea, vomiting, decreased sweating. | Continue. Call doctor when convenient. |
| • Constipation. | Continue. Tell doctor at next visit. |
| • Dryness in ears, nose, throat. | No action necessary. |
| **Infrequent:** | |
| • Nasal congestion, altered taste. | Discontinue. Call doctor right away. |
| • Difficult urination, headache. | Continue. Call doctor when convenient. |
| **Rare:** Rash or hives, pain, blurred vision. | Discontinue. Call doctor right away. |

 **WARNINGS & PRECAUTIONS**

**Don't take if:**
- You are allergic to any anticholinergic.
- You have trouble with stomach bloating.
- You have difficulty emptying your bladder completely.
- You have narrow-angle glaucoma.
- You have severe ulcerative colitis.

**Before you start, consult your doctor:**
- If you have open-angle glaucoma.
- If you have angina.
- If you have chronic bronchitis or asthma.
- If you have hiatal hernia.
- If you have liver disease.
- If you have enlarged prostate.
- If you have myasthenia gravis.
- If you have peptic ulcer.
- If you will have surgery within 2 months, including dental surgery, requiring general or spinal anesthesia.

**Over age 60:**
Adverse reactions and side effects may be more frequent and severe than in younger persons.

**Pregnancy:**
Studies inconclusive on harm to unborn child. Animal studies show fetal abnormalities. Decide with your doctor whether drug benefits justify risk to unborn child.

**Breast-feeding:**
Drug passes into milk and decreases milk flow. Avoid drug or discontinue nursing until you finish medicine. Consult doctor for advice on maintaining milk supply.

**Infants & children:**
Use only under medical supervision.

**Prolonged use:**
Chronic constipation, possible fecal impaction. Consult doctor immediately.

**Skin & sunlight:**
No problems expected.

**Driving, piloting or hazardous work:**
Don't drive or pilot aircraft until you learn how medicine affects you. Don't work around dangerous machinery. Don't climb ladders or work in high places. Danger increases if you drink alcohol or take medicine affecting alertness and reflexes, such as antihistamines, tranquilizers, sedatives, pain medicine, narcotics, or mind-altering drugs.

**Discontinuing:**
May be unnecessary to finish medicine. Follow doctor's instructions.

**Others:**
No problems expected.

## POSSIBLE INTERACTION WITH OTHER DRUGS

| GENERIC NAME OR DRUG CLASS | COMBINED EFFECT |
|---|---|
| Amantadine | Increased clidinium effect. |
| Antacids | Decreased clidinium effect. |
| Anticholinergics (other) | Increased clidinium effect. |
| Antidepressants (tricyclic) | Increased clidinium effect. Increased sedation. |
| Antihistamines | Increased clidinium effect. |
| Haloperidol | Increased internal-eye pressure. |
| MAO inhibitors | Increased clidinium effect. |
| Meperidine | Increased clidinium effect. |
| Methylphenidate | Increased clidinium effect. |
| Molindone | Increased anticholinergic effect. |
| Nitrates | Increased internal-eye pressure. |
| Orphenadrine | Increased clidinium effect. |
| Phenothiazines | Increased clidinium effect. |
| Pilocarpine | Loss of pilocarpine effect in glaucoma treatment. |
| Potassium supplements | Possible intestinal ulcers with oral potassium tablets. |
| Tranquilizers | Decreased clidinium effect. |
| Vitamin C | Decreased clidinium effect. Avoid large doses of vitamin C. |

## POSSIBLE INTERACTION WITH OTHER SUBSTANCES

| INTERACTS WITH | COMBINED EFFECT |
|---|---|
| Alcohol: | None expected. |
| Beverages: | None expected. |
| Cocaine: | Excessively rapid heartbeat. Avoid. |
| Foods: | None expected. |
| Marijuana: | Drowsiness and dry mouth. |
| Tobacco: | None expected. |

# CLINDAMYCIN

## BRAND NAMES

Cleocin                    Dalacin C
Cleocin-T

## BASIC INFORMATION

**Habit forming? No**
**Prescription needed? Yes**
**Available as generic? No**
**Drug class: Antibiotic (lincomycin)**

 **USES**

Treatment of bacterial infections that are
susceptible to clindamycin.

 **DOSAGE & USAGE INFORMATION**

**How to take:**
Capsule or liquid—Swallow with liquid 1 hour
before or 2 hours after eating.

**When to take:**
At the same times each day.

**If you forget a dose:**
Take as soon as you remember up to 2 hours
late. If more than 2 hours, wait for next
scheduled dose (don't double this dose).

**What drug does:**
Destroys susceptible bacteria. Does not kill
viruses.

**Time lapse before drug works:**
3 to 5 days.

**Don't take with:**
See Interaction column and consult doctor.

 **OVERDOSE**

**SYMPTOMS:**
**Severe nausea, vomiting, diarrhea.**
**WHAT TO DO:**
**Overdose unlikely to threaten life. If person
takes much larger amount than prescribed,
call doctor, poison-control center or hospital
emergency room for instructions.**

 **POSSIBLE ADVERSE REACTIONS OR SIDE EFFECTS**

| SYMPTOMS | WHAT TO DO |
|---|---|
| **Life-threatening:** None expected. | |
| **Common:** None expected. | |
| **Infrequent:** | |
| • Unusual thirst; vomiting; stomach cramps; severe and watery diarrhea with blood or mucus; painful, swollen joints; jaundice; fever; tiredness; weakness; weight loss. | Discontinue. Call doctor right away. |
| • White patches in mouth; rash, itch around groin, rectum or armpits; vaginal discharge, itching. | Continue. Call doctor when convenient. |
| **Rare:** None expected. | |

## WARNINGS & PRECAUTIONS

**Don't take if:**
- You are allergic to lincomycins.
- You have had ulcerative colitis.
- Prescribed for infant under 1 month old.

**Before you start, consult your doctor:**
- If you have had yeast infections of mouth, skin or vagina.
- If you will have surgery within 2 months, including dental surgery, requiring general or spinal anesthesia.
- If you have kidney or liver disease.
- If you have allergies of any kind.

**Over age 60:**
Adverse reactions and side effects may be more frequent and severe than in younger persons.

**Pregnancy:**
Risk to unborn child outweighs drug benefits. Don't use.

**Breast-feeding:**
Drug passes into milk. Avoid drug or discontinue nursing until you finish medicine. Consult doctor for advice on maintaining milk supply.

**Infants & children:**
Don't give to infants younger than 1 month. Use for children only under medical supervision.

**Prolonged use:**
- Severe colitis with diarrhea and bleeding.
- You may become more susceptible to infections caused by germs not responsive to clindamycin.

**Skin & sunlight:**
No problems expected.

**Driving, piloting or hazardous work:**
No problems expected.

**Discontinuing:**
Don't discontinue without doctor's advice until you complete prescribed dose, even though symptoms diminish or disappear.

**Others:**
No problems expected.

## POSSIBLE INTERACTION WITH OTHER DRUGS

| GENERIC NAME OR DRUG CLASS | COMBINED EFFECT |
|---|---|
| Antidiarrheal preparations | Decreased clindamycin effect. |
| Chloramphenicol | Decreased clindamycin effect. |
| Erythromycin | Decreased clindamycin effect. |

## POSSIBLE INTERACTION WITH OTHER SUBSTANCES

| INTERACTS WITH | COMBINED EFFECT |
|---|---|
| Alcohol: | None expected. |
| Beverages: | None expected. |
| Cocaine: | None expected. |
| Foods: | None expected. |
| Marijuana: | None expected. |
| Tobacco: | None expected. |

# CLOFIBRATE

## BRAND NAMES

| | |
|---|---|
| Atromid-S | Liprinal |
| Claripex | Novofibrate |

## BASIC INFORMATION

**Habit forming?** No
**Prescription needed?** Yes
**Available as generic?** Yes
**Drug class:** Antihyperlipidemic

## USES

Reduces fatty substances in the blood (cholesterol and triglycerides).

## DOSAGE & USAGE INFORMATION

**How to take:**
Capsule—Swallow with liquid or food to lessen stomach irritation.

**When to take:**
At the same times each day.

**If you forget a dose:**
Take as soon as you remember up to 2 hours late. If more than 2 hours, wait for next scheduled dose (don't double this dose).

**What drug does:**
Inhibits formation of fatty substances.

**Time lapse before drug works:**
3 months or more.

**Don't take with:**
See Interaction column and consult doctor.

## OVERDOSE

**SYMPTOMS:**
Diarrhea, headache, muscle pain.
**WHAT TO DO:**
Overdose unlikely to threaten life. If person takes much larger amount than prescribed, call doctor, poison-control center or hospital emergency room for instructions.

## POSSIBLE ADVERSE REACTIONS OR SIDE EFFECTS

| SYMPTOMS | WHAT TO DO |
|---|---|
| **Life-threatening:** | |
| None expected. | |
| **Common:** | |
| None expected. | |
| **Infrequent:** | |
| • Chest pain, shortness of breath, irregular heartbeat, gallstones. | Discontinue. Call doctor right away. |
| • Nausea, vomiting, diarrhea, stomach pain. | Continue. Call doctor when convenient. |
| **Rare:** | |
| • Rash, itch; mouth or lip sores; sore throat; swollen feet, legs; blood in urine; painful urination; fever; chills. | Discontinue. Call doctor right away. |
| • Dizziness, drowsiness, headache, muscle cramps, backache, diminished sex drive, dryness, hair loss. | Continue. Call doctor when convenient. |

## WARNINGS & PRECAUTIONS

**Don't take if:**
You are allergic to any antihyperlipidemic.

**Before you start, consult your doctor:**
- If you have had liver or kidney disease.
- If you have had peptic-ulcer disease.
- If you have diabetes.

**Over age 60:**
Adverse reactions and side effects may be more frequent and severe than in younger persons. May develop flu-like symptoms.

**Pregnancy:**
Risk to unborn child outweighs drug benefits. Don't use.

**Breast-feeding:**
May harm child. Avoid.

**Infants & children:**
Not recommended.

**Prolonged use:**
No problems expected.

**Skin & sunlight:**
No problems expected.

**Driving, piloting or hazardous work:**
Avoid if you feel drowsy or dizzy. Otherwise, no problems expected.

**Discontinuing:**
Don't discontinue without doctor's advice until you complete prescribed dose, even though symptoms diminish or disappear.

**Others:**
- Periodic blood-cell counts and liver-function studies recommended if you take clofibrate for a long time.
- Some studies question effectiveness. Many studies warn against toxicity.

## POSSIBLE INTERACTION WITH OTHER DRUGS

| GENERIC NAME OR DRUG CLASS | COMBINED EFFECT |
|---|---|
| Anticoagulants (oral) | Increased anticoagulant effect. Dose reduction of anticoagulant necessary. |
| Antidiabetics (oral) | Increased antidiabetic effect. |
| Contraceptives (oral) | Decreased clofibrate effect. |
| Estrogens | Decreased clofibrate effect. |
| Furosemide | Possible toxicity of both drugs. |
| Insulin | Increased insulin effect. |
| Thyroid hormones | Increased clofibrate effect. |

## POSSIBLE INTERACTION WITH OTHER SUBSTANCES

| INTERACTS WITH | COMBINED EFFECT |
|---|---|
| Alcohol: | None expected. |
| Beverages: | None expected. |
| Cocaine: | None expected. |
| Foods: Fatty foods. | Decreased clofibrate effect. |
| Marijuana: | None expected. |
| Tobacco: | None expected. |

# CLOMIPHENE

## BRAND NAMES

Clomid                    Serophene

## BASIC INFORMATION

**Habit forming? No**
**Prescription needed? Yes**
**Available as generic? No**
**Drug class: Gonad stimulant**

 ## USES

- Treatment for men with low sperm counts.
- Treatment for ovulatory failure in women who wish to become pregnant.

 ## DOSAGE & USAGE INFORMATION

**How to take:**
Tablet—Swallow with liquid.

**When to take:**
- Men—Take at the same time each day.
- Women—If you are to begin treatment on "Day 5," count your first menstrual day as "Day 1." Take a tablet each day for 5 days.

**If you forget a dose:**
Take as soon as you remember. If you forget a day, double next dose. If you miss 2 or more doses, consult doctor.

**What drug does:**
Antiestrogen effect stimulates ovulation and sperm production.

**Time lapse before drug works:**
Usually 3 to 6 months. Ovulation may occur 6 to 10 days after last day of treatment in any cycle.

**Don't take with:**
No restrictions.

 ## OVERDOSE

**SYMPTOMS:**
**Increased severity of adverse reactions and side effects.**
**WHAT TO DO:**
**Overdose unlikely to threaten life. If person takes much larger amount than prescribed, call doctor, poison-control center or hospital emergency room for instructions.**

 ## POSSIBLE ADVERSE REACTIONS OR SIDE EFFECTS

| SYMPTOMS | WHAT TO DO |
|---|---|
| **Life-threatening:** | |
| None expected. | |
| **Common:** | |
| • Bloating, stomach pain, pelvic pain. | Discontinue. Call doctor right away. |
| • Hot flashes. | Continue. Tell doctor at next visit. |
| **Infrequent:** | |
| • Rash, itch, jaundice. | Discontinue. Call doctor right away. |
| • Constipation, diarrhea, increased appetite, heavy menstrual flow, frequent urination, breast discomfort, weight change, hair loss. | Continue. Call doctor when convenient. |
| **Rare:** | |
| • Vision changes. | Discontinue. Call doctor right away. |
| • Dizziness, headache, tiredness, depression, nervousness. | Continue. Call doctor when convenient. |

## WARNINGS & PRECAUTIONS

**Don't take if:**
You are allergic to clomiphene.

**Before you start, consult your doctor:**
- If you have an ovarian cyst, fibroid uterine tumors or unusual vaginal bleeding.
- If you have inflamed veins caused by blood clots.
- If you have liver disease.
- If you are depressed.

**Over age 60:**
Not recommended.

**Pregnancy:**
Stop taking at first sign of pregnancy.

**Breast-feeding:**
Not used.

**Infants & children:**
Not used.

**Prolonged use:**
Not recommended.

**Skin & sunlight:**
No problems expected.

**Driving, piloting or hazardous work:**
Avoid if you feel dizzy. Otherwise, no problems expected.

**Discontinuing:**
May be unnecessary to finish medicine. Follow doctor's instructions.

**Others:**
- Have a complete pelvic examination before treatment.
- If you become pregnant, twins or triplets are possible.

## POSSIBLE INTERACTION WITH OTHER DRUGS

| GENERIC NAME OR DRUG CLASS | COMBINED EFFECT |
| --- | --- |
| None | |

## POSSIBLE INTERACTION WITH OTHER SUBSTANCES

| INTERACTS WITH | COMBINED EFFECT |
| --- | --- |
| Alcohol: | None expected. |
| Beverages: | None expected. |
| Cocaine: | None expected. |
| Foods: | None expected. |
| Marijuana: | None expected. |
| Tobacco: | None expected. |

# CLONIDINE

## BRAND NAMES

Catapres                  Combipres
Catapres-TTS

## BASIC INFORMATION

**Habit forming? No**
**Prescription needed? Yes**
**Available as generic? Yes**
**Drug class: Antihypertensive**

 **USES**

- Treatment of high blood pressure.
- Prevention of vascular headaches.
- Treatment of dysmenorrhea and menopausal "hot flashes."
- Treatment of narcotic withdrawal syndrome.
- Treatment of congestive heart failure.

 **DOSAGE & USAGE INFORMATION**

**How to take:**
- Tablet or capsule—Swallow with liquid.
- Patches that attach to skin—Apply to clean, dry, hairless skin on arm or trunk.

**When to take:**
Daily dose at bedtime.

**If you forget a dose:**
Bedtime dose—If you forget your once-a-day dose, take it as soon as you remember. *Don't* double dose.

**What drug does:**
Relaxes and allows expansion of blood vessel walls.

*Continued next column*

 **OVERDOSE**

**SYMPTOMS:**
**Difficult breathing, vomiting, fainting, slow heartbeat, coma, diminished reflexes.**
**WHAT TO DO:**
- **Dial 0 (operator) or 911 (emergency) for an ambulance or medical help. Then give first aid immediately.**
- **If patient is unconscious and not breathing, give mouth-to-mouth breathing. If there is no heartbeat, use cardiac massage and mouth-to-mouth breathing (CPR). Don't try to make patient vomit. If you can't get help quickly, take patient to nearest emergency facility.**
- **See emergency information on inside covers.**

**Time lapse before drug works:**
1 to 3 hours.

**Don't take with:**
- Non-prescription medicines containing alcohol.
- See Interaction column and consult doctor.

 **POSSIBLE ADVERSE REACTIONS OR SIDE EFFECTS**

| SYMPTOMS | WHAT TO DO |
|---|---|
| **Life-threatening:** None expected. | |
| **Common:** | |
| • Dizziness, drowsiness, weight gain, lightheadedness upon rising from sitting or lying, swollen breasts. | Continue. Call doctor when convenient. |
| • Dry mouth. | Continue. Tell doctor at next visit. |
| **Infrequent:** | |
| • Abnormal heart rhythm. | Discontinue. Call doctor right away. |
| • Headache; nightmares; painful glands in neck; nausea; vomiting; cold fingers and toes; dry, burning eyes. | Continue. Call doctor when convenient. |
| • Insomnia, constipation, appetite loss, diminished sex drive. | Continue. Tell doctor at next visit. |
| **Rare:** | |
| • Rash, itch. | Discontinue. Call doctor right away. |
| • Depression. | Continue. Call doctor when convenient. |

 **WARNINGS & PRECAUTIONS**

**Don't take if:**
- You are allergic to any alpha-adrenergic blocker.
- You are under age 12.

**Before you start, consult your doctor:**
- If you will have surgery within 2 months, including dental surgery, requiring general or spinal anesthesia.
- If you have heart disease or chronic kidney disease.
- If you have a peripheral circulation disorder (intermittent claudication, Buerger's disease).
- If you have history of depression.

**Over age 60:**
Adverse reactions and side effects may be more frequent and severe than in younger persons.

**Pregnancy:**
Studies inconclusive on harm to unborn child. Animal studies show fetal abnormalities. Decide with your doctor whether drug benefits justify risk to unborn child.

**Breast-feeding:**
Unknown whether safe or not. Consult doctor.

**Infants & children:**
Use only under careful medical supervision after age 12. Avoid before age 12.

**Prolonged use:**
- Don't discontinue without consulting doctor. Dose may require gradual reduction if you have taken drug for a long time. Doses of other drugs may also require adjustment.
- Continued use may cause fluid retention, requiring addition of diuretic to treatment program.
- Request yearly eye examinations.

**Skin & sunlight:**
No problems expected.

**Driving, piloting or hazardous work:**
Don't drive or pilot aircraft until you learn how medicine affects you. Don't work around dangerous machinery. Don't climb ladders or work in high places. Danger increases if you drink alcohol or take medicine affecting alertness and reflexes.

**Discontinuing:**
Don't discontinue abruptly. May cause rebound high blood pressure, anxiety, chest pain, insomnia, headache, nausea, irregular heartbeat, flushed face, sweating.

**Others:**
No problems expected.

## POSSIBLE INTERACTION WITH OTHER DRUGS

| GENERIC NAME OR DRUG CLASS | COMBINED EFFECT |
|---|---|
| Acebutolol | Increased antihypertensive effect of each. Dosages may require adjustments. |
| Antidepressants (tricyclic) | Decreased clonidine effect. |
| Antihypertensives (other) | Excessive blood-pressure drop. |
| Appetite suppressants | Decreased clonidine effect. |
| Beta-blockers | Blood-pressure control impaired. |

| | |
|---|---|
| Diuretics | Excessive blood-pressure drop. |
| Enalapril | Possible excessive potassium in blood. |
| Fenfluramine | Possible increased clonidine effect. |
| Labetolol | May cause precipitous change in blood pressure if clonidine and labetolol are discontinued simultaneously. |
| Nitrates | Possible excessive blood-pressure drop. |
| Oxprenolol | May cause blood-pressure rise if clonidine is discontinued after simultaneous use with oxprenolol. |
| Pentoxifylline | Increased antihypertensive effect. |

## POSSIBLE INTERACTION WITH OTHER SUBSTANCES

| INTERACTS WITH | COMBINED EFFECT |
|---|---|
| Alcohol: | Increased sensitivity to sedative effect of alcohol and very low blood pressure. Avoid. |
| Beverages: Caffeine-containing drinks. | Decreased clonidine effect. |
| Cocaine: | Blood pressure rise. Avoid. |
| Foods: | No problems expected. |
| Marijuana: | Weakness on standing. |
| Tobacco: | No problems expected. |

# CLONIDINE & CHLORTHALIDONE

## BRAND NAMES

**Combipres**

## BASIC INFORMATION

**Habit forming? No**
**Prescription needed? Yes**
**Available as generic? No**
**Drug class: Antihypertensive**

 ## USES

- Treatment of high blood pressure.
- Reduces fluid retention (edema) caused by conditions such as heart disorders and liver disease.

 ## DOSAGE & USAGE INFORMATION

**How to take:**
Tablet or capsule—Swallow with liquid. If you can't swallow whole, crumble tablet or open capsule and take with liquid or food. Don't exceed dose.

**When to take:**
At the same time each day.

**If you forget a dose:**
Take as soon as you remember up to 2 hours late. If more than 2 hours, wait for next scheduled dose (don't double this dose).

**What drug does:**
- Relaxes and allows expansion of blood vessel walls.

*Continued next column*

 ## OVERDOSE

**SYMPTOMS:**
**Difficult breathing; vomiting; fainting; rapid, irregular, slow heartbeat; diminished reflexes; cramps; weakness; drowsiness; weak pulse; coma.**
**WHAT TO DO:**
- **Dial 0 (operator) or 911 (emergency) for an ambulance or medical help. Then give first aid immediately.**
- **If patient is unconscious and not breathing, give mouth-to-mouth breathing. If there is no heartbeat, use cardiac massage and mouth-to-mouth breathing (CPR). Don't try to make patient vomit. If you can't get help quickly, take patient to nearest emergency facility.**
- **See emergency information on inside covers.**

- Forces sodium and water excretion, reducing body fluid.
- Reduced body fluid and relaxed arteries lower blood pressure.

**Time lapse before drug works:**
4 to 6 hours. May require several weeks to lower blood pressure.

**Don't take with:**
Any medicine that will decrease mental alertness such as alcohol, antihistamines, cold/cough medicines, sedatives, tranquilizers, narcotics, prescription pain medicine, barbiturates, seizure medicine, anesthetics.

 ## POSSIBLE ADVERSE REACTIONS OR SIDE EFFECTS

| SYMPTOMS | WHAT TO DO |
|---|---|
| **Life-threatening:** | |
| Irregular heartbeat, weak pulse. | Discontinue. Seek emergency treatment. |
| **Common:** | |
| Dry mouth, increased thirst, muscle cramps, nausea or vomiting, mood changes, drowsiness. | Discontinue. Call doctor right away. |
| **Infrequent:** | |
| Vomiting, diminished sex desire and performance, insomnia, dizziness, diarrhea, constipaion, appetite loss. | Continue. Call doctor when convenient. |
| **Rare:** | |
| • Jaundice; easy bruising or bleeding; sore throat, fever, mouth ulcers; rash or hives; joint pain; flank pain; abdominal pain. | Discontinue. Call doctor right away. |
| • Cold fingers and toes, nightmares, vomiting. | Continue. Call doctor when convenient. |

 ## WARNINGS & PRECAUTIONS

**Don't take if:**
- You are allergic to any thiazide diuretic drug or alpha-adrenergic blocker.
- You are under age 12.

**Before you start, consult your doctor:**
- If you are allergic to any sulfa drug.
- If you have gout, liver, pancreas or kidney disorder, a peripheral circulation disorder (intermittent claudication, Buerger's disease), history of depression, heart disease.

- If you will have surgery within 2 months, including dental surgery, requiring general or spinal anesthesia.

### Over age 60:
Adverse reactions and side effects may be more frequent and severe than in younger persons, especially dizziness and excessive potassium loss.

### Pregnancy:
Risk to unborn child outweighs drug benefits. Don't use.

### Breast-feeding:
Drug passes into milk. Avoid drug or discontinue nursing until you finish medicine. Consult doctor for advice on maintaining milk supply.

### Infants & children:
Use only after careful medical supervision after age 12. Avoid before age 12.

### Prolonged use:
- Don't discontinue without consulting doctor. Dose may require gradual reduction if you have taken drug for a long time. Doses of other drugs may also require adjustment.
- Continued use may cause fluid retention, requiring addition of diuretic to treatment program.
- Request yearly eye examinations.

### Skin & sunlight:
May cause rash or intensify sunburn in areas exposed to sun or sunlamp.

### Driving, piloting or hazardous work:
Don't drive or pilot aircraft until you learn how medicine affects you. Don't work around dangerous machinery. Don't climb ladders or work in high places. Danger increases if you drink alcohol or take medicine affecting alertness and reflexes, such as antihistamines, tranquilizers, sedatives, pain medicine, narcotics and mind-altering drugs.

### Discontinuing:
Don't discontinue abruptly. May cause rebound high blood pressure, anxiety, chest pain, insomnia, headache, nausea, irregular heartbeat, flushed face, sweating.

### Others:
- Hot weather and fever may cause dehydration and drop in blood pressure. Dose may require temporary adjustment. Weigh daily and report any unexpected weight decreases to your doctor.
- May cause rise in uric acid, leading to gout.
- May cause blood-sugar rise in diabetics.

## POSSIBLE INTERACTION WITH OTHER DRUGS

| GENERIC NAME OR DRUG CLASS | COMBINED EFFECT |
| --- | --- |
| Acebutolol | Increased antihypertensive effect of each. Dosages may require adjustments. |
| Allopurinol | Decreased allopurinol effect. |
| Antidepressants (tricyclic) | Dangerous drop in blood pressure. Avoid combination unless under medical supervision. |
| Antihypertensives (other) | Excessive blood-pressure drop. |
| Appetite suppressants | Decreased clonidine effect. |
| Barbiturates | Increased chlorthalidone effect. |
| Beta-blockers | Blood-pressure control impaired. |
| Cholestyramine | Decreased chlorthalidone effect. |
| Cortisone drugs | Excessive potassium loss that causes dangerous heart rhythms. |

*Continued page 965*

## POSSIBLE INTERACTION WITH OTHER SUBSTANCES

| INTERACTS WITH | COMBINED EFFECT |
| --- | --- |
| Alcohol: | Increased sensitivity to sedative effect of alcohol and very low blood pressure. Avoid. |
| Beverages: Caffeine-containing drinks. | Decreased clonidine effect. |
| Cocaine: | Blood pressure rise. Avoid. |
| Foods: Licorice. | Excessive potassium loss that causes dangerous heart rhythm. |
| Marijuana: | Weakness on standing. May increase blood pressure. |
| Tobacco: | None expected. |

# CLORAZEPATE

## BRAND NAMES

Tranxene          Tranxene-SD

## BASIC INFORMATION

Habit forming? Yes
Prescription needed? Yes
Available as generic? No
Drug class: Tranquilizer (benzodiazepine)

## USES

- Treatment for nervousness or tension.
- Treatment for convulsive disorders.

## DOSAGE & USAGE INFORMATION

**How to take:**
Tablet or capsule—Swallow with liquid. If you
can't swallow whole, crumble tablet or open
capsule and take with liquid or food.

**When to take:**
At the same time each day, according to
instructions on prescription label.

**If you forget a dose:**
Take as soon as you remember up to 2 hours
late. If more than 2 hours, wait for next
scheduled dose (don't double this dose).

**What drug does:**
Affects limbic system of brain—part that
controls emotions.

**Time lapse before drug works:**
2 hours. May take 6 weeks for full benefit.

*Continued next column*

## OVERDOSE

**SYMPTOMS:**
**Drowsiness, weakness, tremor, stupor,**
**coma.**
**WHAT TO DO:**
- **Dial 0 (operator) or 911 (emergency) for an**
  **ambulance or medical help. Then give first**
  **aid immediately.**
- **If patient is unconscious and not**
  **breathing, give mouth-to-mouth breathing.**
  **If there is no heartbeat, use cardiac**
  **massage and mouth-to-mouth breathing**
  **(CPR). Don't try to make patient vomit. If**
  **you can't get help quickly, take patient to**
  **nearest emergency facility.**
- **See emergency information on inside**
  **covers.**

---

**Don't take with:**
See Interaction column and consult doctor.

## POSSIBLE ADVERSE REACTIONS OR SIDE EFFECTS

| SYMPTOMS | WHAT TO DO |
|---|---|
| **Life-threatening:**<br>None expected. | |
| **Common:**<br>Clumsiness,<br>drowsiness, dizziness. | Continue. Call doctor<br>when convenient. |
| **Infrequent:**<br>• Hallucinations,<br>confusion,<br>depression,<br>irritability, rash,<br>itch, vision changes. | Discontinue. Call<br>doctor right away. |
| • Constipation or<br>diarrhea, nausea,<br>vomiting, difficult<br>urination. | Continue. Call doctor<br>when convenient. |
| **Rare:**<br>• Slow heartbeat,<br>breathing difficulty. | Discontinue. Seek<br>emergency treatment. |
| • Mouth, throat<br>ulcers; jaundice. | Discontinue. Call<br>doctor right away. |

## WARNINGS & PRECAUTIONS

**Don't take if:**
- You are allergic to any benzodiazepine.
- You have myasthenia gravis.
- You are active or recovering alcoholic.
- Patient is younger than 6 months.

**Before you start, consult your doctor:**
- If you have liver, kidney or lung disease.
- If you have diabetes, epilepsy or porphyria.

**Over age 60:**
Adverse reactions and side effects may be more frequent and severe than in younger persons. You need smaller doses for shorter periods of time. May develop agitation, rage or "hangover" effect.

**Pregnancy:**
Risk to unborn child outweighs drug benefits. Don't use.

**Breast-feeding:**
Drug passes into milk. Avoid drug or discontinue nursing until you finish medicine. Consult doctor for advice on maintaining milk supply.

**Infants & children:**
Use only under medical supervision for children older than 6 months.

**Prolonged use:**
May impair liver function.

**Skin & sunlight:**
No problems expected.

**Driving, piloting or hazardous work:**
Don't drive or pilot aircraft until you learn how medicine affects you. Don't work around dangerous machinery. Don't climb ladders or work in high places. Danger increases if you drink alcohol or take medicine affecting alertness and reflexes.

**Discontinuing:**
Don't discontinue without consulting doctor. Dose may require gradual reduction if you have taken drug for a long time. Doses of other drugs may also require adjustment.

**Others:**
- Hot weather, heavy exercise and profuse sweat may reduce excretion and cause overdose.
- Blood sugar may rise in diabetics, requiring insulin adjustment.

## POSSIBLE INTERACTION WITH OTHER DRUGS

| GENERIC NAME OR DRUG CLASS | COMBINED EFFECT |
| --- | --- |
| Anticonvulsants | Change in seizure frequency or severity. |
| Antidepressants | Increased sedative effect of both drugs. |
| Antihistamines | Increased sedative effect of both drugs. |
| Antihypertensives | Excessively low blood pressure. |
| Cimetidine | Excess sedation. |
| Disulfiram | Increased clorazepate effect. |
| Dronabinol | Increased effects of both drugs. Avoid. |
| MAO inhibitors | Convulsions, deep sedation, rage. |
| Molindone | Increased tranquilizer effect. |
| Narcotics | Increased sedative effect of both drugs. |
| Sedatives | Increased sedative effect of both drugs. |
| Sleep inducers | Increased sedative effect of both drugs. |
| Tranquilizers | Increased sedative effect of both drugs. |

## POSSIBLE INTERACTION WITH OTHER SUBSTANCES

| INTERACTS WITH | COMBINED EFFECT |
| --- | --- |
| Alcohol: | Heavy sedation. Avoid. |
| Beverages: | None expected. |
| Cocaine: | Decreased clorazepate effect. |
| Foods: | None expected. |
| Marijuana: | Heavy sedation. Avoid. |
| Tobacco: | Decreased clorazepate effect. |

# CLOXACILLIN

## BRAND NAMES

| | |
|---|---|
| Bactopen | Novocloxin |
| Cloxapen | Orbenin |
| Cloxilean | Tegopen |

## BASIC INFORMATION

**Habit forming?** No
**Prescription needed?** Yes
**Available as generic?** Yes
**Drug class:** Antibiotic (penicillin)

## USES

Treatment of bacterial infections that are susceptible to cloxacillin.

## DOSAGE & USAGE INFORMATION

**How to take:**
- Tablets or capsules—Swallow with liquid on an empty stomach 1 hour before or 2 hours after eating.
- Liquid—Take with cold beverage. Liquid form is perishable and effective for only 7 days at room temperature. Effective for 14 days if stored in refrigerator. Don't freeze.

**When to take:**
Follow instructions on prescription label or side of package. Doses should be evenly spaced. For example, 4 times a day means every 6 hours.

**If you forget a dose:**
Take as soon as you remember. Continue regular schedule.

**What drug does:**
Destroys susceptible bacteria. Does not kill viruses.

**Time lapse before drug works:**
May be several days before medicine affects infection.

**Don't take with:**
See Interaction column and consult doctor.

## OVERDOSE

**SYMPTOMS:**
Severe diarrhea, nausea or vomiting.
**WHAT TO DO:**
Overdose unlikely to threaten life. If person takes much larger amount than prescribed, call doctor, poison-control center or hospital emergency room for instructions.

## POSSIBLE ADVERSE REACTIONS OR SIDE EFFECTS

| SYMPTOMS | WHAT TO DO |
|---|---|
| **Life-threatening:** | |
| Hives, rash, intense itching, faintness soon after a dose (anaphylaxis). | Seek emergency treatment immediately. |
| **Common:** | |
| Dark or discolored tongue. | Continue. Tell doctor at next visit. |
| **Infrequent:** | |
| Mild nausea, vomiting, diarrhea. | Continue. Call doctor when convenient. |
| **Rare:** | |
| Unexplained bleeding. | Discontinue. Call doctor right away. |

## WARNINGS & PRECAUTIONS

**Don't take if:**
You are allergic to cloxacillin, cephalosporin antibiotics, other penicillins or penicillamine. Life-threatening reaction may occur.

**Before you start, consult your doctor:**
If you are allergic to any substance or drug.

**Over age 60:**
You may have skin reactions, particularly around genitals and anus.

**Pregnancy:**
Studies inconclusive on harm to unborn child. Animal studies show fetal abnormalities. Decide with your doctor whether drug benefits justify risk to unborn child.

**Breast-feeding:**
Drug passes into milk. Child may become sensitive to penicillins and have allergic reactions to penicillin drugs. Avoid cloxacillin or discontinue nursing until you finish medicine. Consult doctor for advice on maintaining milk supply.

**Infants & children:**
No problems expected.

**Prolonged use:**
You may become more susceptible to infections caused by germs not responsive to cloxacillin.

**Skin & sunlight:**
No problems expected.

**Driving, piloting or hazardous work:**
Usually not dangerous. Most hazardous reactions likely to occur a few minutes after taking cloxacillin.

**Discontinuing:**
Don't discontinue without doctor's advice until you complete prescribed dose, even though symptoms diminish or disappear.

**Others:**
No problems expected.

## POSSIBLE INTERACTION WITH OTHER DRUGS

| GENERIC NAME OR DRUG CLASS | COMBINED EFFECT |
|---|---|
| Beta-adrenergic blockers | Increased chance of anaphylaxis (see emergency information on inside front cover). |
| Chloramphenicol | Decreased effect of both drugs. |
| Erythromycins | Decreased effect of both drugs. |
| Loperamide | Decreased cloxacillin effect. |
| Paromomycin | Decreased effect of both drugs. |
| Tetracyclines | Decreased effect of both drugs. |
| Troleandomycin | Decreased effect of both drugs. |

## POSSIBLE INTERACTION WITH OTHER SUBSTANCES

| INTERACTS WITH | COMBINED EFFECT |
|---|---|
| Alcohol: | Occasional stomach irritation. |
| Beverages: | None expected. |
| Cocaine: | No proven problems. |
| Foods: | None expected. |
| Marijuana: | No proven problems. |
| Tobacco: | None expected. |

# COLCHICINE

## BRAND NAMES

ColBenemid        Novocolchine
Col-Probenecid

## BASIC INFORMATION

**Habit forming? No**
**Prescription needed? Yes**
**Available as generic? Yes**
**Drug class: Antigout**

 **USES**

Relieves joint pain, inflammation, swelling of gout.

 **DOSAGE & USAGE INFORMATION**

**How to take:**
- Tablet—Swallow with liquid or food to lessen stomach irritation.
- Granules—Dissolve in 3 oz. of fluid. Drink all fluid.

**When to take:**
As prescribed. Stop taking when pain stops or at first sign of digestive upset. Wait at least 3 days between treatments.

**If you forget a dose:**
Don't double next dose. Consult doctor.

**What drug does:**
Decreases acidity of joint tissues and prevents deposits of uric-acid crystals.

**Time lapse before drug works:**
12 to 48 hours.

**Don't take with:**
See Interaction column and consult doctor.

 **OVERDOSE**

**SYMPTOMS:**
**Bloody urine, diarrhea, muscle weakness, fever, shortness of breath, stupor, convulsions, coma.**
**WHAT TO DO:**
- **Dial 0 (operator) or 911 (emergency) for an ambulance or medical help. Then give first aid immediately.**
- **See emergency information on inside covers.**

 **POSSIBLE ADVERSE REACTIONS OR SIDE EFFECTS**

| SYMPTOMS | WHAT TO DO |
|---|---|
| **Life-threatening:** | |
| Hives, rash, intense itching, faintness soon after a dose (anaphylaxis). | Seek emergency treatment immediately. |
| **Common:** | |
| Diarrhea, nausea, vomiting, abdominal pain. | Discontinue. Call doctor right away. |
| **Infrequent:** | |
| • Rash, itch, unusual bruising, blood in urine. | Discontinue. Call doctor right away. |
| • Numbness, tingling, pain or weakness in hands or feet; unusual tiredness or weakness; fever. | Continue. Call doctor when convenient. |
| **Rare:** | |
| Jaundice. | Discontinue. Call doctor right away. |

## WARNINGS & PRECAUTIONS

**Don't take if:**
You are allergic to colchicine.

**Before you start, consult your doctor:**
- If you have had peptic ulcers or ulcerative colitis.
- If you have heart, liver or kidney disease.
- If you will have surgery within 2 months, including dental surgery, requiring general or spinal anesthesia.

**Over age 60:**
Adverse reactions and side effects may be more frequent and severe than in younger persons. Colchicine has a narrow margin of safety for people in this age group.

**Pregnancy:**
Risk to unborn child outweighs drug benefits. Don't use.

**Breast-feeding:**
No problems expected, but consult doctor.

**Infants & children:**
Not recommended.

**Prolonged use:**
- Permanent hair loss.
- Anemia. Request blood counts.
- Numbness or tingling in hands and feet.

**Skin & sunlight:**
No problems expected.

**Driving, piloting or hazardous work:**
Don't drive or pilot aircraft until you learn how medicine affects you. Don't work around dangerous machinery. Don't climb ladders or work in high places. Danger increases if you drink alcohol or take medicine affecting alertness and reflexes, such as antihistamines, tranquilizers, sedatives, pain medicine, narcotics and mind-altering drugs.

**Discontinuing:**
- May be unnecessary to finish medicine. Follow doctor's instructions.
- Stop taking if digestive upsets occur before symptoms are relieved.

**Others:**
- Limit each course of treatment to 8 mg. Don't exceed 3 mg. per 24 hours.
- Possible sperm damage. May cause birth defects if child conceived while father taking colchicine.

## POSSIBLE INTERACTION WITH OTHER DRUGS

| GENERIC NAME OR DRUG CLASS | COMBINED EFFECT |
|---|---|
| Amphetamines | Increased amphetamine effect. |
| Anticoagulants | Decreased anticoagulant effect. |
| Antidepressants | Oversedation. |
| Antihistamines | Oversedation. |
| Antihypertensives | Decreased antihypertensive effect. |
| Appetite suppressants | Increased suppressant effect. |
| Mind-altering drugs | Oversedation. |
| Narcotics | Oversedation. |
| Sedatives | Oversedation. |
| Sleep inducers | Oversedation. |
| Tranquilizers | Oversedation. |

## POSSIBLE INTERACTION WITH OTHER SUBSTANCES

| INTERACTS WITH | COMBINED EFFECT |
|---|---|
| Alcohol: | No proven problems. |
| Beverages: Herbal teas. | Increased colchicine effect. Avoid. |
| Cocaine: | Overstimulation. Avoid. |
| Foods: | No proven problems. |
| Marijuana: | Decreased colchicine effect. |
| Tobacco: | No proven problems. |

# COLESTIPOL

## BRAND NAMES

**Colestid**

## BASIC INFORMATION

**Habit forming? No**
**Prescription needed? Yes**
**Available as generic? No**
**Drug class: Antihyperlipidemic**

 **USES**

- Reduces cholesterol level in blood in patients with type IIa hyperlipidemia.
- Treats overdose of digitalis.
- Reduces skin itching associated with some forms of liver disease.
- Treats diarrhea after some surgical operations.

 **DOSAGE & USAGE INFORMATION**

**How to take:**
Mix well with 6 ounces or more or water or liquid, or in soups, pulpy fruits, with milk or in cereals. Will not dissolve.

**When to take:**
Before meals.

**If you forget a dose:**
Take as soon as you remember up to 2 hours late. If more than 2 hours, wait for next scheduled dose (don't double this dose).

**What drug does:**
Binds with bile acids in intestines, preventing reabsorption.

**Time lapse before drug works:**
3 to 12 months.

**Don't take with:**
See Interaction column and consult doctor.

 **OVERDOSE**

**SYMPTOMS:**
Fecal impaction.
**WHAT TO DO:**
Overdose unlikely to threaten life. If person takes much larger amount than prescribed, call doctor, poison-control center or hospital emergency room for instructions.

 **POSSIBLE ADVERSE REACTIONS OR SIDE EFFECTS**

| SYMPTOMS | WHAT TO DO |
|---|---|
| **Life-threatening:** None expected. | |
| **Common:** None expected. | |
| **Infrequent:** | |
| • Black, tarry stools from gastrointestinal bleeding. | Discontinue. Seek emergency treatment. |
| • Severe abdominal pain. | Discontinue. Call doctor right away. |
| • Constipation, belching, diarrhea, nausea, unexpected weight loss. | Continue. Call doctor when convenient. |
| **Rare:** None expected. | |

## WARNINGS & PRECAUTIONS

**Don't take if:**
You are allergic to colestipol.

**Before you start, consult your doctor:**
- If you have liver disease such as cirrhosis.
- If you are jaundiced.
- If you will have surgery within 2 months, including dental surgery, requiring general or spinal anesthesia.
- If you are constipated.
- If you have peptic ulcer.
- If you have coronary artery disease.

**Over age 60:**
Constipation more likely. Other adverse effects more likely.

**Pregnancy:**
No proven harm to unborn child. Avoid if possible.

**Breast-feeding:**
No proven harm to child. Consult doctor.

**Infants & children:**
Only under expert medical supervision.

**Prolonged use:**
Request lab studies to determine serum cholesterol and serum triglycerides.

**Skin & sunlight:**
No problems expected.

**Driving, piloting or hazardous work:**
No problems expected.

**Discontinuing:**
Don't discontinue without consulting doctor. Dose may require gradual reduction if you have taken drug for a long time. Doses of other drugs may also require adjustment, particularly digitalis.

**Others:**
This medicine does not cure disorders, but helps to control them.

## POSSIBLE INTERACTION WITH OTHER DRUGS

| GENERIC NAME OR DRUG CLASS | COMBINED EFFECT |
|---|---|
| Anticoagulants | Decreased anticoagulant effect. |
| Digitalis preparations | Decreased absorption. |
| Diuretics (thiazide) | Decreased absorption. |
| Penicillins | Decreased absorption. |
| Tetracyclines | Decreased absorption. |
| Vitamins | Decreased absorption of fat-soluble vitamins (A,D,E,K) |
| Other medicines | May delay or reduce absorption. |

## POSSIBLE INTERACTION WITH OTHER SUBSTANCES

| INTERACTS WITH | COMBINED EFFECT |
|---|---|
| Alcohol: | None expected. |
| Beverages: | None expected. |
| Cocaine: | None expected. |
| Foods: | Interferes with absorption of vitamins. Take supplements. |
| Marijuana: | None expected. |
| Tobacco: | None expected. |

# CONJUGATED ESTROGENS

## BRAND NAMES

**Premarin**

## BASIC INFORMATION

**Habit forming? No**
**Prescription needed? Yes**
**Available as generic? Yes**
**Drug class: Female sex hormone (estrogen)**

 ## USES

- Treatment for symptoms of menopause and menstrual-cycle irregularity.
- Replacement for female hormone deficiency.
- Treatment for estrogen-deficiency osteoporosis (bone softening from calcium loss).
- Treatment for cancer of prostate and breast.

 ## DOSAGE & USAGE INFORMATION

**How to take:**
- Tablet—Swallow with liquid. If you can't swallow whole, crumble tablet and take with liquid or food.
- Vaginal cream—Use as directed on label.

**When to take:**
At the same time each day.

**If you forget a dose:**
Take as soon as you remember up to 12 hours late. If more than 12 hours, wait for next scheduled dose (don't double this dose).

**What drug does:**
Restores normal estrogen level in tissues.

**Time lapse before drug works:**
10 to 20 days.

**Don't take with:**
See Interaction column and consult doctor.

 ## OVERDOSE

**SYMPTOMS:**
Nausea, vomiting, fluid retention, breast enlargement and discomfort, abnormal vaginal bleeding.
**WHAT TO DO:**
Overdose unlikely to threaten life. If person takes much larger amount than prescribed, call doctor, poison-control center or hospital emergency room for instructions.

 ## POSSIBLE ADVERSE REACTIONS OR SIDE EFFECTS

| SYMPTOMS | WHAT TO DO |
|---|---|
| **Life-threatening:** | |
| None expected. | |
| **Common:** | |
| • Stomach cramps. | Discontinue. Call doctor right away. |
| • Appetite loss. | Continue. Call doctor when convenient. |
| • Nausea; diarrhea; swollen ankles or feet; swollen, tender breasts. | Continue. Tell doctor at next visit. |
| **Infrequent:** | |
| • Rash, stomach or side pain. | Discontinue. Call doctor right away. |
| • Depression, dizziness, irritability, vomiting, breast lumps. | Continue. Call doctor when convenient. |
| • Brown blotches on skin, hair loss, vaginal discharge or bleeding, changes in sex drive. | Continue. Tell doctor at next visit. |
| **Rare:** | |
| Jaundice. | Discontinue. Call doctor right away. |

## WARNINGS & PRECAUTIONS

**Don't take if:**
- You are allergic to any estrogen-containing drugs.
- You have impaired liver function.
- You have had blood clots, stroke or heart attack.
- You have unexplained vaginal bleeding.

**Before you start, consult your doctor:**
- If you have had cancer of breast or reproductive organs, fibrocystic breast disease, fibroid tumors of the uterus or endometriosis.
- If you have had migraine headaches, epilepsy or porphyria.
- If you have diabetes, high blood pressure, asthma, congestive heart failure, kidney disease or gallstones.
- If you plan to become pregnant within 3 months.

**Over age 60:**
Controversial. You and your doctor must decide if drug risks outweigh benefits.

**Pregnancy:**
Risk to unborn child outweighs drug benefits. Don't use.

**Breast-feeding:**
Drug filters into milk. May harm child. Avoid.

**Infants & children:**
Not recommended.

**Prolonged use:**
Increased growth of fibroid tumors of uterus. Possible association with cancer of uterus.

**Skin & sunlight:**
May cause rash or intensify sunburn in areas exposed to sun or sunlamp.

**Driving, piloting or hazardous work:**
No problems expected.

**Discontinuing:**
You may need to discontinue estrogen periodically. Consult your doctor.

**Others:**
In rare instances, may cause blood clot in lung, brain or leg. Symptoms are *sudden* severe headache, coordination loss, vision change, chest pain, breathing difficulty, slurred speech, pain in legs or groin. Seek emergency treatment immediately.

## POSSIBLE INTERACTION WITH OTHER DRUGS

| GENERIC NAME OR DRUG CLASS | COMBINED EFFECT |
|---|---|
| Anticoagulants (oral) | Decreased anticoagulant effect. |
| Anticonvulsants (hydantoin) | Increased seizures. |
| Antidiabetics (oral) | Unpredictable increase or decrease in blood sugar. |
| Carbamazepine | Increased seizures. |
| Clofibrate | Decreased clofibrate effect. |
| Meprobamate | Increased effect of conjugated estrogens. |
| Phenobarbital | Decreased effect of conjugated estrogens. |
| Primidone | Decreased effect of conjugated estrogens. |
| Rifampin | Decreased effect of conjugated estrogens. |
| Thyroid hormones | Decreased thyroid effect. |

## POSSIBLE INTERACTION WITH OTHER SUBSTANCES

| INTERACTS WITH | COMBINED EFFECT |
|---|---|
| Alcohol: | None expected. |
| Beverages: | None expected. |
| Cocaine: | No proven problems. |
| Foods: | None expected. |
| Marijuana: | Possible menstrual irregularities and bleeding between periods. |
| Tobacco: | Increased risk of blood clots leading to stroke or heart attack. |

# CONTRACEPTIVES (ORAL)

## BRAND NAMES

See complete list of brand names in the *Brand Name Directory,* page 947.

## BASIC INFORMATION

**Habit forming? No**
**Prescription needed? Yes**
**Available as generic? Yes**
**Drug class: Female sex hormone,**
        **contraceptive**

 ## USES

- Prevents pregnancy.
- Regulates menstrual periods.

 ## DOSAGE & USAGE INFORMATION

**How to take:**
Tablet or capsule—Swallow with liquid or food to lessen stomach irritation.

**When to take:**
At same time each day according to prescribed instructions, usually for 21 days of 28-day cycle.

**If you forget a dose:**
Call doctor's office for advice about additional protection against pregnancy.

**What drug does:**
- Alters mucus at cervix entrance to prevent sperm entry.
- Alters uterus lining to resist implantation of fertilized egg.
- Creates same chemical atmosphere in blood that exists during pregnancy, suppressing pituitary hormones which stimulate ovulation.

**Time lapse before drug works:**
10 days or more to provide contraception.

**Don't take with:**
- Tobacco
- See Interaction column and consult doctor.

 ## OVERDOSE

**SYMPTOMS:**
**Drowsiness**
**WHAT TO DO:**
**Overdose unlikely to threaten life. If person takes much larger amount than prescribed, call doctor, poison-control center or hospital emergency room for instructions.**

 ## POSSIBLE ADVERSE REACTIONS OR SIDE EFFECTS

| SYMPTOMS | WHAT TO DO |
|---|---|
| **Life-threatening:**<br>Stroke, chest pain. | Seek emergency treatment immediately. |
| **Common:**<br>Brown blotches on skin; vaginal discharge, itch; fluid retention. | Continue. Call doctor when convenient. |
| **Infrequent:**<br>• Headache; depression; blood clots, pain, swelling in leg; muscle, joint pain. | Discontinue. Call doctor right away. |
| • Blue tinge to objects, lights; appetite change; nausea; bloating; vomiting; pain; changed sex drive. | Continue. Call doctor when convenient. |
| **Rare:**<br>• Clotting tendency. | Discontinue. Seek emergency treatment. |
| • Jaundice, rash, hives, itch. | Discontinue. Call doctor right away. |

 ## WARNINGS & PRECAUTIONS

**Don't take if:**
- You are allergic to any female hormone.
- You have had heart disease, blood clots or stroke.
- You have liver disease.
- You have cancer of breast, uterus or ovaries.
- You have unexplained vaginal bleeding.

**Before you start, consult your doctor:**
- If you have fibrocystic disease of breast.
- If you have migraine headaches.
- If you have fibroid tumors of uterus.
- If you have epilepsy.
- If you have asthma.
- If you have high blood pressure.
- If you will have surgery within 2 months, including dental surgery, requiring general or spinal anesthesia.
- If you have endometriosis.
- If you have diabetes.
- If you have sickle-cell anemia.
- If you smoke cigarettes.

**Over age 60:**
Not used.

**Pregnancy:**
May harm child. Discontinue at first sign of pregnancy.

# CONTRACEPTIVES (ORAL)

**Breast-feeding:**
Drug passes into milk. Avoid drug or discontinue nursing.

**Infants & children:**
Not recommended.

**Prolonged use:**
- Gallstones.
- Gradual blood-pressure rise.
- Possible difficulty becoming pregnant after discontinuing.

**Skin & sunlight:**
May cause rash or intensify sunburn in areas exposed to sun or sunlamp.

**Driving, piloting or hazardous work:**
No problems expected.

**Discontinuing:**
Don't become pregnant for 6 months after discontinuing.

**Others:**
Failure to take oral contraceptives for 1 day may cancel pregnancy protection. If you forget a dose, use other contraceptive measures and call doctor for instructions on re-starting oral contraceptive.

 **POSSIBLE INTERACTION WITH OTHER DRUGS**

| GENERIC NAME OR DRUG CLASS | COMBINED EFFECT |
|---|---|
| Ampicillin | Decreased contraceptive effect. |
| Anticoagulants | Decreased anticoagulant effect. |
| Anticonvulsants (hydantoin) | Decreased contraceptive effect. |
| Antidiabetics | Decreased antidiabetic effect. |
| Antihistamines | Decreased contraceptive effect. |
| Anti-inflammatory drugs (non-steroid) | Decreased contraceptive effect. |
| Barbiturates | Decreased contraceptive effect. |
| Chloramphenicol | Decreased contraceptive effect. |
| Clofibrate | Decreased clofibrate effect. |
| Guanethidine | Decreased guanethidine effect. |
| Meperidine | Increased meperidine effect. |

| | |
|---|---|
| Meprobamate | Decreased contraceptive effect. |
| Mineral oil | Decreased contraceptive effect. |
| Phenothiazines | Increased phenothiazine effect. |
| Rifampin | Decreased contraceptive effect. |
| Tetracyclines | Decreased contraceptive effect. |

 **POSSIBLE INTERACTION WITH OTHER SUBSTANCES**

| INTERACTS WITH | COMBINED EFFECT |
|---|---|
| Alcohol: | No proven problems. |
| Beverages: | No proven problems. |
| Cocaine: | No proven problems. |
| Foods: Salt. | Increased edema (fluid retention). |
| Marijuana: | Increased bleeding between periods. Avoid. |
| Tobacco: | Possible heart attack, blood clots and stroke. |

# CORTISONE

## BRAND NAMES

Cortelan                Cortone
Cortistab

## BASIC INFORMATION

**Habit forming? No**
**Prescription needed? Yes**
**Available as generic? Yes**
**Drug class: Cortisone drug (adrenal**
**corticosteroid)**

 ## USES

- Reduces inflammation caused by many different medical problems.
- Treatment for some allergic diseases, blood disorders, kidney diseases, asthma and emphysema.
- Replaces corticosteroid deficiencies.

 ## DOSAGE & USAGE INFORMATION

**How to take:**
Tablet—Swallow with liquid or food to lessen stomach irritation. If you can't swallow whole, crumble tablet and take with liquid or food.

**When to take:**
At the same times each day. Take once-a-day or once-every-other-day doses in mornings.

**If you forget a dose:**
- Several-doses-per-day prescription—Take as soon as you remember up to 2 hours late. If more than 2 hours, wait for next scheduled dose (don't double this dose).
- Once-a-day dose or less—Wait for next dose. Double this dose.

**What drug does:**
Decreases inflammatory responses.

**Time lapse before drug works:**
2 to 4 days.

**Don't take with:**
See Interaction column and consult doctor.

 ## OVERDOSE

**SYMPTOMS:**
**Headache, convulsions, heart failure.**
**WHAT TO DO:**
- **Dial 0 (operator) or 911 (emergency) for an ambulance or medical help. Then give first aid immediately.**
- **See emergency information on inside covers.**

 ## POSSIBLE ADVERSE REACTIONS OR SIDE EFFECTS

| SYMPTOMS | WHAT TO DO |
|---|---|
| **Life-threatening:**<br>None expected. | |
| **Common:**<br>Acne, thirst, indigestion, nausea, vomiting, poor wound healing. | Continue. Call doctor when convenient. |
| **Infrequent:** | |
| • Bloody or black, tarry stool. | Discontinue. Seek emergency treatment. |
| • Blurred vision; halos around lights; sore throat, fever; muscle cramps; swollen legs, feet. | Discontinue. Call doctor right away. |
| • Mood changes, insomnia, restlessness, frequent urination, weight gain, round face, fatigue, weakness, TB recurrence, irregular menstrual periods. | Continue. Call doctor when convenient. |
| **Rare:** | |
| • Irregular heartbeat. | Discontinue. Seek emergency treatment. |
| • Rash. | Discontinue. Call doctor right away. |

 ## WARNINGS & PRECAUTIONS

**Don't take if:**
- You are allergic to any cortisone drug.
- You have tuberculosis or fungus infection.
- You have herpes infection of eyes, lips or genitals.

**Before you start, consult your doctor:**
- If you have had tuberculosis.
- If you have congestive heart failure.
- If you have diabetes.
- If you have peptic ulcer.
- If you have glaucoma.
- If you have underactive thyroid.
- If you have high blood pressure.
- If you have myasthenia gravis.
- If you have blood clots in legs or lungs.

**Over age 60:**
Adverse reactions and side effects may be more frequent and severe than in younger persons. Likely to aggravate edema, diabetes or ulcers. Likely to cause cataracts and osteoporosis (softening of the bones).

**Pregnancy:**
Risk to unborn child outweighs drug benefits. Don't use.

**Breast-feeding:**
Drug passes into milk. Avoid drug or discontinue nursing until you finish medicine. Consult doctor for advice on maintaining milk supply.

**Infants & children:**
Use only under medical supervision.

**Prolonged use:**
- Retards growth in children.
- Possible glaucoma, cataracts, diabetes, fragile bones and thin skin.
- Functional dependence.

**Skin & sunlight:**
No problems expected.

**Driving, piloting or hazardous work:**
No problems expected.

**Discontinuing:**
- Don't discontinue without doctor's advice until you complete prescribed dose, even though symptoms diminish or disappear.
- Drug affects your response to surgery, illness, injury or stress for 2 years after discontinuing. Tell anyone who takes medical care of you within 2 years about drug.

**Others:**
Avoid immunizations if possible.

 ## POSSIBLE INTERACTION WITH OTHER DRUGS

| GENERIC NAME OR DRUG CLASS | COMBINED EFFECT |
|---|---|
| Amphoterecin B | Potassium depletion. |
| Anticholinergics | Possible glaucoma. |
| Anticoagulants (oral) | Decreased anticoagulant effect. |
| Anticonvulsants (hydantoin) | Decreased cortisone effect. |
| Antidiabetics (oral) | Decreased antidiabetic effect. |
| Antihistamines | Decreased cortisone effect. |
| Aspirin | Increased cortisone effect. |
| Barbiturates | Decreased cortisone effect. Oversedation. |
| Beta-adrenergic blockers | Decreased cortisone effect. |
| Chloral hydrate | Decreased cortisone effect. |
| Chlorthalidone | Potassium depletion. |

| | |
|---|---|
| Cholinergics | Decreased cholinergic effect. |
| Contraceptives (oral) | Increased cortisone effect. |
| Digitalis preparations | Dangerous potassium depletion. Possible digitalis toxicity. |
| Diuretics (thiazide) | Potassium depletion. |
| Ephedrine | Decreased cortisone effect. |
| Estrogens | Increased cortisone effect. |
| Ethacrynic acid | Potassium depletion. |
| Furosemide | Potassium depletion. |
| Glutethimide | Decreased cortisone effect. |
| Indapamide | Possible excessive potassium loss, causing dangerous heartbeat irregularity. |
| Indomethacin | Increased cortisone effect. |
| Insulin | Decreased insulin effect. |
| Isoniazid | Decreased isoniazid effect. |
| Ketoprofen | Increased risk of stomach ulcer and bleeding. |
| Oxyphenbutazone | Possible ulcers. |
| Phenylbutazone | Possible ulcers. |
| Potassium supplements | Decreased potassium effect. |
| Rifampin | Decreased cortisone effect. |

*Continued page 965*

 ## POSSIBLE INTERACTION WITH OTHER SUBSTANCES

| INTERACTS WITH | COMBINED EFFECT |
|---|---|
| Alcohol: | Risk of stomach ulcers. |
| Beverages: | No proven problems. |
| Cocaine: | Overstimulation. Avoid. |
| Foods: | No proven problems. |
| Marijuana: | Decreased immunity. |
| Tobacco: | Increased cortisone effect. Possible toxicity. |

# CROMOLYN

## BRAND NAMES

Fivent
Intal
Nalcrom
Nasalcrom

Opticrom
Rynacrom
Sodium
Cromoblycate

## BASIC INFORMATION

**Habit forming? No**
**Prescription needed? Yes**
**Available as generic? No**
**Drug class: Antiasthmatic, anti-inflammatory**

## USES

- Prevents asthma attacks. Will not stop an active asthma attack.
- Treatment for inflammation of covering to eye and cornea.
- Reduces nasal allergic symptoms.

## DOSAGE & USAGE INFORMATION

**How to take:**
- Inhaler—Follow instructions enclosed with inhaler. Don't swallow cartridges for inhaler. Gargle and rinse mouth after inhalations.
- Eye drops—Follow prescription instructions.
- Nasal solution—Follow prescription instructions.

**When to take:**
At the same times each day. If you also use a bronchodilator inhaler, use the bronchodilator before the cromolyn.

**If you forget a dose:**
Take as soon as you remember up to 2 hours late. If more than 2 hours, wait for next scheduled dose (don't double this dose).

**What drug does:**
Blocks histamine release from mast cells.

**Time lapse before drug works:**
- 4 weeks for prevention of asthma attacks.
- 1 to 2 weeks for nasal or eye symptoms.

*Continued next column*

## OVERDOSE

**SYMPTOMS:**
**Increased side effects and adverse reactions listed.**
**WHAT TO DO:**
**Overdose unlikely to threaten life. If person inhales much larger amount than prescribed, call doctor, poison-control center or hospital emergency room for instructions.**

**Don't take with:**
See Interaction column and consult doctor.

## POSSIBLE ADVERSE REACTIONS OR SIDE EFFECTS

| SYMPTOMS | WHAT TO DO |
|---|---|
| **Life-threatening:**<br>Hives, rash, intense itching, faintness soon after a dose (anaphylaxis). | Seek emergency treatment immediately. |
| **Common:**<br>Hoarseness, cough. | Continue. Call doctor when convenient. |
| **Infrequent:**<br>• Rash, hives, swallowing difficulty, nausea, vomiting, increased wheezing, joint pain or swelling, muscle pain, weakness, difficult or painful urination. | Discontinue. Call doctor right away. |
| • Drowsiness, dizziness, headache, watery eyes, stuffy nose, throat irritation. | Continue. Call doctor when convenient. |
| **Rare:**<br>Nosebleed. | Continue. Call doctor when convenient. |

## WARNINGS & PRECAUTIONS

**Don't take if:**
You are allergic to cromolyn, lactose, milk or milk products.

**Before you start, consult your doctor:**
- If you plan to become pregnant within medication period.
- If you have kidney or liver disease.

**Over age 60:**
Adverse reactions and side effects may be more frequent and severe than in younger persons.

**Pregnancy:**
Risk to unborn child outweighs drug benefits. Don't use.

**Breast-feeding:**
Drug passes into milk. Avoid drug or discontinue nursing.

**Infants & children:**
Use only under medical supervision.

**Prolonged use:**
No problems expected.

**Skin & sunlight:**
No problems expected.

**Driving, piloting or hazardous work:**
No problems expected.

**Discontinuing:**
No problems expected.

**Others:**
- Inhaler must be cleaned and work well for drug to be effective.
- This treatment does not stop an acute asthma attack. It may aggravate it.
- Eye drops:
  Wash hands. Apply pressure to inside corner of eye with middle finger. Continue pressure for 1 minute after placing medicine in eye. Tilt head backward. Pull lower lid away from eye with index finger of the same hand. Drop eye drops into pouch and close eye. Don't blink. Keep eyes closed for 1 to 2 minutes. Don't touch applicator tip to any surface (including the eye). If you accidentally touch tip, clean with warm soap and water. Keep container tightly closed. Keep cool, but don't freeze. Wash hands immediately after using.

## POSSIBLE INTERACTION WITH OTHER DRUGS

| GENERIC NAME OR DRUG CLASS | COMBINED EFFECT |
| --- | --- |
| Cortisone drugs | Increased cortisone effect in treating asthma. Cortisone dose may be decreased. |

## POSSIBLE INTERACTION WITH OTHER SUBSTANCES

| INTERACTS WITH | COMBINED EFFECT |
| --- | --- |
| Alcohol: | None expected. |
| Beverages: | None expected. |
| Cocaine: | None expected. |
| Foods: | None expected. |
| Marijuana: | None expected. |
| Tobacco: | None expected, but tobacco smoke aggravates asthma and eye irritation. Avoid. |

# CYCLACILLIN

## BRAND NAMES

Cyclapen-W

## BASIC INFORMATION

**Habit forming? No**
**Prescription needed? Yes**
**Available as generic? Yes**
**Drug class: Antibiotic (penicillin)**

## USES

Treatment of bacterial infections that are susceptible to cyclacillin.

## DOSAGE & USAGE INFORMATION

**How to take:**
- Tablets or capsules—Swallow with liquid on an empty stomach 1 hour before or 2 hours after eating.
- Liquid—Take with cold beverage. Liquid form is perishable and effective for only 7 days at room temperature. Effective for 14 days if stored in refrigerator. Don't freeze.

**When to take:**
Follow instructions on prescription label or side of package. Doses should be evenly spaced. For example, 4 times a day means every 6 hours.

**If you forget a dose:**
Take as soon as you remember. Continue regular schedule.

**What drug does:**
Destroys susceptible bacteria. Does not kill viruses.

**Time lapse before drug works:**
May be several days before medicine affects infection.

**Don't take with:**
See Interaction column and consult doctor.

## OVERDOSE

**SYMPTOMS:**
**Severe diarrhea, nausea or vomiting.**
**WHAT TO DO:**
**Overdose unlikely to threaten life. If person takes much larger amount than prescribed, call doctor, poison-control center or hospital emergency room for instructions.**

## POSSIBLE ADVERSE REACTIONS OR SIDE EFFECTS

| SYMPTOMS | WHAT TO DO |
|---|---|
| **Life-threatening:** | |
| Hives, rash, intense itching, faintness soon after a dose (anaphylaxis). | Seek emergency treatment immediately. |
| **Common:** | |
| Dark or discolored tongue. | Continue. Tell doctor at next visit. |
| **Infrequent:** | |
| Mild nausea, vomiting, diarrhea. | Continue. Call doctor when convenient. |
| **Rare:** | |
| Unexplained bleeding. | Discontinue. Call doctor right away. |

## WARNINGS & PRECAUTIONS

**Don't take if:**
Your are allergic to cyclacillin, cephalosporin antibiotics, other penicillins or penicillamine. Life-threatening reaction may occur.

**Before you start, consult your doctor:**
If you are allergic to any substance or drug.

**Over age 60:**
You may have skin reactions, particularly around genitals and anus.

**Pregnancy:**
Studies inconclusive on harm to unborn child. Animal studies show fetal abnormalities. Decide with your doctor whether drug benefits justify risk to unborn child.

**Breast-feeding:**
Drug passes into milk. Child may become sensitive to penicillins and have allergic reactions to penicillin drugs. Avoid cyclacillin or discontinue nursing until you finish medicine. Consult doctor for advice on maintaining milk supply.

**Infants & children:**
No problems expected.

**Prolonged use:**
You may become more susceptible to infections caused by germs not responsive to cyclacillin.

**Skin & sunlight:**
No problems expected.

**Driving, piloting or hazardous work:**
Usually not dangerous. Most hazardous reactions likely to occur a few minutes after taking cyclacillin.

**Discontinuing:**
Don't discontinue without doctor's advice until you complete prescribed dose, even though symptoms diminish or disappear.

**Others:**
No problems expected.

## POSSIBLE INTERACTION WITH OTHER DRUGS

| GENERIC NAME OR DRUG CLASS | COMBINED EFFECT |
|---|---|
| Beta-adrenergic blockers | Increased chance of anaphylaxis (see emergency information on inside front cover). |
| Chloramphenicol | Decreased effect of both drugs. |
| Erythromycins | Decreased effect of both drugs. |
| Loperamide | Decreased cyclacillin effect. |
| Paromomycin | Decreased effect of both drugs. |
| Tetracyclines | Decreased effect of both drugs. |
| Troleandomycin | Decreased effect of both drugs. |

## POSSIBLE INTERACTION WITH OTHER SUBSTANCES

| INTERACTS WITH | COMBINED EFFECT |
|---|---|
| Alcohol: | Occasional stomach irritation. |
| Beverages: | None expected. |
| Cocaine: | No proven problems. |
| Foods: | Decreased effect of cyclacillin. |
| Marijuana: | No proven problems. |
| Tobacco: | None expected. |

# CYCLANDELATE

## BRAND NAMES

Cyclospasmol          Cyraso-400

## BASIC INFORMATION

Habit forming? No
Prescription needed?
  U.S.: Yes
  Canada: No
Available as generic? Yes
Drug class: Vasodilator

 **USES**

Improves poor blood flow to brain and extremities.

 **DOSAGE & USAGE INFORMATION**

**How to take:**
Tablet or capsule—Swallow with liquid. If you can't swallow whole, crumble tablet or open capsule and take with liquid or food.

**When to take:**
At the same time each day.

**If you forget a dose:**
Take as soon as you remember up to 2 hours late. If more than 2 hours, wait for next scheduled dose (don't double this dose).

**What drug does:**
Increases blood flow by relaxing and expanding blood-vessel walls.

**Time lapse before drug works:**
3 weeks.

**Don't take with:**
See Interaction column and consult doctor.

 **OVERDOSE**

**SYMPTOMS:**
Severe headache, dizziness; nausea, vomiting; flushed, hot face.
**WHAT TO DO:**
Overdose unlikely to threaten life. If person takes much larger amount than prescribed, call doctor, poison-control center or hospital emergency room for instructions.

 **POSSIBLE ADVERSE REACTIONS OR SIDE EFFECTS**

| SYMPTOMS | WHAT TO DO |
|---|---|
| **Life-threatening:**<br>None expected. | |
| **Common:**<br>None expected. | |
| **Infrequent:** | |
| • Rapid heartbeat. | Discontinue. Call doctor right away. |
| • Dizziness; headache; weakness; flushed face; tingling in face, fingers or toes; unusual sweating. | Continue. Call doctor when convenient. |
| • Belching, heartburn, nausea or stomach pain. | Continue. Tell doctor at next visit. |
| **Rare:**<br>None expected. | |

## WARNINGS & PRECAUTIONS

**Don't take if:**
You have had allergic reaction to cyclandelate.

**Before you start, consult your doctor:**
* If you have glaucoma.
* If you have had heart attack or stroke.

**Over age 60:**
Adverse reactions and side effects may be more frequent and severe than in younger persons.

**Pregnancy:**
No proven harm to unborn child. Avoid if possible.

**Breast-feeding:**
No proven problems. Consult doctor.

**Infants & children:**
Not recommended.

**Prolonged use:**
No problems expected.

**Skin & sunlight:**
No problems expected.

**Driving, piloting or hazardous work:**
Avoid if you feel dizzy or weak. Otherwise, no problems expected.

**Discontinuing:**
Don't discontinue without doctor's advice until you complete prescribed dose, even though symptoms diminish or disappear.

**Others:**
Response to drug varies. If your symptoms don't improve after 3 weeks of use, consult doctor.

## POSSIBLE INTERACTION WITH OTHER DRUGS

| GENERIC NAME OR DRUG CLASS | COMBINED EFFECT |
| --- | --- |
| None | |

## POSSIBLE INTERACTION WITH OTHER SUBSTANCES

| INTERACTS WITH | COMBINED EFFECT |
| --- | --- |
| Alcohol: | None expected. |
| Beverages: | None expected. |
| Cocaine: | Decreased cyclandelate effect. Avoid. |
| Foods: | None expected. |
| Marijuana: | None expected. |
| Tobacco: | May decrease cyclandelate effect. |

# CYCLIZINE

## BRAND NAMES

Marezine                    Marzine

## BASIC INFORMATION

**Habit forming? No**
**Prescription needed?**
  **U.S.: No**
  **Canada: Yes**
**Available as generic? No**
**Drug class: Antihistamine, antiemetic**

 ## USES

Prevents motion sickness.

 ## DOSAGE & USAGE INFORMATION

**How to take:**
Tablet—Swallow with liquid or food to lessen
stomach irritation. If you can't swallow whole,
crumble tablet and chew or take with liquid or
food.

**When to take:**
30 minutes to 1 hour before traveling.

**If you forget a dose:**
Take as soon as you remember. Wait 4 hours
for next dose.

**What drug does:**
Reduces sensitivity of nerve endings in inner
ear, blocking messages to brain's vomiting
center.

**Time lapse before drug works:**
30 to 60 minutes.

**Don't take with:**
See Interaction column and consult doctor.

 ## OVERDOSE

**SYMPTOMS:**
**Drowsiness, confusion, incoordination,**
**stupor, coma, weak pulse, shallow**
**breathing.**
**WHAT TO DO:**
- **Dial 0 (operator) or 911 (emergency) for an**
  **ambulance or medical help. Then give first**
  **aid immediately.**
- **See emergency information on inside**
  **covers.**

 ## POSSIBLE ADVERSE REACTIONS OR SIDE EFFECTS

| SYMPTOMS | WHAT TO DO |
|---|---|
| **Life-threatening:** | |
| None expected. | |
| **Common:** | |
| Drowsiness. | Continue. Tell doctor at next visit. |
| **Infrequent:** | |
| • Headache, diarrhea or constipation, fast heartbeat. | Continue. Call doctor when convenient. |
| • Dry mouth, nose, throat. | Continue. Tell doctor at next visit. |
| **Rare:** | |
| • Rash or hives, jaundice. | Discontinue. Call doctor right away. |
| • Restlessness, excitement, insomnia, blurred vision, frequent or difficult urination. | Continue. Call doctor when convenient. |
| • Appetite loss, nausea. | Continue. Tell doctor at next visit. |

## WARNINGS & PRECAUTIONS

**Don't take if:**
- You are allergic to meclizine, buclizine or cyclizine.
- You have taken MAO inhibitors in the past 2 weeks.

**Before you start, consult your doctor:**
- If you have glaucoma.
- If you have prostate enlargement.
- If you have reacted badly to any antihistamine.

**Over age 60:**
Adverse reactions and side effects may be more frequent and severe than in younger persons, especially impaired urination from enlarged prostate gland.

**Pregnancy:**
Studies inconclusive on harm to unborn child. Animal studies show fetal abnormalities. Decide with your doctor whether drug benefits justify risk to unborn child.

**Breast-feeding:**
Drug passes into milk. Avoid drug or discontinue nursing until you finish medicine. Consult doctor for advice on maintaining milk supply.

**Infants & children:**
No problems expected.

**Prolonged use:**
No problems expected.

**Skin & sunlight:**
No problems expected.

**Driving, piloting or hazardous work:**
Don't fly aircraft. Don't drive until you learn how medicine affects you. Don't work around dangerous machinery. Don't climb ladders or work in high places. Danger increases if you drink alcohol or take medicine affecting alertness and reflexes, such as antihistamines, tranquilizers, sedatives, pain medicine, narcotics and mind-altering drugs.

**Discontinuing:**
No problems expected.

**Others:**
No problems expected.

## POSSIBLE INTERACTION WITH OTHER DRUGS

| GENERIC NAME OR DRUG CLASS | COMBINED EFFECT |
|---|---|
| Amphetamines | May decrease drowsiness caused by cyclizine. |
| Anticholinergics | Increased effect of both drugs. |
| Antidepressants (tricyclic) | Increased effect of both drugs. |
| MAO inhibitors | Increased cyclizine effect. |
| Narcotics | Increased effect of both drugs. |
| Pain relievers | Increased effect of both drugs. |
| Sedatives | Increased effect of both drugs. |
| Sleep inducers | Increased effect of both drugs. |
| Tranquilizers | Increased effect of both drugs. |

## POSSIBLE INTERACTION WITH OTHER SUBSTANCES

| INTERACTS WITH | COMBINED EFFECT |
|---|---|
| Alcohol: | Increased sedation. Avoid. |
| Beverages: Caffeine drinks. | May decrease drowsiness. |
| Cocaine: | None expected. |
| Foods: | None expected. |
| Marijuana: | Increased drowsiness, dry mouth. |
| Tobacco: | None expected. |

# CYCLOBENZAPRINE

## BRAND NAMES

**Flexeril**

## BASIC INFORMATION

**Habit forming?** No
**Prescription needed?** Yes
**Available as generic?** No
**Drug class:** Muscle relaxant (skeletal)

## USES

Treatment for pain and limited motion caused by spasms in voluntary muscles.

## DOSAGE & USAGE INFORMATION

**How to take:**
Tablet or capsule—Swallow with liquid.

**When to take:**
At the same time each day or according to label instructions.

**If you forget a dose:**
Take as soon as you remember. Wait 4 hours for next dose.

**What drug does:**
Blocks body's pain messages to brain. May also sedate.

**Time lapse before drug works:**
30 to 60 minutes.

*Continued next column*

## OVERDOSE

**SYMPTOMS:**
**Drowsiness, confusion, difficulty concentrating, visual problems, vomiting, blood-pressure drop, low body temperature, weak and rapid pulse, convulsions, coma.**
**WHAT TO DO:**
- **Dial 0 (operator) or 911 (emergency) for an ambulance or medical help. Then give first aid immediately.**
- **If patient is unconscious and not breathing, give mouth-to-mouth breathing. If there is no heartbeat, use cardiac massage and mouth-to-mouth breathing (CPR). Don't try to make patient vomit. If you can't get help quickly, take patient to nearest emergency facility.**
- **See emergency information on inside covers.**

**Don't take with:**
- Non-prescription drugs without consulting doctor.
- See Interaction column and consult doctor.

## POSSIBLE ADVERSE REACTIONS OR SIDE EFFECTS

| SYMPTOMS | WHAT TO DO |
|---|---|
| **Life-threatening:**<br>None expected. | |
| **Common:**<br>Drowsiness, dizziness, dry mouth. | Continue. Call doctor when convenient. |
| **Infrequent:**<br>• Blurred vision, fast heartbeat. | Discontinue. Call doctor right away. |
| • Insomnia, numbness in extremities, bad taste in mouth. | Continue. Call doctor when convenient. |
| **Rare:**<br>• Unsteadiness, confusion, depression, hallucinations, rash, itch, swelling, breathing difficulty. | Discontinue. Call doctor right away. |
| • Difficult urination. | Continue. Call doctor when convenient. |

## WARNINGS & PRECAUTIONS

**Don't take if:**
- You are allergic to any skeletal-muscle relaxant.
- You have taken MAO inhibitors in last 2 weeks.
- You have had a heart attack within 6 weeks, or suffer from congestive heart failure.
- You have overactive thyroid.

**Before you start, consult your doctor:**
- If you have a heart problem.
- If you have reacted to tricyclic antidepressants.
- If you have glaucoma.
- If you have a prostate condition and urination difficulty.
- If you intend to pilot aircraft.

**Over age 60:**
Adverse reactions and side effects may be more frequent and severe than in younger persons. Avoid extremes of heat and cold.

**Pregnancy:**
Risk to unborn child outweighs drug benefits. Don't use.

**Breast-feeding:**
Drug passes into milk. Avoid drug or discontinue nursing until you finish medicine. Consult doctor for advice on maintaining milk supply.

**Infants & children:**
Don't use for children younger than 15.

**Prolonged use:**
No problems expected.

**Skin & sunlight:**
May cause rash or intensify sunburn in areas exposed to sun or sunlamp.

**Driving, piloting or hazardous work:**
Don't drive or pilot aircraft until you learn how medicine affects you. Don't work around dangerous machinery. Don't climb ladders or work in high places. Danger increases if you drink alcohol or take medicine affecting alertness and reflexes.

**Discontinuing:**
May be unnecessary to finish medicine. Follow doctor's instructions.

**Others:**
No problems expected.

## POSSIBLE INTERACTION WITH OTHER DRUGS

| GENERIC NAME OR DRUG CLASS | COMBINED EFFECT |
|---|---|
| Anticholinergics | Increased anticholinergic effect. |
| Antidepressants | Increased sedation. |
| Antihistamines | Increased antihistamine effect. |
| Clonidine | Decreased clonidine effect. |
| Dronabinol | Increased effect of dronabinol on central nervous system. Avoid combination. |
| Guanethidine | Decreased guanethidine effect. |
| MAO inhibitors | High fever, convulsions, possible death. |
| Mind-altering drugs | Increased mind-altering effect. |
| Narcotics | Increased sedation. |
| Pain relievers | Increased pain reliever effect. |
| Rauwolfia alkaloids | Decreased effect of rauwolfia alkaloids. |
| Sedatives | Increased sedative effect. |
| Sleep inducers | Increased sedation. |
| Tranquilizers | Increased tranquilizer effect. |

## POSSIBLE INTERACTION WITH OTHER SUBSTANCES

| INTERACTS WITH | COMBINED EFFECT |
|---|---|
| Alcohol: | Depressed brain function. Avoid. |
| Beverages: | None expected. |
| Cocaine: | Decreased cyclobenzaprine effect. |
| Foods: | None expected. |
| Marijuana: | Occasional use—Drowsiness. Frequent use—Severe mental and physical impairment. |
| Tobacco: | None expected. |

# CYCLOPHOSPHAMIDE

## BRAND NAMES

Cytoxan       Procytox
Neosar

## BASIC INFORMATION

Habit forming? No
Available as generic? No
Prescription needed? Yes
Drug class: Immunosuppressant

 **USES**

- Treatment for cancer.
- Treatment for severe rheumatoid arthritis.
- Treatment for blood-vessel disease.
- Treatment for skin disease.

 **DOSAGE & USAGE INFORMATION**

**How to take:**
Tablet—Swallow with liquid. If you can't swallow whole, crumble tablet and take with liquid or food.

**When to take:**
Works best if taken first thing in morning. However, may take with food to lessen stomach irritation. Don't take at bedtime.

**If you forget a dose:**
Take as soon as you remember up to 12 hours late. If more than 12 hours, wait for next scheduled dose (don't double this dose).

**What drug does:**
- Kills cancer cells.
- Suppresses spread of cancer cells.
- Suppresses immune system.

**Time lapse before drug works:**
7 to 10 days continual use.

**Don't take with:**
See Interaction column and consult doctor.

 **OVERDOSE**

**SYMPTOMS:**
Bloody urine, water retention, weight gain, severe infection.
**WHAT TO DO:**
Overdose unlikely to threaten life. If person takes much larger amount than prescribed, call doctor, poison-control center or hospital emergency room for instructions.

 **POSSIBLE ADVERSE REACTIONS OR SIDE EFFECTS**

| SYMPTOMS | WHAT TO DO |
|---|---|
| **Life-threatening:** | |
| None expected. | |
| **Common:** | |
| • Sore throat, fever. | Discontinue. Call doctor right away. |
| • Dark skin, nails; nausea; appetite loss; vomiting; missed period. | Continue. Call doctor when convenient. |
| **Infrequent:** | |
| • Rash, hives, itch; shortness of breath; rapid heartbeat; cough; blood in urine, painful urination; pain in side; bleeding; bruising; increased sweating. | Discontinue. Call doctor right away. |
| • Confusion, agitation, headache, dizziness, flushed face, stomach pain, joint pain, fatigue, weakness. | Continue. Call doctor when convenient. |
| **Rare:** | |
| • Mouth, lip sores; black stool; unusual thirst. | Discontinue. Call doctor right away. |
| • Blurred vision, increased urination. | Continue. Call doctor when convenient. |

## WARNINGS & PRECAUTIONS

### Don't take if:
- You are allergic to any alkylating agent.
- You have an infection.
- You have bloody urine.
- You will have surgery within 2 months, including dental surgery, requiring general or spinal anesthesia.

### Before you start, consult your doctor:
- If you have impaired liver or kidney function.
- If you have impaired bone-marrow or blood-cell production.
- If you have had chemotherapy or X-ray therapy.
- If you have taken cortisone drugs in the past year.

### Over age 60:
Adverse reactions and side effects may be more frequent and severe than in younger persons. To reduce risk of chemical bladder inflammation, drink 8 to 10 glasses of water daily.

### Pregnancy:
Risk to unborn child outweighs drug benefits. Don't use.

### Breast-feeding:
Drug passes into milk. Avoid drug or discontinue nursing until you finish medicine. Consult doctor for advice on maintaining milk supply.

### Infants & children:
Use only under medical supervision.

### Prolonged use:
- Development of fibrous lung tissue.
- Possible jaundice.
- Swelling of feet, lower legs.

### Skin & sunlight:
No problems expected.

### Driving, piloting or hazardous work:
Avoid if you feel dizzy or have blurred vision. Otherwise, no problems expected.

### Discontinuing:
Don't discontinue without consulting doctor. Dose may require gradual reduction if you have taken drug for a long time. Doses of other drugs may also require adjustment.

### Others:
Frequently causes hair loss. After treatment ends, hair should grow back.

## POSSIBLE INTERACTION WITH OTHER DRUGS

| GENERIC NAME OR DRUG CLASS | COMBINED EFFECT |
|---|---|
| Allopurinol | Possible anemia. |
| Antidiabetics (oral) | Increased antidiabetic effect. |
| Insulin | Increased insulin effect. |
| Phenobarbital | Increased cyclophosphamide effect. |

## POSSIBLE INTERACTION WITH OTHER SUBSTANCES

| INTERACTS WITH | COMBINED EFFECT |
|---|---|
| Alcohol: | No problems expected. |
| Beverages: | No problems expected. Drink at least 2 quarts fluid every day. |
| Cocaine: | None expected. |
| Foods: | None expected. |
| Marijuana: | Increased impairment of immunity. |
| Tobacco: | None expected. |

# CYCLOTHIAZIDE

## BRAND NAMES

Anhydron               Fluidil

## BASIC INFORMATION

Habit forming? No
Prescription needed? Yes
Available as generic? Yes
Drug class: Antihypertensive, diuretic
          (thiazide)

## USES

- Controls, but doesn't cure, high blood pressure.
- Reduces fluid retention (edema) caused by conditions such as heart disorders and liver disease.

## DOSAGE & USAGE INFORMATION

**How to take:**
Tablet or capsule—Swallow with liquid. If you can't swallow whole, crumble tablet or open capsule and take with liquid or food.

**When to take:**
At the same time each day.

**If you forget a dose:**
Take as soon as you remember up to 2 hours late. If more than 2 hours, wait for next scheduled dose (don't double this dose).

**What drug does:**
- Forces sodium and water excretion, reducing body fluid.
- Relaxes muscle cells of small arteries.
- Reduced body fluid and relaxed arteries lower blood pressure.

**Time lapse before drug works:**
4 to 6 hours. May require several weeks to lower blood pressure.

*Continued next column*

## OVERDOSE

**SYMPTOMS:**
**Cramps, weakness, drowsiness, weak pulse, coma.**
**WHAT TO DO:**
- **Dial 0 (operator) or 911 (emergency) for an ambulance or medical help. Then give first aid immediately.**
- **See emergency information on inside covers.**

**Don't take with:**
- See Interaction column and consult doctor.
- Non-prescription drugs without consulting doctor.

## POSSIBLE ADVERSE REACTIONS OR SIDE EFFECTS

| SYMPTOMS | WHAT TO DO |
|---|---|
| **Life-threatening:** None expected. | |
| **Common:** None expected. | |
| **Infrequent:** | |
| • Blurred vision, severe abdominal pain, nausea, vomiting, irregular heartbeat, weak pulse. | Discontinue. Call doctor right away. |
| • Dizziness, mood changes, headaches, weakness, tiredness, weight changes. | Continue. Call doctor when convenient. |
| • Dry mouth, thirst. | Continue. Tell doctor at next visit. |
| **Rare:** | |
| • Rash or hives. | Discontinue. Seek emergency treatment. |
| • Sore throat, fever, jaundice. | Discontinue. Call doctor right away. |

## WARNINGS & PRECAUTIONS

**Don't take if:**
You are allergic to any thiazide diuretic drugs.

**Before you start, consult your doctor:**
- If you are allergic to any sulfa drug.
- If you have gout.
- If you have liver, pancreas or kidney disorder.

**Over age 60:**
Adverse reactions and side effects may be more frequent and severe than in younger persons, especially dizziness and excessive potassium loss.

**Pregnancy:**
Risk to unborn child outweighs drug benefits. Don't use.

**Breast-feeding:**
Drug passes into milk. Avoid drug or discontinue nursing.

**Infants & children:**
No problems expected.

**Prolonged use:**
You may need medicine to treat high blood pressure for the rest of your life.

**Skin & sunlight:**
May cause rash or intensify sunburn in areas exposed to sun or sunlamp.

**Driving, piloting or hazardous work:**
Don't drive or pilot aircraft until you learn how medicine affects you. Don't work around dangerous machinery. Don't climb ladders or work in high places. Danger increases if you drink alcohol or take medicine affecting alertness and reflexes, such as antihistamines, tranquilizers, sedatives, pain medicine, narcotics and mind-altering drugs.

**Discontinuing:**
Don't discontinue without medical advice.

**Others:**
- Hot weather and fever may cause dehydration and drop in blood pressure. Dose may require temporary adjustment. Weigh daily and report any unexpected weight decreases to your doctor.
- May cause rise in uric acid, leading to gout.
- May cause blood-sugar rise in diabetics.

## POSSIBLE INTERACTION WITH OTHER DRUGS

| GENERIC NAME OR DRUG CLASS | COMBINED EFFECT |
|---|---|
| Acebutolol | Increased antihypertensive effect. Dosages of both drugs may require adjustments. |
| Allopurinol | Decreased allopurinol effect. |
| Amiodarone | Increased risk of heartbeat irregularity due to low potassium. |
| Antidepressants (tricyclic) | Dangerous drop in blood pressure. Avoid combination unless under medical supervision. |
| Barbiturates | Increased cyclothiazide effect. |
| Calcium supplements | Increased calcium in blood. |
| Cholestyramine | Decreased cyclothiazide effect. |
| Cortisone drugs | Excessive potassium loss that causes dangerous heart rhythms. |
| Digitalis preparations | Excessive potassium loss that causes dangerous heart rhythms. |

| | |
|---|---|
| Diuretics (thiazide) | Increased effect of other thiazide diuretics. |
| Indapamide | Increased diuretic effect. |
| Labetolol | Increased antihypertensive effects. |
| Lithium | Increased effect of lithium. |
| MAO inhibitors | Increased cyclothiazide effect. |
| Nitrates | Excessive blood-pressure drop. |
| Oxprenolol | Increased antihypertensive effect. Dosages of both drugs may require adjustments. |
| Pentoxifylline | Increased antihypertensive effect. |
| Potassium supplements | Decreased potassium effect. |
| Probenecid | Decreased probenecid effect. |

## POSSIBLE INTERACTION WITH OTHER SUBSTANCES

| INTERACTS WITH | COMBINED EFFECT |
|---|---|
| Alcohol: | Dangerous blood-pressure drop. |
| Beverages: | None expected. |
| Cocaine: | None expected. |
| Foods: Licorice. | Excessive potassium loss that causes dangerous heart rhythms. |
| Marijuana: | May increase blood pressure. |
| Tobacco: | None expected. |

# CYCRIMINE

## BRAND NAMES

**Pagitane**

## BASIC INFORMATION

**Habit forming? No**
**Prescription needed? Yes**
**Available as generic? No**
**Drug class: Antidyskinetic, antiparkinsonism**

 **USES**

- Treatment of Parkinson's disease.
- Treatment of adverse effects of phenothiazines.

 **DOSAGE & USAGE INFORMATION**

**How to take:**
Tablets or capsules—Take with food to lessen stomach irritation.

**When to take:**
At the same times each day.

**If you forget a dose:**
Take as soon as you remember up to 2 hours late. If more than 2 hours, wait for next scheduled dose (don't double this dose).

**What drug does:**
- Balances chemical reactions necessary to send nerve impulses within base of brain.
- Improves muscle control and reduces stiffness.

**Time lapse before drug works:**
1 to 2 hours.

*Continued next column*

 **OVERDOSE**

**SYMPTOMS:**
**Agitation, dilated pupils, hallucinations, dry mouth, rapid heartbeat, sleepiness.**
**WHAT TO DO:**
- **Dial 0 (operator) or 911 (emergency) for an ambulance or medical help. Then give first aid immediately.**
- **If patient is unconscious and not breathing, give mouth-to-mouth breathing. If there is no heartbeat, use cardiac massage and mouth-to-mouth breathing (CPR). Don't try to make patient vomit. If you can't get help quickly, take patient to nearest emergency facility.**
- **See emergency information on inside covers.**

**Don't take with:**
- Non-prescription drugs for colds, cough or allergy.
- See Interaction column and consult doctor.

 **POSSIBLE ADVERSE REACTIONS OR SIDE EFFECTS**

| SYMPTOMS | WHAT TO DO |
|---|---|
| **Life-threatening:** None expected. | |
| **Common:** | |
| • Blurred vision, light sensitivity, constipation, nausea, vomiting. | Continue. Call doctor when convenient. |
| • Difficult or painful urination. | Continue. Tell doctor at next visit. |
| **Infrequent:** None expected. | |
| **Rare:** | |
| • Rash, eye pain. | Discontinue. Call doctor right away. |
| • Confusion; dizziness; sore mouth or tongue; muscle cramps; numbness, weakness in hands or feet. | Continue. Call doctor when convenient. |

## WARNINGS & PRECAUTIONS

**Don't take if:**
You are allergic to any antidyskinetic.

**Before you start, consult your doctor:**
- If you have had glaucoma.
- If you have had high blood pressure or heart disease.
- If you have had impaired liver function.
- If you have had kidney disease or urination difficulty.

**Over age 60:**
More sensitive to drug. Aggravates symptoms of enlarged prostate. Causes impaired thinking, hallucinations, nightmares. Consult doctor about any of these.

**Pregnancy:**
Studies inconclusive on harm to unborn child. Animal studies show fetal abnormalities. Decide with your doctor whether drug benefits justify risk to unborn child.

**Breast-feeding:**
No problems expected.

**Infants & children:**
Not recommended for children 3 and younger. Use for older children only under doctor's supervision.

**Prolonged use:**
Possible glaucoma.

**Skin & sunlight:**
No problems expected.

**Driving, piloting or hazardous work:**
Don't drive or pilot aircraft until you learn how medicine affects you. Don't work around dangerous machinery. Don't climb ladders or work in high places. Danger increases if you drink alcohol or take medicine affecting alertness and reflexes, such as antihistamines, tranquilizers, sedatives, pain medicine, narcotics and mind-altering drugs.

**Discontinuing:**
Don't discontinue without consulting doctor. Dose may require gradual reduction if you have taken drug for a long time. Doses of other drugs may also require adjustment.

**Others:**
- Internal eye pressure should be measured regularly.
- Avoid becoming overheated.

## POSSIBLE INTERACTION WITH OTHER DRUGS

| GENERIC NAME OR DRUG CLASS | COMBINED EFFECT |
|---|---|
| Amantadine | Increased amantadine effect. |
| Antidepressants (tricyclic) | Increased cycrimine effect. May cause glaucoma. |
| Antihistamines | Increased cycrimine effect. |
| Levodopa | Increased levodopa effect. Improved results in treating Parkinson's disease. |
| Meperidine | Increased cycrimine effect. |
| MAO inhibitors | Increased cycrimine effect. |
| Orphenadrine | Increased cycrimine effect. |
| Phenothiazines | Behavior changes. |
| Primidone | Excessive sedation. |
| Procainamide | Increased procainamide effect. |
| Quinidine | Increased cycrimine effect. |
| Tranquilizers | Excessive sedation. |

## POSSIBLE INTERACTION WITH OTHER SUBSTANCES

| INTERACTS WITH | COMBINED EFFECT |
|---|---|
| Alcohol: | None expected. |
| Beverages: | None expected. |
| Cocaine: | Decreased cycrimine effect. Avoid. |
| Foods: | None expected. |
| Marijuana: | None expected. |
| Tobacco: | None expected. |

# CYPROHEPTADINE

## BRAND NAMES

Cyprodine        Vimicon
Periactin

## BASIC INFORMATION

Habit forming? No
Prescription needed? Yes
Available as generic? Yes
Drug class: Antihistamine

 **USES**

- Reduces allergic symptoms such as hay fever, hives, rash or itching.
- Induces sleep.
- Reduces symptoms of cold urticaria.

 **DOSAGE & USAGE INFORMATION**

**How to take:**
Tablet or syrup—Swallow with liquid or food to lessen stomach irritation.

**When to take:**
Varies with form. Follow label directions.

**If you forget a dose:**
Take as soon as you remember up to 2 hours late. If more than 2 hours, wait for next scheduled dose (don't double this dose).

**What drug does:**
Blocks action of histamine after an allergic response triggers histamine release in sensitive cells.

**Time lapse before drug works:**
30 minutes.

*Continued next column*

 **OVERDOSE**

**SYMPTOMS:**
Convulsions, red face, hallucinations, coma.
**WHAT TO DO:**
- **Dial 0 (operator) or 911 (emergency) for an ambulance or medical help. Then give first aid immediately.**
- **If patient is unconscious and not breathing, give mouth-to-mouth breathing. If there is no heartbeat, use cardiac massage and mouth-to-mouth breathing (CPR). Don't try to make patient vomit. If you can't get help quickly, take patient to nearest emergency facility.**
- **See emergency information on inside covers.**

**Don't take with:**
See Interaction column and consult doctor.

 **POSSIBLE ADVERSE REACTIONS OR SIDE EFFECTS**

| SYMPTOMS | WHAT TO DO |
|---|---|
| **Life-threatening:** None expected. | |
| **Common:** Drowsiness, dizziness, dry mouth, nose, throat, nausea. | Continue. Tell doctor at next visit. |
| **Infrequent:** | |
| • Vision changes. | Discontinue. Call doctor right away. |
| • Less tolerance for contact lenses, difficult urination. | Continue. Call doctor when convenient. |
| • Appetite loss. | Continue. Tell doctor at next visit. |
| **Rare:** Nightmares, agitation, irritability, sore throat, fever, rapid heartbeat, unusual bleeding or bruising, fatigue, weakness. | Discontinue. Call doctor right away. |

## WARNINGS & PRECAUTIONS

**Don't take if:**
You are allergic to any antihistamine.

**Before you start, consult your doctor:**
- If you have glaucoma.
- If you have enlarged prostate.
- If you have asthma.
- If you have kidney disease.
- If you have peptic ulcer.
- If you will have surgery within 2 months, including dental surgery, requiring general or spinal anesthesia.

**Over age 60:**
Don't exceed recommended dose. Adverse reactions and side effects may be more frequent and severe than in younger persons, especially urination difficulty, diminished alertness and other brain and nervous-system symptoms.

**Pregnancy:**
No proven harm to unborn child. Avoid if possible.

**Breast-feeding:**
Drug passes into milk. Avoid drug or discontinue nursing until you finish medicine. Consult doctor for advice on maintaining milk supply.

**Infants & children:**
Not recommended for premature or newborn infants. Otherwise, no problems expected.

**Prolonged use:**
Avoid. May damage bone marrow and nerve cells.

**Skin & sunlight:**
May cause rash or intensify sunburn in areas exposed to sun or sunlamp.

**Driving, piloting or hazardous work:**
Don't drive or pilot aircraft until you learn how medicine affects you. Don't work around dangerous machinery. Don't climb ladders or work in high places. Danger increases if you drink alcohol or take medicine affecting alertness and reflexes, such as antihistamines, tranquilizers, sedatives, pain medicine, narcotics and mind-altering drugs.

**Discontinuing:**
No problems expected.

**Others:**
May mask symptoms of hearing damage from aspirin, other salicylates, cisplatin, paromomycin, vancomycin or anticonvulsants. Consult doctor if you use these.

## POSSIBLE INTERACTION WITH OTHER DRUGS

| GENERIC NAME OR DRUG CLASS | COMBINED EFFECT |
| --- | --- |
| Anticholinergics | Increased anticholinergic effect. |
| Antidepressants | Excess sedation. Avoid. |
| Antihistamines (other) | Excess sedation. Avoid. |
| Dronabinol | Increased effects of both drugs. Avoid. |
| Hypnotics | Excess sedation. Avoid. |
| MAO inhibitors | Increased cyproheptadine effect. |
| Mind-altering drugs | Excess sedation. Avoid. |
| Molindone | Increased antihistamine effect. |
| Narcotics | Excess sedation. Avoid. |
| Sedatives | Excess sedation. Avoid. |
| Sleep inducers | Excess sedation. Avoid. |
| Tranquilizers | Excess sedation. Avoid. |

## POSSIBLE INTERACTION WITH OTHER SUBSTANCES

| INTERACTS WITH | COMBINED EFFECT |
| --- | --- |
| Alcohol: | Excess sedation. Avoid. |
| Beverages: Caffeine drinks. | Less cyproheptadine sedation. |
| Cocaine: | Decreased cyproheptadine effect. Avoid. |
| Foods: | None expected. |
| Marijuana: | Excess sedation. Avoid. |
| Tobacco: | None expected. |

# DANAZOL

## BRAND NAMES

Cyclomen                    Danocrine

## BASIC INFORMATION

Habit forming? No
Prescription needed? Yes
Available as generic? No
Drug class: Gonadotropin inhibitor

 **USES**

Treatment of endometriosis, fibrocystic breast
disease, angioneurotic edema except in
pregnant women, gynecomastia, infertility,
excessive menstruation, precocious puberty.

 **DOSAGE & USAGE INFORMATION**

How to take:
Tablet or capsule—Swallow with liquid or food
to lessen stomach irritation. If you can't swallow
whole, crumble tablet or open capsule and take
with liquid or food.

When to take:
At the same times each day.

If you forget a dose:
Take as soon as you remember (don't double
dose).

What drug does:
Partially prevents output of pituitary
follicle-stimulating hormone and lutenizing
hormone reducing estrogen production.

Time lapse before drug works:
● 2 to 3 months to treat endometriosis.
● 1 to 2 months to treat other disorders.

Don't take with:
● Birth control pills.
● See Interaction column and consult doctor.

 **OVERDOSE**

SYMPTOMS:
None expected.
WHAT TO DO:
Overdose unlikely to threaten life. If person
takes much larger amount than prescribed,
call doctor, poison-control center or hospital
emergency room for instructions.

 **POSSIBLE ADVERSE REACTIONS OR SIDE EFFECTS**

| SYMPTOMS | WHAT TO DO |
|---|---|
| **Life-threatening:** | |
| None expected. | |
| **Common:** | |
| Menstrual irregularities. | Continue. Call doctor when convenient. |
| **Infrequent:** | |
| ● Unnatural hair growth in women, nosebleeds. | Discontinue. Call doctor right away. |
| ● Dizziness; hoarseness; voice deepens; flushed or red skin; muscle cramps; enlarged clitoris; decreased testicle size; vaginal burning, itch; swollen feet; decreased breast size. | Continue. Call doctor when convenient. |
| ● Headache, acne, weight gain. | Continue. Tell doctor at next visit. |
| **Rare:** | |
| Jaundice. | Discontinue. Call doctor right away. |

# DANAZOL

## WARNINGS & PRECAUTIONS

**Don't take if:**
You become pregnant.

**Before you start, consult your doctor:**
- If you take birth control pills.
- If you have diabetes.
- If you have heart disease.
- If you have epilepsy.
- If you have kidney disease.
- If you have liver disease.
- If you have migraine headache.

**Over age 60:**
Adverse reactions and side effects may be more frequent and severe than in younger persons.

**Pregnancy:**
Risk to unborn child outweighs drug benefits. Don't use. Stop if you get pregnant.

**Breast-feeding:**
Unknown whether medicine filters into milk. Consult doctor.

**Infants & children:**
Not recommended.

**Prolonged use:**
Required for full effect. Don't discontinue without consulting doctor.

**Skin & sunlight:**
No problems expected.

**Driving, piloting or hazardous work:**
No problems expected.

**Discontinuing:**
Don't discontinue without consulting doctor. Menstrual periods may be absent for 2 to 3 months after discontinuation.

**Others:**
May alter blood-sugar levels in diabetic persons.

## POSSIBLE INTERACTION WITH OTHER DRUGS

| GENERIC NAME OR DRUG CLASS | COMBINED EFFECT |
|---|---|
| Anticoagulants (oral) | Increased anticoagulant effect. |

## POSSIBLE INTERACTION WITH OTHER SUBSTANCES

| INTERACTS WITH | COMBINED EFFECT |
|---|---|
| Alcohol: | Excessive nervous system depression. Avoid. |
| Beverages: Caffeine. | Rapid, irregular heartbeat. Avoid. |
| Cocaine: | May interfere with expected action of danazol. Avoid. |
| Foods: | No problems expected. |
| Marijuana: | May interfere with expected action of danazol. Avoid. |
| Tobacco: | Rapid, irregular heartbeat. Avoid. Increased leg cramps. |

# DANTHRON

## BRAND NAMES

| | |
|---|---|
| AKshun | Doxidan |
| Dorbane | Modane |
| Dorbantyl L | Roydan |

## BASIC INFORMATION

Habit forming? No
Prescription needed? No
Available as generic? Yes
Drug class: Laxative (stimulant)

 ## USES

Constipation relief.

 ## DOSAGE & USAGE INFORMATION

**How to take:**
- Tablet—Swallow with liquid or food.
- Liquid—Drink 6 to 8 glasses of water each day, in addition to one taken with each dose.

**When to take:**
Usually at bedtime with a snack, unless directed otherwise.

**If you forget a dose:**
Take as soon as you remember.

**What drug does:**
Acts on smooth muscles of intestine wall to cause vigorous bowel movement.

**Time lapse before drug works:**
6 to 10 hours.

**Don't take with:**
- See Interaction column and consult doctor.
- Don't take within 2 hours of taking another medicine. Laxative interferes with medicine absorption.

 ## OVERDOSE

**SYMPTOMS:**
Vomiting, electrolyte depletion.
**WHAT TO DO:**
Overdose unlikely to threaten life. If person takes much larger amount than prescribed, call doctor, poison-control center or hospital emergency room for instructions.

 ## POSSIBLE ADVERSE REACTIONS OR SIDE EFFECTS

| SYMPTOMS | WHAT TO DO |
|---|---|
| **Life-threatening:**<br>None expected. | |
| **Common:**<br>Rectal irritation. | Continue. Call doctor when convenient. |
| **Infrequent:** | |
| • Dangerous potassium loss. | Discontinue. Call doctor right away. |
| • Belching, cramps, nausea. | Continue. Call doctor when convenient. |
| **Rare:** | |
| • Irritability, confusion, headache, rash, breathing difficulty, irregular heartbeat, muscle cramps, unusual tiredness, weakness. | Discontinue. Call doctor right away. |
| • Burning on urination. | Continue. Call doctor when convenient. |

## WARNINGS & PRECAUTIONS

### Don't take if:
- You have symptoms of appendicitis, inflamed bowel or intestinal blockage.
- You are allergic to a stimulant laxative.
- You have missed a bowel movement for only 1 or 2 days.

### Before you start, consult your doctor:
- If you have a colostomy or ileostomy.
- If you have congestive heart disease.
- If you have diabetes.
- If you have high blood pressure.
- If you have a laxative habit.
- If you have rectal bleeding.
- If you take other laxatives.

### Over age 60:
Adverse reactions and side effects may be more frequent and severe than in younger persons.

### Pregnancy:
Risk to mother and unborn child outweighs drug benefits. Don't use.

### Breast-feeding:
Drug passes into milk. Avoid drug or discontinue nursing until you finish medicine. Consult doctor for advice on maintaining milk supply.

### Infants & children:
Use only under medical supervision.

### Prolonged use:
Don't take for more than 1 week unless under a doctor's supervision. May cause laxative dependence.

### Skin & sunlight:
No problems expected.

### Driving, piloting or hazardous work:
No problems expected.

### Discontinuing:
May be unnecessary to finish medicine. Follow doctor's instructions.

### Others:
Don't take to "flush out" your system or as a "tonic."

## POSSIBLE INTERACTION WITH OTHER DRUGS

| GENERIC NAME OR DRUG CLASS | COMBINED EFFECT |
| --- | --- |
| Antihypertensives | May cause dangerous low potassium level. |
| Diuretics | May cause dangerous low potassium level. |
| Docusate calcium | Liver toxicity. |
| Docusate sodium | Liver toxicity. |

## POSSIBLE INTERACTION WITH OTHER SUBSTANCES

| INTERACTS WITH | COMBINED EFFECT |
| --- | --- |
| Alcohol: | None expected. |
| Beverages: | None expected. |
| Cocaine: | None expected. |
| Foods: | None expected. |
| Marijuana: | None expected. |
| Tobacco: | None expected. |

# DANTROLENE

## BRAND NAMES

**Dantrium**

## BASIC INFORMATION

**Habit forming? No**
**Prescription needed? Yes**
**Available as generic? No**
**Drug class: Muscle relaxant, antispastic**

 USES

- Relieves muscle spasticity caused by diseases such as multiple sclerosis, cerebral palsy, stroke.
- Relieves muscle spasticity caused by injury to spinal cord.
- Relieves or prevents excess body temperature brought on by some surgical procedures.

 DOSAGE & USAGE INFORMATION

**How to take:**
Capsules—Swallow with liquid.

**When to take:**
Once a day for muscle spasticity during first 6 days. Later, every 6 hours. For excess temperature, follow label instructions.

**If you forget a dose:**
Take as soon as you remember up to 2 hours late. If more than 2 hours, wait for next scheduled dose (don't double this dose).

*Continued next column*

 OVERDOSE

**SYMPTOMS:**
**Bloody stools, chest pain, convulsive seizures.**
**WHAT TO DO:**
- **Dial 0 (operator) or 911 (emergency) for an ambulance or medical help. Then give first aid immediately.**
- **If patient is unconscious and not breathing, give mouth-to-mouth breathing. If there is no heartbeat, use cardiac massage and mouth-to-mouth breathing (CPR). Don't try to make patient vomit. If you can't get help quickly, take patient to nearest emergency facility.**
- **See emergency information on inside covers.**

**What drug does:**
Acts directly on muscles to prevent excess contractions.

**Time lapse before drug works:**
1 or more weeks.

**Don't take with:**
See Interaction column and consult doctor.

 POSSIBLE ADVERSE REACTIONS OR SIDE EFFECTS

| SYMPTOMS | WHAT TO DO |
|---|---|
| **Life-threatening:** | |
| Seizure. | Seek emergency treatment immediately. |
| **Common:** | |
| None expected. | |
| **Infrequent:** | |
| • Rash, hives; black or bloody stools; chest pain; fast heartbeat; backache; blood in urine; painful, swollen feet; chills; fever. | Discontinue. Call doctor right away. |
| • Depression, confusion, headache, slurred speech, nervousness, insomnia, blurred vision, diarrhea, difficult swallowing, appetite loss, difficult urination, decreased sexual function in males. | Continue. Call doctor when convenient. |
| **Rare:** | |
| Jaundice. | Discontinue. Call doctor right away. |

## WARNINGS & PRECAUTIONS

**Don't take if:**
You are allergic to dantrolene or any muscle relaxant or antispastic medication.

**Before you start, consult your doctor:**
- If you have liver disease.
- If you have heart disease.
- If you have lung disease (especially emphysema).
- If you are over age 35.
- If you will have surgery within 2 months, including dental surgery, requiring general or spinal anesthesia.

**Over age 60:**
Adverse reactions and side effects may be more frequent and severe than in younger persons.

**Pregnancy:**
No proven harm to unborn child. Avoid it possible.

**Breast-feeding:**
Avoid nursing or discontinue until you finish drug.

**Infants & children:**
Only under close medical supervision.

**Prolonged use:**
Blood counts, G6PD tests before treatment begins in Negroes and Caucasians of Mediterranean heritage, liver function studies—all recommended periodically during prolonged use.

**Skin & sunlight:**
May cause rash or intensify sunburn in areas exposed to sun or sunlamp.

**Driving, piloting or hazardous work:**
Don't drive or pilot aircraft until you learn how medicine affects you. Don't work around dangerous machinery. Don't climb ladders or work in high places. Danger increases if you drink alcohol or take medicine affecting alertness and reflexes, such as antihistamines, tranquilizers, sedatives, pain medicine, narcotics and mind-altering drugs.

**Discontinuing:**
Don't discontinue without consulting doctor. Dose may require gradual reduction if you have taken drug for a long time. Doses of other drugs may also require adjustment.

**Others:**
No problems expected.

## POSSIBLE INTERACTION WITH OTHER DRUGS

| GENERIC NAME OR DRUG CLASS | COMBINED EFFECT |
|---|---|
| Central nervous system depressants: Sedatives, sleeping pills, tranquilizers, antidepressants, antihistamines, narcotics, other muscle relaxants | Increased sedation, low blood pressure. Avoid. |
| Dronabinol | Increased effect of dronabinol on central nervous system. Avoid. |

## POSSIBLE INTERACTION WITH OTHER SUBSTANCES

| INTERACTS WITH | COMBINED EFFECT |
|---|---|
| Alcohol: | Increased sedation, low blood pressure. Avoid. |
| Beverages: | No problems expected. |
| Cocaine: | Increased spasticity. Avoid. |
| Foods: | No problems expected. |
| Marijuana: | Increased spasticity. Avoid. |
| Tobacco: | May interfere with absorption of medicine. |

# DAPSONE

## BRAND NAMES

Avlosulfon        DDS

## BASIC INFORMATION

**Habit forming? No**
**Prescription needed? Yes**
**Available as generic? Yes**
**Drug class: Antibacterial (Antileprosy),**
       **Sulfone**

 USES

- Treatment of dermatitis herpetiformis.
- Treatment of leprosy.

 DOSAGE & USAGE INFORMATION

**How to take:**
Tablet or capsule—Swallow with liquid or food to lessen stomach irritation.

**When to take:**
Once a day at same time.

**If you forget a dose:**
Take as soon as you remember up to 2 hours late. If more than 2 hours, wait for next scheduled dose (don't double this dose).

**What drug does:**
Inhibits enzymes. Kills leprosy germs.

**Time lapse before drug works:**
- 3 years for leprosy.
- 1 to 2 weeks for dermatitis herpetiformis.

**Don't take with:**
See Interaction column and consult doctor.

 OVERDOSE

**SYMPTOMS:**
**Bleeding, vomiting, coma.**
**WHAT TO DO:**
- **Dial 0 (operator) or 911 (emergency) for an ambulance or medical help. Then give first aid immediately.**
- **If patient is unconscious and not breathing, give mouth-to-mouth breathing. If there is no heartbeat, use cardiac massage and mouth-to-mouth breathing (CPR). Don't try to make patient vomit. If you can't get help quickly, take patient to nearest emergency facility.**
- **See emergency information on inside covers.**

 POSSIBLE ADVERSE REACTIONS OR SIDE EFFECTS

| SYMPTOMS | WHAT TO DO |
|---|---|
| **Life-threatening:** | |
| None expected. | |
| **Common:** | |
| • Rash. | Discontinue. Call doctor right away. |
| • Abdominal pain, appetite loss. | Continue. Call doctor when convenient. |
| **Infrequent:** | |
| Pale. | Discontinue. Call doctor right away. |
| **Rare:** | |
| • Dizziness; mental changes; sore throat; fever; difficult breathing; bleeding; jaundice; numbness, tingling, pain or burning in hands or feet. | Discontinue. Call doctor right away. |
| • Headache; itching; nausea; vomiting; blue fingernails, lips. | Continue. Call doctor when convenient. |

## WARNINGS & PRECAUTIONS

**Don't take if:**
- You have G6PD deficiency.
- You are allergic to furosemide, thiazide diuretics, sulfonureas, carbonic anhydrase inhibitors, sulfonamides.

**Before you start, consult your doctor:**
- If you are anemic.
- If you have liver or kidney disease.
- If you are Negro or Caucasian with Mediterranean heritage.
- If you will have surgery within 2 months, including dental surgery, requiring general or spinal anesthesia.

**Over age 60:**
Adverse reactions and side effects may be more frequent and severe than in younger persons.

**Pregnancy:**
No problems expected.

**Breast feeding:**
Consult doctor.

**Infants & children:**
Under close medical supervision only.

**Prolonged use:**
Request blood counts, liver function studies.

**Skin & sunlight:**
No problems expected.

**Driving, piloting or hazardous work:**
Don't drive or pilot aircraft until you learn how medicine affects you. Don't work around dangerous machinery. Don't climb ladders or work in high places. Danger increases if you drink alcohol or take medicine affecting alertness and reflexes, such as antihistamines, tranquilizers, sedatives, pain medicine, narcotics and mind-altering drugs.

**Discontinuing:**
Don't discontinue without consulting doctor. Dose may require gradual reduction if you have taken drug for a long time. Doses of other drugs may also require adjustment.

**Others:**
No problems expected.

## POSSIBLE INTERACTION WITH OTHER DRUGS

| GENERIC NAME OR DRUG CLASS | COMBINED EFFECT |
| --- | --- |
| Aminobenzoic acid (PABA) | Decreased dapsone effect. Avoid. |
| Probenecid | Increased toxicity of dapsone. |
| Rifampin | Decreased effect of dapsone. |

## POSSIBLE INTERACTION WITH OTHER SUBSTANCES

| INTERACTS WITH | COMBINED EFFECT |
| --- | --- |
| Alcohol: | Increased chance of toxicity to liver. |
| Beverages: | No problems expected. |
| Cocaine: | Increased chance of toxicity. Avoid. |
| Foods: | No problems expected. |
| Marijuana: | Increased chance of toxicity. Avoid. |
| Tobacco: | May interfere with absorption of medicine. |

# DEHYDROCHOLIC ACID

## BRAND NAMES

| | |
|---|---|
| Bilaz | G.B.S. |
| Cholan-DH | Hepahydrin |
| Cholan-HMB | Neocholan |
| Decholin | Neolax |
| Dycholium | Trilax |

## BASIC INFORMATION

**Habit forming? No**
**Prescription needed? No**
**Available as generic? Yes**
**Drug class: Laxative (stimulant)**

## USES

Constipation relief.

## DOSAGE & USAGE INFORMATION

**How to take:**
Tablet—Swallow with liquid.

**When to take:**
Usually at bedtime with a snack, unless directed otherwise.

**If you forget a dose:**
Take as soon as you remember.

**What drug does:**
Acts on smooth muscles of intestine wall to cause vigorous bowel movement.

**Time lapse before drug works:**
6 to 10 hours.

**Don't take with:**
- See Interaction column and consult doctor.
- Don't take within 2 hours of taking another medicine. Laxative interferes with medicine absorption.

## OVERDOSE

**SYMPTOMS:**
Vomiting, electrolyte depletion.
**WHAT TO DO:**
Overdose unlikely to threaten life. If person takes much larger amount than prescribed, call doctor, poison-control center or hospital emergency room for instructions.

## POSSIBLE ADVERSE REACTIONS OR SIDE EFFECTS

| SYMPTOMS | WHAT TO DO |
|---|---|
| **Life-threatening:**<br>None expected. | |
| **Common:**<br>Rectal irritation. | Continue. Call doctor when convenient. |
| **Infrequent:** | |
| • Dangerous potassium loss. | Discontinue. Call doctor right away. |
| • Belching, cramps, nausea. | Continue. Call doctor when convenient. |
| **Rare:** | |
| • Irritability, confusion, headache, rash, breathing difficulty, irregular heartbeat, muscle cramps, unusual tiredness or weakness. | Discontinue. Call doctor right away. |
| • Burning on urination. | Continue. Call doctor when convenient. |

## WARNINGS & PRECAUTIONS

**Don't take if:**
- You have symptoms of appendicitis, inflamed bowel or intestinal blockage.
- You are allergic to a stimulant laxative.
- You have missed a bowel movement for only 1 or 2 days.
- You have liver disease.

**Before you start, consult your doctor:**
- If you have a colostomy or ileostomy.
- If you have congestive heart disease.
- If you have diabetes.
- If you have enlarged prostate.
- If you have a laxative habit.
- If you have rectal bleeding.
- If you take other laxatives.

**Over age 60:**
Adverse reactions and side effects may be more frequent and severe than in younger persons.

**Pregnancy:**
Risk to mother and unborn child outweighs drug benefits. Don't use.

**Breast-feeding:**
Drug passes into milk. Avoid drug or discontinue nursing until you finish medicine. Consult doctor for advice on maintaining milk supply.

**Infants & children:**
Use only under medical supervision.

**Prolonged use:**
Don't take for more than 1 week unless under a doctor's supervision. May cause laxative dependence.

**Skin & sunlight:**
No problems expected.

**Driving, piloting or hazardous work:**
No problems expected.

**Discontinuing:**
May be unnecessary to finish medicine. Follow doctor's instructions.

**Others:**
Don't take to "flush out" your system or as a "tonic."

## POSSIBLE INTERACTION WITH OTHER DRUGS

| GENERIC NAME OR DRUG CLASS | COMBINED EFFECT |
|---|---|
| Antihypertensives | May cause dangerous low potassium level. |
| Diuretics | May cause dangerous low potassium level. |

## POSSIBLE INTERACTION WITH OTHER SUBSTANCES

| INTERACTS WITH | COMBINED EFFECT |
|---|---|
| Alcohol: | None expected. |
| Beverages: | None expected. |
| Cocaine: | None expected. |
| Foods: | None expected. |
| Marijuana: | None expected. |
| Tobacco: | None expected. |

# DEXAMETHASONE

## BRAND NAMES

See complete list of brand names in the *Brand Name Directory,* page 947.

## BASIC INFORMATION

**Habit forming? No**
**Prescription needed? Yes**
**Available as generic? Yes**
**Drug class: Cortisone drug (adrenal corticosteroid)**

## USES

- Reduces inflammation caused by many different medical problems.
- Treatment for some allergic diseases, blood disorders, kidney diseases, asthma and emphysema.
- Replaces corticosteroid deficiencies.

## DOSAGE & USAGE INFORMATION

**How to take:**
- Tablet or liquid—Swallow with liquid or food to lessen stomach irritation. If you can't swallow whole, crumble tablet and take with liquid or food.
- Inhaler—Follow label instructions.

**When to take:**
At the same times each day. Take once-a-day or once-every-other-day doses in mornings.

**If you forget a dose:**
- Several-doses-per-day prescription—Take as soon as you remember up to 2 hours late. If more than 2 hours, wait for next scheduled dose (don't double this dose).
- Once-a-day dose or less—Wait for next dose. Double this dose.

**What drug does:**
Decreases inflammatory responses.

**Time lapse before drug works:**
2 to 4 days.

*Continued next column*

## OVERDOSE

**SYMPTOMS:**
**Headache, convulsions, heart failure.**
**WHAT TO DO:**
- **Dial 0 (operator) or 911 (emergency) for an ambulance or medical help. Then give first aid immediately.**
- **See emergency information on inside covers.**

**Don't take with:**
See Interaction column and consult doctor.

## POSSIBLE ADVERSE REACTIONS OR SIDE EFFECTS

| SYMPTOMS | WHAT TO DO |
|---|---|
| **Life-threatening:**<br>None expected. | |
| **Common:**<br>Poor wound healing, acne, thirst, indigestion, nausea, vomiting. | Continue. Call doctor when convenient. |
| **Infrequent:** | |
| ● Bloody or black, tarry stool. | Discontinue. Seek emergency treatment. |
| ● Blurred vision; halos around lights; sore throat, fever; muscle cramps; swollen legs, feet. | Discontinue. Call doctor right away. |
| ● Mood changes, insomnia, restlessness, frequent urination, weight gain, round face, fatigue, weakness, TB recurrence, irregular menstrual periods. | Continue. Call doctor when convenient. |
| **Rare:** | |
| ● Irregular heartbeat. | Discontinue. Seek emergency treatment. |
| ● Rash. | Discontinue. Call doctor right away. |

## WARNINGS & PRECAUTIONS

**Don't take if:**
- You are allergic to any cortisone drug.
- You have tuberculosis or fungus infection.
- You have herpes infection of eyes, lips or genitals.

**Before you start, consult your doctor:**
- If you have had tuberculosis.
- If you have congestive heart failure.
- If you have diabetes.
- If you have peptic ulcer.
- If you have glaucoma.
- If you have underactive thyroid.
- If you have high blood pressure.
- If you have myasthenia gravis.
- If you have blood clots in legs or lungs.

**Over age 60:**
Adverse reactions and side effects may be more frequent and severe than in younger persons. Likely to aggravate edema, diabetes or ulcers. Likely to cause cataracts and osteoporosis (softening of the bones).

**Pregnancy:**
Risk to unborn child outweighs drug benefits. Don't use.

**Breast-feeding:**
Drug passes into milk. Avoid drug or discontinue nursing until you finish medicine. Consult doctor for advice on maintaining milk supply.

**Infants & children:**
Use only under medical supervision.

**Prolonged use:**
- Retards growth in children.
- Possible glaucoma, cataracts, diabetes, fragile bones and thin skin.
- Functional dependence.

**Skin & sunlight:**
No problems expected.

**Driving, piloting or hazardous work:**
No problems expected.

**Discontinuing:**
- Don't discontinue without doctor's advice until you complete prescribed dose, even though symptoms diminish or disappear.
- Drug affects your response to surgery, illness, injury or stress for 2 years after discontinuing. Tell anyone who takes medical care of you within 2 years about drug.

**Others:**
Avoid immunizations if possible.

## POSSIBLE INTERACTION WITH OTHER DRUGS

| GENERIC NAME OR DRUG CLASS | COMBINED EFFECT |
|---|---|
| Amphoterecin B | Potassium depletion. |
| Anticholinergics | Possible glaucoma. |
| Anticoagulants (oral) | Decreased anticoagulant effect. |
| Anticonvulsants (hydantoin) | Decreased dexamethasone effect. |
| Antidiabetics (oral) | Decreased antidiabetic effect. |
| Antihistamines | Decreased dexamethasone effect. |
| Aspirin | Increased dexamethasone effect. |
| Barbiturates | Decreased dexamethasone effect. Oversedation. |

| | |
|---|---|
| Beta-adrenergic blockers | Decreased dexamethasone effect. |
| Chloral hydrate | Decreased dexamethasone effect. |
| Chlorthalidone | Potassium depletion. |
| Cholinergics | Decreased cholinergic effect. |
| Contraceptives (oral) | Increased dexamethasone effect. |
| Digitalis preparations | Dangerous potassium depletion. Possible digitalis toxicity. |
| Diuretics (thiazide) | Potassium depletion. |
| Ephedrine | Decreased dexamethasone effect. |
| Estrogens | Increased dexamethasone effect. |
| Ethacrynic acid | Potassium depletion |
| Furosemide | Potassium depletion. |
| Glutethimide | Decreased dexamethasone effect. |
| Indapamide | Possible excessive potassium loss, causing dangerous heartbeat irregularity. |
| Indomethacin | Increased dexamethasone effect. |
| Insulin | Decreased insulin effect. |
| Isoniazid | Decreased isoniazid effect. |
| Oxyphenbutazone | Possible ulcers. |
| Phenylbutazone | Possible ulcers. |
| Potassium supplements | Decreased potassium effect. |

*Continued page 965*

## POSSIBLE INTERACTION WITH OTHER SUBSTANCES

| INTERACTS WITH | COMBINED EFFECT |
|---|---|
| Alcohol: | Risk of stomach ulcers. |
| Beverages: | No proven problems. |
| Cocaine: | Overstimulation. Avoid. |
| Foods: | No proven problems. |
| Marijuana: | Decreased immunity. |
| Tobacco: | Increased dexamethasone effect. Possible toxicity. |

# DEXCHLORPHENIRAMINE

## BRAND NAMES

Dexchlor      Polaramine Repetabs
Polaramine

## BASIC INFORMATION

Habit forming? No
Prescription needed? Yes
Available as generic? No
Drug class: Antihistamine

## USES

- Reduces allergic symptoms such as hay fever, hives, rash or itching.
- Induces sleep.

## DOSAGE & USAGE INFORMATION

**How to take:**
- Tablet or syrup—Swallow with liquid or food to lessen stomach irritation.
- Extended-release tablets or capsules—Swallow each dose whole. If you take regular tablets, you may chew or crush them.

**When to take:**
Varies with form. Follow label directions.

**If you forget a dose:**
Take as soon as you remember up to 2 hours late. If more than 2 hours, wait for next scheduled dose (don't double this dose).

**What drug does:**
Blocks action of histamine after an allergic response triggers histamine release in sensitive cells.

*Continued next column*

## OVERDOSE

**SYMPTOMS:**
Convulsions, red face, hallucinations, coma.
**WHAT TO DO:**
- Dial 0 (operator) or 911 (emergency) for an ambulance or medical help. Then give first aid immediately.
- If patient is unconscious and not breathing, give mouth-to-mouth breathing. If there is no heartbeat, use cardiac massage and mouth-to-mouth breathing (CPR). Don't try to make patient vomit. If you can't get help quickly, take patient to nearest emergency facility.
- See emergency information on inside covers.

**Time lapse before drug works:**
30 minutes.

**Don't take with:**
See Interaction column and consult doctor.

## POSSIBLE ADVERSE REACTIONS OR SIDE EFFECTS

| SYMPTOMS | WHAT TO DO |
|---|---|
| **Life-threatening:** None expected. | |
| **Common:** Drowsiness; dizziness; dry mouth, nose, throat; nausea. | Continue. Tell doctor at next visit. |
| **Infrequent:** | |
| • Vision changes. | Discontinue. Call doctor right away. |
| • Less tolerance for contact lenses, difficult urination. | Continue. Call doctor when convenient. |
| • Appetite loss. | Continue. Tell doctor at next visit. |
| **Rare:** Nightmares, agitation, irritability, sore throat, fever, rapid heartbeat, unusual bleeding or bruising, fatigue, weakness. | Discontinue. Call doctor right away. |

# DEXCHLORPHENIRAMINE

## WARNINGS & PRECAUTIONS

**Don't take if:**
You are allergic to any antihistamine.

**Before you start, consult your doctor:**
- If you have glaucoma.
- If you have enlarged prostate.
- If you have asthma.
- If you have kidney disease.
- If you have peptic ulcer.
- If you will have surgery within 2 months, including dental surgery, requiring general or spinal anesthesia.

**Over age 60:**
Don't exceed recommended dose. Adverse reactions and side effects may be more frequent and severe than in younger persons, especially urination difficulty, diminished alertness and other brain and nervous-system symptoms.

**Pregnancy:**
No proven harm to unborn child. Avoid if possible.

**Breast-feeding:**
Drug passes into milk. Avoid drug or discontinue nursing until you finish medicine. Consult doctor for advice on maintaining milk supply.

**Infants & children:**
Not recommended for premature or newborn infants. Otherwise, no problems expected.

**Prolonged use:**
Avoid. May damage bone marrow and nerve cells.

**Skin & sunlight:**
May cause rash or intensify sunburn in areas exposed to sun or sunlamp.

**Driving, piloting or hazardous work:**
Don't drive or pilot aircraft until you learn how medicine affects you. Don't work around dangerous machinery. Don't climb ladders or work in high places. Danger increases if you drink alcohol or take medicine affecting alertness and reflexes, such as antihistamines, tranquilizers, sedatives, pain medicine, narcotics and mind-altering drugs.

**Discontinuing:**
No problems expected.

**Others:**
May mask symptoms of hearing damage from aspirin, other salicylates, cisplatin, paromomycin, vancomycin or anticonvulsants. Consult doctor if you use these.

## POSSIBLE INTERACTION WITH OTHER DRUGS

| GENERIC NAME OR DRUG CLASS | COMBINED EFFECT |
|---|---|
| Anticholinergics | Increased anticholinergic effect. |
| Antidepressants | Excess sedation. Avoid. |
| Antihistamines (other) | Excess sedation. Avoid. |
| Dronabinol | Increased effects of both drugs. Avoid. |
| Hypnotics | Excess sedation. Avoid. |
| MAO inhibitors | Increased dexchlorpheniramine effect. |
| Mind-altering drugs | Excess sedation. Avoid. |
| Molindone | Increased antihistamine effect. |
| Narcotics | Excess sedation. Avoid. |
| Sedatives | Excess sedation. Avoid. |
| Sleep inducers | Excess sedation. Avoid. |
| Tranquilizers | Excess sedation. Avoid. |

## POSSIBLE INTERACTION WITH OTHER SUBSTANCES

| INTERACTS WITH | COMBINED EFFECT |
|---|---|
| Alcohol: | Excess sedation. Avoid. |
| Beverages: Caffeine drinks. | Decreased dexchlorpheniramine effect. |
| Cocaine: | Decreased dexchlorpheniramine effect. Avoid. |
| Foods: | None expected. |
| Marijuana: | Excess sedation. Avoid. |
| Tobacco: | None expected. |

# DEXTROAMPHETAMINE

## BRAND NAMES

| | |
|---|---|
| Amphaplex | Ferndex |
| Biphetamine | Obetrol |
| Declobese | Obotan |
| Dexampex | Oxydess II |
| Dexedrine | Spancap No. 1 |
| Eskatrol | |

## BASIC INFORMATION

**Habit forming? Yes**
**Prescription needed? Yes**
**Available as generic? Yes**
**Drug class: Central-nervous-system stimulant (amphetamine)**

 **USES**

- Prevents narcolepsy (attacks of uncontrollable sleepiness).
- Controls hyperactivity in children.

 **DOSAGE & USAGE INFORMATION**

**How to take:**
- Tablet or capsule—Swallow with liquid. If you can't swallow whole, crumble tablet or open capsule and take with liquid or food.
- Lozenges or syrups—Take as directed on label.

**When to take:**
- At the same times each day.
- Short-acting form—Don't take later than 6 hours before bedtime.
- Long-acting form—Take on awakening.

**If you forget a dose:**
- Short-acting form—Take up to 2 hours late. If more than 2 hours, wait for next dose (don't double this dose).
- Long-acting form—Take as soon as you remember. Wait 20 hours for next dose.

*Continued next column*

 **OVERDOSE**

**SYMPTOMS:**
**Rapid heartbeat, hyperactivity, high fever, hallucinations, suicidal or homicidal feelings, convulsions, coma.**
**WHAT TO DO:**
- **Dial 0 (operator) or 911 (emergency) for an ambulance or medical help. Then give first aid immediately.**
- **See emergency information on inside covers.**

**What drug does:**
- Narcolepsy—Apparently affects brain centers to decrease fatigue or sleepiness and increase alertness and motor activity.
- Hyperactive children—Calms children, opposite to effect on narcoleptic adults.

**Time lapse before drug works:**
15 to 30 minutes.

**Don't take with:**
See Interaction column and consult doctor.

 **POSSIBLE ADVERSE REACTIONS OR SIDE EFFECTS**

| SYMPTOMS | WHAT TO DO |
|---|---|
| **Life-threatening:**<br>None expected. | |
| **Common:** | |
| • Irritability, nervousness, insomnia. | Continue. Call doctor when convenient. |
| • Dry mouth. | Continue. Tell doctor at next visit. |
| **Infrequent:** | |
| • Dizziness; lack of alertness; blurred vision; fast, pounding heartbeat; unusual sweating. | Discontinue. Call doctor right away. |
| • Headache. | Continue. Call doctor when convenient. |
| • Diarrhea or constipation, appetite loss, stomach pain, nausea, vomiting, weight loss, diminished sex drive, impotence. | Continue. Tell doctor at next visit. |
| **Rare:** | |
| • Rash, hives; chest pain or irregular heartbeat; uncontrollable movements of head, neck, arms, legs. | Discontinue. Call doctor right away. |
| • Mood changes, enlarged breasts. | Continue. Call doctor when convenient. |

## WARNINGS & PRECAUTIONS

**Don't take if:**
- You are allergic to any amphetamine or central-nervous-system stimulant.
- You will have surgery within 2 months, including dental surgery, requiring general or spinal anesthesia.

**Before you start, consult your doctor:**
- If you plan to become pregnant within medication period.
- If you have glaucoma.
- If you have heart or blood-vessel disease, or high blood pressure.
- If you have overactive thyroid, anxiety or tension.
- If you have a severe mental illness (especially children).

**Over age 60:**
Adverse reactions and side effects may be more frequent and severe than in younger persons.

**Pregnancy:**
Risk to unborn child outweighs drug benefits. Don't use.

**Breast-feeding:**
Drug passes into milk. Avoid drug or discontinue nursing.

**Infants & children:**
Not recommended for children under 12.

**Prolonged use:**
Habit forming.

**Skin & sunlight:**
No problems expected.

**Driving, piloting or hazardous work:**
Don't drive or pilot aircraft until you learn how medicine affects you. Don't work around dangerous machinery. Don't climb ladders or work in high places. Danger increases if you drink alcohol or take medicine affecting alertness and reflexes.

**Discontinuing:**
May be unnecessary to finish medicine. Follow doctor's instructions.

**Others:**
- This is a dangerous drug and must be closely supervised. Don't use for appetite control or depression. Potential for damage and abuse.
- During withdrawal phase, may cause prolonged sleep of several days.

## POSSIBLE INTERACTION WITH OTHER DRUGS

| GENERIC NAME OR DRUG CLASS | COMBINED EFFECT |
| --- | --- |
| Anesthesias (general) | Irregular heartbeat. |
| Antidepressants (tricyclic) | Decreased dextroamphetamine effect. |
| Antihypertensives | Decreased antihypertensive effect. |
| Carbonic anhydrase inhibitors | Increased dextroamphetamine effect. |
| Guanethidine | Decreased guanethidine effect. |
| Haloperidol | Decreased dextroamphetamine effect. |
| MAO inhibitors | May severely increase blood pressure. |
| Phenothiazines | Decreased dextroamphetamine effect. |
| Sodium bicarbonate | Increased dextroamphetamine effect. |

## POSSIBLE INTERACTION WITH OTHER SUBSTANCES

| INTERACTS WITH | COMBINED EFFECT |
| --- | --- |
| Alcohol: | Decreased dextroamphetamine effect. Avoid. |
| Beverages: Caffeine drinks. | Overstimulation. Avoid. |
| Cocaine: | Dangerous stimulation of nervous system. Avoid. |
| Foods: | None expected. |
| Marijuana: | Frequent use—Severely impaired mental function. |
| Tobacco: | None expected. |

# DEXTROMETHORPHAN

## BRAND NAMES

See complete list of brand names in the *Brand Name Directory,* page 948.

## BASIC INFORMATION

**Habit forming? No**
**Prescription needed? No**
**Available as generic? Yes**
**Drug class: Cough suppressant**

 ## USES

Suppresses cough associated with allergies or infections such as colds, bronchitis, flu and lung disorders.

 ## DOSAGE & USAGE INFORMATION

**How to take:**
- Tablet or capsule—Swallow with liquid. If you can't swallow whole, crumble tablet or open capsule and take with liquid or food.
- Lozenges or syrups—Take as directed on label.

**When to take:**
As needed, no more often than every 3 hours.

**If you forget a dose:**
Take as soon as you remember. Wait 3 hours for next dose.

**What drug does:**
Reduces sensitivity of brain's cough-control center, suppressing urge to cough.

**Time lapse before drug works:**
15 to 30 minutes.

**Don't take with:**
See Interaction column and consult doctor.

 ## OVERDOSE

**SYMPTOMS:**
**Euphoria, overactivity, sense of intoxication, visual and auditory hallucinations, lack of coordination, stagger, stupor, shallow breathing.**
**WHAT TO DO:**
- **Dial 0 (operator) or 911 (emergency) for an ambulance or medical help. Then give first aid immediately.**
- **See emergency information on inside covers.**

 ## POSSIBLE ADVERSE REACTIONS OR SIDE EFFECTS

| SYMPTOMS | WHAT TO DO |
|---|---|
| **Life-threatening:**<br>None expected. | |
| **Common:**<br>None expected. | |
| **Infrequent:**<br>None expected. | |
| **Rare:**<br>Dizziness, drowsiness, rash, diarrhea, nausea or vomiting, stomach pain. | Discontinue. Call doctor right away. |

## WARNINGS & PRECAUTIONS

**Don't take if:**
You are allergic to any cough syrup containing dextromethorphan.

**Before you start, consult your doctor:**
- If you have asthma attacks.
- If you have impaired liver function.

**Over age 60:**
May become constipated, excessively drowsy or unsteady. If drug is used for cough, other treatment may be necessary to liquefy thick mucus in bronchial tubes.

**Pregnancy:**
No proven harm to unborn child. Avoid if possible.

**Breast-feeding:**
No proven problems. Consult doctor.

**Infants & children:**
Use only as label directs.

**Prolonged use:**
No problems expected.

**Skin & sunlight:**
No problems expected.

**Driving, piloting or hazardous work:**
Don't drive or pilot aircraft until you learn how medicine affects you. Don't work around dangerous machinery. Don't climb ladders or work in high places. Danger increases if you drink alcohol or take medicine affecting alertness and reflexes, such as antihistamines, tranquilizers, sedatives, pain medicine, narcotics and mind-altering drugs.

**Discontinuing:**
May be unnecessary to finish medicine. Follow doctor's instructions.

**Others:**
- If cough persists or if you cough blood or brown-yellow, thick mucus, call your doctor.
- Excessive use may lead to functional dependence.

## POSSIBLE INTERACTION WITH OTHER DRUGS

| GENERIC NAME OR DRUG CLASS | COMBINED EFFECT |
|---|---|
| MAO inhibitors | Disorientation, high fever, drop in blood pressure and loss of consciousness. |

## POSSIBLE INTERACTION WITH OTHER SUBSTANCES

| INTERACTS WITH | COMBINED EFFECT |
|---|---|
| Alcohol: | None expected. |
| Beverages: | None expected. |
| Cocaine: | Decreased dextromethorphan effect. Avoid |
| Foods: | None expected. |
| Marijuana: | None expected. |
| Tobacco: | None expected. |

# DIAZEPAM

## BRAND NAMES

| | |
|---|---|
| Apo-Diazepam | Rival |
| D-Tran | Serenack |
| E-Pam | Stress-Pam |
| Meval | Valium |
| Neo-Calme | Valrelease |
| Novodipam | Vivol |
| Q-Pam | |

## BASIC INFORMATION

**Habit forming? Yes**
**Prescription needed? Yes**
**Available as generic? Yes**
**Drug class: Tranquilizer (benzodiazepine)**

 ## USES

- Treatment for nervousness or tension.
- Treatment for muscle spasm.
- Treatment for convulsive disorders.

 ## DOSAGE & USAGE INFORMATION

**How to take:**
Tablet or capsule—Swallow with liquid. If you can't swallow whole, crumble tablet or open capsule and take with liquid or food.

**When to take:**
At the same time each day, according to instructions on prescription label.

**If you forget a dose:**
Take as soon as you remember up to 2 hours late. If more than 2 hours, wait for next scheduled dose (don't double this dose).

*Continued next column*

 ## OVERDOSE

**SYMPTOMS:**
**Drowsiness, weakness, tremor, stupor, coma.**
**WHAT TO DO:**
- **Dial 0 (operator) or 911 (emergency) for an ambulance or medical help. Then give first aid immediately.**
- **If patient is unconscious and not breathing, give mouth-to-mouth breathing. If there is no heartbeat, use cardiac massage and mouth-to-mouth breathing (CPR). Don't try to make patient vomit. If you can't get help quickly, take patient to nearest emergency facility.**
- **See emergency information on inside covers.**

**What drug does:**
Affects limbic system of brain—part that controls emotions.

**Time lapse before drug works:**
2 hours. May take 6 weeks for full benefit.

**Don't take with:**
See Interaction column and consult doctor.

 ## POSSIBLE ADVERSE REACTIONS OR SIDE EFFECTS

| SYMPTOMS | WHAT TO DO |
|---|---|
| **Life-threatening:**<br>None expected. | |
| **Common:**<br>Clumsiness, drowsiness, dizziness. | Continue. Call doctor when convenient. |
| **Infrequent:**<br>• Hallucinations, confusion, depression, irritability, rash, itch, vision changes. | Discontinue. Call doctor right away. |
| • Constipation or diarrhea, nausea, vomiting, difficult urination. | Continue. Call doctor when convenient. |
| **Rare:**<br>• Slow heartbeat, breathing difficulty. | Discontinue. Seek emergency treatment. |
| • Mouth, throat ulcers; jaundice. | Discontinue. Call doctor right away. |

276

## WARNINGS & PRECAUTIONS

**Don't take if:**
- You are allergic to any benzodiazepine.
- You have myasthenia gravis.
- You are active or recovering alcoholic.
- Patient is younger than 6 months.

**Before you start, consult your doctor:**
- If you have liver, kidney or lung disease.
- If you have diabetes, epilepsy or porphyria.

**Over age 60:**
Adverse reactions and side effects may be more frequent and severe than in younger persons. You need smaller doses for shorter periods of time. May develop agitation, rage or "hangover" effect.

**Pregnancy:**
Risk to unborn child outweighs drug benefits. Don't use.

**Breast-feeding:**
Drug passes into milk. Avoid drug or discontinue nursing until you finish medicine. Consult doctor for advice on maintaining milk supply.

**Infants & children:**
Use only under medical supervision for children older than 6 months.

**Prolonged use:**
May impair liver function.

**Skin & sunlight:**
No problems expected.

**Driving, piloting or hazardous work:**
Don't drive or pilot aircraft until you learn how medicine affects you. Don't work around dangerous machinery. Don't climb ladders or work in high places. Danger increases if you drink alcohol or take medicine affecting alertness and reflexes.

**Discontinuing:**
Don't discontinue without consulting doctor. Dose may require gradual reduction if you have taken drug for a long time. Doses of other drugs may also require adjustment.

**Others:**
- Hot weather, heavy exercise and profuse sweat may reduce excretion and cause overdose.
- Blood sugar may rise in diabetics, requiring insulin adjustment.

## POSSIBLE INTERACTION WITH OTHER DRUGS

| GENERIC NAME OR DRUG CLASS | COMBINED EFFECT |
|---|---|
| Anticonvulsants | Change in seizure frequency or severity. |
| Antidepressants | Increased sedative effect of both drugs. |
| Antihistamines | Increased sedative effect of both drugs. |
| Antihypertensives | Excessively low blood pressure. |
| Cimetidine | Excess sedation. |
| Disulfiram | Increased diazepam effect. |
| Dronabinol | Increased effects of both drugs. Avoid. |
| MAO inhibitors | Convulsions, deep sedation, rage. |
| Molindone | Increased tranquilizer effect. |
| Narcotics | Increased sedative effect of both drugs. |
| Sedatives | Increased sedative effect of both drugs. |
| Sleep inducers | Increased sedative effect of both drugs. |
| Tranquilizers | Increased sedative effect of both drugs. |

## POSSIBLE INTERACTION WITH OTHER SUBSTANCES

| INTERACTS WITH | COMBINED EFFECT |
|---|---|
| Alcohol: | Heavy sedation. Avoid. |
| Beverages: | None expected. |
| Cocaine: | Decreased diazepam effect. |
| Foods: | None expected. |
| Marijuana: | Heavy sedation. Avoid. |
| Tobacco: | Decreased diazepam effect. |

# DICLOXACILLIN

## BRAND NAMES

Dycill             Pathocil
Dynapen

## BASIC INFORMATION

**Habit forming? No**
**Prescription needed? Yes**
**Available as generic? Yes**
**Drug class: Antibiotic (penicillin)**

## USES

Treatment of bacterial infections that are susceptible to dicloxacillin.

## DOSAGE & USAGE INFORMATION

**How to take:**
- Tablets or capsules—Swallow with liquid on an empty stomach 1 hour before or 2 hours after eating.
- Liquid—Take with cold beverage. Liquid form is perishable and effective for only 7 days at room temperature. Effective for 14 days if stored in refrigerator. Don't freeze.

**When to take:**
Follow instructions on prescription label or side of package. Doses should be evenly spaced. For example, 4 times a day means every 6 hours.

**If you forget a dose:**
Take as soon as you remember. Continue regular schedule.

**What drug does:**
Destroys susceptible bacteria. Does not kill viruses.

**Time lapse before drug works:**
May be several days before medicine affects infection.

**Don't take with:**
See Interaction column and consult doctor.

## OVERDOSE

**SYMPTOMS:**
Severe diarrhea, nausea or vomiting.
**WHAT TO DO:**
Overdose unlikely to threaten life. If person takes much larger amount than prescribed, call doctor, poison-control center or hospital emergency room for instructions.

## POSSIBLE ADVERSE REACTIONS OR SIDE EFFECTS

| SYMPTOMS | WHAT TO DO |
|---|---|
| **Life-threatening:** Hives, rash, intense itching, faintness soon after a dose (anaphylaxis). | Seek emergency treatment immediately. |
| **Common:** Dark or discolored tongue. | Continue. Tell doctor at next visit. |
| **Infrequent:** Mild nausea, vomiting, diarrhea. | Continue. Call doctor when convenient. |
| **Rare:** Unexplained bleeding. | Discontinue. Call doctor right away. |

## WARNINGS & PRECAUTIONS

**Don't take if:**
You are allergic to dicloxacillin, cephalosporin antibiotics, other penicillins or penicillamine. Life-threatening reaction may occur.

**Before you start, consult your doctor:**
If you are allergic to any substance or drug.

**Over age 60:**
You may have skin reactions, particularly around genitals and anus.

**Pregnancy:**
Studies inconclusive on harm to unborn child. Animal studies show fetal abnormalities. Decide with your doctor whether drug benefits justify risk to unborn child.

**Breast-feeding:**
Drug passes into milk. Child may become sensitive to penicillins and have allergic reactions to penicillin drugs. Avoid dicloxacillin or discontinue nursing until you finish medicine. Consult doctor for advice on maintaining milk supply.

**Infants & children:**
No problems expected.

**Prolonged use:**
You may become more susceptible to infections caused by germs not responsive to dicloxacillin.

**Skin & sunlight:**
No problems expected.

**Driving, piloting or hazardous work:**
Usually not dangerous. Most hazardous reactions likely to occur a few minutes after taking dicloxacillin.

**Discontinuing:**
Don't discontinue without doctor's advice until you complete prescribed dose, even though symptoms diminish or disappear.

**Others:**
No problems expected.

## POSSIBLE INTERACTION WITH OTHER DRUGS

| GENERIC NAME OR DRUG CLASS | COMBINED EFFECT |
|---|---|
| Beta-adrenergic blockers | Increased chance of anaphylaxis (see emergency information on inside front cover). |
| Chloramphenicol | Decreased effect of both drugs. |
| Erythromycins | Decreased effect of both drugs. |
| Loperamide | Decreased dicloxacillin effect. |
| Paromomycin | Decreased effect of both drugs. |
| Tetracyclines | Decreased effect of both drugs. |
| Troleandomycin | Decreased effect of both drugs. |

## POSSIBLE INTERACTION WITH OTHER SUBSTANCES

| INTERACTS WITH | COMBINED EFFECT |
|---|---|
| Alcohol: | Occasional stomach irritation. |
| Beverages: | None expected. |
| Cocaine: | No proven problems. |
| Foods: | None expected. |
| Marijuana: | No proven problems. |
| Tobacco: | None expected. |

# DICYCLOMINE

## BRAND NAMES

See complete list of brand names in the *Brand Name Directory,* page 948.

## BASIC INFORMATION

**Habit forming? No**
**Prescription needed?**
  **Low strength: No**
  **High strength: Yes**
**Available as generic? Yes**
**Drug class: Antispasmodic, anticholinergic**

## USES

Reduces spasms of digestive system, bladder and urethra.

## DOSAGE & USAGE INFORMATION

**How to take:**
- Tablet, syrup or capsule—Swallow with liquid or food to lessen stomach irritation.
- Drops—Dilute dose in beverage before swallowing.

**When to take:**
30 minutes before meals (unless directed otherwise by doctor).

**If you forget a dose:**
Take as soon as you remember up to 2 hours late. If more than 2 hours, wait for next scheduled dose (don't double this dose).

**What drug does:**
Blocks nerve impulses at parasympathetic nerve endings, preventing muscle contractions and gland secretions of organs involved.

**Time lapse before drug works:**
15 to 30 minutes.

**Don't take with:**
See Interaction column and consult doctor.

## OVERDOSE

**SYMPTOMS:**
**Dilated pupils, rapid pulse and breathing, dizziness, fever, hallucinations, confusion, slurred speech, agitation, flushed face, convulsions, coma.**
**WHAT TO DO:**
- **Dial 0 (operator) or 911 (emergency) for an ambulance or medical help. Then give first aid immediately.**
- **See emergency information on inside covers.**

## POSSIBLE ADVERSE REACTIONS OR SIDE EFFECTS

| SYMPTOMS | WHAT TO DO |
|---|---|
| **Life-threatening:** | |
| None expected. | |
| **Common:** | |
| • Confusion, delirium, rapid heartbeat. | Discontinue. Call doctor right away. |
| • Nausea, vomiting, decreased sweating. | Continue. Call doctor when convenient. |
| • Constipation. | Continue. Tell doctor at next visit. |
| • Dry ears, nose, throat. | No action necessary. |
| **Infrequent:** | |
| Headache, difficult urination. | Continue. Call doctor when convenient. |
| **Rare:** | |
| Rash or hives, pain, blurred vision. | Discontinue. Call doctor right away. |

## WARNINGS & PRECAUTIONS

**Don't take if:**
- You are allergic to any anticholinergic.
- You have trouble with stomach bloating.
- You have difficulty emptying your bladder completely.
- You have narrow-angle glaucoma.
- You have severe ulcerative colitis.

**Before you start, consult your doctor:**
- If you have open-angle glaucoma.
- If you have angina.
- If you have chronic bronchitis or asthma.
- If you have hiatal hernia.
- If you have liver disease.
- If you have enlarged prostate.
- If you have myasthenia gravis.
- If you have peptic ulcer.
- If you will have surgery within 2 months, including dental surgery, requiring general or spinal anesthesia.

**Over age 60:**
Adverse reactions and side effects may be more frequent and severe than in younger persons.

**Pregnancy:**
Studies inconclusive on harm to unborn child. Animal studies show fetal abnormalities. Decide with your doctor whether drug benefits justify risk to unborn child.

**Breast-feeding:**
Drug passes into milk and decreases milk flow. Avoid drug or discontinue nursing until you finish medicine. Consult doctor for advice on maintaining milk supply.

**Infants & children:**
Use only under medical supervision.

**Prolonged use:**
Chronic constipation, possible fecal impaction.
Consult doctor immediately.

**Skin & sunlight:**
No problems expected.

**Driving, piloting or hazardous work:**
Use disqualifies you for piloting aircraft.
Otherwise, no problems expected.

**Discontinuing:**
May be unnecessary to finish medicine. Follow
doctor's instructions.

**Others:**
No problems expected.

## POSSIBLE INTERACTION WITH OTHER DRUGS

| GENERIC NAME OR DRUG CLASS | COMBINED EFFECT |
|---|---|
| Amantadine | Increased dicyclomine effect. |
| Anticholinergics (other) | Increased dicyclomine effect. |
| Antidepressants (tricyclic) | Increased dicyclomine effect. Increased sedation. |
| Antihistamines | Increased dicyclomine effect. |
| Cortisone drugs | Increased internal-eye pressure. |
| Haloperidol | Increased internal-eye pressure. |
| MAO inhibitors | Increased dicyclomine effect. |
| Meperidine | Increased dicyclomine effect. |
| Methylphenidate | Increased dicyclomine effect. |
| Nitrates | Increased internal-eye pressure. |
| Orphenadrine | Increased dicyclomine effect. |
| Phenothiazines | Increased dicyclomine effect. |
| Pilocarpine | Loss of pilocarpine effect in glaucoma treatment. |

| | |
|---|---|
| Potassium supplements | Possible intestinal ulcers with oral potassium tablets. |
| Vitamin C | Decreased dicyclomine effect. Avoid large doses of vitamin C. |

## POSSIBLE INTERACTION WITH OTHER SUBSTANCES

| INTERACTS WITH | COMBINED EFFECT |
|---|---|
| Alcohol: | None expected. |
| Beverages: | None expected. |
| Cocaine: | Excessively rapid heartbeat. Avoid. |
| Foods: | None expected. |
| Marijuana: | Drowsiness and dry mouth. |
| Tobacco: | None expected. |

# DIETHYLSTILBESTROL

## BRAND NAMES

DES                Stilphostrol
Honvol             Stilbilium
Stilbestrol

## BASIC INFORMATION

Habit forming? No
Prescription needed? Yes
Available as generic? Yes
Drug class: Female sex hormone (estrogen)

## USES

- Treatment for symptoms of menopause and menstrual-cycle irregularity.
- Replacement for female hormone deficiency.
- Treatment for cancer of prostate and breast.

## DOSAGE & USAGE INFORMATION

**How to take:**
- Tablet—Swallow with liquid. If you can't swallow whole, crumble tablet and take with liquid or food.
- Vaginal suppositories—Use as directed on label.

**When to take:**
At the same time each day.

**If you forget a dose:**
Take as soon as you remember up to 12 hours late. If more than 12 hours, wait for next scheduled dose (don't double this dose).

**What drug does:**
Restores normal estrogen level in tissues.

**Time lapse before drug works:**
10 to 20 days.

**Don't take with:**
See Interaction column and consult doctor.

## OVERDOSE

**SYMPTOMS:**
Nausea, vomiting, fluid retention, breast enlargement and discomfort, abnormal vaginal bleeding.
**WHAT TO DO:**
Overdose unlikely to threaten life. If person takes much larger amount than prescribed, call doctor, poison-control center or hospital emergency room for instructions.

## POSSIBLE ADVERSE REACTIONS OR SIDE EFFECTS

| SYMPTOMS | WHAT TO DO |
|---|---|
| **Life-threatening:** None expected. | |
| **Common:** | |
| • Stomach cramps. | Discontinue. Call doctor right away. |
| • Appetite loss. | Continue. Call doctor when convenient. |
| • Nausea; diarrhea; swollen ankles and feet; tender, swollen breasts. | Continue. Tell doctor at next visit. |
| **Infrequent:** | |
| • Rash, stomach or side pain. | Discontinue. Call doctor right away. |
| • Depression, dizziness, irritability, vomiting, breast lumps. | Continue. Call doctor when convenient. |
| • Brown blotches, hair loss, vaginal discharge or bleeding, changes in sex drive. | Continue. Tell doctor at next visit. |
| **Rare:** | |
| Jaundice. | Discontinue. Call doctor right away. |

## WARNINGS & PRECAUTIONS

**Don't take if:**
- You are allergic to any estrogen-containing drugs.
- You have impaired liver function.
- You have had blood clots, stroke or heart attack.
- You have unexplained vaginal bleeding.

**Before you start, consult your doctor:**
- If you have had cancer of breast or reproductive organs, fibrocystic breast disease, fibroid tumors of the uterus or endometriosis.
- If you have had migraine headaches, epilepsy or porphyria.
- If you have diabetes, high blood pressure, asthma, congestive heart failure, kidney disease or gallstones.
- If you plan to become pregnant within 3 months.

**Over age 60:**
Controversial. You and your doctor must decide if drug risks outweigh benefits.

**Pregnancy:**
Risk to unborn child outweighs drug benefits. Don't use.

**Breast-feeding:**
Drug filters into milk. May harm child. Avoid.

**Infants & children:**
Not recommended.

**Prolonged use:**
Increased growth of fibroid tumors of uterus. Possible association with cancer of uterus.

**Skin & sunlight:**
May cause rash or intensify sunburn in areas exposed to sun or sunlamp.

**Driving, piloting or hazardous work:**
No problems expected.

**Discontinuing:**
You may need to discontinue diethylstilbestrol periodically. Consult your doctor.

**Others:**
In rare instances, may cause blood clot in lung, brain or leg. Symptoms are *sudden* severe headache, coordination loss, vision change, chest pain, breathing difficulty, slurred speech, pain in legs or groin. Seek emergency treatment immediately.

## POSSIBLE INTERACTION WITH OTHER DRUGS

| GENERIC NAME OR DRUG CLASS | COMBINED EFFECT |
|---|---|
| Anticoagulants (oral) | Decreased anticoagulant effect. |
| Anticonvulsants (hydantoin) | Increased seizures. |
| Antidiabetics (oral) | Unpredictable increase or decrease in blood sugar. |
| Carbamazepine | Increased seizures. |
| Clofibrate | Decreased clofibrate effect. |
| Meprobamate | Increased diethylstilbestrol effect. |
| Phenobarbital | Decreased diethylstilbestrol effect. |
| Primidone | Decreased diethylstilbestrol effect. |
| Rifampin | Decreased diethylstilbestrol effect. |
| Thyroid hormones | Decreased thyroid effect. |

## POSSIBLE INTERACTION WITH OTHER SUBSTANCES

| INTERACTS WITH | COMBINED EFFECT |
|---|---|
| Alcohol: | None expected. |
| Beverages: | None expected. |
| Cocaine: | No proven problems. |
| Foods: | None expected. |
| Marijuana: | Possible menstrual irregularities and bleeding between periods. |
| Tobacco: | Increased risk of blood clots leading to stroke or heart attack. |

# DIFENOXIN & ATROPINE

## BRAND NAMES

Motofen

## BASIC INFORMATION

**Habit forming?** No
**Prescription needed?** Yes
**Available as generic?** No
**Drug class:** Antidiarrheal

 **USES**

- Reduces spasms of digestive system.
- Treats severe diarrhea.

 **DOSAGE & USAGE INFORMATION**

**How to take:**
Tablet—Swallow with liquid or food to lessen stomach irritation.

**When to take:**
After each loose stool or every 3 to 4 hours. No more than 5 tablets in 12 hours.

**If you forget a dose:**
Take as soon as you remember. Don't double this dose.

**What drug does:**
- Blocks nerve impulses at parasympathetic nerve endings, preventing muscle contractions and gland secretions of organs involved.
- Acts on brain to decrease spasm of smooth muscle.

**Time lapse before drug works:**
40 to 60 minutes.

*Continued next column*

 **OVERDOSE**

**SYMPTOMS:**
**Dilated pupils, rapid pulse and breathing, dizziness, fever, hallucinations, confusion, slurred speech, agitation, flushed face, convulsions, coma.**
**WHAT TO DO:**
- **Dial 0 (operator) or 911 (emergency) for an ambulance or medical help. Then give first aid immediately.**
- **See emergency information on inside covers.**

**Don't take with:**
- Any medicine that will decrease mental alertness or reflexes, such as alcohol, other mind-altering drugs, cough/cold medicines, antihistamines, allergy medicine, sedatives, tranquilizers (sleeping pills or "downers") barbiturates, seizure medicine, narcotics, other prescription medicine for pain, muscle relaxants, anesthetics.
- See Interaction column and consult doctor.

 **POSSIBLE ADVERSE REACTIONS OR SIDE EFFECTS**

| SYMPTOMS | WHAT TO DO |
|---|---|
| **Life-threatening:** | |
| Shortness of breath, agitation, nervousness. | Discontinue. Seek emergency treatment. |
| **Common:** | |
| Dizziness, drowsiness. | Continue. Call doctor when convenient. |
| **Infrequent:** | |
| • Bloating; constipation; appetite loss; abdominal pain; blurred vision; warm, flushed skin; fast heartbeat; dry mouth. | Discontinue. Call doctor right away. |
| • Frequent urination, lightheadedness, dry skin, headache, insomnia. | Continue. Call doctor when convenient. |
| **Rare:** | |
| Weakness, confusion, fever. | Continue. Call doctor when convenient. |

 **WARNINGS & PRECAUTIONS**

**Don't take if:**
- You are allergic to any anticholinergic.
- You have trouble with stomach bloating, difficulty emptying your bladder completely, narrow-angle glaucoma, severe ulcerative colitis.
- You are dehydrated.

**Before you start, consult your doctor:**
- If you have open-angle glaucoma, angina, chronic bronchitis, asthma, liver disease, hiatal hernia, enlarged prostate, myasthenia gravis, peptic ulcer.
- If you will have surgery within 2 months, including dental surgery, requiring general or spinal anesthesia.

**Over age 60:**
Adverse reactions and side effects may be more frequent and severe than in younger persons.

**Pregnancy:**
Studies inconclusive on harm to unborn child. Animal studies show fetal abnormalities. Decide with your doctor whether drug benefits justify risk to unborn child.

**Breast-feeding:**
Drug passes into milk. Avoid drug or discontinue nursing until you finish medicine. Consult doctor for advice on maintaining milk supply.

**Infants & children:**
Use only under medical supervision.

**Prolonged use:**
Chronic constipation, possible fecal impaction. Consult doctor immediately.

**Skin & sunlight:**
No problems expected.

**Driving, piloting or hazardous work:**
Use disqualifies you for piloting aircraft. Otherwise, no problems expected.

**Discontinuing:**
May be unnecessary to finish medicine. Follow doctor's instructions.

**Others:**
Atropine included at doses below therapeutic level to prevent abuse.

## POSSIBLE INTERACTION WITH OTHER DRUGS

| GENERIC NAME OR DRUG CLASS | COMBINED EFFECT |
|---|---|
| Addictive substances (narcotics, others) | Increased chance of abuse. |
| Amantadine | Increased atropine effect. |
| Anticholinergics (other) | Increased atropine effect. |
| Antidepressants (tricyclic, see Glossary) | Increased atropine effect. Increased sedation. |
| Antihistamines | Increased atropine effect. |
| Antihypertensive medicines | Increased sedation. |
| Cortisone drugs | Increased internal-eye pressure. |
| Haloperidol | Increased internal-eye pressure. |
| MAO inhibitors | Increased atropine effect. |
| Meperidine | Increased atropine effect. |
| Methylphenidate | Increased atropine effect. |
| Nitrates | Increased internal-eye pressure. |
| Orphenadrine | Increased atropine effect. |
| Phenothiazines | Increased atropine effect. |
| Pilocarpine | Loss of pilocarpine effect in glaucoma treatment. |
| Potassium supplements | Possible intestinal ulcers with oral potassium tablets. |
| Procainamide | Increased atropine effect. |
| Vitamin C | Decreased atropine effect. Avoid large doses of vitamin C. |

## POSSIBLE INTERACTION WITH OTHER SUBSTANCES

| INTERACTS WITH | COMBINED EFFECT |
|---|---|
| Alcohol: | Increased sedation Avoid. |
| Beverages: | None expected. |
| Cocaine: | Excessively rapid heartbeat. Avoid. |
| Foods: | None expected. |
| Marijuana: | Drowsiness and dry mouth. |
| Tobacco: | May increase diarrhea. Avoid. |

# DIFLUNISAL

## BRAND NAMES

Dolobid

## BASIC INFORMATION

**Habit forming? No**
**Prescription needed? Yes**
**Available as generic? Yes**
**Drug class: Anti-inflammatory (non-steroid)**

## USES

- Treatment for joint pain, stiffness, inflammation and swelling of arthritis and gout.
- Pain reliever.

## DOSAGE & USAGE INFORMATION

**How to take:**
Tablet or capsule—Swallow with liquid or food to lessen stomach irritation. If you can't swallow whole, crumble tablet or open capsule and take with liquid or food.

**When to take:**
At the same times each day.

**If you forget a dose:**
Take as soon as you remember up to 2 hours late. If more than 2 hours, wait for next scheduled dose (don't double this dose).

**What drug does:**
Reduces tissue concentration of prostaglandins (hormones which produce inflammation and pain).

**Time lapse before drug works:**
Begins in 4 to 24 hours. May require 3 weeks regular use for maximum benefit.

**Don't take with:**
See Interaction column and consult doctor.

## OVERDOSE

**SYMPTOMS:**
Confusion, agitation, incoherence, convulsions, possible hemorrhage from stomach or intestine, coma.
**WHAT TO DO:**
- Dial 0 (operator) or 911 (emergency) for an ambulance or medical help. Then give first aid immediately.
- See emergency information on inside covers.

## POSSIBLE ADVERSE REACTIONS OR SIDE EFFECTS

| SYMPTOMS | WHAT TO DO |
|---|---|
| **Life-threatening:** None expected. | |
| **Common:** | |
| • Dizziness, nausea, pain. | Continue. Call doctor when convenient. |
| • Headache. | Continue. Tell doctor at next visit. |
| **Infrequent:** Depression; drowsiness; ringing in ears; constipation or diarrhea; vomiting; swollen feet, legs. | Continue. Call doctor when convenient. |
| **Rare:** | |
| • Convulsions; confusion; rash, hives, or itch; blurred vision; bloody or black, tarry stools; difficult breathing; tightness in chest; rapid heartbeat; unusual bleeding or bruising; blood in urine; jaundice. | Discontinue. Call doctor right away. |
| • Urgent, frequent, painful or difficult urination; fatigue; weakness. | Continue. Call doctor when convenient. |

## WARNINGS & PRECAUTIONS

### Don't take if:
- You are allergic to aspirin or any non-steroid, anti-inflammatory drug.
- You have gastritis, peptic ulcer, enteritis, ileitis, ulcerative colitis, asthma, heart failure, high blood pressure or bleeding problems.
- Patient is younger than 15.

### Before you start, consult your doctor:
- If you have epilepsy.
- If you have Parkinson's disease.
- If you have been mentally ill.
- If you have had kidney disease or impaired kidney function.

### Over age 60:
Adverse reactions and side effects may be more frequent and severe than in younger persons.

### Pregnancy:
Studies inconclusive on harm to unborn child. Animal studies show fetal abnormalities. Decide with your doctor whether drug benefits justify risk to unborn child.

### Breast-feeding:
May harm child. Avoid.

### Infants & children:
Not recommended for anyone younger than 15. Use only under medical supervision.

### Prolonged use:
- Eye damage.
- Reduced hearing.
- Sore throat, fever.
- Weight gain.

### Skin & sunlight:
No problems expected.

### Driving, piloting or hazardous work:
Don't drive or pilot aircraft until you learn how medicine affects you. Don't work around dangerous machinery. Don't climb ladders or work in high places. Danger increases if you drink alcohol or take medicine affecting alertness and reflexes, such as antihistamines, tranquilizers, sedatives, pain medicine, narcotics and mind-altering drugs.

### Discontinuing:
Don't discontinue without consulting doctor. Dose may require gradual reduction if you have taken drug for a long time. Doses of other drugs may also require adjustment.

### Others:
No problems expected.

## POSSIBLE INTERACTION WITH OTHER DRUGS

| GENERIC NAME OR DRUG CLASS | COMBINED EFFECT |
|---|---|
| Acebutolol | Decreased antihypertensive effect of acebutolol. |
| Antacids | Decreased diflunisal effect. |
| Anticoagulants (oral) | Decreased effect of anticoagulant. |
| Aspirin, other anti-inflammatory drugs | Increased risk of stomach ulcer. |
| Cortisone drugs | Increased risk of stomach ulcer. |
| Furosemide | Decreased diuretic effect of furosemide. |
| Gold compounds | Possible increased likelihood of kidney damage. |
| Hydrochlorothiazide | Increased risk of severe blood-pressure drop. |
| Indomethacin | Increased possibility of intestinal hemorrhage. |
| Minoxidil | Decreased minoxidil effect. |
| Oxyphenbutazone | Possible stomach ulcer. |
| Oxprenolol | Decreased antihypertensive effect of oxprenolol. |
| Phenylbutazone | Possible stomach ulcer. |
| Probenecid | Increased diflunisal effect. |
| Thyroid hormones | Rapid heartbeat. Blood-pressure rise. |

## POSSIBLE INTERACTION WITH OTHER SUBSTANCES

| INTERACTS WITH | COMBINED EFFECT |
|---|---|
| Alcohol: | Possible stomach ulcer or bleeding. |
| Beverages: | None expected. |
| Cocaine: | Increased cocaine toxicity. Avoid. |
| Foods: | None expected. |
| Marijuana: | Increased pain relief from diflunisal. |
| Tobacco: | Decreased absorption of diflunisal. Avoid. |

# DIGITALIS PREPARATIONS

## BRAND AND GENERIC NAMES

Crystodigin
Crystogin
Digifortis
Digiglusin
DIGITALIS
DIGITOXIN
DIGOXIN

Gitaligen
GITALIN
Lanoxicaps
Lanoxin
Natigozine
Novodigoxin
Purodigin

## BASIC INFORMATION

Habit forming? No
prescription needed? Yes
Available as generic? Yes
Drug class: Digitalis preparations

## USES

- Strengthens weak heart-muscle contractions to prevent congestive heart failure.
- Corrects irregular heartbeat.

## DOSAGE & USAGE INFORMATION

**How to take:**
- Tablet or capsule—Swallow with liquid. If you can't swallow whole, crumble tablet or open capsule and take with liquid or food.
- Liquid—Dilute dose in beverage before swallowing.

**When to take:**
At the same time each day.

**If you forget a dose:**
Take as soon as you remember up to 12 hours late. If more than 12 hours, wait for next scheduled dose (don't double this dose).

**What drug does:**
- Strengthens heart-muscle contraction.
- Delays nerve impulses to heart.

*Continued next column*

## OVERDOSE

**SYMPTOMS:**
Nausea, vomiting, diarrhea, vision disturbances with halos around lights, irregular heartbeat, confusion, hallucinations, convulsions.
**WHAT TO DO:**
- Dial 0 (operator) or 911 (emergency) for an ambulance or medical help. Then give first aid immediately.
- See emergency information on inside covers.

**Time lapse before drug works:**
May require regular use for a week or more.

**Don't take with:**
- Non-prescription drugs without consulting doctor.
- See Interaction column and consult doctor.

## POSSIBLE ADVERSE REACTIONS OR SIDE EFFECTS

| SYMPTOMS | WHAT TO DO |
|---|---|
| **Life-threatening:**<br>None expected. | |
| **Common:**<br>Appetite loss, diarrhea. | Continue. Call doctor when convenient. |
| **Infrequent:**<br>Drowsiness, lethargy, disorientation. | Discontinue. Call doctor right away. |
| **Rare:**<br>• Rash, hives. | Discontinue. Call doctor right away. |
| • Double or yellow-green vision; enlarged, sensitive male breasts; tiredness; weakness. | Continue. Call doctor when convenient. |

## WARNINGS & PRECAUTIONS

**Don't take if:**
- You are allergic to any digitalis preparation.
- Your heartbeat is slower than 50 beats per minute.

**Before you start, consult your doctor:**
- If you have taken another digitalis preparation in past 2 weeks.
- If you have taken a diuretic within 2 weeks.
- If you have liver or kidney disease.
- If you have a thyroid disorder.
- If you will have surgery within 2 months, including dental surgery, requiring general or spinal anesthesia.

**Over age 60:**
Adverse reactions and side effects may be more frequent and severe than in younger persons.

**Pregnancy:**
Studies inconclusive on harm to unborn child. Consult your doctor.

**Breast-feeding:**
Drug filters into milk. May harm child. Avoid.

**Infants & children:**
Use only under medical supervision.

**Prolonged use:**
No problems expected.

**Skin & sunlight:**
No problems expected.

**Driving, piloting or hazardous work:**
Possible vision disturbances. Otherwise, no problems expected.

**Discontinuing:**
Don't stop without doctor's advice.

**Others:**
No problems expected.

## POSSIBLE INTERACTION WITH OTHER DRUGS

| GENERIC NAME OR DRUG CLASS | COMBINED EFFECT |
| --- | --- |
| Albuterol | Increased risk of heartbeat irregularity. |
| Amiodarone | Increased digitalis effect. |
| Antacids | Decreased digitalis effect. |
| Anticonvulsants (hydantoin) | Increased digitalis effect at first, then decreased. |
| Beta-adrenergic blockers | Increased digitalis effect. |
| Calcium supplements | Decreased digitalis effects. |
| Cortisone drugs | Digitalis toxicity. |
| Diuretics | Possible digitalis toxicity. |
| Ephedrine | Disturbed heart rhythm. Avoid. |
| Epinephrine | Disturbed heart rhythm. Avoid. |
| Flecainide | May increase digitalis blood level. |
| Guanethidine | Increased digitalis effect. |
| Indapamide | Excessive potassium loss that may cause irregular heartbeat. |
| Laxatives | Decreased digitalis effect. |
| Oxyphenbutazone | Decreased digitalis effect. |
| Phenobarbital | Decreased digitalis effect. |
| Phenylbutazone | Decreased digitalis effect. |
| Potassium supplements | Overdosage of either drug may cause severe heartbeat irregularity. |
| Quinidine | Increased digitalis effect. |
| Rauwolfia alkaloids | Increased digitalis effect. |
| Thyroid hormones | Digitalis toxicity. |

## POSSIBLE INTERACTION WITH OTHER SUBSTANCES

| INTERACTS WITH | COMBINED EFFECT |
| --- | --- |
| Alcohol: | None expected. |
| Beverages: Caffeine drinks. | Irregular heartbeat. Avoid. |
| Cocaine: | Irregular heartbeat. Avoid. |
| Foods: | None expected. |
| Marijuana: | Decreased digitalis effect. |
| Tobacco: | Irregular heartbeat. Avoid. |

# DILTIAZEM

## BRAND NAMES

Cardizem

## BASIC INFORMATION

**Habit forming? No**
**Prescription needed? Yes**
**Available as generic? No**
**Drug class: Calcium-channel blocker,**
                **antiarrhythmic, antianginal**

 ## USES

- Prevents angina attacks.
- Stabilizes irregular heartbeat.

 ## DOSAGE & USAGE INFORMATION

**How to take:**
Tablet or capsule—Swallow with liquid.

**When to take:**
At the same times each day 1 hour before or 2 hours after eating.

**If you forget a dose:**
Take as soon as you remember up to 2 hours late. If more than 2 hours, wait for next scheduled dose (don't double this dose).

**What drug does:**
- Reduces work that heart must perform.
- Reduces normal artery pressure.
- Increases oxygen to heart muscle.

**Time lapse before drug works:**
1 to 2 hours.

**Don't take with:**
See Interaction column and consult doctor.

 ## OVERDOSE

**SYMPTOMS:**
**Unusually fast or unusually slow heartbeat, loss of consciousness, cardiac arrest.**
**WHAT TO DO:**
- **Dial 0 (operator) or 911 (emergency) for an ambulance or medical help. Then give first aid immediately.**
- **See emergency information on inside covers.**

 ## POSSIBLE ADVERSE REACTIONS OR SIDE EFFECTS

| SYMPTOMS | WHAT TO DO |
|---|---|
| **Life-threatening:** None expected. | |
| **Common:** Tiredness. | Continue. Tell doctor at next visit. |
| **Infrequent:** | |
| ● Unusually slow or fast heartbeat, wheezing, cough, shortness of breath. | Discontinue. Call doctor right away. |
| ● Dizziness; numbness or tingling in hands or feet; swollen ankles, feet or legs; difficult urination. | Continue. Call doctor when convenient. |
| ● Nausea, constipation or diarrhea, vomiting, indigestion. | Continue. Tell doctor at next visit. |
| **Rare:** | |
| ● Fainting, rash, jaundice. | Discontinue. Call doctor right away. |
| ● Headache. | Continue. Tell doctor at next visit. |

## WARNINGS & PRECAUTIONS

**Don't take if:**
You are allergic to any calcium-channel blocker.

**Before you start, consult your doctor:**
- If you have kidney or liver disease.
- If you have high or low blood pressure.
- If you have heart disease other than coronary artery disease.

**Over age 60:**
Adverse reactions and side effects may be more frequent and severe than in younger persons.

**Pregnancy:**
No proven harm to unborn child. Avoid if possible.

**Breast-feeding:**
No problems expected.

**Infants & children:**
Not recommended.

**Prolonged use:**
No problems expected.

**Skin & sunlight:**
May cause rash or intensify sunburn in areas exposed to sun or sunlamp.

**Driving, piloting or hazardous work:**
Avoid if you feel dizzy. Otherwise, no problems expected.

**Discontinuing:**
Don't discontinue without consulting doctor.

**Others:**
Learn to check your own pulse rate. If it drops to 50 beats per minute or lower, don't take diltiazem until your consult your doctor.

## POSSIBLE INTERACTION WITH OTHER DRUGS

| GENERIC NAME OR DRUG CLASS | COMBINED EFFECT |
|---|---|
| Amiodarone | Increased likelihood of slow heartbeat. |
| Antihypertensives | Dangerous blood-pressure drop. |
| Beta-adrenergic blockers | Decreased angina attacks. |
| Diuretics | Dangerous blood-pressure drop. |
| Disopyramide | May cause dangerously slow, fast or irregular heartbeat. |
| Enalapril | Possible excessive potassium in blood. |
| Flecainide | Possible irregular heartbeat. |
| Nitrates | Reduced angina attacks. |
| Quinidine | Increased quinidine effect. |
| Tocainide | Increased likelihood of adverse reactions from either drug. |

## POSSIBLE INTERACTION WITH OTHER SUBSTANCES

| INTERACTS WITH | COMBINED EFFECT |
|---|---|
| Alcohol: | Dangerously low blood pressure. |
| Beverages: | None expected. |
| Cocaine: | Possible irregular heartbeat. Avoid. |
| Foods: | None expected. |
| Marijuana: | Possible irregular heartbeat. Avoid. |
| Tobacco: | Possible rapid heartbeat. Avoid. |

# DIMENHYDRINATE

## BRAND NAMES

See complete list of brand names in the *Brand Name Directory,* page 948.

## BASIC INFORMATION

**Habit forming? No**
**Prescription needed?**
   **High strength: Yes**
   **Low strength: No**
**Available as generic? Yes**
**Drug class: Antihistamine**

## USES

- Reduces allergic symptoms such as hay fever, hives, rash or itching.
- Prevents motion sickness, nausea, vomiting.
- Induces sleep.

## DOSAGE & USAGE INFORMATION

**How to take:**
Tablet or liquid—Swallow with liquid or food to lessen stomach irritation.

**When to take:**
Varies with form. Follow label directions.

**If you forget a dose:**
Take as soon as you remember up to 2 hours late. If more than 2 hours, wait for next scheduled dose (don't double this dose).

**What drug does:**
Blocks action of histamine after an allergic response triggers histamine release in sensitive cells.

*Continued next column*

## OVERDOSE

**SYMPTOMS:**
**Convulsions, red face, hallucinations, coma.**
**WHAT TO DO:**
- **Dial 0 (operator) or 911 (emergency) for an ambulance or medical help. Then give first aid immediately.**
- **If patient is unconscious and not breathing, give mouth-to-mouth breathing. If there is no heartbeat, use cardiac massage and mouth-to-mouth breathing (CPR). Don't try to make patient vomit. If you can't get help quickly, take patient to nearest emergency facility.**
- **See emergency information on inside covers.**

**Time lapse before drug works:**
30 minutes.

**Don't take with:**
See Interaction column and consult doctor.

## POSSIBLE ADVERSE REACTIONS OR SIDE EFFECTS

| SYMPTOMS | WHAT TO DO |
|---|---|
| **Life-threatening:**<br>None expected. | |
| **Common:**<br>Drowsiness; dizziness; dry mouth, eyes and nose; nausea. | Continue. Tell doctor at next visit. |
| **Infrequent:**<br>• Change in vision. | Discontinue. Call doctor right away. |
| • Less tolerance for contact lenses, frequent urination. | Continue. Call doctor when convenient. |
| • Appetite loss. | Continue. Tell doctor at next visit. |
| **Rare:**<br>Nightmares, agitation, irritability, sore throat, fever, rapid heartbeat, unusual bleeding or bruising, fatigue, weakness. | Discontinue. Call doctor right away. |

## WARNINGS & PRECAUTIONS

**Don't take if:**
You are allergic to any antihistamine.

**Before you start, consult your doctor:**
- If you have glaucoma.
- If you have enlarged prostate.
- If you have asthma.
- If you have kidney disease.
- If you have peptic ulcer.
- If you will have surgery within 2 months, including dental surgery, requiring general or spinal anesthesia.

**Over age 60:**
Don't exceed recommended dose. Adverse reactions and side effects may be more frequent and severe than in younger persons, especially urination difficulty, diminished alertness and other brain and nervous-system symptoms.

**Pregnancy:**
No proven harm to unborn child. Avoid if possible.

**Breast-feeding:**
Drug passes into milk. Avoid drug or discontinue nursing until you finish medicine. Consult doctor for advice on maintaining milk supply.

**Infants & children:**
Not recommended for premature or newborn infants. Otherwise, no problems expected.

**Prolonged use:**
Avoid. May damage bone marrow and nerve cells.

**Skin & sunlight:**
May cause rash or intensify sunburn in areas exposed to sun or sunlamp.

**Driving, piloting or hazardous work:**
Don't drive or pilot aircraft until you learn how medicine affects you. Don't work around dangerous machinery. Don't climb ladders or work in high places. Danger increases if you drink alcohol or take medicine affecting alertness and reflexes, such as antihistamines, tranquilizers, sedatives, pain medicine, narcotics and mind-altering drugs.

**Discontinuing:**
No problems expected.

**Others:**
May mask symptoms of hearing damage from aspirin, other salicylates, cisplatin, paromomycin, vancomycin or anticonvulsants. Consult doctor if you use these.

## POSSIBLE INTERACTION WITH OTHER DRUGS

| GENERIC NAME OR DRUG CLASS | COMBINED EFFECT |
|---|---|
| Anticholinergics | Increased anticholinergic effect. |
| Antidepressants | Excess sedation. Avoid. |
| Antihistamines (other) | Excess sedation. Avoid. |
| Dronabinol | Increased effects of both drugs. Avoid. |
| Hypnotics | Excess sedation. Avoid. |
| MAO inhibitors | Increased dimenhydrinate effect. |
| Mind-altering drugs | Excess sedation. Avoid. |
| Molindone | Increased antihistamine effect. |
| Narcotics | Excess sedation. Avoid. |
| Sedatives | Excess sedation. Avoid. |
| Sleep inducers | Excess sedation. Avoid. |
| Tranquilizers | Excess sedation. Avoid. |

## POSSIBLE INTERACTION WITH OTHER SUBSTANCES

| INTERACTS WITH | COMBINED EFFECT |
|---|---|
| Alcohol: | Excess sedation. Avoid. |
| Beverages: Caffeine drinks. | Less dimenhydrinate sedation. |
| Cocaine: | Decreased dimenhydrinate effect. Avoid. |
| Foods: | None expected. |
| Marijuana: | Excess sedation. Avoid. |
| Tobacco: | None expected. |

# DIMETHINDENE

## BRAND NAMES

Forhistal         Triten Tab-In
Triten

## BASIC INFORMATION

**Habit forming?** No
**Prescription needed?** Yes
**Available as generic?** Yes
**Drug class:** Antihistamine

## USES

- Reduces allergic symptoms such as hay fever, hives, rash or itching.
- Induces sleep.

## DOSAGE & USAGE INFORMATION

**How to take:**
Extended-release tablets or capsules—Take with liquid or food. Swallow each dose whole.

**When to take:**
Varies with form. Follow label directions.

**If you forget a dose:**
Take as soon as you remember up to 2 hours late. If more than 2 hours, wait for next scheduled dose (don't double this dose).

**What drug does:**
Blocks action of histamine after an allergic response triggers histamine release in sensitive cells.

**Time lapse before drug works:**
30 minutes.

**Don't take with:**
See Interaction column and consult doctor.

## OVERDOSE

**SYMPTOMS:**
**Convulsions, red face, hallucinations, coma.**
**WHAT TO DO:**
- **Dial 0 (operator) or 911 (emergency) for an ambulance or medical help. Then give first aid immediately.**
- **If patient is unconscious and not breathing, give mouth-to-mouth breathing. If there is no heartbeat, use cardiac massage and mouth-to-mouth breathing (CPR). Don't try to make patient vomit. If you can't get help quickly, take patient to nearest emergency facility.**
- **See emergency information on inside covers.**

## POSSIBLE ADVERSE REACTIONS OR SIDE EFFECTS

| SYMPTOMS | WHAT TO DO |
|---|---|
| **Life-threatening:**<br>None expected. | |
| **Common:**<br>Drowsiness; dizziness; dry mouth, nose, throat; nausea. | Continue. Tell doctor at next visit. |
| **Infrequent:**<br>• Change in vision. | Discontinue. Call doctor right away. |
| • Less tolerance for contact lenses, painful or difficult urination. | Continue. Call doctor when convenient. |
| • Appetite loss. | Continue. Tell doctor at next visit. |
| **Rare:**<br>Nightmares, agitation, irritability, sore throat, fever, rapid heartbeat, unusual bleeding or bruising, fatigue, weakness. | Discontinue. Call doctor right away. |

# DIMETHINDENE

## WARNINGS & PRECAUTIONS

**Don't take if:**
You are allergic to any antihistamine.

**Before you start, consult your doctor:**
- If you have glaucoma.
- If you have enlarged prostate.
- If you have asthma.
- If you have kidney disease.
- If you have peptic ulcer.
- If you will have surgery within 2 months, including dental surgery, requiring general or spinal anesthesia.

**Over age 60:**
Don't exceed recommended dose. Adverse reactions and side effects may be more frequent and severe than in younger persons, especially urination difficulty, diminished alertness and other brain and nervous-system symptoms.

**Pregnancy:**
No proven harm to unborn child. Avoid if possible.

**Breast-feeding:**
Drug passes into milk. Avoid drug or discontinue nursing until you finish medicine. Consult doctor for advice on maintaining milk supply.

**Infants & children:**
Not recommended for premature or newborn infants. Otherwise, no problems expected.

**Prolonged use:**
Avoid. May damage bone marrow and nerve cells.

**Skin & sunlight:**
May cause rash or intensify sunburn in areas exposed to sun or sunlamp.

**Driving, piloting or hazardous work:**
Don't drive or pilot aircraft until you learn how medicine affects you. Don't work around dangerous machinery. Don't climb ladders or work in high places. Danger increases if you drink alcohol or take medicine affecting alertness and reflexes, such as antihistamines, tranquilizers, sedatives, pain medicine, narcotics and mind-altering drugs.

**Discontinuing:**
No problems expected.

**Others:**
May mask symptoms of hearing damage from aspirin, other salicylates, cisplatin, paromomycin, vancomycin or anticonvulsants. Consult doctor if you use these.

## POSSIBLE INTERACTION WITH OTHER DRUGS

| GENERIC NAME OR DRUG CLASS | COMBINED EFFECT |
| --- | --- |
| Anticholinergics | Increased anticholinergic effect. |
| Antidepressants | Excess sedation. Avoid. |
| Antihistamines (other) | Excess sedation. Avoid. |
| Dronabinol | Increased effects of both drugs. Avoid. |
| Hypnotics | Excess sedation. Avoid. |
| MAO inhibitors | Increased dimethindene effect. |
| Mind-altering drugs | Excess sedation. Avoid. |
| Narcotics | Excess sedation. Avoid. |
| Sedatives | Excess sedation. Avoid. |
| Sleep inducers | Excess sedation. Avoid. |
| Tranquilizers | Excess sedation. Avoid. |

## POSSIBLE INTERACTION WITH OTHER SUBSTANCES

| INTERACTS WITH | COMBINED EFFECT |
| --- | --- |
| Alcohol: | Excess sedation. Avoid. |
| Beverages: Caffeine drinks. | Less dimethindene sedation. |
| Cocaine: | Decreased dimethindene effect. Avoid. |
| Foods: | None expected. |
| Marijuana: | Excess sedation. Avoid. |
| Tobacco: | None expected. |

# DIPHENHYDRAMINE

## BRAND NAMES

See complete list of brand names in the
*Brand Name Directory,* page 948.

## BASIC INFORMATION

**Habit forming? No**
**Prescription needed?**
  **High strength: Yes**
  **Low strength: No**
**Available as generic? Yes**
**Drug class: Antihistamine**

## USES

- Reduces allergic symptoms such as hay fever, hives, rash or itching.
- Prevents motion sickness, nausea, vomiting.
- Induces sleep.
- Reduces stiffness and tremors of Parkinson's disease.

## DOSAGE & USAGE INFORMATION

**How to take:**
- Tablet or capsule—Swallow with liquid or food to lessen stomach irritation.
- Extended-release tablets or capsules—Swallow each dose whole.
- Suppositories—Remove wrapper and moisten suppository with water. Gently insert larger end into rectum. Push well into rectum with finger.

**When to take:**
Varies with form. Follow label directions.

**If you forget a dose:**
Take as soon as you remember up to 2 hours late. If more than 2 hours, wait for next scheduled dose (don't double this dose).

**What drug does:**
Blocks action of histamine after an allergic response triggers histamine release in sensitive cells.

*Continued next column*

## OVERDOSE

**SYMPTOMS:**
**Convulsions, red face, hallucinations, coma.**
**WHAT TO DO:**
- **Dial 0 (operator) or 911 (emergency) for an ambulance or medical help. Then give first aid immediately.**
- **See emergency information on inside covers.**

**Time lapse before drug works:**
30 minutes.

**Don't take with:**
See Interaction column and consult doctor.

## POSSIBLE ADVERSE REACTIONS OR SIDE EFFECTS

| SYMPTOMS | WHAT TO DO |
|---|---|
| **Life-threatening:**<br>None expected. | |
| **Common:**<br>Drowsiness; dizziness; dry mouth, nose, throat; nausea. | Continue. Tell doctor at next visit. |
| **Infrequent:**<br>• Change in vision. | Discontinue. Call doctor right away. |
| • Less tolerance for contact lenses, painful or difficult urination. | Continue. Call doctor when convenient. |
| • Appetite loss. | Continue. Tell doctor at next visit. |
| **Rare:**<br>Nightmares, agitation, irritability, sore throat, fever, rapid heartbeat, unusual bleeding or bruising, fatigue, weakness. | Discontinue. Call doctor right away. |

# DIPHENHYDRAMINE

 **WARNINGS & PRECAUTIONS**

**Don't take if:**
You are allergic to any antihistamine.

**Before you start, consult your doctor:**
- If you have glaucoma.
- If you have enlarged prostate.
- If you have asthma.
- If you have kidney disease.
- If you have peptic ulcer.
- If you will have surgery within 2 months, including dental surgery, requiring general or spinal anesthesia.

**Over age 60:**
Don't exceed recommended dose. Adverse reactions and side effects may be more frequent and severe than in younger persons, especially urination difficulty, diminished alertness and other brain and nervous-system symptoms.

**Pregnancy:**
No proven harm to unborn child. Avoid if possible.

**Breast-feeding:**
Drug passes into milk. Avoid drug or discontinue nursing until you finish medicine. Consult doctor for advice on maintaining milk supply.

**Infants & children:**
Not recommended for premature or newborn infants. Otherwise, no problems expected.

**Prolonged use:**
Avoid. May damage bone marrow and nerve cells.

**Skin & sunlight:**
May cause rash or intensify sunburn in areas exposed to sun or sunlamp.

**Driving, piloting or hazardous work:**
Don't drive or pilot aircraft until you learn how medicine affects you. Don't work around dangerous machinery. Don't climb ladders or work in high places. Danger increases if you drink alcohol or take medicine affecting alertness and reflexes, such as antihistamines, tranquilizers, sedatives, pain medicine, narcotics and mind-altering drugs.

**Discontinuing:**
No problems expected.

**Others:**
May mask symptoms of hearing damage from aspirin, other salicylates, cisplatin, paromomycin, vancomycin or anticonvulsants. Consult doctor if you use these.

 **POSSIBLE INTERACTION WITH OTHER DRUGS**

| GENERIC NAME OR DRUG CLASS | COMBINED EFFECT |
| --- | --- |
| Anticholinergics | Increased anticholinergic effect. |
| Antidepressants | Excess sedation. Avoid. |
| Antihistamines (other) | Excess sedation. Avoid. |
| Dronabinol | Increased effects of both drugs. Avoid. |
| Hypnotics | Excess sedation. Avoid. |
| MAO inhibitors | Increased diphenhydramine effect. |
| Mind-altering drugs | Excess sedation. Avoid. |
| Molindone | Increased sedative and antihistamine effect. |
| Narcotics | Excess sedation. Avoid. |
| Sedatives | Excess sedation. Avoid. |
| Sleep inducers | Excess sedation. Avoid. |
| Tranquilizers | Excess sedation. Avoid. |

**POSSIBLE INTERACTION WITH OTHER SUBSTANCES**

| INTERACTS WITH | COMBINED EFFECT |
| --- | --- |
| Alcohol: | Excess sedation. Avoid. |
| Beverages: Caffeine drinks. | Less diphenhydramine sedation. |
| Cocaine: | Decreased diphenhydramine effect. Avoid. |
| Foods: | None expected. |
| Marijuana: | Excess sedation. Avoid. |
| Tobacco: | None expected. |

# DIPHENIDOL

## BRAND NAMES

Vontrol

## BASIC INFORMATION

**Habit forming? No**
**Prescription needed? Yes**
**Available as generic? No**
**Drug class: Antiemetic, antivertigo**

 ## USES

- Prevents motion sickness.
- Controls nausea and vomiting (do not use during pregnancy).

 ## DOSAGE & USAGE INFORMATION

**How to take:**
Tablet—Swallow with liquid or food to lessen stomach irritation. If you can't swallow whole, crumble tablet and chew or take with liquid or food.

**When to take:**
30 to 60 minutes before traveling.

**If you forget a dose:**
Take as soon as you remember. Wait 4 hours for next dose.

**What drug does:**
Reduces sensitivity of nerve endings in inner ear, blocking messages to brain's vomiting center.

**Time lapse before drug works:**
30 to 60 minutes.

**Don't take with:**
See Interaction column and consult doctor.

 ## OVERDOSE

**SYMPTOMS:**
Drowsiness, confusion, incoordination, weak pulse, shallow breathing, stupor, coma.
**WHAT TO DO:**
- **Dial 0 (operator) or 911 (emergency) for an ambulance or medical help. Then give first aid immediately.**
- **See emergency information on inside covers.**

 ## POSSIBLE ADVERSE REACTIONS OR SIDE EFFECTS

| SYMPTOMS | WHAT TO DO |
|---|---|
| **Life-threatening:**<br>None expected. | |
| **Common:**<br>Drowsiness. | Continue. Tell doctor at next visit. |
| **Infrequent:** | |
| ● Headache, diarrhea or constipation, fast heartbeat. | Continue. Call doctor when convenient. |
| ● Dry mouth, nose, throat. | Continue. Tell doctor at next visit. |
| **Rare:** | |
| ● Rash or hives. | Discontinue. Call doctor right away. |
| ● Restlessness; excitement; insomnia; blurred vision; urgent, painful or difficult urination. | Continue. Call doctor when convenient. |
| ● Appetite loss, nausea. | Continue. Tell doctor at next visit. |

## WARNINGS & PRECAUTIONS

**Don't take if:**
- You have severe kidney disease.
- You are allergic to diphenidol or meclizine.

**Before you start, consult your doctor:**
- If you have prostate enlargement.
- If you have glaucoma.
- If you have heart disease.
- If you have intestinal obstruction or ulcers in the gastrointestinal tract.
- If you have kidney disease.
- If you have low blood pressure.
- If you will have surgery within 2 months, including dental surgery, requiring general or spinal anesthesia.

**Over age 60:**
Adverse reactions and side effects may be more frequent and severe than in younger persons.

**Pregnancy:**
Animal studies show fetal abnormalities. Decide with your doctor whether drug benefits justify risk to unborn child.

**Breast-feeding:**
Drug passes into milk. Avoid drug or discontinue nursing until you finish medicine. Consult doctor for advice on maintaining milk supply.

**Infants & children:**
No problems expected.

**Prolonged use:**
No problems expected.

**Skin & sunlight:**
No problems expected.

**Driving, piloting or hazardous work:**
Don't fly aircraft. Don't drive until you learn how medicine affects you. Don't work around dangerous machinery. Don't climb ladders or work in high places. Danger increases if you drink alcohol or take medicine affecting alertness and reflexes, such as antihistamines, tranquilizers, sedatives, pain medicine, narcotics and mind-altering drugs.

**Discontinuing:**
No problems expected.

**Others:**
No problems expected.

## POSSIBLE INTERACTION WITH OTHER DRUGS

| GENERIC NAME OR DRUG CLASS | COMBINED EFFECT |
|---|---|
| Anticonvulsants | Increased effect of both drugs. |
| Antidepressants (tricyclic) | Increased sedative effect of both drugs. |
| Antihistamines | Increased sedative effect of both drugs. |
| Atropine | Increased chance of toxic effect of atropine and atropine-like medicines. |
| Narcotics | Increased sedative effect of both drugs. |
| Sedatives | Increased sedative effect of both drugs. |
| Tranquilizers | Increased sedative effect of both drugs. |

## POSSIBLE INTERACTION WITH OTHER SUBSTANCES

| INTERACTS WITH | COMBINED EFFECT |
|---|---|
| Alcohol: | Increased sedation. Avoid. |
| Beverages: Caffeine. | May decrease drowsiness. |
| Cocaine: | Increased chance of toxic effects of cocaine. Avoid. |
| Foods: | None expected. |
| Marijuana: | Increased drowsiness, dry mouth. |
| Tobacco: | None expected. |

# DIPHENOXYLATE & ATROPINE

## BRAND NAMES

Colonil
Diphenatol
Enoxa
Latropine
Lofene
Lomanate

Lomotil
Lonox
Lo-Trol
Low-Quel
Nor-Mil
SK-Diphenoxylate

## BASIC INFORMATION

**Habit forming? Yes**
**Prescription needed? Yes**
**Available as generic? Yes**
**Drug class: Antidiarrheal**

## USES

Relieves diarrhea and intestinal cramps.

## DOSAGE & USAGE INFORMATION

**How to take:**
- Tablet or capsule—Swallow with liquid or food to lessen stomach irritation.
- Drops or liquid—Follow label instructions and use marked dropper.

**When to take:**
No more often than directed on label.

**If you forget a dose:**
Take as soon as you remember up to 2 hours late. If more than 2 hours, wait for next scheduled dose (don't double this dose).

**What drug does:**
Blocks digestive tract's nerve supply, which reduces propelling movements.

*Continued next column*

## OVERDOSE

**SYMPTOMS:**
**Excitement, constricted pupils, shallow breathing, coma.**
**WHAT TO DO:**
- **Dial 0 (operator) or 911 (emergency) for an ambulance or medical help. Then give first aid immediately.**
- **If patient is unconscious and not breathing, give mouth-to-mouth breathing. If there is no heartbeat, use cardiac massage and mouth-to-mouth breathing (CPR). Don't try to make patient vomit. If you can't get help quickly, take patient to nearest emergency facility.**
- **See emergency information on inside covers.**

**Time lapse before drug works:**
May require 12 to 24 hours of regular doses to control diarrhea.

**Don't take with:**
See Interaction column and consult doctor.

## POSSIBLE ADVERSE REACTIONS OR SIDE EFFECTS

| SYMPTOMS | WHAT TO DO |
|---|---|
| **Life-threatening:**<br>None expected. | |
| **Common:**<br>None expected. | |
| **Infrequent:**<br>• Dry mouth, swollen gums, rapid heartbeat. | Discontinue. Call doctor right away. |
| • Dizziness, depression, drowsiness, rash or itch, blurred vision, decreased urination. | Continue. Call doctor when convenient. |
| **Rare:**<br>Restlessness, flush, fever, headache, stomach pain, nausea, vomiting, bloating, constipation, numbness of hands or feet. | Discontinue. Call doctor right away. |

## WARNINGS & PRECAUTIONS

### Don't take if:
- You are allergic to diphenoxylate & atropine or any narcotic or anticholinergic.
- You have jaundice.
- Patient is younger than 2.

### Before you start, consult your doctor:
- If you have had liver problems.
- If you have ulcerative colitis.
- If you plan to become pregnant within medication period.
- If you have any medical disorder.
- If you take any medication, including non-prescription drugs.

### Over age 60:
Adverse reactions and side effects may be more frequent and severe than in younger persons.

### Pregnancy:
No proven harm to unborn child. Avoid because of many side effects.

### Breast-feeding:
Drug passes into milk. Avoid drug or discontinue nursing until you finish medicine. Consult doctor for advice on maintaining milk supply.

### Infants & children:
Don't give to infants or toddlers. Use only under doctor's supervision for children older than 2.

### Prolonged use:
Habit forming.

### Skin & sunlight:
No problems expected.

### Driving, piloting or hazardous work:
Don't drive or pilot aircraft until you learn how medicine affects you. Don't work around dangerous machinery. Don't climb ladders or work in high places. Danger increases if you drink alcohol or take medicine affecting alertness and reflexes.

### Discontinuing:
- May be unnecessary to finish medicine. Follow doctor's instructions.
- After discontinuing, consult doctor if you experience muscle cramps, nausea, vomiting, trembling, stomach cramps or unusual sweating.

### Others:
If diarrhea lasts longer than 4 days, discontinue and call doctor.

## POSSIBLE INTERACTION WITH OTHER DRUGS

| GENERIC NAME OR DRUG CLASS | COMBINED EFFECT |
|---|---|
| MAO inhibitors | May increase blood pressure excessively. |
| Sedatives | Increased effect of both drugs. |
| Tranquilizers | Increased effect of both drugs. |

## POSSIBLE INTERACTION WITH OTHER SUBSTANCES

| INTERACTS WITH | COMBINED EFFECT |
|---|---|
| Alcohol: | Depressed brain function. Avoid. |
| Beverages: | None expected. |
| Cocaine: | Decreased effect of diphenoxylate and atropine. |
| Foods: | None expected. |
| Marijuana: | None expected. |
| Tobacco: | None expected. |

# DIPHENYLPYRALINE

## BRAND NAMES

Diafen                     Hispril

## BASIC INFORMATION

**Habit forming?** No
**Prescription needed?**
  **High strength:** Yes
  **Low strength:** No
**Available as generic?** No
**Drug class:** Antihistamine

## USES

- Reduces allergic symptoms such as hay fever, hives, rash or itching.
- Induces sleep.

## DOSAGE & USAGE INFORMATION

**How to take:**
Extended-release capsules—Swallow each dose whole with liquid.

**When to take:**
Varies with form. Follow label directions.

**If you forget a dose:**
Take as soon as you remember up to 2 hours late. If more than 2 hours, wait for next scheduled dose (don't double this dose).

**What drug does:**
Blocks action of histamine after an allergic response triggers histamine release in sensitive cells.

**Time lapse before drug works:**
30 minutes.

**Don't take with:**
See Interaction column and consult doctor.

## OVERDOSE

**SYMPTOMS:**
Convulsions, red face, hallucinations, coma.
**WHAT TO DO:**
- **Dial 0 (operator) or 911 (emergency) for an ambulance or medical help. Then give first aid immediately.**
- **If patient is unconscious and not breathing, give mouth-to-mouth breathing. If there is no heartbeat, use cardiac massage and mouth-to-mouth breathing (CPR). Don't try to make patient vomit. If you can't get help quickly, take patient to nearest emergency facility.**
- **See emergency information on inside covers.**

## POSSIBLE ADVERSE REACTIONS OR SIDE EFFECTS

| SYMPTOMS | WHAT TO DO |
|---|---|
| **Life-threatening:** None expected. | |
| **Common:** Drowsiness; dizziness; dry mouth, nose, throat; nausea. | Continue. Tell doctor at next visit. |
| **Infrequent:** | |
| • Change in vision. | Discontinue. Call doctor right away. |
| • Less tolerance for contact lenses, painful or difficult urination. | Continue. Call doctor when convenient. |
| • Appetite loss. | Continue. Tell doctor at next visit. |
| **Rare:** Nightmares, agitation, irritability, sore throat, fever, rapid heartbeat, unusual bleeding or bruising, fatigue, weakness. | Discontinue. Call doctor right away. |

## WARNINGS & PRECAUTIONS

**Don't take if:**
You are allergic to any antihistamine.

**Before you start, consult your doctor:**
- If you have glaucoma.
- If you have enlarged prostate.
- If you have asthma.
- If you have kidney disease.
- If you have peptic ulcer.
- If you will have surgery within 2 months, including dental surgery, requiring general or spinal anesthesia.

**Over age 60:**
Don't exceed recommended dose. Adverse reactions and side effects may be more frequent and severe than in younger persons, especially urination difficulty, diminished alertness and other brain and nervous-system symptoms.

**Pregnancy:**
No proven harm to unborn child. Avoid if possible.

**Breast-feeding:**
Drug passes into milk. Avoid drug or discontinue nursing until you finish medicine. Consult doctor for advice on maintaining milk supply.

**Infants & children:**
Not recommended for premature or newborn infants. Otherwise, no problems expected.

**Prolonged use:**
Avoid. May damage bone marrow and nerve cells.

**Skin & sunlight:**
May cause rash or intensify sunburn in areas exposed to sun or sunlamp.

**Driving, piloting or hazardous work:**
Don't drive or pilot aircraft until you learn how medicine affects you. Don't work around dangerous machinery. Don't climb ladders or work in high places. Danger increases if you drink alcohol or take medicine affecting alertness and reflexes, such as antihistamines, tranquilizers, sedatives, pain medicine, narcotics and mind-altering drugs.

**Discontinuing:**
No problems expected.

**Others:**
May mask symptoms of hearing damage from aspirin, other salicylates, cisplatin, paromomycin, vancomycin or anticonvulsants. Consult doctor if you use these.

## POSSIBLE INTERACTION WITH OTHER DRUGS

| GENERIC NAME OR DRUG CLASS | COMBINED EFFECT |
|---|---|
| Anticholinergics | Increased anticholinergic effect. |
| Antidepressants | Excess sedation. Avoid. |
| Antihistamines (other) | Excess sedation. Avoid. |
| Dronabinol | Increased effects of both drugs. Avoid. |
| Hypnotics | Excess sedation. Avoid. |
| MAO inhibitors | Increased diphenylpyraline effect. |
| Mind-altering drugs | Excess sedation. Avoid. |
| Molindone | Increased antihistamine effect. |
| Narcotics | Excess sedation. Avoid. |
| Sedatives | Excess sedation. Avoid. |
| Sleep inducers | Excess sedation. Avoid. |
| Tranquilizers | Excess sedation. Avoid. |

## POSSIBLE INTERACTION WITH OTHER SUBSTANCES

| INTERACTS WITH | COMBINED EFFECT |
|---|---|
| Alcohol: | Excess sedation. Avoid. |
| Beverages: Caffeine drinks. | Less diphenylpyraline sedation. |
| Cocaine: | Decreased diphenylpyraline effect. Avoid. |
| Foods: | None expected. |
| Marijuana: | Excess sedation. Avoid. |
| Tobacco: | None expected. |

# DIPYRIDAMOLE

## BRAND NAMES

| | |
|---|---|
| Apo-Dipyridamole | Pyridamole |
| Persantine | SK-Dipyridamole |

## BASIC INFORMATION

Habit forming? No
Prescription needed?
  U.S.: Yes
  Canada: No
Available as generic? Yes
Drug class: Coronary vasodilator

## USES

* Reduces frequency and intensity of angina attacks.
* Prevents blood clots after heart surgery.

## DOSAGE & USAGE INFORMATION

**How to take:**
Tablet or capsule—Swallow with liquid. If you can't swallow whole, crumble tablet or open capsule and take with liquid.

**When to take:**
1 hour before meals.

**If you forget a dose:**
Take as soon as you remember up to 2 hours late. If more than 2 hours, wait for next scheduled dose (don't double this dose).

**What drug does:**
* Probably dilates blood vessels to increase oxygen to heart.
* Prevents platelet clumping, which causes blood clots.

*Continued next column*

## OVERDOSE

**SYMPTOMS:**
Decreased blood pressure; weak, rapid pulse; cold, clammy skin; collapse.
**WHAT TO DO:**
* Dial 0 (operator) or 911 (emergency) for an ambulance or medical help. Then give first aid immediately.
* If patient is unconscious and not breathing, give mouth-to-mouth breathing. If there is no heartbeat, use cardiac massage and mouth-to-mouth breathing (CPR). Don't try to make patient vomit. If you can't get help quickly, take patient to nearest emergency facility.
* See emergency information on inside covers.

**Time lapse before drug works:**
3 months of continual use.

**Don't take with:**
See Interaction column and consult doctor.

## POSSIBLE ADVERSE REACTIONS OR SIDE EFFECTS

| SYMPTOMS | WHAT TO DO |
|---|---|
| **Life-threatening:**<br>None expected. | |
| **Common:**<br>None expected. | |
| **Infrequent:** | |
| • Dizziness, fainting, headache. | Discontinue. Call doctor right away. |
| • Red flush, rash, nausea, vomiting, cramps, weakness. | Continue. Call doctor when convenient. |
| **Rare:**<br>None expected. | |

# DISOPYRAMIDE

## BRAND NAMES

Norpace
Norpace CR

Rythmodan
Rythmodan-LA

## BASIC INFORMATION

Habit forming? No
Prescription needed? Yes
Available as generic? Yes
Drug class: Antiarrhythmic

 USES

Corrects heart rhythm disorders.

 DOSAGE & USAGE
INFORMATION

**How to take:**
Tablet or capsule—Swallow with liquid. If you
can't swallow whole, crumble tablet or open
capsule and take with liquid or food.

**When to take:**
At the same times each day.

**If you forget a dose:**
Take as soon as you remember up to 2 hours
late. If more than 2 hours, wait for next
scheduled dose (don't double this dose).

**What drug does:**
Delays nerve impulses to heart to regulate
heartbeat.

**Time lapse before drug works:**
Begins in 30 to 60 minutes. Must use for 5 to 7
days to determine effectiveness.

**Don't take with:**
See Interaction column and consult doctor.

 OVERDOSE

**SYMPTOMS:**
Blood-pressure drop, irregular heartbeat.
**WHAT TO DO:**
- Dial 0 (operator) or 911 (emergency) for an
  ambulance or medical help. Then give first
  aid immediately.
- If patient is unconscious and not
  breathing, give mouth-to-mouth breathing.
  If there is no heartbeat, use cardiac
  massage and mouth-to-mouth breathing
  (CPR). Don't try to make patient vomit. If
  you can't get help quickly, take patient to
  nearest emergency facility.
- See emergency information on inside
  covers.

 POSSIBLE
ADVERSE REACTIONS
OR SIDE EFFECTS

| SYMPTOMS | WHAT TO DO |
|---|---|
| **Life-threatening:** | |
| None expected. | |
| **Common:** | |
| • Hypoglycemia. | Discontinue. Call doctor right away. |
| • Dry mouth, constipation, painful or difficult urination, rapid weight gain. | Continue. Call doctor when convenient. |
| **Infrequent:** | |
| • Dizziness, fainting, confusion, nervousness, depression, chest pain, slow or fast heartbeat. | Discontinue. Call doctor right away. |
| • Swollen feet. | Continue. Call doctor when convenient. |
| **Rare:** | |
| • Sore throat with fever, jaundice. | Discontinue. Call doctor right away. |
| • Eye pain, diminished sex drive. | Continue. Call doctor when convenient. |

# DISOPYRAMIDE

## WARNINGS & PRECAUTIONS

**Don't take if:**
- You are allergic to disopyramide or any antiarrhythmic.
- You have second- or third-degree heart block.

**Before you start, consult your doctor:**
- If you react unfavorably to other antiarrhythmic drugs.
- If you have had heart disease.
- If you have low blood pressure.
- If you have liver disease.
- If you have glaucoma.
- If you have enlarged prostate.
- If you have myasthenia gravis.
- If you take digitalis preparations or diuretics.

**Over age 60:**
- May require reduced dose.
- More likely to have difficulty urinating or be constipated.
- More likely to have blood-pressure drop.

**Pregnancy:**
No proven harm to unborn child. Avoid if possible.

**Breast-feeding:**
Drug passes into milk. Avoid drug or discontinue nursing until you finish medicine. Consult doctor for advice on maintaining milk supply.

**Infants & children:**
Safety not established. Don't use.

**Prolonged use:**
No problems expected.

**Skin & sunlight:**
No problems expected.

**Driving, piloting or hazardous work:**
Don't drive or pilot aircraft until you learn how medicine affects you. Don't work around dangerous machinery. Don't climb ladders or work in high places. Danger increases if you drink alcohol or take medicine affecting alertness and reflexes, such as antihistamines, tranquilizers, sedatives, pain medicine, narcotics, or mind-altering drugs.

**Discontinuing:**
Don't discontinue without doctor's advice until you complete prescribed dose, even though symptoms diminish or disappear.

**Others:**
If new illness, injury or surgery occurs, tell doctors of disopyramide use.

## POSSIBLE INTERACTION WITH OTHER DRUGS

| GENERIC NAME OR DRUG CLASS | COMBINED EFFECT |
|---|---|
| Ambenonium | Decreased ambenonium effect. |
| Anticholinergics | Increased anticholinergic effect. |
| Anticoagulants (oral) | Increased anticoagulant effect. |
| Antihypertensives | Increased antihypertensive effect. |
| Antimyasthenics | Decreased antimyasthenic effect. |
| Flecainide | Possible irregular heartbeat. |
| Tocainide | Increased likelihood of adverse reactions with either drug. |

## POSSIBLE INTERACTION WITH OTHER SUBSTANCES

| INTERACTS WITH | COMBINED EFFECT |
|---|---|
| Alcohol: | Decreased blood pressure and blood sugar. Use caution. |
| Beverages: | None expected. |
| Cocaine: | Irregular heartbeat. |
| Foods: | None expected. |
| Marijuana: | Unpredictable. May decrease disopyramide effect. |
| Tobacco: | May decrease disopyramide effect. |

# DISULFIRAM

## BRAND NAMES

Antabuse

## BASIC INFORMATION

Habit forming? No
Prescription needed? Yes
Available as generic? Yes
Drug class: None

 **USES**

Treatment for alcoholism. Will not cure alcoholism, but is a powerful deterrent to drinking.

 **DOSAGE & USAGE INFORMATION**

**How to take:**
Tablet or capsule—Swallow with liquid.

**When to take:**
Morning or bedtime. Avoid if you have used *any* alcohol, tonics, cough syrups, fermented vinegar, after-shave lotion or backrub solutions within 12 hours.

**If you forget a dose:**
Take as soon as you remember up to 12 hours late. If more than 12 hours, wait for next scheduled dose (don't double this dose).

**What drug does:**
In combination with alcohol, produces a metabolic change that causes severe, temporary toxicity.

**Time lapse before drug works:**
Immediate.

**Don't take with:**
- See Interaction column and consult doctor.
- Non-prescription drugs that contain *any* alcohol.

 **OVERDOSE**

**SYMPTOMS:**
Memory loss, behavior disturbances, lethargy, confusion and headaches; nausea, vomiting, stomach pain and diarrhea; weakness and unsteady walk; temporary paralysis.
**WHAT TO DO:**
- Dial 0 (operator) or 911 (emergency) for an ambulance or medical help. Then give first aid immediately.
- See emergency information on inside covers.

 **POSSIBLE ADVERSE REACTIONS OR SIDE EFFECTS**

| SYMPTOMS | WHAT TO DO |
|---|---|
| **Life-threatening:** None expected. | |
| **Common:** Drowsiness. | Continue. Tell doctor at next visit. |
| **Infrequent:** | |
| • Eye pain, vision changes, stomach discomfort, throbbing headache, numbness in hands and feet. | Continue. Call doctor when convenient. |
| • Mood change, decreased sexual ability in men, tiredness. | Continue. Tell doctor at next visit. |
| • Bad taste in mouth (metal or garlic). | No action necessary. |
| **Rare:** Rash, jaundice. | Discontinue. Call doctor right away. |

## WARNINGS & PRECAUTIONS

### Don't take if:
- You are allergic to disulfiram (alcohol-disulfiram combination is not an allergic reaction).
- You have used alcohol in any form or amount within 12 hours.
- You have taken paraldehyde within 1 week.
- You have heart disease.

### Before you start, consult your doctor:
- If you have allergies.
- If you plan to become pregnant within medication period.
- If no one has explained to you how disulfiram reacts.
- If you think you cannot avoid drinking.
- If you have diabetes, epilepsy, liver or kidney disease.
- If you take other drugs.

### Over age 60:
Adverse reactions and side effects may be more frequent and severe than in younger persons.

### Pregnancy:
Risk to unborn child outweighs drug benefits. Don't use.

### Breast-feeding:
Studies inconclusive. Consult your doctor.

### Infants & children:
Not recommended.

### Prolonged use:
Periodic blood-cell counts and liver-function tests recommended if you take this drug a long time.

### Skin & sunlight:
No problems expected.

### Driving, piloting or hazardous work:
Avoid if you feel drowsy or have vision side effects. Otherwise, no restrictions.

### Discontinuing:
Don't discontinue without consulting doctor. Dose may require gradual reduction if you have taken drug for a long time. Doses of other drugs may also require adjustment. Avoid alcohol at least 14 days following last dose.

### Others:
No problems expected.

## POSSIBLE INTERACTION WITH OTHER DRUGS

| GENERIC NAME OR DRUG CLASS | COMBINED EFFECT |
|---|---|
| Anticoagulants | Possible unexplained bleeding. |
| Anticonvulsants | Excessive sedation. |
| Barbiturates | Excessive sedation. |
| Cephalosporins | Disulfiram reaction (see Glossary). |
| Isoniazid | Unsteady walk and disturbed behavior. |
| Metronidazole | Disulfiram reaction (see Glossary). |
| Sedatives | Excessive sedation. |

## POSSIBLE INTERACTION WITH OTHER SUBSTANCES

| INTERACTS WITH | COMBINED EFFECT |
|---|---|
| **Alcohol:** *Any* form or amount. | Possible life-threatening toxicity. See disulfiram reaction in Glossary. |
| **Beverages:** Punch or fruit drink that may contain alcohol. | Disulfiram reaction. |
| **Cocaine:** | Increased disulfiram effect. |
| **Foods:** Sauces, fermented vinegar, marinades, desserts or other foods prepared with *any* alcohol. | Disulfiram reaction. |
| **Marijuana:** | None expected. |
| **Tobacco:** | None expected. |

# DIVALPOREX

## BRAND NAMES

Depakote            Epival

## BASIC INFORMATION

**Habit forming? No**
**Prescription needed? Yes**
**Available as generic? No**
**Drug class: Anticonvulsant**

## USES

Controls petit mal (absence) seizures in treatment of epilepsy.

## DOSAGE & USAGE INFORMATION

**How to take:**
Tablet or capsule—Swallow with liquid or food to lessen stomach irritation.

**When to take:**
Once a day.

**If you forget a dose:**
Take as soon as you remember. Don't ever double dose.

**What drug does:**
Increases concentration of gamma aminobutyric acid, which inhibits nerve transmission in parts of brain.

**Time lapse before drug works:**
1 to 4 hours.

**Don't take with:**
See Interaction column and consult doctor.

## OVERDOSE

**SYMPTOMS:**
Coma.
**WHAT TO DO:**
- **Dial 0 (operator) or 911 (emergency) for an ambulance or medical help. Then give first aid immediately.**
- **If patient is unconscious and not breathing, give mouth-to-mouth breathing. If there is no heartbeat, use cardiac massage and mouth-to-mouth breathing (CPR). Don't try to make patient vomit. If you can't get help quickly, take patient to nearest emergency facility.**
- **See emergency information on inside covers.**

## POSSIBLE ADVERSE REACTIONS OR SIDE EFFECTS

| SYMPTOMS | WHAT TO DO |
|---|---|
| **Life-threatening:** None expected. | |
| **Common:** Menstrual irregularities. | Continue. Call doctor when convenient. |
| **Infrequent:** | |
| • Rash, bloody spots under skin, hair loss, bleeding, easy bruising. | Discontinue. Call doctor right away. |
| • Drowsiness, weakness, easily upset emotionally, depression, psychic changes, headache, incoordination, nausea, vomiting, abdominal cramps, appetite change. | Continue. Call doctor when convenient. |
| **Rare:** | |
| • Double vision, unusual movements of eyes (nystagmus). | Discontinue. Call doctor right away. |
| • Anemia. | Continue. Call doctor when convenient. |

## WARNINGS & PRECAUTIONS

**Don't take if:**
You are allergic to divalporex.

**Before you start, consult your doctor:**
- If you have blood, kidney or liver disease.
- If you will have surgery within 2 months, including dental surgery, requiring general or spinal anesthesia.

**Over age 60:**
Adverse reactions and side effects may be more frequent and severe than in younger persons.

**Pregnancy:**
No proven harm to unborn child. Avoid if possible.

**Breast-feeding:**
Unknown effect.

**Infants & children:**
Under close medical supervision only.

**Prolonged use:**
Request periodic blood tests, liver and kidney function tests.

**Skin & sunlight:**
No problems expected.

**Driving, piloting or hazardous work:**
Don't drive or pilot aircraft until you learn how medicine affects you. Don't work around dangerous machinery. Don't climb ladders or work in high places. Danger increases if you drink alcohol or take medicine affecting alertness and reflexes, such as antihistamines, tranquilizers, sedatives, pain medicine, narcotics and mind-altering drugs.

**Discontinuing:**
Don't discontinue without consulting doctor. Dose may require gradual reduction if you have taken drug for a long time. Doses of other drugs may also require adjustment.

**Others:**
No problems expected.

## POSSIBLE INTERACTION WITH OTHER DRUGS

| GENERIC NAME OR DRUG CLASS | COMBINED EFFECT |
|---|---|
| Anticoagulants | Increases chance of bleeding. |
| Aspirin | Increases chance of bleeding. |
| Central nervous system depressants: Antidepressants, antihistamines, narcotics, sedatives, sleeping pills, tranquilizers. | Increases sedative effect. |
| Clonazepam | May prolong seizure. |
| Dypiradamole | Increases chance of bleeding. |
| MAO inhibitors | Increases sedative effect. |
| Phenytoin | Unpredictable. May require increased or decreased dosage. |
| Primidone | Increases chance of toxicity. |
| Sulfinpyrazone | Increases chance of bleeding. |

## POSSIBLE INTERACTION WITH OTHER SUBSTANCES

| INTERACTS WITH | COMBINED EFFECT |
|---|---|
| Alcohol: | Deep sedation. Avoid. |
| Beverages: | No problems expected. |
| Cocaine: | Increased brain sensitivity. Avoid. |
| Foods: | No problems expected. |
| Marijuana: | Increased brain sensitivity. Avoid. |
| Tobacco: | Increased brain sensitivity. Avoid. |

# DOCUSATE CALCIUM

## BRAND NAMES

Dioctocal            Pro-Cal-Sof
Doxidan              Surfak
O-C-S

## BASIC INFORMATION

**Habit forming? No**
**Prescription needed? No**
**Available as generic? Yes**
**Drug class: Laxative (emollient)**

 **USES**

Constipation relief.

 **DOSAGE & USAGE INFORMATION**

**How to take:**
- Tablet or capsule—Swallow with liquid. Don't open capsules.
- Drops—Dilute dose in beverage before swallowing.
- Syrup—Take as directed on bottle.

**When to take:**
At the same time each day, preferably bedtime.

**If you forget a dose:**
Take as soon as you remember. Wait 12 hours for next dose. Return to regular schedule.

**What drug does:**
Makes stool hold fluid so it is easier to pass.

**Time lapse before drug works:**
2 to 3 days of continual use.

**Don't take with:**
- Other medicines at same time. Wait 2 hours.
- See Interaction column and consult doctor.

 **OVERDOSE**

**SYMPTOMS:**
**Appetite loss, nausea, vomiting, diarrhea.**
**WHAT TO DO:**
**Overdose unlikely to threaten life. If person takes much larger amount than prescribed, call doctor, poison-control center or hospital emergency room for instructions.**

 **POSSIBLE ADVERSE REACTIONS OR SIDE EFFECTS**

| SYMPTOMS | WHAT TO DO |
| --- | --- |
| **Life-threatening:**<br>None expected. | |
| **Common:**<br>None expected. | |
| **Infrequent:**<br>Throat irritation (liquid only), intestinal and stomach cramps. | Continue. Call doctor when convenient. |
| **Rare:**<br>Rash. | Discontinue. Call doctor right away. |

## WARNINGS & PRECAUTIONS

**Don't take if:**
- You are allergic to any emollient laxative.
- You have abdominal pain and fever that might be appendicitis.

**Before you start, consult your doctor:**
- If you are taking other laxatives.
- To be sure constipation isn't a sign of a serious disorder.

**Over age 60:**
You must drink 6 to 8 glasses of fluid every 24 hours for drug to work.

**Pregnancy:**
No problems expected. Consult doctor.

**Breast-feeding:**
No problems expected.

**Infants & children:**
No problems expected.

**Prolonged use:**
Avoid. Overuse of laxatives may damage intestine lining.

**Skin & sunlight:**
No problems expected.

**Driving, piloting or hazardous work:**
No problems expected.

**Discontinuing:**
May be unnecessary to finish medicine. Follow doctor's instructions.

**Others:**
No problems expected.

## POSSIBLE INTERACTION WITH OTHER DRUGS

| GENERIC NAME OR DRUG CLASS | COMBINED EFFECT |
| --- | --- |
| Danthron | Possible liver damage. |
| Digitalis preparations | Toxic absorption of digitalis. |
| Mineral oil | Increased mineral oil absorption into bloodstream. Avoid. |
| Phenolphthalein | Increased phenolphthalein absorption. Possible toxicity. |

## POSSIBLE INTERACTION WITH OTHER SUBSTANCES

| INTERACTS WITH | COMBINED EFFECT |
| --- | --- |
| Alcohol: | None expected. |
| Beverages: | None expected. |
| Cocaine: | None expected. |
| Foods: | None expected. |
| Marijuana: | None expected. |
| Tobacco: | None expected. |

# DOCUSATE POTASSIUM

## BRAND NAMES

| | |
|---|---|
| Dialose | Pro-Cal-Sof |
| Kasof | Surfac |

## BASIC INFORMATION

**Habit forming? No**
**Prescription needed? No**
**Available as generic? Yes**
**Drug class: Laxative (emollient)**

 **USES**

Constipation relief.

 **DOSAGE & USAGE INFORMATION**

**How to take:**
- Tablet or capsule—Swallow with liquid. Don't open capsules.
- Drops—Dilute dose in beverage before swallowing.
- Syrup—Take as directed on bottle.

**When to take:**
At the same time each day, preferably bedtime.

**If you forget a dose:**
Take as soon as you remember. Wait 12 hours for next dose. Return to regular schedule.

**What drug does:**
Makes stool hold fluid so it is easier to pass.

**Time lapse before drug works:**
2 to 3 days of continual use.

**Don't take with:**
- Other medicines at same time. Wait 2 hours.
- See Interaction column and consult doctor.

 **OVERDOSE**

**SYMPTOMS:**
Appetite loss, nausea, vomiting, diarrhea.
**WHAT TO DO:**
Overdose unlikely to threaten life. If person takes much larger amount than prescribed, call doctor, poison-control center or hospital emergency room for instructions.

 **POSSIBLE ADVERSE REACTIONS OR SIDE EFFECTS**

| SYMPTOMS | WHAT TO DO |
|---|---|
| **Life-threatening:** None expected. | |
| **Common:** None expected. | |
| **Infrequent:** Throat irritation (liquid only), intestinal and stomach cramps. | Continue. Call doctor when convenient. |
| **Rare:** Rash. | Discontinue. Call doctor right away. |

## WARNINGS & PRECAUTIONS

**Don't take if:**
- You are allergic to any emollient laxative.
- You have abdominal pain and fever that might be appendicitis.

**Before you start, consult your doctor:**
- If you are taking other laxatives.
- To be sure constipation isn't a sign of a serious disorder.

**Over age 60:**
You must drink 6 to 8 glasses of fluid every 24 hours for drug to work.

**Pregnancy:**
No problems expected. Consult doctor.

**Breast-feeding:**
No problems expected.

**Infants & children:**
No problems expected.

**Prolonged use:**
Avoid. Overuse of laxatives may damage intestine lining.

**Skin & sunlight:**
No problems expected.

**Driving, piloting or hazardous work:**
No problems expected.

**Discontinuing:**
May be unnecessary to finish medicine. Follow doctor's instructions.

**Others:**
No problems expected.

## POSSIBLE INTERACTION WITH OTHER DRUGS

| GENERIC NAME OR DRUG CLASS | COMBINED EFFECT |
| --- | --- |
| Danthron | Possible liver damage. |
| Digitalis preparations | Toxic absorption of digitalis. |
| Mineral oil | Increased mineral oil absorption into bloodstream. Avoid. |
| Phenolphthalein | Increased phenolphthalein absorption. Possible toxicity. |

## POSSIBLE INTERACTION WITH OTHER SUBSTANCES

| INTERACTS WITH | COMBINED EFFECT |
| --- | --- |
| Alcohol: | None expected. |
| Beverages: | None expected. |
| Cocaine: | None expected. |
| Foods: | None expected. |
| Marijuana: | None expected. |
| Tobacco: | None expected. |

# DOCUSATE SODIUM

## BRAND NAMES

See complete list of brand names in the *Brand Name Directory,* page 948.

## BASIC INFORMATION

**Habit forming? No**
**Prescription needed? No**
**Available as generic? Yes**
**Drug class: Laxative (emollient)**

 ## USES

Constipation relief.

 ## DOSAGE & USAGE INFORMATION

**How to take:**
- Tablet or capsule—Swallow with liquid. Don't open capsules.
- Drops—Dilute dose in beverage before swallowing.
- Syrup—Take as directed on bottle.

**When to take:**
At the same time each day, preferably bedtime.

**If you forget a dose:**
Take as soon as you remember. Wait 12 hours for next dose. Return to regular schedule.

**What drug does:**
Makes stool hold fluid so it is easier to pass.

**Time lapse before drug works:**
2 to 3 days of continual use.

**Don't take with:**
- Other medicines at same time. Wait 2 hours.
- See Interaction column and consult doctor.

 ## OVERDOSE

**SYMPTOMS:**
**Appetite loss, nausea, vomiting, diarrhea.**
**WHAT TO DO:**
**Overdose unlikely to threaten life. If person takes much larger amount than prescribed, call doctor, poison-control center or hospital emergency room for instructions.**

 ## POSSIBLE ADVERSE REACTIONS OR SIDE EFFECTS

| SYMPTOMS | WHAT TO DO |
|---|---|
| **Life-threatening:** None expected. | |
| **Common:** None expected. | |
| **Infrequent:** Throat irritation (liquid only), intestinal and stomach cramps. | Continue. Call doctor when convenient. |
| **Rare:** Rash. | Discontinue. Call doctor right away. |

## WARNINGS & PRECAUTIONS

**Don't take if:**
- You are allergic to any emollient laxative.
- You have abdominal pain and fever that might be appendicitis.

**Before you start, consult your doctor:**
- If you are taking other laxatives.
- To be sure constipation isn't a sign of a serious disorder.

**Over age 60:**
You must drink 6 to 8 glasses of fluid every 24 hours for drug to work.

**Pregnancy:**
No problems expected. Consult doctor.

**Breast-feeding:**
No problems expected.

**Infants & children:**
No problems expected.

**Prolonged use:**
Avoid. Overuse of laxatives may damage intestine lining.

**Skin & sunlight:**
No problems expected.

**Driving, piloting or hazardous work:**
No problems expected.

**Discontinuing:**
May be unnecessary to finish medicine. Follow doctor's instructions.

**Others:**
No problems expected.

## POSSIBLE INTERACTION WITH OTHER DRUGS

| GENERIC NAME OR DRUG CLASS | COMBINED EFFECT |
|---|---|
| Danthron | Possible liver damage. |
| Digitalis preparations | Toxic absorption of digitalis. |
| Mineral oil | Increased mineral oil absorption into bloodstream. Avoid. |
| Phenolphthalein | Increased phenolphthalein absorption. Possible toxicity. |

## POSSIBLE INTERACTION WITH OTHER SUBSTANCES

| INTERACTS WITH | COMBINED EFFECT |
|---|---|
| Alcohol: | None expected. |
| Beverages: | None expected. |
| Cocaine: | None expected. |
| Foods: | None expected. |
| Marijuana: | None expected. |
| Tobacco: | None expected. |

# DOXYLAMINE

## BRAND NAMES

Bendectin
Cremacoat 4
Decapryn

Unisom Nighttime
Sleep Aid

## BASIC INFORMATION

**Habit forming? No**
**Prescription needed? Yes**
**Available as generic? No**
**Drug class: Antihistamine**

## USES

- Reduces allergic symptoms such as hay fever, hives, rash or itching.
- Prevents motion sickness, nausea, vomiting.
- Induces sleep.

## DOSAGE & USAGE INFORMATION

**How to take:**
Tablet or syrup—Swallow with liquid or food to lessen stomach irritation.

**When to take:**
Varies with form. Follow label directions.

**If you forget a dose:**
Take as soon as you remember up to 2 hours late. If more than 2 hours, wait for next scheduled dose (don't double this dose).

**What drug does:**
Blocks action of histamine after an allergic response triggers histamine release in sensitive cells.

**Time lapse before drug works:**
30 minutes.

*Continued next column*

## OVERDOSE

**SYMPTOMS:**
**Convulsions, red face, hallucinations, coma.**
**WHAT TO DO:**
- **Dial 0 (operator) or 911 (emergency) for an ambulance or medical help. Then give first aid immediately.**
- **If patient is unconscious and not breathing, give mouth-to-mouth breathing. If there is no heartbeat, use cardiac massage and mouth-to-mouth breathing (CPR). Don't try to make patient vomit. If you can't get help quickly, take patient to nearest emergency facility.**
- **See emergency information on inside covers.**

**Don't take with:**
See Interaction column and consult doctor.

## POSSIBLE ADVERSE REACTIONS OR SIDE EFFECTS

| SYMPTOMS | WHAT TO DO |
|---|---|
| **Life-threatening:** None expected. | |
| **Common:** Drowsiness; dizziness; nausea; dry mouth, nose, throat. | Continue. Tell doctor at next visit. |
| **Infrequent:** | |
| • Change in vision. | Discontinue. Call doctor right away. |
| • Less tolerance for contact lenses, difficult urination. | Continue. Call doctor when convenient. |
| • Appetite loss. | Continue. Tell doctor at next visit. |
| **Rare:** Nightmares, agitation, irritability, sore throat, fever, rapid heartbeat, unusual bleeding or bruising, fatigue, weakness. | Discontinue. Call doctor right away. |

## WARNINGS & PRECAUTIONS

**Don't take if:**
You are allergic to any antihistamine.

**Before you start, consult your doctor:**
- If you have glaucoma.
- If you have enlarged prostate.
- If you have asthma.
- If you have kidney disease.
- If you have peptic ulcer.
- If you will have surgery within 2 months, including dental surgery, requiring general or spinal anesthesia.

**Over age 60:**
Don't exceed recommended dose. Adverse reactions and side effects may be more frequent and severe than in younger persons, especially urination difficulty, diminished alertness and other brain and nervous-system symptoms.

**Pregnancy:**
No proven harm to unborn child. Avoid if possible.

**Breast-feeding:**
Drug passes into milk. Avoid drug or discontinue nursing until you finish medicine. Consult doctor for advice on maintaining milk supply.

**Infants & children:**
Not recommended for premature or newborn infants. Otherwise, no problems expected.

**Prolonged use:**
Avoid. May damage bone marrow and nerve cells.

**Skin & sunlight:**
May cause rash or intensify sunburn in areas exposed to sun or sunlamp.

**Driving, piloting or hazardous work:**
Don't drive or pilot aircraft until you learn how medicine affects you. Don't work around dangerous machinery. Don't climb ladders or work in high places. Danger increases if you drink alcohol or take medicine affecting alertness and reflexes, such as antihistamines, tranquilizers, sedatives, pain medicine, narcotics and mind-altering drugs.

**Discontinuing:**
No problems expected.

**Others:**
May mask symptoms of hearing damage from aspirin, other salicylates, cisplatin, paromomycin, vancomycin or anticonvulsants. Consult doctor if you use these.

## POSSIBLE INTERACTION WITH OTHER DRUGS

| GENERIC NAME OR DRUG CLASS | COMBINED EFFECT |
| --- | --- |
| Anticholinergics | Increased anticholinergic effect. |
| Antidepressants | Excess sedation. Avoid. |
| Antihistamines (other) | Excess sedation. Avoid. |
| Dronabinol | Increased effects of both drugs. Avoid. |
| Hypnotics | Excess sedation. Avoid. |
| MAO inhibitors | Increased doxylamine effect. |
| Mind-altering drugs | Excess sedation. Avoid. |
| Molindone | Increased sedative and antihistamine effect. |
| Narcotics | Excess sedation. Avoid. |
| Sedatives | Excess sedation. Avoid. |
| Sleep inducers | Excess sedation. Avoid. |
| Tranquilizers | Excess sedation. Avoid. |

## POSSIBLE INTERACTION WITH OTHER SUBSTANCES

| INTERACTS WITH | COMBINED EFFECT |
| --- | --- |
| Alcohol: | Excess sedation. Avoid. |
| Beverages: Caffeine drinks. | Less doxylamine sedation. |
| Cocaine: | Decreased doxylamine effect. Avoid. |
| Foods: | None expected. |
| Marijuana: | Excess sedation. Avoid. |
| Tobacco: | None expected. |

# DRONABINOL

## BRAND NAMES

**Marinol**

## BASIC INFORMATION

**Habit forming? Yes**
**Prescription needed? Yes**
**Available as generic? No**
**Drug class: Antiemetic**

 ## USES

Prevents nausea and vomiting that may accompany taking anticancer medication (cancer chemotherapy). Should not be used unless other antinausea medicines fail.

 ## DOSAGE & USAGE INFORMATION

**How to take:**
Capsule—Swallow with liquid.

**When to take:**
Under supervision, a total of no more than 4 to 6 doses per day, every 2 to 4 hours after cancer chemotherapy for prescribed number of days.

**If you forget a dose:**
Take as soon as you remember up to 2 hours late. If more than 2 hours, wait for next scheduled dose (don't double this dose).

**What drug does:**
Affects nausea and vomiting center in brain to make it less irritable following cancer chemotherapy. Exact mechanism is unknown.

**Time lapse before drug works:**
2 to 4 hours.

**Don't take with:**
- Non-prescription drugs without consulting doctor.
- Drugs in interaction column without consulting doctor.

 ## OVERDOSE

**SYMPTOMS:**
**Pounding, rapid heart rate; high or low blood pressure; confusion; hallucinations; drastic mood changes; nervousness or anxiety.**
**WHAT TO DO:**
**Overdose unlikely to threaten life. If person takes much larger amount than prescribed, call doctor, poison-control center or hospital emergency room for instructions.**

 ## POSSIBLE ADVERSE REACTIONS OR SIDE EFFECTS

| SYMPTOMS | WHAT TO DO |
|---|---|
| **Life-threatening:** | |
| None expected. | |
| **Common:** | |
| • Rapid, pounding heartbeat. | Discontinue. Call doctor right away. |
| • Dizziness, drowsiness, decreased coordination, euphoria. | Continue. Call doctor when convenient. |
| • Red eyes, dry mouth. | No action necessary. |
| **Infrequent:** | |
| • Depression, nervousness, anxiety, hallucinations, dramatic mood changes. | Discontinue. Call doctor right away. |
| • Blurred or changed vision. | Continue. Call doctor when convenient. |
| **Rare:** | |
| None expected. | |

## WARNINGS & PRECAUTIONS

### Don't take if:
- Your nausea and vomiting is caused by anything other than cancer chemotherapy.
- You are sensitive or allergic to any form of marijuana or sesame oil.
- Your cycle of chemotherapy is longer than 7 consecutive days. Harmful side effects may occur.

### Before you start, consult your doctor:
- If you have heart disease or high blood pressure.
- If you are an alcoholic or drug addict.
- If you are pregnant or intend to become pregnant.
- If you are nursing an infant.
- If you have schizophrenia or a manic-depressive disorder.

### Over age 60:
Adverse reactions and side effects may be more frequent and severe than in younger persons.

### Pregnancy:
No studies in humans. Avoid if possible.

### Breast-feeding:
No studies in humans. Avoid if possible.

### Infants & children:
Not recommended.

### Prolonged use:
Avoid. Habit forming.

### Skin & sunlight:
No problems expected.

### Driving, piloting or hazardous work:
Don't drive or pilot aircraft until you learn how medicine affects you. Don't work around dangerous machinery. Don't climb ladders or work in high places. Danger increases if you drink alcohol or take medicine affecting alertness and reflexes, such as antihistamines, tranquilizers, sedatives, pain medicine, narcotics and mind-altering drugs.

### Discontinuing:
Withdrawal effects such as irritability, insomnia, restlessness, sweating, diarrhea, hiccoughs, loss of appetite and "hot flashes" may follow abrupt withdrawal within 12 hours. These symptoms, should they occur, will probably subside within 96 hours.

### Others:
Store in refrigerator.

## POSSIBLE INTERACTION WITH OTHER DRUGS

| GENERIC NAME OR DRUG CLASS | COMBINED EFFECT |
| --- | --- |
| Anesthetics | Oversedation |
| Anticonvulsants | Oversedation |
| Antidepressants (tricyclics) | Oversedation |
| Antihistamines | Oversedation |
| Barbiturates | Oversedation |
| Molindone | Increased effects of both drugs. Avoid. |
| Muscle relaxants | Oversedation |
| Narcotics | Oversedation |
| Sedatives | Oversedation |
| Tranquilizers | Oversedation |

## POSSIBLE INTERACTION WITH OTHER SUBSTANCES

| INTERACTS WITH | COMBINED EFFECT |
| --- | --- |
| Alcohol: | Oversedation |
| Beverages: | No problems expected. |
| Cocaine: | No problems expected. |
| Foods: | No problems expected. |
| Marijuana: | Oversedation |
| Tobacco: | No problems expected. |

# ENALAPRIL

## BRAND NAMES

Vasotec

## BASIC INFORMATION

**Habit forming?** No
**Prescription needed?** Yes
**Available as generic?** No
**Drug class:** Antihypertensive, A.C.E.
         inhibitor

 **USES**

Treatment for high blood pressure and
congestive heart failure.

 **DOSAGE & USAGE
INFORMATION**

**How to take:**
Tablets—Swallow with liquid. These are
long-acting tablets. Food does not alter normal
absorption from the gastrointestinal tract.

**When to take:**
Usually once a day, sometimes twice a day.
Follow doctor's instructions.

**If you forget a dose:**
Take as soon as you remember up to 8 hours
late. If more than 8 hours, wait for next
scheduled dose (don't double this dose).

**What drug does:**
• Reduces resistance in arteries.
• Strengthens heartbeat.

**Time lapse before drug works:**
60 to 90 minutes.

**Don't take with:**
See Interaction column and consult doctor.

 **OVERDOSE**

**SYMPTOMS:**
**Fever, chills, sore throat, fainting,
convulsions, coma.**
**WHAT TO DO:**
• **Dial 0 (operator) or 911 (emergency) for an
ambulance or medical help. Then give first
aid immediately.**
• **See emergency information on inside
covers.**

 **POSSIBLE
ADVERSE REACTIONS
OR SIDE EFFECTS**

| SYMPTOMS | WHAT TO DO |
|---|---|
| **Life-threatening:** None expected. | |
| **Common:** Rash, loss of taste. | Discontinue. Call doctor right away. |
| **Infrequent:** | |
| • Swelling of face, hands, mouth or feet. | Discontinue. Seek emergency treatment. |
| • Dizziness, fainting, chest pain, fast or irregular heartbeat. | Discontinue. Call doctor right away. |
| **Rare:** | |
| • Sore throat, cloudy urine, fever, chills. | Discontinue. Call doctor right away. |
| • Nausea, vomiting, indigestion, abdominal pain. | Continue. Call doctor when convenient. |

## WARNINGS & PRECAUTIONS

**Don't take if:**
- If you are allergic to enalapril or captopril.
- You have any autoimmune disease, including AIDS or lupus.
- You are receiving blood from a blood bank.
- You take drugs for cancer.
- You will have surgery within 2 months, including dental surgery, requiring general or spinal anesthesia.

**Before you start, consult your doctor:**
- If you have had a stroke.
- If you have angina, heart or blood-vessel disease, a high level of potassium in blood, kidney disease, lupus.
- If you are on severe salt-restricted diet.

**Over age 60:**
Adverse reactions and side effects may be more frequent and severe than in younger persons.

**Pregnancy:**
Risk to unborn child outweighs drug benefits. Don't use.

**Breast-feeding:**
Drug passes into milk. Avoid drug or discontinue nursing until you finish medicine. Consult doctor for advice on maintaining milk supply.

**Infants & children:**
Not recommended.

**Prolonged use:**
May decrease white cells in blood or cause protein loss in urine. Request periodic laboratory blood counts and urine tests.

**Skin & sunlight:**
No problems expected.

**Driving, piloting or hazardous work:**
Avoid if you become dizzy or faint. Otherwise, no problems expected.

**Discontinuing:**
Don't discontinue without consulting doctor. Dose may require gradual reduction if you have taken drug for a long time. Doses of other drugs may also require adjustment.

**Others:**
- Stop taking diuretics or increase salt intake 1 week before starting enalapril.
- Avoid exercising in hot weather.

## POSSIBLE INTERACTION WITH OTHER DRUGS

| GENERIC NAME OR DRUG CLASS | COMBINED EFFECT |
|---|---|
| Acebutolol | Increased antihypertensive effect. Dosage of each may require adjustment. |
| Amiloride | Possible excessive potassium in blood. |
| Antihypertensives (other) | Possible excessive blood-pressure drop. |
| Chloramphenicol | Possible blood disorders. |
| Diuretics | Possible severe blood-pressure drop with first dose. |
| Nitrates | Possible excessive blood-pressure drop. |
| Oxprenolol | Increased antihypertensive effect. Dosage of each may require adjustment. |
| Potassium supplements | Excessive potassium in blood. |
| Spironolactone | Possible excessive potassium in blood. |
| Triamterene | Possible excessive potassium in blood. |

## POSSIBLE INTERACTION WITH OTHER SUBSTANCES

| INTERACTS WITH | COMBINED EFFECT |
|---|---|
| Alcohol: | Possible excessive blood-pressure drop. |
| Beverages: Low-salt milk. | Possible excessive potassium in blood. |
| Cocaine: | Increased dizziness and chest pain. |
| Foods: Salt substitutes. | Possible excessive potassium. |
| Marijuana: | Increased dizziness. |
| Tobacco: | May decrease enalapril effect. |

# ENALAPRIL & HYDROCHLOROTHIAZIDE

## BRAND NAMES

**Vaseretic**

## BASIC INFORMATION

**Habit forming?** No
**Prescription needed?** Yes
**Available as generic?** No
**Drug class:** Antihypertensive, diuretic, A.C.E. inhibitor

## USES

- Treatment for high blood pressure and congestive heart failure.
- Reduces fluid retention.

## DOSAGE & USAGE INFORMATION

**How to take:**
Tablets—Swallow with liquid. These tablets are long-acting. Food does not alter normal absorption from the gastrointestinal tract.

**When to take:**
Usually once a day.

**If you forget a dose:**
Take as soon as you remember up to 18 hours late. If more than 18 hours, wait for next scheduled dose (don't double this dose).

**What drug does:**
- Forces sodium and water excretion, reducing body fluid.
- Relaxes muscle cells of small arteries.
- Reduced body fluid and relaxed arteries lower blood pressure.
- Reduces resistance in arteries.
- Strengthens heartbeat.

**Time lapse before drug works:**
4 to 6 hours. May require several weeks to lower blood pressure.

*Continued next column*

## OVERDOSE

**SYMPTOMS:**
**Cramps, weakness, drowsiness, weak pulse, fever, chills, sore throat, fainting, convulsions, coma.**
**WHAT TO DO:**
- **Dial 0 (operator) or 911 (emergency) for an ambulance or medical help. Then give first aid immediately.**
- **See emergency information on inside covers.**

**Don't take with:**
- Non-prescription drugs without consulting doctor.
- See Interaction column and consult doctor.

## POSSIBLE ADVERSE REACTIONS OR SIDE EFFECTS

| SYMPTOMS | WHAT TO DO |
|---|---|
| **Life-threatening:** | |
| Irregular heartbeat (fast or uneven). | Discontinue. Seek emergency treatment. |
| **Common:** | |
| • Dry mouth, thirst, tiredness, weakness, muscle cramps, vomiting, chest pain, skin rash. | Discontinue. Call doctor right away. |
| • Taste loss, dizziness. | Continue. Call doctor when convenient. |
| **Infrequent:** | |
| • Face, mouth, hands swelling. | Discontinue. Call doctor right away. |
| • Nausea, diarrhea. | Continue. Call doctor when convenient. |

**Rare:**
None expected.

## WARNINGS & PRECAUTIONS

**Don't take if:**
- You are allergic to enalapril, captopril, or any thiazide diuretic drug.
- You have any autoimmune disease, including AIDS or lupus.
- You are receiving blood from a blood bank.
- You take drugs for cancer.
- If you will have surgery within 2 months, including dental surgery, requiring general or spinal anesthesia.

**Before you start, consult your doctor:**
- If you have had a stroke.
- If you have angina, heart or blood-vessel disease, a high level of potassium in blood, lupus, gout, liver, pancreas or kidney disorder.
- If you are on a severe salt-restricted diet.
- If you are allergic to any sulfa drug.

**Over age 60:**
Adverse reactions and side effects may be more frequent and severe than in younger persons, especially dizziness and excessive potassium loss.

**Pregnancy:**
Risk to unborn child outweighs drug benefits. Don't use.

**Breast-feeding:**
Drug passes into milk. Avoid drug or discontinue nursing until you finish medicine. Consult doctor for advice on maintaining milk supply.

**Infants & children:**
Not recommended.

**Prolonged use:**
May decrease white cells in blood or cause protein loss in urine. Request periodic laboratory blood counts and urine tests.

**Skin & sunlight:**
May cause rash or intensify sunburn in areas exposed to sun or sunlamp.

**Driving, piloting or hazardous work:**
Don't drive or pilot aircraft until you learn how medicine affects you. Don't work around dangerous machinery. Don't climb ladders or work in high places. Danger increases if you drink alcohol or take medicine affecting alertness and reflexes, such as antihistamines, tranquilizers, sedatives, pain medicine, narcotics and mind-altering drugs.

**Discontinuing:**
Don't discontinue without consulting doctor. Dose may require gradual reduction if you have taken drug for a long time. Doses of other drugs may also require adjustment.

**Others:**
- Hot weather and fever may cause dehydration and drop in blood pressure. Dose may require temporary adjustment. Weigh daily and report any unexpected weight decreases to your doctor.
- May cause rise in uric acid, leading to gout.
- May cause blood-sugar rise in diabetics.

 POSSIBLE INTERACTION
WITH OTHER DRUGS

| GENERIC NAME OR DRUG CLASS | COMBINED EFFECT |
|---|---|
| Acebutolol | Increased antihypertensive effect Dosages of both drugs may require adjustments. |
| Allopurinol | Decreased allopurinol effect. |
| Amiloride | Possible excessive potassium in blood. |
| Antidepressants (tricyclic) | Dangerous drop in blood pressure. Avoid combination unless under medical supervision. |
| Antihypertensives (other) | Possible excessive blood-pressure drop. |

| | |
|---|---|
| Barbiturates | Increased hydrochlorothiazide effect. |
| Chloramphenicol | Possible blood disorders. |
| Cholestyramine | Decreased hydrochlorothiazide effect. |
| Cortisone drugs | Excessive potassium loss that causes dangerous heart rhythms. |
| Digitalis preparations | Excessive potassium loss that causes dangerous heart rhythms. |
| Diuretics (thiazide) | Increased effect of other thiazide diuretics. |
| Indapamide | Increased diuretic effect. |
| Lithium | Increased effect of lithium. |
| MAO inhibitors | Increased hydrochlorothiazide effect. |
| Nitrates | Excessive blood-pressure drop. |
| Oxprenolol | Increased antihypertensive effect. Dosages of both drugs may require adjustments. |

*Continued page 965*

 POSSIBLE INTERACTION
WITH OTHER SUBSTANCES

| INTERACTS WITH | COMBINED EFFECT |
|---|---|
| Alcohol: | Dangerous blood-pressure drop. Avoid. |
| Beverages: Low-salt milk. | Possible excessive potassium in blood. |
| Cocaine: | Increased dizziness, chest pain. |
| Foods: Salt substitutes. | Possible excessive potassium. |
| Marijuana: | Increased dizziness, may increase blood pressure. |
| Tobacco: | May decrease enalapril effect. |

# EPHEDRINE

## BRAND NAMES

See complete list of brand names in the *Brand Name Directory,* page 948.

## BASIC INFORMATION

**Habit forming? No**
**Prescription needed?**
  **Low strength: No**
  **High strength: Yes**
**Available as generic? Yes**
**Drug class: Sympathomimetic**

## USES

- Relieves bronchial asthma.
- Decreases congestion of breathing passages.
- Suppresses allergic reactions.

## DOSAGE & USAGE INFORMATION

**How to take:**
- Tablet or capsule—Swallow with liquid. You may chew or crush tablet.
- Extended-release tablets or capsules—Swallow each dose whole.
- Syrup—Take as directed on bottle.
- Drops—Dilute dose in beverage.

**When to take:**
As needed, no more often than every 4 hours.

**If you forget a dose:**
Take up to 2 hours late. If more than 2 hours, wait for next dose (don't double this dose).

**What drug does:**
- Prevents cells from releasing allergy-causing chemicals (histamines).
- Relaxes muscles of bronchial tubes.
- Decreases blood-vessel size and blood flow, thus causing decongestion.

**Time lapse before drug works:**
30 to 60 minutes.

*Continued next column*

## OVERDOSE

**SYMPTOMS:**
**Severe anxiety, confusion, delirium, muscle tremors, rapid and irregular pulse.**
**WHAT TO DO:**
- **Dial 0 (operator) or 911 (emergency) for an ambulance or medical help. Then give first aid immediately.**
- **See emergency information on inside covers.**

**Don't take with:**
- See Interaction column and consult doctor.
- Non-prescription drugs with ephedrine, pseudoephedrine or epinephrine.
- Non-prescription drugs for cough, cold, allergy or asthma without consulting doctor.

## POSSIBLE ADVERSE REACTIONS OR SIDE EFFECTS

| SYMPTOMS | WHAT TO DO |
|---|---|
| **Life-threatening:** None expected. | |
| **Common:** | |
| • Nervousness, headache, paleness, rapid heartbeat. | Continue. Call doctor when convenient. |
| • Insomnia. | Continue. Tell doctor at next visit. |
| **Infrequent:** | |
| • Irregular heartbeat. | Discontinue. Call doctor right away. |
| • Dizziness, appetite loss, nausea, vomiting, painful or difficult urination. | Continue. Call doctor when convenient. |
| **Rare:** None expected. | |

## WARNINGS & PRECAUTIONS

**Don't take if:**
You are allergic to ephedrine or any sympathomimetic drug.

**Before you start, consult your doctor:**
- If you have high blood pressure.
- If you have diabetes.
- If you have overactive thyroid gland.
- If you have difficulty urinating.
- If you have taken any MAO inhibitor in past 2 weeks
- If you have taken digitalis preparations in the last 7 days.
- If you will have surgery within 2 months, including dental surgery, requiring general or spinal anesthesia.

**Over age 60:**
More likely to develop high blood pressure, heart-rhythm disturbances, angina and to feel drug's stimulant effects.

**Pregnancy:**
No proven harm to unborn child. Avoid if possible.

**Breast-feeding:**
Drug passes into milk. Avoid drug or discontinue nursing until you finish medicine. Consult doctor for advice on maintaining milk supply.

**Infants & children:**
No problems expected.

**Prolonged use:**
- Excessive doses—Rare toxic psychosis.
- Men with enlarged prostate gland may have more urination difficulty.

**Skin & sunlight:**
No problems expected.

**Driving, piloting or hazardous work:**
Avoid if you feel dizzy. Otherwise, no problems expected.

**Discontinuing:**
May be unnecessary to finish medicine. Follow doctor's instructions.

**Others:**
No problems expected.

## POSSIBLE INTERACTION WITH OTHER DRUGS

| GENERIC NAME OR DRUG CLASS | COMBINED EFFECT |
|---|---|
| Albuterol | Increased effect of both drugs, especially harmful side effects. |
| Antidepressants (tricyclic) | Increased effect of ephedrine. Excessive stimulation of heart and blood pressure. |
| Antihypertensives | Decreased antihypertensive effect. |
| Beta-adrenergic blockers | Decreased effects of both drugs. |
| Digitalis preparations | Serious heart-rhythm disturbances. |
| Epinephrine | Increased epinephrine effect. |
| Ergot preparations | Serious blood-pressure rise. |
| Guanethidine | Decreased effect of both drugs. |
| MAO inhibitors | Increased ephedrine effect. Dangerous blood-pressure rise. |
| Nitrates | Possible decreased effects of both drugs. |
| Pseudoephedrine | Increased pseudoephedrine effect. |

## POSSIBLE INTERACTION WITH OTHER SUBSTANCES

| INTERACTS WITH | COMBINED EFFECT |
|---|---|
| Alcohol: | None expected. |
| Beverages: Caffeine drinks. | Nervousness or insomnia. |
| Cocaine: | Rapid heartbeat. Avoid. |
| Foods: | None expected. |
| Marijuana: | Rapid heartbeat, possible heart-rhythm disturbance. |
| Tobacco: | None expected. |

# EPINEPHRINE

## BRAND NAMES

See complete list of brand names in the *Brand Name Directory*, page 948.

## BASIC INFORMATION

**Habit forming?** No
**Prescription needed?** Yes
**Available as generic?**
　Nose drops, aerosol inhaler—No
　Eye drops, injection—Yes
**Drug class:** Sympathomimetic, antiglaucoma

 **USES**

- Relieves allergic symptoms of anaphylaxis.
- Eases symptoms of acute bronchial spasms.
- Relieves congestion of nose, sinuses and throat.
- Reduces internal eye pressure.

 **DOSAGE & USAGE INFORMATION**

**How to take:**
Eyedrops, nose drops, aerosol inhaler, injection—Use as directed on labels.

**When to take:**
As needed, no more often than label directs.

**If you forget a dose:**
If needed, take when you remember. Wait 3 hours for next dose.

**What drug does:**
- Contracts blood-vessel walls and raises blood pressure.
- Inhibits release of histamine.
- Dilates constricted bronchial tubes and decreases volume of blood in nasal tissue.
- Reduces fluid formation within the eye.

**Time lapse before drug works:**
1 to 2 minutes.

*Continued next column*

 **OVERDOSE**

**SYMPTOMS:**
**Tremor, rapid breathing, palpitations, extreme rise in blood pressure, irregular heartbeat, breathing difficulty, convulsions, coma.**
**WHAT TO DO:**
- **Dial 0 (operator) or 911 (emergency) for an ambulance or medical help. Then give first aid immediately.**
- **See emergency information on inside covers.**

**Don't take with:**
- Non-prescription drugs without consulting doctor.
- See Interaction column and consult doctor.

 **POSSIBLE ADVERSE REACTIONS OR SIDE EFFECTS**

| SYMPTOMS | WHAT TO DO |
|---|---|
| **Life-threatening:** | |
| None expected. | |
| **Common:** | |
| • Headache, agitation, dizziness, insomnia, fast or pounding heartbeat. | Continue. Call doctor when convenient. |
| • Dry mouth and throat (inhaler only). | Continue. Tell doctor at next visit. |
| **Infrequent:** | |
| • Difficult breathing. | Discontinue. Call doctor right away. |
| • Shakiness, nausea, vomiting, cough or bronchial irritation (inhaler only), weakness, flushed face or redness. | Continue. Call doctor when convenient. |
| **Rare:** | |
| Chest pain, irregular heartbeat, sweating. | Discontinue. Call doctor right away. |

 **WARNINGS & PRECAUTIONS**

**Don't take if:**
- You are allergic to any sympathomimetic.
- You have narrow-angle glaucoma.
- You have had a stroke or heart attack within 3 weeks.
- You have heart-rhythm disturbance.

**Before you start, consult your doctor:**
- If you have high blood pressure, heart disease or have had a stroke.
- If you have diabetes.
- If you have overactive thyroid.

**Over age 60:**
- Use with caution if you have hardening of the arteries.
- If you have enlarged prostate, drug may increase urination difficulty.
- If you have Parkinson's disease, drug may temporarily increase rigidity and tremor.
- If you see "floaters" in field of vision, tell your doctor.

**Pregnancy:**
No proven harm to unborn child. Avoid if possible.

**Breast-feeding:**
Drug passes into milk. Avoid drug or discontinue nursing until you finish medicine. Consult doctor for advice on maintaining milk supply.

**Infants & children:**
Use only under medical supervision.

**Prolonged use:**
- You may stop responding to drug.
- Drug may reduce blood volume.
- Drug may damage eye retina and impair vision.

**Skin & sunlight:**
No problems expected.

**Driving, piloting or hazardous work:**
No problems expected. Use caution if you feel dizzy or nervous.

**Discontinuing:**
- May be unnecessary to finish medicine. Follow doctor's instructions.
- If drug fails to provide relief after several doses, discontinue. Don't increase dose or frequency.

**Others:**
- May temporarily raise blood sugar in diabetics.
- Excessive use can cause sudden death.
- Discard medicine if cloudy or discolored.

## POSSIBLE INTERACTION WITH OTHER DRUGS

| GENERIC NAME OR DRUG CLASS | COMBINED EFFECT |
|---|---|
| Acebutolol | Decreased effects of both drugs. |
| Albuterol | Increased effect of both drugs, especially harmful side effects. |
| Antidepressants (tricyclic) | Increased epinephrine effect. |
| Antidiabetics (oral) | Decreased antidiabetic effect. |
| Antihistamines | Increased epinephrine effect. |
| Beta-adrenergic blockers | Decreased epinephrine effect. |
| Carbonic anhydrase inhibitors | Increased epinephrine effect. |
| Digitalis preparations | Possible irregular heartbeat. |
| Ephedrine | Increased ephedrine effect. |
| Guanethidine | Decreased guanethidine effect. |

| | |
|---|---|
| Insulin | Decreased insulin effect. |
| Isoproterenol | Dangerous to heart. |
| MAO inhibitors | Dangerous to heart. |
| Minoxidil | Decreased minoxidil effect. |
| Nitrates | Possible decreased effects of both drugs. |
| Oxprenolol | Decreased effects of both drugs. |
| Pilocarpine | Increased pilocarpine effect. |
| Rauwolfia alkaloids | Increased epinephrine effect. |
| Thyroid preparations | Increased epinephrine effect. |

## POSSIBLE INTERACTION WITH OTHER SUBSTANCES

| INTERACTS WITH | COMBINED EFFECT |
|---|---|
| Alcohol: | May increase urinary excretion of drug and reduce effectiveness. |
| Beverages: | None expected. |
| Cocaine: | Dangerous overstimulation. Avoid. |
| Foods: | None expected. |
| Marijuana: | Increase in epinephrine's antiasthmatic effect. |
| Tobacco: | None expected. |

# ERGOLOID MESYLATES

## BRAND NAMES

Circanol
Deapril-ST
Dihydrogenated
  Ergot Alkaloids

Hydergine
Hydergine LC
Trigot

## BASIC INFORMATION

Habit forming? No
Prescription needed? Yes
Available as generic? No
Drug class: Ergot preparation

## USES

Treatment for reduced alertness, poor memory, confusion, depression or lack of motivation in the elderly.

## DOSAGE & USAGE INFORMATION

**How to take:**
- Tablet or capsule—Swallow with liquid. If you can't swallow whole, crumble tablet or open capsule and take with liquid or food.
- Liquid—Take as directed on label.
- Sublingual tablets—Dissolve tablet under tongue.

**When to take:**
At the same times each day.

**If you forget a dose:**
Take as soon as you remember up to 2 hours late. If more than 2 hours, wait for next scheduled dose (don't double this dose).

**What drug does:**
Stimulates brain-cell metabolism to increase use of oxygen and nutrients.

**Time lapse before drug works:**
Gradual improvements over 3 to 4 months.

*Continued next column*

## OVERDOSE

**SYMPTOMS:**
**Headache, flushed face, nasal congestion, nausea, vomiting, blood-pressure drop, weakness, collapse, coma.**
**WHAT TO DO:**
- **Dial 0 (operator) or 911 (emergency) for an ambulance or medical help. Then give first aid immediately.**
- **See emergency information on inside covers.**

**Don't take with:**
- Non-prescription drugs containing alcohol without consulting doctor.
- See Interaction column and consult doctor.

## POSSIBLE ADVERSE REACTIONS OR SIDE EFFECTS

| SYMPTOMS | WHAT TO DO |
|---|---|
| **Life-threatening:** None expected. | |
| **Common:** Runny nose. | Continue. Tell doctor at next visit. |
| **Infrequent:** | |
| • Slow heartbeat, tingling fingers. | Discontinue. Call doctor right away. |
| • Nervousness, hostility, confusion, depression, blurred vision. | Continue. Call doctor when convenient. |
| **Rare:** | |
| • Fainting. | Discontinue. Seek emergency treatment. |
| • Rash, nausea, vomiting, stomach cramps. | Discontinue. Call doctor right away. |
| • Dizziness when getting up, drowsiness, soreness under tongue, appetite loss, fever. | Continue. Call doctor when convenient. |

## WARNINGS & PRECAUTIONS

**Don't use if:**
- If you are allergic to any ergot preparation.
- Your heartbeat is less than 60 beats per minute.
- Your systolic blood pressure is consistently below 100.

**Before you start, consult your doctor:**
If you have had low blood pressure.

**Over age 60:**
Primarily used in persons older than 60. Results unpredictable, but many patients show improved brain function.

**Pregnancy:**
Not recommended.

**Breast-feeding:**
Risk to nursing child outweighs drug benefits. Don't use.

**Infants & children:**
Not recommended.

**Prolonged use:**
No problems expected.

**Skin & sunlight:**
No problems expected.

**Driving, piloting or hazardous work:**
Avoid if you feel dizzy, faint or have blurred vision. Otherwise, no problems expected.

**Discontinuing:**
No problems expected.

**Others:**
No problems expected.

## POSSIBLE INTERACTION WITH OTHER DRUGS

| GENERIC NAME OR DRUG CLASS | COMBINED EFFECT |
|---|---|
| Antihypertensives | Increased antihypertensive effect. |
| Beta-adrenergic blockers | Excessive decrease in heartbeat and/or blood pressure. |
| Digitalis preparations | Excessively slow heartbeat. |

## POSSIBLE INTERACTION WITH OTHER SUBSTANCES

| INTERACTS WITH | COMBINED EFFECT |
|---|---|
| Alcohol: | Use caution. May drop blood pressure excessively. |
| Beverages: | None expected. |
| Cocaine: | Overstimulation. Avoid. |
| Foods: | None expected. |
| Marijuana: | Decreased effect of ergot alkaloids. |
| Tobacco: | None expected. |

# ERGONOVINE

## BRAND NAMES

Ergometrine          Ergotrate

## BASIC INFORMATION

**Habit forming?** No
**Prescription needed?** Yes
**Available as generic?** Yes
**Drug class:** Ergot preparation (uterine stimulant)

 ## USES

Retards excessive post-delivery bleeding.

 ## DOSAGE & USAGE INFORMATION

**How to take:**
Tablet—Swallow with liquid or food to lessen stomach irritation.

**When to take:**
At the same times each day.

**If you forget a dose:**
Don't take missed dose and don't double next one. Wait for next scheduled dose.

**What drug does:**
Causes smooth-muscle cells of uterine wall to contract and surround bleeding blood vessels of relaxed uterus.

**Time lapse before drug works:**
Tablets—20 to 30 minutes.

**Don't take with:**
See Interaction column and consult doctor.

 ## OVERDOSE

**SYMPTOMS:**
Vomiting, diarrhea, weak pulse, low blood pressure, convulsions.
**WHAT TO DO:**
- **Dial 0 (operator) or 911 (emergency) for an ambulance or medical help. Then give first aid immediately.**
- **If patient is unconscious and not breathing, give mouth-to-mouth breathing. If there is no heartbeat, use cardiac massage and mouth-to-mouth breathing (CPR). Don't try to make patient vomit. If you can't get help quickly, take patient to nearest emergency facility.**
- **See emergency information on inside covers.**

 ## POSSIBLE ADVERSE REACTIONS OR SIDE EFFECTS

| SYMPTOMS | WHAT TO DO |
|---|---|
| **Life-threatening:**<br>None expected. | |
| **Common:**<br>Nausea, vomiting. | Discontinue. Call doctor right away. |
| **Infrequent:**<br>• Confusion, ringing in ears, diarrhea, muscle cramps. | Discontinue. Call doctor right away. |
| • Unusual sweating. | Continue. Call doctor when convenient. |
| **Rare:**<br>Sudden, severe headache; shortness of breath; chest pain; numb, cold hands and feet. | Discontinue. Seek emergency treatment. |

# ERGONOVINE

## WARNINGS & PRECAUTIONS

**Don't take if:**
You are allergic to any ergot preparation.

**Before you start, consult your doctor:**
- If you have coronary-artery or blood-vessel disease.
- If you have liver or kidney disease.
- If you have high blood pressure.
- If you have postpartum infection.

**Over age 60:**
Not recommended.

**Pregnancy:**
Risk to unborn child outweighs drug benefits. Don't use.

**Breast-feeding:**
Drug passes into milk. Avoid drug or discontinue nursing until you finish medicine. Consult doctor for advice on maintaining milk supply.

**Infants & children:**
Not recommended.

**Prolonged use:**
Not recommended.

**Skin & sunlight:**
No problems expected.

**Driving, piloting or hazardous work:**
No problems expected.

**Discontinuing:**
May be unnecessary to finish medicine. Follow doctor's instructions.

**Others:**
Drug should be used for short time only following childbirth or miscarriage.

## POSSIBLE INTERACTION WITH OTHER DRUGS

| GENERIC NAME OR DRUG CLASS | COMBINED EFFECT |
| --- | --- |
| Ergot preparations (other) | Increased ergonovine effect. |

## POSSIBLE INTERACTION WITH OTHER SUBSTANCES

| INTERACTS WITH | COMBINED EFFECT |
| --- | --- |
| Alcohol: | None expected. |
| Beverages: | None expected. |
| Cocaine: | None expected. |
| Foods: | None expected. |
| Marijuana: | None expected. |
| Tobacco: | None expected. |

# ERGOTAMINE

## BRAND NAMES

| | |
|---|---|
| Cafetrate-PB | Migral |
| Ergomar | Migrastat |
| Ergostat | Wigraine |
| Gynergen | Wigraine-PB |
| Medihaler-Ergotamine | Wigrettes |
| Migraine | |

## BASIC INFORMATION

**Habit forming? No**
**Prescription needed? Yes**
**Available as generic? Yes**
**Drug class: Vasoconstrictor,**
**ergot preparation**

## USES

Relieves pain of migraines and other headaches caused by dilated blood vessels. Will not prevent headaches.

## DOSAGE & USAGE INFORMATION

**How to take:**
- Tablet or capsule—Swallow with liquid, or let dissolve under tongue. If you can't swallow whole, crumble tablet or open capsule and take with liquid or food.
- Suppositories—Remove wrapper and moisten suppository with water. Gently insert larger end into rectum. Push well into rectum with finger.
- Aerosol inhaler—Use only as directed on prescription label.
- Lie down in quiet, dark room after taking.

**When to take:**
At first sign of vascular or migraine headache.

*Continued next column*

## OVERDOSE

**SYMPTOMS:**
**Tingling, cold extremities and muscle pain.**
**Progresses to nausea, vomiting, diarrhea,**
**cold skin, rapid and weak pulse, severe**
**numbness of extremities, confusion,**
**convulsions, coma.**
**WHAT TO DO:**
- **Dial 0 (operator) or 911 (emergency) for an ambulance or medical help. Then give first aid immediately.**
- **See emergency information on inside covers.**

**If you forget a dose:**
Take as soon as you remember. Wait 4 hours for next dose.

**What drug does:**
Constricts blood vessels in the head.

**Time lapse before drug works:**
30 to 60 minutes.

**Don't take with:**
See Interaction column and consult doctor.

## POSSIBLE ADVERSE REACTIONS OR SIDE EFFECTS

| SYMPTOMS | WHAT TO DO |
|---|---|
| **Life-threatening:**<br>None expected. | |
| **Common:**<br>Dizziness, nausea, diarrhea, vomiting. | Continue. Call doctor when convenient. |
| **Infrequent:**<br>Itchy or swollen skin; cold, pale hands or feet; pain or weakness in arms, legs, back. | Discontinue. Call doctor right away. |
| **Rare:**<br>Anxiety or confusion; red or purple blisters, especially on hands, feet; change in vision; extreme thirst; stomach pain or bloating; unusually fast or slow heartbeat; possible chest pain; numbness or tingling in face, fingers, toes. | Discontinue. Call doctor right away. |

## WARNINGS & PRECAUTIONS

**Don't take if:**
You are allergic to any ergot preparation.

**Before you start, consult your doctor:**
- If you plan to become pregnant within medication period.
- If you have an infection.
- If you have angina, heart problems, high blood pressure, hardening of the arteries or vein problems.
- If you have kidney or liver disease.
- If you are allergic to other spray inhalants.

**Over age 60:**
Adverse reactions and side effects may be more frequent and severe than in younger persons.

**Pregnancy:**
Risk to unborn child outweighs drug benefits. Don't use.

**Breast-feeding:**
Drug filters into milk. May harm child. Avoid.

**Infants & children:**
Studies inconclusive on harm to children. Consult your doctor.

**Prolonged use:**
Cold skin, muscle pain, gangrene of hands and feet. This medicine not intended for uninterrupted use.

**Skin & sunlight:**
No problems expected.

**Driving, piloting or hazardous work:**
Don't drive or pilot aircraft until you learn how medicine affects you. Don't work around dangerous machinery. Don't climb ladders or work in high places. Danger increases if you drink alcohol or take medicine affecting alertness and reflexes, such as antihistamines, tranquilizers, sedatives, pain medicine, narcotics and mind-altering drugs.

**Discontinuing:**
May be unnecessary to finish medicine. Follow doctor's instructions.

**Others:**
Impaired blood circulation can lead to gangrene in intestines or extremities. Never exceed recommended dose.

## POSSIBLE INTERACTION WITH OTHER DRUGS

| GENERIC NAME OR DRUG CLASS | COMBINED EFFECT |
|---|---|
| Amphetamines | Dangerous blood-pressure rise. |
| Ephedrine | Dangerous blood-pressure rise. |
| Epinephrine | Dangerous blood-pressure rise. |
| Pseudoephedrine | Dangerous blood-pressure rise. |
| Troleandomycin | Increased adverse reactions of ergotamine. |

## POSSIBLE INTERACTION WITH OTHER SUBSTANCES

| INTERACTS WITH | COMBINED EFFECT |
|---|---|
| Alcohol: | Dilates blood vessels. Makes headache worse. |
| Beverages: Caffeine drinks. | May help relieve headache. |
| Cocaine: | Decreased ergotamine effect. |
| Foods: Any to which you are allergic. | May make headache worse. Avoid. |
| Marijuana: | Occasional use—Cool extremities. Regular use— Persistent chill. |
| Tobacco: | Decreased effect of ergotamine. Makes headache worse. |

# ERGOTAMINE, BELLADONNA & PHENOBARBITAL

## BRAND NAMES

Bellergal                Bellergal-S

## BASIC INFORMATION

**Habit forming?** Yes
**Prescription needed?** Yes
**Available as generic?** No
**Drug class:** Analgesic, antispasmodic, vasoconstrictor

## USES

Reduces anxiety or nervous tension (low dose).

## DOSAGE & USAGE INFORMATION

**How to take:**
- Tablet or capsule—Swallow with liquid, or let dissolve under tongue. If you can't swallow whole, crumble tablet or open capsule and take with liquid or food.
- Suppositories—Remove wrapper and moisten suppository with water. Gently insert larger end into rectum. Push well into rectum with finger.
- Lie down in quiet, dark room after taking.

**When to take:**
At first sign of vascular or migraine headache.

**If you forget a dose:**
Take as soon as you remember. Wait 4 hours for next dose.

**What drug does:**
- Constricts blood vessels in the head.

*Continued next column*

## OVERDOSE

**SYMPTOMS:**
**Tingling, cold extremities; muscle pain; nausea; vomiting; diarrhea; cold skin; rapid and weak pulse; severe numbness of extremities; confusion; dilated pupils; rapid pulse and breathing; dizziness; fever; hallucinations; slurred speech; agitation; flushed face; convulsions; coma.**
**WHAT TO DO:**
- **Dial 0 (operator) or 911 (emergency) for an ambulance or medical help. Then give first aid immediately.**
- **See emergency information on inside covers.**

- Blocks nerve impulses at parasympathetic nerve endings, preventing muscle contractions and gland secretions of organs involved.

**Time lapse before drug works:**
15 to 30 minutes.

**Don't take with:**
Non-prescription drugs without consulting doctor.

## POSSIBLE ADVERSE REACTIONS OR SIDE EFFECTS

| SYMPTOMS | WHAT TO DO |
|---|---|
| **Life-threatening:** | |
| Fast heartbeat, chest pain. | Discontinue. Seek emergency treatment. |
| **Common:** | |
| • Flushed skin, fever, drowsiness, depression, bloating, frequent urination. | Discontinue. Call doctor right away. |
| • Constipation, dizziness, drowsiness, "hangover" effect. | Continue. Call doctor when convenient. |
| **Infrequent:** | |
| Swollen feet and ankles, numbness or tingling in hands or feet, cold hands and feet, rash. | Discontinue. Call doctor right away. |
| **Rare:** | |
| Jaundice, weak legs, swallowing difficulty, dry mouth, increased sensitivity to sunlight, nausea, vomiting, decreased sweating. | Discontinue. Call doctor right away. |

## WARNINGS & PRECAUTIONS

**Don't take if:**
- You are allergic to any barbiturate, anticholinergic or ergot preparation.
- You have porphyria, trouble with stomach bloating, difficulty emptying your bladder completely, narrow-angle glaucoma, severe ulcerative colitis.

## Before you start, consult your doctor:
- If you have epilepsy, kidney or liver damage, anemia, chronic pain, open-angle glaucoma, angina, heart problems, high blood pressure, hardening of the arteries, vein problems, chronic bronchitis, asthma, hiatal hernia, enlarged prostate, myasthenia gravis, peptic ulcer, an infection.
- If you plan to become pregnant within medication period.
- If you will have surgery within 2 months, including dental surgery, requiring general or spinal anesthesia.

## Over age 60:
Adverse reactions and side effects may be more frequent and severe than in younger persons.

## Pregnancy:
Risk to unborn child outweighs drug benefits. Don't use.

## Breast-feeding:
Drug passes into milk. Avoid drug or discontinue nursing until you finish medicine. Consult doctor for advice on maintaining milk supply.

## Infants & children:
Not recommended.

## Prolonged use:
- May cause addiction, anemia, chronic intoxication.
- May lower body temperature, making exposure to cold temperatures hazardous.
- Chronic constipation, possible fecal impaction.
- Cold skin, muscle pain, gangrene of hands and feet. This medicine not intended for uninterrupted use.

## Skin & sunlight:
May cause rash or intensify sunburn in areas exposed to sun or sunlamp.

## Driving, piloting or hazardous work:
Don't drive or pilot aircraft until you learn how medicine affects you. Don't work around dangerous machinery. Don't climb ladders or work in high places. Danger increases if you drink alcohol or take medicine affecting alertness and reflexes, such as antihistamines, tranquilizers, sedatives, pain medicine, narcotics and mind-altering drugs.

## Discontinuing:
May be unnecessary to finish medicine. Follow doctor's instructions. If you develop withdrawal symptoms of hallucinations, agitation or sleeplessness after discontinuing, call doctor right away.

## Others:
Impaired blood circulation can lead to gangrene in intestines or extremities. Never exceed recommended dose.

 ## POSSIBLE INTERACTION WITH OTHER DRUGS

| GENERIC NAME OR DRUG CLASS | COMBINED EFFECT |
| --- | --- |
| Amantadine | Increased belladonna effect. |
| Amphetamines | Dangerous blood-pressure rise. |
| Anticholinergics (other) | Increased belladonna effect. |
| Anticoagulants (oral) | Decreased anticoagulant effect. |
| Anticonvulsants | Changed seizure patterns. |
| Antidepressants (tricyclics) | Decreased antidepressant effect. Possible dangerous oversedation. |
| Antidiabetics (oral) | Increased phenobarbital effect. |
| Antihistamines | Dangerous sedation. Avoid. |
| Anti-inflammatory drugs (non-steroidal) | Decreased anti-inflammatory effect. |
| Aspirin | Decreased aspirin effect. |
| Beta-adrenergic blockers | Decreased effect of beta-adrenergic blocker. |

*Continued page 965*

 ## POSSIBLE INTERACTION WITH OTHER SUBSTANCES

| INTERACTS WITH | COMBINED EFFECT |
| --- | --- |
| Alcohol: | Possible fatal oversedation. Avoid. |
| Beverages: | None expected. |
| Cocaine: | Excessively rapid heartbeat. Avoid. |
| Foods: | None expected. |
| Marijuana: | Drowsiness and dry mouth, excessive sedation. Avoid. |
| Tobacco: | None expected. |

# ERGOTAMINE & CAFFEINE

## BRAND NAMES

Cafergot
Cafertabs
Cafetrate

Ercaf
Ercatabs
Ergo-Caff

## BASIC INFORMATION

**Habit forming? No**
**Prescription needed? Yes**
**Available as generic? No**
**Drug class: Analgesic, stimulant (xanthine)**
**vasoconstrictor**

## USES

Relieves pain of migraines and other headaches caused by dilated blood vessels. Will not prevent headaches.

## DOSAGE & USAGE INFORMATION

**How to take:**
- Tablet or capsule—Swallow with liquid, or let dissolve under tongue. If you can't swallow whole, crumble tablet or open capsule and take with liquid or food.
- Suppositories—Remove wrapper and moisten suppository with water. Gently insert larger end into rectum. Push well into rectum with finger.
- Extended-release capsules—Swallow whole with liquid.
- Lie down in quiet, dark room after taking.

**When to take:**
At first sign of vascular or migraine headache.

**If you forget a dose:**
Take as soon as you remember up to 2 hours late. If more than 2 hours, wait for next scheduled dose (don't double this dose).

*Continued next column*

## OVERDOSE

**SYMPTOMS:**
Tingling, cold extremities; muscle pain; nausea; vomiting; diarrhea; cold skin; severe numbness of extremities; confusion; excitement; rapid heartbeat; hallucinations; convulsions; coma.
**WHAT TO DO:**
- **Dial 0 (operator) or 911 (emergency) for an ambulance or medical help. Then give first aid immediately.**
- **See emergency information on inside covers.**

**What drug does:**
- Constricts blood vessels in the head.
- Constricts blood-vessel walls.
- Stimulates central nervous system.

**Time lapse before drug works:**
30 to 60 minutes.

**Don't take with:**
- Non-prescription drugs containing alcohol without consulting doctor.
- See Interaction column and consult doctor.

## POSSIBLE ADVERSE REACTIONS OR SIDE EFFECTS

| SYMPTOMS | WHAT TO DO |
|---|---|
| **Life-threatening:** | |
| Slow or fast heartbeat. | Discontinue. Seek emergency treatment. |
| **Common:** | |
| • Fast heartbeat. | Discontinue. Call doctor right away. |
| • Dizziness, nausea, diarrhea, vomiting, nervousness. | Continue. Call doctor when convenient. |
| **Infrequent:** | |
| Itchy skin; abdominal pain; cold hands and feet; weakness in arms, legs, back; confusion; irritability; indigestion; low blood sugar with weakness and trembling. | Discontinue. Call doctor right away. |
| **Rare:** | |
| Anxiety; red or purple blisters, especially on hands and feet; change in vision; extreme thirst; numbness or tingling in hands or feet. | Discontinue. Call doctor right away. |

## WARNINGS & PRECAUTIONS

**Don't take if:**
- You are allergic to any stimulant or any ergot preparation.
- You have heart disease.
- You have active peptic ulcer of stomach or duodenum.

**Before you start, consult your doctor:**
- If you have irregular heartbeat, angina, heart problems, high blood pressure, hardening of the arteries or vein problems.
- If you have hypoglycemia (low blood sugar), epilepsy, an infection, kidney or liver disease.
- If you are allergic to spray inhalants.
- If you plan to become pregnant within medication period.

**Over age 60:**
Adverse reactions and side effects may be more frequent and severe than in younger persons, especially dizziness and excessive potassium loss.

**Pregnancy:**
Risk to unborn child outweighs drug benefits. Don't use.

**Breast-feeding:**
Drug passes into milk. Avoid drug or discontinue nursing until you finish medicine. Consult doctor for advice on maintaining milk supply.

**Infants & children:**
Not recommended.

**Prolonged use:**
Cold skin, muscle pain, stomach ulcers, gangrene of hands and feet. This medicine not intended for uninterrupted use.

**Skin & sunlight:**
No problems expected.

**Driving, piloting or hazardous work:**
Don't drive or pilot aircraft until you learn how medicine affects you. Don't work around dangerous machinery. Don't climb ladders or work in high places. Danger increases if you drink alcohol or take medicine affecting alertness and reflexes, such as antihistamines, tranquilizers, sedatives, pain medicine, narcotics and mind-altering drugs.

**Discontinuing:**
Will cause withdrawal symptoms of headache, irritability, drowsiness. Discontinue gradually if you use caffeine for a month or more.

**Others:**
- May produce or aggravate fibrocystic breast disease in women.
- Impaired blood circulation can lead to gangrene in intestines or extremities. Never exceed recommended dose.

## POSSIBLE INTERACTION WITH OTHER DRUGS

| GENERIC NAME OR DRUG CLASS | COMBINED EFFECT |
|---|---|
| Amphetamines | Dangerous blood-pressure rise. |
| Contraceptives (oral) | Increased caffeine effect. |
| Ephedrine | Dangerous blood-pressure rise. |
| Epinephrine | Dangerous blood-pressure rise. |
| Isoniazid | Increased caffeine effect. |

| | |
|---|---|
| MAO inhibitors | Dangerous blood-pressure rise. |
| Pseudoephedrine | Dangerous blood-pressure rise. |
| Sedatives | Decreased sedative effect. |
| Sleep inducers | Decreased sedative effect. |
| Sympathomimetics | Overstimulation. |
| Thyroid hormones | Increased thyroid effect. |
| Tranquilizers | Decreased tranquilizer effect. |
| Troleandomycin | Increased adverse reactions of ergotamine. |

## POSSIBLE INTERACTION WITH OTHER SUBSTANCES

| INTERACTS WITH | COMBINED EFFECT |
|---|---|
| Alcohol: | Dilates blood vessels. Makes headache worse. |
| Beverages: Caffeine drinks. | May help relieve headache. |
| Cocaine: | Overstimulation. Avoid. |
| Foods: Any to which you are allergic. | May make headache worse. Avoid. |
| Marijuana: | Occasional use—Cool extremities. Regular use—Persistent chill. Increased effect of both drugs. May lead to dangerous, rapid heartbeat. Avoid. |
| Tobacco: | Decreased effect of ergotamine. Makes headache worse. Avoid. |

# ERGOTAMINE, CAFFEINE, BELLADONNA & PENTOBARBITAL

## BRAND NAMES

Cafergot-PB

## BASIC INFORMATION

**Habit forming? Yes**
**Prescription needed? Yes**
**Available as generic? No**
**Drug class: Vasoconstrictor, stimulant (xanthine), sedative, antispasmodic**

## USES

- Relieves pain of migraines and other headaches caused by dilated blood vessels. Will not prevent headaches.
- Reduces anxiety or nervous tension (low dose).

## DOSAGE & USAGE INFORMATION

### How to take:

- Tablet, elixir or capsule—Swallow with liquid or food to lessen stomach irritation.
- Tablet or capsule—Swallow with liquid, or let dissolve under tongue. If you can't swallow whole, crumble tablet or open capsule and take with liquid or food.
- Suppositories—Remove wrapper and moisen suppository with water. Gently insert larger end into rectum. Push well into rectum with finger.
- Lie down in quiet, dark room after taking.

### When to take:

At first sign of vascular or migraine headache.

*Continued next column*

## OVERDOSE

### SYMPTOMS:

**Tingling, cold extremities and muscle pain. Progresses to nausea, vomiting, diarrhea, cold skin, rapid and weak pulse, severe numbness of extremities, confusion, convulsions, coma.**
**WHAT TO DO:**
- **Dial 0 (operator) or 911 (emergency) for an ambulance or medical help. Then give first aid immediately.**
- **See emergency information on inside covers.**

### If you forget a dose:

Take as soon as you remember up to 2 hours late. If more than 2 hours, wait for next scheduled dose (don't double this dose).

### What drug does:

- Blocks nerve impulses at parasympathetic nerve endings, preventing muscle contractions and gland secretions of organs involved.
- May partially block nerve impulses at nerve-cell connections.
- Constricts blood-vessel walls.
- Stimulates central nervous system.

### Time lapse before drug works:

15 to 30 minutes.

### Don't take with:

- Non-prescription drugs without consulting doctor.
- See Interaction column and consult doctor.

## POSSIBLE ADVERSE REACTIONS OR SIDE EFFECTS

| SYMPTOMS | WHAT TO DO |
|---|---|
| **Life-threatening:** | |
| Slow or fast heartbeat. | Discontinue. Seek emergency treatment. |
| **Common:** | |
| • Fast heartbeat. | Discontinue. Call doctor right away. |
| • Dizziness, nausea, diarrhea, vomiting, nervousness, "hangover" effect. | Continue. Call doctor when convenient. |
| **Infrequent:** | |
| Itchy skin; rash; abdominal pain; cold hands and feet; weakness in arms, back, legs; confusion; irritability; indigestion; low blood sugar with weakness and trembling. | Discontinue. Call doctor right away. |
| **Rare:** | |
| Anxiety; red or purple blisters, especially in hands and feet; change in vision; extreme thirst; numbness or tingling in hands or feet; jaundice. | Discontinue. Call doctor right away. |

# ERGOTAMINE, CAFFEINE, BELLADONNA & PENTOBARBITAL

## WARNINGS & PRECAUTIONS

**Don't take if:**

- You are allergic to any stimulant, ergot preparation, barbiturate or anticholinergic.
- You have heart disease, peptic ulcer of stomach or duodenum, porphyria, trouble with stomach bloating, difficulty emptying your bladder completely, narrow-angle glaucoma, severe ulcerative colitis.

**Before you start, consult your doctor:**

- If you have hypoglycemia (low blood sugar), an infection, angina, heart problems, high blood pressure, hardening of the arteries, vein problems, kidney or liver disease, epilepsy, asthma, anemia, chronic pain, open-angle glaucoma, chronic bronchitis, hiatal hernia, enlarged prostate, myasthenia gravis, peptic ulcer.
- If you plan to become pregnant within medication period.
- If you will have surgery within 2 months, including dental surgery, requiring general or spinal anesthesia.

**Over age 60:**
Adverse reactions and side effects may be more frequent and severe than in younger persons, especially dizziness and excessive potassium loss.

**Pregnancy:**
Risk to unborn child outweighs drug benefits. Don't use.

**Breast-feeding:**
Drug filters into milk. May harm child. Avoid.

**Infants & children:**
Not recommended.

**Prolonged use:**

- Stomach ulcers.
- Cold skin, muscle pain, gangrene of hands and feet. This medicine not intended for uninterrupted use.
- May cause addiction, anemia, chronic intoxication.
- May lower body temperature, making exposure to cold temperatures hazardous.
- Chronic constipation, possible fecal impaction.

**Skin & sunlight:**
May cause rash or intensify sunburn in areas exposed to sun or sunlamp.

**Driving, piloting or hazardous work:**
Don't drive or pilot aircraft until you learn how medicine affects you. Don't work around dangerous machinery. Don't climb ladders or work in high places. Danger increases if you drink alcohol or take medicine affecting alertness and reflexes, such as antihistamines, tranquilizers, sedatives, pain medicine, narcotics and mind-altering drugs.

**Discontinuing:**
May be unnecessary to finish medicine. Follow doctor's instructions. If you develop withdrawal symptoms of hallucinations, headache, agitation or sleeplessness after discontinuing, call doctor right away.

**Others:**

- Great potential for abuse.
- May produce or aggravate fibrocystic breast disease in women.
- Impaired blood circulation can lead to gangrene in intestines or extremities. Never exceed recommended dose.

## POSSIBLE INTERACTION WITH OTHER DRUGS

| GENERIC NAME OR DRUG CLASS | COMBINED EFFECT |
|---|---|
| **Amantadine** | Increased belladonna effect. |
| **Amphetamines** | Dangerous blood-pressure rise. |

*Continued page 966*

## POSSIBLE INTERACTION WITH OTHER SUBSTANCES

| INTERACTS WITH | COMBINED EFFECT |
|---|---|
| **Alcohol:** | Dilates blood vessels. Makes headache worse. Possible fatal oversedation. Avoid. |
| **Beverages:** Caffeine drinks. | May help relieve headache. |
| **Cocaine:** | Excessively rapid heartbeat. Avoid. |
| **Foods:** Any to which you are allergic. | May make headache worse. Avoid. |
| **Marijuana:** | Drowsiness and dry mouth, excessive sedation. Avoid. Occasional use—Cool extremities. Regular use—Persistent chill. |
| **Tobacco:** | Decreased effect of ergotamine. Makes headache worse. |

## BRAND AND GENERIC NAMES

See complete list of brand names in the
*Brand Name Directory,* page 949.

## BASIC INFORMATION

**Habit forming? No**
**Prescription needed? Yes**
**Available as generic? Yes**
**Drug class: Antibiotic (erythromycin)**

 ## USES

Treatment of infections responsive to
erythromycin.

 ## DOSAGE & USAGE INFORMATION

**How to take:**
- Tablet or capsule—Swallow with liquid.
- Extended-release tablets or
  capsules—Swallow each dose whole. If you
  take regular tablets, you may chew or crush
  them.
- Liquid, drops, granules, skin ointment, eye
  ointment, skin solution—Follow prescription
  label directions.

**When to take:**
At the same times each day, 1 hour before or 2
hours after eating.

**If you forget a dose:**
- If you take 3 or more doses daily—Take as
  soon as you remember. Return to regular
  schedule.
- If you take 2 doses daily—Take as soon as
  you remember. Wait 5 to 6 hours for next
  dose. Return to regular schedule.

**What drug does:**
Prevents growth and reproduction of susceptible
bacteria.

**Time lapse before drug works:**
2 to 5 days.

*Continued next column*

 ## OVERDOSE

**SYMPTOMS:**
**Nausea, vomiting, abdominal discomfort,**
**diarrhea.**
**WHAT TO DO:**
**Overdose unlikely to threaten life. If person**
**takes much larger amount than prescribed,**
**call doctor, poison-control center or hospital**
**emergency room for instructions.**

**Don't take with:**
See Interaction column and consult doctor.

 ## POSSIBLE ADVERSE REACTIONS OR SIDE EFFECTS

| SYMPTOMS | WHAT TO DO |
|---|---|
| **Life-threatening:**<br>None expected. | |
| **Common:**<br>None expected. | |
| **Infrequent:** | |
| • Diarrhea, nausea, stomach cramps, discomfort, vomiting. | Discontinue. Call doctor right away. |
| • Skin dryness, irritation, itch, stinging with use of skin solution, sore mouth or tongue. | Continue. Call doctor when convenient. |
| **Rare:** | |
| • Jaundice in adults. | Discontinue. Call doctor right away. |
| • Unusual tiredness or weakness. | Continue. Call doctor when convenient. |

*[Handwritten note:]*
3-97- Given to Jessica for
Bowers bad cough-broncits
½ tsp. 3 X Day
Erythrom ETH 400/5ML

---

## WARNINGS & PRECAUTIONS

### Don't take if:
- You are allergic to any erythromycin.
- You have had liver disease or impaired liver function.

### Before you start, consult your doctor:
If you have taken erythromycin estolate in the past.

### Over age 60:
Adverse reactions and side effects may be more frequent and severe than in younger persons, especially skin reactions around genitals and anus.

### Pregnancy:
No proven harm to unborn child. Avoid if possible.

### Breast-feeding:
Drug passes into milk. Avoid drug or discontinue nursing until you finish medicine. Consult doctor for advice on maintaining milk supply.

### Infants & children:
Use only under medical supervision.

### Prolonged use:
You may become more susceptible to infections caused by germs not responsive to erythromycin.

### Skin & sunlight:
No problems expected.

### Driving, piloting or hazardous work:
No problems expected.

### Discontinuing:
You must take full dose at least 10 consecutive days for streptococcal or staphylococcal infections.

### Others:
No problems expected.

## POSSIBLE INTERACTION WITH OTHER DRUGS

| GENERIC NAME OR DRUG CLASS | COMBINED EFFECT |
|---|---|
| Aminophylline | Increased effect of aminophylline in blood. |
| Lincomycins | Decreased lincomycin effect. |
| Oxtriphylline | Increased level of oxtriphylline in blood. |
| Penicillins | Decreased penicillin effect. |
| Theophylline | Increased level of theophylline in blood. |

## POSSIBLE INTERACTION WITH OTHER SUBSTANCES

| INTERACTS WITH | COMBINED EFFECT |
|---|---|
| Alcohol: | Possible liver damage. |
| Beverages: | None expected. |
| Cocaine: | None expected. |
| Foods: | None expected. |
| Marijuana: | None expected. |
| Tobacco: | None expected. |

# ERYTHROMYCIN & SULFISOXAZOLE

## BRAND NAMES

**Pediazole**

## BASIC INFORMATION

**Habit forming? No**
**Prescription needed? Yes**
**Available as generic? Yes**
**Drug class: Antibiotic (erythromycin), sulfa**
**(sulfonamide)**

 ## USES

Treatment of infections responsive to erythromycin and sulfa.

 ## DOSAGE & USAGE INFORMATION

**How to take:**
Suspension—Swallow with liquid. Instructions to take on empty stomach mean 1 hour before or 2 hours after eating. Shake carefully before measuring.

**When to take:**
At the same times each day, 1 hour before or 2 hours after eating.

**If you forget a dose:**
Take as soon as you remember up to 2 hours late. If more than 2 hours, wait for next scheduled dose (don't double this dose).

**What drug does:**
Prevents growth and reproduction of susceptible bacteria.

**Time lapse before drug works:**
2 to 5 days to affect infection.

**Don't take with:**
See Interaction column and consult doctor.

 ## OVERDOSE

**SYMPTOMS:**
**Less urine, bloody urine, nausea, vomiting, abdominal discomfort, diarrhea, coma.**
**WHAT TO DO:**
- **Dial 0 (operator) or 911 (emergency) for an ambulance or medical help. Then give first aid immediately.**
- **See emergency information on inside covers.**

 ## POSSIBLE ADVERSE REACTIONS OR SIDE EFFECTS

| SYMPTOMS | WHAT TO DO |
|---|---|
| **Life-threatening:** None expected. | |
| **Common:** Headache, dizziness, itchy skin, rash, appetite loss, vomiting. | Discontinue. Call doctor right away. |
| **Infrequent:** Dryness, irritation, itch, stinging with use of skin solution, mouth or tongue sore, diarrhea, nausea, abdominal cramps, vomiting, swallowing difficulty. | Continue. Call doctor when convenient. |
| **Rare:** • Jaundice, painful or difficult urination. | Discontinue. Call doctor right away. |
| • Weakness and unusual tiredness. | Continue. Call doctor when convenient. |

 ## WARNINGS & PRECAUTIONS

**Don't take if:**
- You are allergic to any sulfa drug or any erythromycin.
- You have had liver disease or impaired liver function.

**Before you start, consult your doctor:**
- If you are allergic to carbonic anhydrase inhibitors, oral antidiabetics or thiazide diuretics.
- If you are allergic by nature.
- If you have liver or kidney disease, porphyria, developed anemia from use of any drug, taken erythromycin estolate in the past.

**Over age 60:**
Adverse reactions and side effects may be more frequent and severe than in younger persons, especially skin reactions around genitals and anus.

**Pregnancy:**
Risk to unborn child outweighs drug benefits. Don't use.

**Breast-feeding:**
Drug passes into milk. Avoid drug or discontinue nursing until you finish medicine. Consult doctor for advice on maintaining milk supply.

**Infants & children:**
Don't give to infants younger than 1 month.

# ERYTHROMYCIN & SULFISOXAZOLE

**Prolonged use:**
- May enlarge thyroid gland.
- Request frequent blood counts, liver- and kidney-function studies.
- You may become more susceptible to infections caused by germs not responsive to erythromycin or sulfa.

**Skin & sunlight:**
May cause rash or intensify sunburn in areas exposed to sun or sunlamp.

**Driving, piloting or hazardous work:**
Avoid if you feel dizzy. Otherwise, no problems expected.

**Discontinuing:**
Don't discontinue without doctor's advice until you complete prescribed dose, even though symptoms diminish or disappear.

**Others:**
- Drink extra liquid each day to prevent adverse reactions.
- If you require surgery, tell anesthetist you take sulfa.

## POSSIBLE INTERACTION WITH OTHER DRUGS

| GENERIC NAME OR DRUG CLASS | COMBINED EFFECT |
|---|---|
| Aminobenzoate potassium | Possible decreased sulfisoxazole effect. |
| Aminophylline | Increased effect of aminophylline in blood. |
| Anticoagulants (oral) | Increased anticoagulant effect. |
| Anticonvulsants (hydantoin) | Toxic effect on brain. |
| Aspirin | Increased sulfa effect. |
| Flecainide | Possible decreased blood-cell production in bone marrow. |
| Isoniazid | Possible anemia. |
| Lincomycins | Decreased lincomycin effect. |
| Methenamine | Possible kidney blockage. |
| Methotrexate | Increased possibility of toxic side effects from methotrexate. |
| Oxtriphylline | Increased level of oxtriphylline in blood. |
| Oxyphenbutazone | Increased sulfa effect. |
| Para-aminosalicylic acid (PAS) | Decreased sulfa effect. |

| | |
|---|---|
| Penicillins | Decreased penicillin effect. |
| Phenylbutazone | Increased sulfa effect. |
| Probenecid | Increased sulfa effect. |
| Sulfinpyrazone | Increased sulfa effect. |
| Theophylline | Increased level of theophylline in blood. |
| Tocainide | Possible decreased blood-cell production in bone marrow. |
| Trimethoprim | Increased sulfa effect. |

## POSSIBLE INTERACTION WITH OTHER SUBSTANCES

| INTERACTS WITH | COMBINED EFFECT |
|---|---|
| Alcohol: | Increased alcohol effect. Possible liver damage. |
| Beverages: Less than 2 quarts of fluid daily. | Kidney damage. |
| Cocaine: | None expected. |
| Foods: | None expected. |
| Marijuana: | None expected. |
| Tobacco: | None expected. |

# ESTERIFIED ESTROGENS

## BRAND NAMES

| | |
|---|---|
| Amnestrogen | Estromed |
| Climestrone | Evex |
| Estratab | Menest |
| Estratest | Neo-Estrone |

## BASIC INFORMATION

**Habit forming? No**
**Prescription needed? Yes**
**Available as generic? Yes**
**Drug class: Female sex hormone (estrogen)**

 ## USES

- Treatment for symptoms of menopause and menstrual-cycle irregularity.
- Replacement for female hormone deficiency.
- Treatment for cancer of prostate and breast.

 ## DOSAGE & USAGE INFORMATION

**How to take:**
Tablet—Swallow with liquid. If you can't swallow whole, crumble tablet and take with liquid or food.

**When to take:**
At the same time each day.

**If you forget a dose:**
Take as soon as you remember up to 12 hours late. If more than 12 hours, wait for next scheduled dose (don't double this dose).

**What drug does:**
Restores normal estrogen level in tissues.

**Time lapse before drug works:**
10 to 20 days.

**Don't take with:**
See Interaction column and consult doctor.

 ## OVERDOSE

**SYMPTOMS:**
**Nausea, vomiting, fluid retention, breast enlargement and discomfort, abnormal vaginal bleeding.**
**WHAT TO DO:**
**Overdose unlikely to threaten life. If person takes much larger amount than prescribed, call doctor, poison-control center or hospital emergency room for instructions.**

 ## POSSIBLE ADVERSE REACTIONS OR SIDE EFFECTS

| SYMPTOMS | WHAT TO DO |
|---|---|
| **Life-threatening:** | |
| None expected. | |
| **Common:** | |
| ● Stomach cramps. | Discontinue. Call doctor right away. |
| ● Appetite loss. | Continue. Call doctor when convenient. |
| ● Nausea; diarrhea; swollen feet and ankles; tender, swollen breasts. | Continue. Tell doctor at next visit. |
| **Infrequent:** | |
| ● Rash, stomach or side pain. | Discontinue. Call doctor right away. |
| ● Depression, dizziness, irritability, vomiting, breast lumps. | Continue. Call doctor when convenient. |
| ● Brown blotches, hair loss, vaginal discharge or bleeding, changes in sex drive. | Continue. Tell doctor at next visit. |
| **Rare:** | |
| Jaundice. | Discontinue. Call doctor right away. |

## WARNINGS & PRECAUTIONS

**Don't take if:**
- You are allergic to any estrogen-containing drugs.
- You have impaired liver function.
- You have had blood clots, stroke or heart attack.
- You have unexplained vaginal bleeding.

**Before you start, consult your doctor:**
- If you have had cancer of breast or reproductive organs, fibrocystic breast disease, fibroid tumors of the uterus or endometriosis.
- If you have had migraine headaches, epilepsy or porphyria.
- If you have diabetes, high blood pressure, asthma, congestive heart failure, kidney disease or gallstones.
- If you plan to become pregnant within 3 months.

**Over age 60:**
Controversial. You and your doctor must decide if drug risks outweigh benefits.

**Pregnancy:**
Risk to unborn child outweighs drug benefits. Don't use.

**Breast-feeding:**
Drug filters into milk. May harm child. Avoid.

**Infants & children:**
Not recommended.

**Prolonged use:**
Increased growth of fibroid tumors of uterus. Possible association with cancer of uterus.

**Skin & sunlight:**
May cause rash or intensify sunburn in areas exposed to sun or sunlamp.

**Driving, piloting or hazardous work:**
No problems expected.

**Discontinuing:**
You may need to discontinue estrogen periodically. Consult your doctor.

**Others:**
In rare instances, may cause blood clot in lung, brain or leg. Symptoms are *sudden* severe headache, coordination loss, vision change, chest pain, breathing difficulty, slurred speech, pain in legs or groin. Seek emergency treatment immediately.

## POSSIBLE INTERACTION WITH OTHER DRUGS

| GENERIC NAME OR DRUG CLASS | COMBINED EFFECT |
| --- | --- |
| Anticoagulants (oral) | Decreased anticoagulant effect. |
| Anticonvulsants (hydantoin) | Increased seizures. |
| Antidiabetics (oral) | Unpredictable increase or decrease in blood sugar. |
| Carbamazepine | Increased seizures. |
| Clofibrate | Decreased clofibrate effect. |
| Meprobamate | Increased effect of esterified estrogens. |
| Phenobarbital | Decreased effect of esterified estrogens. |
| Primidone | Decreased effect of esterified estrogens. |
| Rifampin | Decreased effect of esterified estrogens. |
| Thyroid hormones | Decreased thyroid effect. |

## POSSIBLE INTERACTION WITH OTHER SUBSTANCES

| INTERACTS WITH | COMBINED EFFECT |
| --- | --- |
| Alcohol: | None expected. |
| Beverages: | None expected. |
| Cocaine: | No proven problems. |
| Foods: | None expected. |
| Marijuana: | Possible menstrual irregularities and bleeding between periods. |
| Tobacco: | Increased risk of blood clots leading to stroke or heart attack. |

# ESTRADIOL

## BRAND NAMES

Delestrogen          Estrace

## BASIC INFORMATION

**Habit forming? No**
**Prescription needed? Yes**
**Available as generic? Yes**
**Drug class: Female sex hormone (estrogen)**

 **USES**

- Treatment for symptoms of menopause and menstrual-cycle irregularity.
- Replacement for female hormone deficiency.
- Treatment for cancer of prostate and breast.

 **DOSAGE & USAGE INFORMATION**

**How to take:**
Tablet—Swallow with liquid. If you can't swallow whole, crumble tablet and take with liquid or food.

**When to take:**
At the same time each day.

**If you forget a dose:**
Take as soon as you remember up to 12 hours late. If more than 12 hours, wait for next scheduled dose (don't double this dose).

**What drug does:**
Restores normal estrogen level in tissues.

**Time lapse before drug works:**
10 to 20 days.

**Don't take with:**
See Interaction column and consult doctor.

 **OVERDOSE**

**SYMPTOMS:**
Nausea, vomiting, fluid retention, breast enlargement and discomfort, abnormal vaginal bleeding.
**WHAT TO DO:**
Overdose unlikely to threaten life. If person takes much larger amount than prescribed, call doctor, poison-control center or hospital emergency room for instructions.

 **POSSIBLE ADVERSE REACTIONS OR SIDE EFFECTS**

| SYMPTOMS | WHAT TO DO |
|---|---|
| **Life-threatening:** None expected. | |
| **Common:** | |
| • Stomach cramps. | Discontinue. Call doctor right away. |
| • Appetite loss. | Continue. Call doctor when convenient. |
| • Nausea; diarrhea; swollen feet and ankles; tender, swollen breasts. | Continue. Tell doctor at next visit. |
| **Infrequent:** | |
| • Rash, stomach or side pain. | Discontinue. Call doctor right away. |
| • Depression, dizziness, irritability, vomiting, breast lumps. | Continue. Call doctor when convenient. |
| • Brown blotches, hair loss, vaginal discharge or bleeding, changes in sex drive. | Continue. Tell doctor at next visit. |
| **Rare:** Jaundice. | Discontinue. Call doctor right away. |

## WARNINGS & PRECAUTIONS

**Don't take if:**
- You are allergic to any estrogen-containing drugs.
- You have impaired liver function.
- You have had blood clots, stroke or heart attack.
- You have unexplained vaginal bleeding.

**Before you start, consult your doctor:**
- If you have had cancer of breast or reproductive organs, fibrocystic breast disease, fibroid tumors of the uterus or endometriosis.
- If you have had migraine headaches, epilepsy or porphyria.
- If you have diabetes, high blood pressure, asthma, congestive heart failure, kidney disease or gallstones.
- If you plan to become pregnant within 3 months.

**Over age 60:**
Controversial. You and your doctor must decide if drug risks outweigh benefits.

**Pregnancy:**
Risk to unborn child outweighs drug benefits. Don't use.

**Breast-feeding:**
Drug filters into milk. May harm child. Avoid.

**Infants & children:**
Not recommended.

**Prolonged use:**
Increased growth of fibroid tumors of uterus. Possible association with cancer of uterus.

**Skin & sunlight:**
May cause rash or intensify sunburn in areas exposed to sun or sunlamp.

**Driving, piloting or hazardous work:**
No problems expected.

**Discontinuing:**
You may need to discontinue estradiol periodically. Consult your doctor.

**Others:**
In rare instances, may cause blood clot in lung, brain or leg. Symptoms are *sudden* severe headache, coordination loss, vision change, chest pain, breathing difficulty, slurred speech, pain in legs or groin. Seek emergency treatment immediately.

## POSSIBLE INTERACTION WITH OTHER DRUGS

| GENERIC NAME OR DRUG CLASS | COMBINED EFFECT |
|---|---|
| Anticoagulants (oral) | Decreased anticoagulant effect. |
| Anticonvulsants (hydantoin) | Increased seizures. |
| Antidiabetics (oral) | Unpredictable increase or decrease in blood sugar. |
| Carbamazepine | Increased seizures. |
| Clofibrate | Decreased clofibrate effect. |
| Meprobamate | Increased estradiol effect. |
| Phenobarbital | Decreased estradiol effect. |
| Primidone | Decreased estradiol effect. |
| Rifampin | Decreased estradiol effect. |
| Thyroid hormones | Decreased thyroid effect. |

## POSSIBLE INTERACTION WITH OTHER SUBSTANCES

| INTERACTS WITH | COMBINED EFFECT |
|---|---|
| Alcohol: | None expected. |
| Beverages: | None expected. |
| Cocaine: | No proven problems. |
| Foods: | None expected. |
| Marijuana: | Possible menstrual irregularities and bleeding between periods. |
| Tobacco: | Increased risk of blood clots leading to stroke or heart attack. |

# ESTROGEN

## BRAND NAMES

See complete list of brand names in the *Brand Name Directory*, page 949.

## BASIC INFORMATION

**Habit forming? No**
**Prescription needed? Yes**
**Available as generic? Yes**
**Drug class: Female sex hormone (estrogen)**

## USES

- Treatment for symptoms of menopause and menstrual-cycle irregularity.
- Treatment for estrogen-deficiency osteoporosis (bone softening from calcium loss).
- Treatment for DES-induced cancer.
- Treatment for atrophic vaginitis.

## DOSAGE & USAGE INFORMATION

**How to take:**
- Tablet or capsule—Swallow with liquid. If you can't swallow whole, crumble tablet or open capsule and take with liquid or food.
- Vaginal cream or suppositories—Use as directed on label.

**When to take:**
At the same time each day.

**If you forget a dose:**
Take as soon as you remember up to 12 hours late. If more than 12 hours, wait for next scheduled dose (don't double this dose).

**What drug does:**
Restores normal estrogen level in tissues.

**Time lapse before drug works:**
10 to 20 days.

**Don't take with:**
See Interaction column and consult doctor.

## OVERDOSE

**SYMPTOMS:**
**Nausea, vomiting, fluid retention, breast enlargement and discomfort, abnormal vaginal bleeding.**
**WHAT TO DO:**
**Overdose unlikely to threaten life. If person takes much larger amount than prescribed, call doctor, poison-control center or hospital emergency room for instructions.**

## POSSIBLE ADVERSE REACTIONS OR SIDE EFFECTS

| SYMPTOMS | WHAT TO DO |
|---|---|
| **Life-threatening:** | |
| None expected. | |
| **Common:** | |
| ● Stomach cramps. | Discontinue. Call doctor right away. |
| ● Appetite loss. | Continue. Call doctor when convenient. |
| ● Nausea; diarrhea; swollen feet and ankles; tender, swollen breasts. | Continue. Tell doctor at next visit. |
| **Infrequent:** | |
| ● Rash, stomach or side pain. | Discontinue. Call doctor right away. |
| ● Depression, dizziness, irritability, vomiting, breast lumps. | Continue. Call doctor when convenient. |
| ● Brown blotches, hair loss, vaginal discharge or bleeding, changes in sex drive. | Continue. Tell doctor at next visit. |
| **Rare:** | |
| Jaundice. | Discontinue. Call doctor right away. |

## WARNINGS & PRECAUTIONS

### Don't take if:
- You are allergic to any estrogen-containing drugs.
- You have impaired liver function.
- You have had blood clots, stroke or heart attack.
- You have unexplained vaginal bleeding.

### Before you start, consult your doctor:
- If you have had cancer of breast or reproductive organs, fibrocystic breast disease, fibroid tumors of the uterus or endometriosis.
- If you have had migraine headaches, epilepsy or porphyria.
- If you have diabetes, high blood pressure, asthma, congestive heart failure, kidney disease or gallstones.
- If you plan to become pregnant within 3 months.

### Over age 60:
Controversial. You and your doctor must decide if drug risks outweigh benefits.

### Pregnancy:
Risk to unborn child outweighs drug benefits. Don't use.

### Breast-feeding:
Drug filters into milk. May harm child. Avoid.

### Infants & children:
Not recommended.

### Prolonged use:
Increased growth of fibroid tumors of uterus. Possible association with cancer of uterus.

### Skin & sunlight:
May cause rash or intensify sunburn in areas exposed to sun or sunlamp.

### Driving, piloting or hazardous work:
No problems expected.

### Discontinuing:
You may need to discontinue estrogens periodically. Consult your doctor.

### Others:
- In rare instances, may cause blood clot in lung, brain or leg. Symptoms are *sudden* severe headache, coordination loss, vision change, chest pain, breathing difficulty, slurred speech, pain in legs or groin. Seek emergency treatment immediately.
- Carefully read the paper called "Information for the Patient" that was given to you with your prescription. If you lose it, ask your pharmacist for a copy.

 ## POSSIBLE INTERACTION WITH OTHER DRUGS

| GENERIC NAME OR DRUG CLASS | COMBINED EFFECT |
| --- | --- |
| Anticoagulants (oral) | Decreased anticoagulant effect. |
| Anticonvulsants (hydantoin) | Increased seizures. |
| Antidiabetics (oral) | Unpredictable increase or decrease in blood sugar. |
| Carbamazepine | Increased seizures. |
| Clofibrate | Decreased clofibrate effect. |
| Meprobamate | Increased estrogen effect. |
| Phenobarbital | Decreased estrogen effect. |
| Primidone | Decreased estrogen effect. |
| Rifampin | Decreased estrogen effect. |
| Thyroid hormones | Decreased thyroid effect. |

 ## POSSIBLE INTERACTION WITH OTHER SUBSTANCES

| INTERACTS WITH | COMBINED EFFECT |
| --- | --- |
| Alcohol: | None expected. |
| Beverages: | None expected. |
| Cocaine: | No proven problems. |
| Foods: | None expected. |
| Marijuana: | Possible menstrual irregularities and bleeding between periods. |
| Tobacco: | Increased risk of blood clots leading to stroke or heart attack. |

# ESTRONE

## BRAND NAMES

| | |
|---|---|
| Besterone | Kestrin |
| Estaqua | Kestrin Aqueous |
| Estrofol | Kestrone |
| Estroject | Natural Estrogenic |
| Estrone-A | Substance |
| Estronol | Ogen |
| Femogen | Theelin |
| Foygen Aqueous | Theogen |
| Gynogen | Unigen |
| Hormogen-A | Wehgen |

## BASIC INFORMATION

**Habit forming? No**
**Prescription needed? Yes**
**Available as generic? Yes**
**Drug class: Female sex hormone (estrogen)**

 ## USES

- Treatment for symptoms of menopause and menstrual-cycle irregularity.
- Replacement for female hormone deficiency.
- Treatment for cancer of prostate.

 ## DOSAGE & USAGE INFORMATION

**How to take:**
By injection under medical supervision.

**When to take:**
Varies according to doctor's instructions.

**If you forget an injection:**
Consult doctor.

**What drug does:**
Restores normal estrogen level in tissues.

**Time lapse before drug works:**
10 to 20 days.

**Don't take with:**
See Interaction column and consult doctor.

 ## OVERDOSE

**SYMPTOMS:**
Nausea, vomiting, fluid retention, breast enlargement and discomfort, abnormal vaginal bleeding.
**WHAT TO DO:**
Overdose unlikely to threaten life. If person takes much larger amount than prescribed, call doctor, poison-control center or hospital emergency room for instructions.

 ## POSSIBLE ADVERSE REACTIONS OR SIDE EFFECTS

| SYMPTOMS | WHAT TO DO |
|---|---|
| **Life-threatening:** | |
| None expected. | |
| **Common:** | |
| ● Stomach cramps. | Discontinue. Call doctor right away. |
| ● Appetite loss. | Continue. Call doctor when convenient. |
| ● Nausea; diarrhea; swollen feet and ankles; tender, swollen breasts. | Continue. Tell doctor at next visit. |
| **Infrequent:** | |
| ● Rash, stomach or side pain. | Discontinue. Call doctor right away. |
| ● Depression, dizziness, irritability, vomiting, breast lumps. | Continue. Call doctor when convenient. |
| ● Brown blotches, hair loss, vaginal discharge or bleeding, changes in sex drive. | Continue. Tell doctor at next visit. |
| **Rare:** | |
| Jaundice. | Discontinue. Call doctor right away. |

## WARNINGS & PRECAUTIONS

### Don't take if:
- You are allergic to any estrogen-containing drugs.
- You have impaired liver function.
- You have had blood clots, stroke or heart attack.
- You have unexplained vaginal bleeding.

### Before you start, consult your doctor:
- If you have had cancer of breast or reproductive organs, fibrocystic breast disease, fibroid tumors of the uterus or endometriosis.
- If you have had migraine headaches, epilepsy or porphyria.
- If you have diabetes, high blood pressure, asthma, congestive heart failure, kidney disease or gallstones.
- If you plan to become pregnant within 3 months.

### Over age 60:
Controversial. You and your doctor must decide if drug risks outweigh benefits.

### Pregnancy:
Risk to unborn child outweighs drug benefits. Don't use.

### Breast-feeding:
Drug filters into milk. May harm child. Avoid.

### Infants & children:
Not recommended.

### Prolonged use:
Increased growth of fibroid tumors of uterus. Possible association with cancer of uterus.

### Skin & sunlight:
May cause rash or intensify sunburn in areas exposed to sun or sunlamp.

### Driving, piloting or hazardous work:
No problems expected.

### Discontinuing:
You may need to discontinue estrone periodically. Consult your doctor.

### Others:
In rare instances, may cause blood clot in lung, brain or leg. Symptoms are *sudden* severe headache, coordination loss, vision change, chest pain, breathing difficulty, slurred speech, pain in legs or groin. Seek emergency treatment immediately.

## POSSIBLE INTERACTION WITH OTHER DRUGS

| GENERIC NAME OR DRUG CLASS | COMBINED EFFECT |
| --- | --- |
| Anticoagulants (oral) | Decreased anticoagulant effect. |
| Anticonvulsants (hydantoin) | Increased seizures. |
| Antidiabetics (oral) | Unpredictable increase or decrease in blood sugar. |
| Carbamazepine | Increased seizures. |
| Clofibrate | Decreased clofibrate effect. |
| Meprobamate | Increased estrone effect. |
| Phenobarbital | Decreased estrone effect. |
| Primidone | Decreased estrone effect. |
| Rifampin | Decreased estrone effect. |
| Thyroid hormones | Decreased thyroid effect. |

## POSSIBLE INTERACTION WITH OTHER SUBSTANCES

| INTERACTS WITH | COMBINED EFFECT |
| --- | --- |
| Alcohol: | None expected. |
| Beverages: | None expected. |
| Cocaine: | No proven problems. |
| Foods: | None expected. |
| Marijuana: | Possible menstrual irregularities and bleeding between periods. |
| Tobacco: | Increased risk of blood clots leading to stroke or heart attack. |

# ESTROPIPATE

## BRAND NAMES

Ogen

Piperazine Estrone Sulfate

## BASIC INFORMATION

Habit forming? No
Prescription needed? Yes
Available as generic? Yes
Drug class: Female sex hormone (estrogen)

 ## USES

- Treatment for symptoms of menopause and menstrual-cycle irregularity.
- Replacement for female hormone deficiency.

 ## DOSAGE & USAGE INFORMATION

**How to take:**
- Tablet—Swallow with liquid. If you can't swallow whole, crumble tablet and take with liquid or food.
- Vaginal cream—Use as directed on label.

**When to take:**
At the same time each day.

**If you forget a dose:**
Take as soon as you remember up to 12 hours late. If more than 12 hours, wait for next scheduled dose (don't double this dose).

**What drug does:**
Restores normal estrogen level in tissues.

**Time lapse before drug works:**
10 to 20 days.

**Don't take with:**
See Interaction column and consult doctor.

 ## OVERDOSE

**SYMPTOMS:**
Nausea, vomiting, fluid retention, breast enlargement and discomfort, abnormal vaginal bleeding.
**WHAT TO DO:**
Overdose unlikely to threaten life. If person takes much larger amount than prescribed, call doctor, poison-control center or hospital emergency room for instructions.

 ## POSSIBLE ADVERSE REACTIONS OR SIDE EFFECTS

| SYMPTOMS | WHAT TO DO |
|---|---|
| **Life-threatening:** | |
| None expected. | |
| **Common:** | |
| • Stomach cramps. | Discontinue. Call doctor right away. |
| • Appetite loss. | Continue. Call doctor when convenient. |
| • Nausea; diarrhea; swollen feet and ankles; tender, swollen breasts. | Continue. Tell doctor at next visit. |
| **Infrequent:** | |
| • Rash, stomach or side pain. | Discontinue. Call doctor right away. |
| • Depression, dizziness, irritability, vomiting, breast lumps. | Continue. Call doctor when convenient. |
| • Brown blotches, hair loss, vaginal discharge or bleeding, changes in sex drive. | Continue. Tell doctor at next visit. |
| **Rare:** | |
| Jaundice. | Discontinue. Call doctor right away. |

## WARNINGS & PRECAUTIONS

### Don't take if:
- You are allergic to any estrogen-containing drugs.
- You have impaired liver function.
- You have had blood clots, stroke or heart attack.
- You have unexplained vaginal bleeding.

### Before you start, consult your doctor:
- If you have had cancer of breast or reproductive organs, fibrocystic breast disease, fibroid tumors of the uterus or endometriosis.
- If you have had migraine headaches, epilepsy or porphyria.
- If you have diabetes, high blood pressure, asthma, congestive heart failure, kidney disease or gallstones.
- If you plan to become pregnant within 3 months.

### Over age 60:
Controversial. You and your doctor must decide if drug risks outweigh benefits.

### Pregnancy:
Risk to unborn child outweighs drug benefits. Don't use.

### Breast-feeding:
Drug filters into milk. May harm child. Avoid.

### Infants & children:
Not recommended.

### Prolonged use:
Increased growth of fibroid tumors of uterus. Possible association with cancer of uterus.

### Skin & sunlight:
May cause rash or intensify sunburn in areas exposed to sun or sunlamp.

### Driving, piloting or hazardous work:
No problems expected.

### Discontinuing:
You may need to discontinue estropipate periodically. Consult your doctor.

### Others:
In rare instances, may cause blood clot in lung, brain or leg. Symptoms are *sudden* severe headache, coordination loss, vision change, chest pain, breathing difficulty, slurred speech, pain in legs or groin. Seek emergency treatment immediately.

## POSSIBLE INTERACTION WITH OTHER DRUGS

| GENERIC NAME OR DRUG CLASS | COMBINED EFFECT |
|---|---|
| Anticoagulants (oral) | Decreased anticoagulant effect. |
| Anticonvulsants (hydantoin) | Increased seizures. |
| Antidiabetics (oral) | Unpredictable increase or decrease in blood sugar. |
| Carbamazepine | Increased seizures. |
| Clofibrate | Decreased clofibrate effect. |
| Meprobamate | Increased estropipate effect. |
| Phenobarbital | Decreased estropipate effect. |
| Primidone | Decreased estropipate effect. |
| Rifampin | Decreased estropipate effect. |
| Thyroid hormones | Decreased thyroid effect. |

## POSSIBLE INTERACTION WITH OTHER SUBSTANCES

| INTERACTS WITH | COMBINED EFFECT |
|---|---|
| Alcohol: | None expected. |
| Beverages: | None expected. |
| Cocaine: | No proven problems. |
| Foods: | None expected. |
| Marijuana: | Possible menstrual irregularities and bleeding between periods. |
| Tobacco: | Increased risk of blood clots leading to stroke or heart attack. |

# ETHACRYNIC ACID

## BRAND NAMES

**Edecrin**

## BASIC INFORMATION

**Habit forming? No**
**Prescription needed? Yes**
**Available as generic? No**
**Drug class:** Diuretic (loop diuretic);
antihypertensive

## USES

- Lowers blood pressure.
- Decreases fluid retention.

## DOSAGE & USAGE INFORMATION

**How to take:**
Tablet or capsule—Swallow with liquid or food to lessen stomach irritation. If you can't swallow whole, crumble tablet or open capsule and take with liquid or food.

**When to take:**
- 1 dose a day—Take after breakfast.
- More than 1 dose a day—Take last dose no later than 6 p.m. unless otherwise directed.

**If you forget a dose:**
- 1 dose a day—Take as soon as you remember up to 12 hours late. If more than 12 hours, wait for next scheduled dose (don't double this dose).
- More than 1 dose a day—Take as soon as you remember up to 2 hours late. If more than 2 hours, wait for next scheduled dose (don't double this dose).

**What drug does:**
Increases elimination of sodium and water from body. Decreased body fluid reduces blood pressure.

*Continued next column*

## OVERDOSE

**SYMPTOMS:**
**Weakness, lethargy, dizziness, confusion, nausea, vomiting, leg-muscle cramps, thirst, stupor, deep sleep, weak and rapid pulse, cardiac arrest.**
**WHAT TO DO:**
- **Dial 0 (operator) or 911 (emergency) for an ambulance or medical help. Then give first aid immediately.**
- **See emergency information on inside covers.**

**Time lapse before drug works:**
1 hour to increase water loss. Requires 2 to 3 weeks to lower blood pressure.

**Don't take with:**
- Non-prescription drugs with aspirin.
- See Interaction column and consult doctor.

## POSSIBLE ADVERSE REACTIONS OR SIDE EFFECTS

| SYMPTOMS | WHAT TO DO |
|---|---|
| **Life-threatening:**<br>None expected. | |
| **Common:**<br>Dizziness. | Continue. Call doctor when convenient. |
| **Infrequent:**<br>Mood change, appetite loss, diarrhea, irregular heartbeat, muscle cramps, fatigue, weakness. | Discontinue. Call doctor right away. |
| **Rare:**<br>Rash or hives, yellow vision, ringing in ears, hearing loss, sore throat, fever, dry mouth, thirst, side or stomach pain, nausea, vomiting, unusual bleeding or bruising, joint pain, jaundice. | Discontinue. Call doctor right away. |

## WARNINGS & PRECAUTIONS

**Don't take if:**
You are allergic to ethacrynic acid.

**Before you start, consult your doctor:**
- If you are allergic to any sulfa drug.
- If you have liver or kidney disease.
- If you have gout.
- If you have diabetes.
- If you have impaired hearing.
- If you will have surgery within 2 months, including dental surgery, requiring general or spinal anesthesia.

**Over age 60:**
Adverse reactions and side effects may be more frequent and severe than in younger persons. Hot weather may cause need to reduce dosage.

**Pregnancy:**
Risk to unborn child outweighs drug benefits. Don't use.

**Breast-feeding:**
Drug filters into milk. May harm child. Avoid.

**Infants & children:**
Use only under medical supervision.

**Prolonged use:**
- Impaired balance of water, salt and potassium in blood and body tissues.
- Possible diabetes.

**Skin & sunlight:**
May cause rash or intensify sunburn in areas exposed to sun or sunlamp.

**Driving, piloting or hazardous work:**
No problems expected.

**Discontinuing:**
Don't discontinue without doctor's advice until you complete prescribed dose, even though symptoms diminish or disappear.

**Others:**
Frequent laboratory studies to monitor potassium level in blood recommended. Eat foods rich in potassium or take potassium supplements. Consult doctor.

 **POSSIBLE INTERACTION WITH OTHER DRUGS**

| GENERIC NAME OR DRUG CLASS | COMBINED EFFECT |
| --- | --- |
| Acebutolol | Increased antihypertensive effect of each. Dosages may require adjustments. |
| Allopurinol | Decreased allopurinol effect. |
| Amiodarone | Increased risk of heartbeat irregularity due to low potassium. |
| Anticoagulants | Abnormal clotting. |
| Antidepressants (tricyclic) | Excessive blood-pressure drop. |
| Antidiabetics (oral) | Decreased antidiabetic effect. |
| Antihypertensives | Increased antihypertensive effect. |
| Anti-inflammatory drugs (non-steroid) | Decreased ethacrynic acid effect. |
| Barbiturates | Low blood pressure. |
| Calcium supplements | Increased calcium in blood. |
| Cortisone drugs | Excessive potassium loss. |
| Digitalis preparations | Serious heart-rhythm disorders. |
| Insulin | Decreased insulin effect. |
| Labetolol | Increased antihypertensive effects. |
| Lithium | Increased lithium toxicity. |
| MAO inhibitors | Increased ethacrynic acid effect. |
| Narcotics | Dangerous low blood pressure. Avoid. |
| Nitrates | Excessive blood-pressure drop. |
| Oxprenolol | Increased antihypertensive effect of each. Dosages may require adjustments. |
| Phenothiazines | Increased phenothiazine effect. |
| Potassium supplements | Decreased potassium effect. |
| Probenecid | Decreased probenecid effect. |
| Salicylates (including aspirin) | Dangerous salicylate retention. |
| Sedatives | Increased ethacrynic acid effect. |

 **POSSIBLE INTERACTION WITH OTHER SUBSTANCES**

| INTERACTS WITH | COMBINED EFFECT |
| --- | --- |
| Alcohol: | Blood-pressure drop. Avoid. |
| Beverages: | None expected. |
| Cocaine: | Dangerous blood-pressure drop. Avoid. |
| Foods: | None expected. |
| Marijuana: | Increased thirst and urinary frequency, fainting. |
| Tobacco: | Decreased ethacrynic acid effect. |

# ETHCHLORVYNOL

## BRAND NAMES

Placidyl

## BASIC INFORMATION

**Habit forming?** Yes
**Prescription needed?** Yes
**Available as generic?** No
**Drug class:** Sleep inducer (hypnotic)

 **USES**

Treatment of insomnia.

 **DOSAGE & USAGE INFORMATION**

**How to take:**
With food or milk to lessen side effects.

**When to take:**
At or near bedtime.

**If you forget a dose:**
Bedtime dose—If you forget your once-a-day bedtime dose, don't take it more than 3 hours late.

**What drug does:**
Affects brain centers that control waking and sleeping.

**Time lapse before drug works:**
30 to 60 minutes.

**Don't take with:**
See Interaction column and consult doctor.

 **OVERDOSE**

**SYMPTOMS:**
Excitement, delirium, incoordination, excessive drowsiness, deep coma.
**WHAT TO DO:**
- **Dial 0 (operator) or 911 (emergency) for an ambulance or medical help. Then give first aid immediately.**
- **If patient is unconscious and not breathing, give mouth-to-mouth breathing. If there is no heartbeat, use cardiac massage and mouth-to-mouth breathing (CPR). Don't try to make patient vomit. If you can't get help quickly, take patient to nearest emergency facility.**
- **See emergency information on inside covers.**

 **POSSIBLE ADVERSE REACTIONS OR SIDE EFFECTS**

| SYMPTOMS | WHAT TO DO |
|---|---|
| **Life-threatening:**<br>None expected. | |
| **Common:** | |
| • Indigestion, nausea, vomiting, stomach pain. | Discontinue. Call doctor right away. |
| • Blurred vision, dizziness. | Continue. Call doctor when convenient. |
| • Unpleasant taste in mouth, fatigue, weakness. | Continue. Tell doctor at next visit. |
| **Infrequent:**<br>Jitters, clumsiness, unsteadiness, drowsiness, confusion, rash, hives, unusual bleeding or bruising. | Discontinue. Call doctor right away. |
| **Rare:**<br>Slow heartbeat, difficult breathing, jaundice. | Discontinue. Call doctor right away. |

## WARNINGS & PRECAUTIONS

**Don't take if:**
- You are allergic to any hypnotic.
- You have porphyria.
- Patient is younger than 12.

**Before you start, consult your doctor:**
- If you plan to become pregnant within medication period.
- If you have kidney or liver disease.

**Over age 60:**
Adverse reactions and side effects, especially a "hangover" effect, may be more frequent and severe than in younger persons.

**Pregnancy:**
Risk to unborn child outweighs drug benefits. Don't use.

**Breast-feeding:**
No problems expected, but observe child and ask doctor for guidance.

**Infants & children:**
Not recommended.

**Prolonged use:**
Impaired vision.

**Skin & sunlight:**
No problems expected.

**Driving, piloting or hazardous work:**
Don't drive or pilot aircraft until you learn how medicine affects you. Don't work around dangerous machinery. Don't climb ladders or work in high places. Danger increases if you drink alcohol or take medicine affecting alertness and reflexes.

**Discontinuing:**
- Don't discontinue without consulting doctor. Dose may require gradual reduction if you have taken drug for a long time. Doses of other drugs may also require adjustment.
- Many side effects may occur when you stop taking this drug, including irritability, muscle twitching, hallucinations or seizures. Consult your doctor.

**Others:**
No problems expected.

## POSSIBLE INTERACTION WITH OTHER DRUGS

| GENERIC NAME OR DRUG CLASS | COMBINED EFFECT |
| --- | --- |
| Anticoagulants (oral) | Decreased anticoagulant effect. |
| Antidepressants (tricyclic) | Delirium and deep sedation. |
| Antihistamines | Increased antihistamine effect. |
| Molindone | Increased sedative effect. |
| Narcotics | Increased narcotic effect. |
| Pain relievers | Increased effect of pain reliever. |
| Sedatives | Increased sedative effect. |
| Tranquilizers | Increased tranquilizer effect. |

## POSSIBLE INTERACTION WITH OTHER SUBSTANCES

| INTERACTS WITH | COMBINED EFFECT |
| --- | --- |
| Alcohol: | Excessive depressant and sedative effect. Avoid. |
| Beverages: | None expected. |
| Cocaine: | Decreased ethchlorvynol effect. |
| Foods: | None expected. |
| Marijuana: | Occasional use—Drowsiness, unsteadiness, depressed function. Frequent use—Severe drowsiness, impaired physical and mental function. |
| Tobacco: | None expected. |

# ETHINYL ESTRADIOL

## BRAND NAMES

| | |
|---|---|
| Brevicon | Norette |
| Demulen | Norinyl |
| Estinyl | Norlestrin |
| Feminone | Ortho-Novum |
| Loestrin | Ovcon |
| Lo-Ovral | Ovral |
| Modicon | Tri-Norinyl |

## BASIC INFORMATION

**Habit forming? No**
**Prescription needed? Yes**
**Available as generic? Yes**
**Drug class: Female sex hormone (estrogen)**

## USES

- Treatment for symptoms of menopause and menstrual-cycle irregularity.
- Replacement for female hormone deficiency.
- Prevention of pregnancy.
- Treatment for cancer of breast and prostate.

## DOSAGE & USAGE INFORMATION

**How to take:**
Tablet—Swallow with liquid. If you can't swallow whole, crumble tablet and take with liquid or food.

**When to take:**
At the same time each day.

**If you forget a dose:**
Take as soon as you remember up to 12 hours late. If more than 12 hours, wait for next scheduled dose (don't double this dose).

**What drug does:**
- Restores normal estrogen level in tissues.
- Prevents pituitary gland from secreting hormone that causes ovary to ripen and release egg.

*Continued next column*

## OVERDOSE

**SYMPTOMS:**
**Nausea, vomiting, fluid retention, breast enlargement and discomfort, abnormal vaginal bleeding.**
**WHAT TO DO:**
**Overdose unlikely to threaten life. If person takes much larger amount than prescribed, call doctor, poison-control center or hospital emergency room for instructions.**

**Time lapse before drug works:**
10 to 20 days.

**Don't take with:**
See Interaction column and consult doctor.

## POSSIBLE ADVERSE REACTIONS OR SIDE EFFECTS

| SYMPTOMS | WHAT TO DO |
|---|---|
| **Life-threatening:**<br>None expected. | |
| **Common:** | |
| • Stomach cramps. | Discontinue. Call doctor right away. |
| • Appetite loss. | Continue. Call doctor when convenient. |
| • Nausea; diarrhea; swollen feet and ankles; tender, swollen breasts. | Continue. Tell doctor at next visit. |
| **Infrequent:** | |
| • Rash, stomach or side pain. | Discontinue. Call doctor right away. |
| • Depression, dizziness, irritability, vomiting, breast lumps. | Continue. Call doctor when convenient. |
| • Brown blotches, hair loss, vaginal discharge or bleeding, changes in sex drive. | Continue. Tell doctor at next visit. |
| **Rare:**<br>Jaundice. | Discontinue. Call doctor right away. |

## WARNINGS & PRECAUTIONS

**Don't take if:**
- You are allergic to any estrogen-containing drugs.
- You have impaired liver function.
- You have had blood clots, stroke or heart attack.
- You have unexplained vaginal bleeding.

**Before you start, consult your doctor:**
- If you have had cancer of breast or reproductive organs, fibrocystic breast disease, fibroid tumors of the uterus or endometriosis.
- If you have had migraine headaches, epilepsy or porphyria.
- If you have diabetes, high blood pressure, asthma, congestive heart failure, kidney disease or gallstones.
- If you plan to become pregnant within 3 months.

**Over age 60:**
Controversial. You and your doctor must decide if drug risks outweigh benefits.

**Pregnancy:**
Risk to unborn child outweighs drug benefits. Don't use.

**Breast-feeding:**
Drug filters into milk. May harm child. Avoid.

**Infants & children:**
Not recommended.

**Prolonged use:**
Increased growth of fibroid tumors of uterus. Possible association with cancer of uterus.

**Skin & sunlight:**
May cause rash or intensify sunburn in areas exposed to sun or sunlamp.

**Driving, piloting or hazardous work:**
No problems expected.

**Discontinuing:**
You may need to discontinue ethinyl estradiol periodically. Consult your doctor.

**Others:**
In rare instances, may cause blood clot in lung, brain or leg. Symptoms are *sudden* severe headache, coordination loss, vision change, chest pain, breathing difficulty, slurred speech, pain in legs or groin. Seek emergency treatment immediately.

## POSSIBLE INTERACTION WITH OTHER DRUGS

| GENERIC NAME OR DRUG CLASS | COMBINED EFFECT |
|---|---|
| Anticoagulants (oral) | Decreased anticoagulant effect. |
| Anticonvulsants (hydantoin) | Increased seizures. |
| Antidiabetics (oral) | Unpredictable increase or decrease in blood sugar. |
| Carbamazepine | Increased seizures. |
| Clofibrate | Decreased clofibrate effect. |
| Meprobamate | Increased effect of ethinyl estradiol. |
| Phenobarbital | Decreased effect of ethinyl estradiol. |
| Primidone | Decreased effect of ethinyl estradiol. |
| Rifampin | Decreased effect of ethinyl estradiol. |
| Thyroid hormones | Decreased thyroid effect. |

## POSSIBLE INTERACTION WITH OTHER SUBSTANCES

| INTERACTS WITH | COMBINED EFFECT |
|---|---|
| Alcohol: | None expected. |
| Beverages: | None expected. |
| Cocaine: | No proven problems. |
| Foods: | None expected. |
| Marijuana: | Possible menstrual irregularities and bleeding between periods. |
| Tobacco: | Increased risk of blood clots leading to stroke or heart attack. |

# ETHOPROPAZINE

## BRAND NAMES

Parsidol          Parsitan

## BASIC INFORMATION

**Habit forming?** No
**Prescription needed?** Yes
**Available as generic?** No
**Drug class:** Antidyskinetic, antiparkinsonism

## USES

- Treatment of Parkinson's disease.
- Treatment of adverse effects of phenothiazines.

## DOSAGE & USAGE INFORMATION

**How to take:**
Tablets or capsules—Take with food to lessen stomach irritation.

**When to take:**
At the same times each day.

**If you forget a dose:**
Take as soon as you remember up to 2 hours late. If more than 2 hours, wait for next scheduled dose (don't double this dose).

**What drug does:**
- Balances chemical reactions necessary to send nerve impulses within base of brain.
- Improves muscle control and reduces stiffness.

**Time lapse before drug works:**
1 to 2 hours.

*Continued next column*

## OVERDOSE

**SYMPTOMS:**
**Agitation, dilated pupils, hallucinations, dry mouth, rapid heartbeat, sleepiness.**
**WHAT TO DO:**
- **Dial 0 (operator) or 911 (emergency) for an ambulance or medical help. Then give first aid immediately.**
- **If patient is unconscious and not breathing, give mouth-to-mouth breathing. If there is no heartbeat, use cardiac massage and mouth-to-mouth breathing (CPR). Don't try to make patient vomit. If you can't get help quickly, take patient to nearest emergency facility.**
- **See emergency information on inside covers.**

**Don't take with:**
- Non-prescription drugs for colds, cough or allergy.
- See Interaction column and consult doctor.

## POSSIBLE ADVERSE REACTIONS OR SIDE EFFECTS

| SYMPTOMS | WHAT TO DO |
|---|---|
| **Life-threatening:** | |
| None expected. | |
| **Common:** | |
| • Blurred vision, light sensitivity, constipation, nausea, vomiting. | Continue. Call doctor when convenient. |
| • Painful or difficult urination. | Continue. Tell doctor at next visit. |
| **Infrequent:** | |
| None expected. | |
| **Rare:** | |
| • Rash, eye pain. | Discontinue. Call doctor right away. |
| • Confusion; dizziness; sore mouth or tongue; muscle cramps; numbness, weakness in hands or feet. | Continue. Call doctor when convenient. |

## WARNINGS & PRECAUTIONS

**Don't take if:**
You are allergic to any antidyskinetic.

**Before you start, consult your doctor:**
- If you have had glaucoma.
- If you have had high blood pressure or heart disease.
- If you have had impaired liver function.
- If you have had kidney disease or urination difficulty.

**Over age 60:**
More sensitive to drug. Aggravates symptoms of enlarged prostate. Causes impaired thinking, hallucinations, nightmares. Consult doctor about any of these.

**Pregnancy:**
Studies inconclusive on harm to unborn child. Animal studies show fetal abnormalities. Decide with your doctor whether drug benefits justify risk to unborn child.

**Breast-feeding:**
No problems expected.

**Infants & children:**
Not recommended for children 3 and younger. Use for older children only under doctor's supervision.

**Prolonged use:**
Possible glaucoma.

**Skin & sunlight:**
No problems expected.

**Driving, piloting or hazardous work:**
Don't drive or pilot aircraft until you learn how medicine affects you. Don't work around dangerous machinery. Don't climb ladders or work in high places. Danger increases if you drink alcohol or take medicine affecting alertness and reflexes, such as antihistamines, tranquilizers, sedatives, pain medicine, narcotics and mind-altering drugs.

**Discontinuing:**
Don't discontinue without consulting doctor. Dose may require gradual reduction if you have taken drug for a long time. Doses of other drugs may also require adjustment.

**Others:**
- Internal eye pressure should be measured regularly.
- Avoid becoming overheated.

## POSSIBLE INTERACTION WITH OTHER DRUGS

| GENERIC NAME OR DRUG CLASS | COMBINED EFFECT |
|---|---|
| Amantadine | Increased amantadine effect. |
| Antidepressants (tricyclic) | Increased ethopropazine effect. May cause glaucoma. |
| Antihistamines | Increased ethopropazine effect. |
| Levodopa | Increased levodopa effect. Improved results in treating Parkinson's disease. |
| MAO inhibitors | Increased ethopropazine effect. |
| Meperidine | Increased ethopropazine effect. |
| Orphenadrine | Increased ethopropazine effect. |
| Phenothiazines | Behavior changes. |
| Primidone | Excessive sedation. |
| Procainamide | Increased procainamide effect. |
| Quinidine | Increased ethopropazine effect. |
| Tranquilizers | Excessive sedation. |

## POSSIBLE INTERACTION WITH OTHER SUBSTANCES

| INTERACTS WITH | COMBINED EFFECT |
|---|---|
| Alcohol: | None expected. |
| Beverages: | None expected. |
| Cocaine: | Decreased ethopropazine effect. Avoid. |
| Foods: | None expected. |
| Marijuana: | None expected. |
| Tobacco: | None expected. |

# ETHOSUXIMIDE

## BRAND NAMES

Zarontin

## BASIC INFORMATION

**Habit forming? No**
**Prescription needed? Yes**
**Available as generic? No**
**Drug class: Anticonvulsant (succinimide)**

## USES

Controls seizures in treatment of epilepsy.

## DOSAGE & USAGE INFORMATION

**How to take:**
Capsule—Swallow with liquid or food to lessen stomach irritation.

**When to take:**
Every day in regularly-spaced doses, according to prescription.

**If you forget a dose:**
Take as soon as you remember up to 2 hours late. If more than 2 hours, wait for next scheduled dose (don't double this dose).

**What drug does:**
Depresses nerve transmissions in part of brain that controls muscles.

**Time lapse before drug works:**
3 hours.

**Don't take with:**
See Interaction column and consult doctor.

## OVERDOSE

**SYMPTOMS:**
Coma
**WHAT TO DO:**
- Dial 0 (operator) or 911 (emergency) for an ambulance or medical help. Then give first aid immediately.
- If patient is unconscious and not breathing, give mouth-to-mouth breathing. If there is no heartbeat, use cardiac massage and mouth-to-mouth breathing (CPR). Don't try to make patient vomit. If you can't get help quickly, take patient to nearest emergency facility.
- See emergency information on inside covers.

## POSSIBLE ADVERSE REACTIONS OR SIDE EFFECTS

| SYMPTOMS | WHAT TO DO |
|---|---|
| **Life-threatening:**<br>None expected. | |
| **Common:**<br>Nausea, vomiting, stomach cramps, appetite loss. | Continue. Call doctor when convenient. |
| **Infrequent:**<br>Dizziness, drowsiness, headache, irritability, mood change. | Continue. Call doctor when convenient. |
| **Rare:**<br>• Sore throat, fever, rash, unusual bleeding or bruising. | Discontinue. Call doctor right away. |
| • Swollen lymph glands. | Continue. Call doctor when convenient. |

## WARNINGS & PRECAUTIONS

**Don't take if:**
You are allergic to any succinimide anticonvulsant.

**Before you start, consult your doctor:**
- If you plan to become pregnant within medication period.
- If you take other anticonvulsants.
- If you have blood disease.
- If you have kidney or liver disease.

**Over age 60:**
Adverse reactions and side effects may be more frequent and severe than in younger persons.

**Pregnancy:**
Risk to unborn child outweighs drug benefits. Don't use.

**Breast-feeding:**
Drug passes into milk. Avoid drug or discontinue nursing.

**Infants & children:**
Use only under medical supervision.

**Prolonged use:**
No problems expected.

**Skin & sunlight:**
No problems expected.

**Driving, piloting or hazardous work:**
Don't drive or pilot aircraft until you learn how medicine affects you. Don't work around dangerous machinery. Don't climb ladders or work in high places. Danger increases if you drink alcohol or take medicine affecting alertness and reflexes, such as antihistamines, tranquilizers, sedatives, pain medicine, narcotics and mind-altering drugs.

**Discontinuing:**
Don't discontinue without doctor's advice until you complete prescribed dose, even though symptoms diminish or disappear.

**Others:**
- Your response to medicine should be checked regularly by your doctor. Dose and schedule may have to be altered frequently to fit individual needs.
- Periodic blood-cell counts, kidney- and liver-function studies recommended.

 ## POSSIBLE INTERACTION WITH OTHER DRUGS

| GENERIC NAME OR DRUG CLASS | COMBINED EFFECT |
|---|---|
| Anticonvulsants (other) | Increased effect of both drugs. |
| Antidepressants (tricyclic) | May provoke seizures. |
| Antipsychotics | May provoke seizures. |

 ## POSSIBLE INTERACTION WITH OTHER SUBSTANCES

| INTERACTS WITH | COMBINED EFFECT |
|---|---|
| Alcohol: | May provoke seizures. |
| Beverages: | None expected. |
| Cocaine: | May provoke seizures. |
| Foods: | None expected. |
| Marijuana: | May provoke seizures. |
| Tobacco: | None expected. |

# ETHOTOIN

## BRAND NAMES

Peganone

## BASIC INFORMATION

**Habit forming? No**
**Prescription needed? Yes**
**Available as generic? Yes**
**Drug class: Anticonvulsant (hydantoin)**

## USES

- Prevents epileptic seizures.
- Stabilizes irregular heartbeat.

## DOSAGE & USAGE INFORMATION

**How to take:**
- Tablet or capsule—Swallow with liquid.
- Extended-release tablets or capsules—Swallow each dose whole. If you take regular tablets, you may chew or crush them.

**When to take:**
At the same time each day.

**If you forget a dose:**
- If drug taken 1 time per day—Take as soon as you remember up to 12 hours late. If more than 12 hours, wait for next scheduled dose (don't double this dose).
- If taken several times per day—Take as soon as possible, then return to regular schedule.

**What drug does:**
Promotes sodium loss from nerve fibers. This lessens excitability and inhibits spread of nerve impulses.

**Time lapse before drug works:**
7 to 10 days continual use.

**Don't take with:**
See Interaction column and consult doctor.

## OVERDOSE

**SYMPTOMS:**
**Jerky eye movements; stagger; slurred speech; imbalance; drowsiness; blood-pressure drop; slow, shallow breathing; coma.**
**WHAT TO DO:**
- **Dial 0 (operator) or 911 (emergency) for an ambulance or medical help. Then give first aid immediately.**
- **See emergency information on inside covers.**

## POSSIBLE ADVERSE REACTIONS OR SIDE EFFECTS

| SYMPTOMS | WHAT TO DO |
|---|---|
| **Life-threatening:**<br>None expected. | |
| **Common:**<br>Mild dizziness, drowsiness, constipation, nausea, vomiting. | Continue. Call doctor when convenient. |
| **Infrequent:** | |
| • Hallucinations, confusion, slurred speech, stagger, rash, change in vision. | Discontinue. Call doctor right away. |
| • Headache, sleeplessness, diarrhea, muscle twitching. | Continue. Call doctor when convenient. |
| • Increased body and facial hair. | Continue. Tell doctor at next visit. |
| **Rare:**<br>Sore throat, fever, unusual bleeding or bruising, stomach pain, jaundice. | Discontinue. Call doctor right away. |

## WARNINGS & PRECAUTIONS

**Don't take if:**
You are allergic to any hydantoin anticonvulsant.

**Before you start, consult your doctor:**
- If you have had impaired liver function or disease.
- If you will have surgery within 2 months, including dental surgery, requiring general or spinal anesthesia.

**Over age 60:**
Adverse reactions and side effects may be more frequent and severe than in younger persons.

**Pregnancy:**
Risk to unborn child outweighs drug benefits. Don't use.

**Breast-feeding:**
Drug passes into milk. Avoid drug or discontinue nursing until you finish medicine. Consult doctor for advice on maintaining milk supply.

**Infants & children:**
Use only under medical supervision.

**Prolonged use:**
- Weakened bones.
- Lymph gland enlargement.
- Possible liver damage.

- Numbness and tingling of hands and feet.
- Continual back-and-forth eye movements.
- Bleeding, swollen or tender gums.

**Skin & sunlight:**
May cause rash or intensify sunburn in areas exposed to sun or sunlamp.

**Driving, piloting or hazardous work:**
Don't drive or pilot aircraft until you learn how medicine affects you. Don't work around dangerous machinery. Don't climb ladders or work in high places. Danger increases if you drink alcohol or take medicine affecting alertness and reflexes.

**Discontinuing:**
Don't discontinue without consulting doctor. Dose may require gradual reduction if you have taken drug for a long time. Doses of other drugs may also require adjustment.

**Others:**
No problems expected.

## POSSIBLE INTERACTION WITH OTHER DRUGS

| GENERIC NAME OR DRUG CLASS | COMBINED EFFECT |
|---|---|
| Anticoagulants | Increased effect of both drugs. |
| Antidepressants (tricyclic) | Need to adjust ethotoin dose. |
| Antihypertensives | Increased effect of antihypertensive. |
| Aspirin | Increased ethotoin effect. |
| Barbiturates | Changed seizure pattern. |
| Carbonic anhydrase inhibitors | Increased chance of bone disease. |
| Chloramphenicol | Increased ethotoin effect. |
| Contraceptives (oral) | Increased seizures. |
| Cortisone drugs | Decreased cortisone effect. |
| Digitalis preparations | Decreased digitalis effect. |
| Disulfiram | Increased ethotoin effect. |
| Estrogens | Increased ethotoin effect. |
| Furosemide | Decreased furosemide effect. |
| Glutethimide | Decreased ethotoin effect. |

| | |
|---|---|
| Griseofulvin | Increased griseofulvin effect. |
| Isoniazid | Increased ethotoin effect. |
| Methadone | Decreased methadone effect. |
| Methotrexate | Increased methotrexate effect. |
| Methylphenidate | Increased ethotoin effect. |
| Oxyphenbutazone | Increased ethotoin effect. |
| Para-aminosalicylic acid (PAS) | Increased ethotoin effect. |
| Phenothiazines | Increased ethotoin effect. |
| Phenylbutazone | Increased ethotoin effect. |
| Propranolol | Increased propranolol effect. |
| Quinidine | Increased quinidine effect. |
| Sedatives | Increased sedative effect. |
| Sulfa drugs | Increased ethotoin effect. |
| Theophylline | Reduced anticonvulsant effect. |

## POSSIBLE INTERACTION WITH OTHER SUBSTANCES

| INTERACTS WITH | COMBINED EFFECT |
|---|---|
| Alcohol: | Possible decreased anticonvulsant effect. Use with caution. |
| Beverages: | None expected. |
| Cocaine: | Possible seizures. |
| Foods: | None expected. |
| Marijuana: | Drowsiness, unsteadiness, decreased anticonvulsant effect. |
| Tobacco: | None expected. |

# FENOPROFEN

## BRAND NAMES

Fenopron          Progesic
Nalfon

## BASIC INFORMATION

Habit forming? No
Available as generic? No
Prescription needed? Yes
Drug class: Anti-inflammatory (non-steroid)

 ## USES

- Treatment for joint pain, stiffness, inflammation and swelling of arthritis and gout.
- Pain reliever.
- Treatment for dysmenorrhea (painful or difficult menstruation).

 ## DOSAGE & USAGE INFORMATION

**How to take:**
Tablet or capsule—Swallow with liquid or food to lessen stomach irritation. If you can't swallow whole, crumble tablet or open capsule and take with liquid or food.

**When to take:**
At the same times each day.

**If you forget a dose:**
Take as soon as you remember up to 2 hours late. If more than 2 hours, wait for next scheduled dose (don't double this dose).

**What drug does:**
Reduces tissue concentration of prostaglandins (hormones which produce inflammation and pain).

**Time lapse before drug works:**
Begins in 4 to 24 hours. May require 3 weeks regular use for maximum benefit.

*Continued next column*

 ## OVERDOSE

**SYMPTOMS:**
Confusion, agitation, incoherence, convulsions, possible hemorrhage from stomach or intestine, coma.
**WHAT TO DO:**
- **Dial 0 (operator) or 911 (emergency) for an ambulance or medical help. Then give first aid immediately.**
- **See emergency information on inside covers.**

---

**Don't take with:**
See Interaction column and consult doctor.

 ## POSSIBLE ADVERSE REACTIONS OR SIDE EFFECTS

| SYMPTOMS | WHAT TO DO |
|---|---|
| **Life-threatening:**<br>None expected. | |
| **Common:** | |
| • Dizziness, nausea, pain. | Continue. Call doctor when convenient. |
| • Headache. | Continue. Tell doctor at next visit. |
| **Infrequent:** | |
| Depression; drowsiness; ringing in ears; swollen feet, legs; constipation or diarrhea; vomiting. | Continue. Call doctor when convenient. |
| **Rare:** | |
| • Convulsions; confusion, rash, hives or itch; black or bloody, tarry stools; difficult breathing; tightness in chest; blurred vision; rapid heartbeat; unusual bleeding or bruising; blood in urine; jaundice. | Discontinue. Call doctor right away. |
| • Urgent, frequent or painful urination; fatigue; weakness. | Continue. Call doctor when convenient. |

# FENOPROFEN

## WARNINGS & PRECAUTIONS

**Don't take if:**
- You are allergic to aspirin or any non-steroid, anti-inflammatory drug.
- You have gastritis, peptic ulcer, enteritis, ileitis, ulcerative colitis, asthma, heart failure, high blood pressure or bleeding problems.
- Patient is younger than 15.

**Before you start, consult your doctor:**
- If you have epilepsy.
- If you have Parkinson's disease.
- If you have been mentally ill.
- If you have had kidney disease or impaired kidney function.

**Over age 60:**
Adverse reactions and side effects may be more frequent and severe than in younger persons.

**Pregnancy:**
Studies inconclusive on harm to unborn child. Decide with your doctor whether drug benefits justify risk to unborn child.

**Breast-feeding:**
May harm child. Avoid.

**Infants & children:**
Not recommended for anyone younger than 15. Use only under medical supervision.

**Prolonged use:**
- Eye damage.
- Reduced hearing.
- Sore throat, fever.
- Weight gain.

**Skin & sunlight:**
No problems expected.

**Driving, piloting or hazardous work:**
Don't drive or pilot aircraft until you learn how medicine affects you. Don't work around dangerous machinery. Don't climb ladders or work in high places. Danger increases if you drink alcohol or take medicine affecting alertness and reflexes, such as antihistamines, tranquilizers, sedatives, pain medicine, narcotics and mind-altering drugs.

**Discontinuing:**
Don't discontinue without consulting doctor. Dose may require gradual reduction if you have taken drug for a long time. Doses of other drugs may also require adjustment.

**Others:**
No problems expected.

## POSSIBLE INTERACTION WITH OTHER DRUGS

| GENERIC NAME OR DRUG CLASS | COMBINED EFFECT |
|---|---|
| Anticoagulants (oral) | Increased risk of bleeding. |
| Aspirin | Increased risk of stomach ulcer. |
| Cortisone drugs | Increased risk of stomach ulcer. |
| Furosemide | Decreased diuretic effect of furosemide. |
| Ketoprofen | Increased possibility of internal bleeding. |
| Oxyphenbutazone | Possible stomach ulcer. |
| Phenylbutazone | Possible stomach ulcer. |
| Probenecid | Increased fenoprofen effect. |
| Thyroid hormones | Rapid heartbeat, blood-pressure rise. |

## POSSIBLE INTERACTION WITH OTHER SUBSTANCES

| INTERACTS WITH | COMBINED EFFECT |
|---|---|
| Alcohol: | Possible stomach ulcer or bleeding. |
| Beverages: | None expected. |
| Cocaine: | None expected. |
| Foods: | None expected. |
| Marijuana: | Increased pain relief from fenoprofen. |
| Tobacco: | None expected. |

# FERROUS FUMARATE

## BRAND NAMES

See complete list of brand names in the *Brand Name Directory,* page 949.

## BASIC INFORMATION

**Habit forming? No**
**Prescription needed?**
   **With folic acid: Yes**
   **Without folic acid: No**
**Available as generic? Yes**
**Drug class: Mineral supplement (iron)**

 ## USES

Treatment for dietary iron deficiency or iron-deficiency anemia from other causes.

 ## DOSAGE & USAGE INFORMATION

**How to take:**
- Tablet, capsule or liquid—Swallow with liquid or food to lessen stomach irritation. If you can't swallow whole, crumble tablet or open capsule and take with liquid or food. Place medicine far back on tongue to avoid staining teeth.
- Drops—Dilute dose in beverage before swallowing and drink through a straw.

**When to take:**
1 hour before or 2 hours after meals.

**If you forget a dose:**
Take up to 2 hours late. If more than 2 hours, wait for next dose (don't double this dose).

**What drug does:**
Stimulates bone-marrow production of hemoglobin (red-blood-cell pigment that carries oxygen to body cells).

**Time lapse before drug works:**
3 to 7 days. May require 3 weeks for maximum benefit.

*Continued next column*

 ## OVERDOSE

**SYMPTOMS:**
**Weakness, collapse; pallor, blue lips, hands and fingernails; weak, rapid heartbeat; shallow breathing; convulsions; coma.**
**WHAT TO DO:**
- **Dial 0 (operator) or 911 (emergency) for an ambulance or medical help. Then give first aid immediately.**
- **See emergency information on inside covers.**

**Don't take with:**
- Multiple vitamin and mineral supplements.
- See Interaction column and consult doctor.

 ## POSSIBLE ADVERSE REACTIONS OR SIDE EFFECTS

| SYMPTOMS | WHAT TO DO |
|---|---|
| **Life-threatening:** | |
| Weak, rapid heartbeat. | Seek emergency treatment immediately. |
| **Always:** | |
| Gray or black stool. | No action necessary. |
| **Common:** | |
| Stained teeth with liquid iron. | No action necessary. |
| **Infrequent:** | |
| • Constipation or diarrhea, heartburn, nausea, vomiting. | Discontinue. Call doctor right away. |
| • Fatigue, weakness. | Continue. Call doctor when convenient. |
| • Dark urine. | Continue. Tell doctor at next visit. |
| **Rare:** | |
| • Throat or chest pain on swallowing, pain, cramps, blood in stool. | Discontinue. Call doctor right away. |
| • Drowsiness. | Continue. Call doctor when convenient. |

## WARNINGS & PRECAUTIONS

**Don't take if:**
- You are allergic to any iron supplement.
- You take iron injections.
- Your daily iron intake is high.
- You plan to take this supplement for a long time.
- You have acute hepatitis.
- You have hemosiderosis or hemochromatosis (conditions involving excess iron in body).
- You have hemolytic anemia.

**Before you start, consult your doctor:**
- If you plan to become pregnant within medication period.
- If you have had stomach surgery.
- If you have had peptic ulcer disease, enteritis or colitis.
- If you have had pancreatitis or hepatitis.

**Over age 60:**
May cause hemochromatosis (iron storage disease) with bronze skin, liver damage, diabetes, heart problems and impotence.

**Pregnancy:**
No proven harm to unborn child. Avoid if possible. Take only if your doctor prescribes supplement during last half of pregnancy.

**Breast-feeding:**
No problems expected. Take only if your doctor confirms you have a dietary deficiency or an iron-deficiency anemia.

**Infants & children:**
Use only under medical supervision. Overdose common and dangerous. Keep out of children's reach.

**Prolonged use:**
May cause hemochromatosis (iron storage disease) with bronze skin, liver damage, diabetes, heart problems and impotence.

**Skin & sunlight:**
No problems expected.

**Driving, piloting or hazardous work:**
No problems expected.

**Discontinuing:**
May be unnecessary to finish medicine. Follow doctor's instructions.

**Others:**
Liquid form stains teeth. Mix with water or juice to lessen the effect. Brush with baking soda or hydrogen peroxide to help remove stain.

## POSSIBLE INTERACTION WITH OTHER DRUGS

| GENERIC NAME OR DRUG CLASS | COMBINED EFFECT |
| --- | --- |
| Acetohydroxamic acid | Decreased effects of both drugs. |
| Allopurinol | Possible excess iron storage in liver. |
| Antacids | Poor iron absorption. |
| Chloramphenicol | Decreased effect of iron. Interferes with red-blood-cell and hemoglobin formation. |
| Cholestyramine | Decreased iron effect. |
| Iron supplements (other) | Possible excess iron storage in liver. |
| Penicillamine | Decreased penicillamine effect. |
| Sulfasalazine | Decreased iron effect. |
| Tetracyclines | Decreased tetracycline effect. Take iron 3 hours before or 2 hours after taking tetracycline. |
| Vitamin C | Increased iron effect. Contributes to red-blood-cell and hemoglobin formation. |
| Vitamin E | Decreased iron effect. |

## POSSIBLE INTERACTION WITH OTHER SUBSTANCES

| INTERACTS WITH | COMBINED EFFECT |
| --- | --- |
| Alcohol: | Increased iron absorption. May cause organ damage. Avoid or use in moderation. |
| Beverages: Milk, tea. | Decreased iron effect. |
| Cocaine: | None expected. |
| Foods: Dairy foods, eggs, whole-grain bread and cereal. | Decreased iron effect. |
| Marijuana: | None expected. |
| Tobacco: | None expected. |

# FERROUS GLUCONATE

## BRAND NAMES

Apo-Ferrous
  Gluconate
Fergon
Ferralet
Ferralet Plus
Ferrous-G
Fertinic
Fosfree

Glytinic
I.L.X. B-12
Iromin-G
Megadose
Mission
Novoferrogluc
Simron

## BASIC INFORMATION

Habit forming? No
Prescription needed?
  With folic acid: Yes
  Without folic acid: No
Available as generic? Yes
Drug class: Mineral supplement (iron)

## USES

Treatment for dietary iron deficiency or
iron-deficiency anemia from other causes.

## DOSAGE & USAGE INFORMATION

How to take:
- Tablet or capsule—Swallow with liquid or
  food to lessen stomach irritation. If you can't
  swallow whole, crumble tablet or open
  capsule and take with liquid or food. Place
  medicine far back on tongue to avoid staining
  teeth.
- Drops—Dilute dose in beverage before
  swallowing and drink through a straw.

When to take:
1 hour before or 2 hours after eating.

If you forget a dose:
Take up to 2 hours late. If more than 2 hours,
wait for next dose (don't double this dose).

*Continued next column*

## OVERDOSE

SYMPTOMS:
- Moderate overdose—Stomach pain,
  vomiting, diarrhea, black stools, lethargy.
- Serious overdose—Weakness and
  collapse; pallor, weak and rapid heartbeat;
  shallow breathing; convulsions and coma.
WHAT TO DO:
- Dial 0 (operator) or 911 (emergency) for an
  ambulance or medical help. Then give first
  aid immediately.
- See emergency information on inside
  covers.

What drug does:
Stimulates bone-marrow production of
hemoglobin (red-blood-cell pigment that carries
oxygen to body cells).

Time lapse before drug works:
3 to 7 days. May require 3 weeks for maximum
benefit.

Don't take with:
- Multiple vitamin and mineral supplements.
- See Interaction column and consult doctor.

## POSSIBLE ADVERSE REACTIONS OR SIDE EFFECTS

| SYMPTOMS | WHAT TO DO |
|---|---|
| **Life-threatening:** | |
| Weak, rapid heartbeat. | Seek emergency treatment immediately. |
| **Always:** | |
| Gray or black stool. | No action necessary. |
| **Common:** | |
| Stained teeth with liquid iron. | No action necessary. |
| **Infrequent:** | |
| • Constipation or diarrhea, heartburn, nausea, vomiting. | Discontinue. Call doctor right away. |
| • Fatigue, weakness. | Continue. Call doctor when convenient. |
| **Rare:** | |
| • Blue lips, fingernails, palms of hands; pale, clammy skin. | Discontinue. Seek emergency treatment. |
| • Throat pain on swallowing, pain, cramps, blood in stool. | Discontinue. Call doctor right away. |
| • Drowsiness. | Continue. Call doctor when convenient. |

## WARNINGS & PRECAUTIONS

### Don't take if:
- You are allergic to any iron supplement.
- You take iron injections.
- You have acute hepatitis, hemosiderosis or hemochromatosis (conditions involving excess iron in body).
- You have hemolytic anemia.

### Before you start, consult your doctor:
- If you plan to become pregnant within medication period.
- If you have had stomach surgery.
- If you have had peptic ulcer, enteritis or colitis.

### Over age 60:
May cause hemochromatosis (iron storage disease) with bronze skin, liver damage, diabetes, heart problems and impotence.

### Pregnancy:
No proven harm to unborn child. Avoid if possible. Take only if your doctor advises supplement during last half of pregnancy.

### Breast-feeding:
No problems expected. Take only if your doctor confirms you have a dietary deficiency or an iron-deficiency anemia.

### Infants & children:
Use only under medical supervision. Overdose common and dangerous. Keep out of children's reach.

### Prolonged use:
May cause hemochromatosis (iron storage disease) with bronze skin, liver damage, diabetes, heart problems and impotence.

### Skin & sunlight:
No problems expected.

### Driving, piloting or hazardous work:
No problems expected.

### Discontinuing:
May be unnecessary to finish medicine. Follow doctor's instructions.

### Others:
Liquid form stains teeth. Mix with water or juice to lessen the effect. Brush with baking soda or hydrogen peroxide to help remove.

## POSSIBLE INTERACTION WITH OTHER DRUGS

| GENERIC NAME OR DRUG CLASS | COMBINED EFFECT |
|---|---|
| Acetohydroxamic acid | Decreased effects of both drugs. |
| Allopurinol | Possible excess iron storage in liver. |
| Antacids | Poor iron absorption. |
| Chloramphenicol | Decreased effect of iron. Interferes with red-blood-cell and hemoglobin formation. |
| Cholestyramine | Decreased iron effect. |
| Iron supplements (other) | Possible excess iron storage in liver. |
| Sulfasalazine | Decreased iron effect. |
| Tetracyclines | Decreased tetracycline effect. Take iron 3 hours before or 2 hours after taking tetracycline. |
| Vitamin C | Increased iron effect. Contributes to red-blood-cell and hemoglobin formation. |
| Vitamin E | Decreased iron effect. |

## POSSIBLE INTERACTION WITH OTHER SUBSTANCES

| INTERACTS WITH | COMBINED EFFECT |
|---|---|
| Alcohol: | Increased iron absorption. May cause organ damage. Avoid or use in moderation. |
| Beverages: Milk, tea. | Decreased iron effect. |
| Cocaine: | None expected. |
| Foods: Dairy foods, eggs, whole-grain bread and cereal. | Decreased iron effect. |
| Marijuana: | None expected. |
| Tobacco: | None expected. |

# FERROUS SULFATE

## BRAND NAMES

See complete list of brand names in the *Brand Name Directory,* page 949.

## BASIC INFORMATION

Habit forming? No
Prescription needed?
  With folic acid: Yes
  Without folic acid: No
Available as generic? Yes
Drug class: Mineral supplement (iron)

## USES

Treatment for dietary iron deficiency or iron-deficiency anemia from other causes.

## DOSAGE & USAGE INFORMATION

**How to take:**
- Tablet, capsule, or liquid—Swallow with liquid or food to lessen stomach irritation. Place medicine far back on tongue to avoid staining teeth.
- Drops—Dilute dose in beverage before swallowing and drink through a straw.
- Extended release tablet or capsule—Swallow whole with liquid.

**When to take:**
1 hour before or 2 hours after meals.

**If you forget a dose:**
Take up to 2 hours late. If more than 2 hours, wait for next dose (don't double this dose).

**What drug does:**
Stimulates bone-marrow production of hemoglobin (red-blood-cell pigment that carries oxygen to body cells).

**Time lapse before drug works:**
3 to 7 days. May require 3 weeks for maximum benefit.

*Continued next column*

## OVERDOSE

**SYMPTOMS:**
**Weakness, collapse; pallor, blue lips, hands and fingernails; weak, rapid heartbeat; shallow breathing; convulsions; coma.**
**WHAT TO DO:**
- **Dial 0 (operator) or 911 (emergency) for an ambulance or medical help. Then give first aid immediately.**
- **See emergency information on inside covers.**

**Don't take with:**
- Multiple vitamin and mineral supplements.
- See Interaction column and consult doctor.

## POSSIBLE ADVERSE REACTIONS OR SIDE EFFECTS

| SYMPTOMS | WHAT TO DO |
|---|---|
| **Life-threatening:** | |
| Weak, rapid heartbeat. | Seek emergency treatment immediately. |
| **Always:** | |
| Gray or black stool. | No action necessary. |
| **Common:** | |
| Stained teeth with liquid iron. | No action necessary. |
| **Infrequent:** | |
| • Constipation or diarrhea, heartburn, nausea, vomiting. | Discontinue. Call doctor right away. |
| • Fatigue, weakness. | Continue. Call doctor when convenient. |
| • Dark urine. | Continue. Tell doctor at next visit. |
| **Rare:** | |
| • Throat or chest pain on swallowing, pain, cramps, blood in stool. | Discontinue. Call doctor right away. |
| • Drowsiness. | Continue. Call doctor when convenient. |

## WARNINGS & PRECAUTIONS

**Don't take if:**
- You are allergic to any iron supplement.
- You take iron injections.
- Your daily iron intake is high.
- You plan to take this supplement for a long time.
- You have acute hepatitis.
- You have hemosiderosis or hemochromatosis (conditions involving excess iron in body).
- You have hemolytic anemia.

**Before you start, consult your doctor:**
- If you plan to become pregnant within medication period.
- If you have had stomach surgery.
- If you have had peptic ulcer disease, enteritis or colitis.
- If you have had pancreatitis or hepatitis.

**Over age 60:**
May cause hemochromatosis (iron storage disease) with bronze skin, liver damage, diabetes, heart problems and impotence.

**Pregnancy:**
No proven harm to unborn child. Avoid if possible. Take only if your doctor prescribes supplement during last half of pregnancy.

**Breast-feeding:**
No problems expected. Take only if your doctor confirms you have a dietary deficiency or an iron-deficiency anemia.

**Infants & children:**
Use only under medical supervision. Overdose common and dangerous. Keep out of children's reach.

**Prolonged use:**
May cause hemochromatosis (iron storage disease) with bronze skin, liver damage, diabetes, heart problems and impotence.

**Skin & sunlight:**
No problems expected.

**Driving, piloting or hazardous work:**
No problems expected.

**Discontinuing:**
May be unnecessary to finish medicine. Follow doctor's instructions.

**Others:**
Liquid form stains teeth. Mix with water or juice to lessen the effect. Brush with baking soda or hydrogen peroxide to help remove stain.

## POSSIBLE INTERACTION WITH OTHER DRUGS

| GENERIC NAME OR DRUG CLASS | COMBINED EFFECT |
|---|---|
| Acetohydroxamic acid | Decreased effects of both drugs. |
| Allopurinol | Possible excess iron storage in liver. |
| Antacids | Poor iron absorption. |
| Chloramphenicol | Decreased effect of iron. Interferes with red-blood-cell and hemoglobin formation. |
| Cholestyramine | Decreased iron effect. |
| Iron supplements (other) | Possible excess iron storage in liver. |
| Penicillamine | Decreased penicillamine effect. |
| Sulfasalazine | Decreased iron effect. |
| Tetracyclines | Decreased tetracycline effect. Take iron 3 hours before or 2 hours after taking tetracycline. |
| Vitamin C | Increased iron effect. Contributes to red-blood-cell and hemoglobin formation. |
| Vitamin E | Decreased iron effect. |

## POSSIBLE INTERACTION WITH OTHER SUBSTANCES

| INTERACTS WITH | COMBINED EFFECT |
|---|---|
| Alcohol: | Increased iron absorption. May cause organ damage. Avoid or use in moderation. |
| Beverages: Milk, tea. | Decreased iron effect. |
| Cocaine: | None expected. |
| Foods: Dairy foods, eggs, whole-grain bread and cereal. | Decreased iron effect. |
| Marijuana: | None expected. |
| Tobacco: | None expected. |

# FLAVOXATE

## BRAND NAMES

**Urispas**

## BASIC INFORMATION

**Habit forming? No**
**Prescription needed? Yes**
**Available as generic? No**
**Drug class: Smooth-muscle relaxant,**
**anticholinergic**

 ## USES

Relieves urinary pain, urgency, nighttime urination, unusual frequency of urination associated with urinary system disorders.

 ## DOSAGE & USAGE INFORMATION

**How to take:**
Tablet or capsule—Swallow with liquid or food to lessen stomach irritation.

**When to take:**
30 minutes before meals (unless directed otherwise by doctor).

**If you forget a dose:**
Take as soon as you remember up to 2 hours late. If more than 2 hours, wait for next scheduled dose (don't double this dose).

**What drug does:**
Blocks nerve impulses at smooth muscle nerve endings, preventing muscle contractions and gland secretions of organs involved.

**Time lapse before drug works:**
15 to 30 minutes.

**Don't take with:**
See Interaction column and consult doctor.

 ## OVERDOSE

**SYMPTOMS:**
**Dilated pupils, rapid pulse and breathing, dizziness, fever, hallucinations, confusion, slurred speech, agitation, flushed face, convulsions, coma.**
**WHAT TO DO:**
- **Dial 0 (operator) or 911 (emergency) for an ambulance or medical help. Then give first aid immediately.**
- **See emergency information on inside covers.**

 ## POSSIBLE ADVERSE REACTIONS OR SIDE EFFECTS

| SYMPTOMS | WHAT TO DO |
|---|---|
| **Life-threatening:** | |
| None expected. | |
| **Common:** | |
| • Confusion, delirium, rapid heartbeat. | Discontinue. Call doctor right away. |
| • Nausea, vomiting, less perspiration. | Continue. Call doctor when convenient. |
| • Constipation. | Continue. Tell doctor at next visit. |
| • Dry ears, nose, throat. | No action necessary. |
| **Infrequent:** | |
| • Unusual excitement, irritability, restlessness. | Discontinue. Call doctor right away. |
| • Headache, increased sensitivity to light, painful or difficult urination. | Continue. Call doctor when convenient. |
| **Rare:** | |
| • Shortness of breath. | Discontinue. Seek emergency treatment. |
| • Rash or hives; pain; blurred vision; sore throat, fever, mouth sores. | Discontinue. Call doctor right away. |

## WARNINGS & PRECAUTIONS

**Don't take if:**
- You are allergic to any anticholinergic.
- You have trouble with stomach bloating.
- You have difficulty emptying your bladder completely.
- You have narrow-angle glaucoma.
- You have severe ulcerative colitis.

**Before you start, consult your doctor:**
- If you have open-angle glaucoma.
- If you have angina.
- If you have chronic bronchitis or asthma.
- If you have liver disease.
- If you have hiatal hernia.
- If you have enlarged prostate.
- If you have myasthenia gravis.
- If you have peptic ulcer.
- If you will have surgery within 2 months, including dental surgery, requiring general or spinal anesthesia.

**Over age 60:**
Adverse reactions and side effects, particularly mental confusion, may be more frequent and severe than in younger persons.

**Pregnancy:**
Studies inconclusive on harm to unborn child. Animal studies show fetal abnormalities. Decide with your doctor whether drug benefits justify risk to unborn child.

**Breast-feeding:**
Drug passes into milk. Avoid drug or discontinue nursing until you finish medicine. Consult doctor for advice on maintaining milk supply.

**Infants & children:**
Use only under medical supervision.

**Prolonged use:**
Chronic constipation, possible fecal impaction. Consult doctor immediately.

**Skin & sunlight:**
No problems expected.

**Driving, piloting or hazardous work:**
Use disqualifies you for piloting aircraft. Otherwise, no problems expected.

**Discontinuing:**
May be unnecessary to finish medicine. Follow doctor's instructions.

**Others:**
No problems expected.

## POSSIBLE INTERACTION WITH OTHER DRUGS

| GENERIC NAME OR DRUG CLASS | COMBINED EFFECT |
|---|---|
| Amantadine | Increased flavoxate effect. |
| Anticholinergics (other) | Increased flavoxate effect. |
| Antidepressants (tricyclic) | Increased flavoxate effect. Increased sedation. |
| Antihistamines | Increased flavoxate effect. |
| Atropine | Increased effect of both drugs. |
| Cortisone drugs | Increased internal-eye pressure. |
| Haloperidol | Increased internal-eye pressure. |
| MAO inhibitors | Increased flavoxate effect. |
| Meperidine | Increased flavoxate effect. |
| Nitrates | Increased internal-eye pressure. |
| Orphenadrine | Increased flavoxate effect. |
| Phenothiazines | Increased flavoxate effect. |
| Pilocarpine | Loss of pilocarpine effect in glaucoma treatment. |
| Potassium supplements | Increased possibility of intestinal ulcers with oral potassium tablets. |
| Vitamin C | Decreased flavoxate effect. Avoid large doses of vitamin C. |

## POSSIBLE INTERACTION WITH OTHER SUBSTANCES

| INTERACTS WITH | COMBINED EFFECT |
|---|---|
| Alcohol: | None expected. |
| Beverages: | None expected. |
| Cocaine: | Excessively rapid heartbeat. Avoid. |
| Foods: | None expected. |
| Marijuana: | Drowsiness, dry mouth. |
| Tobacco: | None expected. |

# FLECAINIDE ACETATE

## BRAND NAMES

Tambocor

## BASIC INFORMATION

Habit forming? No
Prescription needed? Yes
Available as generic? No
Drug class: Antiarrhythmic

## USES

Stabilizes irregular heartbeat.

## DOSAGE & USAGE INFORMATION

**How to take:**
Tablet or capsule—Swallow with liquid. If you can't swallow whole, crumble tablet or open capsule and take with liquid or food.

**When to take:**
At the same time each day, according to instructions on prescription label. Take tablets approximately 12 hours apart.

**If you forget a dose:**
Take as soon as you remember up to 4 hours late. If more than 4 hours, wait for next scheduled dose (don't double this dose).

**What drug does:**
Decreases conduction of abnormal electrical activity in the heart muscle or its regulating systems.

**Time lapse before drug works:**
1 to 6 hours. May need doses daily for 2 to 3 days for maximum effect.

*Continued next column*

## OVERDOSE

**SYMPTOMS:**
**Low blood pressure or unconsciousness, irregular or rapid heartbeat.**
**WHAT TO DO:**
- **Dial 0 (operator) or 911 (emergency) for an ambulance or medical help. Then give first aid immediately.**
- **If patient is unconscious and not breathing, give mouth-to-mouth breathing. If there is no heartbeat, use cardiac massage and mouth-to-mouth breathing (CPR). Don't try to make patient vomit. If you can't get help quickly, take patient to nearest emergency facility.**
- **See emergency information on inside covers.**

**Don't take with:**
See Interaction column and consult doctor.

## POSSIBLE ADVERSE REACTIONS OR SIDE EFFECTS

| SYMPTOMS | WHAT TO DO |
|---|---|
| **Life-threatening:** None expected. | |
| **Common:** Blurred vision. | Continue. Call doctor when convenient. |
| **Infrequent:** | |
| • Chest pain, irregular heartbeat. | Discontinue. Seek emergency treatment. |
| • Shakiness, dizziness, rash, nausea, vomiting. | Discontinue. Call doctor right away. |
| • Anxiety; depression; weakness; headache; appetite loss; weakness in muscles, bones, joints; swollen feet, ankles or legs. | Continue. Call doctor when convenient. |
| • Constipation. | Continue. Tell doctor at next visit. |
| **Rare:** Unusual bleeding or bruising, sore throat, jaundice, fever, chills. | Discontinue. Call doctor right away. |

## WARNINGS & PRECAUTIONS

### Don't take if:
You are allergic to flecainide or a local anesthetic such as novocaine, xylocaine or other drug whose generic name ends with "caine."

### Before you start, consult your doctor:
- If you have kidney disease.
- If you have liver disease.
- If you have had a heart attack in past 3 weeks.
- If you have a pacemaker.

### Over age 60:
Adverse reactions and side effects may be more frequent and severe than in younger persons.

### Pregnancy:
Studies inconclusive on harm to unborn child. Animal studies show fetal abnormalities. Decide with your doctor whether drug benefits justify risk to unborn child.

### Breast-feeding:
No proven problems.

### Infants & children:
Not recommended. Safety and dosage have not been established.

### Prolonged use:
No proven problems.

### Skin & sunlight:
No problems expected.

### Driving, piloting or hazardous work:
Don't drive or pilot aircraft until you learn how medicine affects you. Don't work around dangerous machinery. Don't climb ladders or work in high places. Danger increases if you drink alcohol or take medicine affecting alertness and reflexes, such as antihistamines, tranquilizers, sedatives, pain medicine, narcotics and mind-altering drugs.

### Discontinuing:
Don't discontinue without consulting doctor. Dose may require gradual reduction if you have taken drug for a long time. Doses of other drugs may also require adjustment.

### Others:
Wear identification bracelet or carry an identification card with inscription of medicine you take.

## POSSIBLE INTERACTION WITH OTHER DRUGS

| GENERIC NAME OR DRUG CLASS | COMBINED EFFECT |
| --- | --- |
| Antiarrhythmics (other) | Possible irregular heartbeat. |
| Beta-adrenergic blockers | Possible decreased efficiency of heart-muscle contraction, leading to congestive heart failure. |
| Digitalis preparations | Increased digitalis effect. Possible irregular heartbeat. |
| Drugs that depress bone-marrow function, such as anticancer drugs, antithyroid drugs, azathioprine, carbamazepine, chloramphenicol, flucytosine, penicillamine, phenylbutazone, primaquine, pyrimethamine, rifampin, sulfa drugs, tocainide, trimethoprim, valproic acid. | Possible decreased production of blood cells in bone marrow. |

## POSSIBLE INTERACTION WITH OTHER SUBSTANCES

| INTERACTS WITH | COMBINED EFFECT |
| --- | --- |
| Alcohol: | May further depress normal heart function. |
| Beverages: Caffeine-containing beverages. | Possible decreased flecainide effect. |
| Cocaine: | Possible decreased flecainide effect. |
| Foods: | None expected. |
| Marijuana: | Possible decreased flecainide effect. |
| Tobacco: | Possible decreased flecainide effect. |

# FLUPHENAZINE

## BRAND NAMES

| | |
|---|---|
| Apo-Fluphenazine | Permitil |
| Modecate | Prolixin |
| Moditen | Prolixin Decanoate |
| Moditen Etanthate | Prolixin Enanthate |

## BASIC INFORMATION

**Habit forming?** No
**Prescription needed?** Yes
**Available as generic?** Yes
**Drug class:** Tranquilizer, antiemetic
(phenothiazine)

## USES

- Stops nausea, vomiting.
- Reduces anxiety, agitation.

## DOSAGE & USAGE INFORMATION

**How to take:**
- Tablet or capsule—Swallow with liquid or food to lessen stomach irritation.
- Suppositories—Remove wrapper and moisten suppository with water. Gently insert into rectum, large end first.
- Drops or liquid—Dilute dose in beverage.

**When to take:**
- Nervous and mental disorders—Take at the same times each day.
- Nausea and vomiting—Take as needed, no more often than every 4 hours.

**If you forget a dose:**
- Nervous and mental disorders—Take up to 2 hours late. If more than 2 hours, wait for next scheduled dose (don't double this dose).
- Nausea and vomiting—Take as soon as you remember. Wait 4 hours for next dose.

**What drug does:**
- Suppresses brain's vomiting center.
- Suppresses brain centers that control abnormal emotions and behavior.

*Continued next column*

## OVERDOSE

**SYMPTOMS:**
Stupor, convulsions, coma.
**WHAT TO DO:**
- Dial 0 (operator) or 911 (emergency) for an ambulance or medical help. Then give first aid immediately.
- See emergency information on inside covers.

**Time lapse before drug works:**
- Nausea and vomiting—1 hour or less.
- Nervous and mental disorders—4-6 weeks.

**Don't take with:**
- Antacid or medicine for diarrhea.
- Non-prescription drug for cough, cold or allergy.
- See Interaction column and consult doctor.

## POSSIBLE ADVERSE REACTIONS OR SIDE EFFECTS

| SYMPTOMS | WHAT TO DO |
|---|---|
| **Life-threatening:** | |
| None expected. | |
| **Common:** | |
| • Muscle spasms of face and neck, unsteady gait. | Discontinue. Seek emergency treatment. |
| • Restlessness, tremor, drowsiness. | Discontinue. Call doctor right away. |
| • Decreased sweating, dry mouth, runny nose, constipation. | Continue. Call doctor when convenient. |
| **Infrequent:** | |
| • Fainting. | Discontinue. Seek emergency treatment. |
| • Rash. | Discontinue. Call doctor right away. |
| • Painful or difficult urination, diminished sex drive, swollen breasts, menstrual irregularities. | Continue. Call doctor when convenient. |
| **Rare:** | |
| Change in vision, sore throat, fever, jaundice. | Discontinue. Call doctor right away. |

## WARNINGS & PRECAUTIONS

**Don't take if:**
- You are allergic to any phenothiazine.
- You have a blood or bone-marrow disease.

**Before you start, consult your doctor:**
- If you will have surgery within 2 months, including dental surgery, requiring general or spinal anesthesia.
- If you have asthma, emphysema or other lung disorder.
- If you take non-prescription ulcer medicine, asthma medicine or amphetamines.

**Over age 60:**
Adverse reactions and side effects may be more frequent and severe than in younger persons. More likely to develop involuntary movement of jaws, lips, tongue, chewing. Report this to your doctor immediately. Early treatment can help.

**Pregnancy:**
Risk to unborn child outweighs drug benefits. Don't use.

**Breast-feeding:**
Drug passes into milk. Avoid drug or discontinue nursing until you finish medicine. Consult doctor for advice on maintaining milk supply.

**Infants & children:**
Don't give to children younger than 2.

**Prolonged use:**
May lead to tardive dyskinesia (involuntary movement of jaws, lips, tongue, chewing).

**Skin & sunlight:**
May cause rash or intensify sunburn in areas exposed to sun or sunlamp. Skin may remain sensitive for 3 months after discontinuing.

**Driving, piloting or hazardous work:**
Don't drive or pilot aircraft until you learn how medicine affects you. Don't work around dangerous machinery. Don't climb ladders or work in high places. Danger increases if you drink alcohol or take medicine affecting alertness and reflexes.

**Discontinuing:**
- Nervous and mental disorders—Don't discontinue without doctor's advice until you complete prescribed dose, even though symptoms diminish or disappear.
- Nausea and vomiting—May be unnecessary to finish medicine. Follow doctor's instructions.

**Others:**
No problems expected.

## POSSIBLE INTERACTION WITH OTHER DRUGS

| GENERIC NAME OR DRUG CLASS | COMBINED EFFECT |
|---|---|
| Anticholinergics | Increased anticholinergic effect. |
| Antidepressants (tricyclic) | Increased fluphenazine effect. |
| Antihistamines | Increased antihistamine effect. |
| Appetite suppressants | Decreased suppressant effect. |
| Dronabinol | Increased effects of both drugs. Avoid. |
| Levodopa | Decreased levodopa effect. |
| Mind-altering drugs | Increased effect of mind-altering drugs. |
| Molindone | Increased tranquilizer effect. |
| Narcotics | Increased narcotic effect. |
| Phenytoin | Increased phenytoin effect. |
| Quinidine | Impaired heart function. Dangerous mixture. |
| Sedatives | Increased sedative effect. |
| Tranquilizers (other) | Increased tranquilizer effect. |

## POSSIBLE INTERACTION WITH OTHER SUBSTANCES

| INTERACTS WITH | COMBINED EFFECT |
|---|---|
| Alcohol: | Dangerous oversedation. |
| Beverages: | None expected. |
| Cocaine: | Decreased fluphenazine effect. Avoid. |
| Foods: | None expected. |
| Marijuana: | Drowsiness. May increase antinausea effect. |
| Tobacco: | None expected. |

# FLUPREDNISOLONE

## BRAND NAMES

Alphadrol

## BASIC INFORMATION

Habit forming? No
Prescription needed? Yes
Available as generic? No
Drug class: Cortisone drug (adrenal
    corticosteroid)

## USES

- Reduces inflammation caused by many different medical problems.
- Treatment for some allergic diseases, blood disorders, kidney diseases, asthma and emphysema.
- Replaces corticosteroid deficiencies.

## DOSAGE & USAGE INFORMATION

How to take:
Tablet—Swallow with liquid or food to lessen stomach irritation. If you can't swallow whole, crumble tablet.

When to take:
At the same times each day. Take once-a-day or once-every-other-day doses in mornings.

If you forget a dose:
- Several-doses-per-day prescription—Take as soon as you remember up to 2 hours late. If more than 2 hours, wait for next scheduled dose (don't double this dose).
- Once-a-day dose or less—Wait for next dose. Double this dose.

What drug does:
Decreases inflammatory responses.

Time lapse before drug works:
2 to 4 days.

Don't take with:
See Interaction column and consult doctor.

## OVERDOSE

SYMPTOMS:
Headache, convulsions, heart failure.
WHAT TO DO:
- **Dial 0 (operator) or 911 (emergency) for an ambulance or medical help. Then give first aid immediately.**
- **See emergency information on inside covers.**

## POSSIBLE ADVERSE REACTIONS OR SIDE EFFECTS

| SYMPTOMS | WHAT TO DO |
|---|---|
| **Life-threatening:**<br>None expected. | |
| **Common:**<br>Acne, poor wound healing, thirst, indigestion, nausea, vomiting. | Continue. Call doctor when convenient. |
| **Infrequent:**<br>• Black, bloody or tarry stools. | Discontinue. Seek emergency treatment. |
| • Blurred vision; halos around lights; sore throat; fever; muscle cramps; swollen legs, feet. | Discontinue. Call doctor right away. |
| • Mood changes, insomnia, restlessness, frequent urination, weight gain, round face, fatigue, weakness, TB recurrence, menstrual irregularities. | Continue. Call doctor when convenient. |
| **Rare:**<br>• Irregular heartbeat. | Discontinue. Seek emergency treatment. |
| • Rash. | Discontinue. Call doctor right away. |

## WARNINGS & PRECAUTIONS

Don't take if:
- You are allergic to any cortisone drug.
- You have tuberculosis or fungus infection.
- You have herpes infection of eyes, lips or genitals.

Before you start, consult your doctor:
- If you have had tuberculosis.
- If you have congestive heart failure.
- If you have diabetes.
- If you have peptic ulcer.
- If you have glaucoma.
- If you have underactive thyroid.
- If you have high blood pressure.
- If you have myasthenia gravis.
- If you have blood clots in legs or lungs.

Over age 60:
Adverse reactions and side effects may be more frequent and severe than in younger persons. Likely to aggravate edema, diabetes or ulcers. Likely to cause cataracts and osteoporosis (softening of the bones).

**Pregnancy:**
Risk to unborn child outweighs drug benefits. Don't use.

**Breast-feeding:**
Drug passes into milk. Avoid drug or discontinue nursing until you finish medicine. Consult doctor for advice on maintaining milk supply.

**Infants & children:**
Use only under medical supervision.

**Prolonged use:**
● Retards growth in children.
● Possible glaucoma, cataracts, diabetes, fragile bones and thin skin.
● Functional dependence.

**Skin & sunlight:**
No problems expected.

**Driving, piloting or hazardous work:**
No problems expected.

**Discontinuing:**
● Don't discontinue without doctor's advice until you complete prescribed dose, even though symptoms diminish or disappear.
● Drug affects your response to surgery, illness, injury or stress for 2 years after discontinuing. Tell anyone who takes medical care of you about this drug for 2 years after discontinuing.

**Others:**
Avoid immunizations if possible.

## POSSIBLE INTERACTION WITH OTHER DRUGS

| GENERIC NAME OR DRUG CLASS | COMBINED EFFECT |
|---|---|
| Amphoterecin B | Potassium depletion. |
| Anticholinergics | Possible glaucoma. |
| Anticoagulants (oral) | Decreased anticoagulant effect. |
| Anticonvulsants (hydantoin) | Decreased fluprednisolone effect. |
| Antidiabetics (oral) | Decreased antidiabetic effect. |
| Antihistamines | Decreased fluprednisolone effect. |
| Aspirin | Increased fluprednisolone effect. |
| Barbiturates | Decreased fluprednisolone effect. Oversedation. |
| Beta-adrenergic blockers | Decreased fluprednisolone effect. |
| Chloral hydrate | Decreased fluprednisolone effect. |
| Chlorthalidone | Potassium depletion. |
| Cholinergics | Decreased cholinergic effect. |
| Contraceptives (oral) | Increased fluprednisolone effect. |
| Digitalis preparations | Dangerous potassium depletion. Possible digitalis toxicity. |
| Diuretics (thiazide) | Potassium depletion. |
| Ephedrine | Decreased fluprednisolone effect. |
| Estrogens | Increased fluprednisolone effect. |
| Ethacrynic acid | Potassium depletion. |
| Furosemide | Potassium depletion. |
| Glutethimide | Decreased fluprednisolone effect. |
| Indapamide | Possible excessive potassium loss, causing dangerous heartbeat irregularity. |
| Indomethacin | Increased fluprednisolone effect. |
| Insulin | Decreased insulin effect. |
| Isoniazid | Decreased isoniazid effect. |
| Oxyphenbutazone | Possible ulcers. |
| Phenylbutazone | Possible ulcers. |
| Potassium supplements | Decreased potassium effect. |
| Rifampin | Decreased fluprednisolone effect. |
| Sympathomimetics | Possible glaucoma. |

## POSSIBLE INTERACTION WITH OTHER SUBSTANCES

| INTERACTS WITH | COMBINED EFFECT |
|---|---|
| Alcohol: | Risk of stomach ulcers. |
| Beverages: | No proven problems. |
| Cocaine: | Overstimulation. Avoid. |
| Foods: | No proven problems. |
| Marijuana: | Decreased immunity. |
| Tobacco: | Increased fluprednisolone effect. Possible toxicity. |

# FLURAZEPAM

## BRAND NAMES

| | |
|---|---|
| Apo-Flurazepam | Somnal |
| Dalmane | Som-Pam |
| Novoflupam | |

## BASIC INFORMATION

**Habit forming? Yes**
**Prescription needed? Yes**
**Available as generic? Yes**
**Drug class: Tranquilizer (benzodiazepine)**

## USES

Treatment for insomnia and tension.

## DOSAGE & USAGE INFORMATION

**How to take:**
Tablet or capsule—Swallow with liquid. If you can't swallow whole, crumble tablet or open capsule and take with liquid or food.

**When to take:**
At the same time each day, according to instructions on prescription label.

**If you forget a dose:**
Take as soon as you remember up to 2 hours late. If more than 2 hours, wait for next scheduled dose (don't double this dose).

**What drug does:**
Affects limbic system of brain—part that controls emotions. Induces near-normal sleep pattern.

**Time lapse before drug works:**
30 minutes.

*Continued next column*

## OVERDOSE

**SYMPTOMS:**
**Drowsiness, weakness, tremor, stupor, coma.**
**WHAT TO DO:**
- **Dial 0 (operator) or 911 (emergency) for an ambulance or medical help. Then give first aid immediately.**
- **If patient is unconscious and not breathing, give mouth-to-mouth breathing. If there is no heartbeat, use cardiac massage and mouth-to-mouth breathing (CPR). Don't try to make patient vomit. If you can't get help quickly, take patient to nearest emergency facility.**
- **See emergency information on inside covers.**

**Don't take with:**
See Interaction column and consult doctor.

## POSSIBLE ADVERSE REACTIONS OR SIDE EFFECTS

| SYMPTOMS | WHAT TO DO |
|---|---|
| **Life-threatening:**<br>None expected. | |
| **Common:**<br>Clumsiness, drowsiness, dizziness. | Continue. Call doctor when convenient. |
| **Infrequent:**<br>• Hallucinations, confusion, depression, irritability, rash, itch, change in vision. | Discontinue. Call doctor right away. |
| • Constipation or diarrhea, nausea, vomiting, painful or difficult urination. | Continue. Call doctor when convenient. |
| **Rare:**<br>• Slow heartbeat, difficult breathing. | Discontinue. Seek emergency treatment. |
| • Mouth, throat ulcers, jaundice. | Discontinue. Call doctor right away. |

# FLURAZEPAM

## WARNINGS & PRECAUTIONS

**Don't take if:**
- You are allergic to any benzodiazepine.
- You have myasthenia gravis.
- You are active or recovering alcoholic.
- Patient is younger than 6 months.

**Before you start, consult your doctor:**
- If you have liver, kidney or lung disease.
- If you have diabetes, epilepsy or porphyria.

**Over age 60:**
Adverse reactions and side effects may be more frequent and severe than in younger persons. May develop agitation, rage or "hangover" effect.

**Pregnancy:**
Risk to unborn child outweighs drug benefits. Don't use.

**Breast-feeding:**
Drug passes into milk. Avoid drug or discontinue nursing until you finish medicine. Consult doctor for advice on maintaining milk supply.

**Infants & children:**
Use only under medical supervision for children older than 6 months.

**Prolonged use:**
May impair liver function.

**Skin & sunlight:**
No problems expected.

**Driving, piloting or hazardous work:**
Don't drive or pilot aircraft until you learn how medicine affects you. Don't work around dangerous machinery. Don't climb ladders or work in high places. Danger increases if you drink alcohol or take medicine affecting alertness and reflexes.

**Discontinuing:**
Don't discontinue without doctor's advice until you complete prescribed dose, even though symptoms diminish or disappear.

**Others:**
- Hot weather, heavy exercise and profuse sweat may reduce excretion and cause overdose.
- "Hangover" effect may occur.
- Blood sugar may rise in diabetics, requiring insulin adjustment.

## POSSIBLE INTERACTION WITH OTHER DRUGS

| GENERIC NAME OR DRUG CLASS | COMBINED EFFECT |
|---|---|
| Anticonvulsants | Change in seizure frequency or severity. |
| Antidepressants | Increased sedative effect of both drugs. |
| Antihistamines | Increased sedative effect of both drugs. |
| Antihypertensives | Excessively low blood pressure. |
| Cimetidine | Excess sedation. |
| Disulfiram | Increased flurazepam effect. |
| Dronabinol | Increased effects of both drugs. Avoid. |
| MAO inhibitors | Convulsions, deep sedation, rage. |
| Molindone | Increased sedative effect. |
| Narcotics | Increased sedative effect of both drugs. |
| Sedatives | Increased sedative effect of both drugs. |
| Sleep inducers | Increased sedative effect of both drugs. |
| Tranquilizers | Increased sedative effect of both drugs. |

## POSSIBLE INTERACTION WITH OTHER SUBSTANCES

| INTERACTS WITH | COMBINED EFFECT |
|---|---|
| Alcohol: | Heavy sedation. Avoid. |
| Beverages: | None expected. |
| Cocaine: | Decreased flurazepam effect. |
| Foods: | None expected. |
| Marijuana: | Heavy sedation. Avoid. |
| Tobacco: | Decreased flurazepam effect. |

## BRAND NAMES

Apo-Folic
Folvite
Novofolacid

Numerous other
multiple
vitamin-mineral
supplements.

## BASIC INFORMATION

**Habit forming? No**
**Prescription needed?**
  **High strength: Yes**
  **Vitamin mixtures: No**
**Available as generic? Yes**
**Drug class: Vitamin supplement**

 ## USES

- Dietary supplement to promote normal growth, development and good health.
- Treatment for anemias due to folic-acid deficiency occurring from alcoholism, liver disease, hemolytic anemia, sprue, infants on artificial formula, pregnancy, breast-feeding and oral-contraceptive use.

 ## DOSAGE & USAGE INFORMATION

**How to take:**
Tablet—Swallow with liquid or food to lessen stomach irritation. If you can't swallow whole, crumble tablet and take with liquid or food.

**When to take:**
At the same time each day.

**If you forget a dose:**
Take when you remember. Don't double next dose. Resume regular schedule.

**What drug does:**
Essential to normal red-blood-cell formation.

**Time lapse before drug works:**
Not determined.

**Don't take with:**
See Interaction column and consult doctor.

 ## OVERDOSE

**SYMPTOMS:**
**None expected.**
**WHAT TO DO:**
**Overdose unlikely to threaten life.**

 ## POSSIBLE ADVERSE REACTIONS OR SIDE EFFECTS

| SYMPTOMS | WHAT TO DO |
|---|---|
| **Life-threatening:**<br>None expected. | |
| **Common:**<br>Large dose may produce yellow urine. | Continue. Tell doctor at next visit. |
| **Infrequent:**<br>None expected. | |
| **Rare:**<br>None expected. | |

# FOLIC ACID (VITAMIN B-9)

## WARNINGS & PRECAUTIONS

**Don't take if:**
You are allergic to any B vitamin.

**Before you start, consult your doctor:**
- If you have liver disease.
- If you have pernicious anemia. (Folic acid corrects anemia, but nerve damage of pernicious anemia continues.)

**Over age 60:**
No problems expected.

**Pregnancy:**
No problems expected.

**Breast-feeding:**
No problems expected.

**Infants & children:**
No problems expected.

**Prolonged use:**
No problems expected.

**Skin & sunlight:**
No problems expected.

**Driving, piloting or hazardous work:**
No problems expected.

**Discontinuing:**
Don't discontinue without doctor's advice until you complete prescribed dose, even though symptoms diminish or disappear.

**Others:**
- Folic acid removed by kidney dialysis. Dialysis patients should increase intake to 300% of RDA.
- A balanced diet should provide all the folic acid a healthy person needs and make supplements unnecessary. Best sources are green, leafy vegetables, fruits, liver and kidney.

## POSSIBLE INTERACTION WITH OTHER DRUGS

| GENERIC NAME OR DRUG CLASS | COMBINED EFFECT |
|---|---|
| Analgesics | Decreased effect of folic acid. |
| Anticonvulsants | Decreased effect of folic acid. |
| Contraceptives (oral) | Decreased effect of folic acid. |
| Cortisone drugs | Decreased effect of folic acid. |
| Methotrexate | Decreased effect of folic acid. |
| Pyrimethamine | Decreased effect of folic acid. |
| Quinine | Decreased effect of folic acid. |
| Sulfasalazine | Decreased dietary absorption of folic acid. |
| Triamterene | Decreased effect of folic acid. |
| Trimethoprim | Decreased effect of folic acid. |
| Zinc | Decreased zinc effect. |

## POSSIBLE INTERACTION WITH OTHER SUBSTANCES

| INTERACTS WITH | COMBINED EFFECT |
|---|---|
| Alcohol: | None expected. |
| Beverages: | None expected. |
| Cocaine: | None expected. |
| Foods: | None expected. |
| Marijuana: | None expected. |
| Tobacco: | None expected. |

# FUROSEMIDE

## BRAND NAMES

| | |
|---|---|
| Apo-Furosemide | Novosemide |
| Furoside | SK-Furosemide |
| Lasix | Uritol |
| Neo-Renal | |

## BASIC INFORMATION

**Habit forming? No**
**Prescription needed? Yes**
**Available as generic? Yes**
**Drug class: Diuretic, antihypertensive**

## USES

- Lowers high blood pressure.
- Decreases fluid retention.

## DOSAGE & USAGE INFORMATION

**How to take:**
Tablet, liquid or capsule—Swallow with liquid. If you can't swallow whole, crumble tablet or open capsule and take with liquid or food.

**When to take:**
- 1 dose a day—Take after breakfast.
- More than 1 dose a day—Take last dose no later than 6 p.m. unless otherwise directed.

**If you forget a dose:**
- 1 dose a day—Take as soon as you remember up to 12 hours late. If more than 12 hours, wait for next scheduled dose (don't double this dose).
- More than 1 dose a day—Take as soon as you remember up to 2 hours late. If more than 2 hours, wait for next scheduled dose (don't double this dose).

**What drug does:**
Increases elimination of sodium and water from body. Decreased body fluid reduces blood pressure.

*Continued next column*

## OVERDOSE

**SYMPTOMS:**
**Weakness, lethargy, dizziness, confusion, nausea, vomiting, leg-muscle cramps, thirst, stupor, deep sleep, weak and rapid pulse, cardiac arrest.**
**WHAT TO DO:**
- **Dial 0 (operator) or 911 (emergency) for an ambulance or medical help. Then give first aid immediately.**
- **See emergency information on inside covers.**

---

**Time lapse before drug works:**
1 hour to increase water loss. Requires 2 to 3 weeks to lower blood pressure.

**Don't take with:**
- Non-prescription drugs with aspirin.
- See Interaction column and consult doctor.

## POSSIBLE ADVERSE REACTIONS OR SIDE EFFECTS

| SYMPTOMS | WHAT TO DO |
|---|---|
| **Life-threatening:**<br>None expected. | |
| **Common:**<br>Dizziness. | Continue. Call doctor when convenient. |
| **Infrequent:**<br>Mood change, appetite loss, diarrhea, irregular heartbeat, muscle cramps, fatigue, weakness. | Discontinue. Call doctor right away. |
| **Rare:**<br>Rash or hives, yellow vision, ringing in ears, hearing loss, sore throat, fever, dry mouth, thirst, side or stomach pain, nausea, vomiting, unusual bleeding or bruising, joint pain, jaundice. | Discontinue. Call doctor right away. |

## WARNINGS & PRECAUTIONS

**Don't take if:**
You are allergic to furosemide.

**Before you start, consult your doctor:**
- If you are allergic to any sulfa drug.
- If you have liver or kidney disease.
- If you have gout.
- If you have diabetes.
- If you have impaired hearing.
- If you will have surgery within 2 months, including dental surgery, requiring general or spinal anesthesia.

**Over age 60:**
Adverse reactions and side effects may be more frequent and severe than in younger persons.

**Pregnancy:**
Risk to unborn child outweighs drug benefits. Don't use.

**Breast-feeding:**
Drug filters into milk. May harm child. Avoid.

**Infants & children:**
Use only under medical supervision.

**Prolonged use:**
- Impaired balance of water, salt and potassium in blood and body tissues.
- Possible diabetes.

**Skin & sunlight:**
May cause rash or intensify sunburn in areas exposed to sun or sunlamp.

**Driving, piloting or hazardous work:**
No problems expected.

**Discontinuing:**
Don't discontinue without doctor's advice until you complete prescribed dose, even though symptoms diminish or disappear.

**Others:**
Frequent laboratory studies to monitor potassium level in blood recommended. Eat foods rich in potassium or take potassium supplements. Consult doctor.

## POSSIBLE INTERACTION WITH OTHER DRUGS

| GENERIC NAME OR DRUG CLASS | COMBINED EFFECT |
|---|---|
| Acebutolol | Increased antihypertensive effect. Dosages may require adjustment. |
| Allopurinol | Decreased allopurinol effect. |
| Amiodarone | Increased risk of heartbeat irregularity due to low potassium. |
| Anticoagulants | Abnormal clotting. |
| Antidepressants (tricyclic) | Excessive blood-pressure drop. |
| Antidiabetics (oral) | Decreased antidiabetic effect. |
| Anti-inflammatory drugs (non-steroid) | Decreased furosemide effect. |
| Antihypertensives | Increased antihypertensive effect. |
| Barbiturates | Low blood pressure. |
| Calcium supplements | Increased calcium in blood. |
| Cortisone drugs | Excessive potassium loss. |
| Digitalis preparations | Serious heart-rhythm disorders. |
| Indapamide | Increased diuretic effect. |

| | |
|---|---|
| Insulin | Decreased insulin effect. |
| Ketoprofen | Decreased diuretic effect of furosemide. |
| Labetolol | Increased antihypertensive effects. |
| Lithium | Increased lithium toxicity. |
| MAO inhibitors | Increased furosemide effect. |
| Narcotics | Dangerous low blood pressure. Avoid. |
| Nitrates | Excessive blood-pressure drop. |
| Oxprenolol | Increased antihypertensive effect. Dosages may require adjustment. |
| Phenothiazines | Increased phenothiazine effect. |
| Potassium supplements | Decreased potassium effect. |
| Probenecid | Decreased probenecid effect. |
| Salicylates (including aspirin) | Dangerous salicylate retention. |
| Sedatives | Increased furosemide effect. |
| Suprofen | Decreased diuretic effect of furosemide. |

## POSSIBLE INTERACTION WITH OTHER SUBSTANCES

| INTERACTS WITH | COMBINED EFFECT |
|---|---|
| Alcohol: | Blood-pressure drop. Avoid. |
| Beverages: | None expected. |
| Cocaine: | Dangerous blood-pressure drop. Avoid. |
| Foods: | None expected. |
| Marijuana: | Increased thirst and urinary frequency, fainting. |
| Tobacco: | Decreased furosemide effect. |

# GALLBLADDER X-RAY TEST DRUGS (CHOLECYSTOGRAPHIC AGENTS)

## BRAND AND GENERIC NAMES

Bilivist
Bilopaque
Cholebrine
IOCETAMIC ACID
IOPANOIC ACID

IPODATE
Oragrafin Calcium
Oragrafin Sodium
Telepaque
TYROPANOATE

## BASIC INFORMATION

Habit forming? No
Prescription needed? Yes
Available as generic? No
Drug class: Diagnostic aid, radiopaque

## USES

To check for problems with the gallbladder or
the bile ducts.

## DOSAGE & USAGE INFORMATION

**How to take:**
- Take tablets or liquid as directed after the
  evening meal on the evening before special
  x-rays will be taken.
- Don't eat or drink anything (except water)
  after taking.

**When to take:**
As directed.

**If you forget a dose:**
Take as soon as you remember.

**What drug does:**
These are organic iodine compounds which get
absorbed into the blood stream, get
concentrated in a healthy gallbladder and make
the gallbladder and gallstones (if present) visible
on special x-rays.

**Time lapse before drug works:**
10 to 15 hours.

*Continued next column*

## OVERDOSE

**SYMPTOMS:**
Severe diarrhea, nausea or vomiting; difficult
urination.
**WHAT TO DO:**
Not life-threatening. Discontinue and call
doctor right away.

**Don't take with:**
- Other medicines unless directed by your
  doctor or x-ray specialist.
- If you take cholestyramine, discontinue it for
  48 hours before taking the radiopaque drug.

## POSSIBLE ADVERSE REACTIONS OR SIDE EFFECTS

| SYMPTOMS | WHAT TO DO |
|---|---|
| **Life-threatening:** None expected. | |
| **Common:** None expected. | |
| **Infrequent:** Abdominal cramps, diarrhea, dizziness, headache, indigestion, vomiting. | Discontinue. Call doctor right away. |
| **Rare:** Itching, unusual bleeding or bruising, hives or rash. | Discontinue. Call doctor right away. |

# GALLBLADDER X-RAY TEST DRUGS (CHOLECYSTOGRAPHIC AGENTS)

## WARNINGS & PRECAUTIONS

**Don't take if:**
You are allergic to any iodine compound or other radiopaque chemicals.

**Before you start, consult your doctor:**
If you are allergic to anything, including shellfish, cabbage, kale, turnips, iodized salt.

**Over age 60:**
Adverse reactions and side effects may be more frequent and severe than in younger persons. Ask doctor about smaller doses.

**Pregnancy:**
X-rays should not be taken unless absolutely necessary during pregnancy.

**Breast-feeding:**
No problems expected, but ask doctor.

**Infants & children:**
No problems expected, but ask doctor.

**Prolonged use:**
Not intended for prolonged use.

**Skin & sunlight:**
No problems expected.

**Driving, piloting or hazardous work:**
Don't drive or pilot aircraft until you learn how medicine affects you. Don't work around dangerous machinery. Don't climb ladders or work in high places. Danger increases if you drink alcohol or take medicine affecting alertness and reflexes, such as antihistamines, tranquilizers, sedatives, pain medicine, narcotics and mind-altering drugs.

**Discontinuing:**
No problems expected.

**Others:**
- Special diets and laxatives or enemas before x-rays may be ordered. Follow instructions.
- Tests on your thyroid gland may be made inaccurate for 8 weeks because of the iodine contained in radiopaque substances. Keep this in mind if your doctor orders thyroid tests.

## POSSIBLE INTERACTION WITH OTHER DRUGS

| GENERIC NAME OR DRUG CLASS | COMBINED EFFECT |
| --- | --- |
| None expected. | |

## POSSIBLE INTERACTION WITH OTHER SUBSTANCES

| INTERACTS WITH | COMBINED EFFECT |
| --- | --- |
| **Alcohol:** | None expected. |
| **Beverages:** | None expected. |
| **Cocaine:** | None expected. |
| **Foods:** | None expected. |
| **Marijuana:** | None expected. |
| **Tobacco:** | None expected. |

# GEMFIBROZIL

## BRAND NAMES

Lopid

## BASIC INFORMATION

**Habit forming? No**
**Prescription needed? Yes**
**Available as generic? No**
**Drug class: Antihyperlipidemic**

 ## USES

Reduces fatty substances in the blood
(cholesterol and triglycerides).

 ## DOSAGE & USAGE INFORMATION

**How to take:**
Capsule—Swallow with liquid or food to lessen
stomach irritation.

**When to take:**
At the same times each day.

**If you forget a dose:**
Take as soon as you remember up to 2 hours
late. If more than 2 hours, wait for next
scheduled dose (don't double this dose).

**What drug does:**
Inhibits formation of fatty substances.

**Time lapse before drug works:**
3 months or more.

**Don't take with:**
See Interaction column and consult doctor.

 ## OVERDOSE

**SYMPTOMS:**
**Diarrhea, headache, muscle pain.**
**WHAT TO DO:**
**Overdose unlikely to threaten life. If person
takes much larger amount than prescribed,
call doctor, poison-control center or hospital
emergency room for instructions.**

 ## POSSIBLE ADVERSE REACTIONS OR SIDE EFFECTS

| SYMPTOMS | WHAT TO DO |
|---|---|
| **Life-threatening:** None expected. | |
| **Common:** None expected. | |
| **Infrequent:** | |
| • Chest pain, shortness of breath, irregular heartbeat, gallstones. | Discontinue. Call doctor right away. |
| • Nausea, vomiting, diarrhea, stomach pain. | Continue. Call doctor when convenient. |
| **Rare:** | |
| • Rash, itch; sores in mouth, on lips; sore throat; swollen feet, legs; blood in urine; painful urination; fever; chills. | Discontinue. Call doctor right away. |
| • Dizziness, drowsiness, headache, dryness (skin), hair loss, muscle cramps, backache, diminished sex drive. | Continue. Call doctor when convenient. |

## WARNINGS & PRECAUTIONS

**Don't take if:**
You are allergic to any antihyperlipidemic.

**Before you start, consult your doctor:**
- If you have had liver or kidney disease.
- If you have had peptic-ulcer disease.
- If you have diabetes.

**Over age 60:**
Adverse reactions and side effects may be more frequent and severe than in younger persons.

**Pregnancy:**
Risk to unborn child outweighs drug benefits. Don't use.

**Breast-feeding:**
May harm child. Avoid.

**Infants & children:**
Not recommended.

**Prolonged use:**
Periodic blood-cell counts and liver-function studies recommended if you take gemfibrozil for a long time.

**Skin & sunlight:**
No problems expected.

**Driving, piloting or hazardous work:**
Avoid if you feel drowsy or dizzy. Otherwise, no problems expected.

**Discontinuing:**
Don't discontinue without doctor's advice until you complete prescribed dose, even though symptoms diminish or disappear.

**Others:**
Some studies question effectiveness. Many studies warn against toxicity.

## POSSIBLE INTERACTION WITH OTHER DRUGS

| GENERIC NAME OR DRUG CLASS | COMBINED EFFECT |
| --- | --- |
| Anticoagulants (oral) | Increased anticoagulant effect. Dose reduction of anticoagulant necessary. |
| Antidiabetics (oral) | Increased antidiabetic effect. |
| Contraceptives (oral) | Decreased gemfibrozil effect. |
| Estrogens | Decreased gemfibrozil effect. |
| Furosemide | Possible toxicity of both drugs. |
| Insulin | Increased insulin effect. |
| Thyroid hormones | Increased gemfibrozil effect. |

## POSSIBLE INTERACTION WITH OTHER SUBSTANCES

| INTERACTS WITH | COMBINED EFFECT |
| --- | --- |
| Alcohol: | None expected. |
| Beverages: | None expected. |
| Cocaine: | Decreased effect of gemfibrozil. Avoid cocaine. |
| Foods: Fatty foods. | Decreased gemfibrozil effect. |
| Marijuana: | None expected. |
| Tobacco: | Decreased gemfibrozil absorption. Avoid. |

# GLIPIZIDE

## BRAND NAMES

**Glucotrol**

## BASIC INFORMATION

**Habit forming? No**
**Prescription needed? Yes**
**Available as generic? No**
**Drug class: Antidiabetic (oral), sulfonurea**

 ## USES

Treatment for diabetes in adults who can't control blood sugar by diet, weight loss and exercise.

 ## DOSAGE & USAGE INFORMATION

**How to take:**
Tablet—Swallow with liquid or food to lessen stomach irritation. If you can't swallow whole, crumble tablet and take with liquid or food.

**When to take:**
At the same times each day.

**If you forget a dose:**
Take as soon as you remember up to 2 hours late. If more than 2 hours, wait for next scheduled dose (don't double this dose).

**What drug does:**
Stimulates pancreas to produce more insulin. Insulin in blood forces cells to use sugar in blood.

**Time lapse before drug works:**
3 to 4 hours. May require 2 weeks for maximum benefit.

**Don't take with:**
See Interaction column and consult doctor.

 ## OVERDOSE

**SYMPTOMS:**
**Excessive hunger, nausea, anxiety, cool skin, cold sweats, drowsiness, rapid heartbeat, weakness, unconsciousness, coma.**
**WHAT TO DO:**
- **Dial 0 (operator) or 911 (emergency) for an ambulance or medical help. Then give first aid immediately.**
- **See emergency information on inside covers.**

 ## POSSIBLE ADVERSE REACTIONS OR SIDE EFFECTS

| SYMPTOMS | WHAT TO DO |
|---|---|
| **Life-threatening:** | |
| None expected. | |
| **Common:** | |
| ● Dizziness. | Discontinue. Call doctor right away. |
| ● Diarrhea, appetite loss, nausea, stomach pain, heartburn. | Continue. Call doctor when convenient. |
| **Infrequent:** | |
| Low blood sugar (hunger, anxiety, cold sweats, rapid pulse), drowsiness, nervousness, headache, weakness. | Discontinue. Seek emergency treatment. |
| **Rare:** | |
| Itching or rash, sore throat, fever, ringing in ears, unusual bleeding or bruising, fatigue, jaundice. | Discontinue. Call doctor right away. |

## WARNINGS & PRECAUTIONS

**Don't take if:**
- You are allergic to any sulfonurea.
- You have impaired kidney or liver function.

**Before you start, consult your doctor:**
- If you have a severe infection.
- If you have thyroid disease.
- If you take insulin.
- If you have heart disease.

**Over age 60:**
Dose usually smaller than for younger adults. Avoid "low-blood-sugar" episodes because repeated ones can damage brain permanently.

**Pregnancy:**
No proven harm to unborn child. Avoid if possible.

**Breast-feeding:**
Drug filters into milk. May lower baby's blood sugar. Avoid.

**Infants & children:**
Don't give to infants or children.

**Prolonged use:**
None expected.

**Skin & sunlight:**
May cause rash or intensify sunburn in areas exposed to sun or sunlamp.

**Driving, piloting or hazardous work:**
No problems expected unless you develop hypoglycemia (low blood sugar). If so, avoid driving or hazardous activity.

**Discontinuing:**
Don't discontinue without consulting doctor. Dose may require gradual reduction if you have taken drug for a long time. Doses of other drugs may also require adjustment.

**Others:**
Don't exceed recommended dose. Hypoglycemia (low blood sugar) may occur, even with proper dose schedule. You must balance medicine, diet and exercise.

## POSSIBLE INTERACTION WITH OTHER DRUGS

| GENERIC NAME OR DRUG CLASS | COMBINED EFFECT |
|---|---|
| Androgens | Increased glipizide effect. |
| Anticoagulants (oral) | Unpredictable prothrombin times (see Glossary). |
| Anticonvulsants (hydantoin) | Decreased glipizide effect. |
| Anti-inflammatory drugs (non-steroidal) | Increased glipizide effect. |
| Aspirin | Increased glipizide effect. |
| Beta-adrenergic blockers | Increased glipizide effect. May increase difficulty in regulating blood sugar. |
| Chloramphenicol | Increased glipizide effect. |
| Clofibrate | Increased glipizide effect. |
| Contraceptives (oral) | Decreased glipizide effect. |
| Cortisone drugs | Decreased glipizide effect. |
| Diuretics (thiazide) | Decreased glipizide effect. |
| Epinephrine | Decreased glipizide effect. |
| Estrogens | Increased glipizide effect. |
| Guanethidine | Unpredictable glipizide effect. |
| Labetolol | Increased antidiabetic effect, may mask hypoglycemia. |

## POSSIBLE INTERACTION WITH OTHER SUBSTANCES

| INTERACTS WITH | COMBINED EFFECT |
|---|---|
| Alcohol: | Disulfiram reaction (see Glossary). Avoid. |
| Beverages: | None expected. |
| Cocaine: | No proven problems. |
| Foods: | None expected. |
| Marijuana: | Decreased glipizide effect. Avoid. |
| Tobacco: | None expected. |

# GLYBURIDE

## BRAND NAMES

DiaBeta               Glibenclamide
Euglucon              Micronase

## BASIC INFORMATION

**Habit forming? No**
**Prescription needed? Yes**
**Available as generic? No**
**Drug class: Antidiabetic (oral), sulfonurea**

 **USES**

Treatment for diabetes in adults who can't control blood sugar by diet, weight loss and exercise.

 **DOSAGE & USAGE INFORMATION**

**How to take:**
Tablet—Swallow with liquid or food to lessen stomach irritation. If you can't swallow whole, crumble tablet and take with liquid or food.

**When to take:**
At the same times each day.

**If you forget a dose:**
Take as soon as you remember up to 2 hours late. If more than 2 hours, wait for next scheduled dose (don't double this dose).

**What drug does:**
Stimulates pancreas to produce more insulin. Insulin in blood forces cells to use sugar in blood.

**Time lapse before drug works:**
3 to 4 hours. May require 2 weeks for maximum benefit.

**Don't take with:**
See Interaction column and consult doctor.

 **OVERDOSE**

**SYMPTOMS:**
**Excessive hunger, nausea, anxiety, cool skin, cold sweats, drowsiness, rapid heartbeat, weakness, unconsciousness, coma.**
**WHAT TO DO:**
- **Dial 0 (operator) or 911 (emergency) for an ambulance or medical help. Then give first aid immediately.**
- **See emergency information on inside covers.**

 **POSSIBLE ADVERSE REACTIONS OR SIDE EFFECTS**

| SYMPTOMS | WHAT TO DO |
|---|---|
| **Life-threatening:** None expected. | |
| **Common:** | |
| ● Dizziness. | Discontinue. Call doctor right away. |
| ● Diarrhea, appetite loss, nausea, stomach pain, heartburn. | Continue. Call doctor when convenient. |
| **Infrequent:** Low blood sugar (hunger, anxiety, cold sweats, rapid pulse), drowsiness, nervousness, headache, weakness, rapid heartbeat. | Discontinue. Seek emergency treatment. |
| **Rare:** Itching or rash, sore throat, fever, ringing in ears, unusual bleeding or bruising, fatigue, jaundice. | Discontinue. Call doctor right away. |

# GLYBURIDE

## WARNINGS & PRECAUTIONS

**Don't take if:**
- You are allergic to any sulfonurea.
- You have impaired kidney or liver function.

**Before you start, consult your doctor:**
- If you have a severe infection.
- If you have thyroid disease.
- If you take insulin.
- If you have heart disease.

**Over age 60:**
Dose usually smaller than for younger adults. Avoid "low-blood-sugar" episodes because repeated ones can damage brain permanently.

**Pregnancy:**
No proven harm to unborn child. Avoid if possible.

**Breast-feeding:**
Drug filters into milk. May lower baby's blood sugar. Avoid.

**Infants & children:**
Don't give to infants or children.

**Prolonged use:**
None expected.

**Skin & sunlight:**
May cause rash or intensify sunburn in areas exposed to sun or sunlamp.

**Driving, piloting or hazardous work:**
No problems expected unless you develop hypoglycemia (low blood sugar). If so, avoid driving or hazardous activity.

**Discontinuing:**
Don't discontinue without consulting doctor. Dose may require gradual reduction if you have taken drug for a long time. Doses of other drugs may also require adjustment.

**Others:**
Don't exceed recommended dose. Hypoglycemia (low blood sugar) may occur, even with proper dose schedule. You must balance medicine, diet and exercise.

## POSSIBLE INTERACTION WITH OTHER DRUGS

| GENERIC NAME OR DRUG CLASS | COMBINED EFFECT |
|---|---|
| Androgens | Increased glyburide effect. |
| Anticoagulants (oral) | Unpredictable prothrombin times. |
| Anticonvulsants (hydantoin) | Decreased glyburide effect. |
| Anti-inflammatory drugs (non-steroidal) | Increased glyburide effect. |
| Aspirin | Increased glyburide effect. |
| Beta-adrenergic blockers | Increased glyburide effect. Possible increased difficulty in regulating blood-sugar levels. |
| Chloramphenicol | Increased glyburide offect. |
| Clofibrate | Increased glyburide effect. |
| Contraceptives (oral) | Decreased glyburide effect. |
| Cortisone drugs | Decreased glyburide effect. |
| Diuretics (thiazide) | Decreased glyburide effect. |
| Epinephrine | Decreased glyburide effect. |
| Estrogens | Increased glyburide effect. |
| Guanethidine | Unpredictable glyburide effect. |
| Labetolol | Increased antidiabetic effect, may mask hypoglycemia. |

## POSSIBLE INTERACTION WITH OTHER SUBSTANCES

| INTERACTS WITH | COMBINED EFFECT |
|---|---|
| Alcohol: | Disulfiram reaction (see Glossary). Avoid. |
| Beverages: | None expected. |
| Cocaine: | No proven problems. |
| Foods: | None expected. |
| Marijuana: | Decreased glyburide effect. Avoid. |
| Tobacco: | None expected. |

# GLYCOPYRROLATE

## BRAND NAMES

Robinul              Robinul Forte

## BASIC INFORMATION

Habit forming? No
Prescription needed? Yes
Available as generic? Yes
Drug class: Antispasmodic, anticholinergic

## USES

- Reduces spasms of digestive system.
- Reduces production of saliva during dental procedures.

## DOSAGE & USAGE INFORMATION

**How to take:**
Tablet or capsule—Swallow with liquid. If you can't swallow whole, crumble tablet or open capsule and take with small amount of liquid or food.

**When to take:**
30 minutes before meals (unless directed otherwise by doctor).

**If you forget a dose:**
Wait for next scheduled dose (don't double this dose).

**What drug does:**
Blocks nerve impulses at parasympathetic nerve endings, preventing smooth (involuntary) muscle contractions and gland secretions of organs involved.

**Time lapse before drug works:**
15 to 30 minutes.

**Don't take with:**
See Interaction column and consult doctor.

## OVERDOSE

**SYMPTOMS:**
Dry mouth, low blood pressure, decreased breathing rate, rapid heartbeat, flushed skin, drowsiness.
**WHAT TO DO:**
- Dial 0 (operator) or 911 (emergency) for an ambulance or medical help. Then give first aid immediately.
- See emergency information on inside covers.

## POSSIBLE ADVERSE REACTIONS OR SIDE EFFECTS

| SYMPTOMS | WHAT TO DO |
|---|---|
| **Life-threatening:** None expected. | |
| **Common:** Dry mouth, constipation, difficult urination. | Continue. Call doctor when convenient. |
| **Infrequent:** | |
| • Confusion; dizziness; drowsiness; headache; sleep disturbance such as nightmares, frequent waking; rash; pain in eyes; nausea; vomiting; rapid heartbeat. | Discontinue. Call doctor right away. |
| • Insomnia, blurred vision, diminished sex drive, decreased sweating. | Continue. Call doctor when convenient. |
| **Rare:** None expected. | |

## WARNINGS & PRECAUTIONS

**Don't take if:**
- You are allergic to any anticholinergic.
- You have trouble with stomach bloating.
- You have difficulty emptying your bladder completely.
- You have narrow-angle glaucoma.
- You have severe ulcerative colitis.

**Before you start, consult your doctor:**
- If you have open-angle glaucoma.
- If you have angina.
- If you have chronic bronchitis or asthma.
- If you have liver disease.
- If you have hiatal hernia.
- If you have enlarged prostate.
- If you have myasthenia gravis.
- If you have peptic ulcer.
- If you will have surgery within 2 months, including dental surgery, requiring general or spinal anesthesia.

**Over age 60:**
Adverse reactions and side effects may be more frequent and severe than in younger persons.

**Pregnancy:**
Studies inconclusive on harm to unborn child. Animal studies show fetal abnormalities. Decide with your doctor whether drug benefits justify risk to unborn child.

**Breast-feeding:**
Drug passes into milk and decreases milk flow. Avoid drug or discontinue nursing until you finish medicine. Consult doctor for advice on maintaining milk supply.

**Infants & children:**
Use only under medical supervision.

**Prolonged use:**
Chronic constipation, possible fecal impaction. Consult doctor immediately.

**Skin & sunlight:**
No problems expected.

**Driving, piloting or hazardous work:**
Use disqualifies you for piloting aircraft. Otherwise, no problems expected.

**Discontinuing:**
May be unnecessary to finish medicine. Follow doctor's instructions.

**Others:**
Heatstroke more likely if you become overheated during exertion.

## POSSIBLE INTERACTION WITH OTHER DRUGS

| GENERIC NAME OR DRUG CLASS | COMBINED EFFECT |
|---|---|
| Amantadine | Increased glycopyrrolate effect. |
| Anticholinergics (other) | Increased glycopyrrolate effect. |
| Antidepressants (tricyclics) | Increased glycopyrrolate effect. |
| Cortisone drugs | Increased internal-eye pressure. |
| Haloperidol | Increased internal-eye pressure. |
| MAO inhibitors | Increased glycopyrrolate effect. |
| Meperidine | Increased glycopyrrolate effect. |
| Methylphenidate | Increased glycopyrrolate effect. |
| Molindone | Increased anticholinergic effect. |
| Orphenadrine | Increased glycopyrrolate effect. |
| Phenothiazines | Increased glycopyrrolate effect. |
| Pilocarpine | Increased glycopyrrolate effect. Loss of pilocarpine effect in glaucoma treatment. |

| | |
|---|---|
| **Potassium chloride tabs** | Increased side effects of potassium tablets. |
| **Retocunazole** | Decreased absorption of both. |
| **Vitamin C** | Increased glycopyrrolate effect. Avoid large doses of vitamin C. |

## POSSIBLE INTERACTION WITH OTHER SUBSTANCES

| INTERACTS WITH | COMBINED EFFECT |
|---|---|
| Alcohol: | None expected. |
| Beverages: | None expected. |
| Cocaine: | Excessively rapid heartbeat. Avoid. |
| Foods: | None expected. |
| Marijuana: | Drowsiness and dry mouth. |
| Tobacco: | None expected. |

# GOLD COMPOUNDS

## BRAND AND GENERIC NAMES

AURANOFIN—oral
Aurothioglucose—
   injection
Gold Sodium
   Thiomalate
Myochrysine—
   injection

Myocrisin
Ridaura—oral
SODIUM
   AUROTHIOMALATE
SOLGANAL—
   injection

## BASIC INFORMATION

Habit forming? No
Prescription needed? Yes
Available as generic? No
Drug class: Gold compounds

 ## USES

Treatment for rheumatoid arthritis.

 ## DOSAGE & USAGE INFORMATION

**How to take:**
Swallow with full glass of fluid. Follow
prescription directions. Taking too much can
cause serious adverse reactions.

**When to take:**
Once or twice daily, morning and night.

**If you forget a dose:**
Take as soon as you remember up to 6 hours
late, then go back to usual schedule.

**What drug does:**
Modifies disease activity of rheumatoid arthritis
by mechanisms not yet understood.

**Time lapse before drug works:**
3 to 6 months.

**Don't take with:**
See Interaction column and consult doctor.

 ## OVERDOSE

**SYMPTOMS:**
Confusion, delirium, numbness and tingling
in feet and hands.
**WHAT TO DO:**
- Induce vomiting with syrup of ipecac if
  available.
- Dial 0 (operator) or 911 (emergency) for an
  ambulance or medical help. Then give first
  aid immediately.
- See emergency information on inside
  covers.

 ## POSSIBLE ADVERSE REACTIONS OR SIDE EFFECTS

| SYMPTOMS | WHAT TO DO |
|---|---|
| **Life-threatening:**<br>None expected. | |
| **Common:** | |
| • Itch; rash or hives; sores or white spots in mouth, throat; appetite loss; diarrhea; vomiting; protein in urine; skin rashes; fever. | Discontinue. Call doctor right away. |
| • Abdominal cramps. | Continue. Call doctor when convenient. |
| **Infrequent:** | |
| • Excessive fatigue; sore tongue, mouth or gums; metallic or odd taste; unusual bleeding or bruising; blood in urine; changes in white blood cells, platelets. | Discontinue. Call doctor right away. |
| • Hair loss; pain in muscles, bones and joints (with injections). | Continue. Call doctor when convenient. |
| **Rare:** | |
| • Blood in stool, difficult breathing, coughing. | Discontinue. Seek emergency treatment. |
| • Abdominal pain, jaundice. | Discontinue. Call doctor right away. |
| • "Pink eye." | Continue. Call doctor when convenient. |

## WARNINGS & PRECAUTIONS

### Don't take if:
- You have history of allergy to gold or other metals.
- You have any blood disorder.
- You have kidney disease.

### Before you start, consult your doctor:
- If you are pregnant or may become pregnant.
- If you have lupus erythematosus.
- If you have Schogren's syndrome.
- If you have chronic skin disease.

### Over age 60:
Adverse reactions and side effects may be more frequent and severe than in younger persons.

### Pregnancy:
Avoid if possible. Animal studies show that gold compounds can cause birth defects.

### Breast-feeding:
Drug may filter into milk, causing side effects in infants. Avoid.

### Infants & children:
Not recommended. Safety and dosage have not been established.

### Prolonged use:
Request periodic laboratory studies of blood counts, urine and liver function. These should be done before use and at least once a month during treatment.

### Skin & sunlight:
No problems expected.

### Driving, piloting or hazardous work:
Avoid if you have serious adverse reactions or side effects. Otherwise, no problems expected.

### Discontinuing:
Don't discontinue without doctor's advice until you complete prescribed dose.

### Others:
- Side effects and adverse reactions may appear during treatment or for many months after discontinuing.
- Gold has been shown to cause kidney tumors and kidney cancer in animals given excessive doses.

## POSSIBLE INTERACTION WITH OTHER DRUGS

| GENERIC NAME OR DRUG CLASS | COMBINED EFFECT |
|---|---|
| Ketoprofen | Increased likelihood of kidney damage. |
| Non-steroidal anti-inflammatory drugs | Possible increased likelihood of kidney damage. |
| Penicillamine | Possible increased likelihood of kidney damage. |
| Phenytoin | Increased phenytoin blood levels. Phenytoin dosage may require adjustment. |
| Suprofen | Increased likelihood of kidney damage. |

## POSSIBLE INTERACTION WITH OTHER SUBSTANCES

| INTERACTS WITH | COMBINED EFFECT |
|---|---|
| Alcohol: | None expected. |
| Beverages: | None expected. |
| Cocaine: | None expected. |
| Foods: | None expected. |
| Marijuana: | None expected. |
| Tobacco: | None expected. |

# GRISEOFULVIN

## BRAND NAMES

Fulvicin P/G
Fulvicin U/F
Grifulvin V
Gris-PEG

Grisactin
Grisactin Ultra
Grisovin-FP
grisOwen

## BASIC INFORMATION

**Habit forming?** No
**Prescription needed?** Yes
**Available as generic?** Yes
**Drug class:** Antibiotic (antifungal)

## USES

Treatment for fungal infections susceptible to griseofulvin.

## DOSAGE & USAGE INFORMATION

**How to take:**
- Tablet or capsule—Swallow with liquid or food to lessen stomach irritation. If you can't swallow whole, crumble tablet or open capsule and take with liquid or food.
- Liquid—Follow label instructions.

**When to take:**
With or immediately after meals.

**If you forget a dose:**
Take as soon as you remember up to 2 hours late. If more than 2 hours, wait for next scheduled dose (don't double this dose).

**What drug does:**
Prevents fungi from growing and reproducing.

**Time lapse before drug works:**
2 to 10 days for skin infections. 2 to 4 weeks for infections of fingernails or toenails. Complete cure of either may require several months.

**Don't take with:**
See Interaction column and consult doctor.

## OVERDOSE

**SYMPTOMS:**
Nausea, vomiting, diarrhea. In sensitive individuals, severe diarrhea may occur without overdosing.
**WHAT TO DO:**
Overdose unlikely to threaten life. If person takes much larger amount than prescribed, call doctor, poison-control center or hospital emergency room for instructions.

## POSSIBLE ADVERSE REACTIONS OR SIDE EFFECTS

| SYMPTOMS | WHAT TO DO |
|---|---|
| **Life-threatening:**<br>None expected. | |
| **Common:**<br>Headache. | Continue. Tell doctor at next visit. |
| **Infrequent:** | |
| • Confusion; rash, hives, itch; mouth or tongue irritation; soreness; nausea; vomiting; diarrhea; stomach pain. | Discontinue. Call doctor right away. |
| • Insomnia, tiredness. | Continue. Call doctor when convenient. |
| **Rare:**<br>Sore throat, fever, numbness or tingling in hands or feet. | Discontinue. Call doctor right away. |

## WARNINGS & PRECAUTIONS

**Don't take if:**
- You are allergic to any antifungal medicine.
- You have liver disease.
- You have porphyria.
- The infection is minor and will respond to less-potent drugs.

**Before you start, consult your doctor:**
- If you plan to become pregnant within medication period.
- If you have liver disease.
- If you have lupus.

**Over age 60:**
Adverse reactions and side effects may be more frequent and severe than in younger persons.

**Pregnancy:**
Risk to unborn child outweighs drug benefits. Don't use.

**Breast-feeding:**
No problems expected, but consult your doctor.

**Infants & children:**
Not recommended for children younger than 2.

**Prolonged use:**
You may become susceptible to infections caused by germs not responsive to griseofulvin.

**Skin & sunlight:**
May cause rash or intensify sunburn in areas exposed to sun or sunlamp.

**Driving, piloting or hazardous work:**
- Don't drive if you feel dizzy or have vision problems.
- Don't pilot aircraft.

**Discontinuing:**
Don't discontinue without doctor's advice until you complete prescribed dose, even though symptoms diminish or disappear.

**Others:**
Periodic laboratory blood studies and liver- and kidney-function tests recommended.

## POSSIBLE INTERACTION WITH OTHER DRUGS

| GENERIC NAME OR DRUG CLASS | COMBINED EFFECT |
|---|---|
| Anticoagulants (oral) | Decreased anticoagulant effect. |
| Barbiturates | Decreased griseofulvin effect. |
| Contraceptives (oral) | Decreased contraceptive effect. |

## POSSIBLE INTERACTION WITH OTHER SUBSTANCES

| INTERACTS WITH | COMBINED EFFECT |
|---|---|
| Alcohol: | Increased intoxication. Possible disulfiram reaction (see Glossary). |
| Beverages: | None expected. |
| Cocaine: | None expected |
| Foods: | None expected, but foods high in fat will improve drug absorption. |
| Marijuana: | None expected. |
| Tobacco: | None expected. |

# GUAIFENESIN

## BRAND NAMES

See complete list of brand names in the *Brand Name Directory,* page 949.

## BASIC INFORMATION

**Habit forming? No**
**Prescription needed? No**
**Available as generic? Yes**
**Drug class: Cough/cold preparation**

## USES

Loosens mucus in respiratory passages from allergies and infections (hay fever, cough, cold).

## DOSAGE & USAGE INFORMATION

**How to take:**
- Tablet or capsule—Swallow with liquid. If you can't swallow whole, crumble tablet or open capsule and take with liquid or food.
- Syrup or lozenge—Take as directed on label. Follow with 8 oz. water.

**When to take:**
As needed, no more often than every 3 hours.

**If you forget a dose:**
Take as soon as you remember. Wait 3 hours for next dose.

**What drug does:**
Increases production of watery fluids to thin mucus so it can be coughed out or absorbed.

**Time lapse before drug works:**
15 to 30 minutes. Regular use for 5 to 7 days necessary for maximum benefit.

**Don't take with:**
See Interaction column and consult doctor.

## OVERDOSE

**SYMPTOMS:**
**Drowsiness, mild weakness, nausea, vomiting.**
**WHAT TO DO:**
**Overdose unlikely to threaten life. If person takes much larger amount than prescribed, call doctor, poison-control center or hospital emergency room for instructions.**

## POSSIBLE ADVERSE REACTIONS OR SIDE EFFECTS

| SYMPTOMS | WHAT TO DO |
|---|---|
| **Life-threatening:** None expected. | |
| **Common:** None expected. | |
| **Infrequent:** | |
| • Rash, stomach pain, diarrhea, nausea, vomiting. | Discontinue. Call doctor right away. |
| • Drowsiness. | Continue. Call doctor when convenient. |
| **Rare:** None expected. | |

## WARNINGS & PRECAUTIONS

**Don't take if:**
You are allergic to any cough or cold preparation containing guaifenesin.

**Before you start, consult your doctor:**
See Interaction column and consult doctor.

**Over age 60:**
Adverse reactions and side effects may be more frequent and severe than in younger persons. For drug to work, you must drink 8 to 10 glasses of fluid per day.

**Pregnancy:**
No proven harm to unborn child. Avoid if possible.

**Breast-feeding:**
No proven problems. Consult your doctor.

**Infants & children:**
No problems expected.

**Prolonged use:**
No problems expected.

**Skin & sunlight:**
No problems expected.

**Driving, piloting or hazardous work:**
Avoid if you feel drowsy. Otherwise, no problems expected.

**Discontinuing:**
May be unnecessary to finish medicine. Discontinue when symptoms disappear. If symptoms persist more than 1 week, consult doctor.

**Others:**
No problems expected.

## POSSIBLE INTERACTION WITH OTHER DRUGS

| GENERIC NAME OR DRUG CLASS | COMBINED EFFECT |
|---|---|
| Anticoagulants | Risk of bleeding. |

## POSSIBLE INTERACTION WITH OTHER SUBSTANCES

| INTERACTS WITH | COMBINED EFFECT |
|---|---|
| Alcohol: | No proven problems. |
| Beverages: | You must drink 8 to 10 glasses of fluid per day for drug to work. |
| Cocaine: | No proven problems. |
| Foods: | None expected. |
| Marijuana: | No proven problems. |
| Tobacco: | No proven problems. |

# GUANABENZ

## BRAND NAMES

Wytensin

## BASIC INFORMATION

Habit forming? No
Prescription needed? Yes
Available as generic? No
Drug class: Antihypertensive (alpha
adrenergic stimulant)

 **USES**

Controls, but doesn't cure, high blood pressure.

 **DOSAGE & USAGE INFORMATION**

**How to take:**
Tablet—Swallow with liquid or food to lessen
stomach irritation. If you can't swallow whole,
crumble tablet and take with liquid or food.

**When to take:**
At the same times each day.

**If you forget a dose:**
Take as soon as you remember up to 2 hours
late. If more than 2 hours, wait for next
scheduled dose (don't double this dose).

**What drug does:**
• Relaxes muscle cells of small arteries.
• Slows heartbeat.

**Time lapse before drug works:**
1 hour.

**Don't take with:**
See Interaction column and consult doctor.

 **OVERDOSE**

**SYMPTOMS:**
Severe dizziness, slow heartbeat, pinpoint
pupils, fainting, coma.
**WHAT TO DO:**
• Dial 0 (operator) or 911 (emergency) for an
ambulance or medical help. Then give first
aid immediately.
• If patient is unconscious and not
breathing, give mouth-to-mouth breathing.
If there is no heartbeat, use cardiac
massage and mouth-to-mouth breathing
(CPR). Don't try to make patient vomit. If
you can't get help quickly, take patient to
nearest emergency facility.
• See emergency information on inside
covers.

 **POSSIBLE ADVERSE REACTIONS OR SIDE EFFECTS**

| SYMPTOMS | WHAT TO DO |
|---|---|
| **Life-threatening:**<br>None expected. | |
| **Common:** | |
| • Nervousness, headache, paleness, dry mouth, rapid heartbeat. | Continue. Call doctor when convenient. |
| • Insomnia. | Continue. Tell doctor at next visit. |
| **Infrequent:** | |
| • Irregular heartbeat, shakiness in hands. | Discontinue. Call doctor right away. |
| • Dizziness, appetite loss, nausea, vomiting, painful or difficult urination, diminished sex drive. | Continue. Call doctor when convenient. |
| **Rare:**<br>None expected. | |

## WARNINGS & PRECAUTIONS

**Don't take if:**
You are allergic to any sympathomimetic drug.

**Before you start, consult your doctor:**
- If you have blood disease.
- If you have heart disease.
- If you have liver disease.
- If you have diabetes or overactive thyroid.
- If you will have surgery within 2 months, including dental surgery, requiring general or spinal anesthesia.

**Over age 60:**
Adverse reactions and side effects may be more frequent and severe than in younger persons. Hot weather may cause need to reduce dosage.

**Pregnancy:**
Risk to unborn child outweighs drug benefits. Don't use.

**Breast-feeding:**
Avoid nursing.

**Infants & children:**
Not recommended.

**Prolonged use:**
Side effects tend to diminish. Request uric-acid and kidney-function studies periodically.

**Skin & sunlight:**
No problems expected.

**Driving, piloting or hazardous work:**
Avoid if you feel dizzy; otherwise, no problems expected.

**Discontinuing:**
Don't discontinue without consulting doctor. Dose may require gradual reduction if you have taken drug for a long time. Doses of other drugs may also require adjustment. Abrupt discontinuing may cause anxiety, chest pain, salivation, headache, abdominal cramps, fast heartbeat.

**Others:**
Stay away from high sodium foods. Lose weight if you are overweight.

## POSSIBLE INTERACTION WITH OTHER DRUGS

| GENERIC NAME OR DRUG CLASS | COMBINED EFFECT |
|---|---|
| Antihypertensives (other) | Decreases blood pressure more than either alone. May be beneficial, but requires dosage adjustment. |
| Brain depressants: Sedatives, sleeping pills, tranquilizers, antidepressants, narcotics | Increased brain depression. Avoid. |
| Diuretics | Decreases blood pressure more than either alone. May be beneficial, but requires dosage adjustment. |
| Enalapril | Possible excessive potassium in blood. |

## POSSIBLE INTERACTION WITH OTHER SUBSTANCES

| INTERACTS WITH | COMBINED EFFECT |
|---|---|
| Alcohol: | Oversedation. Avoid. |
| Beverages: Caffeine. | Overstimulation. Avoid. |
| Cocaine: | Overstimulation. Avoid. |
| Foods: Salt. | Decrease salt intake to increase beneficial effects of guanabenz. |
| Marijuana: | Overstimulation. Avoid. |
| Tobacco: | Decreased guanabenz effect. |

# GUANADREL

## BRAND NAMES

Hylorel

## BASIC INFORMATION

Habit forming? No
Prescription needed? Yes
Available as generic? No
Drug class: Antihypertensive

 ## USES

Controls, but doesn't cure, high blood pressure.

 ## DOSAGE & USAGE INFORMATION

**How to take:**
Tablet or capsule—Swallow with liquid or food to lessen stomach irritation. If you can't swallow whole, crumble tablet or open capsule and take with liquid or food.

**When to take:**
At the same time each day.

**If you forget a dose:**
Take as soon as you remember up to 2 hours late. If more than 2 hours, wait for next scheduled dose (don't double this dose).

**What drug does:**
Relaxes muscle cells of small arteries.

**Time lapse before drug works:**
4 to 6 hours. May need to take for lifetime.

**Don't take with:**
See Interaction column and consult doctor.

 ## OVERDOSE

**SYMPTOMS:**
Severe blood-pressure drop; fainting; slow, weak pulse; cold, sweaty skin; loss of consciousness.
**WHAT TO DO:**
- Dial 0 (operator) or 911 (emergency) for an ambulance or medical help. Then give first aid immediately.
- See emergency information on inside covers.

 ## POSSIBLE ADVERSE REACTIONS OR SIDE EFFECTS

| SYMPTOMS | WHAT TO DO |
|---|---|
| **Life-threatening:** | |
| None expected. | |
| **Common:** | |
| ● Diarrhea, more bowel movements, fatigue, weakness. | Continue. Call doctor when convenient. |
| ● Dizziness, headache, lower sex drive. | Continue. Tell doctor at next visit. |
| ● Stuffy nose, dry mouth. | No action necessary. |
| **Infrequent:** | |
| ● Rash, blurred vision, drooping eyelids, chest pain or shortness of breath, muscle pain or tremor. | Discontinue. Call doctor right away. |
| ● Nausea or vomiting. | Continue. Call doctor when convenient. |
| ● Impotence, nighttime urination. | Continue. Tell doctor at next visit. |
| **Rare:** | |
| None expected. | |

## WARNINGS & PRECAUTIONS

### Don't take if:
- You are allergic to guanadrel.
- You have taken MAO inhibitors within 2 weeks.

### Before you start, consult your doctor:
- If you have stroke or heart disease.
- If you have asthma.
- If you have had kidney disease.
- If you have peptic ulcer or chronic acid indigestion.
- If you will have surgery within 2 months, including dental surgery, requiring general or spinal anesthesia.

### Over age 60:
Adverse reactions and side effects may be more frequent and severe than in younger persons. Start with small doses and monitor blood pressure frequently.

### Pregnancy:
No proven harm to unborn child. Avoid if possible.

### Breast-feeding:
No proven harm to nursing infant. Avoid if possible.

### Infants & children:
Not recommended.

### Prolonged use:
Due to drug's cumulative effect, dose will require adjustment to prevent wide fluctuations in blood pressure.

### Skin & sunlight:
No problems expected.

### Driving, piloting or hazardous work:
Don't drive or pilot aircraft until you learn how medicine affects you. Don't work around dangerous machinery. Don't climb ladders or work in high places. Danger increases if you drink alcohol or take medicine affecting alertness and reflexes, such as antihistamines, tranquilizers, sedatives, pain medicine, narcotics and mind-altering drugs.

### Discontinuing:
Don't discontinue without consulting doctor. Dose may require gradual reduction if you have taken drug for a long time. Doses of other drugs may also require adjustment.

### Others:
Hot weather further lowers blood pressure, particularly in patients over 60.

## POSSIBLE INTERACTION WITH OTHER DRUGS

| GENERIC NAME OR DRUG CLASS | COMBINED EFFECT |
|---|---|
| Antidepressants (tricyclic) | Decreased effect of guanadrel. |
| Antihypertensives (other) | Increased effect of guanadrel. |
| Beta blockers | Increased likelihood of dizziness and fainting. |
| CNS depressants: Anticonvulsants, antihistamines, muscle relaxants, narcotics, sedatives, tranquilizers. | Decreased effect of guanadrel. |
| Diuretics | Increased likelihood of dizziness and fainting. |
| Enalapril | Possible excessive potassium in blood. |
| MAO inhibitors | Severe high blood pressure. Avoid. |
| Phenothiazines | Decreased effect of guanadrel. |
| Rauwolfia alkaloids | Increased likelihood of dizziness and fainting. |
| Sympathomimetics | Decreased effect of guanadrel. |

## POSSIBLE INTERACTION WITH OTHER SUBSTANCES

| INTERACTS WITH | COMBINED EFFECT |
|---|---|
| Alcohol: | Decreased effect of guanadrel. Avoid. |
| Beverages: Caffeine. | Decreased effect of guanadrel. |
| Cocaine: | Higher blood pressure. Avoid. |
| Foods: | No problems expected. |
| Marijuana: | Higher blood pressure. Avoid. |
| Tobacco: | Higher blood pressure. Avoid. |

# GUANETHIDINE

## BRAND NAMES

Apo-Guanethidine     Ismelin
Esimil                  Ismelin-Esidrix

## BASIC INFORMATION

**Habit forming? No**
**Prescription needed? Yes**
**Available as generic? Yes**
**Drug class: Antihypertensive**

## USES

Reduces high blood pressure.

## DOSAGE & USAGE INFORMATION

**How to take:**
Tablet or capsule—Swallow with liquid. If you
can't swallow tablet or capsule whole, crumble
or open and take with liquid or food.

**When to take:**
At the same time each day.

**If you forget a dose:**
Take as soon as you remember up to 2 hours
late. If more than 2 hours, wait for next
scheduled dose (don't double this dose).

**What drug does:**
Displaces norepinephrine—hormone necessary
to maintain small blood-vessel tone. Blood
vessels relax and high blood pressure drops.

**Time lapse before drug works:**
Regular use for several weeks may be
necessary to determine effectiveness.

**Don't take with:**
- Non-prescription drugs containing alcohol
  without consulting doctor.
- See Interaction column and consult doctor.

## OVERDOSE

**SYMPTOMS:**
**Severe blood-pressure drop; fainting; slow,**
**weak pulse; cold, sweaty skin; loss of**
**consciousness.**
**WHAT TO DO:**
- **Dial 0 (operator) or 911 (emergency) for an**
  **ambulance or medical help. Then give first**
  **aid immediately.**
- **See emergency information on inside**
  **covers.**

## POSSIBLE ADVERSE REACTIONS OR SIDE EFFECTS

| SYMPTOMS | WHAT TO DO |
|---|---|
| **Life-threatening:** | |
| None expected. | |
| **Common:** | |
| • Unusually slow heartbeat. | Discontinue. Call doctor right away. |
| • Diarrhea; more bowel movements; swollen feet, legs; fatigue, weakness. | Continue. Call doctor when convenient. |
| • Dizziness, headache, lower sex drive. | Continue. Tell doctor at next visit. |
| • Stuffy nose, dry mouth. | No action necessary. |
| **Infrequent:** | |
| • Rash, blurred vision, drooping eyelids, chest pain or shortness of breath, muscle pain or tremor. | Discontinue. Call doctor right away. |
| • Nausea or vomiting. | Continue. Call doctor when convenient. |
| • Impotence, nighttime urination. | Continue. Tell doctor at next visit. |
| **Rare:** | |
| None expected. | |

## WARNINGS & PRECAUTIONS

**Don't take if:**
- You are allergic to guanethidine.
- You have taken MAO inhibitors within 2
  weeks.

**Before you start, consult your doctor:**
- If you have had stroke or heart disease.
- If you have asthma.
- If you have had kidney disease.
- If you have peptic ulcer or chronic acid
  indigestion.
- If you will have surgery within 2 months,
  including dental surgery, requiring general or
  spinal anesthesia.

**Over age 60:**
Adverse reactions and side effects may be
more frequent and severe than in younger
persons. Start with small doses and monitor
blood pressure frequently.

**Pregnancy:**
No proven harm to unborn child. Avoid if
possible.

**Breast-feeding:**
No proven harm to nursing infant. Avoid if
possible.

**Infants & children:**
Not recommended.

**Prolonged use:**
Due to drug's cumulative effect, dose will require adjustment to prevent wide fluctuations in blood pressure.

**Skin & sunlight:**
No problems expected.

**Driving, piloting or hazardous work:**
Don't drive or pilot aircraft until you learn how medicine affects you. Don't work around dangerous machinery. Don't climb ladders or work in high places. Danger increases if you drink alcohol or take medicine affecting alertness and reflexes, such as antihistamines, tranquilizers, sedatives, pain medicine, narcotics and mind-altering drugs.

**Discontinuing:**
Don't discontinue without consulting doctor. Dose may require gradual reduction if you have taken drug for a long time. Doses of other drugs may also require adjustment.

**Others:**
Hot weather further lowers blood pressure.

## POSSIBLE INTERACTION WITH OTHER DRUGS

| GENERIC NAME OR DRUG CLASS | COMBINED EFFECT |
|---|---|
| Amphetamines | Decreased guanethidine effect. |
| Antidepressants (tricyclic) | Decreased guanethidine effect. |
| Antihistamines | Decreased guanethidine effect. |
| Contraceptives (oral) | Decreased guanethidine effect. |
| Digitalis preparations | Slower heartbeat. |
| Diuretics (thiazide) | Increased guanethidine effect. |
| Enalapril | Possible excessive potassium in blood. |
| Indapamide | Possible increased effects of both drugs. When monitored carefully, combination may be beneficial in controlling hypertension. |
| Minoxidil | Dosage adjustments may be necessary to keep blood pressure at proper level. |

| | |
|---|---|
| Pentoxifylline | Increased antihypertensive effect. |
| Rauwolfia alkaloids | Increased guanethidine effect. |

## POSSIBLE INTERACTION WITH OTHER SUBSTANCES

| INTERACTS WITH | COMBINED EFFECT |
|---|---|
| Alcohol: | Use caution. Decreases blood pressure. |
| Beverages: Carbonated drinks. | Use sparingly. Sodium content increases blood pressure. |
| Cocaine: | Raises blood pressure. Avoid. |
| Foods: Spicy or acid foods. | Avoid if subject to indigestion or peptic ulcer. |
| Marijuana: | Excessively low blood pressure. Avoid. |
| Tobacco: | Possible blood-pressure rise. Avoid. |

# GUANETHIDINE & HYDROCHLOROTHIAZIDE

## BRAND NAMES

**Esimil**

## BASIC INFORMATION

**Habit forming? No**
**Prescription needed? Yes**
**Available as generic? No**
**Drug class: Antihypertensive-diuretic**

## USES

- Controls, but doesn't cure, high blood pressure.
- Reduces fluid retention (edema).

## DOSAGE & USAGE INFORMATION

**How to take:**
Tablet or capsule—Swallow with liquid. If you can't swallow whole, crumble tablet or open capsule and take with liquid or food.

**When to take:**
At the same time each day.

**If you forget a dose:**
Take as soon as you remember up to 2 hours late. If more than 2 hours, wait for next scheduled dose (don't double this dose).

**What drug does:**
- Forces sodium and water secretion, reducing body fluid.
- Displaces norepinephrine—hormone necessary to maintain small blood-vessel tone. Blood vessels relax and high blood pressure drops.

**Time lapse before drug works:**
Regular use for several weeks may be necessary to determine effectiveness.

*Continued next column*

## OVERDOSE

**SYMPTOMS:**
**Cramps, weakness, drowsiness, weak pulse, severe blood-pressure drop, fainting, cold and sweaty skin, loss of consciousness, coma.**
**WHAT TO DO:**
- **Dial 0 (operator) or 911 (emergency) for an ambulance or medical help. Then give first aid immediately.**
- **See emergency information on inside covers.**

**Don't take with:**
- Non-prescription drugs containing alcohol without consulting doctor.
- See Interaction column and consult doctor.

## POSSIBLE ADVERSE REACTIONS OR SIDE EFFECTS

| SYMPTOMS | WHAT TO DO |
|---|---|
| **Life-threatening:** | |
| Chest pain, shortness of breath, irregular heartbeat. | Discontinue. Seek emergency treatment. |
| **Common:** | |
| • Slow heartbeat, swollen feet and ankles, fatigue, weakness. | Discontinue. Call doctor right away. |
| • Dizziness, headache, stuffy nose, dry mouth, diarrhea, diminished sex drive. | Continue. Call doctor when convenient. |
| **Infrequent:** | |
| • Mood change, rash or hives, blurred vision, drooping eyelids, muscle pain or tremors. | Discontinue. Call doctor right away. |
| • Increased nighttime urination, abdominal pain, vomiting, nausea, weakness. | Continue. Call doctor when convenient. |
| • Impotence. | Continue. Tell doctor at next visit. |
| **Rare:** | |
| • Sore throat, jaundice. | Discontinue. Call doctor right away. |
| • Weight gain or loss. | Continue. Call doctor when convenient. |

## WARNINGS & PRECAUTIONS

**Don't take if:**
- You are allergic to any thiazide diuretic drug or guanethidine.
- You have taken MAO inhibitors within 2 weeks.

**Before you start, consult your doctor:**
- If you are allergic to any sulfa drug.
- If you have gout, asthma, liver, pancreas or kidney disorder, peptic ulcer or chronic acid indigestion.
- If you have had stroke or heart disease.
- If you will have surgery within 2 months, including dental surgery, requiring general or spinal anesthesia.

**Over age 60:**
Adverse reactions and side effects may be more frequent and severe than in younger persons, especially dizziness and excessive potassium loss.

**Pregnancy:**
Risk to unborn child outweighs drug benefits. Don't use.

**Breast-feeding:**
Drug passes into milk. Avoid drug or discontinue nursing until you finish medicine. Consult doctor for advice on maintaining milk supply.

**Infants & children:**
Not recommended.

**Prolonged use:**
Due to drug's cumulative effect, dose will require adjustment to prevent wide fluctuations in blood pressure.

**Skin & sunlight:**
May cause rash or intensify sunburn in areas exposed to sun or sunlamp.

**Driving, piloting or hazardous work:**
Don't drive or pilot aircraft until you learn how medicine affects you. Don't work around dangerous machinery. Don't climb ladders or work in high places. Danger increases if you drink alcohol or take medicine affecting alertness and reflexes, such as antihistamines, tranquilizers, sedatives, pain medicine, narcotics and mind-altering drugs.

**Discontinuing:**
Don't discontinue without consulting doctor. Dose may require gradual reduction if you have taken drug for a long time. Doses of other drugs may also require adjustment.

**Others:**
- Hot weather and fever may cause dehydration and drop in blood pressure. Dose may require temporary adjustment. Weigh daily and report any unexpected weight decreases to your doctor.
- May cause rise in uric acid, leading to gout.
- May cause blood-sugar rise in diabetics.

## POSSIBLE INTERACTION WITH OTHER DRUGS

| GENERIC NAME OR DRUG CLASS | COMBINED EFFECT |
| --- | --- |
| Acebutolol | Increased antihypertensive effect. Dosages of both drugs may require adjustments. |
| Allopurinol | Decreased allopurinol effect. |

| | |
| --- | --- |
| Amphetamines | Decreased guanethidine effect. |
| Antidepressants (tricyclic) | Dangerous drop in blood pressure. Avoid combination unless under medical supervision. |
| Antihistamines | Decreased guanethidine effect. |
| Barbiturates | Increased hydrochlorothiazide effect. |
| Cholestyramine | Decreased hydrochlorothiazide effect. |
| Contraceptives (oral) | Decreased guanethidine effect. |
| Cortisone drugs | Excessive potassium loss that causes dangerous heart rhythms. |
| Digitalis preparations | Excessive potassium loss that causes dangerous heart rhythms. |
| Diuretics (thiazide) | Increased thiazide and guanethidine effect. |

*Continued page 967*

## POSSIBLE INTERACTION WITH OTHER SUBSTANCES

| INTERACTS WITH | COMBINED EFFECT |
| --- | --- |
| Alcohol: | Use caution. Decreases blood pressure. |
| Beverages: Carbonated drinks. | Use sparingly. Sodium content increases blood pressure. |
| Cocaine: | Raises blood pressure. Avoid. |
| Foods: Spicy or acid foods. | Avoid if subject to indigestion or peptic ulcer. |
| Licorice. | Excessive potassium loss that causes dangerous heart rhythms. |
| Marijuana: | Effect on blood pressure unpredictable. |
| Tobacco: | Possible blood-pressure rise. Avoid. |

# HALAZEPAM

## BRAND NAMES

Paxipam

## BASIC INFORMATION

**Habit forming? Yes**
**Prescription needed? Yes**
**Available as generic? No**
**Drug class: Tranquilizer (benzodiazepine)**

 ## USES

Treatment for nervousness or tension.

 ## DOSAGE & USAGE INFORMATION

**How to take:**
Tablet or capsule—Swallow with liquid. If you can't swallow whole, crumble tablet or open capsule and take with liquid or food.

**When to take:**
At the same time each day, according to instructions on prescription label.

**If you forget a dose:**
Take as soon as you remember up to 2 hours late. If more than 2 hours, wait for next scheduled dose (don't double this dose).

**What drug does:**
Affects limbic system of brain—part that controls emotions.

**Time lapse before drug works:**
2 hours. May take 6 weeks for full benefit.

**Don't take with:**
See Interaction column and consult doctor.

 ## OVERDOSE

**SYMPTOMS:**
**Drowsiness, weakness, tremor, stupor, coma.**
**WHAT TO DO:**
- **Dial 0 (operator) or 911 (emergency) for an ambulance or medical help. Then give first aid immediately.**
- **If patient is unconscious and not breathing, give mouth-to-mouth breathing. If there is no heartbeat, use cardiac massage and mouth-to-mouth breathing (CPR). Don't try to make patient vomit. If you can't get help quickly, take patient to nearest emergency facility.**
- **See emergency information on inside covers.**

 ## POSSIBLE ADVERSE REACTIONS OR SIDE EFFECTS

| SYMPTOMS | WHAT TO DO |
|---|---|
| **Life-threatening:** | |
| None expected. | |
| **Common:** | |
| Clumsiness, drowsiness, dizziness. | Continue. Call doctor when convenient. |
| **Infrequent:** | |
| ● Hallucinations, confusion, depression, irritability, rash, itch, change in vision. | Discontinue. Call doctor right away. |
| ● Constipation or diarrhea, nausea, vomiting, painful or difficult urination. | Continue. Call doctor when convenient. |
| **Rare:** | |
| ● Slow heartbeat, difficult breathing. | Discontinue. Seek emergency treatment. |
| ● Mouth, throat ulcers; jaundice. | Discontinue. Call doctor right away. |

## WARNINGS & PRECAUTIONS

**Don't take if:**
- You are allergic to any benzodiazepine.
- You have myasthenia gravis.
- You are active or recovering alcoholic.
- Patient is younger than 6 months.

**Before you start, consult your doctor:**
- If you have liver, kidney or lung disease.
- If you have diabetes, epilepsy or porphyria.

**Over age 60:**
Adverse reactions and side effects may be more frequent and severe than in younger persons. You need smaller doses for shorter periods of time. May develop agitation, rage or "hangover" effect.

**Pregnancy:**
Risk to unborn child outweighs drug benefits. Don't use.

**Breast-feeding:**
Drug passes into milk. Avoid drug or discontinue nursing until you finish medicine. Consult doctor for advice on maintaining milk supply.

**Infants & children:**
Use only under medical supervision for children older than 6 months.

**Prolonged use:**
May impair liver function.

**Skin & sunlight:**
No problems expected.

**Driving, piloting or hazardous work:**
Don't drive or pilot aircraft until you learn how medicine affects you. Don't work around dangerous machinery. Don't climb ladders or work in high places. Danger increases if you drink alcohol or take medicine affecting alertness and reflexes.

**Discontinuing:**
Don't discontinue without consulting doctor. Dose may require gradual reduction if you have taken drug for a long time. Doses of other drugs may also require adjustment.

**Others:**
- Hot weather, heavy exercise and profuse sweat may reduce excretion and cause overdose.
- Blood sugar may rise in diabetics, requiring insulin adjustment.

## POSSIBLE INTERACTION WITH OTHER DRUGS

| GENERIC NAME OR DRUG CLASS | COMBINED EFFECT |
|---|---|
| Anticonvulsants | Change in seizure frequency or severity. |
| Antidepressants | Increased sedative effect of both drugs. |
| Antihistamines | Increased sedative effect of both drugs. |
| Antihypertensives | Excessively low blood pressure. |
| Cimetidine | Excess sedation. |
| Disulfiram | Increased halazepam effect. |
| Dronabinol | Increased effects of both drugs. Avoid. |
| MAO inhibitors | Convulsions, deep sedation, rage. |
| Molindone | Increased tranquilizer effect. |
| Narcotics | Increased sedative effect of both drugs. |
| Sedatives | Increased sedative effect of both drugs. |
| Sleep inducers | Increased sedative effect of both drugs. |
| Tranquilizers | Increased sedative effect of both drugs. |

## POSSIBLE INTERACTION WITH OTHER SUBSTANCES

| INTERACTS WITH | COMBINED EFFECT |
|---|---|
| Alcohol: | Heavy sedation. Avoid. |
| Beverages: | None expected. |
| Cocaine: | Decreased halazepam effect. |
| Foods: | None expected. |
| Marijuana: | Heavy sedation. Avoid. |
| Tobacco: | Decreased halazepam effect. |

# HALOPERIDOL

## BRAND NAMES

Apo-Haloperidol
Haldol
Haldol Decanoate

Haldol LA
Novoperidol
Peridol

## BASIC INFORMATION

Habit forming? No
Prescription needed? Yes
Available as generic? Yes
Drug class: Tranquilizer (antipsychotic)

## USES

Reduces severe anxiety, agitation and psychotic behavior.

## DOSAGE & USAGE INFORMATION

**How to take:**
- Tablet or capsule—Swallow with liquid. If you can't swallow whole, crumble tablet or open capsule and take with liquid or food.
- Drops—Dilute dose in beverage before swallowing.

**When to take:**
At the same times each day.

**If you forget a dose:**
Take as soon as you remember up to 2 hours late. If more than 2 hours, wait for next scheduled dose (don't double this dose).

**What drug does:**
Corrects an imbalance in nerve impulses from brain.

*Continued next column*

## OVERDOSE

**SYMPTOMS:**
Weak, rapid pulse; shallow, slow breathing; very low blood pressure; convulsions; deep sleep ending in coma.
**WHAT TO DO:**
- Dial 0 (operator) or 911 (emergency) for an ambulance or medical help. Then give first aid immediately.
- If patient is unconscious and not breathing, give mouth-to-mouth breathing. If there is no heartbeat, use cardiac massage and mouth-to-mouth breathing (CPR). Don't try to make patient vomit. If you can't get help quickly, take patient to nearest emergency facility.
- See emergency information on inside covers.

**Time lapse before drug works:**
3 weeks to 2 months for maximum benefit.

**Don't take with:**
- Non-prescription drugs without consulting doctor.
- See Interaction column and consult doctor.

## POSSIBLE ADVERSE REACTIONS OR SIDE EFFECTS

| SYMPTOMS | WHAT TO DO |
|---|---|
| **Life-threatening:** | |
| None expected. | |
| **Common:** | |
| • Blurred vision. | Discontinue. Call doctor right away. |
| • Shuffling, stiffness, jerkiness, shakiness, constipation. | Continue. Call doctor when convenient. |
| • Dry mouth. | No action necessary. |
| **Infrequent:** | |
| • Rash, circling motions of tongue. | Discontinue. Call doctor right away. |
| • Dizziness, faintness, drowsiness, difficult urination, decreased sexual ability, nausea or vomiting. | Continue. Call doctor when convenient. |
| **Rare:** | |
| Sore throat, fever, jaundice. | Discontinue. Call doctor right away. |

## WARNINGS & PRECAUTIONS

### Don't take if:
- You have ever been allergic to haloperidol.
- You are depressed.
- You have Parkinson's disease.
- Patient is younger than 3 years old.

### Before you start, consult your doctor:
- If you take sedatives, sleeping pills, tranquilizers, antidepressants, antihistamines, narcotics or mind-altering drugs.
- If you have a history of mental depression.
- If you have had kidney or liver problems.
- If you have diabetes, epilepsy, glaucoma, high blood pressure or heart disease.
- If you drink alcoholic beverages frequently.

### Over age 60:
Adverse reactions and side effects may be more frequent and severe than in younger persons.

### Pregnancy:
Risk to unborn child outweighs drug benefits. Don't use.

### Breast-feeding:
No proven harm to nursing infant. Avoid if possible.

### Infants & children:
Not recommended.

### Prolonged use:
May develop tardive dyskinesia (involuntary movements of jaws, lips and tongue).

### Skin & sunlight:
May cause rash or intensify sunburn in areas exposed to sun or sunlamp.

### Driving, piloting or hazardous work:
Don't drive or pilot aircraft until you learn how medicine affects you. Don't work around dangerous machinery. Don't climb ladders or work in high places. Danger increases if you drink alcohol or take medicine affecting alertness and reflexes.

### Discontinuing:
Don't discontinue without consulting doctor. Dose may require gradual reduction if you have taken drug for a long time. Doses of other drugs may also require adjustment.

### Others:
No problems expected.

## POSSIBLE INTERACTION WITH OTHER DRUGS

| GENERIC NAME OR DRUG CLASS | COMBINED EFFECT |
|---|---|
| Anticholinergics | Increased anticholinergic effect. May cause pressure within the eye. |
| Anticoagulants (oral) | Decreased anticoagulant effect. |
| Anticonvulsants | Changed seizure pattern. |
| Antidepressants | Excessive sedation. |
| Antihistamines | Excessive sedation. |
| Antihypertensives | May cause severe blood-pressure drop. |
| Barbiturates | Excessive sedation. |
| Bethanidine | Decreased bethanidine effect. |
| Dronabinol | Increased effects of both drugs. Avoid. |
| Guanethidine | Decreased guanethidine effect. |
| Levodopa | Decreased levodopa effect. |
| Methyldopa | Possible psychosis. |
| Narcotics | Excessive sedation. |
| Sedatives | Excessive sedation. |
| Tranquilizers | Excessive sedation. |

## POSSIBLE INTERACTION WITH OTHER SUBSTANCES

| INTERACTS WITH | COMBINED EFFECT |
|---|---|
| Alcohol: | Excessive sedation and depressed brain function. Avoid. |
| Beverages: | None expected. |
| Cocaine: | Decreased effect of haloperidol. Avoid. |
| Foods: | None expected. |
| Marijuana: | Occasional use—Increased sedation. Frequent use—Possible toxic psychosis. |
| Tobacco: | None expected. |

# HETACILLIN

## BRAND NAMES

Versapen                    Versapen-K

## BASIC INFORMATION

**Habit forming?** No
**Prescription needed?** Yes
**Available as generic?** Yes
**Drug class:** Antibiotic (penicillin)

## USES

Treatment of bacterial infections that are susceptible to hetacillin.

## DOSAGE & USAGE INFORMATION

**How to take:**
- Tablets or capsules—Swallow with liquid on an empty stomach 1 hour before or 2 hours after eating.
- Liquid—Take with cold beverage. Liquid form is perishable and effective for only 7 days at room temperature. Effective for 14 days if stored in refrigerator. Don't freeze.

**When to take:**
Follow instructions on prescription label or side of package. Doses should be evenly spaced. For example, 4 times a day means every 6 hours.

**If you forget a dose:**
Take as soon as you remember. Continue regular schedule.

**What drug does:**
Destroys susceptible bacteria. Does not kill viruses.

**Time lapse before drug works:**
May be several days before medicine affects infection.

**Don't take with:**
See Interaction column and consult doctor.

## OVERDOSE

**SYMPTOMS:**
Severe diarrhea, nausea or vomiting.
**WHAT TO DO:**
Overdose unlikely to threaten life. If person takes much larger amount than prescribed, call doctor, poison-control center or hospital emergency room for instructions.

## POSSIBLE ADVERSE REACTIONS OR SIDE EFFECTS

| SYMPTOMS | WHAT TO DO |
|---|---|
| **Life-threatening:** | |
| Hives, rash, intense itching, faintness soon after a dose (anaphylaxis). | Seek emergency treatment immediately. |
| **Common:** | |
| Dark or discolored tongue. | Continue. Tell doctor at next visit. |
| **Infrequent:** | |
| Nausea, vomiting, diarrhea. | Continue. Call doctor when convenient. |
| **Rare:** | |
| Unexplained bleeding. | Discontinue. Call doctor right away. |

## WARNINGS & PRECAUTIONS

**Don't take if:**
You are allergic to hetacillin, cephalosporin antibiotics, other penicillins or penicillamine. Life-threatening reaction may occur.

**Before you start, consult your doctor:**
If you are allergic to any substance or drug.

**Over age 60:**
You may have skin reactions, particularly around genitals and anus.

**Pregnancy:**
Studies inconclusive on harm to unborn child. Animal studies show fetal abnormalities. Decide with your doctor whether drug benefits justify risk to unborn child.

**Breast-feeding:**
Drug passes into milk. Child may become sensitive to penicillins and have allergic reactions to penicillin drugs. Avoid hetacillin or discontinue nursing until you finish medicine. Consult doctor for advice on maintaining milk supply.

**Infants & children:**
No problems expected.

**Prolonged use:**
You may become more susceptible to infections caused by germs not responsive to hetacillin.

**Skin & sunlight:**
No problems expected.

**Driving, piloting or hazardous work:**
Usually not dangerous. Most hazardous reactions likely to occur a few minutes after taking hetacillin.

**Discontinuing:**
Don't discontinue without doctor's advice until you complete prescribed dose, even though symptoms diminish or disappear.

**Others:**
Urine sugar test for diabetes may show false positive result.

## POSSIBLE INTERACTION WITH OTHER DRUGS

| GENERIC NAME OR DRUG CLASS | COMBINED EFFECT |
|---|---|
| Beta-adrenergic blockers | Increased chance of anaphylaxis (see emergency information on inside front cover). |
| Chloramphenicol | Decreased effect of both drugs. |
| Erythromycins | Decreased effect of both drugs. |
| Loperamide | Decreased hetacillin effect. |
| Paromomycin | Decreased effect of both drugs. |
| Tetracyclines | Decreased effect of both drugs. |
| Troleandomycin | Decreased effect of both drugs. |

## POSSIBLE INTERACTION WITH OTHER SUBSTANCES

| INTERACTS WITH | COMBINED EFFECT |
|---|---|
| Alcohol: | Occasional stomach irritation. |
| Beverages: | None expected. |
| Cocaine: | No proven problems. |
| Foods: | None expected. |
| Marijuana: | No proven problems. |
| Tobacco: | None expected. |

# HEXOBARBITAL

## BRAND NAMES

Sombulex

## BASIC INFORMATION

Habit forming? Yes
Prescription needed? Yes
Available as generic? Yes
Drug class: Sedative, hypnotic (barbiturate)

 ## USES

- Reduces anxiety or nervous tension (low dose).
- Relieves insomnia (higher bedtime dose).

 ## DOSAGE & USAGE INFORMATION

**How to take:**
Tablet—Swallow with liquid or food to lessen stomach irritation. If you can't swallow whole, crumble tablet and take with liquid or food.

**When to take:**
At the same times each day.

**If you forget a dose:**
Take as soon as you remember up to 2 hours late. If more than 2 hours, wait for next scheduled dose (don't double this dose).

**What drug does:**
May partially block nerve impulses at nerve-cell connections.

**Time lapse before drug works:**
60 minutes.

**Don't take with:**
- Non-prescription drugs without consulting doctor.
- See Interaction column and consult doctor.

 ## OVERDOSE

**SYMPTOMS:**
Deep sleep, weak pulse, coma.
**WHAT TO DO:**
- Dial 0 (operator) or 911 (emergency) for an ambulance or medical help. Then give first aid immediately.
- If patient is unconscious and not breathing, give mouth-to-mouth breathing. If there is no heartbeat use cardiac massage and mouth-to-mouth breathing (CPR). Don't try to make patient vomit. If you can't get help quickly, take patient to nearest emergency facility.
- See emergency information on inside covers.

 ## POSSIBLE ADVERSE REACTIONS OR SIDE EFFECTS

| SYMPTOMS | WHAT TO DO |
|---|---|
| **Life-threatening:** | |
| None expected. | |
| **Common:** | |
| Dizziness, drowsiness, "hangover" effect. | Continue. Call doctor when convenient. |
| **Infrequent:** | |
| • Rash or hives; face, lip swelling; swollen eyelids; sore throat; fever. | Discontinue. Call doctor right away. |
| • Depression, confusion, slurred speech, diarrhea, nausea, vomiting, joint or muscle pain. | Continue. Call doctor when convenient. |
| **Rare:** | |
| • Agitation, slow heartbeat, difficult breathing, jaundice. | Discontinue. Call doctor right away. |
| • Unusual bleeding or bruising. | Continue. Call doctor when convenient. |

 ## WARNINGS & PRECAUTIONS

**Don't take if:**
- You are allergic to any barbiturate.
- You have porphyria.

**Before you start, consult your doctor:**
- If you have epilepsy.
- If you have kidney or liver damage.
- If you have asthma.
- If you have anemia.
- If you have chronic pain.
- If you will have surgery within 2 months, including dental surgery, requiring general or spinal anesthesia.

**Over age 60:**
Adverse reactions and side effects may be more frequent and severe than in younger persons. Use small doses.

**Pregnancy:**
Risk to unborn child outweighs drug benefits. Don't use.

**Breast-feeding:**
Drug passes into milk. Avoid drug or discontinue nursing until you finish medicine. Consult doctor for advice on maintaining milk supply.

**Infants & children:**
Use only under doctor's supervision.

**Prolonged use:**
- May cause addiction, anemia, chronic intoxication.
- May lower body temperature, making exposure to cold temperatures hazardous.

**Skin & sunlight:**
May cause rash or intensify sunburn in areas exposed to sun or sunlamp.

**Driving, piloting or hazardous work:**
Don't drive or pilot aircraft until you learn how medicine affects you. Don't work around dangerous machinery. Don't climb ladders or work in high places. Danger increases if you drink alcohol or take medicine affecting alertness and reflexes.

**Discontinuing:**
May be unnecessary to finish medicine. Follow doctor's instructions. If you develop withdrawal symptoms of hallucinations, agitation or sleeplessness after discontinuing, call doctor right away.

**Others:**
No problems expected.

## POSSIBLE INTERACTION WITH OTHER DRUGS

| GENERIC NAME OR DRUG CLASS | COMBINED EFFECT |
| --- | --- |
| Anticoagulants (oral) | Decreased anticoagulant effect. |
| Anticonvulsants | Changed seizure patterns. |
| Antidepressants (tricyclics) | Decreased antidepressant effect. Possible dangerous oversedation. |
| Antidiabetics (oral) | Increased hexobarbital effect. |
| Antihistamines | Dangerous sedation. Avoid. |
| Anti-inflammatory drugs (non-steroidal) | Decreased anti-inflammatory effect. |
| Aspirin | Decreased aspirin effect. |
| Beta-adrenergic blockers | Decreased effect of beta-adrenergic blocker. |
| Contraceptives (oral) | Decreased contraceptive effect. |
| Cortisone drugs | Decreased cortisone effect. |
| Digitoxin | Decreased digitoxin effect. |
| Doxycycline | Decreased doxycycline effect. |
| Dronabinol | Increased effects of both drugs. Avoid. |
| Griseofulvin | Decreased griseofulvin effect. |
| Indapamide | Increased indapamide effect. |
| MAO inhibitors | Increased hexobarbital effect. |
| Mind-altering drugs | Dangerous sedation. Avoid. |
| Narcotics | Dangerous sedation. Avoid. |
| Pain relievers | Dangerous sedation. Avoid. |
| Sedatives | Dangerous sedation. Avoid. |
| Sleep inducers | Dangerous sedation. Avoid. |
| Tranquilizers | Dangerous sedation. Avoid. |
| Valproic acid | Increased hexobarbital effect. |

## POSSIBLE INTERACTION WITH OTHER SUBSTANCES

| INTERACTS WITH | COMBINED EFFECT |
| --- | --- |
| Alcohol: | Possible fatal oversedation. Avoid. |
| Beverages: | None expected. |
| Cocaine: | Decreased hexobarbital effect. |
| Foods: | None expected. |
| Marijuana: | Excessive sedation. Avoid. |
| Tobacco: | None expected. |

# HYDRALAZINE

## BRAND NAMES

| | |
|---|---|
| Apresoline | Ser-Ap-Es |
| Dralzine | Serpasil-Apresoline |
| H-H-R | Unipes |
| Hydralazide | Uniserp |
| Rolazine | |

## BASIC INFORMATION

**Habit forming? No**
**Prescription needed? Yes**
**Available as generic? Yes**
**Drug class: Antihypertensive**

## USES

Treatment for high blood pressure and congestive heart failure.

## DOSAGE & USAGE INFORMATION

**How to take:**
Tablet or capsule—Swallow with liquid. If you can't swallow whole, crumble tablet or open capsule and take with liquid or food.

**When to take:**
At the same time each day.

**If you forget a dose:**
Take as soon as you remember up to 2 hours late. If more than 2 hours, wait for next scheduled dose (don't double this dose).

**What drug does:**
Relaxes and expands blood-vessel walls, lowering blood pressure.

*Continued next column*

## OVERDOSE

**SYMPTOMS:**
**Rapid and weak heartbeat, fainting, extreme weakness, cold and sweaty skin.**
**WHAT TO DO:**
- **Dial 0 (operator) or 911 (emergency) for an ambulance or medical help. Then give first aid immediately.**
- **If patient is unconscious and not breathing, give mouth-to-mouth breathing. If there is no heartbeat, use cardiac massage and mouth-to-mouth breathing (CPR). Don't try to make patient vomit. If you can't get help quickly, take patient to nearest emergency facility.**
- **See emergency information on inside covers.**

**Time lapse before drug works:**
Regular use for several weeks may be necessary to determine drug's effectiveness.

**Don't take with:**
- Non-prescription drugs containing alcohol without consulting doctor.
- See Interaction column and consult doctor.

## POSSIBLE ADVERSE REACTIONS OR SIDE EFFECTS

| SYMPTOMS | WHAT TO DO |
|---|---|
| **Life-threatening:** None expected. | |
| **Common:** | |
| • Nausea or vomiting, rapid or irregular heartbeat. | Discontinue. Call doctor right away. |
| • Headache, diarrhea, appetite loss, painful or difficult urination. | Continue. Tell doctor at next visit. |
| **Infrequent:** | |
| • Hives or rash, flushed face, sore throat, fever, chest pain, swelling of lymph gland. | Discontinue. Call doctor right away. |
| • Confusion, dizziness, joint pain, general discomfort or weakness. | Continue. Call doctor when convenient. |
| • Watery eyes and irritation, constipation. | Continue. Tell doctor at next visit. |
| **Rare:** Jaundice. | Discontinue. Call doctor right away. |

# HYDRALAZINE

## WARNINGS & PRECAUTIONS

**Don't take if:**
- You are allergic to hydralazine.
- You have history of coronary-artery disease or rheumatic heart disease.

**Before you start, consult your doctor:**
- If you feel pain in chest, neck or arms on physical exertion.
- If you have had lupus.
- If you have had a stroke.
- If you have had kidney disease or impaired kidney function.
- If you will have surgery within 2 months, including dental surgery, requiring general or spinal anesthesia.

**Over age 60:**
Adverse reactions and side effects may be more frequent and severe than in younger persons.

**Pregnancy:**
Risk to unborn child outweighs drug benefits. Don't use.

**Breast-feeding:**
Drug filters into milk. May harm child. Avoid.

**Infants & children:**
Not recommended.

**Prolonged use:**
- May cause lupus (arthritis-like illness).
- Possible psychosis.
- May cause numbness, tingling in hands or feet.

**Skin & sunlight:**
No problems expected.

**Driving, piloting or hazardous work:**
Don't drive or pilot aircraft until you learn how medicine affects you. Don't work around dangerous machinery. Don't climb ladders or work in high places. Danger increases if you drink alcohol or take medicine affecting alertness and reflexes, such as antihistamines, tranquilizers, sedatives, pain medicine, narcotics and mind-altering drugs.

**Discontinuing:**
Don't discontinue without doctor's advice until you complete prescribed dose, even though symptoms diminish or disappear.

**Others:**
Vitamin B-6 diet supplement may be advisable. Consult doctor.

## POSSIBLE INTERACTION WITH OTHER DRUGS

| GENERIC NAME OR DRUG CLASS | COMBINED EFFECT |
|---|---|
| Albuterol | Decreased hydralazine effect. |
| Amphetamines | Decreased hydralazine effect. |
| Antidepressants (tricyclic) | Increased hydralazine effect. |
| Antihypertensives (other) | Increased antihypertensive effect. |
| Diuretics (oral) | Increased effects of both drugs. When monitored carefully, combination may be beneficial in controlling hypertension. |
| Enalapril | Possible excessive potassium in blood. |
| MAO inhibitors | Increased hydralazine effect. |
| Pentoxifylline | Increased antihypertensive effect. |

## POSSIBLE INTERACTION WITH OTHER SUBSTANCES

| INTERACTS WITH | COMBINED EFFECT |
|---|---|
| Alcohol: | May lower blood pressure excessively. Use extreme caution. |
| Beverages: | None expected. |
| Cocaine: | Dangerous blood-pressure rise. Avoid. |
| Foods: | Increased hydralazine absorption. |
| Marijuana: | Weakness on standing. |
| Tobacco: | Possible angina attacks. |

# HYDRALAZINE & HYDROCHLOROTHIAZIDE

## BRAND NAMES

| | |
|---|---|
| Apresazide | Apresoline-Esidrix |
| Apresodez | Hydral |

## BASIC INFORMATION

**Habit forming? No**
**Prescription needed? Yes**
**Available as generic? Yes**
**Drug class: Antihypertensive-diuretic**

## USES

- Controls, but doesn't cure, high blood pressure.
- Reduces fluid retention (edema).

## DOSAGE & USAGE INFORMATION

**How to take:**
Tablet or capsule—Swallow with liquid. If you can't swallow whole, crumble tablet or open capsule and take with liquid or food.

**When to take:**
At the same time each day.

**If you forget a dose:**
Take as soon as you remember up to 2 hours late. If more than 2 hours, wait for next scheduled dose (don't double this dose).

**What drug does:**
- Forces sodium and water excretion, reducing body fluid.
- Relaxes and expands blood-vessel walls, lowering blood pressure.

*Continued next column*

## OVERDOSE

**SYMPTOMS:**
**Cramps, drowsiness, weak pulse, rapid and weak heartbeat, fainting, extreme weakness, cold and sweaty skin, coma.**
**WHAT TO DO:**
- **Dial 0 (operator) or 911 (emergency) for an ambulance or medical help. Then give first aid immediately.**
- **If patient is unconscious and not breathing, give mouth-to-mouth breathing. If there is no heartbeat, use cardiac massage and mouth-to-mouth breathing (CPR). Don't try to make patient vomit. If you can't get help quickly, take patient to nearest emergency facility.**
- **See emergency information on inside covers.**

- Reduced body fluid and relaxed arteries lower blood pressure.

**Time lapse before drug works:**
Regular use for several weeks may be necessary to determine drug's effectiveness.

**Don't take with:**
- Non-prescription drugs containing alcohol without consulting doctor.
- See Interaction column and consult doctor.

## POSSIBLE ADVERSE REACTIONS OR SIDE EFFECTS

| SYMPTOMS | WHAT TO DO |
|---|---|
| **Life-threatening:** | |
| Chest pain, irregular and fast heartbeat, weak pulse. | Discontinue. Seek emergency treatment. |
| **Common:** | |
| • Nausea, vomiting. | Discontinue. Call doctor right away. |
| • Headache, diarrhea, appetite loss, frequent urination, dry mouth, thirst. | Continue. Call doctor when convenient. |
| **Infrequent:** | |
| • Rash; black, bloody or tarry stool; red or flushed face; sore throat, fever, mouth sores; constipation; lymph glands swelling; blurred vision. | Discontinue. Call doctor right away. |
| • Dizziness, confusion, watery eyes, joint pain, weight gain or loss. | Continue. Call doctor when convenient. |
| **Rare:** | |
| Jaundice. | Discontinue. Call doctor right away. |

## WARNINGS & PRECAUTIONS

**Don't take if:**
- You are allergic to hydralazine or any thiazide diuretic drug.
- You have history of coronary-artery disease or rheumatic heart disease.

**Before you start, consult your doctor:**
- If you feel pain in chest, neck or arms on physical exertion.
- If you are allergic to any sulfa drug.
- If you have had lupus or a stroke.
- If you have gout, liver, pancreas or kidney disorder.

- If you will have surgery within 2 months, including dental surgery, requiring general or spinal anesthesia.

## Over age 60:
Adverse reactions and side effects may be more frequent and severe than in younger persons, especially dizziness and excessive potassium loss.

## Pregnancy:
Risk to unborn child outweighs drug benefits. Don't use.

## Breast-feeding:
Drug passes into milk. Avoid drug or discontinue nursing until you finish medicine. Consult doctor for advice on maintaining milk supply.

## Infants & children:
Not recommended.

## Prolonged use:
- May cause lupus (arthritis-like illness).
- Possible psychosis.
- May cause numbness, tingling in hands or feet.

## Skin & sunlight:
May cause rash or intensify sunburn in areas exposed to sun or sunlamp.

## Driving, piloting or hazardous work:
Don't drive or pilot aircraft until you learn how medicine affects you. Don't work around dangerous machinery. Don't climb ladders or work in high places. Danger increases if you drink alcohol or take medicine affecting alertness and reflexes, such as antihistamines, tranquilizers, sedatives, pain medicine, narcotics and mind-altering drugs.

## Discontinuing:
Don't discontinue without consulting doctor's advice until you complete prescribed dose, even though symptoms diminish or disappear.

## Others:
- Vitamin B-6 diet supplement may be advisable. Consult doctor.
- Hot weather and fever may cause dehydration and drop in blood pressure. Dose may require temporary adjustment. Weigh daily and report any unexpected weight decreases to your doctor.
- May cause rise in uric acid, leading to gout.
- May cause blood-sugar rise in diabetics.

## POSSIBLE INTERACTION WITH OTHER DRUGS

| GENERIC NAME OR DRUG CLASS | COMBINED EFFECT |
| --- | --- |
| Acebutolol | Decreased antihypertensive effect of acebutolol. |
| Allopurinol | Decreased allopurinol effect. |
| Amphetamines | Decreased hydralazine effect. |
| Antidepressants (tricyclic) | Dangerous drop in blood pressure. Avoid combination unless under medical supervision. |
| Antihypertensives (other) | Increased antihypertensive effect. |
| Barbiturates | Increased hydrochlorothiazide effect. |
| Cholestyramine | Decreased hydrochlorothiazide effect. |
| Cortisone drugs | Excessive potassium loss that causes dangerous heart rhythms. |
| Digitalis preparations | Excessive potassium loss that causes dangerous heart rhythms. |
| Diuretics (oral) | Increased effect of both drugs. When monitored carefully, combination may be beneficial in controlling hypertension. |
| Indapamide | Increased diuretic effect. |

*Continued page 967*

## POSSIBLE INTERACTION WITH OTHER SUBSTANCES

| INTERACTS WITH | COMBINED EFFECT |
| --- | --- |
| Alcohol: | May lower blood pressure excessively. Use extreme caution. |
| Beverages: | None expected. |
| Cocaine: | Dangerous blood-pressure rise. Avoid. |
| Foods: Licorice. | Excessive potassium loss that causes dangerous heart rhythms. |
| Marijuana: | Weakness on standing. May increase blood pressure. |
| Tobacco: | Possible angina attacks. |

# HYDROCHLOROTHIAZIDE

## BRAND NAMES

See complete list of brand names in the *Brand Name Directory,* page 950.

## BASIC INFORMATION

**Habit forming? No**
**Prescription needed? Yes**
**Available as generic? Yes**
**Drug class: Antihypertensive, diuretic (thiazide)**

## USES

- Controls, but doesn't cure, high blood pressure.
- Reduces fluid retention (edema).

## DOSAGE & USAGE INFORMATION

**How to take:**
Tablet or capsule—Swallow with liquid. If you can't swallow whole, crumble tablet or open capsule and take with liquid or food.

**When to take:**
At the same time each day.

**If you forget a dose:**
Take as soon as you remember up to 2 hours late. If more than 2 hours, wait for next scheduled dose (don't double this dose).

**What drug does:**
- Forces sodium and water excretion, reducing body fluid.
- Relaxes muscle cells of small arteries.
- Reduced body fluid and relaxed arteries lower blood pressure.

**Time lapse before drug works:**
4 to 6 hours. May require several weeks to lower blood pressure.

*Continued next column*

## OVERDOSE

**SYMPTOMS:**
**Cramps, weakness, drowsiness, weak pulse, coma.**
WHAT TO DO:
- **Dial 0 (operator) or 911 (emergency) for an ambulance or medical help. Then give first aid immediately.**
- **See emergency information on inside covers.**

**Don't take with:**
- See Interaction column and consult doctor.
- Non-prescription drugs without consulting doctor.

## POSSIBLE ADVERSE REACTIONS OR SIDE EFFECTS

| SYMPTOMS | WHAT TO DO |
|---|---|
| **Life-threatening:** None expected. | |
| **Common:** None expected. | |
| **Infrequent:** | |
| • Blurred vision, severe abdominal pain, nausea, vomiting, irregular heartbeat, weak pulse. | Discontinue. Call doctor right away. |
| • Dizziness, mood change, headache, weakness, tiredness, weight changes. | Continue. Call doctor when convenient. |
| • Dry mouth, thirst. | Continue. Tell doctor at next visit. |
| **Rare:** | |
| • Rash or hives. | Discontinue. Seek emergency treatment. |
| • Sore throat, fever, jaundice. | Discontinue. Call doctor right away. |

## WARNINGS & PRECAUTIONS

**Don't take if:**
You are allergic to any thiazide diuretic drug.

**Before you start, consult your doctor:**
- If you are allergic to any sulfa drug.
- If you have gout.
- If you have liver, pancreas or kidney disorder.

**Over age 60:**
Adverse reactions and side effects may be more frequent and severe than in younger persons, especially dizziness and excessive potassium loss.

**Pregnancy:**
Risk to unborn child outweighs drug benefits. Don't use.

**Breast-feeding:**
Drug passes into milk. Avoid drug or discontinue nursing.

**Infants & children:**
No problems expected.

**Prolonged use:**
You may need medicine to treat high blood pressure for the rest of your life.

**Skin & sunlight:**
May cause rash or intensify sunburn in areas exposed to sun or sunlamp.

**Driving, piloting or hazardous work:**
Don't drive or pilot aircraft until you learn how medicine affects you. Don't work around dangerous machinery. Don't climb ladders or work in high places. Danger increases if you drink alcohol or take medicine affecting alertness and reflexes, such as antihistamines, tranquilizers, sedatives, pain medicine, narcotics and mind-altering drugs.

**Discontinuing:**
Don't discontinue without medical advice.

**Others:**
- Hot weather and fever may cause dehydration and drop in blood pressure. Dose may require temporary adjustment. Weigh daily and report any unexpected weight decreases to your doctor.
- May cause rise in uric acid, leading to gout.
- May cause blood-sugar rise in diabetics.

 **POSSIBLE INTERACTION WITH OTHER DRUGS**

| GENERIC NAME OR DRUG CLASS | COMBINED EFFECT |
|---|---|
| Acebutolol | Increased antihypertensive effect. Dosages of both drugs may require adjustments. |
| Allopurinol | Decreased allopurinol effect. |
| Amiodarone | Increased risk of heartbeat irregularity due to low potassium. |
| Antidepressants (tricyclic) | Dangerous drop in blood pressure. Avoid combination unless under medical supervision. |
| Barbiturates | Increased hydrochlorothiazide effect. |
| Calcium supplements | Increased calcium in blood. |
| Cholestyramine | Decreased hydrochlorothiazide effect. |
| Cortisone drugs | Excessive potassium loss that causes dangerous heart rhythms. |
| Digitalis preparations | Excessive potassium loss that causes dangerous heart rhythms. |
| Diuretics (thiazide) | Increased effect of other thiazide diuretics. |
| Indapamide | Increased diuretic effect. |
| Labetolol | Increased antihypertensive effects. |
| Lithium | Increased effect of lithium. |
| MAO inhibitors | Increased hydrochlorothiazide effect. |
| Nitrates | Excessive blood-pressure drop. |
| Oxprenolol | Increased antihypertensive effect. Dosages of both drugs may require adjustments. |
| Potassium supplements | Decreased potassium effect. |
| Probenecid | Decreased probenecid effect. |

 **POSSIBLE INTERACTION WITH OTHER SUBSTANCES**

| INTERACTS WITH | COMBINED EFFECT |
|---|---|
| Alcohol: | Dangerous blood-pressure drop. |
| Beverages: | None expected. |
| Cocaine: | None expected. |
| Foods: Licorice. | Excessive potassium loss that causes dangerous heart rhythms. |
| Marijuana: | May increase blood pressure. |
| Tobacco: | None expected. |

# HYDROCORTISONE (CORTISOL)

## BRAND NAMES

See complete list of brand names in the *Brand Name Directory,* page 950.

## BASIC INFORMATION

**Habit forming? No**
**Prescription needed? Yes**
**Available as generic? Yes**
**Drug class: Cortisone drug (adrenal corticosteroid)**

 ## USES

- Reduces inflammation caused by many different medical problems.
- Treatment for some allergic diseases, blood disorders, kidney diseases, asthma and emphysema.
- Replaces corticosteroid deficiencies.

 ## DOSAGE & USAGE INFORMATION

**How to take:**
- Tablet or liquid—Swallow with liquid or food to lessen stomach irritation. If you can't swallow whole, crumble tablet.
- Other forms—Follow label instructions.

**When to take:**
At the same times each day. Take once-a-day or once-every-other-day doses in mornings.

**If you forget a dose:**
- Several-doses-per-day prescription—Take as soon as you remember up to 2 hours late. If more than 2 hours, wait for next scheduled dose (don't double this dose).
- Once-a-day dose or less—Wait for next dose. Double this dose.

**What drug does:**
Decreases inflammatory responses.

**Time lapse before drug works:**
2 to 4 days.

**Don't take with:**
See Interaction column and consult doctor.

 ## OVERDOSE

**SYMPTOMS:**
**Headache, convulsions, heart failure.**
**WHAT TO DO:**
- **Dial 0 (operator) or 911 (emergency) for an ambulance or medical help. Then give first aid immediately.**
- **See emergency information on inside covers.**

 ## POSSIBLE ADVERSE REACTIONS OR SIDE EFFECTS

| SYMPTOMS | WHAT TO DO |
|---|---|
| **Life-threatening:**<br>None expected. | |
| **Common:**<br>Acne, poor wound healing, thirst, indigestion, nausea, vomiting. | Continue. Call doctor when convenient. |
| **Infrequent:**<br>• Black, bloody or tarry stools. | Discontinue. Seek emergency treatment. |
| • Blurred vision; halos around lights; sore throat; fever; muscle cramps; swollen legs, feet. | Discontinue. Call doctor right away. |
| • Mood change, insomnia, restlessness, frequent urination, weight gain, round face, fatigue, weakness, TB recurrence, irregular menstrual periods. | Continue. Tell doctor at next visit. |
| **Rare:**<br>• Irregular heartbeat. | Discontinue. Seek emergency treatment. |
| • Rash. | Discontinue. Call doctor right away. |

 ## WARNINGS & PRECAUTIONS

**Don't take if:**
- You are allergic to any cortisone drug.
- You have tuberculosis or fungus infection.
- You have herpes infection of eyes, lips or genitals.

**Before you start, consult your doctor:**
- If you have had tuberculosis.
- If you have congestive heart failure.
- If you have diabetes.
- If you have peptic ulcer.
- If you have glaucoma.
- If you have underactive thyroid.
- If you have high blood pressure.
- If you have myasthenia gravis.
- If you have blood clots in legs or lungs.

**Over age 60:**
Adverse reactions and side effects may be more frequent and severe than in younger persons. Likely to aggravate edema, diabetes or ulcers. Likely to cause cataracts and osteoporosis (softening of the bones).

**Pregnancy:**
Risk to unborn child outweighs drug benefits. Don't use.

**Breast-feeding:**
Drug passes into milk. Avoid drug or discontinue nursing until you finish medicine. Consult doctor for advice on maintaining milk supply.

**Infants & children:**
Use only under medical supervision.

**Prolonged use:**
- Retards growth in children.
- Possible glaucoma, cataracts, diabetes, fragile bones and thin skin.
- Functional dependence.

**Skin & sunlight:**
No problems expected.

**Driving, piloting or hazardous work:**
No problems expected.

**Discontinuing:**
- Don't discontinue without doctor's advice until you complete prescribed dose, even though symptoms diminish or disappear.
- Drug affects your response to surgery, illness, injury or stress for 2 years after discontinuing. Tell anyone who takes medical care of you about the drug for up to 2 years after discontinuing.

**Others:**
Avoid immunizations if possible.

## POSSIBLE INTERACTION WITH OTHER DRUGS

| GENERIC NAME OR DRUG CLASS | COMBINED EFFECT |
|---|---|
| Amphoterecin B | Potassium depletion. |
| Anticholinergics | Possible glaucoma. |
| Anticoagulants (oral) | Decreased anticoagulant effect. |
| Anticonvulsants (hydantoin) | Decreased hydrocortisone effect. |
| Antidiabetics (oral) | Decreased antidiabetic effect. |
| Antihistamines | Decreased hydrocortisone effect. |
| Aspirin | Increased hydrocortisone effect. |
| Barbiturates | Decreased hydrocortisone effect. Oversedation. |
| Beta-adrenergic blockers | Decreased hydrocortisone effect. |
| Chloral hydrate | Decreased hydrocortisone effect. |
| Chlorthalidone | Potassium depletion. |
| Cholinergics | Decreased cholinergic effect. |
| Contraceptives (oral) | Increased hydrocortisone effect. |
| Digitalis preparations | Dangerous potassium depletion. Possible digitalis toxicity. |
| Diuretics (thiazide) | Potassium depletion. |
| Ephedrine | Decreased hydrocortisone effect. |
| Estrogens | Increased hydrocortisone effect. |
| Ethacrynic acid | Potassium depletion. |
| Furosemide | Potassium depletion. |
| Glutethimide | Decreased hydrocortisone effect. |
| Indapamide | Possible excessive potassium loss, causing dangerous heartbeat irregularity. |
| Indomethacin | Increased hydrocortisone effect. |
| Insulin | Decreased insulin effect. |
| Isoniazid | Decreased isoniazid effect. |
| Oxyphenbutazone | Possible ulcers. |
| Phenylbutazone | Possible ulcers. |
| Potassium supplements | Decreased potassium effect. |
| Rifampin | Decreased hydrocortisone effect. |
| Sympathomimetics | Possible glaucoma. |

## POSSIBLE INTERACTION WITH OTHER SUBSTANCES

| INTERACTS WITH | COMBINED EFFECT |
|---|---|
| Alcohol: | Risk of stomach ulcers. |
| Beverages: | No proven problems. |
| Cocaine: | Overstimulation. Avoid. |
| Foods: | No proven problems. |
| Marijuana: | Decreased immunity. |
| Tobacco: | Increased hydrocortisone effect. Possible toxicity. |

# HYDROFLUMETHIAZIDE

## BRAND NAMES

Diucardin          Saluron
Hydro-Fluserpine   Salutensin
  #1 & #2

## BASIC INFORMATION

Habit forming? No
Prescription needed? Yes
Available as generic? Yes
Drug class: Antihypertensive, diuretic
            (thiazide)

## USES

- Controls, but doesn't cure, high blood pressure.
- Reduces fluid retention (edema) caused by conditions such as heart disorders and liver disease.

## DOSAGE & USAGE INFORMATION

How to take:
Tablet or capsule—Swallow with liquid. If you can't swallow whole, crumble tablet or open capsule and take with liquid or food. Don't exceed dose.

When to take:
At the same time each day.

If you forget a dose:
Take as soon as you remember up to 2 hours late. If more than 2 hours, wait for next scheduled dose (don't double this dose).

What drug does:
- Forces sodium and water excretion, reducing body fluid.
- Relaxes muscle cells of small arteries.
- Reduced body fluid and relaxed arteries lower blood pressure.

*Continued next column*

## OVERDOSE

SYMPTOMS:
Cramps, weakness, drowsiness, weak pulse, coma.
WHAT TO DO:
- Dial 0 (operator) or 911 (emergency) for an ambulance or medical help. Then give first aid immediately.
- See emergency information on inside covers.

Time lapse before drug works:
4 to 6 hours. May require several weeks to lower blood pressure.

Don't take with:
- See Interaction column and consult doctor.
- Non-prescription drugs without consulting doctor.

## POSSIBLE ADVERSE REACTIONS OR SIDE EFFECTS

| SYMPTOMS | WHAT TO DO |
|---|---|
| **Life-threatening:**<br>None expected. | |
| **Common:**<br>None expected. | |
| **Infrequent:** | |
| • Blurred vision, severe abdominal pain, nausea, vomiting, irregular heartbeat, weak pulse. | Discontinue. Call doctor right away. |
| • Dizziness, mood change, headache, weakness, tiredness, weight changes. | Continue. Call doctor when convenient. |
| • Dry mouth, thirst. | Continue. Tell doctor at next visit. |
| **Rare:** | |
| • Rash or hives. | Discontinue. Seek emergency treatment. |
| • Sore throat, fever, jaundice. | Discontinue. Call doctor right away. |

## WARNINGS & PRECAUTIONS

Don't take if:
You are allergic to any thiazide diuretic drug.

Before you start, consult your doctor:
- If you are allergic to any sulfa drug.
- If you have gout.
- If you have liver, pancreas or kidney disorder.

Over age 60:
Adverse reactions and side effects may be more frequent and severe than in younger persons, especially dizziness and excessive potassium loss.

Pregnancy:
Risk to unborn child outweighs drug benefits. Don't use.

Breast-feeding:
Drug passes into milk. Avoid drug or discontinue nursing.

Infants & children:
No problems expected.

**Prolonged use:**
You may need medicine to treat high blood pressure for the rest of your life.

**Skin & sunlight:**
May cause rash or intensify sunburn in areas exposed to sun or sunlamp.

**Driving, piloting or hazardous work:**
Don't drive or pilot aircraft until you learn how medicine affects you. Don't work around dangerous machinery. Don't climb ladders or work in high places. Danger increases if you drink alcohol or take medicine affecting alertness and reflexes, such as antihistamines, tranquilizers, sedatives, pain medicine, narcotics and mind-altering drugs.

**Discontinuing:**
Don't discontinue without medical advice.

**Others:**
- Hot weather and fever may cause dehydration and drop in blood pressure. Dose may require temporary adjustment. Weigh daily and report any unexpected weight decreases to your doctor.
- May cause rise in uric acid, leading to gout.
- May cause blood-sugar rise in diabetics.

## POSSIBLE INTERACTION WITH OTHER DRUGS

| GENERIC NAME OR DRUG CLASS | COMBINED EFFECT |
|---|---|
| Acebutolol | Increased antihypertensive effect. Dosages of both drugs may require adjustments. |
| Allopurinol | Decreased allopurinol effect. |
| Amiodarone | Increased risk of heartbeat irregularity due to low potassium. |
| Antidepressants (tricyclic) | Dangerous drop in blood pressure. Avoid combination unless under medical supervision. |
| Barbiturates | Increased hydroflumethiazide effect. |
| Calcium supplements | Increased calcium in blood. |
| Cholestyramine | Decreased hydroflumethiazide effect. |
| Cortisone drugs | Excessive potassium loss that causes dangerous heart rhythms. |
| Digitalis preparations | Excessive potassium loss that causes dangerous heart rhythms. |
| Diuretics (thiazide) | Increased effect of other thiazide diuretics. |
| Indapamide | Increased diuretic effect. |
| Labetolol | Increased antihypertensive effects. |
| Lithium | Increased effect of lithium. |
| MAO inhibitors | Increased hydroflumethiazide effect. |
| Nitrates | Excessive blood-pressure drop. |
| Oxprenolol | Increased antihypertensive effect. Dosages of both drugs may require adjustments. |
| Potassium supplements | Decreased potassium effect. |
| Probenecid | Decreased probenecid effect. |

## POSSIBLE INTERACTION WITH OTHER SUBSTANCES

| INTERACTS WITH | COMBINED EFFECT |
|---|---|
| Alcohol: | Dangerous blood-pressure drop. |
| Beverages: | None expected. |
| Cocaine: | None expected. |
| Foods: Licorice. | Excessive potassium loss that causes dangerous heart rhythms. |
| Marijuana: | May increase blood pressure. |
| Tobacco: | None expected. |

# HYDROXYCHLOROQUINE

## BRAND NAMES

Plaquenil

## BASIC INFORMATION

Habit forming? No
Prescription needed? Yes
Available as generic? Yes
Drug class: Antiprotozoal, antirheumatic

 ## USES

- Treatment for protozoal infections, such as malaria and amebiasis.
- Treatment for some forms of arthritis and lupus.

 ## DOSAGE & USAGE INFORMATION

How to take:
Tablet—Swallow with food or milk to lessen stomach irritation.

When to take:
- Depends on condition. Is adjusted during treatment.
- Malaria prevention—Begin taking medicine 2 weeks before entering areas with malaria.

If you forget a dose:
- 1 or more doses a day—Take as soon as you remember up to 2 hours late. If more than 2 hours, wait for next scheduled dose (don't double this dose).
- 1 dose weekly—Take as soon as possible, then return to regular dosing schedule.

What drug does:
- Inhibits parasite multiplication.
- Decreases inflammatory response in diseased joint.

Time lapse before drug works:
1 to 2 hours.

Don't take with:
See Interaction column and consult doctor.

 ## OVERDOSE

SYMPTOMS:
Severe breathing difficulty, drowsiness, faintness.
WHAT TO DO:
- Dial 0 (operator) or 911 (emergency) for an ambulance or medical help. Then give first aid immediately.
- See emergency information on inside covers.

 ## POSSIBLE ADVERSE REACTIONS OR SIDE EFFECTS

| SYMPTOMS | WHAT TO DO |
|---|---|
| **Life-threatening:** None expected. | |
| **Common:** Headache. | Continue. Tell doctor at next visit. |
| **Infrequent:** | |
| • Blurred vision, changes in vision. | Discontinue. Call doctor right away. |
| • Rash or itch, diarrhea, nausea, vomiting. | Continue. Call doctor when convenient. |
| **Rare:** | |
| • Mood or mental changes, seizures, sore throat, fever, unusual bleeding or bruising, muscle weakness. | Discontinue. Call doctor right away. |
| • Ringing or buzzing in ears, hearing loss. | Continue. Call doctor when convenient. |

## WARNINGS & PRECAUTIONS

**Don't take if:**
You are allergic to chloroquine or hydroxychloroquine.

**Before you start, consult your doctor:**
- If you plan to become pregnant within the medication period.
- If you have blood disease.
- If you have eye or vision problems.
- If you have a G6PD deficiency.
- If you have liver disease.
- If you have nerve or brain disease (including seizure disorders).
- If you have porphyria.
- If you have psoriasis.
- If you have stomach or intestinal disease.
- If you drink more than 3 oz. of alcohol daily.

**Over age 60:**
Adverse reactions and side effects may be more frequent and severe than in younger persons.

**Pregnancy:**
Risk to unborn child outweighs drug benefits. Don't use.

**Breast-feeding:**
Drug passes into milk. Avoid drug or discontinue nursing.

**Infants & children:**
Not recommended. Dangerous.

**Prolonged use:**
Permanent damage to the retina (back part of the eye) or nerve deafness.

**Skin & sunlight:**
May cause rash or intensify sunburn in areas exposed to sun or sunlamp.

**Driving, piloting or hazardous work:**
Don't drive or pilot aircraft until you learn how medicine affects you. Don't work around dangerous machinery. Don't climb ladders or work in high places. Danger increases if you drink alcohol or take medicine affecting alertness and reflexes.

**Discontinuing:**
Don't discontinue without doctor's advice until you complete prescribed dose, even though symptoms diminish or disappear.

**Others:**
- Periodic physical and blood examinations recommended.
- If you are in a malaria area for a long time, you may need to change to another preventive drug every 2 years.

## POSSIBLE INTERACTION WITH OTHER DRUGS

| GENERIC NAME OR DRUG CLASS | COMBINED EFFECT |
|---|---|
| Estrogens | Possible liver toxicity. |
| Gold compounds | Risk of severe rash and itch. |
| Oxyphenbutazone | Risk of severe rash and itch. |
| Penicillamine | Possible blood or kidney toxicity. |
| Phenylbutazone | Risk of severe rash and itch. |
| Sulfa drugs | Possible liver toxicity. |

## POSSIBLE INTERACTION WITH OTHER SUBSTANCES

| INTERACTS WITH | COMBINED EFFECT |
|---|---|
| Alcohol: | Possible liver toxicity. Avoid. |
| Beverages: | None expected. |
| Cocaine: | None expected. |
| Foods: | None expected. |
| Marijuana: | None expected. |
| Tobacco: | None expected. |

# HYDROXYZINE

## BRAND NAMES

See complete list of brand names in the
*Brand Name Directory,* page 950.

## BASIC INFORMATION

**Habit forming? No**
**Prescription needed? Yes**
**Available as generic? Yes**
**Drug class: Tranquilizer, antihistamine**

 **USES**

- Treatment for anxiety, tension and agitation.
- Relieves itching from allergic reactions.

## DOSAGE & USAGE INFORMATION

**How to take:**
- Tablet or capsule—Swallow with liquid. If you can't swallow whole, crumble tablet or open capsule and take with liquid or food.
- Liquid—If desired, dilute dose in beverage before swallowing.

**When to take:**
At the same times each day.

**If you forget a dose:**
Take as soon as you remember up to 2 hours late. If more than 2 hours, wait for next scheduled dose (don't double this dose).

**What drug does:**
May reduce activity in areas of the brain that influence emotional stability.

**Time lapse before drug works:**
15 to 30 minutes.

**Don't take with:**
- Non-prescription drugs without consulting doctor.
- See Interaction column and consult doctor.

 **OVERDOSE**

**SYMPTOMS:**
**Drowsiness, unsteadiness, agitation, purposeless movements, tremor, convulsions.**
**WHAT TO DO:**
- **Dial 0 (operator) or 911 (emergency) for an ambulance or medical help. Then give first aid immediately.**
- **See emergency information on inside covers.**

 **POSSIBLE ADVERSE REACTIONS OR SIDE EFFECTS**

| SYMPTOMS | WHAT TO DO |
|---|---|
| **Life-threatening:** None expected. | |
| **Common:** Drowsiness, difficult urination, dry mouth. | Continue. Tell doctor at next visit. |
| **Infrequent:** Headache. | Continue. Tell doctor at next visit. |
| **Rare:** Tremor, rash. | Discontinue. Call doctor right away. |

## WARNINGS & PRECAUTIONS

**Don't take if:**
You are allergic to any antihistamine.

**Before you start, consult your doctor:**
- If you have epilepsy.
- If you will have surgery within 2 months, including dental surgery, requiring general or spinal anesthesia.

**Over age 60:**
Adverse reactions and side effects may be more frequent and severe than in younger persons. Drug likely to increase urination difficulty caused by enlarged prostate gland.

**Pregnancy:**
Studies inconclusive on harm to unborn child. Animal studies show fetal abnormalities. Decide with your doctor whether drug benefits justify risk to unborn child.

**Breast-feeding:**
Drug passes into milk. Avoid drug or discontinue nursing until you finish medicine. Consult doctor for advice on maintaining milk supply.

**Infants & children:**
Use only under medical supervision.

**Prolonged use:**
Tolerance develops and reduces effectiveness.

**Skin & sunlight:**
No problems expected.

**Driving, piloting or hazardous work:**
Don't drive or pilot aircraft until you learn how medicine affects you. Don't work around dangerous machinery. Don't climb ladders or work in high places. Danger increases if you drink alcohol or take medicine affecting alertness and reflexes, such as antihistamines, tranquilizers, sedatives, pain medicine, narcotics and mind-altering drugs.

**Discontinuing:**
Don't discontinue without consulting doctor. Dose may require gradual reduction if you have taken drug for a long time. Doses of other drugs may also require adjustment.

**Others:**
No problems expected.

## POSSIBLE INTERACTION WITH OTHER DRUGS

| GENERIC NAME OR DRUG CLASS | COMBINED EFFECT |
|---|---|
| Anticoagulants (oral) | Increased anticoagulant effect. |
| Anticonvulsants (hydantoin) | Decreased anticonvulsant effect. |
| Antidepressants (tricyclic) | Increased effect of both drugs. |
| Antihistamines | Increased hydroxyzine effect. |
| Dronabinol | Increased effects of both drugs. Avoid. |
| Molindone | Increased tranquilizer and antihistamine effect. |
| Narcotics | Increased effect of both drugs. |
| Pain relievers | Increased effect of both drugs. |
| Sedatives | Increased effect of both drugs. |
| Sleep inducers | Increased effect of both drugs. |
| Tranquilizers | Increased effect of both drugs. |

## POSSIBLE INTERACTION WITH OTHER SUBSTANCES

| INTERACTS WITH | COMBINED EFFECT |
|---|---|
| Alcohol: | Increased sedation and intoxication. Use with caution. |
| Beverages: Caffeine drinks. | Decreased tranquilizer effect of hydroxyzine. |
| Cocaine: | Decreased hydroxyzine effect. Avoid. |
| Foods: | None expected. |
| Marijuana: | None expected. |
| Tobacco: | None expected. |

# HYOSCYAMINE

## BRAND NAMES

See complete list of brand names in the
*Brand Name Directory,* page 950.

## BASIC INFORMATION

**Habit forming? No**
**Prescription needed?**
**Low strength: No**
**High strength: Yes**
**Available as generic? Yes**
**Drug class: Antispasmodic, anticholinergic**

## USES

Reduces spasms of digestive system, bladder
and urethra.

## DOSAGE & USAGE INFORMATION

**How to take:**
- Tablet or liquid—Swallow with liquid or food
  to lessen stomach irritation.
- Extended-release tablets or
  capsules—Swallow each dose whole. If you
  take regular tablets, you may chew or crush
  them.
- Drops—Dilute dose in beverage before
  swallowing.

**When to take:**
30 minutes before meals (unless directed
otherwise by doctor).

**If you forget a dose:**
Take as soon as you remember up to 2 hours
late. If more than 2 hours, wait for next
scheduled dose (don't double this dose).

**What drug does:**
Blocks nerve impulses at parasympathetic nerve
endings, preventing muscle contractions and
gland secretions of organs involved.

*Continued next column*

## OVERDOSE

**SYMPTOMS:**
**Dilated pupils, rapid pulse and breathing,**
**dizziness, fever, hallucinations, confusion,**
**slurred speech, agitation, flushed face,**
**convulsions, coma.**
**WHAT TO DO:**
- **Dial 0 (operator) or 911 (emergency) for an**
  **ambulance or medical help. Then give first**
  **aid immediately.**
- **See emergency information on inside**
  **covers.**

**Time lapse before drug works:**
15 to 30 minutes.

**Don't take with:**
See Interaction column and consult doctor.

## POSSIBLE ADVERSE REACTIONS OR SIDE EFFECTS

| SYMPTOMS | WHAT TO DO |
|---|---|
| **Life-threatening:** None expected. | |
| **Common:** | |
| • Confusion, delirium, rapid heartbeat. | Discontinue. Call doctor right away. |
| • Nausea, vomiting, decreased sweating. | Continue. Call doctor when convenient. |
| • Constipation. | Continue. Tell doctor at next visit. |
| • Dryness in ears, nose, throat. | No action necessary. |
| **Infrequent:** Headache, painful or difficult urination. | Continue. Call doctor when convenient. |
| **Rare:** Rash or hives, pain, blurred vision. | Discontinue. Call doctor right away. |

## WARNINGS & PRECAUTIONS

**Don't take if:**
- You are allergic to any anticholinergic.
- You have trouble with stomach bloating.
- You have difficulty emptying your bladder completely.
- You have narrow-angle glaucoma.
- You have severe ulcerative colitis.

**Before you start, consult your doctor:**
- If you have open-angle glaucoma.
- If you have angina.
- If you have chronic bronchitis or asthma.
- If you have hiatal hernia.
- If you have liver disease.
- If you have enlarged prostate.
- If you have myasthenia gravis.
- If you have peptic ulcer.
- If you will have surgery within 2 months, including dental surgery, requiring general or spinal anesthesia.

**Over age 60:**
Adverse reactions and side effects may be more frequent and severe than in younger persons.

**Pregnancy:**
Studies inconclusive on harm to unborn child. Animal studies show fetal abnormalities. Decide with your doctor whether drug benefits justify risk to unborn child.

**Breast-feeding:**
Drug passes into milk and decreases milk flow. Avoid drug or discontinue nursing until you finish medicine. Consult doctor for advice on maintaining milk supply.

**Infants & children:**
Use only under medical supervision.

**Prolonged use:**
Chronic constipation, possible fecal impaction. Consult doctor immediately.

**Skin & sunlight:**
No problems expected.

**Driving, piloting or hazardous work:**
Use disqualifies you for piloting aircraft. Otherwise, no problems expected.

**Discontinuing:**
May be unnecessary to finish medicine. Follow doctor's instructions.

**Others:**
No problems expected.

## POSSIBLE INTERACTION WITH OTHER DRUGS

| GENERIC NAME OR DRUG CLASS | COMBINED EFFECT |
|---|---|
| Amantadine | Increased hyoscyamine effect. |
| Anticholinergics (other) | Increased hyoscyamine effect. |
| Antidepressants (tricyclic) | Increased hyoscyamine effect. |
| Antihistamines | Increased hyoscyamine effect. |
| Cortisone drugs | Increased internal-eye pressure. |
| Haloperidol | Increased internal-eye pressure. |
| MAO inhibitors | Increased hyoscyamine effect. |
| Meperidine | Increased hyoscyamine effect. |
| Methylphenidate | Increased hyoscyamine effect. |
| Molindone | Increased anticholinergic effect. |
| Orphenadrine | Increased hyoscyamine effect. |
| Phenothiazines | Increased hyoscyamine effect. |
| Pilocarpine | Loss of pilocarpine effect in glaucoma treatment. |
| Vitamin C | Decreased hyoscyamine effect. Avoid large doses of vitamin C. |

## POSSIBLE INTERACTION WITH OTHER SUBSTANCES

| INTERACTS WITH | COMBINED EFFECT |
|---|---|
| Alcohol: | None expected. |
| Beverages: | None expected. |
| Cocaine: | Excessively rapid heartbeat. Avoid. |
| Foods: | None expected. |
| Marijuana: | Drowsiness and dry mouth. |
| Tobacco: | None expected. |

# IBUPROFEN

## BRAND NAMES

| | |
|---|---|
| Advil | Haltran |
| Amersol | Medipren |
| Apo-Ibuprofen | Motrin |
| Apsifen | Novoprofen |
| Apsifen-F | Nuprin |
| Brufen | Rufen |

## BASIC INFORMATION

**Habit forming? No**
**Prescription needed? No**
**Available as generic? Yes**
**Drug class: Anti-inflammatory (non-steroid)**

## USES

- Treatment for joint pain, stiffness, inflammation and swelling of arthritis and gout.
- Pain reliever.
- Treatment for dysmenorrhea (painful or difficult menstruation).

## DOSAGE & USAGE INFORMATION

**How to take:**
Tablet—Swallow with liquid or food to lessen stomach irritation. If you can't swallow whole, crumble tablet and take with liquid or food.

**When to take:**
At the same times each day.

**If you forget a dose:**
Take as soon as you remember up to 2 hours late. If more than 2 hours, wait for next scheduled dose (don't double this dose).

**What drug does:**
Reduces tissue concentration of prostaglandins (hormones which produce inflammation and pain).

*Continued next column*

## OVERDOSE

**SYMPTOMS:**
**Confusion, agitation, incoherence, convulsions, possible hemorrhage from stomach or intestine, coma.**
**WHAT TO DO:**
- **Dial 0 (operator) or 911 (emergency) for an ambulance or medical help. Then give first aid immediately.**
- **See emergency information on inside covers.**

**Time lapse before drug works:**
Begins in 4 to 24 hours. May require 3 weeks regular use for maximum benefit.

**Don't take with:**
See Interaction column and consult doctor.

## POSSIBLE ADVERSE REACTIONS OR SIDE EFFECTS

| SYMPTOMS | WHAT TO DO |
|---|---|
| **Life-threatening:**<br>None expected. | |
| **Common:**<br>• Dizziness, nausea, pain. | Continue. Call doctor when convenient. |
| • Headache. | Continue. Tell doctor at next visit. |
| **Infrequent:**<br>Depression; drowsiness; ringing in ears; swollen feet, legs; constipation or diarrhea; vomiting. | Continue. Call doctor when convenient. |
| **Rare:**<br>• Convulsions; confusion; rash, hives or itch; blurred vision; black, bloody, tarry stool; difficult breathing; tightness in chest; rapid heartbeat; unusual bleeding or bruising; blood in urine; jaundice. | Discontinue. Call doctor right away. |
| • Frequent, painful, or difficult urination; fatigue; weakness. | Continue. Call doctor when convenient. |

# IBUPROFEN

## WARNINGS & PRECAUTIONS

**Don't take if:**
- You are allergic to aspirin or any non-steroid, anti-inflammatory drug.
- You have gastritis, peptic ulcer, enteritis, ileitis, ulcerative colitis, asthma, heart failure, high blood pressure or bleeding problems.
- Patient is younger than 15.

**Before you start, consult your doctor:**
- If you have epilepsy.
- If you have Parkinson's disease.
- If you have been mentally ill.
- If you have had kidney disease or impaired kidney function.

**Over age 60:**
Adverse reactions and side effects may be more frequent and severe than in younger persons.

**Pregnancy:**
Studies inconclusive on harm to unborn child. Decide with your doctor whether drug benefits justify risk to unborn child.

**Breast-feeding:**
May harm child. Avoid.

**Infants & children:**
Not recommended for anyone younger than 15. Use only under medical supervision.

**Prolonged use:**
- Eye damage.
- Reduced hearing.
- Sore throat, fever.
- Weight gain.

**Skin & sunlight:**
No problems expected.

**Driving, piloting or hazardous work:**
Don't drive or pilot aircraft until you learn how medicine affects you. Don't work around dangerous machinery. Don't climb ladders or work in high places. Danger increases if you drink alcohol or take medicine affecting alertness and reflexes, such as antihistamines, tranquilizers, sedatives, pain medicine, narcotics and mind-altering drugs.

**Discontinuing:**
Don't discontinue without consulting doctor. Dose may require gradual reduction if you have taken drug for a long time. Doses of other drugs may also require adjustment.

**Others:**
No problems expected.

## POSSIBLE INTERACTION WITH OTHER DRUGS

| GENERIC NAME OR DRUG CLASS | COMBINED EFFECT |
| --- | --- |
| Acebutolol | Decreased antihypertensive effect of acebutolol. |
| Anticoagulants (oral) | Increased risk of bleeding. |
| Aspirin | Increased risk of stomach ulcer. |
| Cortisone drugs | Increased risk of stomach ulcer. |
| Furosemide | Decreased diuretic effect of furosemide. |
| Gold compounds | Possible increased likelihood of kidney damage. |
| Ketoprofen | Increased possibility of internal bleeding. |
| Minoxidil | Decreased minoxidil effect. |
| Oxprenolol | Decreased antihypertensive effect of oxprenolol. |
| Oxyphenbutazone | Possible stomach ulcer. |
| Phenylbutazone | Possible stomach ulcer. |
| Probenecid | Increased ibuprofen effect. |
| Thyroid hormones | Rapid heartbeat, blood-pressure rise. |

## POSSIBLE INTERACTION WITH OTHER SUBSTANCES

| INTERACTS WITH | COMBINED EFFECT |
| --- | --- |
| Alcohol: | Possible stomach ulcer or bleeding. |
| Beverages: | None expected. |
| Cocaine: | None expected. |
| Foods: | None expected. |
| Marijuana: | Increased pain relief from ibuprofen. |
| Tobacco: | None expected. |

# INDAPAMIDE

## BRAND NAMES

Lozide                Lozol

## BASIC INFORMATION

**Habit forming? No**
**Prescription needed? Yes**
**Available as generic? No**
**Drug class: Antihypertensive, diuretic**

## USES

- Controls, but doesn't cure, high blood pressure.
- Reduces fluid retention (edema) caused by conditions such as heart disorders.

## DOSAGE & USAGE INFORMATION

**How to take:**
Tablet or capsule—Swallow with liquid or food to lessen stomach irritation.

**When to take:**
At the same times each day, usually at bedtime.

**If you forget a dose:**
Bedtime dose—If you forget your once-a-day bedtime dose, don't take it more than 3 hours late. Never double dose.

**What drug does:**
Forces kidney to excrete more sodium and causes excess salt and fluid to be excreted.

**Time lapse before drug works:**
2 hours for effect to begin. May require 1 to 4 weeks for full effects.

*Continued next column*

## OVERDOSE

**SYMPTOMS:**
**Nausea, vomiting, diarrhea, very dry mouth, thirst, weakness, excessive fatigue, very rapid heart rate, weak pulse.**
**WHAT TO DO:**
- **Dial 0 (operator) or 911 (emergency) for an ambulance or medical help. Then give first aid immediately.**
- **If patient is unconscious and not breathing, give mouth-to-mouth breathing. If there is no heartbeat, use cardiac massage and mouth-to-mouth breathing (CPR). Don't try to make patient vomit. If you can't get help quickly, take patient to nearest emergency facility.**
- **See emergency information on inside covers.**

**Don't take with:**
See Interaction column and consult doctor.

## POSSIBLE ADVERSE REACTIONS OR SIDE EFFECTS

| SYMPTOMS | WHAT TO DO |
|---|---|
| **Life-threatening:** None expected. | |
| **Common:** | |
| • Excessive tiredness or weakness, muscle cramps. | Discontinue. Call doctor right away. |
| • Frequent urination. | Continue. Tell doctor at next visit. |
| **Infrequent:** | |
| • Gouty arthritis. | Discontinue. Call doctor right away. |
| • Insomnia, mood change, dizziness on changing position, headache, excessive thirst, diarrhea, appetite loss, nausea. | Continue. Call doctor when convenient. |
| **Rare:** | |
| • Weak pulse. | Discontinue. Seek emergency treatment. |
| • Itching, rash, hives, irregular heartbeat. | Discontinue. Call doctor right away. |

## WARNINGS & PRECAUTIONS

**Don't take if:**
- You are allergic to indapamide or to any sulfa drug or thiazide diuretic (see index).
- You have severe kidney disease.

**Before you start, consult your doctor:**
- If you have severe kidney disease.
- If you have diabetes.
- If you have gout.
- If you have liver disease.
- If you will have surgery within 2 months, including dental surgery, requiring general or spinal anesthesia.
- If you have lupus erythematosus.
- If you are pregnant or plan to become pregnant.

**Over age 60:**
Adverse reactions and side effects may be more frequent and severe than in younger persons.

**Pregnancy:**
Risk to unborn child outweighs drug benefits. Don't use.

**Breast-feeding:**
Unknown effect on child. Consult doctor.

**Infants & children:**
Use only under close medical supervision.

# INDAPAMIDE

**Prolonged use:**
Request laboratory studies for blood sugar, BUN, uric acid and serum electrolytes (potassium and sodium).

**Skin & sunlight:**
May cause rash or intensify sunburn in areas exposed to sun or sunlamp.

**Driving, piloting or hazardous work:**
Don't drive or pilot aircraft until you learn how medicine affects you. Don't work around dangerous machinery. Don't climb ladders or work in high places. Danger increases if you drink alcohol or take medicine affecting alertness and reflexes, such as antihistamines, tranquilizers, sedatives, pain medicine, narcotics and mind-altering drugs.

**Discontinuing:**
Don't discontinue without consulting doctor. Dose may require gradual reduction if you have taken drug for a long time. Doses of other drugs may also require adjustment.

**Others:**
No problems expected.

 ## POSSIBLE INTERACTION WITH OTHER DRUGS

| GENERIC NAME OR DRUG CLASS | COMBINED EFFECT |
|---|---|
| Antihypertensives (other) | Increased antihypertensive effect. |
| Allopurinol | Decreased allopurinol effect. |
| Amiodarone | Increased risk of heartbeat irregularity due to low potassium. |
| Antidepressants (tricyclic) | Dangerous drop in blood pressure. |
| Barbiturates | Increased indapamide effect. |
| Calcium supplements | Increased calcium in blood. |
| Cholestyramine | Decreased indapamide effect. |
| Cortisone drugs | Excessive potassium loss that may cause dangerous heart rhythms. |
| Digitalis preparations | Excessive potassium loss that may cause dangerous heart rhythms. |
| Diuretics (thiazide) | Increased effect of thiazide diuretics. |

| | |
|---|---|
| Enalapril | Possible excessive potassium in blood. |
| Labetolol | Increased antihypertensive effects. |
| Lithium | High risk of lithium toxicity. |
| MAO inhibitors | Increased indapamide effect. |
| Probenecid | Decreased probenecid effect. |

 ## POSSIBLE INTERACTION WITH OTHER SUBSTANCES

| INTERACTS WITH | COMBINED EFFECT |
|---|---|
| Alcohol: | Dangerous blood-pressure drop. Avoid. |
| Beverages: | No problems expected. |
| Cocaine: | Reduced effectiveness of indapamide. Avoid. |
| Foods: Licorice. | Excessive potassium loss that may cause dangerous heart rhythms. |
| Marijuana: | Reduced effectiveness of indapamide. Avoid. |
| Tobacco: | Reduced effectiveness of indapamide. Avoid. |

# INDOMETHACIN

## BRAND NAMES

| | |
|---|---|
| Apo-Indomethacin | Indocin-SR |
| Imbrilon | Indolar SR |
| Indocid | Indo-Lemmon |
| Indocid R | Indometacin |
| Indocid-SR | Novomethacin |
| Indocin | Zendole |

## BASIC INFORMATION

Habit forming? No
Prescription needed? Yes
Available as generic? Yes
Drug class: Anti-inflammatory (non-steroid)

## USES

- Treatment for joint pain, stiffness, inflammation and swelling of arthritis and gout.
- Pain reliever.
- Treatment for dysmenorrhea (painful or difficult menstruation).

## DOSAGE & USAGE INFORMATION

**How to take:**
- Tablet or capsule—Swallow with liquid or food to lessen stomach irritation. If you can't swallow whole, crumble tablet or open capsule and take with liquid or food.
- Extended release tablets or capsules—Swallow whole with liquid or food to lessen stomach irritation.

**When to take:**
At the same times each day.

**If you forget a dose:**
Take as soon as you remember up to 2 hours late. If more than 2 hours, wait for next scheduled dose (don't double this dose).

*Continued next column*

## OVERDOSE

**SYMPTOMS:**
Confusion, agitation, incoherence, convulsions, possible hemorrhage from stomach or intestine, coma.
**WHAT TO DO:**
- Dial 0 (operator) or 911 (emergency) for an ambulance or medical help. Then give first aid immediately.
- See emergency information on inside covers.

**What drug does:**
Reduces tissue concentration of prostaglandins (hormones which produce inflammation and pain).

**Time lapse before drug works:**
Begins in 4 to 24 hours. May require 3 weeks regular use for maximum benefit.

**Don't take with:**
See Interaction column and consult doctor.

## POSSIBLE ADVERSE REACTIONS OR SIDE EFFECTS

| SYMPTOMS | WHAT TO DO |
|---|---|
| **Life-threatening:**<br>None expected. | |
| **Common:**<br>• Dizziness, nausea, pain. | Continue. Call doctor when convenient. |
| • Headache. | Continue. Tell doctor at next visit. |
| **Infrequent:**<br>Depression; drowsiness; ringing in ears; constipation or diarrhea; vomiting; swollen feet, legs. | Continue. Call doctor when convenient. |
| **Rare:**<br>• Convulsions; confusion; rash, hives or itch; blurred vision; black, bloody, tarry stool; difficult breathing; tightness in chest; rapid heartbeat; unusual bleeding or bruising; blood in urine; jaundice. | Discontinue. Call doctor right away. |
| • Frequent, painful or difficult urination; fatigue; weakness. | Continue. Call doctor when convenient. |

## WARNINGS & PRECAUTIONS

### Don't take if:
- You are allergic to aspirin or any non-steroid, anti-inflammatory drug.
- You have gastritis, peptic ulcer, enteritis, ileitis, ulcerative colitis, asthma, heart failure, high blood pressure or bleeding problems.
- Patient is younger than 15.

### Before you start, consult your doctor:
- If you have epilepsy.
- If you have Parkinson's disease.
- If you have been mentally ill.
- If you have had kidney disease or impaired kidney function.

### Over age 60:
Adverse reactions and side effects may be more frequent and severe than in younger persons.

### Pregnancy:
Studies inconclusive on harm to unborn child. Decide with your doctor whether drug benefits justify risk to unborn child.

### Breast-feeding:
May harm child. Avoid.

### Infants & children:
Not recommended for anyone younger than 15. Use only under medical supervision.

### Prolonged use:
- Eye damage.
- Reduced hearing.
- Sore throat, fever.
- Weight gain.

### Skin & sunlight:
No problems expected.

### Driving, piloting or hazardous work:
Don't drive or pilot aircraft until you learn how medicine affects you. Don't work around dangerous machinery. Don't climb ladders or work in high places. Danger increases if you drink alcohol or take medicine affecting alertness and reflexes, such as antihistamines, tranquilizers, sedatives, pain medicine, narcotics and mind-altering drugs.

### Discontinuing:
Don't discontinue without consulting doctor. Dose may require gradual reduction if you have taken drug for a long time. Doses of other drugs may also require adjustment.

### Others:
No problems expected.

## POSSIBLE INTERACTION WITH OTHER DRUGS

| GENERIC NAME OR DRUG CLASS | COMBINED EFFECT |
|---|---|
| Acebutolol | Decreased antihypertensive effect of acebutolol. |
| Anticoagulants (oral) | Increased risk of bleeding. |
| Aspirin | Increased risk of stomach ulcer. |
| Cortisone drugs | Increased risk of stomach ulcer. |
| Furosemide | Decreased diuretic effect of furosemide. |
| Gold compounds | Possible increased likelihood of kidney damage. |
| Ketoprofen | Increased possibility of internal bleeding. |
| Lithium | Increased lithium effect. |
| Minoxidil | Reduced minoxidil effect. |
| Oxprenolol | Decreased antihypertensive effect of oxprenolol. |
| Oxyphenbutazone | Possible stomach ulcer. |
| Phenylbutazone | Possible stomach ulcer. |
| Probenecid | Increased indomethacin effect. |
| Thyroid hormones | Rapid heartbeat, blood-pressure rise. |

## POSSIBLE INTERACTION WITH OTHER SUBSTANCES

| INTERACTS WITH | COMBINED EFFECT |
|---|---|
| Alcohol: | Possible stomach ulcer or bleeding. |
| Beverages: | None expected. |
| Cocaine: | None expected. |
| Foods: | None expected. |
| Marijuana: | Increased pain relief from indomethacin. |
| Tobacco: | None expected. |

# INSULIN

## BRAND NAMES

See complete list of brand names in the *Brand Name Directory,* page 951.

## BASIC INFORMATION

**Habit forming? No**
**Prescription needed? No**
**Available as generic? Yes**
**Drug class: Antidiabetic**

 **USES**

Controls diabetes, a complex metabolic disorder, in which the body does not manufacture insulin.

 **DOSAGE & USAGE INFORMATION**

**How to take:**
Must be taken by injection under the skin. Use disposable, sterile needles. Rotate injection sites.

**When to take:**
At the same time each day.

**If you forget a dose:**
Take as soon as you remember. Wait at least 4 hours for next dose. Resume regular schedule.

**What drug does:**
Facilitates passage of blood sugar through cell membranes so sugar is usable.

*Continued next column*

 **OVERDOSE**

**SYMPTOMS:**
**Low blood sugar (hypoglycemia)—Anxiety; chills, cold sweats, pale skin; drowsiness; excess hunger; headache; nausea; nervousness; fast heartbeat; shakiness; unusual tiredness or weakness.**
**WHAT TO DO:**
- **Eat some type of sugar immediately, such as orange juice, honey, sugar cubes, crackers, sandwich.**
- **If patient loses consciousness, give glucagon if you have it and know how to use it.**
- **Otherwise, dial 0 (operator) or 911 (emergency) for an ambulance or medical help. Then give first aid immediately.**
- **See emergency information on inside covers.**

**Time lapse before drug works:**
30 minutes to 8 hours, depending on type of insulin used.

**Don't take with:**
See Interaction column and consult doctor.

 **POSSIBLE ADVERSE REACTIONS OR SIDE EFFECTS**

| SYMPTOMS | WHAT TO DO |
|---|---|
| **Life-threatening:** | |
| Hives, rash, intense itching, faintness soon after a dose (anaphylaxis). | Seek emergency treatment immediately. |
| **Common:** | |
| None expected. | |
| **Infrequent:** | |
| • Hives. | Discontinue. Call doctor right away. |
| • Swelling, redness, itch at injection site. | Continue. Call doctor when convenient. |
| **Rare:** | |
| None expected. | |

## WARNINGS & PRECAUTIONS

**Don't take if:**
- Your diagnosis and dose schedule is not established.
- You don't know how to deal with overdose emergencies.

**Before you start, consult your doctor:**
- If you are allergic to insulin.
- If you take MAO inhibitors.
- If you have liver or kidney disease or low thyroid function.

**Over age 60:**
Guard against hypoglycemia. Repeated episodes can cause permanent confusion and abnormal behavior.

**Pregnancy:**
Possible drug benefits outweigh risk to unborn child. Adhere rigidly to diabetes treatment program.

**Breast-feeding:**
No problems expected.

**Infants & children:**
Use only under medical supervision.

**Prolonged use:**
No problems expected.

**Skin & sunlight:**
No problems expected.

**Driving, piloting or hazardous work:**
No problems expected after dose is established.

**Discontinuing:**
Don't discontinue without doctor's advice until you complete prescribed dose, even though symptoms diminish or disappear.

**Others:**
- Diet and exercise affect how much insulin you need. Work with your doctor to determine accurate dose.
- Notify your doctor if you skip a dose, overeat, have fever or infection.
- Notify doctor if you develop symptoms of high blood sugar: drowsiness, dry skin, orange fruit-like odor to breath, increased urination, appetite loss, unusual thirst.

## POSSIBLE INTERACTION WITH OTHER DRUGS

| GENERIC NAME OR DRUG CLASS | COMBINED EFFECT |
|---|---|
| Anticoagulants (oral) | Increased anticoagulant effect. |
| Anticonvulsants (hydantoin) | Decreased insulin effect. |
| Antidiabetics (oral) | Increased antibiabetic effect. |
| Beta-adrenergic blockers | Possible increased difficulty in regulating blood-sugar levels. |
| Contraceptives (oral) | Decreased insulin effect. |
| Cortisone drugs | Decreased insulin effect. |
| Diuretics | Decreased insulin effect. |
| Furosemide | Decreased insulin effect. |
| MAO inhibitors | Increased insulin effect. |
| Oxyphenbutazone | Increased insulin effect. |
| Phenylbutazone | Increased insulin effect. |
| Salicylates | Increased insulin effect. |
| Sulfa drugs | Increased insulin effect. |
| Tetracyclines | Increased insulin effect. |
| Thyroid hormones | Decreased insulin effect. |

## POSSIBLE INTERACTION WITH OTHER SUBSTANCES

| INTERACTS WITH | COMBINED EFFECT |
|---|---|
| Alcohol: | Increased insulin effect. May cause hypoglycemia and brain damage. |
| Beverages: | None expected. |
| Cocaine: | May cause brain damage. |
| Foods: | None expected. |
| Marijuana: | Possible increase in blood sugar. |
| Tobacco: | None expected. |

# IODOQUINOL

## BRAND NAMES

| | |
|---|---|
| Diiodohydroxyquin | Diquinol |
| Diodoquin | Yodoxin |

## BASIC INFORMATION

**Habit forming? No**
**Prescription needed? Yes**
**Available as generic? Yes**
**Drug class: Antiprotozoal**

## USES

Treatment for intestinal amebiasis.

## DOSAGE & USAGE INFORMATION

**How to take:**
Tablets—Mix with applesauce or chocolate syrup if unable to swallow tablets.

**When to take:**
Three times daily after meals for 20 days. Treatment may be repeated after 2 to 3 weeks.

**If you forget a dose:**
Take as soon as you remember up to 2 hours late. If more than 2 hours, wait for next scheduled dose (don't double this dose).

**What drug does:**
Kills amoeba (microscopic parasites) in intestinal tract.

**Time lapse before drug works:**
May require full course of treatment (20 days) to cure.

**Don't take with:**
See Interaction column and consult doctor.

## OVERDOSE

**SYMPTOMS:**
- **Prolonged dosing at high level may produce blurred vision, muscle pain, eye pain, numbness and tingling in hands or feet.**
- **Single overdosage unlikely to threaten life.**

**WHAT TO DO:**
If person takes much larger amount than prescribed, call doctor, poison-control center or hospital emergency room for instructions.

## POSSIBLE ADVERSE REACTIONS OR SIDE EFFECTS

| SYMPTOMS | WHAT TO DO |
|---|---|
| **Life-threatening:**<br>None expected. | |
| **Common:** | |
| • Diarrhea, nausea, vomiting, stomach pain. | Discontinue. Call doctor right away. |
| • Dizziness, headache. | Continue. Call doctor when convenient. |
| **Infrequent:**<br>Clumsiness, rash, hives, itching, blurred vision, muscle pain, numbness or tingling in hands or feet, chills, fever, weakness. | Discontinue. Call doctor right away. |
| **Rare:**<br>None expected. | |

## WARNINGS & PRECAUTIONS

**Don't take if:**
You have kidney or liver disease.

**Before you start, consult your doctor:**
If you have optic atrophy thyroid disease.

**Over age 60:**
Adverse reactions and side effects may be more frequent and severe than in younger persons.

**Pregnancy:**
No proven problems, but avoid if possible.

**Breast-feeding:**
No proven problems, but avoid if possible. Discontinue nursing until you finish medicine. Consult doctor for advice on maintaining milk supply.

**Infants & children:**
Not recommended. Safety and dosage has not been established.

**Prolonged use:**
Not recommended.

**Skin & sunlight:**
No problems expected.

**Driving, piloting or hazardous work:**
No problems expected.

**Discontinuing:**
Don't discontinue without consulting doctor.

**Others:**
Thyroid tests may be inaccurate for as long as 6 months after discontinuing iodoquinol treatment.

## POSSIBLE INTERACTION WITH OTHER DRUGS

| GENERIC NAME OR DRUG CLASS | COMBINED EFFECT |
|---|---|
| None expected. | |

## POSSIBLE INTERACTION WITH OTHER SUBSTANCES

| INTERACTS WITH | COMBINED EFFECT |
|---|---|
| Alcohol: | None expected. |
| Beverages: | None expected. |
| Cocaine: | None expected. |
| Foods: | Taking with food may decrease gastrointestinal side effects. |
| Marijuana: | None expected. |
| Tobacco: | None expected. |

# IRON-POLYSACCHARIDE

## BRAND NAMES

Hytinic       Nu-Iron
Niferex

## BASIC INFORMATION

**Habit forming? No**
**Prescription needed?**
  **With folic acid: Yes**
  **Without folic acid: No**
**Available as generic? Yes**
**Drug class: Mineral supplement (iron)**

## USES

Treatment for dietary iron deficiency or
iron-deficiency anemia from other causes.

## DOSAGE & USAGE INFORMATION

**How to take:**
Tablet, capsule or liquid—Swallow with liquid or
food to lessen stomach irritation. If you can't
swallow whole, crumble tablet or open capsule
and take with liquid or food. Place medicine far
back on tongue to avoid staining teeth.

**When to take:**
1 hour before or 2 hours after meals.

**If you forget a dose:**
Take up to 2 hours late. If more than 2 hours,
wait for next dose (don't double this dose).

**What drug does:**
Stimulates bone-marrow production of
hemoglobin (red-blood-cell pigment that carries
oxygen to body cells).

**Time lapse before drug works:**
3 to 7 days. May require 3 weeks for maximum
benefit.

**Don't take with:**
- Multiple vitamin and mineral supplements.
- See Interaction column and consult doctor.

## OVERDOSE

**SYMPTOMS:**
**Weakness, collapse; pallor, blue lips, hands
and fingernails; weak, rapid heartbeat;
shallow breathing; convulsions; coma.**
**WHAT TO DO:**
- **Dial 0 (operator) or 911 (emergency) for an
  ambulance or medical help. Then give first
  aid immediately.**
- **See emergency information on inside
  covers.**

## POSSIBLE ADVERSE REACTIONS OR SIDE EFFECTS

| SYMPTOMS | WHAT TO DO |
|---|---|
| **Life-threatening:**<br>Weak, rapid heartbeat. | Seek emergency treatment immediately. |
| **Common:**<br>Stained teeth with liquid iron. | No action necessary. |
| **Always:**<br>Gray or black stool. | No action necessary. |
| **Infrequent:**<br>• Constipation or diarrhea, heartburn, nausea, vomiting. | Discontinue. Call doctor right away. |
| • Fatigue, weakness. | Continue. Call doctor when convenient. |
| • Dark urine. | Continue. Tell doctor at next visit. |
| **Rare:**<br>• Throat or chest pain on swallowing, pain, cramps, blood in stool. | Discontinue. Call doctor right away. |
| • Drowsiness. | Continue. Call doctor when convenient. |

## WARNINGS & PRECAUTIONS

### Don't take if:
- You are allergic to any iron supplement.
- You take iron injections.
- Your daily iron intake is high.
- You plan to take this supplement for a long time.
- You have acute hepatitis.
- You have hemosiderosis or hemochromatosis (conditions involving excess iron in body).
- You have hemolytic anemia.

### Before you start, consult your doctor:
- If you plan to become pregnant within medication period.
- If you have had stomach surgery.
- If you have had peptic ulcer disease, enteritis or colitis.
- If you have had pancreatitis or hepatitis.

### Over age 60:
May cause hemochromatosis (iron storage disease) with bronze skin, liver damage, diabetes, heart problems and impotence.

### Pregnancy:
No proven harm to unborn child. Avoid if possible. Take only if your doctor prescribes supplement during last half of pregnancy.

### Breast-feeding:
No problems expected. Take only if your doctor confirms you have a dietary deficiency or an iron-deficiency anemia.

### Infants & children:
Use only under medical supervision. Overdose common and dangerous. Keep out of children's reach.

### Prolonged use:
May cause hemochromatosis (iron storage disease) with bronze skin, liver damage, diabetes, heart problems and impotence.

### Skin & sunlight:
No problems expected.

### Driving, piloting or hazardous work:
No problems expected.

### Discontinuing:
May be unnecessary to finish medicine. Follow doctor's instructions.

### Others:
Liquid form stains teeth. Mix with water or juice to lessen the effect. Brush with baking soda or hydrogen peroxide to help remove stain.

## POSSIBLE INTERACTION WITH OTHER DRUGS

| GENERIC NAME OR DRUG CLASS | COMBINED EFFECT |
|---|---|
| Allopurinol | Possible excess iron storage in liver. |
| Antacids | Poor iron absorption. |
| Calcium supplements | Decreased iron effect. |
| Chloramphenicol | Decreased effect of iron. Interferes with red-blood-cell and hemoglobin formation. |
| Cholestyramine | Decreased iron effect. |
| Iron supplements (other) | Possible excess iron storage in liver. |
| Penicillamine | Decreased penicillamine effect. |
| Sulfasalazine | Decreased iron effect. |
| Tetracyclines | Decreased tetracycline effect. Take iron 3 hours before or 2 hours after taking tetracycline. |
| Vitamin C | Increased iron effect. Contributes to red-blood-cell and hemoglobin formation. |
| Vitamin E | Decreased iron effect. |

## POSSIBLE INTERACTION WITH OTHER SUBSTANCES

| INTERACTS WITH | COMBINED EFFECT |
|---|---|
| Alcohol: | Increased iron absorption. May cause organ damage. Avoid or use in moderation. |
| Beverages: Milk, tea. | Decreased iron effect. |
| Cocaine: | None expected. |
| Foods: Dairy foods, eggs, whole-grain bread and cereal. | Decreased iron effect. |
| Marijuana: | None expected. |
| Tobacco: | None expected. |

# ISOETHARINE

## BRAND NAMES

Arm-a-Med      Dey-Lute Isoetharine
   Isoetharine    Dilabron
Beta-2           Disorine
Bronkometer     Dispos-a Med
Bronkosol       Isoetharine
Dey-Dose Isoetharine

## BASIC INFORMATION

Habit forming? No
Prescription needed? Yes
Available as generic? Yes
Drug class: Sympathomimetic
           (bronchodilator)

## USES

Eases breathing difficulty from bronchial asthma attacks, bronchitis and emphysema.

## DOSAGE & USAGE INFORMATION

**How to take:**
Aerosol—Use only as directed on label. Don't inhale medicine more than twice per dose unless otherwise directed by doctor.

**When to take:**
As needed, no more often than every 3 hours.

**If you forget a dose:**
Take as soon as you remember if you need it. Never double dose.

**What drug does:**
Dilates constricted bronchial tubes so air can pass.

*Continued next column*

## OVERDOSE

**SYMPTOMS:**
Nervousness, anxiety, dizziness, palpitations, tremor, rapid heartbeat, spasm of bronchial tubes, cardiac arrest.
**WHAT TO DO:**
- **Dial 0 (operator) or 911 (emergency) for an ambulance or medical help. Then give first aid immediately.**
- **If patient is unconscious and not breathing, give mouth-to-mouth breathing. If there is no heartbeat, use cardiac massage and mouth-to-mouth breathing (CPR). Don't try to make patient vomit. If you can't get help quickly, take patient to nearest emergency facility.**
- **See emergency information on inside covers.**

**Time lapse before drug works:**
1 to 2 minutes.

**Don't take with:**
- Non-prescription drugs containing caffeine without consulting doctor.
- See Interaction column and consult doctor.

## POSSIBLE ADVERSE REACTIONS OR SIDE EFFECTS

| SYMPTOMS | WHAT TO DO |
|---|---|
| **Life-threatening:**<br>None expected. | |
| **Common:**<br>Dizziness, agitation, headache, insomnia, nausea, fast or pounding heartbeat. | Continue. Call doctor when convenient. |
| **Infrequent:**<br>• Constriction of bronchial tubes, particularly after overuse. | Discontinue. Call doctor right away. |
| • Weakness. | Continue. Call doctor when convenient. |
| **Rare:**<br>None expected. | |

## WARNINGS & PRECAUTIONS

### Don't take if:
- You are allergic to any sympathomimetic drug.
- You have a heart-rhythm disorder.
- You have taken MAO inhibitors in past 2 weeks.

### Before you start, consult your doctor:
- If you use epinephrine for asthma.
- If you have diabetes.
- If you have an overactive thyroid gland.
- If you take a digitalis preparation, have high blood pressure or heart disease.

### Over age 60:
- If you have hardening of the arteries, use with caution.
- If you have enlarged prostate gland, drug may increase urination difficulty.
- If you have Parkinson's disease, drug may temporarily increase rigidity and tremor in extremities.

### Pregnancy:
No proven harm to unborn child. Avoid if possible.

### Breast-feeding:
No problems expected, but consult doctor.

### Infants & children:
Don't give to infants younger than 2. For older children, use only under medical supervision.

### Prolonged use:
No problems expected.

### Skin & sunlight:
No problems expected.

### Driving, piloting or hazardous work:
No problems expected. Use caution if you feel nervous or dizzy.

### Discontinuing:
Discontinue if drug fails to provide relief. Don't increase dose or frequency.

### Others:
May increase blood- and urine-sugar levels, particularly in diabetics.

## POSSIBLE INTERACTION WITH OTHER DRUGS

| GENERIC NAME OR DRUG CLASS | COMBINED EFFECT |
| --- | --- |
| Antidepressants (tricyclic) | Increased isoetharine effect. |
| Beta-adrenergic blockers | Decreased effects of both drugs. |
| Ephedrine | Increased ephedrine effect. Excessive heart stimulation. |
| Epinephrine | Excessive heart stimulation. |
| Isoproterenol | Excessive heart stimulation. |
| MAO inhibitors | Dangerous mixture. Avoid. |
| Minoxidil | Decreased minoxidil effect. |
| Nitrates | Possible decreased effects of both drugs. |

## POSSIBLE INTERACTION WITH OTHER SUBSTANCES

| INTERACTS WITH | COMBINED EFFECT |
| --- | --- |
| Alcohol: | None expected. |
| Beverages: Caffeine drinks. | May cause irregular or fast heartbeat. |
| Cocaine: | Excessive stimulation. Avoid. |
| Foods: Chocolates. | May cause irregular or fast heartbeat. |
| Marijuana: | Improves drug's antiasthmatic effect. |
| Tobacco: | None expected. |

# ISOMETHAPRINE, DICHLORALPHENAZONE & ACETAMINOPHEN

## BRAND NAMES

Midrin

## BASIC INFORMATION

**Habit forming? No**
**Prescription needed? Yes**
**Available as generic? No**
**Drug class: Analgesic, sedative**

## USES

Treatment of vascular (throbbing or migraine type) and tension headaches.

## DOSAGE & USAGE INFORMATION

**How to take:**
Capsules—Take with fluid. Usual dose—2 capsules at start, then 1 every hour until fully relieved. Don't exceed 5 capsules in 12 hours.

**When to take:**
At first sign of headache.

**If you forget a dose:**
Use as soon as you remember.

**What drug does:**
Causes blood vessels in head to constrict or become narrower. Acetaminophen relieves pain by effects on hypothalamus—the part of the brain that helps regulate body heat and receives body's pain messages.

**Time lapse before drug works:**
30-60 minutes.

*Continued next column*

## OVERDOSE

**SYMPTOMS:**
**Stomach upsets, irritability, convulsions, coma.**
**WHAT TO DO:**
- **Dial 0 (operator) or 911 (emergency) for an ambulance or medical help. Then give first aid immediately.**
- **See emergency information on inside covers.**

**Don't take with:**
- Any medicine that will decrease mental alertness or reflexes, such as alcohol, other mind-altering drugs, cough/cold medicines, antihistamines, allergy medicine, sedatives, tranquilizers (sleeping pills or "downers") barbiturates, seizure medicine, narcotics, other prescription medicine for pain, muscle relaxants, anesthetics.
- See Interaction column and consult doctor.

## POSSIBLE ADVERSE REACTIONS OR SIDE EFFECTS

| SYMPTOMS | WHAT TO DO |
|---|---|
| **Life-threatening:** | |
| Fast heartbeat. | Discontinue. Seek emergency treatment. |
| **Common:** | |
| Dizziness. | Continue. Call doctor when convenient. |
| **Infrequent:** | |
| Diarrhea, vomiting, nausea, abdominal cramps. | Discontinue. Call doctor right away. |
| **Rare:** | |
| Rash; itchy skin; sore throat, fever, mouth sores; unusual bleeding or bruising; weakness; jaundice. | Discontinue. Call doctor right away. |

## WARNINGS & PRECAUTIONS

**Don't take if:**
- You are allergic to acetaminophen or any other component of this combination medicine.
- Your symptoms don't improve after 2 days use. Call your doctor.

**Before you start, consult your doctor:**
If you have bronchial asthma, kidney disease, liver damage, glaucoma, heart or blood vessel disorder, hypertension.

**Over age 60:**
Don't exceed recommended dose. You can't eliminate drug as efficiently as younger persons.

**Pregnancy:**
No proven harm to unborn child. Avoid if possible.

**Breast-feeding:**
No proven harm to nursing infant.

**Infants & children:**
Not recommended.

**Prolonged use:**
May affect blood system and cause anemia. Limit use to 5 days for children 12 and under, and 10 days for adults.

**Skin & sunlight:**
No problems expected.

**Driving, piloting or hazardous work:**
Avoid if you feel drowsy. Otherwise, no restrictions.

**Discontinuing:**
Discontinue in 2 days if symptoms don't improve.

**Others:**
No problems expected.

## POSSIBLE INTERACTION WITH OTHER DRUGS

| GENERIC NAME OR DRUG CLASS | COMBINED EFFECT |
|---|---|
| Anticoagulants (oral) | May increase anticoagulant effect. If combined frequently, prothrombin time should be monitored. |
| Anti-inflammatory agents (non-steroidal) | Long-term combined effect (3 years or longer) increases chance of damage to kidney, including malignancy. |
| Aspirin or other salicylates | Long-term combined effect (3 years or longer) increases chance of damage to kidney, including malignancy. |
| MAO inhibitors | Sudden increase in blood pressure. |
| Phenacetin | Long-term combined effect (3 years or longer) increases chance of damage to kidney, including malignancy. |
| Phenobarbital | Quicker elimination and decreased effect of acetaminophen. |
| Tetracyclines (effervescent granules or tablets) | May slow tetracycline absorption. Space doses 2 hours apart. |

## POSSIBLE INTERACTION WITH OTHER SUBSTANCES

| INTERACTS WITH | COMBINED EFFECT |
|---|---|
| Alcohol: | Drowsiness. Toxicity to liver. |
| Beverages: | None expected. |
| Cocaine: | None expected. However, cocaine may slow body's recovery. Avoid. |
| Foods: | None expected. |
| Marijuana: | Increased pain relief. However, marijuana may slow body's recovery. Avoid. |
| Tobacco: | May decrease effectiveness of Midrin. |

# ISONIAZID

## BRAND NAMES

DOW-Isoniazid
Ethionamide
INH
Isotamine
Laniazid
Laniazid C.P.

Nydrazid
PMS Isoniazid
Rifamate
Rimifon
Trecator-SC

## BASIC INFORMATION

**Habit forming? No**
**Prescription needed? Yes**
**Available as generic? Yes**
**Drug class: Antitubercular (antimicrobial)**

## USES

Kills tuberculosis germs.

## DOSAGE & USAGE INFORMATION

**How to take:**
- Tablet or capsule—Swallow with liquid to lessen stomach irritation.
- Syrup—Follow label directions.

**When to take:**
At the same time each day.

**If you forget a dose:**
Take as soon as you remember up to 12 hours late. If more than 12 hours, wait for next scheduled dose (don't double this dose).

**What drug does:**
Interferes with TB germ metabolism. Eventually destroys the germ.

*Continued next column*

## OVERDOSE

**SYMPTOMS:**
Difficult breathing, convulsions, coma.
**WHAT TO DO:**
- Dial 0 (operator) or 911 (emergency) for an ambulance or medical help. Then give first aid immediately.
- If patient is unconscious and not breathing, give mouth-to-mouth breathing. If there is no heartbeat, use cardiac massage and mouth-to-mouth breathing (CPR). Don't try to make patient vomit. If you can't get help quickly, take patient to nearest emergency facility.
- See emergency information on inside covers.

**Time lapse before drug works:**
3 to 6 months. You may need to take drug as long as 2 years.

**Don't take with:**
See Interaction column and consult doctor.

## POSSIBLE ADVERSE REACTIONS OR SIDE EFFECTS

| SYMPTOMS | WHAT TO DO |
|---|---|
| **Life-threatening:** | |
| None expected. | |
| **Common:** | |
| • Muscle pain and pain in joints, tingling or numbness in extremities, jaundice. | Discontinue. Call doctor right away. |
| • Confusion, unsteady walk. | Continue. Call doctor when convenient. |
| **Infrequent:** | |
| • Swollen glands, nausea, indigestion, vomiting, appetite loss. | Discontinue. Call doctor right away. |
| • Dizziness, increase in blood sugar. | Continue. Call doctor when convenient. |
| **Rare:** | |
| • Rash, fever, impaired vision, anemia with fatigue, weakness, fever, sore throat, unusual bleeding or bruising. | Discontinue. Call doctor right away. |
| • Breast enlargement or discomfort. | Continue. Tell doctor at next visit. |

## WARNINGS & PRECAUTIONS

**Don't take if:**
You are allergic to isoniazid.

**Before you start, consult your doctor:**
- If you plan to become pregnant within medication period.
- If you are allergic to athionamide, pyrazinamide or nicotinic acid.
- If you drink alcohol.
- If you have liver or kidney disease.
- If you have epilepsy, diabetes or lupus.

**Over age 60:**
Adverse reactions and side effects, especially jaundice, may be more frequent and severe than in younger persons. Kidneys may be less efficient.

**Pregnancy:**
No proven harm to unborn child. Avoid if possible, especially in the first 6 months of pregnancy. Consult doctor about use in last 3 months.

**Breast-feeding:**
Drug passes into milk. Avoid drug or discontinue nursing until you finish medicine. Consult doctor for advice on maintaining milk supply.

**Infants & children:**
Use only under medical supervision.

**Prolonged use:**
Numbness and tingling of hands and feet.

**Skin & sunlight:**
No problems expected.

**Driving, piloting or hazardous work:**
Avoid if you feel dizzy. Otherwise, no problems expected.

**Discontinuing:**
Don't discontinue without doctor's advice until you complete prescribed dose, even though symptoms diminish or disappear.

**Others:**
- Diabetic patients may have false blood-sugar tests.
- Periodic liver-function tests and laboratory blood studies recommended.
- Prescription for vitamin B-6 (pyridoxine) recommended to prevent nerve damage.

## POSSIBLE INTERACTION WITH OTHER DRUGS

| GENERIC NAME OR DRUG CLASS | COMBINED EFFECT |
|---|---|
| Antacids | Decreased absorption of isoniazid. |
| Anticholinergics | May increase pressure within eyeball. |
| Anticoagulants | Increased anticoagulant effect. |
| Antidiabetics | Increased antidiabetic effect. |
| Antihypertensives | Increased antihypertensive effect. |
| Disulfiram | Increased effect of disulfiram. |
| Laxatives | Decreased absorption and effect of isoniazid. |
| Narcotics | Increased narcotic effect. |
| Phenytoin | Increased phenytoin effect. |
| Pyridoxine (Vitamin B-6) | Decreased chance of nerve damage in extremities. |
| Rifampin | Increased isoniazid toxicity to liver. |
| Sedatives | Increased sedative effect. |
| Stimulants | Increased stimulant effect. |

## POSSIBLE INTERACTION WITH OTHER SUBSTANCES

| INTERACTS WITH | COMBINED EFFECT |
|---|---|
| Alcohol: | Decreased isoniazid effect. Avoid. |
| Beverages: | None expected. |
| Cocaine: | None expected. |
| Foods: | Decreased absorption of isoniazid. |
| Marijuana: | No interactions expected, but marijuana may slow body's recovery. |
| Tobacco: | No interactions expected, but tobacco may slow body's recovery. |

# ISOPROPAMIDE

## BRAND NAMES

Allergine
Allernade
Capade
Combid
Darbid

Oraminic
Ornade
Prochlor-Iso
Pro-Iso

## BASIC INFORMATION

Habit forming? No
Prescription needed?
  Low strength: No
  High strength: Yes
Available as generic? Yes
Drug class: Antispasmodic, anticholinergic

## USES

Reduces spasms of digestive system, bladder and urethra.

## DOSAGE & USAGE INFORMATION

How to take:
- Tablet or capsule—Swallow with liquid or food to lessen stomach irritation.
- Extended-release tablets or capsules—Swallow each dose whole. If you take regular tablets, you may chew or crush them.

When to take:
30 minutes before meals (unless directed otherwise by doctor).

If you forget a dose:
Take as soon as you remember up to 2 hours late. If more than 2 hours, wait for next scheduled dose (don't double this dose).

What drug does:
Blocks nerve impulses at parasympathetic nerve endings, preventing muscle contractions and gland secretions of organs involved.

*Continued next column*

## OVERDOSE

SYMPTOMS:
Dilated pupils, rapid pulse and breathing, dizziness, fever, hallucinations, confusion, slurred speech, agitation, flushed face, convulsions, coma.
WHAT TO DO:
- Dial 0 (operator) or 911 (emergency) for an ambulance or medical help. Then give first aid immediately.
- See emergency information on inside covers.

Time lapse before drug works:
15 to 30 minutes.

Don't take with:
See Interaction column and consult doctor.

## POSSIBLE ADVERSE REACTIONS OR SIDE EFFECTS

| SYMPTOMS | WHAT TO DO |
|---|---|
| **Life-threatening:**<br>None expected. | |
| **Common:** | |
| • Confusion, delirium, rapid heartbeat. | Discontinue. Call doctor right away. |
| • Nausea, vomiting, decreased sweating. | Continue. Call doctor when convenient. |
| • Constipation. | Continue. Tell doctor at next visit. |
| • Dryness in ears, nose, throat. | No action necessary. |
| **Infrequent:**<br>Headache, difficult urination. | Continue. Call doctor when convenient. |
| **Rare:**<br>Rash or hives, pain, blurred vision. | Discontinue. Call doctor right away. |

# ISOPROPAMIDE

## WARNINGS & PRECAUTIONS

**Don't take if:**
- You are allergic to any anticholinergic.
- You have trouble with stomach bloating.
- You have difficulty emptying your bladder completely.
- You have narrow-angle glaucoma.
- You have severe ulcerative colitis.

**Before you start, consult your doctor:**
- If you have open-angle glaucoma.
- If you have angina.
- If you have chronic bronchitis or asthma.
- If you have hiatal hernia.
- If you have liver disease.
- If you have enlarged prostate.
- If you have myasthenia gravis.
- If you have peptic ulcer.
- If you will have surgery within 2 months, including dental surgery, requiring general or spinal anesthesia.

**Over age 60:**
Adverse reactions and side effects may be more frequent and severe than in younger persons.

**Pregnancy:**
Studies inconclusive on harm to unborn child. Animal studies show fetal abnormalities. Decide with your doctor whether drug benefits justify risk to unborn child.

**Breast-feeding:**
Drug passes into milk and decreases milk flow. Avoid drug or discontinue nursing until you finish medicine. Consult doctor for advice on maintaining milk supply.

**Infants & children:**
Use only under medical supervision.

**Prolonged use:**
Chronic constipation, possible fecal impaction. Consult doctor immediately.

**Skin & sunlight:**
No problems expected.

**Driving, piloting or hazardous work:**
Use disqualifies you for piloting aircraft. Otherwise, no problems expected.

**Discontinuing:**
May be unnecessary to finish medicine. Follow doctor's instructions.

**Others:**
No problems expected.

## POSSIBLE INTERACTION WITH OTHER DRUGS

| GENERIC NAME OR DRUG CLASS | COMBINED EFFECT |
|---|---|
| Amantadine | Increased isopropamide effect. |
| Anticholinergics (other) | Increased isopropamide effect |
| Antidepressants (tricyclic) | Increased atropine effect. Increased sedation. |
| Antihistamines | Increased isopropamide effect. |
| Cortisone drugs | Increased internal-eye pressure. |
| Haloperidol | Increased internal-eye pressure. |
| MAO inhibitors | Increased isopropamide effect. |
| Meperidine | Increased isopropamide effect. |
| Methylphenidate | Increased isopropamide effect. |
| Nitrates | Increased internal-eye pressure. |
| Orphenadrine | Increased isopropamide effect. |
| Phenothiazines | Increased isopropamide effect. |
| Pilocarpine | Loss of pilocarpine effect in glaucoma treatment. |
| Potassium supplements | Possible intestinal ulcers with oral potassium tablets. |
| Vitamin C | Decreased isopropamide effect. Avoid large doses of vitamin C. |

## POSSIBLE INTERACTION WITH OTHER SUBSTANCES

| INTERACTS WITH | COMBINED EFFECT |
|---|---|
| Alcohol: | None expected. |
| Beverages: | None expected. |
| Cocaine: | Excessively rapid heartbeat. Avoid. |
| Foods: | None expected. |
| Marijuana: | Drowsiness and dry mouth. |
| Tobacco: | None expected. |

# ISOPROTERENOL

## BRAND NAMES

| | |
|---|---|
| Aerolone | Medihaler-Iso |
| Brondilate | Norisodrine |
| Duo-Medihaler | Norisodrine Aerotrol |
| Iprenol | Proternol |
| Isuprel | Vapo-Iso |

## BASIC INFORMATION

Habit forming? No
Prescription needed? Yes
Available as generic? Yes
Drug class: Sympathomimetic,
            bronchodilator

## USES

Treatment for breathing difficulty from acute asthma, bronchitis and emphysema.

## DOSAGE & USAGE INFORMATION

**How to take:**
- Tablet—Swallow with liquid or food to lessen stomach irritation.
- Extended-release tablets—Swallow each dose whole.
- Sublingual tablets—Dissolve under tongue.
- Aerosol inhaler—Don't inhale more than twice per dose.

**When to take:**
As needed, no more often than every 4 hours.

**If you forget a dose:**
Take as soon as you remember. Wait 4 hours for next dose.

**What drug does:**
- Dilates constricted bronchial tubes, improving air flow.
- Stimulates heart muscle and dilates blood vessels.

*Continued next column*

## OVERDOSE

**SYMPTOMS:**
Nervousness, rapid or irregular heartbeat, fainting, sweating, headache, tremor, vomiting, chest pain, blood-pressure drop.
**WHAT TO DO:**
- Dial 0 (operator) or 911 (emergency) for an ambulance or medical help. Then give first aid immediately.
- See emergency information on inside covers.

**Time lapse before drug works:**
2 to 4 minutes.

**Don't take with:**
See Interaction column and consult doctor.

## POSSIBLE ADVERSE REACTIONS OR SIDE EFFECTS

| SYMPTOMS | WHAT TO DO |
|---|---|
| **Life-threatening:**<br>None expected. | |
| **Common:** | |
| • Nervousness, insomnia. | Continue. Call doctor when convenient. |
| • Dry mouth, dry throat. | Continue. Tell doctor at next visit. |
| **Infrequent:** | |
| • Chest pain; irregular, fast or pounding heartbeat; unusual sweating. | Discontinue. Call doctor right away. |
| • Dizziness, headache, shakiness, weakness, flushed face, nausea, vomiting. | Continue. Call doctor when convenient. |
| **Rare:**<br>None expected. | |

## WARNINGS & PRECAUTIONS

### Don't take if:
- You are allergic to any sympathomimetic, including some diet pills.
- You have serious heart-rhythm disorder.
- You have taken MAO inhibitors in past 2 weeks.

### Before you start, consult your doctor:
- If you are sensitive to sympathomimetics.
- If you use epinephrine.
- If you have high blood pressure, heart disease, or take a digitalis preparation.
- If you have diabetes.
- If you have overactive thyroid.
- If your heartbeat is faster than 100 beats per minute.

### Over age 60:
You may be more sensitive to drug's stimulant effects. Use with caution if you have hardening of the arteries.

### Pregnancy:
Studies inconclusive on harm to unborn child. Animal studies show fetal abnormalities. Decide with your doctor whether drug benefits justify risk to unborn child.

### Breast-feeding:
Drug does not appear in milk. Consult doctor.

### Infants & children:
Not recommended.

### Prolonged use:
- Salivary glands may swell.
- Mouth ulcers (sublingual tablets).

### Skin & sunlight:
No problems expected.

### Driving, piloting or hazardous work:
Use caution if you feel dizzy or nervous.

### Discontinuing:
Discontinue if drug fails to provide relief after 2 or 3 days. Consult doctor.

### Others:
No problems expected.

## POSSIBLE INTERACTION WITH OTHER DRUGS

| GENERIC NAME OR DRUG CLASS | COMBINED EFFECT |
|---|---|
| Albuterol | Increased effect of both drugs, especially harmful side effects. |
| Antidepressants (tricyclic) | Increased effect of both drugs. |
| Beta-adrenergic blockers | Decreased effects of both drugs. |
| Ephedrine | Increased ephedrine effect. |
| Epinephrine | Increased chance of serious heart disturbances. |
| Minoxidil | Decreased minoxidil effect. |
| Nitrates | Possible decreased effects of both drugs. |
| Sympathomimetics (other) | Increased effect of both drugs, especially harmful side effects. |

## POSSIBLE INTERACTION WITH OTHER SUBSTANCES

| INTERACTS WITH | COMBINED EFFECT |
|---|---|
| Alcohol: | Decreased isoproterenol effect. |
| Beverages: Caffeine drinks. | Overstimulation. Avoid. |
| Cocaine: | Overstimulation of brain and heart. Avoid. |
| Foods: | None expected. |
| Marijuana: | Increased antiasthmatic effect of isoproterenol. |
| Tobacco: | None expected. |

# ISOPROTERENOL & PHENYLEPHRINE

## BRAND NAMES

**Duo-Medihaler**

## BASIC INFORMATION

**Habit forming? No**
**Prescription needed? Yes**
**Available as generic? No**
**Drug class: Sympathomimetic,
            bronchodilator**

## USES

- Temporary relief of congestion of nose, sinuses and throat caused by allergies, colds or sinusitis.
- Treatment for breathing difficulty from acute asthma, bronchitis and emphysema.

## DOSAGE & USAGE INFORMATION

**How to take:**
Aerosol inhaler—Don't inhale more than twice per dose. Follow package instructions.

**When to take:**
As needed, no more often than every 4 hours.

**If you forget a dose:**
Take as soon as you remember. Wait 4 hours for next dose. Don't double this dose.

**What drug does:**
- Dilates constricted bronchial tubes, improving air flow.
- Stimulates heart muscle and dilates blood vessels.

**Time lapse before drug works:**
2 to 4 minutes.

*Continued next column*

## OVERDOSE

**SYMPTOMS:**
**Headache, blood-pressure rise, slow and forceful pulse, nervousness, rapid or irregular heartbeat, fainting, sweating, tremor, vomiting, chest pain, convulsions, coma.**
**WHAT TO DO:**
- **Dial 0 (operator) or 911 (emergency) for an ambulance or medical help. Then give first aid immediately.**
- **See emergency information on inside covers.**

**Don't take with:**
Non-prescription drugs for asthma, cough, cold, allergy, appetite suppressants, sleeping pills or drugs containing caffeine without consulting doctor.

## POSSIBLE ADVERSE REACTIONS OR SIDE EFFECTS

| SYMPTOMS | WHAT TO DO |
|---|---|
| **Life-threatening:**<br>None expected. | |
| **Common:**<br>Chest pain; irregular, fast heartbeat; dry mouth. | Discontinue. Call doctor right away. |
| **Infrequent:**<br>• Increased sweating. | Discontinue. Call doctor right away. |
| • Nervousness, insomnia, dizziness, headache, shakiness, weakness, red or flushed face, vomiting, nausea, pale skin. | Continue. Call doctor when convenient. |
| **Rare:**<br>None expected. | |

## WARNINGS & PRECAUTIONS

**Don't take if:**
- You are allergic to any sympathomimetic, including some diet pills.
- You have serious heart-rhythm disorder.
- You have taken MAO inhibitors in past 2 weeks.

**Before you start, consult your doctor:**
- If you have high blood pressure, heart disease, or take a digitalis preparation.
- If you have diabetes or overactive thyroid.
- If you have taken MAO inhibitors in past 2 weeks.
- If you are sensitive to sympathomimetics.
- If you use epinephrine.
- If your heartbeat is faster than 100 beats per minute.

**Over age 60:**
You may be more sensitive to drug's stimulant effects. Use with caution if you have hardening of the arteries.

**Pregnancy:**
Risk to unborn child outweighs drug benefits. Don't use.

**Breast-feeding:**
Drug passes into milk. Avoid drug or discontinue nursing until you finish medicine. Consult doctor for advice on maintaining milk supply.

**Infants & children:**
Use only under close supervision.

**Prolonged use:**
- May cause functional dependence.
- Salivary glands may swell.

**Skin & sunlight:**
No problems expected.

**Driving, piloting or hazardous work:**
Use caution if you feel dizzy or nervous.

**Discontinuing:**
Discontinue if drug fails to provide relief after 2 or 3 days. Consult doctor.

**Others:**
No problems expected.

## POSSIBLE INTERACTION WITH OTHER DRUGS

| GENERIC NAME OR DRUG CLASS | COMBINED EFFECT |
|---|---|
| Acebutolol | Decreased effect of both drugs. |
| Amphetamines | Increased nervousness. |
| Antiasthmatics | Nervous stimulation. |
| Antidepressants | Increased effect of both drugs. |
| Antihypertensives | Increased antihypertensive effect. |
| Beta-adrenergic blockers | Decreased effect of both drugs. |
| Ephedrine | Increased ephedrine effect. |
| Epinephrine | Increased chance of serious heart disturbances. |
| MAO inhibitors | Dangerous blood-pressure rise. |
| Minoxidil | Increased minoxidil effect. |
| Nitrates | Possible decreased effect of both drugs. |
| Oxprenolol | Decreased effect of both drugs. |
| Sedatives | Decreased sedative effect. |
| Sympathomimetics (other) | Increased effect of both drugs, especially harmful side effects. |
| Tranquilizers | Decreased tranquilizer effect. |

## POSSIBLE INTERACTION WITH OTHER SUBSTANCES

| INTERACTS WITH | COMBINED EFFECT |
|---|---|
| Alcohol: | Decreased isoproterenol effect. |
| Beverages: Caffeine drinks. | Overstimulation. Avoid. |
| Cocaine: | Overstimulation of brain and heart. Avoid. |
| Foods: | None expected. |
| Marijuana: | Increased antiasthmatic effect of isoproterenol. |
| Tobacco: | None expected. |

# ISOTRETINOIN

## BRAND NAMES

**Accutane**

## BASIC INFORMATION

**Habit forming? No**
**Prescription needed? Yes**
**Available as generic? No**
**Drug classification: Antiacne**

 **USES**

- Decreases cystic acne formation in severe cases.
- Certain other skin disorders involving an overabundance of outer skin layer.

 **DOSAGE & USAGE INFORMATION**

**How to take:**
Tablet or capsule—Swallow with liquid or food to lessen stomach irritation. If you can't swallow whole, crumble tablet or open capsule and take with liquid or food.

**When to take:**
Twice a day. Follow prescription directions.

**If you forget a dose:**
Take as soon as you remember up to 2 hours late. If more than 2 hours, wait for next scheduled dose and double dose.

**What drug does:**
Reduces sebaceous gland activity and size.

**Time lapse before drug works:**
May require 15 to 20 weeks to experience full benefit.

**Don't take with:**
Vitamin A or supplements containing Vitamin A.

 **OVERDOSE**

**SYMPTOMS:**
**None reported.**
**WHAT TO DO:**
**Overdose unlikely to threaten life. If person takes much larger amount than prescribed, call doctor, poison-control center or hospital emergency room for instructions.**

 **POSSIBLE ADVERSE REACTIONS OR SIDE EFFECTS**

| SYMPTOMS | WHAT TO DO |
|---|---|
| **Life-threatening:** None expected. | |
| **Common:** | |
| • Burning, red, itching eyes; lip scaling; burning pain. | Discontinue. Call doctor right away. |
| • Itchy skin. | Continue. Call doctor when convenient. |
| **Frequent:** Dry mouth. | Continue. Tell doctor at next visit. (Suck ice or chew gum.) |
| **Infrequent:** | |
| • Rash, infection, nausea, vomiting. | Discontinue. Call doctor right away. |
| • Headache; pain in muscles, bones, joints; hair thinning; tiredness. | Continue. Call doctor when convenient. |
| **Rare:** None expected. | |

## WARNINGS & PRECAUTIONS

**Don't take if:**
- You are allergic to isotretinoin.
- You are pregnant or plan pregnancy.

**Before you start, consult your doctor:**
- If you have diabetes.
- If you or any member of family have high triglyceride levels in blood.

**Over age 60:**
Adverse reactions and side effects may be more frequent and severe than in younger persons.

**Pregnancy:**
Risk to unborn child outweighs drug benefits. Don't use.

**Breast-feeding:**
Drug filters into milk. May harm child. Avoid.

**Infants & children:**
Not recommended.

**Prolonged use:**
Possible damage to cornea.

**Skin & sunlight:**
May cause rash or intensify sunburn in areas exposed to sun or sunlamp.

**Driving, piloting or hazardous work:**
No problems expected.

**Discontinuing:**
Single course of treatment usually all needed. If second course required, wait 8 weeks after completing first course.

**Others:**
Use only for severe cases of cystic acne that have not responded to less hazardous forms of acne treatment.

## POSSIBLE INTERACTION WITH OTHER DRUGS

| GENERIC NAME OR DRUG CLASS | COMBINED EFFECT |
|---|---|
| Vitamin A | Additive toxic effect of each. Avoid. |

## POSSIBLE INTERACTION WITH OTHER SUBSTANCES

| INTERACTS WITH | COMBINED EFFECT |
|---|---|
| Alcohol: | Significant increase in triglycerides in blood. Avoid. |
| Beverages: | No problems expected. |
| Cocaine: | Increased chance of toxicity of isotretinoin. Avoid. |
| Foods: | No problems expected. |
| Marijuana: | Increased chance of toxicity of isotretinoin. Avoid. |
| Tobacco: | May decrease absorption of medicine. Avoid tobacco while in treatment. |

# ISOXSUPRINE

## BRAND NAMES

Vasodilan

Vasoprine

## BASIC INFORMATION

Habit forming? No
Prescription needed? Yes
Available as generic? Yes
Drug class: Vasodilator

 **USES**

Improves poor blood circulation.

 **DOSAGE & USAGE INFORMATION**

**How to take:**
Tablet—Swallow with liquid or food to lessen stomach irritation. If you can't swallow whole, crumble tablet and take with liquid or food.

**When to take:**
At the same times each day.

**If you forget a dose:**
Take as soon as you remember up to 2 hours late. If more than 2 hours, wait for next scheduled dose (don't double this dose).

**What drug does:**
Expands blood vessels, increasing flow and permitting distribution of oxygen and nutrients.

**Time lapse before drug works:**
1 hour.

**Don't take with:**
See Interaction column and consult doctor.

 **OVERDOSE**

**SYMPTOMS:**
Headache, dizziness, flush, vomiting, weakness, sweating, fainting, shortness of breath, coma.
**WHAT TO DO:**
● Dial 0 (operator) or 911 (emergency) for an ambulance or medical help. Then give first aid immediately.
● If patient is unconscious and not breathing, give mouth-to-mouth breathing. If there is no heartbeat, use cardiac massage and mouth-to-mouth breathing (CPR). Don't try to make patient vomit. If you can't get help quickly, take patient to nearest emergency facility.
● See emergency information on inside covers.

 **POSSIBLE ADVERSE REACTIONS OR SIDE EFFECTS**

| SYMPTOMS | WHAT TO DO |
|---|---|
| **Life-threatening:** | |
| None expected. | |
| **Common:** | |
| ● Appetite loss, nausea, vomiting. | Discontinue. Call doctor right away. |
| ● Dizziness, faintness. | Continue. Call doctor when convenient. |
| ● Weakness, lethargy. | Continue. Tell doctor at next visit. |
| **Infrequent:** | |
| Rash. | Discontinue. Call doctor right away. |
| **Rare:** | |
| Rapid or irregular heartbeat. | Discontinue. Call doctor right away. |

# ISOXSUPRINE

## WARNINGS & PRECAUTIONS

**Don't take if:**
- You are allergic to any vasodilator.
- You have any bleeding disease.

**Before you start, consult your doctor:**
- If you have high blood pressure, hardening of the arteries or heart disease.
- If you plan to become pregnant within medication period.
- If you have glaucoma.

**Over age 60:**
Adverse reactions and side effects may be more frequent and severe than in younger persons.

**Pregnancy:**
Studies inconclusive on harm to unborn child. Decide with your doctor whether drug benefits justify risk to unborn child.

**Breast-feeding:**
No problems expected, but consult doctor.

**Infants & children:**
Not recommended.

**Prolonged use:**
No problems expected.

**Skin & sunlight:**
No problems expected.

**Driving, piloting or hazardous work:**
Avoid if you feel dizzy or faint. Otherwise, no problems expected.

**Discontinuing:**
Don't discontinue without doctor's advice until you complete prescribed dose, even though symptoms diminish or disappear.

**Others:**
Be cautious when arising from lying or sitting position, when climbing stairs, or if dizziness occurs.

## POSSIBLE INTERACTION WITH OTHER DRUGS

| GENERIC NAME OR DRUG CLASS | COMBINED EFFECT |
| --- | --- |
| None | |

## POSSIBLE INTERACTION WITH OTHER SUBSTANCES

| INTERACTS WITH | COMBINED EFFECT |
| --- | --- |
| Alcohol: | None expected. |
| Beverages: Milk. | Decreased stomach irritation. |
| Cocaine: | Decreased blood circulation to extremities. Avoid. |
| Foods: | None expected. |
| Marijuana: | Rapid heartbeat. |
| Tobacco: | Decreased isoxsuprine effect. |

# KAOLIN & PECTIN

## BRAND NAMES

| | |
|---|---|
| Donnagel-MB | K-C |
| Donnagel-PG | K-P |
| Kao-Con | K-Pek |
| Kaopectate | Parepectolin |
| Kapectolin | Pecto Kay |
| Kaypectol | |

## BASIC INFORMATION

**Habit forming? No**
**Prescription needed? No**
**Available as generic? Yes**
**Drug class: Antidiarrheal**

 **USES**

Reduces intestinal cramps and diarrhea.

 **DOSAGE & USAGE INFORMATION**

**How to take:**
Liquid—Swallow prescribed dosage (without diluting) after each loose bowel movement.

**When to take:**
After each loose bowel movement.

**If you forget a dose:**
Take when you remember.

**What drug does:**
Makes loose stools less watery, but may not prevent loss of fluids.

**Time lapse before drug works:**
15 to 30 minutes.

**Don't take with:**
See Interaction column and consult doctor.

 **OVERDOSE**

**SYMPTOMS:**
Fecal impaction.
**WHAT TO DO:**
Overdose unlikely to threaten life. If person takes much larger amount than prescribed, call doctor, poison-control center or hospital emergency room for instructions.

 **POSSIBLE ADVERSE REACTIONS OR SIDE EFFECTS**

| SYMPTOMS | WHAT TO DO |
|---|---|
| **Life-threatening:**<br>None expected. | |
| **Common:**<br>None expected. | |
| **Infrequent:**<br>None expected. | |
| **Rare:**<br>Constipation (mild). | Continue. Call doctor when convenient. |

## WARNINGS & PRECAUTIONS

**Don't take if:**
You are allergic to kaolin or pectin.

**Before you start, consult your doctor:**
• If patient is child or infant.
• If you have any chronic medical problem with heart disease, peptic ulcer, asthma or others.
• If you have fever over 101F.

**Over age 60:**
Fluid loss caused by diarrhea, especially if taking other medicines, may lead to serious disability. Consult doctor.

**Pregnancy:**
No problems expected.

**Breast-feeding:**
No problems expected.

**Infants & children:**
Fluid loss caused by diarrhea in infants and children can cause serious dehydration. Consult doctor before giving any medicine for diarrhea.

**Prolonged use:**
Not recommended.

**Skin & sunlight:**
No problems expected.

**Driving, piloting or hazardous work:**
No problems expected.

**Discontinuing:**
May be unnecessary to finish medicine. Follow doctor's instructions.

**Others:**
Consult doctor about fluids, diet and rest.

## POSSIBLE INTERACTION WITH OTHER DRUGS

| GENERIC NAME OR DRUG CLASS | COMBINED EFFECT |
| --- | --- |
| Digoxin | Decreases absorption of digoxin. Separate doses by at least 2 hours. |
| Lincomycin | Decreases absorption of lincomycin. Separate doses by at least 2 hours. |
| All other oral medicines. | Decreases absorption of other medicines. Separate doses by at least 2 hours. |

## POSSIBLE INTERACTION WITH OTHER SUBSTANCES

| INTERACTS WITH | COMBINED EFFECT |
| --- | --- |
| Alcohol: | Increased diarrhea. Prevents action of kaolin and pectin. |
| Beverages: | No problems expected. |
| Cocaine: | Aggravates underlying disease. Avoid. |
| Foods: | No problems expected. |
| Marijuana: | Aggravates underlying disease. Avoid. |
| Tobacco: | Aggravates underlying disease. Avoid. |

# KAOLIN, PECTIN, BELLADONNA & OPIUM

## BRAND NAMES

Donnagel-PG

## BASIC INFORMATION

**Habit forming? Yes**
**Prescription needed? Yes**
**Available as generic? No**
**Drug class: Narcotic, antidiarrheal,**
**antispasmodic**

## USES

Reduces intestinal cramps and diarrhea.

## DOSAGE & USAGE INFORMATION

**How to take:**
Liquid—Swallow prescribed dosage (without diluting) after each loose bowel movement.

**When to take:**
As needed for diarrhea, no more often than every 4 hours.

**If you forget a dose:**
Take when you remember.

**What drug does:**
- Blocks nerve impulses at parasympathetic nerve endings, preventing muscle contractions and gland secretions of organs involved.
- Makes loose stools less watery, but may not prevent loss of fluids.

*Continued next column*

## OVERDOSE

**SYMPTOMS:**
**Fecal impaction, rapid pulse, dizziness, fever, hallucinations, confusion, slurred speech, agitation, flushed face, convulsions, deep sleep, slow breathing, slow pulse, warm skin, constricted pupils, coma.**
**WHAT TO DO:**
- **Dial 0 (operator) or 911 (emergency) for an ambulance or medical help. Then give first aid immediately.**
- **If patient is unconscious and not breathing, give mouth-to-mouth breathing. If there is no heartbeat, use cardiac massage and mouth-to-mouth breathing (CPR). Don't try to make patient vomit. If you can't get help quickly, take patient to nearest emergency facility.**
- **See emergency information on inside covers.**

- Anesthetizes surface membranes of intestines and blocks nerve impulses.

**Time lapse before drug works:**
15 to 30 minutes.

**Don't take with:**
See Interaction column and consult doctor.

## POSSIBLE ADVERSE REACTIONS OR SIDE EFFECTS

| SYMPTOMS | WHAT TO DO |
|---|---|
| **Life-threatening:** | |
| Unusually rapid heartbeat (over 100), difficult breathing, slow heartbeat (under 50/minute). | Discontinue. Seek emergency treatment. |
| **Common:** | |
| (with large dosage) Weakness, increased sweating, red or flushed face, lightheadedness, headache, dry mouth, dry skin, drowsiness, dizziness, frequent urination, decreased sweating, constipation, confusion. | Continue. Call doctor when convenient. |
| **Infrequent:** | |
| • Taste sense reduced, nervousness, sunlight hurts eyes, blurred vision. | Discontinue. Call doctor right away. |
| • Diminished sex drive. | Continue. Call doctor when convenient. |
| **Rare:** | |
| Bloating, abdominal cramps and vomiting, eye pain, hallucinations, shortness of breath, rash, itchy skin. | Discontinue. Call doctor right away. |

## WARNINGS & PRECAUTIONS

**Don't take if:**
- You are allergic to any anticholinergic, narcotic, kaolin or pectin.
- You have trouble with stomach bloating, difficulty emptying your bladder completely, narrow-angle glaucoma, severe ulcerative colitis.

# KAOLIN, PECTIN, BELLADONNA & OPIUM

**Before you start, consult your doctor:**
- If you have open-angle glaucoma, angina, chronic bronchitis or asthma, hiatal hernia, liver disease, enlarged prostate, myasthenia gravis, peptic ulcer, impaired liver or kidney function, fever over 101F, any chronic medical problem with heart disease, peptic ulcer, asthma or others.
- If patient is child or infant.
- If you will have surgery within 2 months, including dental surgery, requiring general or spinal anesthesia.

**Over age 60:**
- Adverse reactions and side effects may be more frequent and severe than in younger persons.
- More likely to be drowsy, dizzy, unsteady or constipated.
- Fluid loss caused by diarrhea, especially if taking other medicines, may lead to serious disability. Consult doctor.

**Pregnancy:**
No proven harm to unborn child. Avoid if possible.

**Breast-feeding:**
Drug passes into milk. Avoid drug or discontinue nursing until you finish medicine. Consult doctor for advice on maintaining milk supply.

**Infants & children:**
Fluid loss caused by diarrhea in infants and children can cause serious dehydration. Consult doctor before giving any medicine for diarrhea.

**Prolonged use:**
Causes psychological and physical dependence. Not recommended.

**Skin & sunlight:**
No problems expected.

**Driving, piloting or hazardous work:**
Don't drive or pilot aircraft until you learn how medicine affects you. Don't work around dangerous machinery. Don't climb ladders or work in high places. Danger increases if you drink alcohol or take medicine affecting alertness and reflexes, such as antihistamines, tranquilizers, sedatives, pain medicine, narcotics and mind-altering drugs.

**Discontinuing:**
May be unnecessary to finish medicine. Follow doctor's instructions.

**Others:**
- Great potential for abuse.
- Consult doctor about fluids, diet and rest.

## POSSIBLE INTERACTION WITH OTHER DRUGS

| GENERIC NAME OR DRUG CLASS | COMBINED EFFECT |
|---|---|
| Amantadine | Increased belladonna effect. |
| Analgesics | Increased analgesic effect. |
| Antidepressants | Increased sedative effect. |
| Antihistamines | Increased sedative effect. |
| Cortisone drugs | Increased internal-eye pressure. |
| Digoxin | Decreases absorption of digoxin. Separate doses by at least 2 hours. |
| Haloperidol | Increased internal-eye pressure. |
| Lincomycin | Decreases absorption of lincomycin. Separate doses by at least 2 hours. |
| MAO inhibitors | Increased belladonna effect. |
| Meperidine | Increased belladonna effect. |
| Methylphenidate | Increased belladonna effect. |

*Continued page 968*

## POSSIBLE INTERACTION WITH OTHER SUBSTANCES

| INTERACTS WITH | COMBINED EFFECT |
|---|---|
| Alcohol: | Increases alcohol's intoxicating effect, increased diarrhea, prevents action of kaolin and pectin. Avoid. |
| Beverages: | No problems expected. |
| Cocaine: | Aggravates underlying disease. Avoid. |
| Foods: | No problems expected. |
| Marijuana: | Impairs physical and mental performance, aggravates underlying disease. Avoid. |
| Tobacco: | Aggravates underlying disease. Avoid. |

# KAOLIN, PECTIN & PAREGORIC

## BRAND NAMES

Parepectolin

## BASIC INFORMATION

**Habit forming? Yes**
**Prescription needed? Yes**
**Available as generic? Yes**
**Drug class: Narcotic, antidiarrheal,**
**antispasmodic**

 ## USES

- Reduces intestinal cramps and diarrhea.
- Relieves pain.

 ## DOSAGE & USAGE INFORMATION

**How to take:**
Liquid—Swallow prescribed dosage (without diluting) after each loose bowel movement.

**When to take:**
After each loose bowel movement. No more often then every 4 hours.

**If you forget a dose:**
Take when you remember.

**What drug does:**
Makes loose stools less watery, but may not prevent loss of fluids.

**Time lapse before drug works:**
15 to 30 minutes.

**Don't take with:**
See Interaction column and consult doctor.

 ## OVERDOSE

**SYMPTOMS:**
**Deep sleep; slow breathing; slow pulse; flushed, warm skin.**
**WHAT TO DO:**
- **Dial 0 (operator) or 911 (emergency) for an ambulance or medical help. Then give first aid immediately.**
- **If patient is unconscious and not breathing, give mouth-to-mouth breathing. If there is no heartbeat, use cardiac massage and mouth-to-mouth breathing (CPR). Don't try to make patient vomit. If you can't get help quickly, take patient to nearest emergency facility.**
- **See emergency information on inside covers.**

 ## POSSIBLE ADVERSE REACTIONS OR SIDE EFFECTS

| SYMPTOMS | WHAT TO DO |
|---|---|
| **Life-threatening:** | |
| Unusually rapid heartbeat (over 100), difficult breathing, slow heartbeat (under 50/minute). | Discontinue. Seek emergency treatment. |
| **Common:** | |
| (with large dosage) Weakness, increased sweating, red or flushed face, lightheadedness, headache, dry mouth, dry skin, drowsiness, dizziness, frequent urination, decreased sweating, constipation, confusion. | Continue. Call doctor when convenient. |
| **Infrequent:** | |
| • Taste sense reduced, nervousness, sunlight hurts eyes, blurred vision. | Discontinue. Call doctor right away. |
| • Diminished sex drive. | Continue. Call doctor when convenient. |
| **Rare:** | |
| Bloating, abdominal cramps and vomiting, eye pain, hallucinations, shortness of breath, rash, itchy skin. | Discontinue. Call doctor right away. |

## WARNINGS & PRECAUTIONS

**Don't take if:**
You are allergic to any narcotic, kaolin or pectin.

**Before you start, consult your doctor:**
- If you have impaired liver or kidney function, chronic medical problem with heart disease, peptic ulcer, asthma or others, fever over 101F.
- If patient is child or infant.
- If you will have surgery within 2 months, including dental surgery, requiring general or spinal anesthesia.

**Over age 60:**
Fluid loss caused by diarrhea, especially if taking other medicines, may lead to serious disability. Consult doctor.

**Pregnancy:**
Abuse by pregnant woman will result in addicted newborn. Withdrawal of newborn can be life-threatening.

**Breast-feeding:**
Drug filters into milk. May harm child. Avoid.

**Infants & children:**
Fluid loss caused by diarrhea in infants and children can cause serious dehydration. Consult doctor before giving any medicine for diarrhea.

**Prolonged use:**
Causes psychological and physical dependence. Not recommended.

**Skin & sunlight:**
May cause rash or intensify sunburn in areas exposed to sun or sunlamp.

**Driving, piloting or hazardous work:**
Don't drive or pilot aircraft until you learn how medicine affects you. Don't work around dangerous machinery. Don't climb ladders or work in high places. Danger increases if you drink alcohol or take medicine affecting alertness and reflexes, such as antihistamines, tranquilizers, sedatives, pain medicine, narcotics and mind-altering drugs.

**Discontinuing:**
May be unnecessary to finish medicine. Follow doctor's instructions.

**Others:**
Consult doctor about fluids, diet and rest.

## POSSIBLE INTERACTION WITH OTHER DRUGS

| GENERIC NAME OR DRUG CLASS | COMBINED EFFECT |
| --- | --- |
| Analgesics (other) | Increased analgesic effect. |
| Anticholinergics | Increased anticholinergic effect. |
| Antidepressants | Increased sedative effect. |
| Antihistamines | Increased sedative effect. |
| Digoxin | Decreases absorption of digoxin. Separate doses by at least 2 hours. |
| Lincomycin | Decreases absorption of lincomycin. Separate doses by at least 2 hours. |
| Mind-altering drugs | Increased sedative effect. |
| Narcotics (other) | Increased narcotic effect. |
| Phenothiazines | Increased phenothiazine effect. |
| Sedatives | Increased sedative effect. |
| Sleep inducers | Increased sedative effect. |
| Terfenadine | Possible oversedation. |
| Tranquilizers | Increased sedative effect. |
| All other oral medicines | Decreases absorption of other medicines. Separate doses by at least 2 hours. |

## POSSIBLE INTERACTION WITH OTHER SUBSTANCES

| INTERACTS WITH | COMBINED EFFECT |
| --- | --- |
| Alcohol: | Increases alcohol's intoxicating effect, increased diarrhea, prevents action of kaolin and pectin. Avoid. |
| Beverages: | No problems expected. |
| Cocaine: | Increased cocaine toxic effects, aggravates underlying disease. Avoid. |
| Foods: | No problems expected. |
| Marijuana: | Aggravates underlying disease. Avoid. |
| Tobacco: | Aggravates underlying disease. Avoid. |

# KETOCONAZOLE

## BRAND NAMES

**Nizoral**

## BASIC INFORMATION

**Habit forming? No**
**Prescription needed? Yes**
**Available as generic? No**
**Drug class: Antifungal**

 ## USES

Treatment of fungus infections susceptible to ketoconazole.

 ## DOSAGE & USAGE INFORMATION

**How to take:**
Tablet or capsule—Swallow with liquid or food to lessen stomach irritation. If you can't swallow whole, crumble tablet or open capsule and take with liquid or food.

**When to take:**
At same time once a day.

**If you forget a dose:**
Take as soon as you remember up to 2 hours late. If more than 2 hours, wait for next scheduled dose (don't double this dose).

**What drug does:**
Prevents fungi from growing and reproducing.

**Time lapse before drug works:**
8 to 10 months or longer.

**Don't take with:**
See Interaction column and consult doctor.

 ## OVERDOSE

**SYMPTOMS:**
**Nausea, vomiting, diarrhea.**
**WHAT TO DO:**
**Overdose unlikely to threaten life. If person takes much larger amount than prescribed, call doctor, poison-control center or hospital emergency room for instructions.**

 ## POSSIBLE ADVERSE REACTIONS OR SIDE EFFECTS

| SYMPTOMS | WHAT TO DO |
|---|---|
| **Life-threatening:**<br>None expected. | |
| **Common:**<br>Nausea or vomiting. | Discontinue. Call doctor right away. |
| **Infrequent:** | |
| • Rash or itchy skin, increased sensitivity to light. | Discontinue. Call doctor right away. |
| • Drowsiness, insomnia, diarrhea. | Continue. Call doctor when convenient. |
| **Rare:** | |
| • Pale stools, abdominal pain, dark or amber urine. | Discontinue. Call doctor right away. |
| • Diminished sex drive in males, tiredness, weakness. | Continue. Call doctor when convenient. |

## WARNINGS & PRECAUTIONS

**Don't take if:**
You are allergic to ketoconazole.

**Before you start, consult your doctor:**
- If you have absence of stomach acid (achlorhydria).
- If you have liver disease.

**Over age 60:**
Adverse reactions and side effects may be more frequent and severe than in younger persons.

**Pregnancy:**
Risk to unborn child outweighs drug benefits. Don't use.

**Breast-feeding:**
Drug passes into milk. Avoid drug or discontinue nursing until you finish medicine. Consult doctor for advice on maintaining milk supply.

**Infants & children:**
Only under close medical supervision.

**Prolonged use:**
Request liver-function studies.

**Skin & sunlight:**
No problems expected.

**Driving, piloting or hazardous work:**
Don't drive or pilot aircraft until you learn how medicine affects you. Don't work around dangerous machinery. Don't climb ladders or work in high places. Danger increases if you drink alcohol or take medicine affecting alertness and reflexes, such as antihistamines, tranquilizers, sedatives, pain medicine, narcotics and mind-altering drugs.

**Discontinuing:**
May be unnecessary to finish medicine. Follow doctor's instructions.

**Others:**
No problems expected.

## POSSIBLE INTERACTION WITH OTHER DRUGS

| GENERIC NAME OR DRUG CLASS | COMBINED EFFECT |
|---|---|
| Antacids | Decreased absorption of ketoconazole. |
| Anticholinergics | Decreased absorption of ketoconazole. |
| Atropine | Decreased absorption of ketoconazole. |
| Belladonna | Decreased absorption of ketoconazole. |
| Cimetidine | Decreased absorption of ketoconazole. |
| Clidinium | Decreased absorption of ketoconazole. |
| Glycopyrrolate | Decreased absorption of ketoconazole. |
| Hyoscyamine | Decreased absorption of ketoconazole. |
| Methscopolamine | Decreased absorption of ketoconazole. |
| Propantheline | Decreased absorption of ketoconazole. |
| Ranitidine | Decreased absorption of ketoconazole. |
| Scopolamine | Decreased absorption of ketoconazole. |

## POSSIBLE INTERACTION WITH OTHER SUBSTANCES

| INTERACTS WITH | COMBINED EFFECT |
|---|---|
| Alcohol: | Increased chance of liver damage. |
| Beverages: | No problems expected. |
| Cocaine: | Decreased ketoconazole effect. Avoid cocaine. |
| Foods: | No problems expected. |
| Marijuana: | Decreased ketoconazole effect. Avoid marijuana. |
| Tobacco: | Decreased ketoconazole effect. Avoid tobacco. |

# KETOPROFEN

## BRAND NAMES

Alrheumat          Orudis-E
Orudis             Profenid

## BASIC INFORMATION

**Habit forming? No**
**Prescription needed? Yes**
**Available as generic? No**
**Drug class: Analgesic, antidysmenorreal**
          **(non-steroidal anti-inflammatory**
          **analgesic [NSAIA])**

## USES

- Treatment of pain.
- Treatment of soft-tissue athletic injuries.
- Treats dysmenorrhea.

## DOSAGE & USAGE INFORMATION

**How to take:**
- Extended-release tablets or capsules—Swallow dose whole. If you take regular tablets, you may chew or crush them.
- Tablets or capsules—Swallow whole with liquid or food to lessen stomach irritation.
- Suppositories—Remove wrapper and moisten suppository with water. Gently insert into rectum, large end first. If suppository is too soft, chill in refrigerator or cool water before removing wrapper.
- Capsule—Take with full glass of water while sitting or standing upright. Take on any empty stomach either 1/2 hour before or 2 hours after meals. If stomach irritation occurs, may take with food or aluminum hydroxide or magnesium hydroxide antacids.

**When to take:**
At the same times each day.

**If you forget a dose:**
Take as soon as you remember up to 2 hours late. If more than 2 hours, wait for next scheduled dose (don't double this dose).

*Continued next column*

## OVERDOSE

**SYMPTOMS:**
**Confusion, agitation, incoherence, convulsions, possible hemorrhage from stomach or intestine, coma.**
**WHAT TO DO:**
- **Dial 0 (operator) or 911 (emergency) for an ambulance or medical help. Then give first aid immediately.**
- **See emergency information on inside covers.**

**What drug does:**
Reduces tissue concentration of prostaglandins (hormones which produce inflammation and pain).

**Time lapse before drug works:**
Begins in 4 to 24 hours. May require 3 weeks regular use for maximum benefit.

**Don't take with:**
- Large doses of acetaminophen. Combination increases possibility of kidney damage.
- See Interaction column and consult doctor.

## POSSIBLE ADVERSE REACTIONS OR SIDE EFFECTS

| SYMPTOMS | WHAT TO DO |
|---|---|
| **Life-threatening:** | |
| Hives, rash, intense itching, faintness soon after a dose (anaphylaxis); breathing difficulty; tightness in chest; rapid heartbeat. | Discontinue. Seek emergency treatment. |
| **Common:** | |
| Dizziness, headache, nausea, pain, depression, drowsiness, ringing in ears. | Continue. Call doctor when convenient. |
| **Infrequent:** | |
| • Flank pain. | Discontinue. Call doctor right away. |
| • Constipation or diarrhea, vomiting. | Continue. Call doctor when convenient. |
| **Rare:** | |
| • Bloody or black, tarry stools; convulsions; confusion; rash, hives or itch; blurred vision; unusual bleeding or bruising; jaundice; blood in urine; difficult, painful or frequent urination. | Discontinue. Call doctor right away. |
| • Fatigue, weakness. | Continue. Call doctor when convenient. |

## WARNINGS & PRECAUTIONS

**Don't take if:**
- You are allergic to ketoprofen, aspirin or any non-steroid, anti-inflammatory drug.
- You have gastritis, peptic ulcer, enteritis, ileitis, ulcerative colitis, asthma, heart failure, high blood pressure or bleeding problems.
- Patient is younger than 15.

**Before you start, consult your doctor:**
- If you have epilepsy or Parkinson's disease.
- If you have been mentally ill.
- If you have had kidney disease or impaired kidney function.

**Over age 60:**
Adverse reactions and side effects may be more frequent and severe than in younger persons.

**Pregnancy:**
Studies inconclusive on harm to unborn child. Decide with your doctor whether drug benefits justify risk to unborn child.

**Breast-feeding:**
May harm child. Avoid.

**Infants & children:**
Not recommended for anyone younger than 15. Use only under medical supervision.

**Prolonged use:**
- Eye damage.
- Reduced hearing.
- Sore throat, fever.
- Weight gain.

**Skin & sunlight:**
No problems expected.

**Driving, piloting or hazardous work:**
Don't drive or pilot aircraft until you learn how medicine affects you. Don't work around dangerous machinery. Don't climb ladders or work in high places. Danger increases if you drink alcohol or take medicine affecting alertness and reflexes, such as antihistamines, tranquilizers, sedatives, pain medicine, narcotics and mind-altering drugs.

**Discontinuing:**
Don't discontinue without consulting doctor. Dose may require gradual reduction if you have taken drug for a long time. Doses of other drugs may also require adjustment.

**Others:**
No problems expected.

## POSSIBLE INTERACTION WITH OTHER DRUGS

| GENERIC NAME OR DRUG CLASS | COMBINED EFFECT |
|---|---|
| Acebutolol | Decreased antihypertensive effect of acebutolol. |
| Anticoagulants (oral) | Increased risk of bleeding. |
| Any other non-steroidal anti-inflammatory analgesic, such as: fenoprofen, ibuprofen, indomethacin, meclofenamate, naproxen, oxyphenbutazone, phenylbutazone, salicylates, sulindac, tolmetin | Increased possibility of internal bleeding. |
| Aspirin | Increased risk of stomach ulcer. |
| Cortisone drugs | Increased risk of stomach ulcer and bleeding. |
| Furosemide | Decreased diuretic effect of furosemide. |
| Gold compounds | Possible increased likelihood of kidney damage. |
| Lithium | May increase lithium in blood. |
| Minoxidil | Decreased minoxidil effect. |
| Nifedipine | Increases chance of nifedipine toxicity. |
| Oxprenolol | Increased antihypertensive effect of oxprenolol. |
| Oxyphenbutazone | Possible stomach ulcer. |
| Phenylbutazone | Possible stomach ulcer. |
| Probenecid | Increased ketoprofen effect. |
| Thyroid hormones | Rapid heartbeat, blood-pressure rise. |
| Verapamil | Increases chance of verapamil toxicity. |

## POSSIBLE INTERACTION WITH OTHER SUBSTANCES

| INTERACTS WITH | COMBINED EFFECT |
|---|---|
| Alcohol: | Possible stomach ulcer or bleeding. Avoid. |
| Beverages: | None expected. |
| Cocaine: | None expected. |
| Foods: | None expected. |
| Marijuana: | Increased pain relief from ketoprofen. |
| Tobacco: | None expected. |

# LABETOLOL

## BRAND NAMES

Normodyne          Trandate

## BASIC INFORMATION

Habit forming? No
Prescription needed? Yes
Available as generic? No
Drug class: Antihypertensive (beta- and
              alpha-adrenergic blocker)

 USES

Controls, but doesn't cure, high blood pressure.

 DOSAGE & USAGE
INFORMATION

**How to take:**
Tablets or capsules—Swallow whole with liquid
or food to lessen stomach irritation.

**When to take:**
With meals or milk at same times each day.

**If you forget a dose:**
Take as soon as you remember up to 3 hours
late. If more than 3 hours, wait for next
scheduled dose (don't double this dose).

**What drug does:**
• Blocks transmission of impulses in
  sympathetic nervous system.
• Slows nerve impulses through heart.

**Time lapse before drug works:**
1 to 4 hours.

**Don't take with:**
See Interaction column and consult doctor.

 OVERDOSE

**SYMPTOMS:**
Fainting, convulsions, coma.
**WHAT TO DO:**
• Dial 0 (operator) or 911 (emergency) for an
  ambulance or medical help. Then give first
  aid immediately.
• See emergency information on inside
  covers.

 POSSIBLE
ADVERSE REACTIONS
OR SIDE EFFECTS

| SYMPTOMS | WHAT TO DO |
|---|---|
| **Life-threatening:**<br>Congestive heart failure (weight gain, rapid pulse, breathlessness on exertion, swelling of feet and abdomen). | Discontinue. Seek emergency treatment. |
| **Common:**<br>None expected. | |
| **Infrequent:**<br>Taste change, diminished sex drive, dizziness, drowsiness, headache, itchy skin, skin and scalp numbness and tingling, abdominal pain, stuffy nose, vomiting. | Discontinue. Call doctor right away. |
| **Rare:**<br>Jaundice. | Discontinue. Call doctor right away. |

## WARNINGS & PRECAUTIONS

**Don't take if:**
- You are allergic to any alpha- or beta-blocking agent.
- You have asthma, congestive heart failure, heart block.

**Before you start, consult your doctor:**
- If you have allergies, coronary artery disease, liver disease, overactive thyroid function, chronic kidney disease.
- If you will have surgery within 2 months, including dental surgery, requiring general or spinal anesthesia.

**Over age 60:**
Adverse reactions and side effects may be more frequent and severe than in younger persons. Ask doctor about smaller doses.

**Pregnancy:**
Risk to unborn child outweighs drug benefits. Don't use.

**Breast-feeding:**
Risk to unborn child outweighs drug benefits. Don't use.

**Infants & children:**
Use only under close medical supervision.

**Prolonged use:**
Weakens heart muscle contractions.

**Skin & sunlight:**
No problems expected.

**Driving, piloting or hazardous work:**
Don't drive or pilot aircraft until you learn how medicine affects you. Don't work around dangerous machinery. Don't climb ladders or work in high places. Danger increases if you drink alcohol or take medicine affecting alertness and reflexes, such as antihistamines, tranquilizers, sedatives, pain medicine, narcotics and mind-altering drugs.

**Discontinuing:**
- Don't discontinue without consulting doctor. Dose may require gradual reduction if you have taken drug for a long time. Doses of other drugs may also require adjustment.
- These symptoms may occur if you stop taking labetolol abruptly—Chest pain, headache, sweating, weakness, trembling, fast or irregular heartbeat.

**Others:**
- You may need to take some form of antihypertensive treatment for the remainder of your life.
- May mask hypoglycemia.
- Get up slowly after sitting or lying to prevent fainting or dizziness.

## POSSIBLE INTERACTION WITH OTHER DRUGS

| GENERIC NAME OR DRUG CLASS | COMBINED EFFECT |
|---|---|
| Antidiabetics | Increased antidiabetic effect, may mask hypoglycemia. |
| Cimetidine | Increased antihypertensive effect of labetolol. |
| Clonidine | May cause precipitous change in blood pressure if clonidine and labetolol are discontinued simultaneously. |
| Diuretics | Increased antihypertensive effect. |
| Insulin | Increased antidiabetic effect, may mask hypoglycemia. |
| Nitroglycerin | Increased antihypertensive effect. |
| Phentolamine | Increased antihypertensive effect. |

## POSSIBLE INTERACTION WITH OTHER SUBSTANCES

| INTERACTS WITH | COMBINED EFFECT |
|---|---|
| Alcohol: | Excessive blood pressure drop. Avoid. |
| Beverages: | No problems expected. |
| Cocaine: | Irregular heartbeat, unusual anxiety. Avoid. |
| Foods: | No problems expected. |
| Marijuana: | Daily use—Impaired circulation to hands and feet. |
| Tobacco: | Irregular heartbeat. Avoid. |

# LACTULOSE

## BRAND NAMES

Cephalac                Chronulac

## BASIC INFORMATION

**Habit forming? No**
**Prescription needed? No**
**Available as generic? No**
**Drug class: Laxative (hyperosmotic)**

 ## USES

Constipation relief.

 ## DOSAGE & USAGE INFORMATION

**How to take:**
Liquid—Dilute dose in beverage before swallowing.

**When to take:**
Usually once a day, preferably in the morning.

**If you forget a dose:**
Take as soon as you remember up to 8 hours before bedtime. If later, wait for next scheduled dose (don't double this dose). Don't take at bedtime.

**What drug does:**
Draws water into bowel from other body tissues. Causes distention through fluid accumulation, which promotes soft stool and accelerates bowel motion.

**Time lapse before drug works:**
30 minutes to 3 hours.

**Don't take with:**
Another medicine. Space 2 hours apart.

 ## OVERDOSE

**SYMPTOMS:**
**Fluid depletion, weakness, vomiting, fainting.**
**WHAT TO DO:**
**Overdose unlikely to threaten life. If person takes much larger amount than prescribed, call doctor, poison-control center or hospital emergency room for instructions.**

 ## POSSIBLE ADVERSE REACTIONS OR SIDE EFFECTS

| SYMPTOMS | WHAT TO DO |
|---|---|
| **Life-threatening:** None expected. | |
| **Common:** None expected. | |
| **Infrequent:** | |
| • Irregular heartbeat. | Discontinue. Call doctor right away. |
| • Increased thirst, cramps, nausea, diarrhea, gaseousness. | Continue. Tell doctor at next visit. |
| **Rare:** Dizziness, confusion, fatigue, weakness. | Continue. Call doctor when convenient. |

## WARNINGS & PRECAUTIONS

**Don't take if:**
- You are allergic to any hyperosmotic laxative.
- You have symptoms of appendicitis, inflamed bowel or intestinal blockage.
- You have missed a bowel movement for only 1 or 2 days.

**Before you start, consult your doctor:**
- If you have congestive heart disease.
- If you have diabetes.
- If you have high blood pressure.
- If you have a colostomy or ileostomy.
- If you have kidney disease.
- If you have a laxative habit.
- If you have rectal bleeding.
- If you take another laxative.
- If you require a low-galactose diet.

**Over age 60:**
Adverse reactions and side effects may be more frequent and severe than in younger persons.

**Pregnancy:**
No proven problems. Avoid if possible.

**Breast-feeding:**
No problems expected.

**Infants & children:**
Use only under medical supervision.

**Prolonged use:**
Don't take for more than 1 week unless under a doctor's supervision. May cause laxative dependence.

**Skin & sunlight:**
No problems expected.

**Driving, piloting or hazardous work:**
No problems expected.

**Discontinuing:**
May be unnecessary to finish medicine. Follow doctor's instructions.

**Others:**
Don't take to "flush out" your system or as a "tonic."

## POSSIBLE INTERACTION WITH OTHER DRUGS

| GENERIC NAME OR DRUG CLASS | COMBINED EFFECT |
|---|---|
| None | |

## POSSIBLE INTERACTION WITH OTHER SUBSTANCES

| INTERACTS WITH | COMBINED EFFECT |
|---|---|
| Alcohol: | None expected. |
| Beverages: | None expected. |
| Cocaine: | None expected. |
| Foods: | None expected. |
| Marijuana: | None expected. |
| Tobacco: | None expected. |

# LEVODOPA

## BRAND NAMES

Bendopa      Levopa
Dopar        Sinemet
Larodopa

## BASIC INFORMATION

Habit forming? No
Prescription needed? Yes
Available as generic? Yes
Drug class: Antiparkinsonism

## USES

Controls Parkinson's disease symptoms such as rigidity, tremor and unsteady gait.

## DOSAGE & USAGE INFORMATION

**How to take:**
Tablet or capsule—Swallow with liquid or food to lessen stomach irritation. If you can't swallow whole, crumble tablet or open capsule and take with liquid or food.

**When to take:**
At the same times each day.

**If you forget a dose:**
Take as soon as you remember up to 2 hours late. If more than 2 hours, wait for next scheduled dose (don't double this dose).

**What drug does:**
Restores chemical balance necessary for normal nerve impulses.

*Continued next column*

## OVERDOSE

**SYMPTOMS:**
Muscle twitch, spastic eyelid closure, nausea, vomiting, diarrhea, irregular and rapid pulse, weakness, fainting, confusion, agitation, hallucination, coma.
**WHAT TO DO:**
- Dial 0 (operator) or 911 (emergency) for an ambulance or medical help. Then give first aid immediately.
- If patient is unconscious and not breathing, give mouth-to-mouth breathing. If there is no heartbeat, use cardiac massage and mouth-to-mouth breathing (CPR). Don't try to make patient vomit. If you can't get help quickly, take patient to nearest emergency facility.
- See emergency information on inside covers.

**Time lapse before drug works:**
2 to 3 weeks to improve; 6 weeks or longer for maximum benefit.

**Don't take with:**
See Interaction column and consult doctor.

## POSSIBLE ADVERSE REACTIONS OR SIDE EFFECTS

| SYMPTOMS | WHAT TO DO |
|---|---|
| **Life-threatening:** None expected. | |
| **Common:** | |
| • Mood change, uncontrollable body movements, diarrhea. | Continue. Call doctor when convenient. |
| • Dry mouth, body odor. | No action necessary. |
| **Infrequent:** | |
| • Fainting, severe dizziness, headache, insomnia, nightmares, itchy skin, rash, nausea, vomiting, irregular heartbeat. | Discontinue. Call doctor right away. |
| • Flushed face, muscle twitching, discolored or dark urine, difficult urination, blurred vision. | Continue. Call doctor when convenient. |
| • Constipation, tiredness. | Continue. Tell doctor at next visit. |
| **Rare:** | |
| • High blood pressure. | Discontinue. Call doctor right away. |
| • Duodenal ulcer, anemia. | Continue. Call doctor when convenient. |

## WARNINGS & PRECAUTIONS

**Don't take if:**
- You are allergic to levodopa or carbidopa.
- You have taken MAO inhibitors in past 2 weeks.
- You have glaucoma (narrow-angle type).

**Before you start, consult your doctor:**
- If you have diabetes or epilepsy.
- If you have had high blood pressure, heart or lung disease.
- If you have had liver or kidney disease.
- If you have a peptic ulcer.
- If you have malignant melanoma.
- If you will have surgery within 2 months, including dental surgery, requiring general or spinal anesthesia.

**Over age 60:**
Adverse reactions and side effects may be more frequent and severe than in younger persons.

**Pregnancy:**
Risk to unborn child outweighs drug benefits. Don't use.

**Breast-feeding:**
Drug filters into milk. May harm child. Avoid.

**Infants & children:**
Not recommended.

**Prolonged use:**
May lead to uncontrolled movements of head, face, mouth, tongue, arms or legs.

**Skin & sunlight:**
No problems expected.

**Driving, piloting or hazardous work:**
Don't drive or pilot aircraft until you learn how medicine affects you. Don't work around dangerous machinery. Don't climb ladders or work in high places. Danger increases if you drink alcohol or take medicine affecting alertness and reflexes, such as antihistamines, tranquilizers, sedatives, pain medicine, narcotics and mind-altering drugs.

**Discontinuing:**
Don't discontinue without doctor's advice until you complete prescribed dose, even though symptoms diminish or disappear.

**Others:**
Expect to start with small dose and increase gradually to lessen frequency and severity of adverse reactions.

## POSSIBLE INTERACTION WITH OTHER DRUGS

| GENERIC NAME OR DRUG CLASS | COMBINED EFFECT |
|---|---|
| Albuterol | Increased risk of heartbeat irregularity. |
| Antiparkinsonism drugs (other) | Increased levodopa effect. |
| Haloperidol | Decreased levodopa effect. |
| MAO inhibitors | Dangerous rise in blood pressure. |
| Methyldopa | Decreased levodopa effect. |
| Molindone | Decreased levodopa effect. |
| Papaverine | Decreased levodopa effect. |
| Phenothiazines | Decreased levodopa effect. |
| Pyridoxine (Vitamin B-6) | Decreased levodopa effect. |
| Rauwolfia alkaloids | Decreased levodopa effect. |

## POSSIBLE INTERACTION WITH OTHER SUBSTANCES

| INTERACTS WITH | COMBINED EFFECT |
|---|---|
| Alcohol: | None expected. |
| Beverages: | None expected. |
| Cocaine: | Decreased levodopa effect. |
| Foods: | None expected. |
| Marijuana: | Increased fatigue, lethargy, fainting. |
| Tobacco: | None expected. |

# LINCOMYCIN

## BRAND AND GENERIC NAMES

Cleocin

CLINDAYCIN

Dalacin C

Lincocin

LINCOMYCIN

## BASIC INFORMATION

**Habit forming?** No
**Prescription needed?** Yes
**Available as generic?** No
**Drug class:** Antibiotic (lincomycin)

 ## USES

Treatment of bacterial infections that are susceptible to lincomycin.

 ## DOSAGE & USAGE INFORMATION

**How to take:**
Capsule or liquid—Swallow with liquid 1 hour before or 2 hours after eating.

**When to take:**
At the same times each day.

**If you forget a dose:**
Take as soon as you remember up to 2 hours late. If more than 2 hours, wait for next scheduled dose (don't double this dose).

**What drug does:**
Destroys susceptible bacteria. Does not kill viruses.

**Time lapse before drug works:**
3 to 5 days.

**Don't take with:**
See Interaction column and consult doctor.

 ## OVERDOSE

**SYMPTOMS:**
Severe nausea, vomiting, diarrhea.
**WHAT TO DO:**
Overdose unlikely to threaten life. If person takes much larger amount than prescribed, call doctor, poison-control center or hospital emergency room for instructions.

 ## POSSIBLE ADVERSE REACTIONS OR SIDE EFFECTS

| SYMPTOMS | WHAT TO DO |
|---|---|
| **Life-threatening:** None expected. | |
| **Common:** None expected. | |
| **Infrequent:** Unusual thirst; vomiting; stomach cramps; severe and watery diarrhea with blood or mucus; painful, swollen joints; jaundice; fever; tiredness; weakness; weight loss; rash; itch around groin, rectum or armpits; white patches in mouth; vaginal discharge, itching. | Discontinue. Call doctor right away. |
| **Rare:** None expected. | |

## WARNINGS & PRECAUTIONS

**Don't take if:**
- You are allergic to lincomycins.
- You have had ulcerative colitis.
- Prescribed for infant under 1 month old.

**Before you start, consult your doctor:**
- If you have had yeast infections of mouth, skin or vagina.
- If you will have surgery within 2 months, including dental surgery, requiring general or spinal anesthesia.
- If you have kidney or liver disease.
- If you have allergies of any kind.

**Over age 60:**
Adverse reactions and side effects may be more frequent and severe than in younger persons.

**Pregnancy:**
Risk to unborn child outweighs drug benefits. Don't use.

**Breast-feeding:**
Drug passes into milk. Avoid drug or discontinue nursing until you finish medicine. Consult doctor for advice on maintaining milk supply.

**Infants & children:**
Don't give to infants younger than 1 month. Use for children only under medical supervision.

**Prolonged use:**
- Severe colitis with diarrhea and bleeding.
- You may become more susceptible to infections caused by germs not responsive to lincomycin.

**Skin & sunlight:**
No problems expected.

**Driving, piloting or hazardous work:**
No problems expected.

**Discontinuing:**
Don't discontinue without doctor's advice until you complete prescribed dose, even though symptoms diminish or disappear.

**Others:**
No problems expected.

 ## POSSIBLE INTERACTION WITH OTHER DRUGS

| GENERIC NAME OR DRUG CLASS | COMBINED EFFECT |
| --- | --- |
| Antidiarrheal preparations | Decreased lincomycin effect. |
| Chloramphenicol | Decreased lincomycin effect. |
| Erythromycin | Decreased lincomycin effect. |
| Loperamide | May delay removal of toxins from colon in cases of diarrhea caused by side effects of lincomycin. |

## POSSIBLE INTERACTION WITH OTHER SUBSTANCES

| INTERACTS WITH | COMBINED EFFECT |
| --- | --- |
| Alcohol: | None expected. |
| Beverages: | None expected. |
| Cocaine: | None expected. |
| Foods: | None expected. |
| Marijuana: | None expected. |
| Tobacco: | None expected. |

# LIOTHYRONINE

## BRAND NAMES

Cytomel                    Tertroxin
Ro-Thyronine

## BASIC INFORMATION

**Habit forming? No**
**Prescription needed? Yes**
**Available as generic? Yes**
**Drug class: Thyroid hormone**

## USES

Replacement for thyroid hormone deficiency.

## DOSAGE & USAGE INFORMATION

**How to take:**
- Tablet or capsule—Swallow with liquid.
- Extended-release tablets or capsules—Swallow each dose whole. If you take regular tablets, you may chew or crush them.

**When to take:**
At the same time each day before a meal or on awakening.

**If you forget a dose:**
Take as soon as you remember up to 12 hours late. If more than 12 hours, wait for next scheduled dose (don't double this dose).

**What drug does:**
Increases cell metabolism rate.

**Time lapse before drug works:**
48 hours.

**Don't take with:**
See Interaction column and consult doctor.

## OVERDOSE

**SYMPTOMS:**
**"Hot" feeling, heart palpitations, nervousness, sweating, hand tremors, insomnia, rapid and irregular pulse, headache, irritability, diarrhea, weight loss, muscle cramps.**
**WHAT TO DO:**
**Overdose unlikely to threaten life. If person takes much larger amount than prescribed, call doctor, poison-control center or hospital emergency room for instructions.**

## POSSIBLE ADVERSE REACTIONS OR SIDE EFFECTS

| SYMPTOMS | WHAT TO DO |
|---|---|
| **Life-threatening:**<br>None expected. | |
| **Common:** | |
| • Tremor, headache, irritability, insomnia. | Discontinue. Call doctor right away. |
| • Appetite change, diarrhea, leg cramps, menstrual irregularities, fever, heat sensitivity, unusual sweating, weight loss. | Continue. Call doctor when convenient. |
| **Infrequent:**<br>Hives, rash, chest pain, rapid and irregular heartbeat, shortness of breath, vomiting. | Discontinue. Call doctor right away. |
| **Rare:**<br>None expected. | |

# LIOTHYRONINE

## WARNINGS & PRECAUTIONS

**Don't take if:**
- You have had a heart attack within 6 weeks.
- You have no thyroid deficiency, but use this to lose weight.

**Before you start, consult your doctor:**
- If you have heart disease or high blood pressure.
- If you have diabetes.
- If you have Addison's disease, have had adrenal gland deficiency or use epinephrine, ephedrine or isoproterenol for asthma.

**Over age 60:**
More sensitive to thyroid hormone. May need smaller doses.

**Pregnancy:**
Considered safe if for thyroid deficiency only.

**Breast-feeding:**
Present in milk. Considered safe if dose is correct.

**Infants & children:**
Use only under medical supervision.

**Prolonged use:**
No problems expected, if dose is correct.

**Skin & sunlight:**
No problems expected.

**Driving, piloting or hazardous work:**
No problems expected.

**Discontinuing:**
Don't discontinue without consulting doctor. Dose may require gradual reduction if you have taken drug for a long time. Doses of other drugs may also require adjustment.

**Others:**
Digestive upsets, tremors, cramps, nervousness, insomnia or diarrhea may indicate need for dose adjustment.

## POSSIBLE INTERACTION WITH OTHER DRUGS

| GENERIC NAME OR DRUG CLASS | COMBINED EFFECT |
|---|---|
| Amphetamines | Increased amphetamine effect. |
| Anticoagulants (oral) | Increased anticoagulant effect. |
| Antidepressants (tricyclic) | Irregular heartbeat. |
| Antidiabetics | Antidiabetic may require adjustment. |
| Aspirin (large doses, continuous use) | Increased liothyronine effect. |
| Barbiturates | Decreased barbiturate effect. |
| Cholestyramine | Decreased liothyronine effect. |
| Contraceptives (oral) | Decreased liothyronine effect. |
| Cortisone drugs | Requires dose adjustment to prevent cortisone deficiency. |
| Digitalis preparations | Increased digitalis effect. |
| Ephedrine | Increased ephedrine effect. |
| Epinephrine | Increased epinephrine effect. |
| Methylphenidate | Increased methylphenidate effect. |
| Phenytoin | Increased liothyronine effect. |

## POSSIBLE INTERACTION WITH OTHER SUBSTANCES

| INTERACTS WITH | COMBINED EFFECT |
|---|---|
| Alcohol: | None expected. |
| Beverages: | None expected. |
| Cocaine: | Excess stimulation. Avoid. |
| Foods: Soybeans. | Heavy consumption interferes with thyroid function. |
| Marijuana: | None expected. |
| Tobacco: | None expected. |

# LIOTRIX

## BRAND NAMES

Euthroid          Thyrolar

## BASIC INFORMATION

**Habit forming?** No
**Prescription needed?** Yes
**Available as generic?** Yes
**Drug class:** Thyroid hormone

## USES

Replacement for thyroid hormone deficiency.

## DOSAGE & USAGE INFORMATION

**How to take:**
- Tablet or capsule—Swallow with liquid.
- Extended-release tablets or capsules—Swallow each dose whole. If you take regular tablets, you may chew or crush them.

**When to take:**
At the same time each day before a meal or on awakening.

**If you forget a dose:**
Take as soon as you remember up to 12 hours late. If more than 12 hours, wait for next scheduled dose (don't double this dose).

**What drug does:**
Increases cell metabolism rate.

**Time lapse before drug works:**
48 hours.

**Don't take with:**
See Interaction column and consult doctor.

## OVERDOSE

**SYMPTOMS:**
**"Hot" feeling, heart palpitations, nervousness, sweating, hand tremors, insomnia, rapid and irregular pulse, headache, irritability, diarrhea, weight loss, muscle cramps.**
**WHAT TO DO:**
**Overdose unlikely to threaten life. If person takes much larger amount than prescribed, call doctor, poison-control center or hospital emergency room for instructions.**

## POSSIBLE ADVERSE REACTIONS OR SIDE EFFECTS

| SYMPTOMS | WHAT TO DO |
|---|---|
| **Life-threatening:** None expected. | |
| **Common:** | |
| • Tremor, headache, irritability, insomnia. | Discontinue. Call doctor right away. |
| • Appetite change, diarrhea, leg cramps, menstrual irregularities, fever, heat sensitivity, unusual sweating, weight loss. | Continue. Call doctor when convenient. |
| **Infrequent:** Hives, itchy skin, vomiting, chest pain, rapid and irregular heartbeat, shortness of breath. | Discontinue. Call doctor right away. |
| **Rare:** None expected. | |

# WARNINGS & PRECAUTIONS

**Don't take if:**
- You have had a heart attack within 6 weeks.
- You have no thyroid deficiency, but use this to lose weight.

**Before you start, consult your doctor:**
- If you have heart disease or high blood pressure.
- If you have diabetes.
- If you have Addison's disease, have had adrenal gland deficiency or use epinephrine, ephedrine or isoproterenol for asthma.

**Over age 60:**
More sensitive to thyroid hormone. May need smaller doses.

**Pregnancy:**
Considered safe if for thyroid deficiency only.

**Breast-feeding:**
Present in milk. Considered safe if dose is correct.

**Infants & children:**
Use only under medical supervision.

**Prolonged use:**
No problems expected, if dose is correct.

**Skin & sunlight:**
No problems expected.

**Driving, piloting or hazardous work:**
No problems expected.

**Discontinuing:**
Don't discontinue without consulting doctor. Dose may require gradual reduction if you have taken drug for a long time. Doses of other drugs may also require adjustment.

**Others:**
Digestive upsets, tremors, cramps, nervousness, insomnia or diarrhea may indicate need for dose adjustment.

# POSSIBLE INTERACTION WITH OTHER DRUGS

| GENERIC NAME OR DRUG CLASS | COMBINED EFFECT |
|---|---|
| Amphetamines | Increased amphetamine effect. |
| Anticoagulants (oral) | Increased anticoagulant effect. |
| Antidepressants (tricyclic) | Irregular heartbeat. |
| Antidiabetics | Antidiabetic may require adjustment. |
| Aspirin (large doses, continuous use) | Increased liotrix effect. |
| Barbiturates | Decreased barbiturate effect. |
| Cholestyramine | Decreased liotrix effect. |
| Contraceptives (oral) | Decreased liotrix effect. |
| Cortisone drugs | Requires dose adjustment to prevent cortisone deficiency. |
| Digitalis preparations | Increased digitalis effect. |
| Ephedrine | Increased ephedrine effect. |
| Epinephrine | Increased epinephrine effect. |
| Methylphenidate | Increased methylphenidate effect. |
| Phenytoin | Increased liotrix effect. |

# POSSIBLE INTERACTION WITH OTHER SUBSTANCES

| INTERACTS WITH | COMBINED EFFECT |
|---|---|
| Alcohol: | None expected. |
| Beverages: | None expected. |
| Cocaine: | Excess stimulation. Avoid. |
| Foods: Soybeans. | Heavy consumption interferes with thyroid function. |
| Marijuana: | None expected. |
| Tobacco: | None expected. |

# LITHIUM

## BRAND NAMES

| | |
|---|---|
| Carbolith | Lithizine |
| Cibalith-S | Lithobid |
| Duralith | Lithonate |
| Eskalith | Lithotabs |
| Eskalith CR | Pfi-Lithium |
| Lithane | |

## BASIC INFORMATION

**Habit forming? No**
**Prescription needed? Yes**
**Available as generic? Yes**
**Drug class: Tranquilizer**

 **USES**

Normalizes mood and behavior in manic-depressive illness.

 **DOSAGE & USAGE INFORMATION**

**How to take:**
- Tablet or capsule—Swallow with liquid or food to lessen stomach irritation. If you can't swallow whole, crumble tablet or open capsule and take with liquid or food. Drink 2 or 3 quarts liquid per day.
- Extended-release tablets or capsules—Swallow each dose whole.
- Syrup—Take at mealtime. Follow with 8 oz. water.

**When to take:**
At the same times each day, preferably mealtime.

**If you forget a dose:**
Take as soon as you remember up to 2 hours late. If more than 2 hours, wait for next scheduled dose (don't double this dose).

*Continued next column*

 **OVERDOSE**

**SYMPTOMS:**
**Moderate overdose increases some side effects. Large overdose may cause convulsions, stupor and coma.**
**WHAT TO DO:**
- **Dial 0 (operator) or 911 (emergency) for an ambulance or medical help. Then give first aid immediately.**
- **See emergency information on inside covers.**

**What drug does:**
May correct chemical imbalance in brain's transmission of nerve impulses that influence mood and behavior.

**Time lapse before drug works:**
1 to 3 weeks. May require 3 months before depressive phase of illness improves.

**Don't take with:**
See Interaction column and consult doctor.

 **POSSIBLE ADVERSE REACTIONS OR SIDE EFFECTS**

| SYMPTOMS | WHAT TO DO |
|---|---|
| **Life-threatening:**<br>None expected. | |
| **Common:** | |
| • Dizziness, diarrhea, nausea, vomiting, shakiness, tremor. | Continue. Call doctor when convenient. |
| • Dry mouth, thirst, decreased sexual ability, increased urination. | Continue. Tell doctor at next visit. |
| **Infrequent:** | |
| • Rash, stomach pain. | Discontinue. Call doctor right away. |
| • Swollen hands, feet; slurred speech; thyroid impairment (coldness, dry, puffy skin); muscle aches; headache; weight gain; fatigue; menstrual irregularities. | Continue. Call doctor when convenient. |
| • Drowsiness, confusion, weakness. | Continue. Tell doctor at next visit. |
| **Rare:** | |
| • Blurred vision. | Discontinue. Call doctor right away. |
| • Jerking of arms and legs. | Continue. Call doctor when convenient. |

## WARNINGS & PRECAUTIONS

**Don't take if:**
- You are allergic to lithium.
- You have kidney or heart disease.
- Patient is younger than 12.

**Before you start, consult your doctor:**
- About all medications you take.
- If you plan to become pregnant within medication period.
- If you have diabetes, low thyroid function, epilepsy or any significant medical problem.
- If you are on a low-salt diet or drink more than 4 cups of coffee per day.
- If you plan surgery within 2 months.

**Over age 60:**
Adverse reactions and side effects may be more frequent and severe than in younger persons.

**Pregnancy:**
Risk to unborn child outweighs drug benefits. Don't use.

**Breast-feeding:**
Drug passes into milk. Avoid drug or discontinue nursing until you finish medicine. Consult doctor for advice on maintaining milk supply.

**Infants & children:**
Don't give to children younger than 12.

**Prolonged use:**
Enlarged thyroid with possible impaired function.

**Skin & sunlight:**
No problems expected.

**Driving, piloting or hazardous work:**
Don't drive or pilot aircraft until you learn how medicine affects you. Don't work around dangerous machinery. Don't climb ladders or work in high places. Danger increases if you drink alcohol or take medicine affecting alertness and reflexes.

**Discontinuing:**
Don't discontinue without consulting doctor. Dose may require gradual reduction if you have taken drug for a long time. Doses of other drugs may also require adjustment.

**Others:**
- Regular checkups, periodic blood tests, and tests of lithium levels and thyroid function recommended.
- Avoid exercise in hot weather and other activities that cause heavy sweating. This contributes to lithium poisoning.

## POSSIBLE INTERACTION WITH OTHER DRUGS

| GENERIC NAME OR DRUG CLASS | COMBINED EFFECT |
|---|---|
| Acetazolamide | Decreased lithium effect. |
| Aminophylline | Decreased lithium effect. |
| Diuretics | Increased lithium effect. |
| Dronabinol | Increased effects of both drugs. Avoid. |
| Haloperidol | Increased toxicity of both drugs. |
| Indomethacin | Increased lithium effect. |
| Ketoprofen | May increase lithium in blood. |
| Methyldopa | Increased lithium effect. |
| Muscle relaxants (skeletal) | Increased skeletal-muscle relaxation. |
| Oxyphenbutazone | Increased lithium effect. |
| Phenothiazines | Decreased lithium effect. |
| Phentyoin | Increased lithium effect. |
| Phenylbutazone | Increased lithium effect. |
| Potassium iodide | Increased potassium iodide effect. |
| Sodium bicarbonate | Decreased lithium effect. |
| Suprofen | May increase lithium in blood. |
| Terfenadine | Possible excessive sedation. |
| Tetracyclines | Increased lithium effect. |

## POSSIBLE INTERACTION WITH OTHER SUBSTANCES

| INTERACTS WITH | COMBINED EFFECT |
|---|---|
| Alcohol: | Possible lithium poisoning. |
| Beverages: Caffeine drinks. | Increased lithium effect. |
| Cocaine: | Possible psychosis. |
| Foods: Salt. | *Don't* restrict intake. |
| Marijuana: | Increased tremor and possible psychosis. |
| Tobacco: | None expected. |

# LOPERAMIDE

## BRAND NAMES

Imodium

## BASIC INFORMATION

**Habit forming?** No, unless taken in high doses for long periods.
**Prescription needed?** Yes
**Available as generic?** No
**Drug class:** Antidiarrheal

 **USES**

Relieves diarrhea and reduces volume of discharge from ileostomies and colostomies.

 **DOSAGE & USAGE INFORMATION**

**How to take:**
- Tablet or capsule—Swallow with food to lessen stomach irritation.
- Liquid—Follow label instructions and use marked dropper.

**When to take:**
No more often than directed on label.

**If you forget a dose:**
Take as soon as you remember up to 2 hours late. If more than 2 hours, wait for next scheduled dose (don't double this dose).

**What drug does:**
Blocks digestive tract's nerve supply, which reduces irritability and contractions in intestinal tract.

**Time lapse before drug works:**
1 to 2 hours.

**Don't take with:**
See Interaction column and consult doctor.

 **OVERDOSE**

**SYMPTOMS:**
**Constipation, lethargy, drowsiness or unconsciousness.**
**WHAT TO DO:**
**Overdose unlikely to threaten life. If person takes much larger amount than prescribed, call doctor, poison-control center or hospital emergency room for instructions.**

 **POSSIBLE ADVERSE REACTIONS OR SIDE EFFECTS**

| SYMPTOMS | WHAT TO DO |
|---|---|
| **Life-threatening:** None expected. | |
| **Common:** None expected. | |
| **Infrequent:** | |
| • Rash. | Discontinue. Call doctor right away. |
| • Drowsiness, dry mouth, bloating, constipation, appetite loss, stomach pain. | Continue. Call doctor when convenient. |
| **Rare:** Unexplained fever. | Discontinue. Call doctor right away. |

## WARNINGS & PRECAUTION

### Don't take if:
- You have severe colitis.
- You have colitis resulting from antibiotic treatment.

### Before you start, consult your doctor:
- If you are dehydrated from fluid loss caused by diarrhea.
- If you have liver disease.

### Over age 60:
Adverse reactions and side effects may be more frequent and severe than in younger persons.

### Pregnancy:
No proven harm. Avoid if possible.

### Breast-feeding:
No proven problems, but avoid if possible or discontinue nursing until you finish medicine. Consult doctor for advice on maintaining milk supply.

### Infants & children:
Don't give to infants or toddlers. Use only under doctor's supervision for children older than 2.

### Prolonged use:
Habit forming at high dose.

### Skin & sunlight:
No problems expected.

### Driving, piloting or hazardous work:
Don't drive or pilot aircraft until you learn how medicine affects you. Don't work around dangerous machinery. Don't climb ladders or work in high places. Danger increases if you drink alcohol or take medicine affecting alertness and reflexes.

### Discontinuing:
- May be unnecessary to finish medicine. Follow doctor's instructions.
- After discontinuing, consult doctor if you experience muscle cramps, nausea, vomiting, trembling, stomach cramps or unusual sweating.

### Others:
If acute diarrhea lasts longer than 48 hours, discontinue and call doctor. In chronic diarrhea, loperamide is unlikely to be effective if diarrhea doesn't improve in 10 days.

 ## POSSIBLE INTERACTION WITH OTHER DRUGS

| GENERIC NAME OR DRUG CLASS | COMBINED EFFECT |
| --- | --- |
| Antibiotics (cephalosporins, clindamycin, lincomycins, penicillins). | May delay removal of toxins from colon in cases of diarrhea caused by side effects of these antibiotics. |

 ## POSSIBLE INTERACTION WITH OTHER SUBSTANCES

| INTERACTS WITH | COMBINED EFFECT |
| --- | --- |
| Alcohol: | Depressed brain function. Avoid. |
| Beverages: | None expected. |
| Cocaine: | Decreased loperamide effect. |
| Foods: | None expected. |
| Marijuana: | None expected. |
| Tobacco: | None expected. |

# LORAZEPAM

## BRAND NAMES

Apo-Lorazepam    Loraz
Ativan    Novolorazem

## BASIC INFORMATION

**Habit forming? Yes**
**Prescription needed? Yes**
**Available as generic? Yes**
**Drug class: Tranquilizer (benzodiazepine)**

## USES

Treatment for nervousness or tension.

## DOSAGE & USAGE INFORMATION

**How to take:**
Tablet or capsule—Swallow with liquid. If you can't swallow whole, crumble tablet or open capsule and take with liquid or food.

**When to take:**
At the same time each day, according to instructions on prescription label.

**If you forget a dose:**
Take as soon as you remember up to 2 hours late. If more than 2 hours, wait for next scheduled dose (don't double this dose).

**What drug does:**
Affects limbic system of brain—part that controls emotions.

**Time lapse before drug works:**
2 hours. May take 6 weeks for full benefit.

**Don't take with:**
See Interaction column and consult doctor.

## OVERDOSE

**SYMPTOMS:**
**Drowsiness, weakness, tremor, stupor, coma.**
**WHAT TO DO:**
- **Dial 0 (operator) or 911 (emergency) for an ambulance or medical help. Then give first aid immediately.**
- **If patient is unconscious and not breathing, give mouth-to-mouth breathing. If there is no heartbeat, use cardiac massage and mouth-to-mouth breathing (CPR). Don't try to make patient vomit. If you can't get help quickly, take patient to nearest emergency facility.**
- **See emergency information on inside covers.**

## POSSIBLE ADVERSE REACTIONS OR SIDE EFFECTS

| SYMPTOMS | WHAT TO DO |
|---|---|
| **Life-threatening:**<br>None expected. | |
| **Common:**<br>Clumsiness, drowsiness, dizziness. | Continue. Call doctor when convenient. |
| **Infrequent:**<br>● Hallucinations, confusion, depression, irritability, itchy skin, rash, change in vision. | Discontinue. Call doctor right away. |
| ● Constipation or diarrhea, nausea, vomiting, difficult urination. | Continue. Call doctor when convenient. |
| **Rare:**<br>● Slow heartbeat, difficult breathing. | Discontinue. Seek emergency treatment. |
| ● Mouth, throat ulcers; jaundice. | Discontinue. Call doctor right away. |

## WARNINGS & PRECAUTIONS

**Don't take if:**
- You are allergic to any benzodiazepine.
- You have myasthenia gravis.
- You are active or recovering alcoholic.
- Patient is younger than 6 months.

**Before you start, consult your doctor:**
- If you have liver, kidney or lung disease.
- If you have diabetes, epilepsy or porphyria.

**Over age 60:**
Adverse reactions and side effects may be more frequent and severe than in younger persons. You need smaller doses for shorter periods of time. May develop agitation, rage or "hangover" effect.

**Pregnancy:**
Risk to unborn child outweighs drug benefits. Don't use.

**Breast-feeding:**
Drug passes into milk. Avoid drug or discontinue nursing until you finish medicine. Consult doctor for advice on maintaining milk supply.

**Infants & children:**
Use only under medical supervision for children older than 6 months.

**Prolonged use:**
May impair liver function.

**Skin & sunlight:**
No problems expected.

**Driving, piloting or hazardous work:**
Don't drive or pilot aircraft until you learn how medicine affects you. Don't work around dangerous machinery. Don't climb ladders or work in high places. Danger increases if you drink alcohol or take medicine affecting alertness and reflexes.

**Discontinuing:**
Don't discontinue without consulting doctor. Dose may require gradual reduction if you have taken drug for a long time. Doses of other drugs may also require adjustment.

**Others:**
- Hot weather, heavy exercise and profuse sweat may reduce excretion and cause overdose.
- Blood sugar may rise in diabetics, requiring insulin adjustment.

## POSSIBLE INTERACTION WITH OTHER DRUGS

| GENERIC NAME OR DRUG CLASS | COMBINED EFFECT |
|---|---|
| Anticonvulsants | Change in seizure frequency or severity. |
| Antidepressants | Increased sedative effect of both drugs. |
| Antihistamines | Increased sedative effect of both drugs. |
| Antihypertensives | Excessively low blood pressure. |
| Cimetidine | Excess sedation. |
| Disulfiram | Increased lorazepam effect. |
| Dronabinol | Increased effects of both drugs. Avoid. |
| MAO inhibitors | Convulsions, deep sedation, rage. |
| Molindone | Increased tranquilizer effect. |
| Narcotics | Increased sedative effect of both drugs. |
| Sedatives | Increased sedative effect of both drugs. |
| Sleep inducers | Increased sedative effect of both drugs. |
| Tranquilizers | Increased sedative effect of both drugs. |

## POSSIBLE INTERACTION WITH OTHER SUBSTANCES

| INTERACTS WITH | COMBINED EFFECT |
|---|---|
| Alcohol: | Heavy sedation. Avoid. |
| Beverages: | None expected. |
| Cocaine: | Decreased lorazepam effect. |
| Foods: | None expected. |
| Marijuana: | Heavy sedation. Avoid. |
| Tobacco: | Decreased lorazepam effect. |

# MAGNESIUM CARBONATE

## BRAND NAMES

| | |
|---|---|
| Alkets | Gaviscon |
| Bisodol | Magnagel |
| De Witt's | Marblen |
| Di-Gel | Osti-Derm |
| Estomul-M | Silain-Gel |

## BASIC INFORMATION

**Habit forming? No**
**Prescription needed? No**
**Available as generic? Yes**
**Drug class: Antacid, laxative**

## USES

- Treatment for hyperacidity in upper gastrointestinal tract, including stomach and esophagus. Symptoms may be heartburn or acid indigestion. Diseases include peptic ulcer, gastritis, esophagitis, hiatal hernia.
- Constipation relief.

## DOSAGE & USAGE INFORMATION

**How to take:**
- Tablet or capsule—Swallow with liquid.
- Chewable tablets or wafers—Chew well before swallowing.
- Liquid—Shake well and take undiluted.
- Powder—Mix with water and drink all liquid.

**When to take:**
1 to 3 hours after meals unless directed otherwise by your doctor.

**If you forget a dose:**
Take as soon as you remember.

**What drug does:**
- Neutralizes some of the hydrochloric acid in the stomach.
- Reduces action of pepsin, a digestive enzyme.
- Stimulates muscles in lower bowel wall.

*Continued next column*

## OVERDOSE

**SYMPTOMS:**
Dry mouth, diarrhea, shallow breathing, stupor.
**WHAT TO DO:**
- **Dial 0 (operator) or 911 (emergency) for an ambulance or medical help. Then give first aid immediately.**
- **See emergency information on inside covers.**

**Time lapse before drug works:**
15 minutes.

**Don't take with:**
Other medicines at the same time. Decreases absorption of other drugs.

## POSSIBLE ADVERSE REACTIONS OR SIDE EFFECTS

| SYMPTOMS | WHAT TO DO |
|---|---|
| **Life-threatening:**<br>None expected. | |
| **Common:**<br>Constipation, appetite loss. | Continue. Call doctor when convenient. |
| **Infrequent:**<br>• Lower abdominal pain and swelling, bone pain, muscle weakness, swollen wrists or ankles. | Discontinue. Call doctor right away. |
| • Weight loss, mood change, nausea, vomiting. | Continue. Call doctor when convenient. |
| **Rare:**<br>Unusual weakness or tiredness. | Discontinue. Call doctor right away. |

## WARNINGS & PRECAUTIONS

**Don't take if:**
You are allergic to any antacid.

**Before you start, consult your doctor:**
- If you have kidney disease.
- If you have chronic constipation, colitis or diarrhea.
- If you have symptoms of appendicitis.
- If you have stomach or intestinal bleeding.

**Over age 60:**
Adverse reactions and side effects may be more frequent and severe than in younger persons. Diarrhea or constipation particularly likely.

**Pregnancy:**
Risk to unborn child outweighs drug benefits. Don't use.

**Breast-feeding:**
Drug passes into milk. Avoid drug or discontinue nursing until you finish medicine. Consult doctor for advice on maintaining milk supply.

**Infants & children:**
Use only under medical supervision.

**Prolonged use:**
No problems expected.

**Skin & sunlight:**
No problems expected.

**Driving, piloting or hazardous work:**
No problems expected.

**Discontinuing:**
May be unnecessary to finish medicine. Follow doctor's instructions.

**Others:**
Don't take longer than 2 weeks unless under medical supervision.

## POSSIBLE INTERACTION WITH OTHER DRUGS

| GENERIC NAME OR DRUG CLASS | COMBINED EFFECT |
|---|---|
| Anticoagulants | Decreased anticoagulant effect. |
| Chlorpromazine | Decreased chlorpromazine effect. |
| Digitalis preparations | Decreased digitalis effect. |
| Iron supplements | Decreased iron effect. |
| Isoniazid | Decreased isoniazid effect. |
| Levodopa | Increased levodopa effect. |
| Meperidine | Increased meperidine effect. |
| Mexiletine | May slow elimination of mexiletine and cause need to adjust dosage. |
| Nalidixic acid | Decreased effect of nalidixic acid. |
| Oxyphenbutazone | Decreased oxyphenbutazone effect. |
| Para-aminosalicylic acid (PAS) | Decreased PAS effect. |
| Penicillins | Decreased penicillin effect. |
| Pentobarbital | Decreased pentobarbital effect. |
| Phenylbutazone | Decreased phenylbutazone effect. |
| Pseudoephedrine | Increased pseudoephedrine effect. |
| Sulfa drugs | Decreased sulfa effect. |
| Tetracyclines | Decreased tetracycline effect. |
| Vitamins A and C | Decreased vitamin effect. |
| Vitamin D | Too much calcium in blood. |

## POSSIBLE INTERACTION WITH OTHER SUBSTANCES

| INTERACTS WITH | COMBINED EFFECT |
|---|---|
| Alcohol: | Decreased antacid effect. |
| Beverages: | No proven problems. |
| Cocaine: | No proven problems. |
| Foods: | Decreased antacid effect if taken with food. Wait 1 hour after eating. |
| Marijuana: | No proven problems. |
| Tobacco: | Decreased antacid effect. |

# MAGNESIUM CITRATE

## BRAND NAMES

Citrate of Magnesia
Citro-Mag
Citro-Nesia
Citroma

Evac-Q-Kit
Evac-Q-Kwik
National

## BASIC INFORMATION

**Habit forming? No**
**Prescription needed? No**
**Available as generic? Yes**
**Drug class: Laxative (hyperosmotic)**

## USES

Constipation relief.

## DOSAGE & USAGE INFORMATION

**How to take:**
Liquid—Dilute dose in beverage before swallowing.

**When to take:**
Usually once a day, preferably in the morning.

**If you forget a dose:**
Take as soon as you remember up to 8 hours before bedtime. If later, wait for next scheduled dose (don't double this dose). Don't take at bedtime.

**What drug does:**
Draws water into bowel from other body tissues. Causes distention through fluid accumulation, which promotes soft stool and accelerates bowel motion.

**Time lapse before drug works:**
30 minutes to 3 hours.

**Don't take with:**
See Interaction column and consult doctor.

## OVERDOSE

**SYMPTOMS:**
**Fluid depletion, weakness, vomiting, fainting.**
**WHAT TO DO:**
**Overdose unlikely to threaten life. If person takes much larger amount than prescribed, call doctor, poison-control center or hospital emergency room for instructions.**

## POSSIBLE ADVERSE REACTIONS OR SIDE EFFECTS

| SYMPTOMS | WHAT TO DO |
|---|---|
| **Life-threatening:** None expected. | |
| **Common:** None expected. | |
| **Infrequent:** | |
| • Irregular heartbeat. | Discontinue. Call doctor right away. |
| • Increased thirst, cramps, nausea, diarrhea, gaseousness. | Continue. Tell doctor at next visit. |
| **Rare:** Dizziness, confusion, tiredness or weakness. | Continue. Call doctor when convenient. |

## WARNINGS & PRECAUTIONS

**Don't take if:**
- You are allergic to any hyperosmotic laxative.
- You have symptoms of appendicitis, inflamed bowel or intestinal blockage.
- You have missed a bowel movement for only 1 or 2 days.

**Before you start, consult your doctor:**
- If you have congestive heart disease.
- If you have diabetes.
- If you have high blood pressure.
- If you have a colostomy or ileostomy.
- If you have kidney disease.
- If you have a laxative habit.
- If you have rectal bleeding.
- If you take another laxative.

**Over age 60:**
Adverse reactions and side effects may be more frequent and severe than in younger persons.

**Pregnancy:**
Salt content may cause fluid retention and swelling. Avoid if possible.

**Breast-feeding:**
No problems expected.

**Infants & children:**
Use only under medical supervision.

**Prolonged use:**
Don't take for more than 1 week unless under a doctor's supervision. May cause laxative dependence.

**Skin & sunlight:**
No problems expected.

**Driving, piloting or hazardous work:**
No problems expected.

**Discontinuing:**
May be unnecessary to finish medicine. Follow doctor's instructions.

**Others:**
- Don't take to "flush out" your system or as a "tonic."
- Don't take within 2 hours of taking another medicine.

## POSSIBLE INTERACTION WITH OTHER DRUGS

| GENERIC NAME OR DRUG CLASS | COMBINED EFFECT |
|---|---|
| Chlordiazepoxide | Decreased chlordiazepoxide effect. |
| Chlorpromazine | Decreased chlorpromazine effect. |
| Dicumarol | Decreased dicumarol effect. |
| Digoxin | Decreased digoxin effect. |
| Isoniazid | Decreased isoniazid effect. |
| Mexiletine | May slow elimination of mexiletine and cause need to adjust dosage. |
| Tetracyclines | Possible intestinal blockage. |

## POSSIBLE INTERACTION WITH OTHER SUBSTANCES

| INTERACTS WITH | COMBINED EFFECT |
|---|---|
| Alcohol: | None expected. |
| Beverages: | None expected. |
| Cocaine: | None expected. |
| Foods: | None expected. |
| Marijuana: | None expected. |
| Tobacco: | None expected. |

# MAGNESIUM HYDROXIDE

## BRAND NAMES

See complete list of brand names in the *Brand Name Directory,* page 951.

## BASIC INFORMATION

**Habit forming? No**
**Prescription needed? No**
**Available as generic? Yes**
**Drug class: Antacid, laxative**

 ## USES

- Treatment for hyperacidity in upper gastrointestinal tract, including stomach and esophagus. Symptoms may be heartburn or acid indigestion. Diseases include peptic ulcer, gastritis, esophagitis, hiatal hernia.
- Constipation relief.

 ## DOSAGE & USAGE INFORMATION

**How to take:**
- Tablet—Swallow with liquid.
- Liquid—Shake well and take undiluted.

**When to take:**
1 to 3 hours after meals unless directed otherwise by your doctor.

**If you forget a dose:**
Take as soon as you remember.

**What drug does:**
- Neutralizes some of the hydrochloric acid in the stomach.
- Reduces action of pepsin, a digestive enzyme.
- Stimulates muscles in lower bowel wall.

**Time lapse before drug works:**
15 minutes.

**Don't take with:**
Other medicines at the same time. Decreases absorption of other drugs.

 ## OVERDOSE

**SYMPTOMS:**
**Dry mouth, shallow breathing, diarrhea, stupor.**
**WHAT TO DO:**
- **Dial 0 (operator) or 911 (emergency) for an ambulance or medical help. Then give first aid immediately.**
- **See emergency information on inside covers.**

 ## POSSIBLE ADVERSE REACTIONS OR SIDE EFFECTS

| SYMPTOMS | WHAT TO DO |
|---|---|
| **Life-threatening:** None expected. | |
| **Common:** Constipation, appetite loss. | Continue. Call doctor when convenient. |
| **Infrequent:** | |
| • Lower abdominal pain and swelling, bone pain, muscle weakness, swollen wrists or ankles. | Discontinue. Call doctor right away. |
| • Mood change, nausea, vomiting, weight loss. | Continue. Call doctor when convenient. |
| **Rare:** None expected. | |

## WARNINGS & PRECAUTIONS

**Don't take if:**
You are allergic to any antacid.

**Before you start, consult your doctor:**
- If you have kidney disease.
- If you have chronic constipation, colitis or diarrhea.
- If you have symptoms of appendicitis.
- If you have stomach or intestinal bleeding.

**Over age 60:**
Adverse reactions and side effects may be more frequent and severe than in younger persons. Diarrhea or constipation particularly likely.

**Pregnancy:**
Risk to unborn child outweighs drug benefits. Don't use.

**Breast-feeding:**
Drug passes into milk. Avoid drug or discontinue nursing until you finish medicine. Consult doctor for advice on maintaining milk supply.

**Infants & children:**
Use only under medical supervision.

**Prolonged use:**
No problems expected.

**Skin & sunlight:**
No problems expected.

**Driving, piloting or hazardous work:**
No problems expected.

**Discontinuing:**
May be unnecessary to finish medicine. Follow doctor's instructions.

**Others:**
Don't take longer than 2 weeks unless under medical supervision.

## POSSIBLE INTERACTION WITH OTHER DRUGS

| GENERIC NAME OR DRUG CLASS | COMBINED EFFECT |
|---|---|
| Anticoagulants | Decreased anticoagulant effect. |
| Chlorpromazine | Decreased chlorpromazine effect. |
| Digitalis preparations | Decreased digitalis effect. |
| Iron supplements | Decreased iron effect. |
| Isoniazid | Decreased isoniazid effect. |
| Levodopa | Increased levodopa effect. |

| | |
|---|---|
| Meperidine | Increased meperidine effect. |
| Mexiletine | May slow elimination of mexiletine and cause need to adjust dosage. |
| Nalidixic acid | Decreased effect of nalidixic acid. |
| Oxyphenbutazone | Decreased oxyphenbutazone effect. |
| Para-aminosalicylic acid (PAS) | Decreased PAS effect. |
| Penicillins | Decreased penicillin effect. |
| Pentobarbital | Decreased pentobarbital effect. |
| Phenylbutazone | Decreased phenylbutazone effect. |
| Pseudoephedrine | Increased pseudoephedrine effect. |
| Sulfa drugs | Decreased sulfa effect. |
| Tetracyclines | Decreased tetracycline effect. |
| Vitamins A and C | Decreased vitamin effect. |
| Vitamin D | Too much calcium in blood. |

## POSSIBLE INTERACTION WITH OTHER SUBSTANCES

| INTERACTS WITH | COMBINED EFFECT |
|---|---|
| Alcohol: | Decreased antacid effect. |
| Beverages: | No proven problems. |
| Cocaine: | No proven problems. |
| Foods: | Decreased antacid effect if taken with food. Wait 1 hour after eating. |
| Marijuana: | No proven problems. |
| Tobacco: | Decreased antacid effect. |

# MAGNESIUM SULFATE

## BRAND NAMES

| | |
|---|---|
| Bilagog | Epsom Salts |
| Eldercaps | Glutofac |
| Eldertonic | Vicon |

## BASIC INFORMATION

**Habit forming? No**
**Prescription needed? No**
**Available as generic? Yes**
**Drug class: Laxative (hyperosmotic)**

## USES

Constipation relief.

## DOSAGE & USAGE INFORMATION

**How to take:**
Powder or solid form—Dilute dose in beverage before swallowing. Solid form must be dissolved.

**When to take:**
Usually once a day, preferably in the morning.

**If you forget a dose:**
Take as soon as you remember up to 8 hours before bedtime. If later, wait for next scheduled dose (don't double this dose). Don't take at bedtime.

**What drug does:**
Draws water into bowel from other body tissues. Causes distention through fluid accumulation, which promotes soft stool and accelerates bowel motion.

**Time lapse before drug works:**
30 minutes to 3 hours.

**Don't take with:**
See Interaction column and consult doctor.

## OVERDOSE

**SYMPTOMS:**
Fluid depletion, weakness, vomiting, fainting.
**WHAT TO DO:**
Overdose unlikely to threaten life. If person takes much larger amount than prescribed, call doctor, poison-control center or hospital emergency room for instructions.

## POSSIBLE ADVERSE REACTIONS OR SIDE EFFECTS

| SYMPTOMS | WHAT TO DO |
|---|---|
| **Life-threatening:** None expected. | |
| **Common:** None expected. | |
| **Infrequent:** | |
| • Irregular heartbeat. | Discontinue. Call doctor right away. |
| • Increased thirst, cramps, nausea, diarrhea, gaseousness. | Continue. Tell doctor at next visit. |
| **Rare:** Dizziness, confusion, tiredness or weakness. | Continue. Call doctor when convenient. |

## WARNINGS & PRECAUTIONS

### Don't take if:
- You are allergic to any hyperosmotic laxative.
- You have symptoms of appendicitis, inflamed bowel or intestinal blockage.
- You have missed a bowel movement for only 1 or 2 days.

### Before you start, consult your doctor:
- If you have congestive heart disease.
- If you have diabetes.
- If you have high blood pressure.
- If you have a colostomy or ileostomy.
- If you have kidney disease.
- If you have a laxative habit.
- If you have rectal bleeding.
- If you take another laxative.

### Over age 60:
Adverse reactions and side effects may be more frequent and severe than in younger persons.

### Pregnancy:
Salt content may cause fluid retention and swelling. Avoid if possible.

### Breast-feeding:
No problems expected.

### Infants & children:
Use only under medical supervision.

### Prolonged use:
Don't take for more than 1 week unless under a doctor's supervision. May cause laxative dependence.

### Skin & sunlight:
No problems expected.

### Driving, piloting or hazardous work:
No problems expected.

### Discontinuing:
May be unnecessary to finish medicine. Follow doctor's instructions.

### Others:
- Don't take to "flush out" your system or as a "tonic."
- Don't take within 2 hours of taking another medicine.

## POSSIBLE INTERACTION WITH OTHER DRUGS

| GENERIC NAME OR DRUG CLASS | COMBINED EFFECT |
|---|---|
| Chlordiazepoxide | Decreased chlordiazepoxide effect. |
| Chlorpromazine | Decreased chlorpromazine effect. |
| Dicumarol | Decreased dicumarol effect. |
| Digoxin | Decreased digoxin effect. |
| Isoniazid | Decreased isoniazid effect. |
| Mexiletine | May slow elimination of mexiletine and cause need to adjust dosage. |
| Tetracyclines | Possible intestinal blockage. |

## POSSIBLE INTERACTION WITH OTHER SUBSTANCES

| INTERACTS WITH | COMBINED EFFECT |
|---|---|
| Alcohol: | None expected. |
| Beverages: | None expected. |
| Cocaine: | None expected. |
| Foods: | None expected. |
| Marijuana: | None expected. |
| Tobacco: | None expected. |

# MAGNESIUM TRISILICATE

## BRAND NAMES

| | |
|---|---|
| A-M-T | Magnatril |
| Alma-Mag | Mucotin |
| Gaviscon | Neutrocomp |
| Gelusil | Sterazolidin |
| Gelusil-M | Trisogel |

## BASIC INFORMATION

**Habit forming? No**
**Prescription needed? No**
**Available as generic? Yes**
**Drug class: Antacid, laxative**

## USES

- Treatment for hyperacidity in upper gastrointestinal tract, including stomach and esophagus. Symptoms may be heartburn or acid indigestion. Diseases include peptic ulcer, gastritis, esophagitis, hiatal hernia.
- Constipation relief.

## DOSAGE & USAGE INFORMATION

**How to take:**
- Tablet or capsule—Swallow with liquid.
- Chewable tablets or wafers—Chew well before swallowing.
- Liquid—Shake well and take undiluted.

**When to take:**
1 to 3 hours after meals unless directed otherwise by your doctor.

**If you forget a dose:**
Take as soon as you remember.

**What drug does:**
- Neutralizes some of the hydrochloric acid in the stomach.
- Reduces action of pepsin, a digestive enzyme.
- Stimulates muscles in lower bowel wall.

*Continued next column*

## OVERDOSE

**SYMPTOMS:**
Dry mouth, diarrhea, shallow breathing, stupor.
**WHAT TO DO:**
- Dial 0 (operator) or 911 (emergency) for an ambulance or medical help. Then give first aid immediately.
- See emergency information on inside covers.

**Time lapse before drug works:**
15 minutes.

**Don't take with:**
Other medicines at the same time. Decreases absorption of other drugs.

## POSSIBLE ADVERSE REACTIONS OR SIDE EFFECTS

| SYMPTOMS | WHAT TO DO |
|---|---|
| **Life-threatening:**<br>None expected. | |
| **Common:**<br>Constipation, appetite loss. | Continue. Call doctor when convenient. |
| **Infrequent:** | |
| • Lower abdominal pain and swelling, bone pain, muscle weakness, swollen wrists or ankles. | Discontinue. Call doctor right away. |
| • Mood change, nausea, vomiting, weight loss. | Continue. Call doctor when convenient. |
| **Rare:**<br>None expected. | |

502

## WARNINGS & PRECAUTIONS

**Don't take if:**
You are allergic to any antacid.

**Before you start, consult your doctor:**
- If you have kidney disease.
- If you have chronic constipation, colitis or diarrhea.
- If you have symptoms of appendicitis.
- If you have stomach or intestinal bleeding.

**Over age 60:**
Adverse reactions and side effects may be more frequent and severe than in younger persons. Diarrhea or constipation particularly likely.

**Pregnancy:**
Risk to unborn child outweighs drug benefits. Don't use.

**Breast-feeding:**
Drug passes into milk. Avoid drug or discontinue nursing until you finish medicine. Consult doctor for advice on maintaining milk supply.

**Infants & children:**
Use only under medical supervision.

**Prolonged use:**
No problems expected.

**Skin & sunlight:**
No problems expected.

**Driving, piloting or hazardous work:**
No problems expected.

**Discontinuing:**
May be unnecessary to finish medicine. Follow doctor's instructions.

**Others:**
Don't take longer than 2 weeks unless under medical supervision.

## POSSIBLE INTERACTION WITH OTHER DRUGS

| GENERIC NAME OR DRUG CLASS | COMBINED EFFECT |
| --- | --- |
| Anticoagulants | Decreased anticoagulant effect. |
| Chlorpromazine | Decreased chlorpromazine effect. |
| Digitalis preparations | Decreased digitalis effect. |
| Iron supplements | Decreased iron effect. |
| Isoniazid | Decreased isoniazid effect. |
| Levodopa | Increased levodopa effect. |
| Meperidine | Increased meperidine effect. |
| Mexiletine | May slow elimination of mexiletine and cause need to adjust dosage. |
| Nalidixic acid | Decreased effect of nalidixic acid. |
| Oxyphenbutazone | Decreased oxyphenbutazone effect. |
| Para-aminosalicylic acid (PAS) | Decreased PAS effect. |
| Penicillins | Decreased penicillin effect. |
| Pentobarbital | Decreased pentobarbital effect. |
| Phenylbutazone | Decreased phenylbutazone effect. |
| Pseudoephedrine | Increased pseudoephedrine effect. |
| Sulfa drugs | Decreased sulfa effect. |
| Tetracyclines | Decreased tetracycline effect. |
| Vitamins A and C | Decreased vitamin effect. |
| Vitamin D | Too much calcium in blood. |

## POSSIBLE INTERACTION WITH OTHER SUBSTANCES

| INTERACTS WITH | COMBINED EFFECT |
| --- | --- |
| Alcohol: | Decreased antacid effect. |
| Beverages: | No proven problems. |
| Cocaine: | No proven problems. |
| Foods: | Decreased antacid effect if taken with food. Wait 1 hour after eating. |
| Marijuana: | No proven problems. |
| Tobacco: | Decreased antacid effect. |

# MALT SOUP EXTRACT

## BRAND NAMES

Maltsupex

## BASIC INFORMATION

Habit forming? No
Prescription needed? No
Available as generic? Yes
Drug class: Laxative (bulk-forming)

## USES

Relieves constipation and prevents straining for bowel movement.

## DOSAGE & USAGE INFORMATION

**How to take:**
- Liquid or powder—Dilute dose in 8 oz. cold water or fruit juice.
- Tablets—Swallow with 8 oz. cold liquid. Drink 6 to 8 glasses of water each day in addition to the one with each dose.

**When to take:**
At the same time each day, preferably morning.

**If you forget a dose:**
Take as soon as you remember. Resume regular schedule.

**What drug does:**
Absorbs water, stimulating the bowel to form a soft, bulky stool.

**Time lapse before drug works:**
May require 2 or 3 days to begin, then works in 12 to 24 hours.

**Don't take with:**
- See Interaction column and consult doctor.
- Don't take within 2 hours of taking another medicine.

## OVERDOSE

**SYMPTOMS:**
None expected.
**WHAT TO DO:**
Overdose unlikely to threaten life. If person takes much larger amount than prescribed, call doctor, poison-control center or hospital emergency room for instructions.

## POSSIBLE ADVERSE REACTIONS OR SIDE EFFECTS

| SYMPTOMS | WHAT TO DO |
|---|---|
| **Life-threatening:** None expected. | |
| **Common:** None expected. | |
| **Infrequent:** Swallowing difficulty, "lump in throat" sensation, nausea, vomiting, diarrhea. | Continue. Call doctor when convenient. |
| **Rare:** Itchy skin, rash, asthma, intestinal blockage. | Discontinue. Call doctor right away. |

## WARNINGS & PRECAUTIONS

### Don't take if:
- You are allergic to any bulk-forming laxative.
- You have symptoms of appendicitis, inflamed bowel or intestinal blockage.
- You have missed a bowel movement for only 1 or 2 days.

### Before you start, consult your doctor:
- If you have diabetes.
- If you have a laxative habit.
- If you have rectal bleeding.
- If you have difficulty swallowing.
- If you take other laxatives.

### Over age 60:
Adverse reactions and side effects may be more frequent and severe than in younger persons.

### Pregnancy:
Most bulk-forming laxatives contain sodium or sugars which may cause fluid retention. Avoid if possible.

### Breast-feeding:
No problems expected.

### Infants & children:
Use only under medical supervision.

### Prolonged use:
Don't take for more than 1 week unless under a doctor's supervision. May cause laxative dependence.

### Skin & sunlight:
No problems expected.

### Driving, piloting or hazardous work:
No problems expected.

### Discontinuing:
May be unnecessary to finish medicine. Follow doctor's instructions.

### Others:
Don't take to "flush out" your system or as a "tonic."

## POSSIBLE INTERACTION WITH OTHER DRUGS

| GENERIC NAME OR DRUG CLASS | COMBINED EFFECT |
|---|---|
| Antibiotics | Decreased antibiotic effect. |
| Anticoagulants | Decreased anticoagulant effect. |
| Digitalis preparations | Decreased digitalis effect. |
| Salicylates (including aspirin) | Decreased salicylate effect. |

## POSSIBLE INTERACTION WITH OTHER SUBSTANCES

| INTERACTS WITH | COMBINED EFFECT |
|---|---|
| Alcohol: | None expected. |
| Beverages: | None expected. |
| Cocaine: | None expected. |
| Foods: | None expected. |
| Marijuana: | None expected. |
| Tobacco: | None expected. |

# MAPROTILINE

## BRAND NAMES

Ludiomil

## BASIC INFORMATION

**Habit forming? No**
**Prescription needed? Yes**
**Available as generic? No**
**Drug class: Antidepressant**

 ## USES

Treatment for depression or anxiety associated with depression.

 ## DOSAGE & USAGE INFORMATION

**How to take:**
Tablet or capsule—Swallow with liquid.

**When to take:**
At the same time each day, usually bedtime.

**If you forget a dose:**
Bedtime dose—If you forget your once-a-day bedtime dose, don't take it more than 3 hours late. If more than 3 hours, wait for next scheduled dose. Don't double this dose.

**What drug does:**
Probably affects part of brain that controls messages between nerve cells.

**Time lapse before drug works:**
Begins in 1 to 2 weeks. May require 4 to 6 weeks for maximum benefit.

**Don't take with:**
- Non-prescription drugs without consulting doctor.
- See Interaction column and consult doctor.

 ## OVERDOSE

**SYMPTOMS:**
Hallucinations, convulsions, coma.
**WHAT TO DO:**
- **Dial 0 (operator) or 911 (emergency) for an ambulance or medical help. Then give first aid immediately.**
- **If patient is unconscious and not breathing, give mouth-to-mouth breathing. If there is no heartbeat, use cardiac massage and mouth-to-mouth breathing (CPR). Don't try to make patient vomit. If you can't get help quickly, take patient to nearest emergency facility.**
- **See emergency information on inside covers.**

 ## POSSIBLE ADVERSE REACTIONS OR SIDE EFFECTS

| SYMPTOMS | WHAT TO DO |
|---|---|
| **Life-threatening:** | |
| Seizures. | Seek emergency treatment immediately. |
| **Common:** | |
| • Headache, dry mouth or unpleasant taste, constipation or diarrhea, nausea, indigestion, fatigue, weakness. | Continue. Call doctor when convenient. |
| • Insomnia, craving sweets. | Continue. Tell doctor at next visit. |
| **Infrequent:** | |
| • Hallucinations, shakiness, dizziness, fainting, blurred vision, eye pain, vomiting, irregular heartbeat or slow pulse. | Discontinue. Call doctor right away. |
| • Painful or difficult urination. | Continue. Call doctor when convenient. |
| **Rare:** | |
| Itchy skin, rash, sore throat, jaundice, fever. | Discontinue. Call doctor right away. |

 ## WARNINGS & PRECAUTIONS

**Don't take if:**
- You are allergic to any tricyclic antidepressant.
- You drink alcohol.
- You have had a heart attack within 6 weeks.
- You have glaucoma.
- You have taken MAO inhibitors within 2 weeks.
- Patient is younger than 12.

**Before you start, consult your doctor:**
- If you will have surgery within 2 months, including dental surgery, requiring general or spinal anesthesia.
- If you have an enlarged prostate.
- If you have heart disease or high blood pressure.
- If you have stomach or intestinal problems.
- If you have overactive thyroid.
- If you have asthma.
- If you have liver disease.

**Over age 60:**
More likely to develop urination difficulty and side effects such as hallucinations, shakiness, dizziness, fainting, headache or insomnia.

## Pregnancy:
Studies inconclusive on harm to unborn child. Animal studies show fetal abnormalities. Decide with your doctor whether drug benefits justify risk to unborn child.

## Breast-feeding:
Drug passes into milk. Avoid drug or discontinue nursing until you finish medicine. Consult doctor for advice on maintaining milk supply.

## Infants & children:
Don't give to children younger than 12.

## Prolonged use:
Request blood cell counts, liver-function studies, monitor blood pressure closely.

## Skin & sunlight:
May cause rash or intensify sunburn in areas exposed to sun or sunlamp.

## Driving, piloting or hazardous work:
Don't drive or pilot aircraft until you learn how medicine affects you. Don't work around dangerous machinery. Don't climb ladders or work in high places. Danger increases if you drink alcohol or take medicine affecting alertness and reflexes.

## Discontinuing:
Don't discontinue without consulting doctor. Dose may require gradual reduction if you have taken drug for a long time. Doses of other drugs may also require adjustment.

## Others:
No problems expected.

# POSSIBLE INTERACTION WITH OTHER DRUGS

| GENERIC NAME OR DRUG CLASS | COMBINED EFFECT |
| --- | --- |
| Anticoagulants | Increased anticoagulant effect. |
| Anticholinergics | Increased sedation. |
| Antihistamines | Increased antihistamine effect. |
| Barbiturates | Decreased antidepressant effect. |
| Clonidine | Decreased clonidine effect. |
| Ethchlorvynol | Delirium. |
| Guanethidine | Decreased guanethidine effect. |
| MAO inhibitors | Fever, delirium, convulsions. |
| Methyldopa | Decreased methyldopa effect. |

| | |
| --- | --- |
| Molindone | Increased tranquilizer effect. |
| Narcotics | Dangerous oversedation. |
| Phenytoin | Decreased phenytoin effect. |
| Quinidine | Irregular heartbeat. |
| Sedatives | Dangerous oversedation. |
| Sympathomimetics | Increased sympathomimetic effect. |
| Thiazide diuretics | Increased maprotiline effect. |
| Thyroid hormones | Irregular heartbeat. |

# POSSIBLE INTERACTION WITH OTHER SUBSTANCES

| INTERACTS WITH | COMBINED EFFECT |
| --- | --- |
| Alcohol: Beverages or medicines with alcohol. | Excessive intoxication. Avoid. |
| Beverages: | None expected. |
| Cocaine: | Excessive intoxication. Avoid. |
| Foods: | None expected. |
| Marijuana: | Excessive drowsiness. Avoid. |
| Tobacco: | May decrease absorption of maprotiline. Avoid. |

# MECLIZINE

## BRAND NAMES

| | |
|---|---|
| Antivert | Motion Cure |
| Bonamine | Ru-Vert-M |
| Bonine | Wehvert |

## BASIC INFORMATION

**Habit forming?** No
**Prescription needed?**
  U.S.—Tablets: No
       Liquid: Yes
  Canada: Yes
**Available as generic?** Yes
**Drug class:** Antihistamine, antiemetic

 USES

Prevents motion sickness.

 DOSAGE & USAGE INFORMATION

**How to take:**
Tablet—Swallow with liquid or food to lessen stomach irritation. If you can't swallow whole, crumble tablet and chew or take with liquid or food.

**When to take:**
30 minutes to 1 hour before traveling.

**If you forget a dose:**
Take as soon as you remember. Wait 4 hours for next dose.

**What drug does:**
Reduces sensitivity of nerve endings in inner ear, blocking messages to brain's vomiting center.

**Time lapse before drug works:**
30 to 60 minutes.

**Don't take with:**
See Interaction column and consult doctor.

 OVERDOSE

**SYMPTOMS:**
Drowsiness, confusion, incoordination, stupor, coma, weak pulse, shallow breathing.
**WHAT TO DO:**
- **Dial 0 (operator) or 911 (emergency) for an ambulance or medical help. Then give first aid immediately.**
- **See emergency information on inside covers.**

 POSSIBLE ADVERSE REACTIONS OR SIDE EFFECTS

| SYMPTOMS | WHAT TO DO |
|---|---|
| **Life-threatening:** None expected. | |
| **Common:** Drowsiness. | Continue. Tell doctor at next visit. |
| **Infrequent:** | |
| ● Headache, diarrhea or constipation, fast heartbeat. | Continue. Call doctor when convenient. |
| ● Dry mouth, nose, throat. | Continue. Tell doctor at next visit. |
| **Rare:** | |
| ● Rash, hives. | Discontinue. Call doctor right away. |
| ● Restlessness, excitement, insomnia, blurred vision, frequent and difficult urination. | Continue. Call doctor when convenient. |
| ● Appetite loss, nausea. | Continue. Tell doctor at next visit. |

## WARNINGS & PRECAUTIONS

**Don't take if:**
- You are allergic to meclizine, buclizine or cyclizine.
- You have taken MAO inhibitors in the past 2 weeks.

**Before you start, consult your doctor:**
- If you have glaucoma.
- If you have prostate enlargement.
- If you have reacted badly to any antihistamine.

**Over age 60:**
Adverse reactions and side effects may be more frequent and severe than in younger persons, especially impaired urination from enlarged prostate gland.

**Pregnancy:**
Studies inconclusive on harm to unborn child. Animal studies show fetal abnormalities. Decide with your doctor whether drug benefits justify risk to unborn child.

**Breast-feeding:**
Drug passes into milk. Avoid drug or discontinue nursing until you finish medicine. Consult doctor for advice on maintaining milk supply.

**Infants & children:**
No problems expected.

**Prolonged use:**
No problems expected.

**Skin & sunlight:**
No problems expected.

**Driving, piloting or hazardous work:**
Don't fly aircraft. Don't drive until you learn how medicine affects you. Don't work around dangerous machinery. Don't climb ladders or work in high places. Danger increases if you drink alcohol or take medicine affecting alertness and reflexes, such as antihistamines, tranquilizers, sedatives, pain medicine, narcotics and mind-altering drugs.

**Discontinuing:**
No problems expected.

**Others:**
No problems expected.

## POSSIBLE INTERACTION WITH OTHER DRUGS

| GENERIC NAME OR DRUG CLASS | COMBINED EFFECT |
|---|---|
| Amphetamines | May decrease drowsiness caused by meclizine. |
| Anticholinergics | Increased effect of both drugs. |
| Antidepressants (tricyclic) | Increased effect of both drugs. |
| MAO inhibitors | Increased meclizine effect. |
| Narcotics | Increased effect of both drugs. |
| Pain relievers | Increased effect of both drugs. |
| Sedatives | Increased effect of both drugs. |
| Sleep inducers | Increased effect of both drugs. |
| Tranquilizers | Increased effect of both drugs. |

## POSSIBLE INTERACTION WITH OTHER SUBSTANCES

| INTERACTS WITH | COMBINED EFFECT |
|---|---|
| Alcohol: | Increased sedation. Avoid. |
| Beverages: Caffeine drinks. | May decrease drowsiness. |
| Cocaine: | None expected. |
| Foods: | None expected. |
| Marijuana: | Increased drowsiness, dry mouth. |
| Tobacco: | None expected. |

# MECLOFENAMATE

## BRAND NAMES

Meclomen

## BASIC INFORMATION

**Habit forming?** No
**Prescription needed?** Yes
**Available as generic?** No
**Drug class:** Anti-inflammatory (non-steroid)

 **USES**

Treatment for joint pain, stiffness, inflammation and swelling of arthritis and gout.

 **DOSAGE & USAGE INFORMATION**

**How to take:**
Capsule—Swallow with liquid or food to lessen stomach irritation. If you can't swallow whole, open capsule and take with liquid or food.

**When to take:**
At the same times each day.

**If you forget a dose:**
Take as soon as you remember up to 2 hours late. If more than 2 hours, wait for next scheduled dose (don't double this dose).

**What drug does:**
Reduces tissue concentration of prostaglandins (hormones which produce inflammation and pain).

**Time lapse before drug works:**
Begins in 4 to 24 hours. May require 3 weeks regular use for maximum benefit.

**Don't take with:**
See Interaction column and consult doctor.

 **OVERDOSE**

**SYMPTOMS:**
**Confusion, agitation, incoherence, convulsions, possible hemorrhage from stomach or intestine, coma.**
**WHAT TO DO:**
- **Dial 0 (operator) or 911 (emergency) for an ambulance or medical help. Then give first aid immediately.**
- **See emergency information on inside covers.**

 **POSSIBLE ADVERSE REACTIONS OR SIDE EFFECTS**

| SYMPTOMS | WHAT TO DO |
|---|---|
| **Life-threatening:** None expected. | |
| **Common:** | |
| • Dizziness, nausea, pain. | Continue. Call doctor when convenient. |
| • Headache. | Continue. Tell doctor at next visit. |
| **Infrequent:** Depression; drowsiness; ringing in ears; constipation or diarrhea; vomiting; swollen feet, legs. | Continue. Call doctor when convenient. |
| **Rare:** | |
| • Convulsions; confusion; rash, hives or itchy skin; blurred vision; black, bloody or tarry stool; difficult breathing; tightness in chest; rapid heartbeat; unusual bleeding or bruising; blood in urine; jaundice. | Discontinue. Call doctor right away. |
| • Frequent, painful or difficult urination; fatigue, weakness. | Continue. Call doctor when convenient. |

## WARNINGS & PRECAUTIONS

**Don't take if:**
- You are allergic to aspirin or any non-steroid, anti-inflammatory drug.
- You have gastritis, peptic ulcer, enteritis, ileitis, ulcerative colitis, asthma, heart failure, high blood pressure or bleeding problems.
- Patient is younger than 15.

**Before you start, consult your doctor:**
- If you have epilepsy.
- If you have Parkinson's disease.
- If you have been mentally ill.
- If you have had kidney disease or impaired kidney function.

**Over age 60:**
Adverse reactions and side effects may be more frequent and severe than in younger persons.

**Pregnancy:**
Studies inconclusive on harm to unborn child. Decide with your doctor whether drug benefits justify risk to unborn child.

**Breast-feeding:**
May harm child. Avoid.

**Infants & children:**
Not recommended for anyone younger than 15. Use only under medical supervision.

**Prolonged use:**
- Eye damage.
- Reduced hearing.
- Sore throat, fever.
- Weight gain.

**Skin & sunlight:**
No problems expected.

**Driving, piloting or hazardous work:**
Don't drive or pilot aircraft until you learn how medicine affects you. Don't work around dangerous machinery. Don't climb ladders or work in high places. Danger increases if you drink alcohol or take medicine affecting alertness and reflexes, such as antihistamines, tranquilizers, sedatives, pain medicine, narcotics and mind-altering drugs.

**Discontinuing:**
Don't discontinue without consulting doctor. Dose may require gradual reduction if you have taken drug for a long time. Doses of other drugs may also require adjustment.

**Others:**
No problems expected.

## POSSIBLE INTERACTION WITH OTHER DRUGS

| GENERIC NAME OR DRUG CLASS | COMBINED EFFECT |
| --- | --- |
| Acebutolol | Decreased antihypertensive effect of acebutolol. |
| Anticoagulants (oral) | Increased risk of bleeding. |
| Aspirin | Increased risk of stomach ulcer. |
| Cortisone drugs | Increased risk of stomach ulcer. |
| Furosemide | Decreased diuretic effect of furosemide. |
| Gold compounds | Possible increased likelihood of kidney damage. |
| Ketoprofen | Increased possibility of internal bleeding. |
| Minoxidil | Decreased minoxidil effect. |
| Oxprenolol | Decreased antihypertensive effect of oxprenolol. |
| Oxyphenbutazone | Possible stomach ulcer. |
| Phenylbutazone | Possible stomach ulcer. |
| Probenecid | Increased meclofenamate effect. |
| Thyroid hormones | Rapid heartbeat, blood-pressure rise. |

## POSSIBLE INTERACTION WITH OTHER SUBSTANCES

| INTERACTS WITH | COMBINED EFFECT |
| --- | --- |
| Alcohol: | Possible stomach ulcer or bleeding. |
| Beverages: | None expected. |
| Cocaine: | None expected. |
| Foods: | None expected. |
| Marijuana: | Increased pain relief from meclofenamate. |
| Tobacco: | None expected. |

# MEDROXYPROGESTERONE

## BRAND NAMES

| | |
|---|---|
| Amen | Depo-Provera |
| Curretab | Provera |

## BASIC INFORMATION

**Habit forming? No**
**Prescription needed? Yes**
**Available as generic? Yes**
**Drug class: Female sex hormone (progestin)**

## USES

- Treatment for menstrual or uterine disorders caused by progestin imbalance.
- Contraceptive.
- Treatment for cancer of breast and uterus.

## DOSAGE & USAGE INFORMATION

**How to take:**
- Tablet or capsule—Swallow with liquid or food to lessen stomach irritation. You may crumble tablet or open capsule.
- Injection—Take under doctor's supervision.

**When to take:**
Tablet, capsule—At the same time each day.

**If you forget a dose:**
- Menstrual disorders—Take up to 2 hours late. If more than 2 hours, wait for next dose (don't double this dose).
- Contraceptive—Consult your doctor. You may need to use another birth-control method until next period.

**What drug does:**
- Creates a uterine lining similar to pregnancy that prevents bleeding.
- Suppresses a pituitary gland hormone responsible for ovulation.
- Stimulates cervical mucus, which stops sperm penetration and prevents pregnancy.

*Continued next column*

## OVERDOSE

**SYMPTOMS:**
**Nausea, vomiting, fluid retention, breast discomfort or enlargement, vaginal bleeding.**
**WHAT TO DO:**
**Overdose unlikely to threaten life. If person takes much larger amount than prescribed, call doctor, poison-control center or hospital emergency room for instructions.**

**Time lapse before drug works:**
- Menstrual disorders—24 to 48 hours.
- Contraception—3 weeks.
- Cancer—May require 2 to 3 months regular use for maximum benefit.

**Don't take with:**
See Interaction column and consult doctor.

## POSSIBLE ADVERSE REACTIONS OR SIDE EFFECTS

| SYMPTOMS | WHAT TO DO |
|---|---|
| **Life-threatening:** | |
| Blood clot in leg, brain or lung. | Seek emergency treatment immediately. |
| **Common:** | |
| Appetite or weight changes, swollen feet or ankles, unusual tiredness or weakness. | Continue. Tell doctor at next visit. |
| **Infrequent:** | |
| • Prolonged vaginal bleeding. | Discontinue. Call doctor right away. |
| • Depression. | Continue. Call doctor when convenient. |
| • Acne, increased facial or body hair, nausea, tender breasts. | Continue. Tell doctor at next visit. |
| **Rare:** | |
| Rash, stomach or side pain, jaundice. | Discontinue. Call doctor right away. |

## WARNINGS & PRECAUTIONS

**Don't take if:**
- You are allergic to any progestin hormone.
- You may be pregnant.
- You have liver or gallbladder disease.
- You have had thrombophlebitis, embolism or stroke.
- You have unexplained vaginal bleeding.
- You have had breast or uterine cancer.

**Before you start, consult your doctor:**
- If you have heart or kidney disease.
- If you have diabetes.
- If you have a seizure disorder.
- If you suffer migraines.
- If you are easily depressed.

**Over age 60:**
Not recommended.

**Pregnancy:**
May harm child. Discontinue at first sign of pregnancy.

**Breast-feeding:**
Drug passes into milk. Avoid drug or discontinue nursing until you finish medicine. Consult doctor for advice on maintaining milk supply.

**Infants & children:**
Use only for female children under medical supervision.

**Prolonged use:**
No problems expected.

**Skin & sunlight:**
No problems expected.

**Driving, piloting or hazardous work:**
No problems expected.

**Discontinuing:**
Consult doctor. This medicine stays in the body and causes fetal abnormalities. Wait at least 3 months before becoming pregnant.

**Others:**
- Patients with diabetes must be monitored closely.
- Symptoms of blood clot in leg, brain or lung are: chest, groin, leg pain; sudden, severe headache; loss of coordination; vision change; shortness of breath; slurred speech.

## POSSIBLE INTERACTION WITH OTHER DRUGS

| GENERIC NAME OR DRUG CLASS | COMBINED EFFECT |
|---|---|
| Antihistamines | Decreased medroxyprogesterone effect. |
| Oxyphenbutazone | Decreased medroxyprogesterone effect. |
| Phenobarbital | Decreased medroxyprogesterone effect. |
| Phenothiazines | Increased phenothiazine effect. |
| Phenylbutazone | Decreased medroxyprogesterone effect. |
| Rifampin | Decreased contraceptive effect. |

## POSSIBLE INTERACTION WITH OTHER SUBSTANCES

| INTERACTS WITH | COMBINED EFFECT |
|---|---|
| Alcohol: | None expected. |
| Beverages: | None expected. |
| Cocaine: | Decreased medroxyprogesterone effect. |
| Foods: Salt. | Fluid retention. |
| Marijuana: | Possible menstrual irregularities or bleeding between periods. |
| Tobacco: All forms. | Possible blood clots in lung, brain, legs. Avoid. |

# MEFENAMIC ACID

## BRAND NAMES

Ponstan        Ponstel

## BASIC INFORMATION

**Habit forming? No**
**Prescription needed? Yes**
**Available as generic? No**
**Drug class: Anti-inflammatory (non-steroid)**

## USES

- Pain reliever.
- Treatment for dysmenorrhea (painful or difficult menstruation).

## DOSAGE & USAGE INFORMATION

**How to take:**
Capsule—Swallow with liquid or food to lessen stomach irritation. If you can't swallow whole, open capsule and take with liquid or food.

**When to take:**
At the same times each day.

**If you forget a dose:**
Take as soon as you remember up to 2 hours late. If more than 2 hours, wait for next scheduled dose (don't double this dose).

**What drug does:**
Reduces tissue concentration of prostaglandins (hormones which produce inflammation and pain).

**Time lapse before drug works:**
Begins in 4 to 24 hours. May require 3 weeks regular use for maximum benefit.

**Don't take with:**
See Interaction column and consult doctor.

## OVERDOSE

**SYMPTOMS:**
**Confusion, agitation, incoherence, convulsions, possible hemorrhage from stomach or intestine, coma.**
**WHAT TO DO:**
- **Dial 0 (operator) or 911 (emergency) for an ambulance or medical help. Then give first aid immediately.**
- **See emergency information on inside covers.**

## POSSIBLE ADVERSE REACTIONS OR SIDE EFFECTS

| SYMPTOMS | WHAT TO DO |
|---|---|
| **Life-threatening:**<br>None expected. | |
| **Common:**<br>• Dizziness, nausea, pain. | Continue. Call doctor when convenient. |
| • Headache. | Continue. Tell doctor at next visit. |
| **Infrequent:**<br>Depression, drowsiness, ringing in ears, constipation or diarrhea, vomiting, swollen feet or legs. | Continue. Call doctor when convenient. |
| **Rare:**<br>• Convulsions; confusion; rash, hives or itchy skin; blurred vision; black, bloody or tarry stool; difficult breathing; tightness in chest; rapid heartbeat; unusual bleeding or bruising; blood in urine; jaundice. | Discontinue. Call doctor right away. |
| • Frequent, painful or difficult urination; fatigue, weakness. | Continue. Call doctor when convenient. |

## WARNINGS & PRECAUTIONS

**Don't take if:**
- You are allergic to aspirin or any non-steroid, anti-inflammatory drug.
- You have gastritis, peptic ulcer, enteritis, ileitis, ulcerative colitis, asthma, heart failure, high blood pressure or bleeding problems.
- Patient is younger than 15.

**Before you start, consult your doctor:**
- If you have epilepsy.
- If you have Parkinson's disease.
- If you have been mentally ill.
- If you have had kidney disease or impaired kidney function.

**Over age 60:**
Adverse reactions and side effects may be more frequent and severe than in younger persons.

**Pregnancy:**
Studies inconclusive on harm to unborn child. Decide with your doctor whether drug benefits justify risk to unborn child.

**Breast-feeding:**
May harm child. Avoid.

**Infants & children:**
Not recommended for anyone younger than 15. Use only under medical supervision.

**Prolonged use:**
- Eye damage.
- Reduced hearing.
- Sore throat, fever.
- Weight gain.

**Skin & sunlight:**
No problems expected.

**Driving, piloting or hazardous work:**
Don't drive or pilot aircraft until you learn how medicine affects you. Don't work around dangerous machinery. Don't climb ladders or work in high places. Danger increases if you drink alcohol or take medicine affecting alertness and reflexes, such as antihistamines, tranquilizers, sedatives, pain medicine, narcotics and mind-altering drugs.

**Discontinuing:**
Don't discontinue without consulting doctor. Dose may require gradual reduction if you have taken drug for a long time. Doses of other drugs may also require adjustment.

**Others:**
Don't take for more than 1 week.

## POSSIBLE INTERACTION WITH OTHER DRUGS

| GENERIC NAME OR DRUG CLASS | COMBINED EFFECT |
| --- | --- |
| Acebutolol | Decreased antihypertensive effect of acebutolol. |
| Anticoagulants (oral) | Increased risk of bleeding. |
| Aspirin | Increased risk of stomach ulcer. |
| Cortisone drugs | Increased risk of stomach ulcer. |
| Furosemide | Decreased diuretic effect of furosemide. |
| Gold compounds | Possible increased likelihood of kidney damage. |
| Minoxidil | Decreased minoxidil effect. |
| Oxprenolol | Decreased antihypertensive effect of oxprenolol. |
| Oxyphenbutazone | Possible stomach ulcer. |
| Phenylbutazone | Possible stomach ulcer. |
| Probenecid | Increased effect of mefenamic acid. |
| Thyroid hormones | Rapid heartbeat, blood-pressure rise. |

## POSSIBLE INTERACTION WITH OTHER SUBSTANCES

| INTERACTS WITH | COMBINED EFFECT |
| --- | --- |
| Alcohol: | Possible stomach ulcer or bleeding. |
| Beverages: | None expected. |
| Cocaine: | None expected. |
| Foods: | None expected. |
| Marijuana: | Increased pain relief from mefenamic acid. |
| Tobacco: | None expected. |

# MELPHALAN (PAM, L-PAM, PHENYLALANINE MUSTARD)

## BRAND NAMES

Alkeran
L-PAM

Phenylalanine
Mustard

## BASIC INFORMATION

Habit forming? No
Prescription needed? Yes
Available as generic? No
Drug class: Antineoplastic,
              immunosuppressant

 ## USES

- Treatment for some kinds of cancer.
- Suppresses immune response after transplant and in immune disorders.

 ## DOSAGE & USAGE INFORMATION

**How to take:**
Tablet or capsule—Swallow with liquid after light meal. Don't drink fluids with meals. Drink extra fluids between meals. Avoid sweet or fatty foods.

**When to take:**
At the same time each day.

**If you forget a dose:**
Take as soon as you remember. Don't ever double dose.

**What drug does:**
Inhibits abnormal cell reproduction. May suppress immune system.

*Continued next column*

 ## OVERDOSE

**SYMPTOMS:**
Bleeding, chills, fever, collapse, stupor, seizure.
**WHAT TO DO:**
- Dial 0 (operator) or 911 (emergency) for an ambulance or medical help. Then give first aid immediately.
- If patient is unconscious and not breathing, give mouth-to-mouth breathing. If there is no heartbeat, use cardiac massage and mouth-to-mouth breathing (CPR). Don't try to make patient vomit. If you can't get help quickly, take patient to nearest emergency facility.
- See emergency information on inside covers.

**Time lapse before drug works:**
Up to 6 weeks for full effect.

**Don't take with:**
See Interaction column and consult doctor.

 ## POSSIBLE ADVERSE REACTIONS OR SIDE EFFECTS

| SYMPTOMS | WHAT TO DO |
|---|---|
| **Life-threatening:** | |
| None expected. | |
| **Common:** | |
| • Unusual bleeding or bruising, mouth sores with sore throat, chills and fever, black stools, sores in mouth and lips, menstrual irregularities. | Discontinue. Call doctor right away. |
| • Hair loss, joint pain. | Continue. Call doctor when convenient. |
| • Nausea, vomiting, diarrhea (unavoidable), tiredness, weakness. | Continue. Tell doctor at next visit. |
| **Infrequent:** | |
| • Mental confusion, shortness of breath, may increase chance of developing leukemia. | Continue. Call doctor when convenient. |
| • Cough. | Continue. Tell doctor at next visit. |
| **Rare:** | |
| Jaundice. | Discontinue. Call doctor right away. |

# MELPHALAN (PAM, L-PAM, PHENYLALANINE MUSTARD)

## WARNINGS & PRECAUTIONS

**Don't take if:**
- You have had hypersensitivity to alkylating antineoplastic drugs.
- Your physician has not explained serious nature of your medical problem and risks of taking this medicine.

**Before you start, consult your doctor:**
- If you have gout.
- If you have had kidney stones.
- If you have active infection.
- If you have impaired kidney or liver function.
- If you have taken other antineoplastic drugs or had radiation treatment in last 3 weeks.

**Over age 60:**
Adverse reactions and side effects may be more frequent and severe than in younger persons.

**Pregnancy:**
Consult doctor. Risk to child is significant.

**Breast-feeding:**
Drug passes into milk. Don't nurse.

**Infants & children:**
Use only under special medical supervision at center experienced in anticancer drugs.

**Prolonged use:**
Adverse reactions more likely the longer drug is required.

**Skin & sunlight:**
No problems expected.

**Driving, piloting or hazardous work:**
No problems expected.

**Discontinuing:**
Don't discontinue without doctor's advice until you complete prescribed dose, even though symptoms diminish or disappear. Some side effects may follow discontinuing. Report to doctor blurred vision, convulsions, confusion, persistent headache.

**Others:**
May cause sterility.

## POSSIBLE INTERACTION WITH OTHER DRUGS

| GENERIC NAME OR DRUG CLASS | COMBINED EFFECT |
|---|---|
| Antigout drugs | Decreased antigout effect. |
| Antineoplastic drugs (other) | Increased effect of all drugs (may be beneficial). |
| Chloramphenicol | Increased likelihood of toxic effects of both drugs. |

## POSSIBLE INTERACTION WITH OTHER SUBSTANCES

| INTERACTS WITH | COMBINED EFFECT |
|---|---|
| Alcohol: | May increase chance of intestinal bleeding. |
| Beverages: | No problems expected. |
| Cocaine: | Increases chance of toxicity. |
| Foods: | Reduces irritation in stomach. |
| Marijuana: | No problems expected. |
| Tobacco: | Increases lung toxicity. |

# MEPHENYTOIN

## BRAND NAMES

Mesantoin         Methoin

## BASIC INFORMATION

**Habit forming? No**
**Prescription needed? Yes**
**Available as generic? Yes**
**Drug class: Anticonvulsant (hydantoin)**

 ## USES

- Prevents epileptic seizures.
- Stabilizes irregular heartbeat.

 ## DOSAGE & USAGE INFORMATION

**How to take:**
- Tablet or capsule—Swallow with liquid.
- Extended-release tablets or capsules—Swallow each dose whole. If you take regular tablets, you may chew or crush them.

**When to take:**
At the same time each day.

**If you forget a dose:**
- If drug taken 1 time per day—Take as soon as you remember up to 12 hours late. If more than 12 hours, wait for next scheduled dose (don't double this dose).
- If taken several times per day—Take as soon as possible, then return to regular schedule.

**What drug does:**
Promotes sodium loss from nerve fibers. This lessens excitability and inhibits spread of nerve impulses.

**Time lapse before drug works:**
7 to 10 days continual use.

**Don't take with:**
See Interaction column and consult doctor.

 ## OVERDOSE

**SYMPTOMS:**
**Jerky eye movements; stagger; slurred speech; imbalance; drowsiness; blood-pressure drop; slow, shallow breathing; coma.**
**WHAT TO DO:**
- **Dial 0 (operator) or 911 (emergency) for an ambulance or medical help. Then give first aid immediately.**
- **See emergency information on inside covers.**

 ## POSSIBLE ADVERSE REACTIONS OR SIDE EFFECTS

| SYMPTOMS | WHAT TO DO |
|---|---|
| **Life-threatening:** None expected. | |
| **Common:** Mild dizziness, drowsiness, constipation, nausea, vomiting. | Continue. Call doctor when convenient. |
| **Infrequent:** | |
| • Hallucinations, confusion, slurred speech, stagger, rash, change in vision. | Discontinue. Call doctor right away. |
| • Headache, sleeplessness, diarrhea, muscle twitching. | Continue. Call doctor when convenient. |
| • Increased body and facial hair. | Continue. Tell doctor at next visit. |
| **Rare:** Sore throat, fever, stomach pain, unusual bleeding or bruising, jaundice. | Discontinue. Call doctor right away. |

 ## WARNINGS & PRECAUTIONS

**Don't take if:**
You are allergic to any hydantoin anticonvulsant.

**Before you start, consult your doctor:**
- If you have had impaired liver function or disease.
- If you will have surgery within 2 months, including dental surgery, requiring general or spinal anesthesia.

**Over age 60:**
Adverse reactions and side effects may be more frequent and severe than in younger persons.

**Pregnancy:**
Risk to unborn child outweighs drug benefits. Don't use.

**Breast-feeding:**
Drug passes into milk. Avoid drug or discontinue nursing until you finish medicine. Consult doctor for advice on maintaining milk supply.

**Infants & children:**
Use only under medical supervision.

**Prolonged use:**
- Weakened bones.
- Lymph gland enlargement.
- Possible liver damage.
- Numbness and tingling of hands and feet.
- Continual back-and-forth eye movements.
- Bleeding, swollen or tender gums.

**Skin & sunlight:**
May cause rash or intensify sunburn in areas exposed to sun or sunlamp.

**Driving, piloting or hazardous work:**
Don't drive or pilot aircraft until you learn how medicine affects you. Don't work around dangerous machinery. Don't climb ladders or work in high places. Danger increases if you drink alcohol or take medicine affecting alertness and reflexes.

**Discontinuing:**
Don't discontinue without consulting doctor. Dose may require gradual reduction if you have taken drug for a long time. Doses of other drugs may also require adjustment.

**Others:**
No problems expected.

## POSSIBLE INTERACTION WITH OTHER DRUGS

| GENERIC NAME OR DRUG CLASS | COMBINED EFFECT |
|---|---|
| Anticoagulants | Increased effect of both drugs. |
| Antidepressants (tricyclic) | Need to adjust mephenytoin dose. |
| Antihypertensives | Increased effect of antihypertensive. |
| Aspirin | Increased mephenytoin effect. |
| Barbiturates | Changed seizure pattern. |
| Carbonic anhydrase inhibitors | Increased chance of bone disease. |
| Chloramphenicol | Increased mephenytoin effect. |
| Contraceptives (oral) | Increased seizures. |
| Cortisone drugs | Decreased cortisone effect. |
| Digitalis preparations | Decreased digitalis effect. |
| Disulfiram | Increased mephenytoin effect. |
| Estrogens | Increased mephenytoin effect. |
| Furosemide | Decreased furosemide effect. |
| Glutethimide | Decreased mephenytoin effect. |
| Griseofulvin | Increased griseofulvin effect. |
| Isoniazid | Increased mephenytoin effect. |
| Methadone | Decreased methadone effect. |
| Methotrexate | Increased methotrexate effect. |
| Methylphenidate | Increased mephenytoin effect. |
| Oxyphenbutazone | Increased mephenytoin effect. |
| Para-aminosalicylic acid (PAS) | Increased mephenytoin effect. |
| Phenothlazines | Increased mephenytoin effect. |
| Phenylbutazone | Increased mephonytoin effect. |
| Propranolol | Increased propranolol effect. |
| Quinidine | Increased quinidine effect. |
| Sedatives | Increased sedative effect. |
| Sulfa drugs | Increased mephenytoin effect. |
| Theophylline | Reduced anticonvulsant effect. |

## POSSIBLE INTERACTION WITH OTHER SUBSTANCES

| INTERACTS WITH | COMBINED EFFECT |
|---|---|
| Alcohol: | Possible decreased anticonvulsant effect. Use with caution. |
| Beverages: | None expected. |
| Cocaine: | Possible seizures. |
| Foods: | None expected. |
| Marijuana: | Drowsiness, unsteadiness, decreased anticonvulsant effect. |
| Tobacco: | None expected. |

# MEPHOBARBITAL

## BRAND NAMES

**Mebaral**

## BASIC INFORMATION

**Habit forming? Yes**
**Prescription needed? Yes**
**Available as generic? Yes**
**Drug class: Sedative, hypnotic (barbiturate)**

## USES

- Reduces anxiety or nervous tension (low dose).
- Relieves insomnia (higher bedtime dose).
- Prevents seizures in epilepsy.

## DOSAGE & USAGE INFORMATION

**How to take:**
Tablet—Swallow with liquid or food to lessen stomach irritation. If you can't swallow whole, crumble tablet and take with liquid or food.

**When to take:**
At the same times each day.

**If you forget a dose:**
Take as soon as you remember up to 2 hours late. If more than 2 hours, wait for next scheduled dose (don't double this dose).

**What drug does:**
May partially block nerve impulses at nerve-cell connections.

**Time lapse before drug works:**
60 minutes.

*Continued next column*

## OVERDOSE

**SYMPTOMS:**
**Deep sleep, weak pulse, coma.**
**WHAT TO DO:**
- **Dial 0 (operator) or 911 (emergency) for an ambulance or medical help. Then give first aid immediately.**
- **If patient is unconscious and not breathing, give mouth-to-mouth breathing. If there is no heartbeat use cardiac massage and mouth-to-mouth breathing (CPR). Don't try to make patient vomit. If you can't get help quickly, take patient to nearest emergency facility.**
- **See emergency information on inside covers.**

**Don't take with:**
- Non-prescription drugs without consulting doctor.
- See Interaction column and consult doctor.

## POSSIBLE ADVERSE REACTIONS OR SIDE EFFECTS

| SYMPTOMS | WHAT TO DO |
|---|---|
| **Life-threatening:**<br>None expected. | |
| **Common:**<br>Dizziness, drowsiness, "hangover" effect. | Continue. Call doctor when convenient. |
| **Infrequent:** | |
| • Rash or hives; face, lip or eyelid swelling; sore throat; fever. | Discontinue. Call doctor right away. |
| • Depression, confusion, diarrhea, nausea, vomiting, joint or muscle pain, slurred speech. | Continue. Call doctor when convenient. |
| **Rare:** | |
| • Agitation, slow heartbeat, difficult breathing, jaundice. | Discontinue. Call doctor right away. |
| • Unexplained bleeding or bruising. | Continue. Call doctor when convenient. |

## WARNINGS & PRECAUTIONS

**Don't take if:**
- You are allergic to any barbiturate.
- You have porphyria.

**Before you start, consult your doctor:**
- If you have epilepsy.
- If you have kidney or liver damage.
- If you have asthma.
- If you have anemia.
- If you have chronic pain.
- If you will have surgery within 2 months, including dental surgery, requiring general or spinal anesthesia.

**Over age 60:**
Adverse reactions and side effects may be more frequent and severe than in younger persons. Use small doses.

**Pregnancy:**
Risk to unborn child outweighs drug benefits. Don't use.

**Breast-feeding:**
Drug passes into milk. Avoid drug or discontinue nursing until you finish medicine. Consult doctor for advice on maintaining milk supply.

**Infants & children:**
Use only under doctor's supervision.

**Prolonged use:**
- May cause addiction, anemia, chronic intoxication.
- May lower body temperature, making exposure to cold temperatures hazardous.

**Skin & sunlight:**
May cause rash or intensify sunburn in areas exposed to sun or sunlamp.

**Driving, piloting or hazardous work:**
Don't drive or pilot aircraft until you learn how medicine affects you. Don't work around dangerous machinery. Don't climb ladders or work in high places. Danger increases if you drink alcohol or take medicine affecting alertness and reflexes.

**Discontinuing:**
May be unnecessary to finish medicine. Follow doctor's instructions. If you develop withdrawal symptoms of hallucinations, agitation or sleeplessness after discontinuing, call doctor right away.

**Others:**
No problems expected.

## POSSIBLE INTERACTION WITH OTHER DRUGS

| GENERIC NAME OR DRUG CLASS | COMBINED EFFECT |
|---|---|
| Anticoagulants (oral) | Decreased effect of anticoagulant. |
| Anticonvulsants | Changed seizure patterns. |
| Antidepressants (tricyclics) | Decreased antidepressant effect. Possible dangerous oversedation. |
| Antidiabetics (oral) | Increased effect of mephobarbital. |
| Antihistamines | Dangerous sedation. Avoid. |
| Anti-inflammatory drugs (non-steroidal) | Decreased anti-inflammatory effect. |
| Aspirin | Decreased aspirin effect. |
| Beta-adrenergic blockers | Decreased effect of beta-adrenergic blocker. |
| Contraceptives (oral) | Decreased contraceptive effect. |
| Cortisone drugs | Decreased cortisone effect. |
| Digitoxin | Decreased digitoxin effect. |
| Doxycycline | Decreased doxycycline effect. |
| Dronabinol | Increased effects of both drugs. Avoid. |
| Griseofulvin | Decreased griseofulvin effect. |
| Indapamide | Increased indapamide effect. |
| MAO inhibitors | Increased mephobarbital effect. |
| Mind-altering drugs | Dangerous sedation. Avoid. |
| Molindone | Increased sedative effect. |
| Narcotics | Dangerous sedation. Avoid. |
| Pain relievers | Dangerous sedation. Avoid. |
| Sedatives | Dangerous sedation. Avoid. |
| Sleep inducers | Dangerous sedation. Avoid. |
| Tranquilizers | Dangerous sedation. Avoid. |
| Valproic acid | Increased mephobarbital effect. |

## POSSIBLE INTERACTION WITH OTHER SUBSTANCES

| INTERACTS WITH | COMBINED EFFECT |
|---|---|
| Alcohol: | Possible fatal oversedation. Avoid. |
| Beverages: | None expected. |
| Cocaine: | Decreased mephobarbital effect. |
| Foods: | None expected. |
| Marijuana: | Excessive sedation. Avoid. |
| Tobacco: | None expected. |

# MEROBAMATE

## BRAND NAMES

See complete list of brand names in the *Brand Name Directory*, page 951.

## BASIC INFORMATION

**Habit forming? Yes**
**Prescription needed? Yes**
**Available as generic? Yes**
**Drug class: Tranquilizer**

## USES

Reduces mild anxiety, tension and insomnia.

## DOSAGE & USAGE INFORMATION

**How to take:**
- Tablet or capsule—Swallow with liquid.
- Extended-release tablets or capsules—Swallow each dose whole. If you take regular tablets, you may chew or crush them.
- Liquid—Take as directed on label.

**When to take:**
At the same time each day.

**If you forget a dose:**
Take as soon as you remember up to 2 hours late. If more than 2 hours, wait for next scheduled dose (don't double this dose).

**What drug does:**
Sedates brain centers which control behavior and emotions.

**Time lapse before drug works:**
1 to 2 hours.

**Don't take with:**
- Non-prescription drugs containing alcohol or caffeine without consulting doctor.
- See Interaction column and consult doctor.

## OVERDOSE

**SYMPTOMS:**
**Dizziness, slurred speech, stagger, depressed breathing and heart function, stupor, coma.**
**WHAT TO DO:**
- **Dial 0 (operator) or 911 (emergency) for an ambulance or medical help. Then give first aid immediately.**
- **See emergency information on inside covers.**

## POSSIBLE ADVERSE REACTIONS OR SIDE EFFECTS

| SYMPTOMS | WHAT TO DO |
|---|---|
| **Life-threatening:**<br>None expected. | |
| **Common:**<br>Dizziness, confusion, agitation, drowsiness, unsteadiness, fatigue, weakness. | Continue. Tell doctor at next visit. |
| **Infrequent:**<br>• Rash, hives, itchy skin; change in vision; diarrhea, nausea or vomiting. | Discontinue. Call doctor right away. |
| • False sense of well-being, headache, slurred speech. | Continue. Call doctor when convenient. |
| **Rare:**<br>Sore throat; fever; rapid, pounding, unusually slow or irregular heartbeat; difficult breathing; unusual bleeding or bruising. | Discontinue. Call doctor right away. |

## WARNINGS & PRECAUTIONS

**Don't take if:**
- You are allergic to meprobamate, tybanate, carbromal or carisoprodol.
- You have had porphyria.
- Patient is younger than 6.

**Before you start, consult your doctor:**
- If you have epilepsy.
- If you have impaired liver or kidney function.

**Over age 60:**
Adverse reactions and side effects may be more frequent and severe than in younger persons.

**Pregnancy:**
Risk to unborn child outweighs drug benefits. Don't use.

**Breast-feeding:**
Drug filters into milk. May harm child. Avoid.

**Infants & children:**
Not recommended.

**Prolonged use:**
- Habit forming.
- May impair blood-cell production.

**Skin & sunlight:**
No problems expected.

**Driving, piloting or hazardous work:**
Don't drive or pilot aircraft until you learn how medicine affects you. Don't work around dangerous machinery. Don't climb ladders or work in high places. Danger increases if you drink alcohol or take medicine affecting alertness and reflexes, such as antihistamines, tranquilizers, sedatives, pain medicine, narcotics and mind-altering drugs.

**Discontinuing:**
Don't discontinue without consulting doctor. Dose may require gradual reduction if you have taken drug for a long time. Doses of other drugs may also require adjustment.

**Others:**
No problems expected.

## POSSIBLE INTERACTION WITH OTHER DRUGS

| GENERIC NAME OR DRUG CLASS | COMBINED EFFECT |
|---|---|
| Anticoagulants | Decreased anticoagulant effect. |
| Anticonvulsants | Change in seizure pattern. |
| Antidepressants | Increased antidepressant effect. |
| Contraceptives (oral) | Decreased contraceptive effect. |
| Dronabinol | Increased effects of both drugs. Avoid. |
| Estrogens | Decreased estrogen effect. |
| MAO inhibitors | Increased meprobamate effect. |
| Molindone | Increased tranquilizer effect. |
| Narcotics | Increased narcotic effect. |
| Sedatives | Increased sedative effect. |
| Sleep inducers | Increased effect of sleep inducer. |
| Terfenadine | Possible excessive sedation. |
| Tranquilizers | Increased tranquilizer effect. |

## POSSIBLE INTERACTION WITH OTHER SUBSTANCES

| INTERACTS WITH | COMBINED EFFECT |
|---|---|
| Alcohol: | Dangerous increased effect of meprobamate. |
| Beverages: Caffeine drinks. | Decreased calming effect of meprobamate. |
| Cocaine: | Decreased meprobamate effect. |
| Foods: | None expected. |
| Marijuana: | Increased sedative effect of meprobamate. |
| Tobacco: | None expected. |

# MEPROBAMATE & ASPIRIN

## BRAND NAMES

**Equagesic**          **Micrainin**

## BASIC INFORMATION

**Habit forming? Yes**
**Prescription needed? Yes**
**Available as generic? No**
**Drug class: Anti-inflammatory, analgesic,
          tranquilizer**

## USES

- Reduces mild anxiety, tension and insomnia.
- Reduces pain, fever, inflammation.
- Relieves swelling, stiffness, joint pain.

## DOSAGE & USAGE INFORMATION

**How to take:**
- Tablet or capsule—Swallow with liquid.
- Extended-release tablets or capsules—Swallow each dose whole. If you take regular tablets, you may chew or crush them.
- Liquid—Take as directed on label.

**When to take:**
Pain, fever, inflammation—As needed, no more often than every 4 hours.

**If you forget a dose:**
Take as soon as you remember up to 2 hours late. If more than 2 hours, wait for next scheduled dose (don't double this dose).

**What drug does:**
- Sedates brain centers which control behavior and emotions.
- Affects hypothalamus, the part of the brain which regulates temperature by dilating small blood vessels in skin.

*Continued next column*

## OVERDOSE

**SYMPTOMS:**
**Dizziness; slurred speech; stagger; depressed heart function; ringing in ears; nausea; vomiting; fever; deep, rapid breathing; hallucinations; convulsions; stupor; coma.**
**WHAT TO DO:**
- **Dial 0 (operator) or 911 (emergency) for an ambulance or medical help. Then give first aid immediately.**
- **See emergency information on inside covers.**

- Prevents clumping of platelets (small blood cells) so blood vessels remain open.
- Decreases prostaglandin effect.
- Suppresses body's pain messages.

**Time lapse before drug works:**
1 to 2 hours.

**Don't take with:**
- Tetracyclines.
- Non-prescription drugs containing alcohol or caffeine without consulting doctor.
- See Interaction column and consult doctor.

## POSSIBLE ADVERSE REACTIONS OR SIDE EFFECTS

| SYMPTOMS | WHAT TO DO |
|---|---|
| **Life-threatening:** | |
| Hives, rash, intense itching, faintness soon after a dose (anaphylaxis). | Seek emergency treatment immediately. |
| **Common:** | |
| • Nausea, vomiting. | Discontinue. Call doctor right away. |
| • Dizziness, confusion, agitation, drowsiness, unsteadiness, fatigue, weakness, ears ringing, heartburn, indigestion. | Continue. Call doctor when convenient. |
| **Infrequent:** | |
| None expected. | |
| **Rare:** | |
| • Black, bloody or tarry stool; vomiting blood or black material; blood in urine. | Discontinue. Seek emergency treatment. |
| • Rash, hives, itchy skin, change in vision, fever, jaundice. | Discontinue. Call doctor right away. |

## WARNINGS & PRECAUTIONS

**Don't take if:**
- You are allergic to meprobamate, tybanate, carbromal or carisoprodol.
- You have had porphyria.
- You have a peptic ulcer of stomach or duodenum or a bleeding disorder.
- Patient is younger than 6.

**Before you start, consult your doctor:**
- If you have epilepsy, impaired liver or kidney function, asthma or nasal polyps.
- If you have had gout, stomach or duodenal ulcers.

**Over age 60:**
Adverse reactions and side effects may be more frequent and severe than in younger

persons. More likely to cause hidden bleeding in stomach or intestines. Watch for dark stools.

**Pregnancy:**
Risk to unborn child outweighs drug benefits. Don't use.

**Breast-feeding:**
Drug passes into milk. Avoid drug or discontinue nursing until you finish medicine. Consult doctor for advice on maintaining milk supply.

**Infants & children:**
Not recommended.

**Prolonged use:**
- Habit forming.
- May impair blood-cell production.
- Kidney damage. Periodic kidney-function test recommended.

**Skin & sunlight:**
Aspirin combined with sunscreen may decrease sunburn.

**Driving, piloting or hazardous work:**
Don't drive or pilot aircraft until you learn how medicine affects you. Don't work around dangerous machinery. Don't climb ladders or work in high places. Danger increases if you drink alcohol or take medicine affecting alertness and reflexes, such as antihistamines, tranquilizers, sedatives, pain medicine, narcotics and mind-altering drugs.

**Discontinuing:**
Don't discontinue without consulting doctor. Dose may require gradual reduction if you have taken drug for a long time. Doses of other drugs may also require adjustment.

**Others:**
- Aspirin can complicate surgery, pregnancy, labor and delivery, and illness.
- Urine tests for blood sugar may be inaccurate.

# POSSIBLE INTERACTION WITH OTHER DRUGS

| GENERIC NAME OR DRUG CLASS | COMBINED EFFECT |
|---|---|
| Acebutolol | Decreased antihypertensive effect of acebutolol. |
| Allopurinol | Decreased allopurinol effect. |
| Antacids | Decreased aspirin effect. |
| Anticoagulants | Increased anticoagulant effect. Abnormal bleeding. |
| Anticonvulsants | Change in seizure pattern. |
| Antidepressants | Increased antidepressant effect. |
| Antidiabetics (oral) | Low blood sugar. |
| Anti-inflammatory drugs (non-steroid) | Risk of stomach bleeding and ulcers. |
| Aspirin (other) | Likely aspirin toxicity. |
| Contraceptives (oral) | Decreased contraceptive effect. |
| Cortisone drugs | Increased cortisone effect. Risk of ulcers and stomach bleeding. |
| Dronabinol | Increased effect of both drugs. |
| Estrogens | Decreased estrogen effect. |
| Furosemide | Possible aspirin toxicity. |
| Gold compounds | Increased likelihood of kidney damage. |
| Indomethacin | Risk of stomach bleeding and ulcers. |
| MAO inhibitors | Increased meprobamate effect. |
| Methotrexate | Increased methotrexate effect. |
| Minoxidil | Decreased minoxidil effect. |
| Narcotics | Increased narcotic effect. |
| Oxprenolol | Decreased antihypertensive effect of oxprenolol. |

*Continued page 968*

# POSSIBLE INTERACTION WITH OTHER SUBSTANCES

| INTERACTS WITH | COMBINED EFFECT |
|---|---|
| Alcohol: | Possible stomach irritation and bleeding. Dangerous increased effect of meprobamate. Avoid. |
| Beverages: Caffeine drinks. | Decreased calming effect of meprobamate. |
| Cocaine: | Decreased meprobamate effect. |
| Foods: | None expected. |
| Marijuana: | Possible increased pain relief, but marijuana may slow body's recovery. Avoid. |
| Tobacco: | None expected. |

# MERCAPTOPURINE

## BRAND NAMES

Purinethol

## BASIC INFORMATION

**Habit forming? No**
**Prescription needed? Yes**
**Available as generic? Yes**
**Drug class: Antineoplastic,**
**immunosuppressant**

 ## USES

- Treatment for some kinds of cancer.
- Treatment for regional enteritis and ulcerative colitis and other immune disorders.

 ## DOSAGE & USAGE INFORMATION

**How to take:**
Tablet—Swallow with liquid.

**When to take:**
At the same time each day.

**If you forget a dose:**
Skip the missed dose. Don't double the next dose.

**What drug does:**
Inhibits abnormal-cell reproduction.

**Time lapse before drug works:**
May require 6 weeks for maximum effect.

**Don't take with:**
See Interaction column and consult doctor.

 ## OVERDOSE

**SYMPTOMS:**
**Headache, stupor, seizures.**
**WHAT TO DO:**
- Dial 0 (operator) or 911 (emergency) for an ambulance or medical help. Then give first aid immediately.
- If patient is unconscious and not breathing, give mouth-to-mouth breathing. If there is no heartbeat, use cardiac massage and mouth-to-mouth breathing (CPR). Don't try to make patient vomit. If you can't get help quickly, take patient to nearest emergency facility.
- See emergency information on inside covers.

 ## POSSIBLE ADVERSE REACTIONS OR SIDE EFFECTS

| SYMPTOMS | WHAT TO DO |
|---|---|
| **Life-threatening:** | |
| None expected. | |
| **Common:** | |
| • Black stools or bloody vomit. | Discontinue. Seek emergency treatment. |
| • Mouth sores, sore throat, fever, chills, unusual bleeding or bruising. | Discontinue. Call doctor right away. |
| • Stomach pain, nausea, vomiting. | Continue. Call doctor when convenient. |
| **Infrequent:** | |
| • Seizures. | Discontinue. Seek emergency treatment. |
| • Dizziness, drowsiness, headache, confusion, blurred vision, shortness of breath, joint pain, blood in urine, jaundice. | Discontinue. Call doctor right away. |
| • Cough. | Continue. Call doctor when convenient. |
| • Acne, boils, hair loss, itchy skin. | Continue. Tell doctor at next visit. |
| **Rare:** | |
| None expected. | |

## WARNINGS & PRECAUTIONS

**Don't take if:**
You are allergic to any antineoplastic.

**Before you start, consult your doctor:**
- If you are alcoholic.
- If you have blood, liver or kidney disease.
- If you have colitis or peptic ulcer.
- If you have gout.
- If you have an infection.
- If you plan to become pregnant within 3 months.

**Over age 60:**
Adverse reactions and side effects may be more frequent and severe than in younger persons.

**Pregnancy:**
Consult doctor.

**Breast-feeding:**
Drug passes into milk. Avoid drug or discontinue nursing.

**Infants & children:**
Use only under special medical supervision.

**Prolonged use:**
Adverse reactions more likely the longer drug is required.

**Skin & sunlight:**
No problems expected.

**Driving, piloting or hazardous work:**
Avoid if you feel dizzy, drowsy or confused. Otherwise, no problems expected.

**Discontinuing:**
Don't discontinue without doctor's advice until you complete prescribed dose, even though symptoms diminish or disappear. Some side effects may follow discontinuing. Report to doctor blurred vision, convulsions, confusion, persistent headache.

**Others:**
- Drink more water than usual to cause frequent urination.
- Don't give this medicine to anyone else for any purpose. It is a strong drug that requires close medical supervision.
- Report for frequent medical follow-up and laboratory studies.

## POSSIBLE INTERACTION WITH OTHER DRUGS

| GENERIC NAME OR DRUG CLASS | COMBINED EFFECT |
|---|---|
| Acetaminophen | Increased likelihood of liver toxicity. |
| Allopurinol | Increased toxic effect of mercaptopurine. |
| Antineoplastic drugs (other) | Increased effect of both (may be desirable) or increase toxicity of each. |
| Chloramphenicol | Increased toxicity of each. |
| Isoniazid | Increased likelihood of liver toxicity. |

## POSSIBLE INTERACTION WITH OTHER SUBSTANCES

| INTERACTS WITH | COMBINED EFFECT |
|---|---|
| Alcohol: | May increase chance of intestinal bleeding. |
| Beverages: | No problems expected. |
| Cocaine: | Increases chance of toxicity. |
| Foods: | Reduced irritation in stomach. |
| Marijuana: | No problems expected. |
| Tobacco: | Increases lung toxicity. |

# MESORIDAZINE

## BRAND NAMES

**Serentil**

## BASIC INFORMATION

**Habit forming? No**
**Prescription needed? Yes**
**Available as generic? Yes**
**Drug class: Tranquilizer, antiemetic**
**(phenothiazine)**

 ## USES

- Stops nausea, vomiting.
- Reduces anxiety, agitation.

 ## DOSAGE & USAGE INFORMATION

**How to take:**
- Tablet or capsule—Swallow with liquid or food to lessen stomach irritation.
- Suppositories—Remove wrapper and moisten suppository with water. Gently insert into rectum, large end first.
- Drops or liquid—Dilute dose in beverage.

**When to take:**
- Nervous and mental disorders—Take at the same times each day.
- Nausea and vomiting—Take as needed, no more often than every 4 hours.

**If you forget a dose:**
- Nervous and mental disorders—Take up to 2 hours late. If more than 2 hours, wait for next scheduled dose (don't double this dose).
- Nausea and vomiting—Take as soon as you remember. Wait 4 hours for next dose.

**What drug does:**
- Suppresses brain's vomiting center.
- Suppresses brain centers that control abnormal emotions and behavior.

**Time lapse before drug works:**
- Nausea and vomiting—1 hour or less.
- Nervous and mental disorders—4-6 weeks.

*Continued next column*

 ## OVERDOSE

**SYMPTOMS:**
**Stupor, convulsions, coma.**
**WHAT TO DO:**
- **Dial 0 (operator) or 911 (emergency) for an ambulance or medical help. Then give first aid immediately.**
- **See emergency information on inside covers.**

**Don't take with:**
- Antacid or medicine for diarrhea.
- Non-prescription drug for cough, cold or allergy.
- See Interaction column and consult doctor.

 ## POSSIBLE ADVERSE REACTIONS OR SIDE EFFECTS

| SYMPTOMS | WHAT TO DO |
|---|---|
| **Life-threatening:** | |
| None expected. | |
| **Common:** | |
| • Muscle spasms of face and neck, unsteady gait. | Discontinue. Seek emergency treatment. |
| • Restlessness, tremor, drowsiness. | Discontinue. Call doctor right away. |
| • Decreased sweating, dry mouth, runny nose, constipation. | Continue. Call doctor when convenient. |
| **Infrequent:** | |
| • Fainting. | Discontinue. Seek emergency treatment. |
| • Rash. | Discontinue. Call doctor right away. |
| • Difficult urination, diminished sex drive, swollen breasts, menstrual irregularities. | Continue. Call doctor when convenient. |
| **Rare:** | |
| Change in vision, jaundice, sore throat, fever. | Discontinue. Call doctor right away. |

## WARNINGS & PRECAUTIONS

**Don't take if:**
- You are allergic to any phenothiazine.
- You have a blood or bone-marrow disease.

**Before you start, consult your doctor:**
- If you will have surgery within 2 months, including dental surgery, requiring general or spinal anesthesia.
- If you have asthma, emphysema or other lung disorder.
- If you take non-prescription ulcer medicine, asthma medicine or amphetamines.

**Over age 60:**
Adverse reactions and side effects may be more frequent and severe than in younger persons. More likely to develop involuntary movement of jaws, lips, tongue, chewing. Report this to your doctor immediately. Early treatment can help.

**Pregnancy:**
Risk to unborn child outweighs drug benefits. Don't use.

**Breast-feeding:**
Drug passes into milk. Avoid drug or discontinue nursing until you finish medicine. Consult doctor for advice on maintaining milk supply.

**Infants & children:**
Don't give to children younger than 2.

**Prolonged use:**
May lead to tardive dyskinesia (involuntary movement of jaws, lips, tongue, chewing).

**Skin & sunlight:**
May cause rash or intensify sunburn in areas exposed to sun or sunlamp. Skin may remain sensitive for 3 months after discontinuing.

**Driving, piloting or hazardous work:**
Don't drive or pilot aircraft until you learn how medicine affects you. Don't work around dangerous machinery. Don't climb ladders or work in high places. Danger increases if you drink alcohol or take medicine affecting alertness and reflexes.

**Discontinuing:**
- Nervous and mental disorders—Don't discontinue without doctor's advice until you complete prescribed dose, even though symptoms diminish or disappear.
- Nausea and vomiting—May be unnecessary to finish medicine. Follow doctor's instructions.

**Others:**
No problems expected.

## POSSIBLE INTERACTION WITH OTHER DRUGS

| GENERIC NAME OR DRUG CLASS | COMBINED EFFECT |
|---|---|
| Anticholinergics | Increased anticholinergic effect. |
| Antidepressants (tricyclic) | Increased mesoridazine effect. |
| Antihistamines | Increased antihistamine effect. |
| Appetite suppressants | Decreased suppressant effect. |
| Dronabinol | Increased effects of both drugs. Avoid. |
| Levodopa | Decreased levodopa effect. |
| Mind-altering drugs | Increased effect of mind-altering drugs. |
| Molindone | Increased tranquilizer effect. |
| Narcotics | Increased narcotic effect. |
| Phenytoin | Increased phenytoin effect. |
| Quinidine | Impaired heart function. Dangerous mixture. |
| Sedatives | Increased sedative effect. |
| Tranquilizers (other) | Increased tranquilizer effect. |

## POSSIBLE INTERACTION WITH OTHER SUBSTANCES

| INTERACTS WITH | COMBINED EFFECT |
|---|---|
| Alcohol: | Dangerous oversedation. |
| Beverages: | None expected. |
| Cocaine: | Decreased effect of mesoridazine. Avoid. |
| Foods: | None expected. |
| Marijuana: | Drowsiness. May increase antinausea effect. |
| Tobacco: | None expected. |

# METAPROTERENOL

## BRAND NAMES

Alupent                    Metaprel

## BASIC INFORMATION

**Habit forming?** No
**Prescription needed?** Yes
**Available as generic?** No
**Drug class:** Bronchodilator,
                   sympathomimetic

 **USES**

Relieves wheezing and shortness of breath in
bronchial asthma attacks, bronchitis and
emphysema.

 **DOSAGE & USAGE INFORMATION**

**How to take:**
- Tablet or liquid—Swallow with liquid or food
  to lessen stomach irritation.
- Inhaler—Follow instructions on package.

**When to take:**
When needed, according to doctor's
instructions. Don't take more than 2 doses 1
hour apart.

**If you forget a dose:**
Take when you remember. Wait 2 hours for
next dose.

**What drug does:**
Relaxes smooth muscles to relieve constriction
of bronchial tubes.

**Time lapse before drug works:**
5 to 30 minutes.

**Don't take with:**
See Interaction column and consult doctor.

 **OVERDOSE**

**SYMPTOMS:**
**Chest pain, irregular heartbeat, convulsions,
coma.**
**WHAT TO DO:**
- **Dial 0 (operator) or 911 (emergency) for an
  ambulance or medical help. Then give first
  aid immediately.**
- **If patient is unconscious and not
  breathing, give mouth-to-mouth breathing.
  If there is no heartbeat, use cardiac
  massage and mouth-to-mouth breathing
  (CPR). Don't try to make patient vomit. If
  you can't get help quickly, take patient to
  nearest emergency facility.**
- **See emergency information on inside
  covers.**

 **POSSIBLE ADVERSE REACTIONS OR SIDE EFFECTS**

| SYMPTOMS | WHAT TO DO |
|---|---|
| **Life-threatening:** | |
| None expected. | |
| **Common:** | |
| • Rapid or pounding heartbeat. | Discontinue. Call doctor right away. |
| • Nervousness, restlessness, dizziness, weakness, headache, shakiness. | Continue. Call doctor when convenient. |
| **Infrequent:** | |
| Chest pain; muscle cramps in arms, hands, legs; unusual sweating; paleness; bad taste in mouth; nausea or vomiting. | Discontinue. Call doctor right away. |
| **Rare:** | |
| None expected. | |

## WARNINGS & PRECAUTIONS

**Don't take if:**
You are allergic to any sympathomimetic.

**Before you start, consult your doctor:**
- If you have irregular or rapid heartbeat, congestive heart failure, coronary-artery disease or high blood pressure.
- If you have diabetes.
- If you have overactive thyroid.

**Over age 60:**
Adverse reactions and side effects may be more frequent and severe than in younger persons.

**Pregnancy:**
Risk to unborn child outweighs drug benefits. Don't use.

**Breast-feeding:**
Drug passes into milk. Avoid drug or discontinue nursing until you finish medicine. Consult doctor for advice on maintaining milk supply.

**Infants & children:**
Use only under medical supervision.

**Prolonged use:**
No problems expected.

**Skin & sunlight:**
No problems expected.

**Driving, piloting or hazardous work:**
Don't drive or pilot aircraft until you learn how medicine affects you. Don't work around dangerous machinery. Don't climb ladders or work in high places. Danger increases if you drink alcohol or take medicine affecting alertness and reflexes, such as antihistamines, tranquilizers, sedatives, pain medicine, narcotics and mind-altering drugs.

**Discontinuing:**
No problems expected.

**Others:**
Consult doctor immediately if breathing difficulty continues or worsens after using metaproterenol.

 ## POSSIBLE INTERACTION WITH OTHER DRUGS

| GENERIC NAME OR DRUG CLASS | COMBINED EFFECT |
|---|---|
| Albuterol | Increased effect of both drugs, especially harmful side effects. |
| Antidepressants (tricyclic) | Increased effect of both drugs. |
| Beta-adrenergic blockers | Decreased effects of both drugs. |
| Hydralazine | Decreased hydralazine effect. |
| Minoxidil | Decreased minoxidil effect. |
| Nitrates | Possible decreased effects of both drugs. |
| Sympathomimetics (other) | Increased effect of both drugs, especially harmful side effects. |

 ## POSSIBLE INTERACTION WITH OTHER SUBSTANCES

| INTERACTS WITH | COMBINED EFFECT |
|---|---|
| Alcohol: | Decreased metaproterenol effect. |
| Beverages: | None expected. |
| Cocaine: | Possible metaproterenol toxicity. |
| Foods: | None expected. |
| Marijuana: | Overstimulation. Avoid. |
| Tobacco: | No proven problems. |

# METAXALONE

## BRAND NAMES

Skelaxin

## BASIC INFORMATION

**Habit forming? No**
**Prescription needed? Yes**
**Available as generic? Yes**
**Drug class: Muscle relaxant (skeletal)**

 ## USES

Treatment for sprains, strains and muscle spasms.

 ## DOSAGE & USAGE INFORMATION

**How to take:**
Tablet or capsule—Swallow with liquid.

**When to take:**
As needed, no more often than every 4 hours.

**If you forget a dose:**
Take as soon as you remember. Wait 4 hours for next dose.

**What drug does:**
Blocks body's pain messages to brain. May also sedate.

**Time lapse before drug works:**
60 minutes.

**Don't take with:**
See Interaction column and consult doctor.

 ## OVERDOSE

**SYMPTOMS:**
**Nausea, vomiting, diarrhea, headache. May progress to severe weakness, difficult breathing, sensation of paralysis, coma.**
**WHAT TO DO:**
- **Dial 0 (operator) or 911 (emergency) for an ambulance or medical help. Then give first aid immediately.**
- **If patient is unconscious and not breathing, give mouth-to-mouth breathing. If there is no heartbeat, use cardiac massage and mouth-to-mouth breathing (CPR). Don't try to make patient vomit. If you can't get help quickly, take patient to nearest emergency facility.**
- **See emergency information on inside covers.**

 ## POSSIBLE ADVERSE REACTIONS OR SIDE EFFECTS

| SYMPTOMS | WHAT TO DO |
|---|---|
| **Life-threatening:**<br>None expected. | |
| **Common:**<br>• Drowsiness, fainting, dizziness. | Continue. Call doctor when convenient. |
| • Orange or red-purple urine. | No action necessary. |
| **Infrequent:**<br>Agitation, constipation or diarrhea, nausea, cramps, vomiting, wheezing, shortness of breath. | Discontinue. Call doctor right away. |
| **Rare:**<br>• Black, bloody or tarry stools. | Discontinue. Seek emergency treatment. |
| • Rash, hives or itch; sore throat; fever; jaundice; tiredness; weakness. | Discontinue. Call doctor right away. |

## WARNINGS & PRECAUTIONS

**Don't take if:**
- You are allergic to any skeletal-muscle relaxant.
- You have porphyria.

**Before you start, consult your doctor:**
- If you have had liver or kidney disease.
- If you plan pregnancy within medication period.

**Over age 60:**
Adverse reactions and side effects may be more frequent and severe than in younger persons.

**Pregnancy:**
No proven harm to unborn child. Avoid if possible.

**Breast-feeding:**
Drug passes into milk. Avoid drug or discontinue nursing until you finish medicine. Consult doctor for advice on maintaining milk supply.

**Infants & children:**
Not recommended.

**Prolonged use:**
Periodic liver-function tests recommended if you use this drug for a long time.

**Skin & sunlight:**
No problems expected.

**Driving, piloting or hazardous work:**
Don't drive or pilot aircraft until you learn how medicine affects you. Don't work around dangerous machinery. Don't climb ladders or work in high places. Danger increases if you drink alcohol or take medicine affecting alertness and reflexes, such as antihistamines, tranquilizers, sedatives, pain medicine, narcotics and mind-altering drugs.

**Discontinuing:**
Don't discontinue without doctor's advice until you complete prescribed dose, even though symptoms diminish or disappear.

**Others:**
No problems expected.

## POSSIBLE INTERACTION WITH OTHER DRUGS

| GENERIC NAME OR DRUG CLASS | COMBINED EFFECT |
|---|---|
| Antidepressants | Increased sedation. |
| Antihistamines | Increased sedation. |
| Dronabinol | Increased effect of dronabinol on central nervous system. Avoid combination. |
| Mind-altering drugs | Increased sedation. |
| Muscle relaxants (other) | Increased sedation. |
| Narcotics | Increased sedation. |
| Sedatives | Increased sedation. |
| Sleep inducers | Increased sedation. |
| Testosterone | Decreased metaxalone effect. |
| Tranquilizers | Increased sedation. |

## POSSIBLE INTERACTION WITH OTHER SUBSTANCES

| INTERACTS WITH | COMBINED EFFECT |
|---|---|
| Alcohol: | Increased sedation. |
| Beverages: | None expected. |
| Cocaine: | Lack of coordination, increased sedation. |
| Foods: | None expected. |
| Marijuana: | Lack of coordination, drowsiness, fainting. |
| Tobacco: | None expected. |

# METHAMPHETAMINE

## BRAND NAMES

Desoxyn          Methampex

## BASIC INFORMATION

**Habit forming?** Yes
**Prescription needed?** Yes
**Available as generic?** Yes
**Drug class:** Central-nervous-system
stimulant (amphetamine)

## USES

- Prevents narcolepsy (attacks of uncontrollable sleepiness).
- Controls hyperactivity in children.

## DOSAGE & USAGE INFORMATION

**How to take:**
- Tablet—Swallow with liquid.
- Extended-release tablets—Swallow each dose whole with liquid.

**When to take:**
- At the same times each day.
- Short-acting form—Don't take later than 6 hours before bedtime.
- Long-acting form—Take on awakening.

**If you forget a dose:**
- Short-acting form—Take up to 2 hours late. If more than 2 hours, wait for next dose (don't double this dose).
- Long-acting form—Take as soon as you remember. Wait 20 hours for next dose.

**What drug does:**
- Narcolepsy—Apparently affects brain centers to decrease fatigue or sleepiness and increase alertness and motor activity.
- Hyperactive children—Calms children, opposite to effect on narcoleptic adults.

*Continued next column*

## OVERDOSE

**SYMPTOMS:**
Rapid heartbeat, hyperactivity, high fever, hallucinations, suicidal or homicidal feelings, convulsions, coma.
**WHAT TO DO:**
- Dial 0 (operator) or 911 (emergency) for an ambulance or medical help. Then give first aid immediately.
- See emergency information on inside covers.

**Time lapse before drug works:**
15 to 30 minutes.

**Don't take with:**
See Interaction column and consult doctor.

## POSSIBLE ADVERSE REACTIONS OR SIDE EFFECTS

| SYMPTOMS | WHAT TO DO |
|---|---|
| **Life-threatening:**<br>None expected. | |
| **Common:** | |
| • Irritability, nervousness, insomnia. | Continue. Call doctor when convenient. |
| • Dry mouth. | Continue. Tell doctor at next visit. |
| **Infrequent:** | |
| • Dizziness; lack of alertness; blurred vision; fast, pounding heartbeat; unusual sweating. | Discontinue. Call doctor right away. |
| • Headache. | Continue. Call doctor when convenient. |
| • Diarrhea or constipation, appetite loss, stomach pain, nausea, vomiting, weight loss, diminished sex drive, impotence. | Continue. Tell doctor at next visit. |
| **Rare:** | |
| • Rash; hives; chest pain or irregular heartbeat; uncontrollable movements of head, neck, arms, legs. | Discontinue. Call doctor right away. |
| • Swollen breasts, mood change. | Continue. Call doctor when convenient. |

## WARNINGS & PRECAUTIONS

**Don't take if:**
- You are allergic to any methamphetamine.
- You will have surgery within 2 months, including dental surgery, requiring general or spinal anesthesia.

**Before you start, consult your doctor:**
- If you plan to become pregnant within medication period.
- If you have glaucoma.
- If you have heart or blood-vessel disease, or high blood pressure.
- If you have overactive thyroid, anxiety or tension.
- If you have a severe mental illness (especially children).

**Over age 60:**
Adverse reactions and side effects may be more frequent and severe than in younger persons.

**Pregnancy:**
Risk to unborn child outweighs drug benefits. Don't use.

**Breast-feeding:**
Drug passes into milk. Avoid drug or discontinue nursing.

**Infants & children:**
Not recommended for children under 12.

**Prolonged use:**
Habit forming.

**Skin & sunlight:**
No problems expected.

**Driving, piloting or hazardous work:**
Don't drive or pilot aircraft until you learn how medicine affects you. Don't work around dangerous machinery. Don't climb ladders or work in high places. Danger increases if you drink alcohol or take medicine affecting alertness and reflexes.

**Discontinuing:**
May be unnecessary to finish medicine. Follow doctor's instructions.

**Others:**
- This is a dangerous drug and must be closely supervised. Don't use for appetite control or depression. Potential for damage and abuse.
- During withdrawal phase, may cause prolonged sleep of several days.

## POSSIBLE INTERACTION WITH OTHER DRUGS

| GENERIC NAME OR DRUG CLASS | COMBINED EFFECT |
|---|---|
| Anesthesias (general) | Irregular heartbeat. |
| Antidepressants (tricyclic) | Decreased methamphetamine effect. |
| Antihypertensives | Decreased antihypertensive effect. |
| Carbonic anhydrase inhibitors | Increased methamphetamine effect. |
| Guanethidine | Decreased guanethidine effect. |
| Haloperidol | Decreased methamphetamine effect. |
| MAO inhibitors | May severely increase blood pressure. |
| Phenothiazines | Decreased methamphetamine effect. |
| Sodium bicarbonate | Increased methamphetamine effect. |

## POSSIBLE INTERACTION WITH OTHER SUBSTANCES

| INTERACTS WITH | COMBINED EFFECT |
|---|---|
| Alcohol: | Decreased methamphetamine effect. Avoid. |
| Beverages: Caffeine drinks. | Overstimulation. Avoid. |
| Cocaine: | Dangerous stimulation of nervous system. Avoid. |
| Foods: | None expected. |
| Marijuana: | Frequent use— Severely impaired mental function. |
| Tobacco: | None expected. |

# METHAQUALONE

## BRAND NAMES

| | |
|---|---|
| Mandrax | Sedalone |
| Mequelon | Sopor |
| Mequin | Triador |
| Methadorm | Tualone |
| Parest | Tualone-300 |
| Quaalude | Vitalone |
| Rouqualone-300 | |

## BASIC INFORMATION

**Habit forming?** Yes
**Prescription needed?** Yes
**Available as generic?** No
**Drug class:** Hypnotic

## USES

Decreases anxiety, tension or insomnia.

## DOSAGE & USAGE INFORMATION

**How to take:**
Tablet or capsule—Swallow with liquid. If you can't swallow whole, crumble tablet or open capsule and take with liquid or food.

**When to take:**
At the same time each day.

**If you forget a dose:**
Don't take missed dose. Wait for next scheduled dose. Don't double this dose.

**What drug does:**
Undetermined.

*Continued next column*

## OVERDOSE

**SYMPTOMS:**
**Drowsiness, confusion, delirium, incoordination, vomiting, convulsions, abnormal bleeding, stupor, coma.**
**WHAT TO DO:**
- **Dial 0 (operator) or 911 (emergency) for an ambulance or medical help. Then give first aid immediately.**
- **If patient is unconscious and not breathing, give mouth-to-mouth breathing. If there is no heartbeat, use cardiac massage and mouth-to-mouth breathing (CPR). Don't try to make patient vomit. If you can't get help quickly, take patient to nearest emergency facility.**
- **See emergency information on inside covers.**

**Time lapse before drug works:**
20 to 30 minutes.

**Don't take with:**
- Alcohol or mind-altering drugs. Combinations can be fatal.
- Non-prescription drugs without consulting doctor.
- See Interaction column and consult doctor.

## POSSIBLE ADVERSE REACTIONS OR SIDE EFFECTS

| SYMPTOMS | WHAT TO DO |
|---|---|
| **Life-threatening:** None expected. | |
| **Common:** | |
| • Diarrhea, nausea, vomiting, stomach pain. | Discontinue. Call doctor right away. |
| • Drowsiness. | Continue. Call doctor when convenient. |
| • Tiredness or weakness. | Continue. Tell doctor at next visit. |
| • "Hangover" effect. | No action necessary. |
| **Infrequent:** | |
| • Unusually slow heartbeat, difficult breathing. | Discontinue. Seek emergency treatment. |
| • Agitation; skin rash or hives; numbness, tingling, pain or weakness in hands or feet; sweating. | Discontinue. Call doctor right away. |
| **Rare:** None expected. | |

## WARNINGS & PRECAUTIONS

**Don't take if:**
- You are allergic to any hypnotic drug.
- You plan to become pregnant within medication period.
- Patient is younger than 12.

**Before you start, consult your doctor:**
- If you have had liver disease or impaired liver function.
- If you will have surgery within 2 months, including dental surgery, requiring general or spinal anesthesia.

**Over age 60:**
Adverse reactions and side effects may be more frequent and severe than in younger persons.

**Pregnancy:**
Risk to unborn child outweighs drug benefits. Don't use.

**Breast-feeding:**
Drug may filter into milk and harm child. Don't use.

**Infants & children:**
Not recommended.

**Prolonged use:**
Psychological and physical dependence.

**Skin & sunlight:**
No problems expected.

**Driving, piloting or hazardous work:**
Don't drive or pilot aircraft until you learn how medicine affects you. Don't work around dangerous machinery. Don't climb ladders or work in high places. Danger increases if you drink alcohol or take medicine affecting alertness and reflexes, such as antihistamines, tranquilizers, sedatives, pain medicine, narcotics and mind-altering drugs.

**Discontinuing:**
Don't discontinue without consulting doctor. Dose may require gradual reduction if you have taken drug for a long time. Doses of other drugs may also require adjustment.

**Others:**
No problems expected.

## POSSIBLE INTERACTION WITH OTHER DRUGS

| GENERIC NAME OR DRUG CLASS | COMBINED EFFECT |
|---|---|
| Anticoagulants | Decreased anticoagulant effect. |
| Antihistamines | Increased sedation. |
| Narcotics | Increased narcotic effect. |
| Pain relievers | Increased effect of pain reliever. |
| Sedatives | Increased sedative effect. |
| Sleep inducers | Increased effect of sleep inducer. |
| Tranquilizers | Increased tranquilizer effect. |

## POSSIBLE INTERACTION WITH OTHER SUBSTANCES

| INTERACTS WITH | COMBINED EFFECT |
|---|---|
| Alcohol: | Dangerous depression of brain function. Avoid. |
| Beverages: | None expected. |
| Cocaine: | Decreased effect of both drugs. Avoid. |
| Foods: | None expected. |
| Marijuana: | Impairs physical performance. Avoid. |
| Tobacco: | None expected. |

# METHARBITAL

## BRAND NAMES

Gemonil

## BASIC INFORMATION

**Habit forming? Yes**
**Prescription needed? Yes**
**Available as generic? Yes**
**Drug class: Sedative, hypnotic (barbiturate)**

## USES

Prevents convulsions.

## DOSAGE & USAGE INFORMATION

**How to take:**
Tablet—Swallow with liquid or food to lessen stomach irritation. If you can't swallow whole, crumble tablet and take with liquid or food.

**When to take:**
At the same times each day.

**If you forget a dose:**
Take as soon as you remember up to 2 hours late. If more than 2 hours, wait for next scheduled dose (don't double this dose).

**What drug does:**
May partially block nerve impulses at nerve-cell connections.

**Time lapse before drug works:**
60 minutes.

**Don't take with:**
- Non-prescription drugs without consulting doctor.
- See Interaction column and consult doctor.

## OVERDOSE

**SYMPTOMS:**
**Deep sleep, weak pulse, coma.**
**WHAT TO DO:**
- **Dial 0 (operator) or 911 (emergency) for an ambulance or medical help. Then give first aid immediately.**
- **If patient is unconscious and not breathing, give mouth-to-mouth breathing. If there is no heartbeat use cardiac massage and mouth-to-mouth breathing (CPR). Don't try to make patient vomit. If you can't get help quickly, take patient to nearest emergency facility.**
- **See emergency information on inside covers.**

## POSSIBLE ADVERSE REACTIONS OR SIDE EFFECTS

| SYMPTOMS | WHAT TO DO |
|---|---|
| **Life-threatening:**<br>None expected. | |
| **Common:**<br>Dizziness, drowsiness, "hangover" effect. | Continue. Call doctor when convenient. |
| **Infrequent:**<br>• Rash or hives; face, lip or eyelid swelling; sore throat; fever. | Discontinue. Call doctor right away. |
| • Depression, confusion, slurred speech, diarrhea, nausea, vomiting, joint or muscle pain. | Continue. Call doctor when convenient. |
| **Rare:**<br>• Agitation, slow heartbeat, difficult breathing, jaundice. | Discontinue. Call doctor right away. |
| • Unusual bleeding or bruising. | Continue. Call doctor when convenient. |

## WARNINGS & PRECAUTIONS

**Don't take if:**
- You are allergic to any barbiturate.
- You have porphyria.

**Before you start, consult your doctor:**
- If you have epilepsy.
- If you have kidney or liver damage.
- If you have asthma.
- If you have anemia.
- If you have chronic pain.
- If you will have surgery within 2 months, including dental surgery, requiring general or spinal anesthesia.

**Over age 60:**
Adverse reactions and side effects may be more frequent and severe than in younger persons. Use small doses.

**Pregnancy:**
Risk to unborn child outweighs drug benefits. Don't use.

**Breast-feeding:**
Drug passes into milk. Avoid drug or discontinue nursing until you finish medicine. Consult doctor for advice on maintaining milk supply.

**Infants & children:**
Use only under doctor's supervision.

**Prolonged use:**
- May cause addiction, anemia, chronic intoxication.
- May lower body temperature, making exposure to cold temperatures hazardous.

**Skin & sunlight:**
May cause rash or intensify sunburn in areas exposed to sun or sunlamp.

**Driving, piloting or hazardous work:**
Don't drive or pilot aircraft until you learn how medicine affects you. Don't work around dangerous machinery. Don't climb ladders or work in high places. Danger increases if you drink alcohol or take medicine affecting alertness and reflexes.

**Discontinuing:**
May be unnecessary to finish medicine. Follow doctor's instructions. If you develop withdrawal symptoms of hallucinations, agitation or sleeplessness after discontinuing, call doctor right away.

**Others:**
Great potential for abuse.

 **POSSIBLE INTERACTION WITH OTHER DRUGS**

| GENERIC NAME OR DRUG CLASS | COMBINED EFFECT |
| --- | --- |
| Anticoagulants (oral) | Decreased anticoagulant effect. |
| Anticonvulsants | Changed seizure patterns. |
| Antidepressants (tricyclics) | Decreased antidepressant effect. Possible dangerous oversedation. |
| Antidiabetics (oral) | Increased metharbital effect. |
| Antihistamines | Dangerous sedation. Avoid. |
| Anti-inflammatory drugs (non-steroidal) | Decreased anti-inflammatory effect. |
| Aspirin | Decreased aspirin effect. |
| Beta-adrenergic blockers | Decreased effect of beta-adrenergic blocker. |

| Contraceptives (oral) | Decreased contraceptive effect. |
| --- | --- |
| Cortisone drugs | Decreased cortisone effect. |
| Digitoxin | Decreased digitoxin effect. |
| Doxycycline | Decreased doxycycline effect. |
| Dronabinol | Increased effects of both drugs. Avoid. |
| Griseofulvin | Decreased griseofulvin effect. |
| Indapamide | Increased indapamide effect. |
| MAO inhibitors | Increased metharbital effect. |
| Mind-altering drugs | Dangerous sedation. Avoid. |
| Narcotics | Dangerous sedation. Avoid. |
| Pain relievers | Dangerous sedation. Avoid. |
| Sedatives | Dangerous sedation. Avoid. |
| Sleep inducers | Dangerous sedation. Avoid. |
| Tranquilizers | Dangerous sedation. Avoid. |
| Valproic acid | Increased metharbital effect. |

 **POSSIBLE INTERACTION WITH OTHER SUBSTANCES**

| INTERACTS WITH | COMBINED EFFECT |
| --- | --- |
| Alcohol: | Possible fatal oversedation. Avoid. |
| Beverages: | None expected. |
| Cocaine: | Decreased metharbital effect. |
| Foods: | None expected. |
| Marijuana: | Excessive sedation. Avoid. |
| Tobacco: | None expected. |

# METHENAMINE

## BRAND NAMES

| | |
|---|---|
| Azo-Mandelamine | Renalgin |
| Hexamine | Sterine |
| Hip-Rex | Trac 2X |
| Hiprex | Urex |
| Mandelamine | Urised |
| Mandelets | Uroblue |
| Methandine | Uro-phosphate |
| Prov-U-Sep | Uroquid-Acid |

## BASIC INFORMATION

Habit forming? No
Prescription needed? Yes
Available as generic? Yes
Drug class: Anti-infective (urinary)

 ## USES

Suppresses chronic urinary-tract infections.

 ## DOSAGE & USAGE INFORMATION

**How to take:**
- Tablet—Swallow with liquid or food to lessen stomach irritation. If you can't swallow whole, crumble tablet and take with liquid or food.
- Liquid form—Use a measuring spoon to ensure correct dose.
- Granules—Dissolve dose in 4 oz. of water. Drink all the liquid.

**When to take:**
At the same times each day.

**If you forget a dose:**
Take as soon as you remember up to 8 hours late. If more than 8 hours, wait for next scheduled dose (don't double this dose).

**What drug does:**
A chemical reaction in the urine changes methenamine into formaldehyde, which destroys certain bacteria.

*Continued next column*

 ## OVERDOSE

**SYMPTOMS:**
Bloody urine, weakness, deep breathing, stupor, coma.
**WHAT TO DO:**
- Dial 0 (operator) or 911 (emergency) for an ambulance or medical help. Then give first aid immediately.
- See emergency information on inside covers.

**Time lapse before drug works:**
Continual use for 3 to 6 months.

**Don't take with:**
See Interaction column and consult doctor.

 ## POSSIBLE ADVERSE REACTIONS OR SIDE EFFECTS

| SYMPTOMS | WHAT TO DO |
|---|---|
| **Life-threatening:** None expected. | |
| **Common:** | |
| • Rash. | Discontinue. Call doctor right away. |
| • Nausea, difficult urination. | Continue. Call doctor when convenient. |
| **Infrequent:** | |
| • Blood in urine. | Discontinue. Call doctor right away. |
| • Burning on urination, lower back pain. | Continue. Call doctor when convenient. |
| **Rare:** None expected. | |

## WARNINGS & PRECAUTIONS

### Don't take if:
- You are allergic to methenamine.
- You have a severe impairment of kidney or liver function.
- The urine cannot or should not be acidified (check with your doctor).

### Before you start, consult your doctor:
- If you have had kidney or liver disease.
- If you plan to become pregnant within medication period.
- If you have had gout.

### Over age 60:
Don't exceed recommended dose.

### Pregnancy:
Studies inconclusive on harm to unborn child. Avoid if possible, especially first 3 months.

### Breast-feeding:
Drug passes into milk in small amounts. Consult doctor.

### Infants & children:
Use only under medical supervision.

### Prolonged use:
No problems expected.

### Skin & sunlight:
No problems expected.

### Driving, piloting or hazardous work:
No problems expected.

### Discontinuing:
Don't discontinue without doctor's advice until you complete prescribed dose, even though symptoms diminish or disappear.

### Others:
Requires an acid urine to be effective. Eat more protein foods, cranberries, cranberry juice with vitamin C, plums, prunes.

## POSSIBLE INTERACTION WITH OTHER DRUGS

| GENERIC NAME OR DRUG CLASS | COMBINED EFFECT |
|---|---|
| Antacids | Decreased methenamine effect. |
| Carbonic anhydrase inhibitors | Decreased methenamine effect. |
| Citrates | Decreases effects of methenamine. |
| Diuretics (thiazide) | Decreased urine acidity. |
| Sodium bicarbonate | Decreased methenamine effect. |
| Sulfa drugs | Possible kidney damage. |
| Vitamin C (1 to 4 grams per day) | Increased effect of methenamine, contributing to urine's acidity. |

## POSSIBLE INTERACTION WITH OTHER SUBSTANCES

| INTERACTS WITH | COMBINED EFFECT |
|---|---|
| Alcohol: | Possible brain depression. Avoid or use with caution. |
| Beverages: Milk. | Decreased methenamine effect. |
| Cocaine: | None expected. |
| Foods: | None expected. |
| Marijuana: | Drowsiness, muscle weakness or blood-pressure drop. |
| Tobacco: | None expected. |

# METHICILLIN

## BRAND NAMES

Azapen
Celbenin

Staphcillin

## BASIC INFORMATION

**Habit forming? No**
**Prescription needed? Yes**
**Available as generic? Yes**
**Drug class: Antibiotic (penicillin)**

 ## USES

Treatment of bacterial infections that are susceptible to methicillin.

 ## DOSAGE & USAGE INFORMATION

**How to take:**
By injection only.

**When to take:**
Follow doctor's instructions.

**If you forget a dose:**
Consult doctor.

**What drug does:**
Destroys susceptible bacteria. Does not kill viruses.

**Time lapse before drug works:**
May be several days before medicine affects infection.

**Don't take with:**
See Interaction column and consult doctor.

## OVERDOSE

**SYMPTOMS:**
**Severe diarrhea, nausea or vomiting.**
**WHAT TO DO:**
**Overdose unlikely to threaten life. If person takes much larger amount than prescribed, call doctor, poison-control center or hospital emergency room for instructions.**

 ## POSSIBLE ADVERSE REACTIONS OR SIDE EFFECTS

| SYMPTOMS | WHAT TO DO |
|---|---|
| **Life-threatening:** Hives, rash, intense itching, faintness soon after a dose (anaphylaxis). | Seek emergency treatment immediately. |
| **Common:** Dark or discolored tongue. | Continue. Tell doctor at next visit. |
| **Infrequent:** Mild nausea, vomiting, diarrhea. | Continue. Call doctor when convenient. |
| **Rare:** Unexplained bleeding. | Discontinue. Call doctor right away. |

## WARNINGS & PRECAUTIONS

**Don't take if:**
You are allergic to methicillin, cephalosporin antibiotics, other penicillins or penicillamine. Life-threatening reaction may occur.

**Before you start, consult your doctor:**
If you are allergic to any substance or drug.

**Over age 60:**
You may have skin reactions, particularly around genitals and anus.

**Pregnancy:**
Studies inconclusive on harm to unborn child. Animal studies show fetal abnormalities. Decide with your doctor whether drug benefits justify risk to unborn child.

**Breast-feeding:**
Drug passes into milk. Child may become sensitive to penicillins and have allergic reactions to penicillin drugs. Avoid methicillin or discontinue nursing until you finish medicine. Consult doctor for advice on maintaining milk supply.

**Infants & children:**
No problems expected.

**Prolonged use:**
• You may become more susceptible to infections caused by germs not responsive to methicillin.
• May cause kidney damage. Laboratory studies to detect damage recommended if you take for a long time.

**Skin & sunlight:**
No problems expected.

**Driving, piloting or hazardous work:**
Usually not dangerous. Most hazardous reactions likely to occur a few minutes after taking methicillin.

**Discontinuing:**
Don't discontinue without doctor's advice until you complete prescribed dose, even though symptoms diminish or disappear.

**Others:**
No problems expected.

## POSSIBLE INTERACTION WITH OTHER DRUGS

| GENERIC NAME OR DRUG CLASS | COMBINED EFFECT |
|---|---|
| Beta-adrenergic blockers | Increased chance of anaphylaxis (see emergency information on inside front cover). |
| Chloramphenicol | Decreased effect of both drugs. |
| Erythromycins | Decreased effect of both drugs. |
| Loperamide | Decreased methicillin effect. |
| Paromomycin | Decreased effect of both drugs. |
| Tetracyclines | Decreased effect of both drugs. |
| Troleandomycin | Decreased effect of both drugs. |

## POSSIBLE INTERACTION WITH OTHER SUBSTANCES

| INTERACTS WITH | COMBINED EFFECT |
|---|---|
| Alcohol: | Occasional stomach irritation. |
| Beverages: | None expected. |
| Cocaine: | No proven problems. |
| Foods: | None expected. |
| Marijuana: | No proven problems. |
| Tobacco: | None expected. |

# METHOCARBAMOL

## BRAND NAMES

| | |
|---|---|
| Delaxin | Robamol |
| Forbaxin | Robaxin |
| Marbaxin | Robaxisal |
| Marbaxin-750 | Spinaxin |
| Metho-500 | Tumol |

## BASIC INFORMATION

**Habit forming? No**
**Prescription needed? Yes**
**Available as generic? Yes**
**Drug class: Muscle relaxant (skeletal)**

 USES

Pain reliever for skeletal-muscle spasms.

 DOSAGE & USAGE INFORMATION

**How to take:**
Tablet—Swallow with liquid. If you can't swallow whole, crumble tablet and take with liquid or food.

**When to take:**
As directed on label.

**If you forget a dose:**
Take as soon as you remember up to 2 hours late. If more than 2 hours, wait for next scheduled dose (don't double this dose).

**What drug does:**
Blocks reflex nerve impulses in brain and spinal cord.

*Continued next column*

 OVERDOSE

**SYMPTOMS:**
**Unsteadiness, lack of coordination, extreme weakness, paralysis, weak and rapid pulse, shallow breathing, cold and sweaty skin.**
**WHAT TO DO:**
- **Dial 0 (operator) or 911 (emergency) for an ambulance or medical help. Then give first aid immediately.**
- **If patient is unconscious and not breathing, give mouth-to-mouth breathing. If there is no heartbeat, use cardiac massage and mouth-to-mouth breathing (CPR). Don't try to make patient vomit. If you can't get help quickly, take patient to nearest emergency facility.**
- **See emergency information on inside covers.**

**Time lapse before drug works:**
30 to 45 minutes.

**Don't take with:**
- Non-prescription drugs containing alcohol without consulting doctor.
- See Interaction column and consult doctor.

 POSSIBLE ADVERSE REACTIONS OR SIDE EFFECTS

| SYMPTOMS | WHAT TO DO |
|---|---|
| **Life-threatening:** | |
| None expected. | |
| **Common:** | |
| • Blurred or double vision. | Discontinue. Call doctor right away. |
| • Dizziness, drowsiness, lightheadedness. | Continue. Call doctor when convenient. |
| **Infrequent:** | |
| • Rash, itchy skin. | Discontinue. Call doctor right away. |
| • Headache, bloodshot eyes, metallic taste, fever. | Continue. Call doctor when convenient. |
| • Stuffy nose, nausea. | Continue. Tell doctor at next visit. |
| **Rare:** | |
| None expected. | |

## WARNINGS & PRECAUTIONS

**Don't take if:**
You are allergic to any muscle relaxant.

**Before you start, consult your doctor:**
- If you have epilepsy.
- If you have myasthenia gravis.
- If you have impaired kidney function.

**Over age 60:**
Adverse reactions and side effects may be more frequent and severe than in younger persons.

**Pregnancy:**
No proven harm to unborn child. Avoid if possible.

**Breast-feeding:**
Drug filters into milk. May harm child. Avoid.

**Infants & children:**
Not recommended.

**Prolonged use:**
No problems expected.

**Skin & sunlight:**
No problems expected.

**Driving, piloting or hazardous work:**
Don't drive or pilot aircraft until you learn how medicine affects you. Don't work around dangerous machinery. Don't climb ladders or work in high places. Danger increases if you drink alcohol or take medicine affecting alertness and reflexes, such as antihistamines, tranquilizers, sedatives, pain medicine, narcotics and mind-altering drugs.

**Discontinuing:**
May be unnecessary to finish medicine. Follow doctor's instructions.

**Others:**
No problems expected.

## POSSIBLE INTERACTION WITH OTHER DRUGS

| GENERIC NAME OR DRUG CLASS | COMBINED EFFECT |
|---|---|
| Antidepressants (tricyclic) | Increased effect of both drugs. |
| Antimyasthenics | Decreased antimyasthenic effect. |
| Dronabinol | Increased effect of dronabinol on central nervous system. Avoid combination. |
| Narcotics | Increased sedative effect. |
| Sedatives | Increased sedative effect. |
| Sleep inducers | Increased effect of sleep inducer. |
| Tranquilizers | Increased tranquilizer effect. |

## POSSIBLE INTERACTION WITH OTHER SUBSTANCES

| INTERACTS WITH | COMBINED EFFECT |
|---|---|
| Alcohol: | Depressed brain function. Avoid. |
| Beverages: | None expected. |
| Cocaine: | May increase muscle spasms. |
| Foods: | None expected. |
| Marijuana: | Drowsiness, muscle weakness, lack of coordination, fainting. |
| Tobacco: | None expected. |

# METHOTREXATE

## BRAND NAMES

| | |
|---|---|
| Folex | Mexate |
| Folex PFS | Mexate AQ |

## BASIC INFORMATION

**Habit forming?** No
**Prescription needed?** Yes
**Available as generic?** Yes
**Drug class:** Antimetabolite, antipsoriatic

 **USES**

- Treatment for some kinds of cancer.
- Treatment for psoriasis in patients with severe problems.

 **DOSAGE & USAGE INFORMATION**

**How to take:**
Tablet—Swallow with liquid.

**When to take:**
At the same time each day.

**If you forget a dose:**
Skip the missed dose. Don't double the next dose.

**What drug does:**
Inhibits abnormal-cell reproduction.

**Time lapse before drug works:**
May require 6 weeks for maximum effect.

**Don't take with:**
See Interaction column and consult doctor.

 **OVERDOSE**

**SYMPTOMS:**
Headache, stupor, seizures.
**WHAT TO DO:**
- Dial 0 (operator) or 911 (emergency) for an ambulance or medical help. Then give first aid immediately.
- If patient is unconscious and not breathing, give mouth-to-mouth breathing. If there is no heartbeat, use cardiac massage and mouth-to-mouth breathing (CPR). Don't try to make patient vomit. If you can't get help quickly, take patient to nearest emergency facility.
- See emergency information on inside covers.

 **POSSIBLE ADVERSE REACTIONS OR SIDE EFFECTS**

| SYMPTOMS | WHAT TO DO |
|---|---|
| **Life-threatening:**<br>None expected. | |
| **Common:** | |
| • Black stools or bloody vomit. | Discontinue. Seek emergency treatment. |
| • Sore throat, fever, mouth sores; chills; unusual bleeding or bruising. | Discontinue. Call doctor right away. |
| • Stomach pain, nausea, vomiting. | Continue. Call doctor when convenient. |
| **Infrequent:** | |
| • Seizures. | Discontinue. Seek emergency treatment. |
| • Dizziness when standing after sitting or lying, drowsiness, headache, confusion, blurred vision, shortness of breath, joint pain, blood in urine, jaundice. | Discontinue. Call doctor right away. |
| • Cough. | Continue. Call doctor when convenient. |
| • Acne, boils, hair loss, itchy skin. | Continue. Tell doctor at next visit. |
| **Rare:**<br>None expected. | |

## WARNINGS & PRECAUTIONS

**Don't take if:**
You are allergic to any antimetabolite.

**Before you start, consult your doctor:**
• If you are alcoholic.
• If you have blood, liver or kidney disease.
• If you have colitis or peptic ulcer.
• If you have gout.
• If you have an infection.
• If you plan to become pregnant within 3 months.

**Over age 60:**
Adverse reactions and side effects may be more frequent and severe than in younger persons.

**Pregnancy:**
• Psoriasis—Risk to unborn child outweighs drug benefits. Don't use.
• Cancer—Consult doctor.

**Breast-feeding:**
Drug passes into milk. Avoid drug or discontinue nursing.

**Infants & children:**
Use only under special medical supervision.

**Prolonged use:**
Adverse reactions more likely the longer drug is required.

**Skin & sunlight:**
No problems expected.

**Driving, piloting or hazardous work:**
Avoid if you feel dizzy, drowsy or confused. Otherwise, no problems expected.

**Discontinuing:**
Don't discontinue without doctor's advice until you complete prescribed dose, even though symptoms diminish or disappear. Some side effects may follow discontinuing. Report to doctor blurred vision, convulsions, confusion, persistent headache.

**Others:**
• Drink more water than usual to cause frequent urination.
• Don't give this medicine to anyone else for any purpose. It is a strong drug that requires close medical supervision.
• Report for frequent medical follow-up and laboratory studies.

## POSSIBLE INTERACTION WITH OTHER DRUGS

| GENERIC NAME OR DRUG CLASS | COMBINED EFFECT |
|---|---|
| Anticoagulants (oral) | Increased anticoagulant effect. |
| Anticonvulsants (hydantoin) | Possible methotrexate toxicity. |
| Antigout drugs | Decreased antigout effect. |
| Asparaginase | Decreased methotrexate effect. |
| Flurouracil | Decreased methotrexate effect. |
| Oxyphenbutazone | Possible methotrexate toxicity. |
| Phenylbutazone | Possible methotrexate toxicity. |
| Probenecid | Possible methotrexate toxicity. |
| Pyrimethamine | Increased toxic effect of methotrexate. |
| Salicylates (including aspirin) | Possible methotrexate toxicity. |
| Sulfa drugs | Possible methotrexate toxicity. |
| Tetracyclines | Possible methotrexate toxicity. |

## POSSIBLE INTERACTION WITH OTHER SUBSTANCES

| INTERACTS WITH | COMBINED EFFECT |
|---|---|
| Alcohol: | Likely liver damage. Avoid. |
| Beverages: | Extra fluid intake decreases chance of methotrexate toxicity. |
| Cocaine: | Increased chance of methotrexate adverse reactions. Avoid. |
| Foods: | None expected. |
| Marijuana: | None expected. |
| Tobacco: | None expected. |

# METHSUXIMIDE

## BRAND NAMES

**Celontin**

## BASIC INFORMATION

**Habit forming? No**
**Prescription needed? Yes**
**Available as generic? No**
**Drug class: Anticonvulsant (succinimide)**

 USES

Controls seizures in treatment of epilepsy.

 DOSAGE & USAGE INFORMATION

**How to take:**
Capsule—Swallow with liquid or food to lessen stomach irritation.

**When to take:**
Every day in regularly spaced doses, according to prescription.

**If you forget a dose:**
Take as soon as you remember up to 2 hours late. If more than 2 hours, wait for next scheduled dose (don't double this dose).

**What drug does:**
Depresses nerve transmissions in part of brain that controls muscles.

**Time lapse before drug works:**
3 hours.

**Don't take with:**
See Interaction column and consult doctor.

 OVERDOSE

**SYMPTOMS:**
Coma
**WHAT TO DO:**
- **Dial 0 (operator) or 911 (emergency) for an ambulance or medical help. Then give first aid immediately.**
- **If patient is unconscious and not breathing, give mouth-to-mouth breathing. If there is no heartbeat, use cardiac massage and mouth-to-mouth breathing (CPR). Don't try to make patient vomit. If you can't get help quickly, take patient to nearest emergency facility.**
- **See emergency information on inside covers.**

 POSSIBLE ADVERSE REACTIONS OR SIDE EFFECTS

| SYMPTOMS | WHAT TO DO |
|---|---|
| **Life-threatening:** None expected. | |
| **Common:** Nausea, vomiting, stomach cramps, appetite loss. | Continue. Call doctor when convenient. |
| **Infrequent:** Dizziness, drowsiness, headache, irritability, mood change. | Continue. Call doctor when convenient. |
| **Rare:**  • Rash, sore throat, fever, unusual bleeding or bruising. | Discontinue. Call doctor right away. |
| • Swollen lymph glands. | Continue. Call doctor when convenient. |

## WARNINGS & PRECAUTIONS

**Don't take if:**
You are allergic to any succinimide anticonvulsant.

**Before you start, consult your doctor:**
- If you plan to become pregnant within medication period.
- If you take other anticonvulsants.
- If you have blood disease.
- If you have kidney or liver disease.

**Over age 60:**
Adverse reactions and side effects may be more frequent and severe than in younger persons.

**Pregnancy:**
Risk to unborn child outweighs drug benefits. Don't use.

**Breast-feeding:**
Drug passes into milk. Avoid drug or discontinue nursing.

**Infants & children:**
Use only under medical supervision.

**Prolonged use:**
No problems expected.

**Skin & sunlight:**
No problems expected.

**Driving, piloting or hazardous work:**
Don't drive or pilot aircraft until you learn how medicine affects you. Don't work around dangerous machinery. Don't climb ladders or work in high places. Danger increases if you drink alcohol or take medicine affecting alertness and reflexes, such as antihistamines, tranquilizers, sedatives, pain medicine, narcotics and mind-altering drugs.

**Discontinuing:**
Don't discontinue without doctor's advice until you complete prescribed dose, even though symptoms diminish or disappear.

**Others:**
- Your response to medicine should be checked regularly by your doctor. Dose and schedule may have to be altered frequently to fit individual needs.
- Periodic blood-cell counts, kidney- and liver-function studies recommended.

## POSSIBLE INTERACTION WITH OTHER DRUGS

| GENERIC NAME OR DRUG CLASS | COMBINED EFFECT |
| --- | --- |
| Anticonvulsants (other) | Increased effect of both drugs. |
| Antidepressants (tricyclic) | May provoke seizures. |
| Antipsychotics | May provoke seizures. |

## POSSIBLE INTERACTION WITH OTHER SUBSTANCES

| INTERACTS WITH | COMBINED EFFECT |
| --- | --- |
| Alcohol: | May provoke seizures. |
| Beverages: | None expected. |
| Cocaine: | May provoke seizures. |
| Foods: | None expected. |
| Marijuana: | May provoke seizures. |
| Tobacco: | None expected. |

# METHYCLOTHIAZIDE

## BRAND NAMES

Aquatensen      Enduron
Diutensen      Enduronyl
Duretic

## BASIC INFORMATION

**Habit forming? No**
**Prescription needed? Yes**
**Available as generic? Yes**
**Drug class: Antihypertensive, diuretic
(thiazide)**

## USES

- Controls, but doesn't cure, high blood pressure.
- Reduces fluid retention (edema) caused by conditions such as heart disorders and liver disease.

## DOSAGE & USAGE INFORMATION

**How to take:**
Tablet or capsule—Swallow with liquid. If you can't swallow whole, crumble tablet or open capsule and take with liquid or food. Don't exceed dose.

**When to take:**
At the same time each day.

**If you forget a dose:**
Take as soon as you remember up to 2 hours late. If more than 2 hours, wait for next scheduled dose (don't double this dose).

**What drug does:**
- Forces sodium and water excretion, reducing body fluid.
- Relaxes muscle cells of small arteries.
- Reduced body fluid and relaxed arteries lower blood pressure.

*Continued next column*

## OVERDOSE

**SYMPTOMS:**
**Cramps, weakness, drowsiness, weak pulse, coma.**
**WHAT TO DO:**
- **Dial 0 (operator) or 911 (emergency) for an ambulance or medical help. Then give first aid immediately.**
- **See emergency information on inside covers.**

**Time lapse before drug works:**
4 to 6 hours. May require several weeks to lower blood pressure.

**Don't take with:**
- See Interaction column and consult doctor.
- Non-prescription drugs without consulting doctor.

## POSSIBLE ADVERSE REACTIONS OR SIDE EFFECTS

| SYMPTOMS | WHAT TO DO |
|---|---|
| **Life-threatening:**<br>None expected. | |
| **Common:**<br>None expected. | |
| **Infrequent:** | |
| • Blurred vision, severe abdominal pain, nausea, vomiting, irregular heartbeat, weak pulse. | Discontinue. Call doctor right away. |
| • Dizziness, mood change, headache, weakness, tiredness, weight changes. | Continue. Call doctor when convenient. |
| • Dry mouth, thirst. | Continue. Tell doctor at next visit. |
| **Rare:** | |
| • Rash or hives. | Discontinue. Seek emergency treatment. |
| • Jaundice, sore throat, fever. | Discontinue. Call doctor right away. |

## WARNINGS & PRECAUTIONS

**Don't take if:**
You are allergic to any thiazide diuretic drug.

**Before you start, consult your doctor:**
- If you are allergic to any sulfa drug.
- If you have gout.
- If you have liver, pancreas or kidney disorder.

**Over age 60:**
Adverse reactions and side effects may be more frequent and severe than in younger persons, especially dizziness and excessive potassium loss.

**Pregnancy:**
Risk to unborn child outweighs drug benefits. Don't use.

**Breast-feeding:**
Drug passes into milk. Avoid drug or discontinue nursing.

**Infants & children:**
No problems expected.

**Prolonged use:**
You may need medicine to treat high blood pressure for the rest of your life.

**Skin & sunlight:**
May cause rash or intensify sunburn in areas exposed to sun or sunlamp.

**Driving, piloting or hazardous work:**
Don't drive or pilot aircraft until you learn how medicine affects you. Don't work around dangerous machinery. Don't climb ladders or work in high places. Danger increases if you drink alcohol or take medicine affecting alertness and reflexes, such as antihistamines, tranquilizers, sedatives, pain medicine, narcotics and mind-altering drugs.

**Discontinuing:**
Don't discontinue without medical advice.

**Others:**
- Hot weather and fever may cause dehydration and drop in blood pressure. Dose may require temporary adjustment. Weigh daily and report any unexpected weight decreases to your doctor.
- May cause rise in uric acid, leading to gout.
- May cause blood-sugar rise in diabetics.

## POSSIBLE INTERACTION WITH OTHER DRUGS

| GENERIC NAME OR DRUG CLASS | COMBINED EFFECT |
|---|---|
| Acebutolol | Increased antihypertensive effect. Dosages of both drugs may require adjustments. |
| Allopurinol | Decreased allopurinol effect. |
| Amiodarone | Increased risk of heartbeat irregularity due to low potassium. |
| Antidepressants (tricyclic) | Dangerous drop in blood pressure. Avoid combination unless under medical supervision. |
| Barbiturates | Increased methyclothiazide effect. |
| Calcium supplements | Increased calcium in blood. |
| Cholestyramine | Decreased methyclothiazide effect. |
| Cortisone drugs | Excessive potassium loss that causes dangerous heart rhythms. |

| | |
|---|---|
| Digitalis preparations | Excessive potassium loss that causes dangerous heart rhythms. |
| Diuretics (thiazide) | Increased effect of other thiazide diuretics. |
| Indapamide | Increased diuretic effect. |
| Labetolol | Increased antihypertensive effects. |
| Lithium | Increased effect of lithium. |
| MAO inhibitors | Increased metolazone effect. |
| Nitrates | Excessive blood-pressure drop. |
| Oxprenolol | Increased antihypertensive effect. Dosages of both drugs may require adjustments. |
| Potassium supplements | Decreased potassium effect. |
| Probenecid | Decreased probenecid effect. |

## POSSIBLE INTERACTION WITH OTHER SUBSTANCES

| INTERACTS WITH | COMBINED EFFECT |
|---|---|
| Alcohol: | Dangerous blood-pressure drop. |
| Beverages: | None expected. |
| Cocaine: | None expected. |
| Foods: Licorice. | Excessive potassium loss that causes dangerous heart rhythms. |
| Marijuana: | May increase blood pressure. |
| Tobacco: | None expected. |

# METHYLCELLULOSE

## BRAND NAMES

Anorex-CCK
Cellothyl
Citrucel
Cologel

Gonio-Gel
Hydrolose
Lacril
Murocel

## BASIC INFORMATION

**Habit forming? No**
**Prescription needed? No**
**Available as generic? Yes**
**Drug class: Laxative (bulk-forming)**

## USES

Relieves constipation and prevents straining for bowel movement.

## DOSAGE & USAGE INFORMATION

**How to take:**
- Liquid, powder, flakes, granules—Dilute dose in 8 oz. cold water or fruit juice.
- Capsules—Swallow with 8 oz. cold liquid. Drink 6 to 8 glasses of water each day in addition to the one with each dose.

**When to take:**
At the same time each day, preferably morning.

**If you forget a dose:**
Take as soon as you remember. Resume regular schedule.

**What drug does:**
Absorbs water, stimulating the bowel to form a soft, bulky stool.

**Time lapse before drug works:**
May require 2 or 3 days to begin, then works in 12 to 24 hours.

**Don't take with:**
- See Interaction column and consult doctor.
- Don't take within 2 hours of taking another medicine. Laxative interferes with medicine absorption.

## OVERDOSE

**SYMPTOMS:**
**None expected.**
**WHAT TO DO:**
**Overdose unlikely to threaten life. If person takes much larger amount than prescribed, call doctor, poison-control center or hospital emergency room for instructions.**

## POSSIBLE ADVERSE REACTIONS OR SIDE EFFECTS

| SYMPTOMS | WHAT TO DO |
|---|---|
| **Life-threatening:**<br>None expected. | |
| **Common:**<br>None expected. | |
| **Infrequent:**<br>Swallowing difficulty, "lump in throat" sensation, nausea, vomiting, diarrhea. | Continue. Call doctor when convenient. |
| **Rare:**<br>Itchy skin, rash, intestinal blockage, asthma. | Discontinue. Call doctor right away. |

## WARNINGS & PRECAUTIONS

**Don't take if:**
- You are allergic to any bulk-forming laxative.
- You have symptoms of appendicitis, inflamed bowel or intestinal blockage.
- You have missed a bowel movement for only 1 or 2 days.

**Before you start, consult your doctor:**
- If you have diabetes.
- If you have a laxative habit.
- If you have rectal bleeding.
- If you have difficulty swallowing.
- If you take other laxatives.

**Over age 60:**
Adverse reactions and side effects may be more frequent and severe than in younger persons.

**Pregnancy:**
Most bulk-forming laxatives contain sodium or sugars which may cause fluid retention. Avoid if possible.

**Breast-feeding:**
No problems expected.

**Infants & children:**
Use only under medical supervision.

**Prolonged use:**
Don't take for more than 1 week unless under a doctor's supervision. May cause laxative dependence.

**Skin & sunlight:**
No problems expected.

**Driving, piloting or hazardous work:**
No problems expected.

**Discontinuing:**
May be unnecessary to finish medicine. Follow doctor's instructions.

**Others:**
Don't take to "flush out" your system or as a "tonic."

## POSSIBLE INTERACTION WITH OTHER DRUGS

| GENERIC NAME OR DRUG CLASS | COMBINED EFFECT |
| --- | --- |
| Antibiotics | Decreased antibiotic effect. |
| Anticoagulants | Decreased anticoagulant effect. |
| Digitalis preparations | Decreased digitalis effect. |
| Salicylates (including aspirin) | Decreased salicylate effect. |

## POSSIBLE INTERACTION WITH OTHER SUBSTANCES

| INTERACTS WITH | COMBINED EFFECT |
| --- | --- |
| Alcohol: | None expected. |
| Beverages: | None expected. |
| Cocaine: | None expected. |
| Foods: | None expected. |
| Marijuana: | None expected. |
| Tobacco: | None expected. |

# METHYLDOPA

## BRAND NAMES

| | |
|---|---|
| Aldoclor | Aldoril-25 |
| Aldoril D30 | Apo-Methyldopa |
| Aldoril D50 | Medimet |
| Aldoril-15 | PMS Dopazide |

## BASIC INFORMATION

Habit forming? No
Prescription needed? Yes
Available as generic? Yes
Drug class: Antihypertensive

## USES

Reduces high blood pressure.

## DOSAGE & USAGE INFORMATION

**How to take:**
Liquid or tablet—Swallow with liquid. If you can't swallow whole, crumble tablet and take with liquid or food.

**When to take:**
At the same times each day.

**If you forget a dose:**
Take as soon as you remember up to 2 hours late. If more than 2 hours, wait for next scheduled dose (don't double this dose).

**What drug does:**
Relaxes walls of small arteries to decrease blood pressure.

*Continued next column*

## OVERDOSE

**SYMPTOMS:**
Drowsiness; exhaustion; stupor; confusion; slow, weak pulse.
**WHAT TO DO:**
- Dial 0 (operator) or 911 (emergency) for an ambulance or medical help. Then give first aid immediately.
- If patient is unconscious and not breathing, give mouth-to-mouth breathing. If there is no heartbeat, use cardiac massage and mouth-to-mouth breathing (CPR). Don't try to make patient vomit. If you can't get help quickly, take patient to nearest emergency facility.
- See emergency information on inside covers.

**Time lapse before drug works:**
Continual use for 2 to 4 weeks may be necessary to determine effectiveness.

**Don't take with:**
See Interaction column and consult doctor.

## POSSIBLE ADVERSE REACTIONS OR SIDE EFFECTS

| SYMPTOMS | WHAT TO DO |
|---|---|
| **Life-threatening:** None expected. | |
| **Common:** Depression, nightmares, drowsiness, weakness, stuffy nose, dry mouth, fluid retention, swollen feet or legs. | Continue. Call doctor when convenient. |
| **Infrequent:** | |
| • Fast heartbeat. | Discontinue. Call doctor right away. |
| • Insomnia, nausea, vomiting, diarrhea. | Continue. Call doctor when convenient. |
| • Swollen breasts, diminished sex drive. | Continue. Tell doctor at next visit. |
| **Rare:** Rash, jaundice, unexplained fever. | Discontinue. Call doctor right away. |

554

## WARNINGS & PRECAUTIONS

**Don't take if:**
You will have surgery within 2 months, including dental surgery, requiring general or spinal anesthesia.

**Before you start, consult your doctor:**
If you have liver disease.

**Over age 60:**
- Increased susceptibility to dizziness, unsteadiness, fainting, falling.
- Drug can produce or intensify Parkinson's disease.

**Pregnancy:**
No proven problems. Consult doctor.

**Breast-feeding:**
No proven problems. Consult doctor.

**Infants & children:**
Not used.

**Prolonged use:**
- May cause anemia.
- Severe edema (fluid retention).

**Skin & sunlight:**
No problems expected.

**Driving, piloting or hazardous work:**
Don't drive or pilot aircraft until you learn how medicine affects you. Don't work around dangerous machinery. Don't climb ladders or work in high places. Danger increases if you drink alcohol or take medicine affecting alertness and reflexes, such as antihistamines, tranquilizers, sedatives, pain medicine, narcotics and mind-altering drugs.

**Discontinuing:**
Don't discontinue without consulting doctor. Dose may require gradual reduction if you have taken drug for a long time. Doses of other drugs may also require adjustment.

**Others:**
Avoid heavy exercise, exertion, sweating.

## POSSIBLE INTERACTION WITH OTHER DRUGS

| GENERIC NAME OR DRUG CLASS | COMBINED EFFECT |
|---|---|
| Amphetamines | Decreased methyldopa effect. |
| Anticoagulants (oral) | Increased anticoagulant effect. |
| Antidepressants (tricyclic) | Dangerous blood-pressure rise. Decreased methyldopa effect. |
| Antihypertensives | Increased antihypertensive effect. |
| Digitalis preparations | Excessively slow heartbeat. |
| Diuretics (thiazide) | Increased methyldopa effect. |
| Enalapril | Possible excessive potassium in blood. |
| Levodopa | Decreased levodopa effect. |
| MAO inhibitors | Dangerous blood-pressure rise. |
| Pentoxifylline | Increased antihypertensive effect. |

## POSSIBLE INTERACTION WITH OTHER SUBSTANCES

| INTERACTS WITH | COMBINED EFFECT |
|---|---|
| Alcohol: | Increased sedation. Excessive blood-pressure drop. Avoid. |
| Beverages: | None expected. |
| Cocaine: | Decreased methyldopa effect. |
| Foods: | None expected. |
| Marijuana: | Possible fainting. |
| Tobacco: | Possible increased blood pressure. |

## BRAND NAMES

Aldomet      Medimet-250
Dopamet      Novomedopa

## BASIC INFORMATION

**Habit forming?** No
**Prescription needed?** Yes
**Available as generic?** Yes
**Drug class:** Antihypertensive, diuretic
        (thiazide)

 **USES**

- Controls, but doesn't cure, high blood pressure.
- Reduces fluid retention (edema).

 **DOSAGE & USAGE INFORMATION**

**How to take:**
Tablet or capsule—Swallow with liquid. If you can't swallow whole, crumble tablet or open capsule and take with liquid or food.

**When to take:**
At the same times each day.

**If you forget a dose:**
Take as soon as you remember up to 2 hours late. If more than 2 hours, wait for next scheduled dose (don't double this dose).

*Continued next column*

 **OVERDOSE**

**SYMPTOMS:**
**Drowsiness; exhaustion; cramps; weakness; stupor; confusion; slow, weak pulse; coma.**
**WHAT TO DO:**
- **Dial 0 (operator) or 911 (emergency) for an ambulance or medical help. Then give first aid immediately.**
- **If patient is unconscious and not breathing, give mouth-to-mouth breathing. If there is no heartbeat, use cardiac massage and mouth-to-mouth breathing (CPR). Don't try to make patient vomit. If you can't get help quickly, take patient to nearest emergency facility.**
- **See emergency information on inside covers.**

**What drug does:**
- Relaxes walls of small arteries to decrease blood pressure.
- Forces sodium and water excretion, reducing body fluid.
- Reduced body fluid and relaxed arteries lower blood pressure.

**Time lapse before drug works:**
Continual use for 2 to 4 weeks may be necessary to determine effectiveness.

**Don't take with:**
- Non-prescription drugs without consulting doctor.
- See Interaction column and consult doctor.

 **POSSIBLE ADVERSE REACTIONS OR SIDE EFFECTS**

| SYMPTOMS | WHAT TO DO |
|---|---|
| **Life-threatening:** | |
| Irregular heartbeat, weak pulse. | Discontinue. Seek emergency treatment. |
| **Common:** | |
| Depression, nightmares, drowsiness, weakness, stuffy nose, dry mouth, swollen feet and ankles, dizziness. | Continue. Call doctor when convenient. |
| **Infrequent:** | |
| • Fast heartbeat, change in vision, abdominal pain, nervousness. | Discontinue. Call doctor right away. |
| • Insomnia, nausea, vomiting, diarrhea, headache. | Continue. Call doctor when convenient. |
| **Rare:** | |
| • Rash; jaundice; hives; sore throat, fever, mouth sores. | Discontinue. Call doctor right away. |
| • Weight gain or loss. | Continue. Call doctor when convenient. |

 **WARNINGS & PRECAUTIONS**

**Don't take if:**
- You are allergic to any thiazide diuretic drug.
- If you will have surgery within 2 months, including dental surgery, requiring general or spinal anesthesia.

**Before you start, consult your doctor:**
- If you are allergic to any sulfa drug.
- If you have gout, liver, pancreas or kidney disorder.

**Over age 60:**
- Increased susceptibility to dizziness, unsteadiness, fainting, falling.

- Drug can produce or intensify Parkinson's disease.

**Pregnancy:**
Risk to unborn child outweighs drug benefits. Don't use.

**Breast-feeding:**
Drug passes into milk. Avoid drug or discontinue nursing until you finish medicine. Consult doctor for advice on maintaining milk supply.

**Infants & children:**
Not recommended.

**Prolonged use:**
- May cause anemia.
- Severe edema (fluid retention).

**Skin & sunlight:**
May cause rash or intensify sunburn in areas exposed to sun or sunlamp.

**Driving, piloting or hazardous work:**
Don't drive or pilot aircraft until you learn how medicine affects you. Don't work around dangerous machinery. Don't climb ladders or work in high places. Danger increases if you drink alcohol or take medicine affecting alertness and reflexes, such as antihistamines, tranquilizers, sedatives, pain medicine, narcotics and mind-altering drugs.

**Discontinuing:**
Don't discontinue without consulting doctor. Dose may require gradual reduction if you have taken drug for a long time. Doses of other drugs may also require adjustment.

**Others:**
- Hot weather and fever may cause dehydration and drop in blood pressure. Dose may require temporary adjustment. Weigh daily and report any unexpected weight decreases to your doctor.
- May cause rise in uric acid, leading to gout.
- May cause blood-sugar rise in diabetics.
- Avoid heavy exercise, exertion, sweating.

 **POSSIBLE INTERACTION WITH OTHER DRUGS**

| GENERIC NAME OR DRUG CLASS | COMBINED EFFECT |
|---|---|
| Acebutolol | Increased antihypertensive effect. Dosages of both drugs may require adjustments. |
| Allopurinol | Decreased allopurinol effect. |
| Amphetamines | Decreased methyldopa effect. |

| | |
|---|---|
| Anticoagulants (oral) | Increased anticoagulant effect. |
| Antidepressants (tricyclic) | Dangerous changes in blood pressure. Avoid combination unless under medical supervision. |
| Antihypertensives | Increased antihypertensive effect. |
| Barbiturates | Increased hydrochlorothiazide effect. |
| Cholestyamine | Decreased hydrochlorothiazide effect. |
| Cortisone drugs | Excessive potassium loss that causes dangerous heart rhythms. |
| Digitalis preparations | Excessive potassium loss that causes dangerous heart rhythms. |
| Diuretics (thiazide) | Increased effect of both drugs. |
| Indapamide | Increased diuretic effect. |
| Levodopa | Decreased levodopa effect. |
| Lithium | Increased lithium effect. |

*Continued page 968*

 **POSSIBLE INTERACTION WITH OTHER SUBSTANCES**

| INTERACTS WITH | COMBINED EFFECT |
|---|---|
| Alcohol: | Increased sedation. Excessive blood-pressure drop. Avoid. |
| Beverages: | None expected. |
| Cocaine: | Decreased methyldopa effect. |
| Foods: Licorice. | Excessive potassium loss that causes dangerous heart rhythms. |
| Marijuana: | May increase blood pressure. |
| Tobacco: | Possible increased blood pressure. |

# METHYLERGONOVINE

## BRAND NAMES

Methergine      Methylergometrine
Methylergobasine-
  Sandoz

## BASIC INFORMATION

**Habit forming?** No
**Prescription needed?** Yes
**Available as generic?** Yes
**Drug class:** Ergot preparation (uterine
            stimulant)

## USES

Retards excessive post-delivery bleeding.

## DOSAGE & USAGE INFORMATION

**How to take:**
Tablet—Swallow with liquid or food to lessen
stomach irritation.

**When to take:**
At the same times each day.

**If you forget a dose:**
Don't take missed dose and don't double next
one. Wait for next scheduled dose.

**What drug does:**
Causes smooth-muscle cells of uterine wall to
contract and surround bleeding blood vessels of
relaxed uterus.

**Time lapse before drug works:**
Tablets—20 to 30 minutes.

**Don't take with:**
See Interaction column and consult doctor.

## OVERDOSE

**SYMPTOMS:**
**Vomiting, diarrhea, weak pulse, low blood
pressure, convulsions.**
**WHAT TO DO:**
- **Dial 0 (operator) or 911 (emergency) for an
  ambulance or medical help. Then give first
  aid immediately.**
- **If patient is unconscious and not
  breathing, give mouth-to-mouth breathing.
  If there is no heartbeat, use cardiac
  massage and mouth-to-mouth breathing
  (CPR). Don't try to make patient vomit. If
  you can't get help quickly, take patient to
  nearest emergency facility.**
- **See emergency information on inside
  covers.**

## POSSIBLE ADVERSE REACTIONS OR SIDE EFFECTS

| SYMPTOMS | WHAT TO DO |
|---|---|
| **Life-threatening:**<br>None expected. | |
| **Common:**<br>Nausea, vomiting. | Discontinue. Call doctor right away. |
| **Infrequent:**<br>• Confusion, ringing in ears, diarrhea, muscle cramps. | Discontinue. Call doctor right away. |
| • Unusual sweating. | Continue. Call doctor when convenient. |
| **Rare:**<br>Sudden, severe headache; shortness of breath; chest pain; numb, cold hands and feet. | Discontinue. Seek emergency treatment. |

558

## WARNINGS & PRECAUTIONS

**Don't take if:**
You are allergic to any ergot preparation.

**Before you start, consult your doctor:**
- If you have coronary-artery or blood-vessel disease.
- If you have liver or kidney disease.
- If you have high blood pressure.
- If you have postpartum infection.

**Over age 60:**
Not recommended.

**Pregnancy:**
Risk to unborn child outweighs drug benefits. Don't use.

**Breast-feeding:**
Drug passes into milk. Avoid drug or discontinue nursing until you finish medicine. Consult doctor for advice on maintaining milk supply.

**Infants & children:**
Not recommended.

**Prolonged use:**
Not recommended.

**Skin & sunlight:**
No problems expected.

**Driving, piloting or hazardous work:**
No problems expected.

**Discontinuing:**
May be unnecessary to finish medicine. Follow doctor's instructions.

**Others:**
Drug should be used for short time only following childbirth or miscarriage.

## POSSIBLE INTERACTION WITH OTHER DRUGS

| GENERIC NAME OR DRUG CLASS | COMBINED EFFECT |
|---|---|
| Ergot preparations (other) | Increased methylergonovine effect. |

## POSSIBLE INTERACTION WITH OTHER SUBSTANCES

| INTERACTS WITH | COMBINED EFFECT |
|---|---|
| Alcohol: | None expected. |
| Beverages: | None expected. |
| Cocaine: | None expected. |
| Foods: | None expected. |
| Marijuana: | None expected. |
| Tobacco: | None expected. |

# METHYLPHENIDATE

## BRAND NAMES

Methldate                    Ritalin SR
Ritalin

## BASIC INFORMATION

**Habit forming? Yes**
**Available as generic? Yes**
**Prescription needed? Yes**
**Drug class: Sympathomimetic**

 ## USES

- Treatment for hyperactive children.
- Treatment for drowsiness and fatigue in adults.
- Treatment for narcolepsy (uncontrollable attacks of sleepiness).

 ## DOSAGE & USAGE INFORMATION

**How to take:**
Tablet or capsule—Swallow with liquid or food to lessen stomach irritation. If you can't swallow whole, crumble tablet or open capsule and take with liquid or food.

**When to take:**
At the same times each day.

**If you forget a dose:**
Take as soon as you remember up to 2 hours late. If more than 2 hours, wait for next scheduled dose (don't double this dose).

*Continued next column*

 ## OVERDOSE

**SYMPTOMS:**
**Rapid heartbeat, fever, confusion, hallucinations, convulsions, coma.**
**WHAT TO DO:**
- **Dial 0 (operator) or 911 (emergency) for an ambulance or medical help. Then give first aid immediately.**
- **If patient is unconscious and not breathing, give mouth-to-mouth breathing. If there is no heartbeat, use cardiac massage and mouth-to-mouth breathing (CPR). Don't try to make patient vomit. If you can't get help quickly, take patient to nearest emergency facility.**
- **See emergency information on inside covers.**

**What drug does:**
Stimulates brain to improve alertness, concentration and attention span. Calms the hyperactive child.

**Time lapse before drug works:**
- 1 month or more for maximum effect on child.
- 30 minutes to stimulate adults.

**Don't take with:**
See Interaction column and consult doctor.

 ## POSSIBLE ADVERSE REACTIONS OR SIDE EFFECTS

| SYMPTOMS | WHAT TO DO |
|---|---|
| **Life-threatening:** | |
| None expected. | |
| **Common:** | |
| • Mood change. | Continue. Call doctor when convenient. |
| • Nervousness, insomnia, dizziness, headache, appetite loss. | Continue. Tell doctor at next visit. |
| **Infrequent:** | |
| • Rash or hives; chest pain; fast, irregular heartbeat; unusual bruising; joint pain; uncontrollable movements; unexplained fever. | Discontinue. Call doctor right away. . |
| • Nausea, abdominal pain. | Continue. Call doctor when convenient. |
| **Rare:** | |
| • Blurred vision, sore throat, fever. | Discontinue. Call doctor right away. |
| • Unusual tiredness. | Continue. Call doctor when convenient. |

## WARNINGS & PRECAUTIONS

**Don't take if:**
- You are allergic to methylphenidate.
- You have glaucoma.
- Patient is younger than 6.

**Before you start, consult your doctor:**
- If you have epilepsy.
- If you have high blood pressure.
- If you take MAO inhibitors.

**Over age 60:**
Adverse reactions and side effects may be more frequent and severe than in younger persons.

**Pregnancy:**
No proven harm to unborn child. Avoid if possible.

**Breast-feeding:**
No proven problems. Consult doctor.

**Infants & children:**
Use only under medical supervision for children 6 or older.

**Prolonged use:**
Rare possibility of physical growth retardation.

**Skin & sunlight:**
No problems expected.

**Driving, piloting or hazardous work:**
No problems expected.

**Discontinuing:**
Don't discontinue abruptly. Don't discontinue without doctor's advice until you complete prescribed dose, even though symptoms diminish or disappear.

**Others:**
Dose must be carefully adjusted by doctor.

## POSSIBLE INTERACTION WITH OTHER DRUGS

| GENERIC NAME OR DRUG CLASS | COMBINED EFFECT |
|---|---|
| Acebutolol | Decreased effects of both drugs. |
| Anticholinergics | Increased anticholinergic effect. |
| Anticoagulants (oral) | Increased anticoagulant effect. |
| Anticonvulsants | Increased anticonvulsant effect. |
| Antidepressants (tricyclic) | Increased antidepressant effect. Decreased methylphenidate effect. |
| Guanethidine | Decreased guanethidine effect. |
| MAO inhibitors | Dangerous rise in blood pressure. |
| Minoxidil | Decreased minoxidil effect. |
| Nitrates | Possible decreased effects of both drugs. |
| Oxprenolol | Decreased effects of both drugs. |
| Oxyphenbutazone | Increased oxyphenbutazone effect. |
| Phenylbutazone | Increased phenylbutazone effect. |

## POSSIBLE INTERACTION WITH OTHER SUBSTANCES

| INTERACTS WITH | COMBINED EFFECT |
|---|---|
| Alcohol: | None expected. |
| Beverages: Caffeine drinks. | May raise blood pressure. |
| Cocaine: | Overstimulation. Avoid. |
| Foods: Foods containing tyramine (see Glossary). | May raise blood pressure. |
| Marijuana: | None expected. |
| Tobacco: | None expected. |

# METHYLPREDNISOLONE

## BRAND NAMES

See complete list of brand names in the *Brand Name Directory,* page 951.

## BASIC INFORMATION

**Habit forming? No**
**Prescription needed? Yes**
**Available as generic? Yes**
**Drug class: Cortisone drug (adrenal corticosteroid)**

## USES

- Reduces inflammation caused by many different medical problems.
- Treatment for some allergic diseases, blood disorders, kidney diseases, asthma and emphysema.
- Replaces corticosteroid deficiencies.

## DOSAGE & USAGE INFORMATION

**How to take:**
Tablet—Swallow with liquid or food to lessen stomach irritation. If you can't swallow whole, crumble tablet and take with liquid or food.

**When to take:**
At the same times each day. Take once-a-day or once-every-other-day doses in mornings.

**If you forget a dose:**
- Several-doses-per-day prescription—Take as soon as you remember up to 2 hours late. If more than 2 hours, wait for next scheduled dose (don't double this dose).
- Once-a-day dose or less—Wait for next dose. Double this dose.

**What drug does:**
Decreases inflammatory responses.

**Time lapse before drug works:**
2 to 4 days.

**Don't take with:**
See Interaction column and consult doctor.

## OVERDOSE

**SYMPTOMS:**
**Headache, convulsions, heart failure.**
**WHAT TO DO:**
- **Dial 0 (operator) or 911 (emergency) for an ambulance or medical help. Then give first aid immediately.**
- **See emergency information on inside covers.**

## POSSIBLE ADVERSE REACTIONS OR SIDE EFFECTS

| SYMPTOMS | WHAT TO DO |
|---|---|
| **Life-threatening:**<br>None expected. | |
| **Common:**<br>Acne, poor wound healing, thirst, indigestion, nausea, vomiting. | Continue. Call doctor when convenient. |
| **Infrequent:** | |
| • Black, bloody or tarry stools. | Discontinue. Seek emergency treatment. |
| • Blurred vision, halos around lights, sore throat, fever, muscle cramps, swollen legs or feet. | Discontinue. Call doctor right away. |
| • Mood change, insomnia, restlessness, frequent urination, weight gain, round face, fatigue, weakness, TB recurrence, irregular menstrual periods. | Continue. Call doctor when convenient. |
| **Rare:** | |
| • Irregular heartbeat. | Discontinue. Seek emergency treatment. |
| • Rash. | Discontinue. Call doctor right away. |

## WARNINGS & PRECAUTIONS

**Don't take if:**
- You are allergic to any cortisone drug.
- You have tuberculosis or fungus infection.
- You have herpes infection of eyes, lips or genitals.

**Before you start, consult your doctor:**
- If you have had tuberculosis.
- If you have congestive heart failure.
- If you have diabetes.
- If you have peptic ulcer.
- If you have glaucoma.
- If you have underactive thyroid.
- If you have high blood pressure.
- If you have myasthenia gravis.
- If you have blood clots in legs or lungs.

**Over age 60:**
Adverse reactions and side effects may be more frequent and severe than in younger persons. Likely to aggravate edema, diabetes or ulcers. Likely to cause cataracts and osteoporosis (softening of the bones).

**Pregnancy:**
Risk to unborn child outweighs drug benefits. Don't use.

**Breast-feeding:**
Drug passes into milk. Avoid drug or discontinue nursing until you finish medicine. Consult doctor for advice on maintaining milk supply.

**Infants & children:**
Use only under medical supervision.

**Prolonged use:**
- Retards growth in children.
- Possible glaucoma, cataracts, diabetes, fragile bones and thin skin.
- Functional dependence.

**Skin & sunlight:**
No problems expected.

**Driving, piloting or hazardous work:**
No problems expected.

**Discontinuing:**
- Don't discontinue without doctor's advice until you complete prescribed dose, even though symptoms diminish or disappear.
- Drug affects your response to surgery, illness, injury or stress for 2 years after discontinuing. Tell anyone who takes medical care of you within 2 years about drug.

**Others:**
Avoid immunizations if possible.

## POSSIBLE INTERACTION WITH OTHER DRUGS

| GENERIC NAME OR DRUG CLASS | COMBINED EFFECT |
|---|---|
| Amphoterecin B | Potassium depletion. |
| Anticholinergics | Possible glaucoma. |
| Anticoagulants (oral) | Decreased anticoagulant effect. |
| Anticonvulsants (hydantoin) | Decreased methylprednisolone effect. |
| Antidiabetics (oral) | Decreased antidiabetic effect. |
| Antihistamines | Decreased methylprednisolone effect. |
| Aspirin | Increased methylprednisolone effect. |
| Barbiturates | Decreased methylprednisolone effect. Oversedation. |
| Beta-adrenergic blockers | Decreased methylprednisolone effect. |

| | |
|---|---|
| Chloral hydrate | Decreased methylprednisolone effect. |
| Chlorthalidone | Potassium depletion. |
| Cholinergics | Decreased cholinergic effect. |
| Contraceptives (oral) | Increased methylprednisolone effect. |
| Digitalis preparations | Dangerous potassium depletion. Possible digitalis toxicity. |
| Diuretics (thiazide) | Potassium depletion. |
| Ephedrine | Decreased methylprednisolone effect. |
| Estrogens | Increased methylprednisolone effect. |
| Ethacrynic acid | Potassium depletion. |
| Furosemide | Potassium depletion. |
| Glutethimide | Decreased methylprednisolone effect. |
| Indapamide | Possible excessive potassium loss, causing dangerous heartbeat irregularity. |
| Indomethacin | Increased methylprednisolone effect. |
| Insulin | Decreased insulin effect. |
| Isoniazid | Decreased isoniazid effect. |
| Oxyphenbutazone | Possible ulcers. |
| Phenylbutazone | Possible ulcers. |

*Continued page 969*

## POSSIBLE INTERACTION WITH OTHER SUBSTANCES

| INTERACTS WITH | COMBINED EFFECT |
|---|---|
| Alcohol: | Risk of stomach ulcers. |
| Beverages: | No proven problems. |
| Cocaine: | Overstimulation. Avoid. |
| Foods: | No proven problems. |
| Marijuana: | Decreased immunity. |
| Tobacco: | Increased methylprednisolone effect. Possible toxicity. |

# METHYSERGIDE

## BRAND NAMES

Sansert

## BASIC INFORMATION

**Habit forming? Yes**
**Prescription needed? Yes**
**Available as generic? No**
**Drug class: Vasoconstrictor (antiserotonin)**

 USES

Prevents migraine and other recurring vascular headaches.

 DOSAGE & USAGE INFORMATION

**How to take:**
Tablet—Swallow with liquid or with food to lessen stomach irritation. If you can't swallow whole, crumble tablet and take with liquid or food.

**When to take:**
At the same times each day.

**If you forget a dose:**
Don't take missed dose. Wait for next scheduled dose (don't double this dose).

**What drug does:**
Blocks the action of serotonin, a chemical that constricts blood vessels.

**Time lapse before drug works:**
About 3 weeks.

**Don't take with:**
See Interaction column and consult doctor.

 OVERDOSE

**SYMPTOMS:**
Nausea, vomiting, abdominal pain, severe diarrhea, lack of coordination, extreme thirst.
**WHAT TO DO:**
Overdose unlikely to threaten life. If person takes much larger amount than prescribed, call doctor, poison-control center or hospital emergency room for instructions.

 POSSIBLE ADVERSE REACTIONS OR SIDE EFFECTS

| SYMPTOMS | WHAT TO DO |
|---|---|
| **Life-threatening:** | |
| None expected. | |
| **Common:** | |
| • Itchy skin. | Discontinue. Call doctor right away. |
| • Nausea, vomiting, diarrhea, numbness or tingling of extremities, leg weakness. | Continue. Call doctor when convenient. |
| • Drowsiness. | Continue. Tell doctor at next visit. |
| **Infrequent:** | |
| • Anxiety, agitation, hallucinations, unusually fast or slow heartbeat. | Discontinue. Call doctor right away. |
| • Change in vision. | Continue. Call doctor when convenient. |
| **Rare:** | |
| • Extreme thirst, chest pain, shortness of breath, fever, pale or swollen extremities, leg cramps, lower back pain, side or groin pain, appetite loss. | Discontinue. Call doctor right away. |
| • Painful or difficult urination. | Continue. Call doctor when convenient. |
| • Weight change, hair loss. | Continue. Tell doctor at next visit. |

## WARNINGS & PRECAUTIONS

**Don't take if:**
- You are allergic to any antiserotonin.
- You plan to become pregnant within medication period.
- You have an infection.
- You have a heart or blood-vessel disease.
- You have a chronic lung disease.
- You have a collagen (connective tissue) disorder.
- You have impaired liver or kidney function.

**Before you start, consult your doctor:**
- If you have been allergic to any ergot preparation.
- If you have had a peptic ulcer.

**Over age 60:**
Adverse reactions and side effects may be more frequent and severe than in younger persons.

**Pregnancy:**
Manufacturer suggests risk to unborn child outweighs drug benefits, even though studies are inconclusive.

**Breast-feeding:**
Drug probably passes into milk. Avoid drug or discontinue nursing until you finish medicine. Consult doctor for advice on maintaining milk supply.

**Infants & children:**
Not recommended.

**Prolonged use:**
Possible fibrosis, a condition in which scar tissue is deposited on heart valves, in lung tissue, blood vessels and internal organs. After 6 months, decrease dose over 2 to 3 weeks. Then discontinue for at least 2 months for re-evaluation.

**Skin & sunlight:**
No problems expected.

**Driving, piloting or hazardous work:**
Avoid if you feel drowsy or dizzy. Otherwise, no problems expected.

**Discontinuing:**
- Don't discontinue without consulting doctor. Dose may require gradual reduction if you have taken drug for a long time. Doses of other drugs may also require adjustment.
- Probably should discontinue drug if you don't improve after 3 weeks' use.

**Others:**
- Periodic laboratory tests for liver function and blood counts recommended.
- Potential for abuse.

## POSSIBLE INTERACTION WITH OTHER DRUGS

| GENERIC NAME OR DRUG CLASS | COMBINED EFFECT |
| --- | --- |
| Ergot preparations | Unpredictable increased or decreased effect of either drug. |
| Narcotics | Decreased narcotic effect. |

## POSSIBLE INTERACTION WITH OTHER SUBSTANCES

| INTERACTS WITH | COMBINED EFFECT |
| --- | --- |
| Alcohol: | None expected. However, alcohol may trigger a migraine headache. |
| Beverages: Caffeine drinks. | Decreased methysergide effect. |
| Cocaine: | May make headache worse. |
| Foods: | None expected. Avoid foods to which you are allergic. |
| Marijuana: | No proven problems. |
| Tobacco: | Blood-vessel constriction. Makes headache worse. |

# METOCLOPRAMIDE

## BRAND NAMES

| | |
|---|---|
| Emex | Maxolon |
| Maxeran | Reglan |

## BASIC INFORMATION

Habit forming? No
Prescription needed? Yes
Available as generic? Yes
Drug class: Antiemetic; dopaminergic
      blocker

## USES

- Relieves nausea and vomiting caused by chemotherapy and drug related postoperative factors.
- Relieves symptoms of esophagitis.

## DOSAGE & USAGE INFORMATION

**How to take:**
Tablet or capsule—Swallow with liquid or food to lessen stomach irritation.

**When to take:**
30 minutes before symptoms expected, up to 4 times a day.

**If you forget a dose:**
Take as soon as you remember up to 2 hours late. If more than 2 hours, wait for next scheduled dose (don't double this dose).

**What drug does:**
- Prevents smooth muscle in stomach from relaxing.
- Affects vomiting center in brain.

*Continued next column*

## OVERDOSE

**SYMPTOMS:**
Severe drowsiness, mental confusion, trembling, seizure, coma.
**WHAT TO DO:**
- Dial 0 (operator) or 911 (emergency) for an ambulance or medical help. Then give first aid immediately.
- If patient is unconscious and not breathing, give mouth-to-mouth breathing. If there is no heartbeat, use cardiac massage and mouth-to-mouth breathing (CPR). Don't try to make patient vomit. If you can't get help quickly, take patient to nearest emergency facility.
- See emergency information on inside covers.

**Time lapse before drug works:**
30 to 60 minutes.

**Don't take with:**
See Interaction column and consult doctor.

## POSSIBLE ADVERSE REACTIONS OR SIDE EFFECTS

| SYMPTOMS | WHAT TO DO |
|---|---|
| **Life-threatening:** None expected. | |
| **Common:** Drowsiness, restlessness. | Continue. Call doctor when convenient. |
| **Frequent** Rash. | Continue. Call doctor when convenient. |
| **Infrequent:** | |
| • Wheezing, shortness of breath. | Discontinue. Call doctor right away. |
| • Dizziness; headache; insomnia; tender, swollen breasts; increased milk flow. | Continue. Call doctor when convenient. |
| **Rare:** Constipation, diarrhea, nausea. | Continue. Call doctor when convenient. |

## WARNINGS & PRECAUTIONS

**Don't take if:**
You are allergic to procaine, procainamide or metoclopramide.

**Before you start, consult your doctor:**
• If you have Parkinson's disease.
• If you have liver or kidney disease.
• If you have epilepsy.
• If you have bleeding from gastrointestinal tract or intestinal obstruction.
• If you will have surgery within 2 months, including dental surgery, requiring general or spinal anesthesia.

**Over age 60:**
Adverse reactions and side effects may be more frequent and severe than in younger persons.

**Pregnancy:**
No proven harm to unborn child. Avoid if possible.

**Breast-feeding:**
Unknown effect.

**Infants & children:**
Adverse reactions more likely to occur than in adults.

**Prolonged use:**
Adverse reactions including muscle spasms and trembling hands more likely to occur.

**Skin & sunlight:**
No problems expected.

**Driving, piloting or hazardous work:**
Don't drive or pilot aircraft until you learn how medicine affects you. Don't work around dangerous machinery. Don't climb ladders or work in high places. Danger increases if you drink alcohol or take medicine affecting alertness and reflexes, such as antihistamines, tranquilizers, sedatives, pain medicine, narcotics and mind-altering drugs.

**Discontinuing:**
May be unnecessary to finish medicine. Follow doctor's instructions.

**Others:**
No problems expected.

## POSSIBLE INTERACTION WITH OTHER DRUGS

| GENERIC NAME OR DRUG CLASS | COMBINED EFFECT |
|---|---|
| Acetaminophen | Slow stomach emptying. |
| Bromocriptine | Decreased bromocriptine effect. |
| Central nervous system depressants: antidepressants, antihistamines, muscle relaxants, narcotics, sedatives, sleeping pills, tranquilizers. | Excess sedation. |
| Digitalis preparations | Decreased absorption of digitalis. |
| Levodopa | Slow stomach emptying. |
| Phenothiazines | Increased chance of muscle spasm and trembling. |
| Tetracycline | Slow stomach emptying. |

## POSSIBLE INTERACTION WITH OTHER SUBSTANCES

| INTERACTS WITH | COMBINED EFFECT |
|---|---|
| Alcohol: | Excess sedation. Avoid. |
| Beverages: Coffee. | Decreased metoclopramide effect. |
| Cocaine: | Decreased metoclopramide effect. |
| Foods: | No problems expected. |
| Marijuana: | Decreased metoclopramide effect. |
| Tobacco: | Decreased metoclopramide effect. |

# METOLAZONE

## BRAND NAMES

Diulo                     Zaroxolyn

## BASIC INFORMATION

**Habit forming?** No
**Prescription needed?** Yes
**Available as generic?** Yes
**Drug class:** Antihypertensive, diuretic
(thiazide)

## USES

- Controls, but doesn't cure, high blood pressure.
- Reduces fluid retention (edema) caused by conditions such as heart disorders and liver disease.

## DOSAGE & USAGE INFORMATION

**How to take:**
Tablet or capsule—Swallow with 8 oz. of liquid. If you can't swallow whole, crumble tablet or open capsule and take with liquid or food. Don't exceed dose.

**When to take:**
At the same time each day.

**If you forget a dose:**
Take as soon as you remember up to 2 hours late. If more than 2 hours, wait for next scheduled dose (don't double this dose).

**What drug does:**
- Forces sodium and water excretion, reducing body fluid.
- Relaxes muscle cells of small arteries.
- Reduced body fluid and relaxed arteries lower blood pressure.

**Time lapse before drug works:**
4 to 6 hours. May require several weeks to lower blood pressure.

*Continued next column*

## OVERDOSE

**SYMPTOMS:**
**Cramps, weakness, drowsiness, weak pulse, coma.**
**WHAT TO DO:**
- **Dial 0 (operator) or 911 (emergency) for an ambulance or medical help. Then give first aid immediately.**
- **See emergency information on inside covers.**

**Don't take with:**
- See Interaction column and consult doctor.
- Non-prescription drugs without consulting doctor.

## POSSIBLE ADVERSE REACTIONS OR SIDE EFFECTS

| SYMPTOMS | WHAT TO DO |
|---|---|
| **Life-threatening:** None expected. | |
| **Common:** None expected. | |
| **Infrequent:** | |
| • Blurred vision, severe abdominal pain, nausea, vomiting, irregular heartbeat, weak pulse. | Discontinue. Call doctor right away. |
| • Dizziness, mood change, headache, weakness, tiredness, weight changes. | Continue. Call doctor when convenient. |
| • Dry mouth, thirst. | Continue. Tell doctor at next visit. |
| **Rare:** | |
| • Rash or hives. | Discontinue. Seek emergency treatment. |
| • Jaundice, sore throat, fever. | Discontinue. Call doctor right away. |

## WARNINGS & PRECAUTIONS

**Don't take if:**
You are allergic to any thiazide diuretic drug.

**Before you start, consult your doctor:**
- If you are allergic to any sulfa drug.
- If you have gout.
- If you have liver, pancreas or kidney disorder.

**Over age 60:**
Adverse reactions and side effects may be more frequent and severe than in younger persons, especially dizziness and excessive potassium loss.

**Pregnancy:**
Risk to unborn child outweighs drug benefits. Don't use.

**Breast-feeding:**
Drug passes into milk. Avoid this medicine or discontinue nursing.

**Infants & children:**
No problems expected.

**Prolonged use:**
You may need medicine to treat high blood pressure for the rest of your life.

**Skin & sunlight:**
May cause rash or intensify sunburn in areas exposed to sun or sunlamp.

**Driving, piloting or hazardous work:**
Don't drive or pilot aircraft until you learn how medicine affects you. Don't work around dangerous machinery. Don't climb ladders or work in high places. Danger increases if you drink alcohol or take medicine affecting alertness and reflexes, such as antihistamines, tranquilizers, sedatives, pain medicine, narcotics and mind-altering drugs.

**Discontinuing:**
Don't discontinue without medical advice.

**Others:**
- Hot weather and fever may cause dehydration and drop in blood pressure. Dose may require temporary adjustment. Weigh daily and report any unexpected weight decreases to your doctor.
- May cause rise in uric acid, leading to gout.
- May cause blood-sugar rise in diabetics.

## POSSIBLE INTERACTION WITH OTHER DRUGS

| GENERIC NAME OR DRUG CLASS | COMBINED EFFECT |
|---|---|
| Acebutolol | Increased antihypertensive effect. Dosages of both drugs may require adjustments. |
| Allopurinol | Decreased allopurinol effect. |
| Amiodarone | Increased risk of heartbeat irregularity due to low potassium. |
| Antidepressants (tricyclic) | Dangerous drop in blood pressure. Avoid combination unless under medical supervision. |
| Barbiturates | Increased metolazone effect. |
| Calcium supplements | Increased calcium in blood. |
| Cholestyramine | Decreased metolazone effect. |
| Cortisone drugs | Excessive potassium loss that causes dangerous heart rhythms. |

| Digitalis preparations | Excessive potassium loss that causes dangerous heart rhythms. |
|---|---|
| Diuretics (thiazide) | Increased effect of other thiazide diuretics. |
| Enalapril | Possible excessive potassium in blood. |
| Indapamide | Increased diuretic effect. |
| Labetolol | Increased antihypertensive effects. |
| Lithium | Increased effect of lithium. |
| MAO inhibitors | Increased metolazone effect. |
| Nitrates | Excessive blood-pressure drop. |
| Oxprenolol | Increased antihypertensive effect. Dosages of both drugs may require adjustments. |
| Potassium supplements | Decreased potassium effect. |
| Probenecid | Decreased probenecid effect. |

## POSSIBLE INTERACTION WITH OTHER SUBSTANCES

| INTERACTS WITH | COMBINED EFFECT |
|---|---|
| Alcohol: | Dangerous blood-pressure drop. |
| Beverages: | None expected. |
| Cocaine: | None expected. |
| Foods: Licorice. | Excessive potassium loss that causes dangerous heart rhythms. |
| Marijuana: | May increase blood pressure. |
| Tobacco: | None expected. |

# METOPROLOL

## BRAND NAMES

| | |
|---|---|
| Apo-metoprolol | Lopressor |
| Betaloc | Lopressor SR |
| Betaloc Durules | Novometoprol |

## BASIC INFORMATION

**Habit forming? No**
**Prescription needed? Yes**
**Available as generic? No**
**Drug class: Beta-adrenergic blocker**

## USES

- Reduces angina attacks.
- Stabilizes irregular heartbeat.
- Lowers blood pressure.
- Reduces frequency of migraine headaches. (Does not relieve headache pain.)
- Other uses prescribed by your doctor.

## DOSAGE & USAGE INFORMATION

**How to take:**
Tablet or capsule—Swallow with liquid. If you can't swallow whole, crumble tablet or open capsule and take with liquid or food.

**When to take:**
With meals or immediately after.

**If you forget a dose:**
Take as soon as you remember. Return to regular schedule, but allow 3 hours between doses.

**What drug does:**
- Blocks certain actions of sympathetic nervous system.
- Lowers heart's oxygen requirements.
- Slows nerve impulses through heart.
- Reduces blood vessel contraction in heart, scalp and other body parts.

*Continued next column*

## OVERDOSE

**SYMPTOMS:**
**Weakness, slow or weak pulse, blood-pressure drop, fainting, convulsions, cold and sweaty skin.**
**WHAT TO DO:**
- **Dial 0 (operator) or 911 (emergency) for an ambulance or medical help. Then give first aid immediately.**
- **See emergency information on inside covers.**

**Time lapse before drug works:**
1 to 4 hours.

**Don't take with:**
Non-prescription drugs or drugs in Interaction column without consulting doctor.

## POSSIBLE ADVERSE REACTIONS OR SIDE EFFECTS

| SYMPTOMS | WHAT TO DO |
|---|---|
| **Life-threatening:** None expected. | |
| **Common:** | |
| • Pulse slower than 50 beats per minute. | Discontinue. Call doctor right away. |
| • Drowsiness, numbness or tingling of fingers or toes, dizziness, diarrhea, nausea, fatigue, weakness. | Continue. Call doctor when convenient. |
| • Cold hands, feet; dry mouth, eyes, skin. | Continue. Tell doctor at next visit. |
| **Infrequent:** | |
| • Hallucinations, nightmares, insomnia, headache, difficult breathing, joint pain. | Discontinue. Call doctor right away. |
| • Confusion, depression, reduced alertness. | Continue. Call doctor when convenient. |
| • Constipation. | Continue. Tell doctor at next visit. |
| **Rare:** | |
| • Rash, sore throat, fever. | Discontinue. Call doctor right away. |
| • Unusual bleeding or bruising. | Continue. Call doctor when convenient. |

## WARNINGS & PRECAUTIONS

**Don't take if:**
- You are allergic to any beta-adrenergic blocker.
- You have asthma or hay fever symptoms.
- You have taken MAO inhibitors in past 2 weeks.

**Before you start, consult your doctor:**
- If you have heart disease or poor circulation to the extremities.
- If you have hay fever, asthma, chronic bronchitis, emphysema.
- If you have overactive thyroid function.
- If you have impaired liver or kidney function.
- If you will have surgery within 2 months, including dental surgery, requiring general or spinal anesthesia.
- If you have diabetes or hypoglycemia.

**Over age 60:**
Adverse reactions and side effects may be more frequent and severe than in younger persons.

**Pregnancy:**
Risk to unborn child outweighs drug benefits. Don't use.

**Breast-feeding:**
Drug passes into milk. Avoid drug or discontinue nursing until you finish medicine. Consult doctor for advice on maintaining milk supply.

**Infants & children:**
Not recommended.

**Prolonged use:**
Weakens heart muscle contractions.

**Skin & sunlight:**
No problems expected.

**Driving, piloting or hazardous work:**
Don't drive or pilot aircraft until you learn how medicine affects you. Don't work around dangerous machinery. Don't climb ladders or work in high places. Danger increases if you drink alcohol or take medicine affecting alertness and reflexes.

**Discontinuing:**
Don't discontinue without consulting doctor. Dose may require gradual reduction if you have taken drug for a long time. Doses of other drugs may also require adjustment.

**Others:**
May mask hypoglycemia.

## POSSIBLE INTERACTION WITH OTHER DRUGS

| GENERIC NAME OR DRUG CLASS | COMBINED EFFECT |
| --- | --- |
| Acebutolol | Increased antihypertensive effects of both drugs. Dosages may require adjustment. |
| Albuterol | Decreased albuterol effect and beta-adrenergic blocking effect. |
| Antidiabetics | Increased antidiabetic effect. |
| Antihistamines | Decreased antihistamine effect. |
| Antihypertensives | Increased antihypertensive effect. |
| Anti-inflammatory drugs | Decreased anti-inflammatory effect. |
| Barbiturates | Increased barbiturate effect. Dangerous sedation. |

| | |
| --- | --- |
| Digitalis preparations | Can either increase or decrease heart rate. Improves irregular heartbeat. |
| Indapamide | Increased effects of both drugs. Can help control high blood pressure. |
| Molindone | Increased tranquilizer effect. |
| Narcotics | Increased narcotic effect. Dangerous sedation. |
| Nitrates | Possible excessive blood-pressure drop. |
| Pentoxifylline | Increased antihypertensive effect. |
| Phenytoin | Increased metoprolol effect. |
| Quinidine | Slows heart excessively. |
| Reserpine | Possible increased effects of both drugs. Slow heartbeat and low blood pressure may result. |
| Tocainide | May worsen congestive heart failure. |

## POSSIBLE INTERACTION WITH OTHER SUBSTANCES

| INTERACTS WITH | COMBINED EFFECT |
| --- | --- |
| Alcohol: | Excessive blood pressure drop. Avoid. |
| Beverages: | None expected. |
| Cocaine: | Irregular heartbeat. Avoid. |
| Foods: | None expected. |
| Marijuana: | Daily use—Impaired circulation to hands and feet. |
| Tobacco: | Possible irregular heartbeat. |

# METRONIDAZOLE

## BRAND NAMES

| | |
|---|---|
| Apo-Metronidazole | Metryl IV |
| Flagyl | Neo-Tric |
| Flagyl I.V. | Novonidazol |
| Flagyl I.V. RTU | PMS Metronidazole |
| Metric 21 | Protostat |
| Metro I.V. | Satric |
| Metronid | SK-Metronidazole |
| Metryl | Trikacide |

## BASIC INFORMATION

Habit forming? No
Prescription needed? Yes
Available as generic? Yes
Drug class: Antiprotozoal

## USES

Treatment for infections susceptible to metronidazole, such as trichomoniasis and amebiasis.

## DOSAGE & USAGE INFORMATION

**How to take:**
- Tablet or capsule—Swallow with liquid or food to lessen stomach irritation. If you can't swallow whole, crumble tablet or open capsule and take with liquid or food.
- Suppositories—Remove wrapper and moisten suppository with water. Gently insert larger end into vagina. Push well into vagina with finger or applicator.

**When to take:**
At the same times each day.

**If you forget a dose:**
Take as soon as you remember up to 2 hours late. If more than 2 hours, wait for next scheduled dose (don't double this dose).

**What drug does:**
Kills organisms causing the infection.

*Continued next column*

## OVERDOSE

**SYMPTOMS:**
**Weakness, nausea, vomiting, diarrhea, confusion, seizures.**
**WHAT TO DO:**
**Overdose unlikely to threaten life. If person takes much larger amount than prescribed, call doctor, poison-control center or hospital emergency room for instructions.**

**Time lapse before drug works:**
Begins in 1 hour. May require regular use for 10 days to cure infection.

**Don't take with:**
- See Interaction column and consult doctor.
- Non-prescription medicines containing alcohol.

## POSSIBLE ADVERSE REACTIONS OR SIDE EFFECTS

| SYMPTOMS | WHAT TO DO |
|---|---|
| **Life-threatening:** | |
| None expected. | |
| **Common:** | |
| • Appetite loss, nausea, stomach pain, diarrhea, vomiting. | Discontinue. Call doctor right away. |
| • Unpleasant taste. | Continue. Tell doctor at next visit. |
| **Infrequent:** | |
| • Dizziness; headache; rash; hives; skin redness; itchy skin; mouth irritation, soreness or infection; sore throat; fever. | Discontinue. Call doctor right away. |
| • Vaginal irritation, discharge, dryness; fatigue; weakness. | Continue. Call doctor when convenient. |
| • Constipation. | Continue. Tell doctor at next visit. |
| **Rare:** | |
| Mood change; unsteadiness; numbness, tingling, weakness or pain in hands or feet. | Discontinue. Call doctor right away. |

## WARNINGS & PRECAUTIONS

**Don't take if:**
- You are allergic to metronidazole.
- You have had a blood-cell or bone-marrow disorder.

**Before you start, consult your doctor:**
- If you plan to become pregnant within medication period.
- If you have a brain or nervous-system disorder.
- If you have liver or heart disease.
- If you drink alcohol.

**Over age 60:**
Adverse reactions and side effects may be more frequent and severe than in younger persons.

**Pregnancy:**
Risk to unborn child outweighs drug benefits. Manufacturer advises against use during first 3 months and only limited use after that. Don't use.

**Breast-feeding:**
Drug passes into milk. Avoid drug or discontinue nursing until you finish medicine. Consult doctor for advice on maintaining milk supply.

**Infants & children:**
Use in children for amoeba infection only under close medical supervision.

**Prolonged use:**
No problems expected.

**Skin & sunlight:**
No problems expected.

**Driving, piloting or hazardous work:**
Avoid if you feel dizzy or unsteady. Otherwise, no problems expected.

**Discontinuing:**
Don't discontinue without doctor's advice until you complete prescribed dose, even though symptoms diminish or disappear.

**Others:**
No problems expected.

## POSSIBLE INTERACTION WITH OTHER DRUGS

| GENERIC NAME OR DRUG CLASS | COMBINED EFFECT |
|---|---|
| Anticoagulants (oral) | Decreased anticoagulant effect. Possible bleeding or bruising. |
| Disulfiram | Disulfiram reaction (see Glossary). Avoid. |
| Oxytetracycline | Decreased metronidazole effect. |

## POSSIBLE INTERACTION WITH OTHER SUBSTANCES

| INTERACTS WITH | COMBINED EFFECT |
|---|---|
| Alcohol: | Possible disulfiram reaction (see Glossary). Avoid alcohol in *any* form or amount. |
| Beverages: | None expected. |
| Cocaine: | Decreased metronidazole effect. Avoid. |
| Foods: | None expected. |
| Marijuana: | None expected. |
| Tobacco: | None expected. |

# MEXILETINE

## BRAND NAMES

Mexitil

## BASIC INFORMATION

**Habit forming? No**
**Prescription needed? Yes**
**Available as generic? No**
**Drug class: Antiarrhythmic**

 **USES**

Stabilizes irregular heartbeat.

 **DOSAGE & USAGE INFORMATION**

**How to take:**
Swallow whole with food, milk or antacid to lessen stomach irritation.

**When to take:**
At the same times each day as directed by your doctor.

**If you forget a dose:**
Take as soon as you remember up to 4 hours late. If more than 4 hours, wait for next scheduled dose (don't double this dose).

**What drug does:**
Blocks the fast sodium channel in heart tissue.

**Time lapse before drug works:**
30 minutes to 2 hours.

**Don't take with:**
See Interaction column and consult doctor.

 **OVERDOSE**

**SYMPTOMS:**
**Nausea, vomiting, seizures, cardiac arrest.**
**WHAT TO DO:**
- **Dial 0 (operator) or 911 (emergency) for an ambulance or medical help. Then give first aid immediately.**
- **See emergency information on inside covers.**

 **POSSIBLE ADVERSE REACTIONS OR SIDE EFFECTS**

| SYMPTOMS | WHAT TO DO |
|---|---|
| **Life-threatening:** Chest pain, shortness of breath, irregular or fast heartbeat. | Discontinue. Seek emergency treatment. |
| **Common:** Dizziness, anxiety, shakiness, unsteadiness when walking, heartburn, nausea, vomiting. | Discontinue. Call doctor right away. |
| **Infrequent:** Sore throat, fever, mouth sores; blurred vision; confusion; constipation; diarrhea; headache; numbness or tingling in hands or feet; ringing in ears; unexplained bleeding or bruising; rash; slurred speech; insomnia; weakness. | Discontinue. Call doctor right away. |
| **Rare:** Jaundice. | Discontinue. Call doctor right away. |

## WARNINGS & PRECAUTIONS

**Don't take if:**
- If you are allergic to mexiletine, lidocaine or tocainide.
- If you take other heart medicine such as digitalis.

**Before you start, consult your doctor:**
- If you have had liver or kidney disease or impaired kidney function.
- If you have had lupus.
- If you have a history of seizures.
- If you will have surgery within 2 months, including dental surgery, requiring general or spinal anesthesia.

**Over age 60:**
Adverse reactions and side effects may be more frequent and severe than in younger persons. Ask doctor about smaller doses.

**Pregnancy:**
Risk to unborn child outweighs drug benefits. Don't use.

**Breast-feeding:**
Drug passes into milk. Avoid drug or discontinue nursing until you finish medicine. Consult doctor for advice on maintaining milk supply.

**Infants & children:**
Use only under close medical supervision.

**Prolonged use:**
May possibly cause lupus-like illness.

**Skin & sunlight:**
No problems expected.

**Driving, piloting or hazardous work:**
Use caution if you feel dizzy or weak. Otherwise, no problems expected.

**Discontinuing:**
Don't discontinue without consulting doctor. Dose may require gradual reduction if you have taken drug for a long time. Doses of other drugs may also require adjustment.

**Others:**
No problems expected.

## POSSIBLE INTERACTION WITH OTHER DRUGS

| GENERIC NAME OR DRUG CLASS | COMBINED EFFECT |
|---|---|
| **Urinary acidifiers (ammonium chloride, ascorbic acid, potassium or sodium phosphate)** | May decrease effectiveness of medicine. |
| **Urinary alkalizers (acetazolamide, antacids with calcium or magnesium, methazolamide, dichlorphenamide, sodium bicarbonate, citric acid, potassium citrate, sodium citrate)** | May slow elimination of mexiletine and cause need to adjust dosage. |

## POSSIBLE INTERACTION WITH OTHER SUBSTANCES

| INTERACTS WITH | COMBINED EFFECT |
|---|---|
| **Alcohol:** | Causes irregular effectiveness of mexiletine. Avoid. |
| **Beverages:** Caffeine drinks, iced drinks. | Irregular heartbeat. |
| **Cocaine:** | Decreased mexiletine effect. |
| **Foods:** | None expected. |
| **Marijuana:** | Irregular heartbeat. Avoid. |
| **Tobacco:** | Dangerous combination. May lead to liver problems and reduce effectiveness of mexiletine. |

# MINOXIDIL

## BRAND NAMES

Loniten

## BASIC INFORMATION

Habit forming? No
Prescription needed? Yes
Available as generic? No
Drug class: Antihypertensive

## USES

- Treatment for high blood pressure in conjunction with other drugs, such as beta-adrenergic blockers and diuretics.
- Treatment for congestive heart failure.
- Can stimulate hair growth.

## DOSAGE & USAGE INFORMATION

**How to take:**
Tablet or capsule—Swallow with liquid. If you can't swallow whole, crumble tablet or open capsule and take with liquid or food.

**When to take:**
At the same time each day, according to instructions on prescription label.

**If you forget a dose:**
Take as soon as you remember up to 2 hours late. If more than 2 hours, wait for next scheduled dose (don't double this dose).

**What drug does:**
Relaxes small blood vessels (arterioles) so blood can pass through more easily.

**Time lapse before drug works:**
2 to 3 hours for effect to begin; 3 to 7 days of continuous use may be necessary for maximum blood-pressure response.

**Don't take with:**
See Interaction column and consult doctor.

## OVERDOSE

**SYMPTOMS:**
Low blood pressure, fainting, coma.
**WHAT TO DO:**
- Dial 0 (operator) or 911 (emergency) for an ambulance or medical help. Then give first aid immediately.
- See emergency information on inside covers.

## POSSIBLE ADVERSE REACTIONS OR SIDE EFFECTS

| SYMPTOMS | WHAT TO DO |
|---|---|
| **Life-threatening:**<br>None expected. | |
| **Common:**<br>Excessive hair growth. | Continue. Call doctor when convenient. |
| **Frequent:**<br>Flushed skin or redness. | Continue. Call doctor when convenient. |
| **Infrequent:**<br>• Chest pain, irregular or slow heartbeat, shortness of breath, swollen feet or legs, rapid weight gain. | Discontinue. Call doctor right away. |
| • Numbness of hands, feet, or face; headache; tender breasts. | Continue. Call doctor when convenient. |
| **Rare:**<br>Rash. | Discontinue. Call doctor right away. |

## WARNINGS & PRECAUTIONS

**Don't take if:**
You are allergic to minoxidil.

**Before you start, consult your doctor:**
• If you have had recent stroke, heart attack or angina pectoris in past 3 weeks.
• If you have impaired kidney function.

**Over age 60:**
Adverse reactions and side effects may be more frequent and severe than in younger persons.

**Pregnancy:**
Human studies not available. Avoid if possible.

**Breast-feeding:**
Human studies not available. Avoid if possible.

**Infants & children:**
Not recommended. Safety and dosage have not been established.

**Prolonged use:**
Request periodic blood examinations that include potassium levels.

**Skin & sunlight:**
No problems expected.

**Driving, piloting or hazardous work:**
Avoid if you become dizzy or faint. Otherwise, no problems expected.

**Discontinuing:**
Don't discontinue without consulting doctor. Dose may require gradual reduction if you have taken drug for a long time. Doses of other drugs may also require adjustment.

**Others:**
• Check pulse regularly. If it exceeds 20 or more beats per minute over your normal rate, consult doctor immediately.
• Check blood pressure frequently.

## POSSIBLE INTERACTION WITH OTHER DRUGS

| GENERIC NAME OR DRUG CLASS | COMBINED EFFECT |
|---|---|
| Anesthesia | Drastic drop in blood pressure. |
| Antihypertensives (other) | Dosage adjustments may be necessary to keep blood pressure at desired level. |
| Anti-inflammatory drugs (non-steroidal) | Decreased minoxidil effect. |
| Diuretics | Dosage adjustments may be necessary to keep blood pressure at desired level. |
| Enalapril | Possible excessive potassium in blood. |
| Ketoprofen | Decreased minoxidil effect. |
| Nitrates | Drastic drop in blood pressure. |
| Suprofen | Decreased minoxidil effect. |
| Sympathomimetics | Decreased minoxidil effect. |

## POSSIBLE INTERACTION WITH OTHER SUBSTANCES

| INTERACTS WITH | COMBINED EFFECT |
|---|---|
| Alcohol: | Possible excessive blood-pressure drop. |
| Beverages: | None expected. |
| Cocaine: | Increased dizziness. Avoid. |
| Foods: Salt substitutes. | Possible excessive potassium levels in blood. |
| Marijuana: | Increased dizziness. |
| Tobacco: | May decrease minoxidil effect. Avoid. |

# MITOTANE

## BRAND NAMES

Lysodren

## BASIC INFORMATION

Habit forming? No
Prescription needed? Yes
Available as generic? No
Drug class: Antineoplastic

 **USES**

- Treatment for some kinds of cancer.
- Treatment of Cushing's disease.

 **DOSAGE & USAGE INFORMATION**

**How to take:**
Tablet or capsule—Take with liquid after light meal. Don't drink fluid with meals. Drink extra fluids between meals. Avoid sweet and fatty foods.

**When to take:**
At the same time each day.

**If you forget a dose:**
Take as soon as you remember. Don't ever double dose.

**What drug does:**
Suppresses adrenal cortex to prevent manufacture of excess cortisone.

**Time lapse before drug works:**
2 to 3 weeks for full effect.

**Don't take with:**
See Interaction column and consult doctor.

 **OVERDOSE**

**SYMPTOMS:**
Headache, vomiting blood, stupor, seizure.
**WHAT TO DO:**
- Dial 0 (operator) or 911 (emergency) for an ambulance or medical help. Then give first aid immediately.
- If patient is unconscious and not breathing, give mouth-to-mouth breathing. If there is no heartbeat, use cardiac massage and mouth-to-mouth breathing (CPR). Don't try to make patient vomit. If you can't get help quickly, take patient to nearest emergency facility.
- See emergency information on inside covers.

 **POSSIBLE ADVERSE REACTIONS OR SIDE EFFECTS**

| SYMPTOMS | WHAT TO DO |
|---|---|
| **Life-threatening:** | |
| None expected. | |
| **Common:** | |
| • Darkened skin, appetite loss, nausea, vomiting. | Continue. Call doctor when convenient. |
| • Mental depression. | Continue. Tell doctor at next visit. |
| **Infrequent:** | |
| • Fever, chills, sore throat. | Discontinue. Seek emergency treatment. |
| • Unusual bleeding or bruising. | Discontinue. Call doctor right away. |
| • Rash, hair loss, purple bands on nails, blurred vision, seeing double, cough, difficult breathing, numbness or tingling in feet and toes, tiredness, weakness, dizziness when standing after sitting or lying. | Continue. Call doctor when convenient. |
| **Rare:** | |
| Blood in urine. | Continue. Call doctor when convenient. |

## WARNINGS & PRECAUTIONS

**Don't take if:**
You are allergic to adrenocorticosteroids or any antineoplastic drug.

**Before you start, consult your doctor:**
- If you have liver disease.
- If you have infection.

**Over age 60:**
Adverse reactions and side effects may be more frequent and severe than in younger persons.

**Pregnancy:**
Consult doctor. Risk to child is significant.

**Breast-feeding:**
Drug passes into milk. Don't nurse.

**Infants & children:**
Use only under care of medical supervisors who are experienced in anticancer drugs.

**Prolonged use:**
Adverse reactions more likely the longer drug is required.

**Skin & sunlight:**
No problems expected.

**Driving, piloting or hazardous work:**
No problems expected.

**Discontinuing:**
- Don't discontinue without consulting doctor. Dose may require gradual reduction if you have taken drug for a long time. Doses of other drugs may also require adjustment.
- Some side effects may follow discontinuing. Report any new symptoms.

**Others:**
No problems expected.

## POSSIBLE INTERACTION WITH OTHER DRUGS

| GENERIC NAME OR DRUG CLASS | COMBINED EFFECT |
|---|---|
| Antidepressants | Increased central nervous system depression. |
| Antihistamines | Increased central nervous system depression. |
| Corticosteroids | Decreased effect of corticosteroid. |
| Mind-altering drugs (LSD, etc.) | Increased central nervous system depression. |
| Narcotics | Increased central nervous system depression. |
| Sedatives | Increased central nervous system depression, |
| Sleeping pills | Increased central nervous system depression. |
| Tranquilizers | Increased central nervous system depression. |

## POSSIBLE INTERACTION WITH OTHER SUBSTANCES

| INTERACTS WITH | COMBINED EFFECT |
|---|---|
| Alcohol: | Increased depression. Avoid. |
| Beverages: | No problems expected. |
| Cocaine: | Increased toxicity. Avoid. |
| Foods: | Reduced irritation in stomach. |
| Marijuana: | No problems expected. |
| Tobacco: | Increased possibility of lung toxicity. |

# MOLINDONE

## BRAND NAMES

Moban

## BASIC INFORMATION

Habit forming? No
Prescription needed? Yes
Available as generic? No
Drug class: Antipsychotic

 **USES**

Treats severe emotional, mental or nervous problems.

 **DOSAGE & USAGE INFORMATION**

**How to take:**
Tablet or capsule—Swallow with liquid or food to lessen stomach irritation. If you can't swallow whole, crumble tablet and take with food or liquid.

**When to take:**
Follow instructions on prescription label or side of package. Doses should be evenly spaced. For example, 4 times a day means every 6 hours.

**If you forget a dose:**
Take as soon as you remember up to 2 hours late. If more than 2 hours, wait for next scheduled dose (don't double this dose).

**What drug does:**
Corrects an imbalance in nerve impulses from the brain.

**Time lapse before drug works:**
- Nausea and vomiting—1 hour or less.
- Nervous and mental disorders—4-6 weeks.

**Don't take with:**
- Antacid or medicine for diarrhea.
- Non-prescription drug for cough, cold or allergy.
- See Interaction column and consult doctor.

 **OVERDOSE**

**SYMPTOMS:**
Stupor, convulsions, coma.
**WHAT TO DO:**
- Dial 0 (operator) or 911 (emergency) for an ambulance or medical help. Then give first aid immediately.
- See emergency information on inside covers.

 **POSSIBLE ADVERSE REACTIONS OR SIDE EFFECTS**

| SYMPTOMS | WHAT TO DO |
|---|---|
| **Life-threatening:**<br>None expected. | |
| **Common:** | |
| • Muscle spasms of face and neck, unsteady gait. | Discontinue. Seek emergency treatment. |
| • Restlessness, tremor, drowsiness. | Discontinue. Call doctor right away. |
| • Decreased sweating, dry mouth, runny nose, constipation. | Continue. Call doctor when convenient. |
| **Infrequent:** | |
| • Fainting. | Discontinue. Seek emergency treatment. |
| • Rash. | Discontinue. Call doctor right away. |
| • Frequent urination, diminished sex drive, swollen breasts, menstrual irregularities. | Continue. Call doctor when convenient. |
| **Rare:** | |
| Change in vision, sore throat, fever, jaundice. | Discontinue. Call doctor right away. |

# MOLINDONE

## WARNINGS & PRECAUTIONS

**Don't take if:**
- You are allergic to any phenothiazine.
- You have a blood or bone-marrow disease.

**Before you start, consult your doctor:**
- If you will have surgery within 2 months, including dental surgery, requiring general or spinal anesthesia.
- If you have asthma, emphysema or other lung disorder.
- If you take non-prescription ulcer medicine, asthma medicine or amphetamines.

**Over age 60:**
Adverse reactions and side effects may be more frequent and severe than in younger persons. More likely to develop involuntary movement of jaws, lips, tongue, chewing. Report this to your doctor immediately. Early treatment can help.

**Pregnancy:**
Risk to unborn child outweighs drug benefits. Don't use.

**Breast-feeding:**
Drug passes into milk. Avoid drug or discontinue nursing until you finish medicine. Consult doctor for advice on maintaining milk supply.

**Infants & children:**
Don't give to children younger than 2.

**Prolonged use:**
May lead to tardive dyskinesia (involuntary movement of jaws, lips, tongue, chewing).

**Skin & sunlight:**
May cause rash or intensify sunburn in areas exposed to sun or sunlamp. Skin may remain sensitive for 3 months after discontinuing.

**Driving, piloting or hazardous work:**
Don't drive or pilot aircraft until you learn how medicine affects you. Don't work around dangerous machinery. Don't climb ladders or work in high places. Danger increases if you drink alcohol or take medicine affecting alertness and reflexes.

**Discontinuing:**
- Nervous and mental disorders—Don't discontinue without doctor's advice until you complete prescribed dose, even though symptoms diminish or disappear.
- Nausea and vomiting—May be unnecessary to finish medicine. Follow doctor's instructions.

**Others:**
No problems expected.

## POSSIBLE INTERACTION WITH OTHER DRUGS

| GENERIC NAME OR DRUG CLASS | COMBINED EFFECT |
|---|---|
| Anticholinergics | Increased anticholinergic effect. |
| Antidepressants (tricyclic) | Increased fluphenazine effect. |
| Antihistamines | Increased antihistamine effect. |
| Appetite suppressants | Decreased suppressant effect. |
| Dronabinol | Increased effects of both drugs. Avoid. |
| Levodopa | Decreased levodopa effect. |
| Mind-altering drugs | Increased effect of mind-altering drugs. |
| Narcotics | Increased narcotic effect. |
| Phenytoin | Increased phenytoin effect. |
| Quinidine | Impaired heart function. Dangerous mixture. |
| Sedatives | Increased sedative effect. |
| Tranquilizers (other) | Increased tranquilizer effect. |

## POSSIBLE INTERACTION WITH OTHER SUBSTANCES

| INTERACTS WITH | COMBINED EFFECT |
|---|---|
| Alcohol: | Dangerous oversedation. |
| Beverages: | None expected. |
| Cocaine: | Decreased fluphenazine effect. Avoid. |
| Foods: | None expected. |
| Marijuana: | Drowsiness. May increase antinausea effect. |
| Tobacco: | None expected. |

# MONAMINE OXIDASE (MAO) INHIBITORS

## BRAND AND GENERIC NAMES

Eutonyl
ISOCARBOXAZID
Marplan
Nardil
PARGYLINE
Parnate
PHENELZINE
TRANYLCYPROMINE

## BASIC INFORMATION

Habit forming? No
Prescription needed? Yes
Available as generic? No
Drug class: MAO (monamine oxidase)
    inhibitor, antidepressant

## USES

- Treatment for depression.
- Pargyline sometimes used to lower blood pressure.

## DOSAGE & USAGE INFORMATION

**How to take:**
Tablet—Swallow with liquid. If you can't swallow whole, crumble tablet and take with liquid or food.

**When to take:**
At the same times each day.

**If you forget a dose:**
Take as soon as you remember up to 2 hours late. If more than 2 hours, wait for next scheduled dose (don't double this dose).

**What drug does:**
Inhibits nerve transmissions in brain that may cause depression.

**Time lapse before drug works:**
4 to 6 weeks for maximum effect.

*Continued next column*

## OVERDOSE

**SYMPTOMS:**
Restlessness, agitation, fever, convulsions, coma.
**WHAT TO DO:**
- Dial 0 (operator) or 911 (emergency) for an ambulance or medical help. Then give first aid immediately.
- See emergency information on inside covers.

**Don't take with:**
- Non-prescription diet pills, nose drops, medicine for asthma, cough, cold or allergy, or medicine containing caffeine or alcohol.
- See Interaction column and consult doctor.

## POSSIBLE ADVERSE REACTIONS OR SIDE EFFECTS

| SYMPTOMS | WHAT TO DO |
|---|---|
| **Life-threatening:** None expected. | |
| **Common:** Fatigue, weakness. | Continue. Call doctor when convenient. |
| Dizziness when changing position, dry mouth, constipation, difficult urination. | Continue. Tell doctor at next visit. |
| **Infrequent:** Fainting. | Discontinue. Seek emergency treatment. |
| Severe headache, chest pain. | Discontinue. Call doctor right away. |
| Hallucinations, insomnia, nightmares, diarrhea, rapid or pounding heartbeat, swollen feet or legs. | Continue. Call doctor when convenient. |
| Diminished sex drive. | Continue. Tell doctor at next visit. |
| **Rare:** Rash, nausea, vomiting, stiff neck, jaundice, fever. | Discontinue. Call doctor right away. |

## WARNINGS & PRECAUTIONS

**Don't take if:**
- You are allergic to any MAO inhibitor.
- You have heart disease, congestive heart failure, heart-rhythm irregularities or high blood pressure.
- You have liver or kidney disease.

**Before you start, consult your doctor:**
- If you are alcoholic.
- If you have asthma.
- If you have had a stroke.
- If you have diabetes or epilepsy.
- If you have overactive thyroid.
- If you have schizophrenia.
- If you have Parkinson's disease.
- If you have adrenal-gland tumor.
- If you will have surgery within 2 months, including dental surgery, requiring general or spinal anesthesia.

**Over age 60:**
Not recommended.

**Pregnancy:**
No proven harm to unborn child. Avoid if possible.

**Breast-feeding:**
Safety not established. Consult doctor.

**Infants & children:**
Not recommended.

**Prolonged use:**
May be toxic to liver.

**Skin & sunlight:**
May cause rash or intensify sunburn in areas exposed to sun or sunlamp.

**Driving, piloting or hazardous work:**
Don't drive or pilot aircraft until you learn how medicine affects you. Don't work around dangerous machinery. Don't climb ladders or work in high places. Danger increases if you drink alcohol or take medicine affecting alertness and reflexes.

**Discontinuing:**
- Don't discontinue without doctor's advice until you complete prescribed dose, even though symptoms diminish or disappear.
- Follow precautions regarding foods, drinks and other medicines for 2 weeks after discontinuing.

**Others:**
- May affect blood-sugar levels in patients with diabetes.
- Fever may indicate that MAO inhibitor dose requires adjustment.

## POSSIBLE INTERACTION WITH OTHER DRUGS

| GENERIC NAME OR DRUG CLASS | COMBINED EFFECT |
|---|---|
| Acebutolol | Possible blood-pressure rise if MAO inhibitor is discontinued after simultaneous use with acebutolol. |
| Amphetamines | Blood-pressure rise to life-threatening level. |
| Anticholinergics | Increased anticholinergic effect. |
| Anticonvulsants | Changed seizure pattern. |
| Antidepressants (tricyclic) | Blood-pressure rise to life-threatening level. Possible fever, convulsions, delirium. |

| Antidiabetics (oral and insulin) | Excessively low blood sugar. |
|---|---|
| Antihypertensives | Excessively low blood pressure. |
| Caffeine | Irregular heartbeat or high blood pressure. |
| Carbamazepine | Fever, seizures. Avoid. |
| Cyclobenzaprine | Fever, seizures. Avoid. |
| Diuretics | Excessively low blood pressure. |
| Guanethidine | Blood-pressure rise to life-threatening level. |
| Indapamide | Increased indapamide effect. |
| Levodopa | Sudden, severe blood-pressure rise. |
| MAO inhibitors (others, when taken together) | High fever, convulsions, death. |
| Oxprenolol | Possible blood-pressure rise if MAO inhibitor is discontinued after simultaneous use with oxprenolol. |
| Terfenadine | Increased side effects of MAO inhibitors. |

## POSSIBLE INTERACTION WITH OTHER SUBSTANCES

| INTERACTS WITH | COMBINED EFFECT |
|---|---|
| Alcohol: | Increased sedation to dangerous level. |
| Beverages: Caffeine drinks. | Irregular heartbeat or high blood pressure. |
| Drinks containing tyramine (see Glossary). | Blood-pressure rise to life-threatening level. |
| Cocaine: | Overstimulation. Possibly fatal. |
| Foods: Foods containing tyramine (see Glossary). | Blood-pressure rise to life-threatening level. |
| Marijuana: | Overstimulation. Avoid. |
| Tobacco: | No proven problems. |

# NADOLOL

## BRAND NAMES

Corgard                    Corzide

## BASIC INFORMATION

**Habit forming?** No
**Prescription needed?** Yes
**Available as generic?** No
**Drug class:** Beta-adrenergic blocker

## USES

- Reduces angina attacks.
- Stabilizes irregular heartbeat.
- Lowers blood pressure.
- Reduces frequency of migraine headaches. (Does not relieve headache pain.)
- Other uses prescribed by your doctor.

## DOSAGE & USAGE INFORMATION

**How to take:**
Tablet or capsule—Swallow with liquid. If you can't swallow whole, crumble tablet or open capsule and take with liquid or food.

**When to take:**
With meals or immediately after.

**If you forget a dose:**
Take as soon as you remember. Return to regular schedule, but allow 3 hours between doses.

**What drug does:**
- Blocks certain actions of sympathetic nervous system.
- Lowers heart's oxygen requirements.
- Slows nerve impulses through heart.
- Reduces blood vessel contraction in heart, scalp and other body parts.

**Time lapse before drug works:**
1 to 4 hours.

*Continued next column*

## OVERDOSE

**SYMPTOMS:**
**Weakness, slow or weak pulse, blood-pressure drop, fainting, convulsions, cold and sweaty skin.**
**WHAT TO DO:**
- **Dial 0 (operator) or 911 (emergency) for an ambulance or medical help. Then give first aid immediately.**
- **See emergency information on inside covers.**

**Don't take with:**
Non-prescription drugs or drugs in Interaction column without consulting doctor.

## POSSIBLE ADVERSE REACTIONS OR SIDE EFFECTS

| SYMPTOMS | WHAT TO DO |
|---|---|
| **Life-threatening:** | |
| None expected. | |
| **Common:** | |
| • Pulse lower than 50 beats per minute. | Discontinue. Call doctor right away. |
| • Drowsiness, numbness or tingling in fingers or toes, dizziness, nausea, diarrhea, fatigue, weakness. | Continue. Call doctor when convenient. |
| • Cold hands, feet; dry mouth, eyes, skin. | Continue. Tell doctor at next visit. |
| **Infrequent:** | |
| • Hallucinations, nightmares, insomnia, headache, difficult breathing, joint pain. | Discontinue. Call doctor right away. |
| • Confusion, depression, reduced alertness. | Continue. Call doctor when convenient. |
| • Constipation. | Continue. Tell doctor at next visit. |
| **Rare:** | |
| • Rash, sore throat, fever. | Discontinue. Call doctor right away. |
| • Unusual bleeding or bruising. | Continue. Call doctor when convenient. |

## WARNINGS & PRECAUTIONS

**Don't take if:**
- You are allergic to any beta-adrenergic blocker.
- You have asthma.
- You have hay fever symptoms.
- You have taken MAO inhibitors in past 2 weeks.

**Before you start, consult your doctor:**
- If you have heart disease or poor circulation to the extremities.
- If you have hay fever, asthma, chronic bronchitis, emphysema.
- If you have overactive thyroid function.
- If you have impaired liver or kidney function.
- If you will have surgery within 2 months, including dental surgery, requiring general or spinal anesthesia.
- If you have diabetes or hypoglycemia.

**Over age 60:**
Adverse reactions and side effects may be more frequent and severe than in younger persons.

**Pregnancy:**
Risk to unborn child outweighs drug benefits. Don't use.

**Breast-feeding:**
Drug passes into milk. Avoid drug or discontinue nursing until you finish medicine. Consult doctor for advice on maintaining milk supply.

**Infants & children:**
Not recommended.

**Prolonged use:**
Weakens heart muscle contractions.

**Skin & sunlight:**
No problems expected.

**Driving, piloting or hazardous work:**
Don't drive or pilot aircraft until you learn how medicine affects you. Don't work around dangerous machinery. Don't climb ladders or work in high places. Danger increases if you drink alcohol or take medicine affecting alertness and reflexes.

**Discontinuing:**
Don't discontinue without consulting doctor. Dose may require gradual reduction if you have taken drug for a long time. Doses of other drugs may also require adjustment.

**Others:**
May mask hypoglycemia.

## POSSIBLE INTERACTION WITH OTHER DRUGS

| GENERIC NAME OR DRUG CLASS | COMBINED EFFECT |
| --- | --- |
| Acebutolol | Increased antihypertensive effects of both drugs. Dosages may require adjustment. |
| Albuterol | Decreased albuterol effect and beta-adrenergic blocking effect |
| Antidiabetics | Increased antidiabetic effect. |
| Antihistamines | Decreased antihistamine effect. |
| Antihypertensives | Increased antihypertensive effect. |
| Anti-inflammatory drugs | Decreased effect of anti-inflammatory. |

| | |
| --- | --- |
| Barbiturates | Increased barbiturate effect. Dangerous sedation. |
| Digitalis preparations | Increased or decreased heart rate. Improves irregular heartbeat. |
| Narcotics | Increased narcotic effect. Dangerous sedation. |
| Nitrates | Possible excessive blood-pressure drop. |
| Pentoxifylline | Increased antihypertensive effect. |
| Phenytoin | Increased nadolol effect. |
| Quinidine | Slows heart excessively. |
| Reserpine | Increased reserpine effect. Oversedation, depression. |
| Tocainide | May worsen congestive heart failure. |

## POSSIBLE INTERACTION WITH OTHER SUBSTANCES

| INTERACTS WITH | COMBINED EFFECT |
| --- | --- |
| Alcohol: | Excessive blood-pressure drop. Avoid. |
| Beverages: | None expected. |
| Cocaine: | Irregular heartbeat. Avoid. |
| Foods: | None expected. |
| Marijuana: | Daily use—Impaired circulation to hands and feet. |
| Tobacco: | Possible irregular heartbeat. |

# NAFCILLIN

## BRAND NAMES

Nafcil
Nallpen
Unipen

## BASIC INFORMATION

**Habit forming? No**
**Prescription needed? Yes**
**Available as generic? Yes**
**Drug class: Antibiotic (penicillin)**

## USES

Treatment of bacterial infections that are susceptible to nafcillin.

## DOSAGE & USAGE INFORMATION

**How to take:**
- Tablets or capsules—Swallow with liquid on an empty stomach 1 hour before or 2 hours after eating.
- Liquid—Take with cold beverage. Liquid form is perishable and effective for only 7 days at room temperature. Effective for 14 days if stored in refrigerator. Don't freeze.

**When to take:**
Follow instructions on prescription label or side of package. Doses should be evenly spaced. For example, 4 times a day means every 6 hours.

**If you forget a dose:**
Take as soon as you remember. Continue regular schedule.

**What drug does:**
Destroys susceptible bacteria. Does not kill viruses.

**Time lapse before drug works:**
May be several days before medicine affects infection.

**Don't take with:**
See Interaction column and consult doctor.

## OVERDOSE

**SYMPTOMS:**
Severe diarrhea, nausea or vomiting.
**WHAT TO DO:**
Overdose unlikely to threaten life. If person takes much larger amount than prescribed, call doctor, poison-control center or hospital emergency room for instructions.

## POSSIBLE ADVERSE REACTIONS OR SIDE EFFECTS

| SYMPTOMS | WHAT TO DO |
|---|---|
| **Life-threatening:**<br>Hives, rash, intense itching, faintness soon after a dose (anaphylaxis). | Seek emergency treatment immediately. |
| **Common:**<br>Dark or discolored tongue. | Continue. Tell doctor at next visit. |
| **Infrequent:**<br>Mild nausea, vomiting, diarrhea. | Continue. Call doctor when convenient. |
| **Rare:**<br>Unexplained bleeding. | Discontinue. Call doctor right away. |

## WARNINGS & PRECAUTIONS

**Don't take if:**
You are allergic to nafcillin, cephalosporin antibiotics, other penicillins or penicillamine. Life-threatening reaction may occur.

**Before you start, consult your doctor:**
If you are allergic to any substance or drug.

**Over age 60:**
You may have skin reactions, particularly around genitals and anus.

**Pregnancy:**
Studies inconclusive on harm to unborn child. Animal studies show fetal abnormalities. Decide with your doctor whether drug benefits justify risk to unborn child.

**Breast-feeding:**
Drug passes into milk. Child may become sensitive to penicillins and have allergic reactions to penicillin drugs. Avoid nafcillin or discontinue nursing until you finish medicine. Consult doctor for advice on maintaining milk supply.

**Infants & children:**
No problems expected.

**Prolonged use:**
You may become more susceptible to infections caused by germs not responsive to nafcillin.

**Skin & sunlight:**
No problems expected.

**Driving, piloting or hazardous work:**
Usually not dangerous. Most hazardous reactions likely to occur a few minutes after taking nafcillin.

**Discontinuing:**
Don't discontinue without doctor's advice until you complete prescribed dose, even though symptoms diminish or disappear.

**Others:**
Absorption of this drug in oral form is unpredictable. Injections are more reliable.

## POSSIBLE INTERACTION WITH OTHER DRUGS

| GENERIC NAME OR DRUG CLASS | COMBINED EFFECT |
|---|---|
| Beta-adrenergic blockers | Increased chance of anaphylaxis (see emergency information on inside front cover). |
| Chloramphenicol | Decreased effect of both drugs. |
| Erythromycins | Decreased effect of both drugs. |
| Loperamide | Decreased nafcillin effect. |
| Paromomycin | Decreased effect of both drugs. |
| Tetracyclines | Decreased effect of both drugs. |
| Troleandomycin | Decreased effect of both drugs. |

## POSSIBLE INTERACTION WITH OTHER SUBSTANCES

| INTERACTS WITH | COMBINED EFFECT |
|---|---|
| Alcohol: | Occasional stomach irritation. |
| Beverages: | None expected. |
| Cocaine: | No proven problems. |
| Foods: | None expected. |
| Marijuana: | No proven problems. |
| Tobacco: | None expected. |

# NALIDIXIC ACID

## BRAND NAMES

NegGram

## BASIC INFORMATION

Habit forming? No
Prescription needed? Yes
Available as generic? No
Drug class: Antimicrobial

## USES

Treatment for urinary-tract infections.

## DOSAGE & USAGE INFORMATION

**How to take:**
- Tablet—Swallow with food or milk to lessen stomach irritation. If you can't swallow whole, crumble tablet and take with liquid or food.
- Liquid—Take with liquid or food.

**When to take:**
At the same times each day.

**If you forget a dose:**
Take as soon as you remember up to 2 hours late. If more than 2 hours, wait for next scheduled dose (don't double this dose).

**What drug does:**
Destroys bacteria susceptible to nalidixic acid.

**Time lapse before drug works:**
1 to 2 weeks.

**Don't take with:**
See Interaction column and consult doctor.

## OVERDOSE

**SYMPTOMS:**
Lethargy, stomach upset, behavioral changes, convulsions and stupor.
**WHAT TO DO:**
- Dial 0 (operator) or 911 (emergency) for an ambulance or medical help. Then give first aid immediately.
- If patient is unconscious and not breathing, give mouth-to-mouth breathing. If there is no heartbeat, use cardiac massage and mouth-to-mouth breathing (CPR). Don't try to make patient vomit. If you can't get help quickly, take patient to nearest emergency facility.
- See emergency information on inside covers.

## POSSIBLE ADVERSE REACTIONS OR SIDE EFFECTS

| SYMPTOMS | WHAT TO DO |
|---|---|
| **Life-threatening:**<br>None expected. | |
| **Common:**<br>Rash; itchy skin; decreased, blurred or double vision; halos around lights or excess brightness; changes in color vision; nausea; vomiting; diarrhea. | Discontinue. Call doctor right away. |
| **Infrequent:**<br>Dizziness, drowsiness. | Continue. Call doctor when convenient. |
| **Rare:**<br>Paleness, sore throat or fever, severe stomach pain, pale stool, unusual bleeding or bruising, jaundice, fatigue, weakness. | Discontinue. Call doctor right away. |

## WARNINGS & PRECAUTIONS

**Don't take if:**
- You are allergic to nalidixic acid.
- You have a seizure disorder (epilepsy, convulsions).

**Before you start, consult your doctor:**
- If you plan to become pregnant within medication period.
- If you have or have had kidney or liver disease.
- If you have impaired circulation of the brain (hardened arteries).
- If you have Parkinson's disease.
- If you have diabetes (it may affect urine-sugar tests).

**Over age 60:**
Adverse reactions and side effects may be more frequent and severe than in younger persons.

**Pregnancy:**
Risk to unborn child outweighs drug benefits. Don't use, especially during first 3 months.

**Breast-feeding:**
No problems expected, unless you have impaired kidney function. Consult doctor.

**Infants & children:**
Don't give to infants younger than 3 months.

**Prolonged use:**
No problems expected.

**Skin & sunlight:**
May cause rash or intensify sunburn in areas exposed to sun or sunlamp.

**Driving, piloting or hazardous work:**
Avoid if you feel drowsy, dizzy or have vision problems. Otherwise, no problems expected.

**Discontinuing:**
Don't discontinue without consulting doctor. Dose may require gradual reduction if you have taken drug for a long time. Doses of other drugs may also require adjustment.

**Others:**
Periodic blood counts and liver- and kidney-function tests recommended.

## POSSIBLE INTERACTION WITH OTHER DRUGS

| GENERIC NAME OR DRUG CLASS | COMBINED EFFECT |
|---|---|
| Antacids | Decreased absorption of nalidixic acid. |
| Anticoagulants (oral) | Increased anticoagulant effect. |
| Calcium supplements | Decreased effect of nalidixic acid. |
| Nitrofurantoin | Decreased effect of nalidixic acid. |
| Probenecid | Decreased effect of nalidixic acid. |
| Vitamin C (in large doses) | Increased effect of nalidixic acid. |

## POSSIBLE INTERACTION WITH OTHER SUBSTANCES

| INTERACTS WITH | COMBINED EFFECT |
|---|---|
| Alcohol: | Impaired alertness, judgment and coordination. |
| Beverages: | None expected. |
| Cocaine: | Impaired judgment and coordination. |
| Foods: | None expected. |
| Marijuana: | Impaired alertness, judgment and coordination. |
| Tobacco: | None expected. |

# NAPROXEN

## BRAND NAMES

| | |
|---|---|
| Anaprox | Naxen |
| Apo-Naproxen | Novonaprox |
| Naprosyn | Synflex |

## BASIC INFORMATION

**Habit forming? No**
**Prescription needed? Yes**
**Available as generic? No**
**Drug class: Anti-inflammatory (non-steroid)**

## USES

- Treatment for joint pain, stiffness, inflammation and swelling of arthritis and gout.
- Pain reliever.
- Treatment for dysmenorrhea (painful or difficult menstruation).

## DOSAGE & USAGE INFORMATION

**How to take:**
Tablet—Swallow with liquid or food to lessen stomach irritation. If you can't swallow whole, crumble tablet and take with liquid or food.

**When to take:**
At the same times each day.

**If you forget a dose:**
Take as soon as you remember up to 2 hours late. If more than 2 hours, wait for next scheduled dose (don't double this dose).

**What drug does:**
Reduces tissue concentration of prostaglandins (hormones which produce inflammation and pain).

**Time lapse before drug works:**
Begins in 4 to 24 hours. May require 3 weeks regular use for maximum benefit.

*Continued next column*

## OVERDOSE

**SYMPTOMS:**
Confusion, agitation, incoherence, convulsions, possible hemorrhage from stomach or intestine, coma.
**WHAT TO DO:**
- Dial 0 (operator) or 911 (emergency) for an ambulance or medical help. Then give first aid immediately.
- See emergency information on inside covers.

**Don't take with:**
See Interaction column and consult doctor.

## POSSIBLE ADVERSE REACTIONS OR SIDE EFFECTS

| SYMPTOMS | WHAT TO DO |
|---|---|
| **Life-threatening:** | |
| None expected. | |
| **Common:** | |
| • Dizziness, nausea, pain. | Continue. Call doctor when convenient. |
| • Headache. | Continue. Tell doctor at next visit. |
| **Infrequent:** | |
| Depression, drowsiness, ringing in ears, constipation or diarrhea, vomiting, swollen feet or legs. | Continue. Call doctor when convenient. |
| **Rare:** | |
| • Convulsions; confusion; rash, hives or itchy skin; blurred vision; black, bloody or tarry stool; difficult breathing; tightness in chest; rapid heartbeat; unusual bleeding or bruising; blood in urine; jaundice. | Discontinue. Call doctor right away. |
| • Urgent, frequent, painful or difficult urination; fatigue; weakness. | Continue. Call doctor when convenient. |

## WARNINGS & PRECAUTIONS

### Don't take if:
- You are allergic to aspirin or any non-steroid, anti-inflammatory drug.
- You have gastritis, peptic ulcer, enteritis, ileitis, ulcerative colitis, asthma, heart failure, high blood pressure or bleeding problems.
- You have had recent rectal bleeding and suppository form has been prescribed.
- Patient is younger than 15.

### Before you start, consult your doctor:
- If you have epilepsy.
- If you have Parkinson's disease.
- If you have been mentally ill.
- If you have had kidney disease or impaired kidney function.

### Over age 60:
Adverse reactions and side effects may be more frequent and severe than in younger persons.

### Pregnancy:
Studies inconclusive on harm to unborn child. Decide with your doctor whether drug benefits justify risk to unborn child.

### Breast-feeding:
May harm child. Avoid.

### Infants & children:
Not recommended for anyone younger than 15. Use only under medical supervision.

### Prolonged use:
- Eye damage.
- Reduced hearing.
- Sore throat, fever.
- Weight gain.

### Skin & sunlight:
No problems expected.

### Driving, piloting or hazardous work:
Don't drive or pilot aircraft until you learn how medicine affects you. Don't work around dangerous machinery. Don't climb ladders or work in high places. Danger increases if you drink alcohol or take medicine affecting alertness and reflexes, such as antihistamines, tranquilizers, sedatives, pain medicine, narcotics and mind-altering drugs.

### Discontinuing:
Don't discontinue without consulting doctor. Dose may require gradual reduction if you have taken drug for a long time. Doses of other drugs may also require adjustment.

### Others:
No problems expected.

## POSSIBLE INTERACTION WITH OTHER DRUGS

| GENERIC NAME OR DRUG CLASS | COMBINED EFFECT |
|---|---|
| Acebutolol | Decreased antihypertensive effect of acebutolol. |
| Anticoagulants, (oral) | Increased risk of bleeding. |
| Aspirin | Increased risk of stomach ulcer. |
| Cortisone drugs | Increased risk of stomach ulcer. |
| Furosemide | Decreased diuretic effect of furosemide. |
| Gold compounds | Possible increased likelihood of kidney damage. |
| Ketoprofen | Increased possibility of internal bleeding. |
| Minoxidil | Decreased minoxidil effect. |
| Oxprenolol | Decreased antihypertensive effect of oxprenolol. |
| Oxyphenbutazone | Possible stomach ulcer. |
| Phenylbutazone | Possible stomach ulcer. |
| Probenecid | Increased naproxen effect. |
| Thyroid hormones | Rapid heartbeat, blood-pressure rise. |

## POSSIBLE INTERACTION WITH OTHER SUBSTANCES

| INTERACTS WITH | COMBINED EFFECT |
|---|---|
| Alcohol: | Possible stomach ulcer or bleeding. |
| Beverages: | None expected. |
| Cocaine: | None expected. |
| Foods: | None expected. |
| Marijuana: | Increased pain relief from naproxen. |
| Tobacco: | None expected. |

# NARCOTIC & ACETAMINOPHEN

## BRAND NAMES

See complete list of brand names in the *Brand Name Directory,* page 951.

## BASIC INFORMATION

**Habit forming? Yes**
**Prescription needed? Yes**
**Available as generic? Yes**
**Drug class: Narcotic, analgesic, fever-reducer**

## USES

- Relieves pain.
- Suppresses cough.

## DOSAGE & USAGE INFORMATION

**How to take:**
- Tablet or capsule—Swallow with liquid. If you can't swallow whole, crumble tablet or open capsule and take with liquid or food.
- Drops or liquid—Dilute dose in beverage before swallowing.

**When to take:**
When needed. No more often than every 4 hours.

**If you forget a dose:**
Take as soon as you remember. Wait 4 hours for next dose.

*Continued next column*

## OVERDOSE

**SYMPTOMS:**
**Stomach upset; irritability; convulsions; deep sleep; slow breathing; slow pulse; flushed, warm skin; constricted pupils; coma.**
**WHAT TO DO:**
- **Dial 0 (operator) or 911 (emergency) for an ambulance or medical help. Then give first aid immediately.**
- **If patient is unconscious and not breathing, give mouth-to-mouth breathing. If there is no heartbeat, use cardiac massage and mouth-to-mouth breathing (CPR). Don't try to make patient vomit. If you can't get help quickly, take patient to nearest emergency facility.**
- **See emergency information on inside covers.**

**What drug does:**
- May affect hypothalamus—the part of the brain that helps regulate body heat and receives body's pain messages.
- Blocks pain messages to brain and spinal cord.
- Reduces sensitivity of brain's cough-control center.

**Time lapse before drug works:**
15 to 30 minutes. May last 4 hours.

**Don't take with:**
- Other drugs with acetaminophen. Too much acetaminophen can damage liver and kidneys.
- See Interaction column and consult doctor.

## POSSIBLE ADVERSE REACTIONS OR SIDE EFFECTS

| SYMPTOMS | WHAT TO DO |
|---|---|
| **Life-threatening:** | |
| Irregular or slow heartbeat, difficult breathing. | Discontinue. Seek emergency treatment. |
| **Common:** | |
| Dizziness, agitation, tiredness. | Continue. Call doctor when convenient. |
| **Infrequent:** | |
| Abdominal pain, constipation, vomiting. | Discontinue. Call doctor right away. |
| **Rare:** | |
| • Fatigue; itchy skin; rash; sore throat, fever, mouth sores; bruising and bleeding increased; painful or difficult urination; blood in urine; anemia; blurred vision. | Discontinue. Call doctor right away. |
| • Depression. | Continue. Call doctor when convenient. |

## WARNINGS & PRECAUTIONS

**Don't take if:**
- You are allergic to any narcotic or acetaminophen.
- Your symptoms don't improve after 2 days use. Call your doctor.

**Before you start, consult your doctor:**
- If you have bronchial asthma, kidney disease or liver damage.
- If you will have surgery within 2 months, including dental surgery, requiring general or spinal anesthesia.

**Over age 60:**
More likely to be drowsy, dizzy, unsteady or constipated. Don't exceed recommended dose. You can't eliminate drug as efficiently as younger persons. Use only if absolutely necessary.

**Pregnancy:**
Decide with your doctor whether drug benefits justify risk to unborn child. Abuse by pregnant woman will result in addicted newborn. Withdrawal of newborn can be life-threatening.

**Breast-feeding:**
Drug filters into milk. May harm child. Avoid.

**Infants & children:**
Not recommended.

**Prolonged use:**
- Causes psychological and physical dependence (addiction).
- May affect blood stream and cause anemia. Limit use to 5 days for children 12 and under, and 10 days for adults.

**Skin & sunlight:**
May cause rash or intensify sunburn in areas exposed to sun or sunlamp.

**Driving, piloting or hazardous work:**
Don't drive or pilot aircraft until you learn how medicine affects you. Don't work around dangerous machinery. Don't climb ladders or work in high places. Danger increases if you drink alcohol or take medicine affecting alertness and reflexes, such as antihistamines, tranquilizers, sedatives, pain medicine, narcotics and mind-altering drugs.

**Discontinuing:**
Discontinue in 2 days if symptoms don't improve.

**Others:**
No problems expected.

## POSSIBLE INTERACTION WITH OTHER DRUGS

| GENERIC NAME OR DRUG CLASS | COMBINED EFFECT |
|---|---|
| Analgesics (other) | Increased analgesic effect. |
| Anticoagulants (other) | May increase anticoagulant effect. Prothrombin times should be monitored. |
| Anticholinergics | Increased anticholinergic effect. |
| Antidepressants | Increased sedative effect. |
| Antihistamines | Increased sedative effect. |
| Mind-altering drugs | Increased sedative effect. |
| Narcotics (other) | Increased narcotic effect. |
| Nitrates | Excessive blood-pressure drop. |
| Phenobarbital and other barbiturates | Quicker elimination and decreased effect of acetaminophen. |
| Phenothiazines | Increased phenothiazine effect. |
| Sedatives | Increased sedative effect. |
| Sleep inducers | Increased sedative effect. |
| Terfenadine | Possible oversedation. |
| Tetracyclines | May slow tetracycline absorption. Space doses 2 hours apart. |
| Tranquilizers | Increased sedative effect. |

## POSSIBLE INTERACTION WITH OTHER SUBSTANCES

| INTERACTS WITH | COMBINED EFFECT |
|---|---|
| Alcohol: | Increases alcohol's intoxicating effect. Avoid. |
| Beverages: | None expected. |
| Cocaine: | Increased cocaine toxic effects. Avoid. |
| Foods: | None expected. |
| Marijuana: | Impairs physical and mental performance. Avoid. |
| Tobacco: | None expected. |

## BRAND AND GENERIC NAMES

See complete list of brand names in the *Brand Name Directory,* page 952.

## BASIC INFORMATION

**Habit forming? Yes**
**Prescription needed? Yes**
**Available as generic? Yes**
**Drug class: Narcotic**

## USES

- Relieves pain.
- Suppresses cough.

## DOSAGE & USAGE INFORMATION

**How to take:**
- Tablet or capsule—Swallow with liquid. If you can't swallow whole, crumble tablet or open capsule and take with liquid or food.
- Drops or liquid—Dilute dose in beverage before swallowing.

**When to take:**
When needed. No more often than every 4 hours.

**If you forget a dose:**
Take as soon as you remember. Wait 4 hours for next dose.

**What drug does:**
- Blocks pain messages to brain and spinal cord.
- Reduces sensitivity of brain's cough-control center.

*Continued next column*

## OVERDOSE

**SYMPTOMS:**
**Deep sleep, slow breathing; slow pulse; flushed, warm skin; constricted pupils.**
**WHAT TO DO:**
- **Dial 0 (operator) or 911 (emergency) for an ambulance or medical help. Then give first aid immediately.**
- **If patient is unconscious and not breathing, give mouth-to-mouth breathing. If there is no heartbeat, use cardiac massage and mouth-to-mouth breathing (CPR). Don't try to make patient vomit. If you can't get help quickly, take patient to nearest emergency facility.**
- **See emergency information on inside covers.**

**Time lapse before drug works:**
30 minutes.

**Don't take with:**
See Interaction column and consult doctor.

## POSSIBLE ADVERSE REACTIONS OR SIDE EFFECTS

| SYMPTOMS | WHAT TO DO |
|---|---|
| **Life-threatening:** None expected. | |
| **Common:** Dizziness, flushed face, difficult urination, unusual tiredness. | Continue. Call doctor when convenient. |
| **Infrequent:** Severe constipation, abdominal pain, vomiting. | Discontinue. Call doctor right away. |
| **Rare:** <br>• Hives, rash, itchy skin, face swelling, slow heartbeat, irregular breathing. | Discontinue. Call doctor right away. |
| • Depression, blurred vision. | Continue. Call doctor when convenient. |

# NARCOTIC ANALGESICS

## WARNINGS & PRECAUTIONS

**Don't take if:**
You are allergic to any narcotic.

**Before you start, consult your doctor:**
- If you have impaired liver or kidney function.
- If you will have surgery within 2 months, including dental surgery, requiring general or spinal anesthesia.

**Over age 60:**
More likely to be drowsy, dizzy, unsteady or constipated. Use only if absolutely necessary.

**Pregnancy:**
Decide with your doctor whether drug benefits justify risk to unborn child. Abuse by pregnant woman will result in addicted newborn. Withdrawal of newborn can be life-threatening.

**Breast-feeding:**
Drug filters into milk. May harm child. Avoid.

**Infants & children:**
Not recommended.

**Prolonged use:**
Causes psychological and physical dependence (addiction).

**Skin & sunlight:**
May cause rash or intensify sunburn in areas exposed to sun or sunlamp.

**Driving, piloting or hazardous work:**
Don't drive or pilot aircraft until you learn how medicine affects you. Don't work around dangerous machinery. Don't climb ladders or work in high places. Danger increases if you drink alcohol or take medicine affecting alertness and reflexes, such as antihistamines, tranquilizers, sedatives, pain medicine, narcotics and mind-altering drugs.

**Discontinuing:**
May be unnecessary to finish medicine. Follow doctor's instructions.

**Others:**
No problems expected.

## POSSIBLE INTERACTION WITH OTHER DRUGS

| GENERIC NAME OR DRUG CLASS | COMBINED EFFECT |
|---|---|
| Analgesics (other) | Increased analgesic effect. |
| Anticholinergics | Increased anticholinergic effect. |
| Antidepressants | Increased sedative effect. |
| Antihistamines | Increased sedative effect. |
| Mind-altering drugs | Increased sedative effect. |
| Molindone | Increased narcotic effect. |
| Narcotics (other) | Increased narcotic effect. |
| Nitrates | Excessive blood-pressure drop. |
| Phenothiazines | Increased phenothiazine effect. |
| Sedatives | Increased sedative effect. |
| Sleep inducers | Increased sedative effect. |
| Terfenadine | Possible oversedation. |
| Tranquilizers | Increased sedative effect. |

## POSSIBLE INTERACTION WITH OTHER SUBSTANCES

| INTERACTS WITH | COMBINED EFFECT |
|---|---|
| Alcohol: | Increases alcohol's intoxicating effect. Avoid. |
| Beverages: | None expected. |
| Cocaine: | Increased cocaine toxic effects. Avoid. |
| Foods: | None expected. |
| Marijuana: | Impairs physical and mental performance. Avoid. |
| Tobacco: | None expected. |

## BRAND NAMES

See complete list of brand names in the *Brand Name Directory,* page 952.

## BASIC INFORMATION

**Habit forming? Yes**
**Prescription needed? Yes**
**Available as generic? Yes**
**Drug class: Narcotic, analgesic,**
           **anti-inflammatory**

 ## USES

- Reduces pain, fever, inflammation.
- Suppresses cough.

 ## DOSAGE & USAGE INFORMATION

**How to take:**
Tablet or capsule—Swallow with liquid. If you can't swallow whole, crumble tablet or open capsule and take with liquid or food.

**When to take:**
When needed. No more often than every 4 hours.

**If you forget a dose:**
Take as soon as you remember. Wait 4 hours for next dose.

**What drug does:**
- Affects hypothalamus, the part of the brain which regulates temperature by dilating small blood vessels in skin.

*Continued next column*

 ## OVERDOSE

**SYMPTOMS:**
**Ringing in ears; nausea; vomiting; dizziness; fever; deep sleep; slow breathing; slow pulse; flushed, warm skin; constricted pupils; hallucinations; convulsions; coma.**
**WHAT TO DO:**
- **Dial 0 (operator) or 911 (emergency) for an ambulance or medical help. Then give first aid immediately.**
- **If patient is unconscious and not breathing, give mouth-to-mouth breathing. If there is no heartbeat, use cardiac massage and mouth-to-mouth breathing (CPR). Don't try to make patient vomit. If you can't get help quickly, take patient to nearest emergency facility.**
- **See emergency information on inside covers.**

- Prevents clumping of platelets (small blood cells) so blood vessels remain open.
- Decreases prostaglandin effect.
- Suppresses body's pain messages.
- Reduces sensitivity of brain's cough-control center.

**Time lapse before drug works:**
30 minutes.

**Don't take with:**
- Tetracyclines. Space doses 1 hour apart.
- See Interaction column and consult doctor.

 ## POSSIBLE ADVERSE REACTIONS OR SIDE EFFECTS

| SYMPTOMS | WHAT TO DO |
|---|---|
| **Life-threatening:** | |
| • Hives, rash, intense itching, faintness soon after a dose (anaphylaxis). | Seek emergency treatment immediately. |
| • Clot or pain over blood vessel, cold hands, feet. | Discontinue. Seek emergency treatment. |
| **Common:** | |
| • Nausea, abdominal cramps or pain. | Discontinue. Call doctor right away. |
| • Dizziness, red or flushed face, frequent urination, unusual tiredness, ringing in ears, heartburn, indigestion. | Continue. Call doctor when convenient. |
| **Infrequent:** | |
| Constipation, abdominal pain or cramps, vomiting. | Discontinue. Call doctor right away. |
| **Rare:** | |
| • Slow heartbeat; change in vision; black, bloody or tarry stool; blood in urine; jaundice. | Discontinue. Call doctor right away. |
| • Depression, blurred vision. | Continue. Call doctor when convenient. |

 ## WARNINGS & PRECAUTIONS

**Don't take if:**
- You are allergic to any narcotic or subject to any substance abuse.
- You have a peptic ulcer of stomach or duodenum or a bleeding disorder.

**Before you start, consult your doctor:**
- If you have impaired liver or kidney function, asthma or nasal polyps.
- If you have had stomach or duodenal ulcers, gout.

- If you will have surgery within 2 months, including dental surgery, requiring general or spinal anesthesia.

### Over age 60:
- More likely to be drowsy, dizzy, unsteady or constipated. Use only if absolutely necessary.
- More likely to cause hidden bleeding in stomach or intestines. Watch for dark stools.

### Pregnancy:
Risk to unborn child outweighs drug benefits. Don't use.

### Breast-feeding:
Drug passes into milk and may harm child. Avoid drug or discontinue nursing until you finish medicine. Consult doctor for advice on maintaining milk supply.

### Infants & children:
Not recommended.

### Prolonged use:
- Causes psychological and physical dependence (addiction).
- Kidney damage. Periodic kidney-function test recommended.

### Skin & sunlight:
May cause rash or intensify sunburn in areas exposed to sun or sunlamp.

### Driving, piloting or hazardous work:
Don't drive or pilot aircraft until you learn how medicine affects you. Don't work around dangerous machinery. Don't climb ladders or work in high places. Danger increases if you drink alcohol or take medicine affecting alertness and reflexes, such as antihistamines, tranquilizers, sedatives, pain medicine, narcotics and mind-altering drugs.

### Discontinuing:
May be unnecessary to finish medicine. Follow doctor's instructions.

### Others:
- Aspirin can complicate surgery, pregnancy, labor and delivery, and illness.
- Urine tests for blood sugar may be inaccurate.

## POSSIBLE INTERACTION WITH OTHER DRUGS

| GENERIC NAME OR DRUG CLASS | COMBINED EFFECT |
|---|---|
| Acebutolol | Decreased antihypertensive effect of acebutolol. |
| Allopurinol | Decreased allopurinol effect. |
| Antacids | Decreased aspirin effect. |
| Anticoagulants | Increased anticoagulant effect. Abnormal bleeding. |
| Antidepressants | Increased sedative effect. |
| Antidiabetics (oral) | Low blood sugar. |
| Anti-inflammatory drugs (non-steroid) | Risk of stomach bleeding and ulcers. |
| Aspirin (other) | Likely aspirin toxicity. |
| Cortisone drugs | Increased cortisone effect. Risk of ulcers and stomach bleeding. |
| Furosemide | Possible aspirin toxicity. |
| Gold compounds | Increased likelihood of kidney damage. |
| Indomethacin | Risk of stomach bleeding and ulcers. |
| Methotrexate | Increased methotrexate effect. |
| Minoxidil | Decreased minoxidil effect. |
| Narcotics (other) | Increased narcotic effect. |
| Nitrates | Excessive blood-pressure drop. |
| Oxprenolol | Decreased antihypertensive effect of oxprenolol. |
| Para-aminosalicylic acid (PAS) | Possible aspirin toxicity. |
| Penicillins | Increased effect of both drugs. |

*Continued page 969*

## POSSIBLE INTERACTION WITH OTHER SUBSTANCES

| INTERACTS WITH | COMBINED EFFECT |
|---|---|
| Alcohol: | Possible stomach irritation and bleeding. Increases alcohol's intoxicating effect. Avoid. |
| Beverages: | None expected. |
| Cocaine: | Decreased cocaine toxic effects. Avoid. |
| Foods: | None expected. |
| Marijuana: | Impairs physical and mental performance. Avoid. |
| Tobacco: | None expected. |

# NEOMYCIN (ORAL)

## BRAND NAMES

Mycifradin      Neobiotic

## BASIC INFORMATION

Habit forming? No
Prescription needed? Yes
Available as generic? Yes
Drug class: Antibiotic

## USES

- Clears intestinal tract of germs prior to surgery.
- Treats some causes of diarrhea.
- Lowers blood cholesterol.
- Lessens symptoms of hepatic coma.

## DOSAGE & USAGE INFORMATION

**How to take:**
Tablet or capsule—Swallow with liquid or food to lessen stomach irritation. If you can't swallow whole, crumble tablet or open capsule and take with liquid or food.

**When to take:**
According to directions on prescription.

**If you forget a dose:**
Take as soon as you remember up to 2 hours late. If more than 2 hours, wait for next scheduled dose (don't double this dose).

**What drug does:**
Kills germs susceptible to neomycin.

**Time lapse before drug works:**
2 to 3 days.

*Continued next column*

## OVERDOSE

**SYMPTOMS:**
Loss of hearing, difficulty breathing, respiratory paralysis.
**WHAT TO DO:**
- Dial 0 (operator) or 911 (emergency) for an ambulance or medical help. Then give first aid immediately.
- If patient is unconscious and not breathing, give mouth-to-mouth breathing. If there is no heartbeat, use cardiac massage and mouth-to-mouth breathing (CPR). Don't try to make patient vomit. If you can't get help quickly, take patient to nearest emergency facility.
- See emergency information on inside covers.

**Don't take with:**
See Interaction column and consult doctor.

## POSSIBLE ADVERSE REACTIONS OR SIDE EFFECTS

| SYMPTOMS | WHAT TO DO |
|---|---|
| **Life-threatening:**<br>None expected. | |
| **Common:**<br>Sore mouth, nausea, vomiting. | Continue. Call doctor when convenient. |
| **Infrequent:**<br>None expected. | |
| **Rare:**<br>Clumsiness, dizziness, rash, hearing loss, ringing or noises in ear, frothy stools, gaseousness, decreased frequency of urination. | Discontinue. Call doctor right away. |

## WARNINGS & PRECAUTIONS

**Don't take if:**
You are allergic to neomycin or any aminoglycoside. (See Interactions column.)

**Before you start, consult your doctor:**
- If you will have surgery within 2 months, including dental surgery, requiring general or spinal anesthesia.
- If you have hearing loss or loss of balance secondary to 8th cranial nerve disease.
- If you have intestinal obstruction.
- If you have myasthenia gravis, Parkinson's disease, kidney disease, ulcers in intestines.

**Over age 60:**
Adverse reactions and side effects may be more frequent and severe than in younger persons.

**Pregnancy:**
No proven harm to unborn child. Avoid if possible.

**Breast-feeding:**
Avoid if possible.

**Infants & children:**
Only under close medical supervision.

**Prolonged use:**
Adverse effects more likely.

**Skin & sunlight:**
No problems expected.

**Driving, piloting or hazardous work:**
No problems expected.

**Discontinuing:**
May be unnecessary to finish medicine. Follow doctor's instructions.

**Others:**
No problems expected.

## POSSIBLE INTERACTION WITH OTHER DRUGS

| GENERIC NAME OR DRUG CLASS | COMBINED EFFECT |
|---|---|
| **Aminoglycosides: Amikacin, Gentamicin, Kanamycin, Streptomycin, Tobramycin** | Increases chance of toxic effect on hearing, kidney, muscles. |
| **Capreomycin Cisplatin Ethacrynic acid Furosemide Mercaptomerin Vancomycin** | Increases chance of toxic effects on hearing, kidneys. |
| **Cephalothin** | Increased chance of toxic effect on kidneys. |

## POSSIBLE INTERACTION WITH OTHER SUBSTANCES

| INTERACTS WITH | COMBINED EFFECT |
|---|---|
| **Alcohol:** | Increased chance of toxicity. Avoid. |
| **Beverages:** | No problems expected. |
| **Cocaine:** | Increased chance of toxicity. Avoid. |
| **Foods:** | No problems expected. |
| **Marijuana:** | Increased chance of toxicity. Avoid. |
| **Tobacco:** | No problems expected. |

# NEOSTIGMINE

## BRAND NAMES

Prostigmin

## BASIC INFORMATION

Habit forming? No
Prescription needed? Yes
Available as generic? Yes
Drug class: Cholinergic (anticholinesterase)

 **USES**

- Treatment of myasthenia gravis.
- Treatment of urinary retention and abdominal distention.
- Antidote to adverse effects of muscle relaxants used in surgery.

 **DOSAGE & USAGE INFORMATION**

**How to take:**
Tablet—Swallow with liquid or food to lessen stomach irritation.

**When to take:**
As directed, usually 3 or 4 times a day.

**If you forget a dose:**
Take as soon as you remember up to 2 hours late. If more than 2 hours, wait for next scheduled dose (don't double this dose).

**What drug does:**
Inhibits the chemical activity of an enzyme (cholinesterase) so nerve impulses can cross the junction of nerves and muscles.

**Time lapse before drug works:**
3 hours.

**Don't take with:**
See Interaction column and consult doctor.

 **OVERDOSE**

**SYMPTOMS:**
**Muscle weakness, cramps, twitching or clumsiness; severe diarrhea, nausea, vomiting, stomach cramps or pain; breathing difficulty; confusion, irritability, nervousness, restlessness, fear; unusually slow heartbeat; seizures.**
**WHAT TO DO:**
- **Dial 0 (operator) or 911 (emergency) for an ambulance or medical help. Then give first aid immediately.**
- **See emergency information on inside covers.**

 **POSSIBLE ADVERSE REACTIONS OR SIDE EFFECTS**

| SYMPTOMS | WHAT TO DO |
|---|---|
| **Life-threatening:** | |
| None expected. | |
| **Common:** | |
| • Mild diarrhea, nausea, vomiting, stomach cramps or pain. | Discontinue. Call doctor right away. |
| • Excess saliva, unusual sweating. | Continue. Call doctor when convenient. |
| **Infrequent:** | |
| • Confusion, irritability. | Discontinue. Seek emergency treatment. |
| • Constricted pupils, watery eyes, lung congestion, frequent urge to urinate. | Continue. Call doctor when convenient. |
| **Rare:** | |
| None expected. | |

## WARNINGS & PRECAUTIONS

**Don't take if:**
- You are allergic to any cholinergic or bromide.
- You take mecamylamine.

**Before you start, consult your doctor:**
- If you plan to become pregnant within medication period.
- If you have bronchial asthma.
- If you have heartbeat irregularities.
- If you have urinary obstruction or urinary-tract infection.

**Over age 60:**
Adverse reactions and side effects may be more frequent and severe than in younger persons.

**Pregnancy:**
No proven harm to unborn child. Avoid if possible. May increase uterus contractions close to delivery.

**Breast-feeding:**
No problems expected, but consult doctor.

**Infants & children:**
Not recommended.

**Prolonged use:**
Medication may lose effectiveness. Discontinuing for a few days may restore effect.

**Skin & sunlight:**
No problems expected.

**Driving, piloting or hazardous work:**
Don't drive or pilot aircraft until you learn how medicine affects you. Don't work around dangerous machinery. Don't climb ladders or work in high places. Danger increases if you drink alcohol or take medicine affecting alertness and reflexes, such as antihistamines, tranquilizers, sedatives, pain medicine, narcotics and mind-altering drugs.

**Discontinuing:**
Don't discontinue without doctor's advice until you complete prescribed dose, even though symptoms diminish or disappear.

**Others:**
No problems expected.

## POSSIBLE INTERACTION WITH OTHER DRUGS

| GENERIC NAME OR DRUG CLASS | COMBINED EFFECT |
|---|---|
| Anesthetics (local or general) | Decreased neostigmine effect. |
| Antiarrhythmics | Decreased neostigmine effect. |
| Antibiotics | Decreased neostigmine effect. |
| Anticholinergics | Decreased neostigmine effect. May mask severe side effects. |
| Cholinergics (other) | Reduced intestinal-tract function. Possible brain and nervous-system toxicity. |
| Mecamylamine | Decreased neostigmine effect. |
| Nitrates | Decreased neostigmine effect. |
| Quinidine | Decreased neostigmine effect. |

## POSSIBLE INTERACTION WITH OTHER SUBSTANCES

| INTERACTS WITH | COMBINED EFFECT |
|---|---|
| Alcohol: | No proven problems with small doses. |
| Beverages: | None expected. |
| Cocaine: | Decreased neostigmine effect. Avoid. |
| Foods: | None expected. |
| Marijuana: | No proven problems. |
| Tobacco: | No proven problems. |

# NIACIN (NICOTINIC ACID)

## BRAND NAMES

See complete list of brand names in the *Brand Name Directory,* page 953.

**There are numerous other multiple vitamin-mineral supplements available.**

## BASIC INFORMATION

**Habit forming? No**
**Prescription needed?**
   **Tablets: No**
   **Liquid, capsules: Yes**
**Available as generic? Yes**
**Drug class: Vitamin supplement, vasodilator, antihyperlipidemic**

## USES

- Replacement for niacin deficiency caused by inadequate diet.
- Treatment for vertigo (dizziness) and ringing in ears.
- Prevention of premenstrual headache.
- Reduction of blood levels of cholesterol and triglycerides.
- Treatment for pellagra.

## DOSAGE & USAGE INFORMATION

**How to take:**
- Tablet, capsule or liquid—Swallow with liquid or food to lessen stomach irritation.
- Extended-release tablets or capsules—Swallow each dose whole.

**When to take:**
At the same times each day.

**If you forget a dose:**
Take as soon as you remember. Wait 4 hours for next dose.

**What drug does:**
- Corrects niacin deficiency.
- Dilates blood vessels.
- In large doses, decreases cholesterol production.

*Continued next column*

## OVERDOSE

**SYMPTOMS:**
**Body flush, nausea, vomiting, abdominal cramps, diarrhea, weakness, lightheadedness, fainting, sweating.**
**WHAT TO DO:**
**Overdose unlikely to threaten life. If person takes much larger amount than prescribed, call doctor, poison-control center or hospital emergency room for instructions.**

**Time lapse before drug works:**
15 to 20 minutes.

**Don't take with:**
See Interaction column and consult doctor.

## POSSIBLE ADVERSE REACTIONS OR SIDE EFFECTS

| SYMPTOMS | WHAT TO DO |
|---|---|
| **Life-threatening:** None expected. | |
| **Common:** None expected. | |
| **Infrequent:** | |
| • Headache, dizziness, faintness, temporary numbness and tingling in hands and feet. | Continue. Call doctor when convenient. |
| • "Hot" feeling, flush. | No action necessary. |
| **Rare:** Jaundice. | Discontinue. Call doctor right away. |

## WARNINGS & PRECAUTIONS

**Don't take if:**
- You are allergic to niacin or any niacin-containing vitamin mixtures.
- You have impaired liver function.
- You have active peptic ulcer.

**Before you start, consult your doctor:**
- If you have diabetes.
- If you have gout.
- If you have gallbladder or liver disease.

**Over age 60:**
Response to drug cannot be predicted. Dose must be individualized.

**Pregnancy:**
Risk to unborn child outweighs drug benefits. Don't use.

**Breast-feeding:**
Studies inconclusive. Consult doctor.

**Infants & children:**
- Use only under supervision.
- Keep vitamin-mineral supplements out of children's reach.

**Prolonged use:**
Possible impaired liver function.

**Skin & sunlight:**
No problems expected.

**Driving, piloting or hazardous work:**
Avoid if you feel dizzy or faint. Otherwise, no problems expected.

**Discontinuing:**
May be unnecessary to finish medicine. Follow doctor's instructions.

**Others:**
- A balanced diet should provide all the niacin a healthy person needs and make supplements unnecessary. Best sources are meat, eggs and dairy products.
- Store in original container in cool, dry, dark place. Bathroom medicine chest too moist.
- Obesity reduces effectiveness.

## POSSIBLE INTERACTION WITH OTHER DRUGS

| GENERIC NAME OR DRUG CLASS | COMBINED EFFECT |
|---|---|
| Antidiabetics | Decreased antidiabetic effect. |
| Beta-adrenergic blockers | Excessively low blood pressure. |
| Guanethidine | Increased guanethidine effect. |
| Isoniazid | Decreased niacin effect. |
| Mecamylamine | Excessively low blood pressure. |
| Methyldopa | Excessively low blood pressure. |
| Pargyline | Excessively low blood pressure. |

## POSSIBLE INTERACTION WITH OTHER SUBSTANCES

| INTERACTS WITH | COMBINED EFFECT |
|---|---|
| Alcohol: | Excessively low blood pressure. Use caution. |
| Beverages: | None expected. |
| Cocaine: | Increased flushing. |
| Foods: | None expected. |
| Marijuana: | None expected. |
| Tobacco: | Decreased niacin effect. |

# NICOTINE RESIN COMPLEX

## BRAND NAMES

**Nicorette**

## BASIC INFORMATION

**Habit forming? Yes**
**Prescription needed? Yes**
**Available as generic? No**
**Drug class: Antismoking agent**

 ## USES

Treats smoking addiction.

 ## DOSAGE & USAGE INFORMATION

**How to take:**
Follow detailed instructions on patient instruction sheet provided with prescription.

**When to take:**
Follow detailed instructions on patient instruction sheet provided with prescription.

**If you forget a dose:**
Follow detailed instructions on patient instruction sheet provided with prescription.

**What drug does:**
Satisfies physical craving for nicotine in addicted persons and avoids peaks in blood nicotine level resulting from smoking.

**Time lapse before drug works:**
30 minutes.

**Don't take with:**
See Interaction column and consult doctor.

 ## OVERDOSE

**SYMPTOMS:**
**Vomiting, irregular heartbeat.**
**WHAT TO DO:**
**Overdose unlikely to threaten life. If person takes much larger amount than prescribed, call doctor, poison-control center or hospital emergency room for instructions.**

 ## POSSIBLE ADVERSE REACTIONS OR SIDE EFFECTS

| SYMPTOMS | WHAT TO DO |
|---|---|
| **Life-threatening:**<br>None expected. | |
| **Frequent:**<br>Increased irritability causing heartbeat irregularity. | Continue. Call doctor when convenient. |
| **Common:** | |
| • Injury to loose teeth, jaw muscle ache. | Continue. Call doctor when convenient. |
| • Belching, mouth irritation or tingling, excessive salivation. | Continue. Tell doctor at next visit. |
| **Infrequent:** | |
| • Nausea and vomiting, abdominal pain. | Discontinue. Call doctor right away. |
| • Lightheadedness, headache, hiccups. | Continue. Call doctor when convenient. |
| **Rare:**<br>None expected. | |

## WARNINGS & PRECAUTIONS

**Don't take if:**
- You are a non-smoker.
- You are pregnant or intend to become pregnant.
- You recently suffered a heart attack.

**Before you start, consult your doctor:**
- If you have coronary artery disease.
- If you have active temperomandibular joint disease.
- If you have severe angina.
- If you have peptic ulcer.

**Over age 60:**
Adverse reactions and side effects may be more frequent and severe than in younger persons.

**Pregnancy:**
Risk to unborn child outweighs drug benefits. Don't use.

**Breast-feeding:**
Drug passes into milk. Avoid drug or discontinue nursing until you finish medicine. Consult doctor for advice on maintaining milk supply.

**Infants & children:**
Don't use.

**Prolonged use:**
May cause addiction and greater likelihood of toxicity.

**Skin & sunlight:**
No problems expected.

**Driving, piloting or hazardous work:**
No problems expected.

**Discontinuing:**
May be unnecessary to finish medicine. Follow doctor's instructions.

**Others:**
No problems expected.

## POSSIBLE INTERACTION WITH OTHER DRUGS

| GENERIC NAME OR DRUG CLASS | COMBINED EFFECT |
| --- | --- |
| Beta-adrenergic blockers | Decreased blood pressure (slight). |
| Caffeine | Increased effect of caffeine. |
| Cortisone drugs | Increased cortisone circulating in blood. |
| Furosemide | Increased effect of furosemide. |
| Glutethimide | Increased absorption of glutethimide. |
| Imipramine | Increased effect of imipramine. |
| Pentazocine | Increased effect of pentazocine. |
| Phenacetin | Increased effect of phenacetin. |
| Propoxyphene | Decreased blood level of propoxyphene. |
| Theophylline | Increased effect of theophylline. |

## POSSIBLE INTERACTION WITH OTHER SUBSTANCES

| INTERACTS WITH | COMBINED EFFECT |
| --- | --- |
| Alcohol: | Increased cardiac irritability. Avoid. |
| Beverages: Caffeine. | Increased cardiac irritability. Avoid any beverage with caffeine. |
| Cocaine: | Increased cardiac irritability. Avoid. |
| Foods: | No problems expected. |
| Marijuana: | Increased toxic effects. Avoid. |
| Tobacco: | Increased toxic effects. Avoid. |

# NIFEDIPINE

## BRAND NAMES

Adalat                    Procardia

## BASIC INFORMATION

Habit forming? No
Prescription needed? Yes
Available as generic? No
Drug class: Calcium-channel blocker,
           antiarrhythmic, antianginal

 **USES**

Prevents angina attacks.

 **DOSAGE & USAGE INFORMATION**

**How to take:**
Capsule—Swallow with liquid.

**When to take:**
At the same times each day 1 hour before or 2 hours after eating.

**If you forget a dose:**
Take as soon as you remember up to 2 hours late. If more than 2 hours, wait for next scheduled dose (don't double this dose).

**What drug does:**
- Reduces work that heart must perform.
- Reduces normal artery pressure.
- Increases oxygen to heart muscle.

**Time lapse before drug works:**
1 to 2 hours.

**Don't take with:**
See Interaction column and consult doctor.

 **OVERDOSE**

**SYMPTOMS:**
Unusually fast or unusually slow heartbeat, loss of consciousness, cardiac arrest.
**WHAT TO DO:**
- Dial 0 (operator) or 911 (emergency) for an ambulance or medical help. Then give first aid immediately.
- If patient is unconscious and not breathing, give mouth-to-mouth breathing. If there is no heartbeat, use cardiac massage and mouth-to-mouth breathing (CPR). Don't try to make patient vomit. If you can't get help quickly, take patient to nearest emergency facility.
- See emergency information on inside covers.

 **POSSIBLE ADVERSE REACTIONS OR SIDE EFFECTS**

| SYMPTOMS | WHAT TO DO |
|---|---|
| **Life-threatening:**<br>None expected. | |
| **Common:**<br>Tiredness. | Continue. Tell doctor at next visit. |
| **Infrequent:**<br>• Unusually fast or unusually slow heartbeat, wheezing, cough, shortness of breath. | Discontinue. Call doctor right away. |
| • Dizziness; numbness or tingling in hands or feet; swelling of ankles, feet, legs; difficult urination. | Continue. Call doctor when convenient. |
| • Nausea, constipation. | Continue. Tell doctor at next visit. |
| **Rare:**<br>• Fainting, chest pain. | Discontinue. Call doctor right away. |
| • Headache. | Continue. Tell doctor at next visit. |

 **WARNINGS & PRECAUTIONS**

**Don't take if:**
- You are allergic to nifedipine.
- You have very low blood pressure.

**Before you start, consult your doctor:**
- If you have kidney or liver disease.
- If you have high blood pressure.
- If you have heart disease other than coronary-artery disease.

**Over age 60:**
Adverse reactions and side effects may be more frequent and severe than in younger persons.

**Pregnancy:**
No proven harm to unborn child: Avoid if possible.

**Breast-feeding:**
Safety not established. Avoid if possible.

**Infants & children:**
Not recommended.

**Prolonged use:**
No problems expected.

**Skin & sunlight:**
No problems expected.

**Driving, piloting or hazardous work:**
Avoid if you feel dizzy. Otherwise, no problems expected.

**Discontinuing:**
Don't discontinue without doctor's advice until you complete prescribed dose, even though symptoms diminish or disappear.

**Others:**
* Learn to check your own pulse rate. If it drops to 50 beats per minute or lower, don't take nifedipine until you consult your doctor.
* Drug may lower blood-sugar level if daily dose is more than 60 mg.

## POSSIBLE INTERACTION WITH OTHER DRUGS

| GENERIC NAME OR DRUG CLASS | COMBINED EFFECT |
|---|---|
| Amiodarone | Increased likelihood of slow heartbeat. |
| Anticoagulants (oral) | Increased anticoagulant effect. |
| Anticonvulsants (hydantoin) | Increased anticonvulsant effect. |
| Antihypertensives | Dangerous blood-pressure drop. |
| Beta-adrenergic blockers | Possible irregular heartbeat. May worsen congestive heart failure. |
| Calcium (large doses) | Decreased nifedipine effect. |
| Digitalis preparations | Increased digitalis effect. May need to reduce dose. |
| Disopyramide | May cause dangerously slow, fast or irregular heartbeat. |
| Diuretics | Dangerous blood-pressure drop. |
| Enalapril | Possible excessive potassium in blood. |
| Flecainide | Possible irregular heartbeat. |
| Ketoprofen | Increases chance of toxicity of nifedipine. |
| Nitrates | Reduced angina attacks. |
| Quinidine | Increased quinidine effect. |
| Suprofen | Increases chances of toxicity of nifedipine. |

| | |
|---|---|
| Tocainide | Increased likelihood of adverse reactions from either drug. |
| Vitamin D (large doses) | Decreased nifedipine effect. |

## POSSIBLE INTERACTION WITH OTHER SUBSTANCES

| INTERACTS WITH | COMBINED EFFECT |
|---|---|
| Alcohol: | Dangerously low blood pressure. Avoid. |
| Beverages: | None expected. |
| Cocaine: | Possible irregular heartbeat. Avoid. |
| Foods: | None expected. |
| Marijuana: | Possible irregular heartbeat. Avoid. |
| Tobacco: | Possible rapid heartbeat. Avoid. |

## BRAND NAMES

See complete list of brand names in the *Brand Name Directory,* page 953.

## BASIC INFORMATION

**Habit forming? No**
**Prescription needed? Yes**
**Available as generic? Yes**
**Drug class: Antianginal (nitrate)**

## USES

Reduces frequency and severity of angina attacks.

## DOSAGE & USAGE INFORMATION

**How to take:**
- Extended-release tablets or capsules—Swallow each dose whole with liquid.
- Chewable tablet—Chew tablet at earliest sign of angina, and hold in mouth for 2 minutes.
- Regular tablet or capsule—Swallow whole with liquid. Don't crush, chew or open.
- Ointment—Apply as directed.
- Sublingual tablets—Place under tongue every 3 to 5 minutes at earliest sign of angina. If you don't have complete relief with 3 or 4 tablets, call doctor.

**When to take:**
- Swallowed tablets—Take at the same times each day, 1 or 2 hours after meals.
- Ointment—Follow prescription directions.

**If you forget a dose:**
Take as soon as you remember up to 2 hours late. If more than 2 hours, wait for next scheduled dose (don't double this dose).

*Continued next column*

## OVERDOSE

**SYMPTOMS:**
**Dizziness; blue fingernails and lips; fainting; shortness of breath; weak, fast heartbeat; convulsions.**
**WHAT TO DO:**
- **Dial 0 (operator) or 911 (emergency) for an ambulance or medical help. Then give first aid immediately.**
- **See emergency information on inside covers.**

**What drug does:**
Relaxes blood vessels, increasing blood flow to heart muscle.

**Time lapse before drug works:**
- Sublingual tablets—1 to 3 minutes.
- Other forms—15 to 30 minutes. Will not stop an attack, but may prevent attacks.

**Don't take with:**
See Interaction column and consult doctor.

## POSSIBLE ADVERSE REACTIONS OR SIDE EFFECTS

| SYMPTOMS | WHAT TO DO |
|---|---|
| **Life-threatening:** None expected. | |
| **Common:** Headache, flushed face and neck, dry mouth, nausea, vomiting, rapid heartbeat. | Continue. Tell doctor at next visit. |
| **Infrequent:** | |
| • Fainting. | Discontinue. Call doctor right away. |
| • Restlessness, blurred vision. | Continue. Call doctor when convenient. |
| **Rare:** | |
| • Rash. | Discontinue. Call doctor right away. |
| • Severe irritation, peeling. | Continue. Call doctor when convenient. |

# NITRATES

## WARNINGS & PRECAUTIONS

**Don't take if:**
You are allergic to nitrates, including nitroglycerin.

**Before you start, consult your doctor:**
- If you are taking non-prescription drugs.
- If you plan to become pregnant within medication period.
- If you have glaucoma.
- If you have reacted badly to any vasodilator drug.
- If you drink alcoholic beverages or smoke marijuana.

**Over age 60:**
Adverse reactions and side effects may be more frequent and severe than in younger persons.

**Pregnancy:**
No proven harm to unborn child. Avoid if possible.

**Breast-feeding:**
No problems expected. Consult your doctor.

**Infants & children:**
Not recommended.

**Prolonged use:**
Drug may become less effective and require higher doses.

**Skin & sunlight:**
No problems expected.

**Driving, piloting or hazardous work:**
Don't drive or pilot aircraft until you learn how medicine affects you. Don't work around dangerous machinery. Don't climb ladders or work in high places. Danger increases if you drink alcohol or take medicine affecting alertness and reflexes.

**Discontinuing:**
Except for sublingual tablets, don't discontinue without doctor's advice until you complete prescribed dose, even though symptoms diminish or disappear.

**Others:**
- If discomfort is not caused by angina, nitrate medication will not bring relief. Call doctor if discomfort persists.
- Periodic urine and laboratory blood studies of white cell counts recommended if you take nitrates.
- Keep sublingual tablets in original container. Always carry them with you, but keep from body heat if possible.

## POSSIBLE INTERACTION WITH OTHER DRUGS

| GENERIC NAME OR DRUG CLASS | COMBINED EFFECT |
| --- | --- |
| Anticholinergics | Increased internal-eye pressure. |
| Antidepressants (tricyclic) | Excessive blood-pressure drop. |
| Antihypertensives | Excessive blood-pressure drop. |
| Beta-adrenergic blockers | Excessive blood-pressure drop. |
| Cholinergics | Decreased cholinergic effect. |
| Ephedrine | Decreased nitrate effect. |
| Labetolol | Increased antihypertensive effects. |
| Narcotics | Excessive blood-pressure drop. |
| Sympathomimetics | Possible reduced effects of both medicines. |

## POSSIBLE INTERACTION WITH OTHER SUBSTANCES

| INTERACTS WITH | COMBINED EFFECT |
| --- | --- |
| Alcohol: | Excessive blood-pressure drop. |
| Beverages: | None expected. |
| Cocaine: | Flushed face and headache. Avoid. |
| Foods: | None expected. |
| Marijuana: | Decreased nitrate effect. |
| Tobacco: | Decreased nitrate effect. |

609

# NITROFURANTOIN

## BRAND NAMES

| | |
|---|---|
| Apo-Nitrofurantoin | Nephronex |
| Cyantin | Nifuran |
| Furadantin | Nitrex |
| Furalan | Nitrodan |
| Furaloid | Novofuran |
| Furantoin | Sarodant |
| Furatine | Trantoin |
| Macrodantin | Urotoin |

## BASIC INFORMATION

**Habit forming?** No
**Prescription needed?** Yes
**Available as generic?** Yes
**Drug class:** Antimicrobial

## USES

Treatment for urinary-tract infections.

## DOSAGE & USAGE INFORMATION

**How to take:**
- Tablet or capsule—Swallow with food or milk to lessen stomach irritation. If you can't swallow whole, crumble tablet or open capsule and take with liquid or food.
- Liquid—Shake well and take with food. Use a measuring spoon to ensure accuracy.

**When to take:**
At the same times each day.

**If you forget a dose:**
Take as soon as you remember up to 2 hours late. If more than 2 hours, wait for next scheduled dose (don't double this dose).

**What drug does:**
Prevents susceptible bacteria in the urinary tract from growing and multiplying.

**Time lapse before drug works:**
1 to 2 weeks.

**Don't take with:**
See Interaction column and consult doctor.

## OVERDOSE

**SYMPTOMS:**
Nausea, vomiting, abdominal pain, diarrhea.
**WHAT TO DO:**
Overdose unlikely to threaten life. If person takes much larger amount than prescribed, call doctor, poison-control center or hospital emergency room for instructions.

## POSSIBLE ADVERSE REACTIONS OR SIDE EFFECTS

| SYMPTOMS | WHAT TO DO |
|---|---|
| **Life-threatening:** | |
| Hives, rash, intense itching, faintness soon after a dose (anaphylaxis). | Seek emergency treatment immediately. |
| **Common:** | |
| • Diarrhea, appetite loss, nausea, vomiting, chest pain, cough, difficult breathing, chills or unexplained fever. | Discontinue. Call doctor right away. |
| • Rusty colored or brown urine. | No action necessary. |
| **Infrequent:** | |
| • Rash, itchy skin, numbness, tingling or burning of face or mouth, fatigue, weakness. | Discontinue. Call doctor right away. |
| • Dizziness, drowsiness, headache, paleness (in children), discolored teeth (from liquid form). | Continue. Call doctor when convenient. |
| **Rare:** | |
| Jaundice. | Discontinue. Call doctor right away. |

## WARNINGS & PRECAUTIONS

**Don't take if:**
- You are allergic to nitrofurantoin.
- You have impaired kidney function.
- You drink alcohol.

**Before you start, consult your doctor:**
- If you are prone to allergic reactions.
- If you are pregnant and within 2 weeks of delivery.
- If you have had kidney disease, lung disease, anemia, nerve damage, or G6PD deficiency (a metabolic deficiency).
- If you have diabetes. Drug may affect urine sugar tests.

**Over age 60:**
Adverse reactions and side effects may be more frequent and severe than in younger persons.

**Pregnancy:**
Risk to unborn child outweighs drug benefits, especially in last month of pregnancy. Don't use.

**Breast-feeding:**
Drug passes into milk. Avoid drug or discontinue nursing until you finish medicine. Consult doctor for advice on maintaining milk supply.

**Infants & children:**
Don't give to infants younger than 1 month. Use only under medical supervision for older children.

**Prolonged use:**
Chest pain, cough, shortness of breath.

**Skin & sunlight:**
No problems expected.

**Driving, piloting or hazardous work:**
Avoid if you feel dizzy or drowsy. Otherwise, no problems expected.

**Discontinuing:**
Don't discontinue without consulting doctor. Dose may require gradual reduction if you have taken drug for a long time. Doses of other drugs may also require adjustment.

**Others:**
Periodic blood counts, liver-function tests, and chest X-rays recommended.

## POSSIBLE INTERACTION WITH OTHER DRUGS

| GENERIC NAME OR DRUG CLASS | COMBINED EFFECT |
|---|---|
| Nalidixic acid | Decreased nitrofurantoin effect. |
| Phenobarbital | Decreased nitrofurantoin effect. |
| Probenecid | Increased nitrofurantoin effect. |
| Sulfinpyrazone | Possible nitrofurantoin toxicity. |

## POSSIBLE INTERACTION WITH OTHER SUBSTANCES

| INTERACTS WITH | COMBINED EFFECT |
|---|---|
| Alcohol: | Possible disulfiram reaction (see Glossary). Avoid. |
| Beverages: | None expected. |
| Cocaine: | No proven problems. |
| Foods: | None expected. |
| Marijuana: | None expected. |
| Tobacco: | None expected. |

# NORETHINDRONE

## BRAND NAMES

| | |
|---|---|
| Micronor | Norlutin |
| Modicon 21 | Nor-Q.D. |
| Norinyl 1 + 35 | Ortho-Novum 1/35 |
|   21-Day Tablets | Ovcon |
| Norlestrin | Tri-Norinyl |
| Norlutate | |

## BASIC INFORMATION

**Habit forming? No**
**Prescription needed? Yes**
**Available as generic? No**
**Drug class: Female sex hormone (progestin)**

 **USES**

- Treatment for menstrual or uterine disorders caused by progestin imbalance.
- Contraceptive.

 **DOSAGE & USAGE INFORMATION**

**How to take:**
Tablet or capsule—Swallow with liquid or food to lessen stomach irritation. You may crumble tablet or open capsule.

**When to take:**
At the same time each day.

**If you forget a dose:**
- Menstrual disorders—Take up to 2 hours late. If more than 2 hours, wait for next dose (don't double this dose).
- Contraceptive—Consult your doctor. You may need to use another birth-control method until next period.

**What drug does:**
- Creates a uterine lining similar to pregnancy that prevents bleeding.
- Suppresses a pituitary gland hormone responsible for ovulation.
- Stimulates cervical mucus, which stops sperm penetration and prevents pregnancy.

*Continued next column*

 **OVERDOSE**

**SYMPTOMS:**
Nausea, vomiting, fluid retention, breast discomfort or enlargement, vaginal bleeding.
**WHAT TO DO:**
Overdose unlikely to threaten life. If person takes much larger amount than prescribed, call doctor, poison-control center or hospital emergency room for instructions.

**Time lapse before drug works:**
- Menstrual disorders—24 to 48 hours.
- Contraception—3 weeks.

**Don't take with:**
See Interaction column and consult doctor.

 **POSSIBLE ADVERSE REACTIONS OR SIDE EFFECTS**

| SYMPTOMS | WHAT TO DO |
|---|---|
| **Life-threatening:** | |
| Blood clot in leg, brain or lung. | Seek emergency treatment immediately. |
| **Common:** | |
| Appetite or weight changes, swollen ankles or feet, unusual tiredness or weakness. | Continue. Tell doctor at next visit. |
| **Infrequent:** | |
| • Prolonged vaginal bleeding. | Discontinue. Call doctor right away. |
| • Depression. | Continue. Call doctor when convenient. |
| • Acne, increased facial or body hair, nausea, breast tenderness. | Continue. Tell doctor at next visit. |
| **Rare:** | |
| Rash, stomach or side pain, jaundice. | Discontinue. Call doctor right away. |

## WARNINGS & PRECAUTIONS

**Don't take if:**
- You are allergic to any progestin hormone.
- You may be pregnant.
- You have liver or gallbladder disease.
- You have had thrombophlebitis, embolism or stroke.
- You have unexplained vaginal bleeding.
- You have had breast or uterine cancer.

**Before you start, consult your doctor:**
- If you have heart or kidney disease.
- If you have diabetes.
- If you have a seizure disorder.
- If you suffer migraines.
- If you are easily depressed.

**Over age 60:**
Not recommended.

**Pregnancy:**
May harm child. Discontinue at first sign of pregnancy.

**Breast-feeding:**
Drug passes into milk. Avoid drug or discontinue nursing until you finish medicine. Consult doctor for advice on maintaining milk supply.

**Infants & children:**
Use only for female children under medical supervision.

**Prolonged use:**
No problems expected.

**Skin & sunlight:**
No problems expected.

**Driving, piloting or hazardous work:**
No problems expected.

**Discontinuing:**
Consult doctor. This medicine stays in the body and causes fetal abnormalities. Wait at least 3 months before becoming pregnant.

**Others:**
- Patients with diabetes must be monitored closely.
- Symptoms of blood clot in leg, brain or lung are: chest, groin, leg pain; sudden, severe headache; loss of coordination; vision change; shortness of breath; slurred speech.

## POSSIBLE INTERACTION WITH OTHER DRUGS

| GENERIC NAME OR DRUG CLASS | COMBINED EFFECT |
| --- | --- |
| Antihistamines | Decreased norethindrone effect. |
| Oxyphenbutazone | Decreased norethindrone effect. |
| Phenobarbital | Decreased norethindrone effect. |
| Phenothiazines | Increased phenothiazine effect. |
| Phenylbutazone | Decreased norethindrone effect. |

## POSSIBLE INTERACTION WITH OTHER SUBSTANCES

| INTERACTS WITH | COMBINED EFFECT |
| --- | --- |
| Alcohol: | None expected. |
| Beverages: | None expected. |
| Cocaine: | Decreased norethindrone effect. |
| Foods: Salt. | Fluid retention. |
| Marijuana: | Possible menstrual irregularities or bleeding between periods. |
| Tobacco: | Possible blood clots in lung, brain, legs. Avoid. |

# NORETHINDRONE ACETATE

## BRAND NAMES

| | |
|---|---|
| Aygestin | Norlutate Acetate |
| Micronor | Norlutin |
| Norlutate | Nor-O.-D. |

## BASIC INFORMATION

**Habit forming? No**
**Prescription needed? Yes**
**Available as generic? No**
**Drug class: Female sex hormone (progestin)**

## USES

- Treatment for menstrual or uterine disorders caused by progestin imbalance.
- Contraceptive.
- Treatment for cancer of breast and uterus.

## DOSAGE & USAGE INFORMATION

**How to take:**
Tablet or capsule—Swallow with liquid or food to lessen stomach irritation. You may crumble tablet or open capsule.

**When to take:**
At the same time each day.

**If you forget a dose:**
- Menstrual disorders—Take up to 2 hours late. If more than 2 hours, wait for next dose (don't double this dose).
- Contraceptive—Consult your doctor. You may need to use another birth-control method until next period.

**What drug does:**
- Creates a uterine lining similar to pregnancy that prevents bleeding.
- Suppresses a pituitary gland hormone responsible for ovulation.
- Stimulates cervical mucus, which stops sperm penetration and prevents pregnancy.

*Continued next column*

## OVERDOSE

**SYMPTOMS:**
Nausea, vomiting, fluid retention, breast discomfort or enlargement, vaginal bleeding.
**WHAT TO DO:**
Overdose unlikely to threaten life. If person takes much larger amount than prescribed, call doctor, poison-control center or hospital emergency room for instructions.

**Time lapse before drug works:**
- Menstrual disorders—24 to 48 hours.
- Contraception—3 weeks.
- Cancer—May require 2 to 3 months.

**Don't take with:**
See Interaction column and consult doctor.

## POSSIBLE ADVERSE REACTIONS OR SIDE EFFECTS

| SYMPTOMS | WHAT TO DO |
|---|---|
| **Life-threatening:** | |
| Blood clot in leg, brain or lung. | Seek emergency treatment immediately. |
| **Common:** | |
| Appetite or weight changes, swollen ankles or feet, unusual tiredness or weakness. | Continue. Tell doctor at next visit. |
| **Infrequent:** | |
| • Prolonged vaginal bleeding. | Discontinue. Call doctor right away. |
| • Depression. | Continue. Call doctor when convenient. |
| • Acne, increased facial or body hair, nausea, breast tenderness. | Continue. Tell doctor at next visit. |
| **Rare:** | |
| Rash, stomach or side pain, jaundice. | Discontinue. Call doctor right away. |

# NORETHINDRONE ACETATE

## WARNINGS & PRECAUTIONS

**Don't take if:**
- You are allergic to any progestin hormone.
- You may be pregnant.
- You have liver or gallbladder disease.
- You have had thrombophlebitis, embolism or stroke.
- You have unexplained vaginal bleeding.
- You have had breast or uterine cancer.

**Before you start, consult your doctor:**
- If you have heart or kidney disease.
- If you have diabetes.
- If you have a seizure disorder.
- If you suffer migraines.
- If you are easily depressed.

**Over age 60:**
Not recommended.

**Pregnancy:**
May harm child. Discontinue at first sign of pregnancy.

**Breast-feeding:**
Drug passes into milk. Avoid drug or discontinue nursing until you finish medicine. Consult doctor for advice on maintaining milk supply.

**Infants & children:**
Use only for female children under medical supervision.

**Prolonged use:**
No problems expected.

**Skin & sunlight:**
No problems expected.

**Driving, piloting or hazardous work:**
No problems expected.

**Discontinuing:**
Consult doctor. This medicine stays in the body and causes fetal abnormalities. Wait at least 3 months before becoming pregnant.

**Others:**
- Patients with diabetes must be monitored closely.
- Symptoms of blood clot in leg, brain or lung are: chest, groin, leg pain; sudden, severe headache; loss of coordination; vision change; shortness of breath; slurred speech.

## POSSIBLE INTERACTION WITH OTHER DRUGS

| GENERIC NAME OR DRUG CLASS | COMBINED EFFECT |
|---|---|
| Antihistamines | Decreased norethindrone acetate effect. |
| Oxyphenbutazone | Decreased norethindrone acetate effect. |
| Phenobarbital | Decreased norethindrone acetate effect. |
| Phenothiazines | Increased phenothiazine effect. |
| Phenylbutazone | Decreased norethindrone acetate effect. |

## POSSIBLE INTERACTION WITH OTHER SUBSTANCES

| INTERACTS WITH | COMBINED EFFECT |
|---|---|
| Alcohol: | None expected. |
| Beverages: | None expected. |
| Cocaine: | Decreased norethindrone acetate effect. |
| Foods: Salt. | Fluid retention. |
| Marijuana: | Possible menstrual irregularities or bleeding between periods. |
| Tobacco: | Possible blood clots in lung, brain, legs. Avoid. |

# NORFLOXACIN

## BRAND NAMES

Noroxin

## BASIC INFORMATION

**Habit forming? No**
**Prescription needed? Yes**
**Available as generic? No**
**Drug class: Antibacterial, fluoroquinolones**

 ## USES

- Treats infections of the kidney, ureter, bladder and urethra. Cure rate reported to be about 95%.
- Treats traveler's diarrhea, gonorrhea, bacterial gastroenteritis.

 ## DOSAGE & USAGE INFORMATION

**How to take:**
Tablets or capsules—On an empty stomach 1 hour before or 2 hours after meals. Take with lots of water.

**When to take:**
As directed. Usually every 12 hours on empty stomach.

**If you forget a dose:**
Take as soon as you remember up to 6 hours late. If more than 6 hours, wait for next scheduled dose (don't double this dose).

**What drug does:**
Interferes with nutrient necessary for growth and reproduction of bacteria. Will not kill viruses.

**Time lapse before drug works:**
2 hours to peak level in blood. May require 7 to 21 days of treatment to cure infections.

**Don't take with:**
- Food, antacids.
- See Interaction column and consult doctor.

 ## OVERDOSE

**SYMPTOMS:**
**Seizures**
**WHAT TO DO:**
- Dial 0 (operator) or 911 (emergency) for an ambulance or medical help. Then give first aid immediately.
- See emergency information on inside covers.

 ## POSSIBLE ADVERSE REACTIONS OR SIDE EFFECTS

| SYMPTOMS | WHAT TO DO |
|---|---|
| **Life-threatening:** None expected. | |
| **Common:** None expected. | |
| **Infrequent:** Nausea, abdominal pain, heartburn, insomnia, diarrhea, dizziness, fatigue, rash, vulvar irritation, crystals in urine. | Discontinue. Call doctor right away. |
| **Rare:** Anemia, joint pain, joint swelling. | Discontinue. Call doctor right away. |

## WARNINGS & PRECAUTIONS

**Don't take if:**
You are allergic to any fluoroquinolone.

**Before you start, consult your doctor:**
If you have chronic kidney disease with loss of kidney function.

**Over age 60:**
Adverse reactions and side effects may be more frequent and severe than in younger persons. Ask doctor about smaller doses.

**Pregnancy:**
Safety to unborn child unestablished. Avoid if possible.

**Breast-feeding:**
Drug passes into milk. Avoid drug or discontinue nursing until you finish medicine. Consult doctor for advice on maintaining milk supply.

**Infants & children:**
Use only under close medical supervision.

**Prolonged use:**
No problems expected.

**Skin & sunlight:**
No problems expected.

**Driving, piloting or hazardous work:**
Avoid if you feel drowsy or dizzy.

**Discontinuing:**
No problems expected.

**Others:**
No problems expected.

## POSSIBLE INTERACTION WITH OTHER DRUGS

| GENERIC NAME OR DRUG CLASS | COMBINED EFFECT |
| --- | --- |
| Antacids | Decreased absorption of norfloxacin. |
| Probenecid | Enhances effect of norfloxacin. |

## POSSIBLE INTERACTION WITH OTHER SUBSTANCES

| INTERACTS WITH | COMBINED EFFECT |
| --- | --- |
| Alcohol: | Decreased effect of norfloxacin. |
| Beverages: | None expected. |
| Cocaine: | Decreased effect of norfloxacin. |
| Foods: | None expected. |
| Marijuana: | Decreased effect of norfloxacin. |
| Tobacco: | May stimulate irritated gastrointestinal tract. Avoid. |

# NORGESTREL

## BRAND NAMES

Lo-Ovral       Ovrette
Ovral

## BASIC INFORMATION

Habit forming? No
Prescription needed? Yes
Available as generic? No
Drug class: Female sex hormone (progestin)

## USES

Contraceptive.

## DOSAGE & USAGE INFORMATION

**How to take:**
Tablet or capsule—Swallow with liquid or food to lessen stomach irritation. You may crumble tablet or open capsule.

**When to take:**
At the same time each day.

**If you forget a dose:**
Consult your doctor. You may need to use another birth-control method until next period, then resume norgestrel.

**What drug does:**
- Creates a uterine lining similar to pregnancy that prevents bleeding.
- Suppresses a pituitary gland hormone responsible for ovulation.
- Stimulates cervical mucus, which stops sperm penetration and prevents pregnancy.

**Time lapse before drug works:**
3 weeks. Use another method of birth control until then.

**Don't take with:**
See Interaction column and consult doctor.

## OVERDOSE

**SYMPTOMS:**
Nausea, vomiting, fluid retention, breast discomfort or enlargement, vaginal bleeding.
**WHAT TO DO:**
Overdose unlikely to threaten life. If person takes much larger amount than prescribed, call doctor, poison-control center or hospital emergency room for instructions.

## POSSIBLE ADVERSE REACTIONS OR SIDE EFFECTS

| SYMPTOMS | WHAT TO DO |
|---|---|
| **Life-threatening:** Blood clot in leg, brain or lung. | Seek emergency treatment immediately. |
| **Common:** Appetite or weight changes, swollen ankles or feet, unusual tiredness or weakness. | Continue. Tell doctor at next visit. |
| **Infrequent:** | |
| • Prolonged vaginal bleeding. | Discontinue. Call doctor right away. |
| • Depression. | Continue. Call doctor when convenient. |
| • Acne, increased facial or body hair, nausea, breast tenderness. | Continue. Tell doctor at next visit. |
| **Rare:** Rash, stomach or side pain, jaundice. | Discontinue. Call doctor right away. |

## WARNINGS & PRECAUTIONS

**Don't take if:**
- You are allergic to any progestin hormone.
- You may be pregnant.
- You have liver or gallbladder disease.
- You have had thrombophlebitis, embolism or stroke.
- You have unexplained vaginal bleeding.
- You have had breast or uterine cancer.

**Before you start, consult your doctor:**
- If you have heart or kidney disease.
- If you have diabetes.
- If you have a seizure disorder.
- If you suffer migraines.
- If you are easily depressed.

**Over age 60:**
Not recommended.

**Pregnancy:**
May harm child. Discontinue at first sign of pregnancy.

**Breast feeding:**
Drug passes into milk. Avoid drug or discontinue nursing until you finish medicine. Consult doctor for advice on maintaining milk supply.

**Infants & children:**
Use only for female children under medical supervision.

**Prolonged use:**
No problems expected.

**Skin & sunlight:**
No problems expected.

**Driving, piloting or hazardous work:**
No problems expected.

**Discontinuing:**
Consult doctor. This medicine stays in the body and causes fetal abnormalities. Wait at least 3 months before becoming pregnant.

**Others:**
- Patients with diabetes must be monitored closely.
- Symptoms of blood clot in leg, brain or lung are: chest, groin, leg pain; sudden, severe headache; loss of coordination; vision change; shortness of breath; slurred speech.

## POSSIBLE INTERACTION WITH OTHER DRUGS

| GENERIC NAME OR DRUG CLASS | COMBINED EFFECT |
|---|---|
| Antihistamines | Decreased norgestrel effect. |
| Oxyphenbutazone | Decreased norgestrel effect. |
| Phenobarbital | Decreased norgestrel effect. |
| Phenothiazines | Increased phenothiazine effect. |
| Phenylbutazone | Decreased norgestrel effect. |

## POSSIBLE INTERACTION WITH OTHER SUBSTANCES

| INTERACTS WITH | COMBINED EFFECT |
|---|---|
| Alcohol: | None expected. |
| Beverages: | None expected. |
| Cocaine: | Decreased norgestrel effect. |
| Foods: Salt. | Fluid retention. |
| Marijuana: | Possible menstrual irregularities or bleeding between periods. |
| Tobacco: | Possible blood clots in lung, brain, legs. Avoid. |

# NYLIDRIN

## BRAND NAMES

| | |
|---|---|
| Arlidin | Pervadil |
| Arlidin Forte | PMS Nylidrin |
| Circlidrin | Rolidrin |

## BASIC INFORMATION

**Habit forming?** No
**Prescription needed?** Yes
**Available as generic?** Yes
**Drug class:** Vasodilator

 **USES**

- Improves poor circulation in extremities.
- Reduces dizziness caused by poor circulation in inner ear.

 **DOSAGE & USAGE INFORMATION**

**How to take:**
Tablet—Swallow with liquid or food to lessen stomach irritation. If you can't swallow whole, crumble tablet and take with liquid or food.

**When to take:**
At the same times each day.

**If you forget a dose:**
Take as soon as you remember up to 2 hours late. If more than 2 hours, wait for next scheduled dose (don't double this dose).

**What drug does:**
Stimulates nerves that dilate blood vessels, increasing oxygen and nutrients.

*Continued next column*

 **OVERDOSE**

**SYMPTOMS:**
**Blood-pressure drop; nausea, vomiting; rapid, irregular heartbeat, chest pain; blurred vision; metallic taste.**
**WHAT TO DO:**
- **Dial 0 (operator) or 911 (emergency) for an ambulance or medical help. Then give first aid immediately.**
- **If patient is unconscious and not breathing, give mouth-to-mouth breathing. If there is no heartbeat, use cardiac massage and mouth-to-mouth breathing (CPR). Don't try to make patient vomit. If you can't get help quickly, take patient to nearest emergency facility.**
- **See emergency information on inside covers.**

**Time lapse before drug works:**
10 to 30 minutes.

**Don't take with:**
See Interaction column and consult doctor.

 **POSSIBLE ADVERSE REACTIONS OR SIDE EFFECTS**

| SYMPTOMS | WHAT TO DO |
|---|---|
| **Life-threatening:**<br>None expected. | |
| **Common:** | |
| • Chest pain. | Discontinue. Call doctor right away. |
| • Blurred vision, fever, low blood pressure on standing, decreased or difficult urination. | Continue. Call doctor when convenient. |
| • Metallic taste. | Continue. Tell doctor at next visit. |
| **Infrequent:** | |
| • Rapid or irregular heartbeat. | Discontinue. Call doctor right away. |
| • Dizziness, weakness, tiredness. | Continue. Call doctor when convenient. |
| **Rare:** | |
| • Shakiness, chills. | Discontinue. Call doctor right away. |
| • Headache, flushed face, nausea, vomiting, nervousness. | Continue. Call doctor when convenient. |

## WARNINGS & PRECAUTIONS

**Don't take if:**
- You are allergic to any vasodilator drugs.
- You have had a heart attack or stroke within 4 weeks.
- You have an active peptic ulcer.

**Before you start, consult your doctor:**
- If you have had heart disease, heart-rhythm disorders (especially rapid heartbeat), a stroke or poor circulation to the brain.
- If you have glaucoma.
- If you have an overactive thyroid gland.
- If you plan to become pregnant within medication period.
- If you use tobacco.

**Over age 60:**
Adverse reactions and side effects may be more frequent and severe than in younger persons.

**Pregnancy:**
No proven harm to unborn child. Avoid if possible.

**Breast-feeding:**
No proven problems. Consult doctor.

**Infants & children:**
Not recommended.

**Prolonged use:**
No problems expected.

**Skin & sunlight:**
No problems expected.

**Driving, piloting or hazardous work:**
Don't drive or pilot aircraft until you learn how medicine affects you. Don't work around dangerous machinery. Don't climb ladders or work in high places. Danger increases if you drink alcohol or take medicine affecting alertness and reflexes, such as antihistamines, tranquilizers, sedatives, pain medicine, narcotics and mind-altering drugs.

**Discontinuing:**
Don't discontinue without consulting doctor. If your condition worsens, contact your doctor immediately. Dose may require gradual reduction if you have taken drug for a long time. Doses of other drugs may also require adjustment.

**Others:**
No problems expected.

## POSSIBLE INTERACTION WITH OTHER DRUGS

| GENERIC NAME OR DRUG CLASS | COMBINED EFFECT |
| --- | --- |
| Beta-adrenergic blockers | Decreased effect of nylidrin. |
| Phenothiazines | Increased blood level of phenothiazines. |

## POSSIBLE INTERACTION WITH OTHER SUBSTANCES

| INTERACTS WITH | COMBINED EFFECT |
| --- | --- |
| Alcohol: | Possible increased stomach-acid secretion. Use with caution. |
| Beverages: | None expected. |
| Cocaine: | Increased adverse effects of nylidrin. |
| Foods: | None expected. |
| Marijuana: | None expected. |
| Tobacco: | Decreased nylidrin effect. Worsens circulation. Avoid. |

# NYSTATIN

## BRAND NAMES

| | |
|---|---|
| Achrostatin V | Mytrex |
| Candex | Nadostine |
| Declostatin | Nilstat |
| Korostatin | Nyaderm |
| Mycolog | Nystaform |
| Mycostatin | Nystex |
| Myco-Triacet | O-V statin |
| Mykinac | Terrastatin |

## BASIC INFORMATION

**Habit forming? No**
**Prescription needed? Yes**
**Available as generic? Yes**
**Drug class: Antifungal**

## USES

Treatment of fungus infections susceptible to nystatin.

## DOSAGE & USAGE INFORMATION

**How to take:**
- Tablet or capsule—Swallow with liquid. If you can't swallow whole, crumble tablet or open capsule and take with liquid or food.
- Suppositories—Remove wrapper and moisten suppository with water. Gently insert larger end into vagina. Push well into vagina with finger.
- Ointment, cream or lotion—Use as directed by doctor and label.
- Liquid—Take as directed. Instruction varies by preparation.

**When to take:**
At the same time each day.

**If you forget a dose:**
Take as soon as you remember up to 2 hours late. If more than 2 hours, wait for next scheduled dose (don't double this dose).

*Continued next column*

## OVERDOSE

**SYMPTOMS:**
**Mild overdose may cause nausea, vomiting, diarrhea.**
**WHAT TO DO:**
**Overdose unlikely to threaten life. If person takes much larger amount than prescribed, call doctor, poison-control center or hospital emergency room for instructions.**

**What drug does:**
Prevents growth and reproduction of fungus.

**Time lapse before drug works:**
Begins immediately. May require 3 weeks for maximum benefit, depending on location and severity of infection.

**Don't take with:**
See Interaction column and consult doctor.

## POSSIBLE ADVERSE REACTIONS OR SIDE EFFECTS

| SYMPTOMS | WHAT TO DO |
|---|---|
| **Life-threatening:**<br>None expected. | |
| **Common:**<br>(at high doses)<br>Nausea, stomach pain, vomiting, diarrhea. | Discontinue. Call doctor right away. |
| **Infrequent:**<br>Mild irritation, itch at application site. | Discontinue. Call doctor right away. |
| **Rare:**<br>None expected. | |

## WARNINGS & PRECAUTIONS

**Don't take if:**
You are allergic to nystatin.

**Before you start, consult your doctor:**
If you plan to become pregnant within medication period.

**Over age 60:**
No problems expected.

**Pregnancy:**
No proven harm to unborn child. Avoid if possible.

**Breast-feeding:**
No proven problems. Consult doctor.

**Infants & children:**
No problems expected.

**Prolonged use:**
No problems expected.

**Skin & sunlight:**
No problems expected.

**Driving, piloting or hazardous work:**
No problems expected.

**Discontinuing:**
Don't discontinue without doctor's advice until you complete prescribed dose, even though symptoms diminish or disappear.

**Others:**
No problems expected.

## POSSIBLE INTERACTION WITH OTHER DRUGS

| GENERIC NAME OR DRUG CLASS | COMBINED EFFECT |
|---|---|
| None | |

## POSSIBLE INTERACTION WITH OTHER SUBSTANCES

| INTERACTS WITH | COMBINED EFFECT |
|---|---|
| Alcohol: | None expected. |
| Beverages: | None expected. |
| Cocaine: | None expected. |
| Foods: | None expected. |
| Marijuana: | None expected. |
| Tobacco: | None expected. |

# ORPHENADRINE

## BRAND NAMES

| | |
|---|---|
| Banflex | Neocyten |
| Disipal | Norflex |
| Flexoject | O-Flex |
| Flexon | Orflagen |
| K-Flex | Orphenate |
| Marflex | Ro-Orphena |
| Myolin | Tega-Flex |
| Myotrol | X-Otag |

## BASIC INFORMATION

**Habit forming? No**
**Prescription needed?**
  **U.S.: Yes**
  **Canada: No**
**Available as generic? Yes**
**Drug class: Muscle relaxant, anticholinergic, antihistamine, antiparkinsonism**

## USES

* Reduces muscle-strain discomfort.
* Relieves symptoms of Parkinson's disease.

## DOSAGE & USAGE INFORMATION

**How to take:**
Tablet—Swallow with liquid. If you can't swallow whole, crumble tablet and take with liquid or food.

**When to take:**
At the same times each day.

**If you forget a dose:**
Take as soon as you remember up to 6 hours late. If more than 6 hours, wait for next scheduled dose (don't double this dose).

**What drug does:**
Sedative and analgesic effects reduce spasm and pain in skeletal muscles.

*Continued next column*

## OVERDOSE

**SYMPTOMS:**
**Fainting, confusion, widely dilated pupils, rapid pulse, convulsions, coma.**
**WHAT TO DO:**
* **Dial 0 (operator) or 911 (emergency) for an ambulance or medical help. Then give first aid immediately.**
* **See emergency information on inside covers.**

**Time lapse before drug works:**
1 to 2 hours.

**Don't take with:**
See Interaction column and consult doctor.

## POSSIBLE ADVERSE REACTIONS OR SIDE EFFECTS

| SYMPTOMS | WHAT TO DO |
|---|---|
| **Life-threatening:** None expected. | |
| **Common:** None expected. | |
| **Infrequent:** | |
| • Weakness, headache, dizziness, drowsiness, agitation, tremor, confusion, rapid or pounding heartbeat. | Discontinue. Call doctor right away. |
| • Dry mouth, nausea, vomiting, constipation, urinary hesitancy or retention. | Continue. Call doctor when convenient. |
| **Rare:** Rash, itchy skin, blurred vision, dilated pupils. | Discontinue. Call doctor right away. |

## WARNINGS & PRECAUTIONS

**Don't take if:**
You are allergic to orphenadrine.

**Before you start, consult your doctor:**
- If you have glaucoma.
- If you have myasthenia gravis.
- If you have difficulty emptying bladder.
- If you have had heart disease or heart-rhythm disturbance.
- If you have had a peptic ulcer.

**Over age 60:**
Adverse reactions and side effects may be more frequent and severe than in younger persons.

**Pregnancy:**
No proven harm to unborn child. Avoid if possible.

**Breast-feeding:**
No proven problems. Consult doctor.

**Infants & children:**
Not recommended for children younger than 12.

**Prolonged use:**
Increased internal-eye pressure.

**Skin & sunlight:**
No problems expected.

**Driving, piloting or hazardous work:**
Don't drive or pilot aircraft until you learn how medicine affects you. Don't work around dangerous machinery. Don't climb ladders or work in high places. Danger increases if you drink alcohol or take medicine affecting alertness and reflexes, such as antihistamines, tranquilizers, sedatives, pain medicine, narcotics and mind-altering drugs.

**Discontinuing:**
May be unnecessary to finish medicine. Follow doctor's instructions.

**Others:**
No problems expected.

## POSSIBLE INTERACTION WITH OTHER DRUGS

| GENERIC NAME OR DRUG CLASS | COMBINED EFFECT |
|---|---|
| Anticholinergics | Increased anticholinergic effect. |
| Antidepressants (tricyclic) | Increased sedation. |
| Chlorpromazine | Hypoglycemia (low blood sugar). |
| Griseofulvin | Decreased griseofulvin effect. |
| Levodopa | Increased effect of levodopa. (Improves effectiveness in treating Parkinson's disease.) |
| Nitrates | Increased internal-eye pressure. |
| Phenylbutazone | Decreased phenylbutazone effect. |
| Potassium supplements | Increased possibility of intestinal ulcers with oral potassium tablets. |
| Propoxyphene | Possible confusion, nervousness, tremors. |
| Terfenadine | Possible increased orphenadrine effect. |

## POSSIBLE INTERACTION WITH OTHER SUBSTANCES

| INTERACTS WITH | COMBINED EFFECT |
|---|---|
| Alcohol: | Increased drowsiness. Avoid. |
| Beverages: | None expected. |
| Cocaine: | Decreased orphenadrine effect. Avoid. |
| Foods: | None expected. |
| Marijuana: | Increased drowsiness, mouth dryness, muscle weakness, fainting. |
| Tobacco: | None expected. |

# ORPHENADRINE, ASPIRIN & CAFFEINE

## BRAND NAMES

Back-Ese      Norgesic Forte
Norgesic

## BASIC INFORMATION

**Habit forming? Yes**
**Prescription needed? Yes**
**Available as generic? No**
**Drug class: Stimulant, vasoconstrictor, muscle relaxant, analgesic, anti-inflammatory**

## USES

- Reduces muscle-strain discomfort.
- Reduces pain, fever, inflammation.
- Relieves swelling, stiffness, joint pain.
- Treatment for drowsiness and fatigue.

## DOSAGE & USAGE INFORMATION

**How to take:**
Tablet or capsule—Swallow with liquid. If you can't swallow whole, crumble tablet or open capsule and take with liquid or food.

**When to take:**
At the same times each day.

**If you forget a dose:**
Take as soon as you remember up to 2 hours late. If more than 2 hours, wait for next scheduled dose (don't double this dose).

**What drug does:**
- Sedative and analgesic effects reduce spasm and pain in skeletal muscles.
- Affects hypothalamus, the part of the brain which regulates temperature by dilating small blood vessels in skin.
- Prevents clumping of platelets (small blood cells) so blood vessels remain open.

*Continued next column*

## OVERDOSE

**SYMPTOMS:**
**Fainting, confusion, widely dilated pupils, rapid pulse, ringing in ears, nausea, vomiting, dizziness, fever, deep and rapid breathing, excitement, rapid heartbeat, hallucinations, coma.**
**WHAT TO DO:**
- **Dial 0 (operator) or 911 (emergency) for an ambulance or medical help. Then give first aid immediately.**
- **See emergency information on inside covers.**

- Decreases prostaglandin effect.
- Suppresses body's pain messages.
- Constricts blood-vessel walls.
- Stimulates central nervous system.

**Time lapse before drug works:**
1 hour.

**Don't take with:**
- Tetracyclines. Space doses 1 hour apart.
- Non-prescription drugs without consulting doctor.
- See Interaction column and consult doctor.

## POSSIBLE ADVERSE REACTIONS OR SIDE EFFECTS

| SYMPTOMS | WHAT TO DO |
|---|---|
| **Life-threatening:** | |
| Hives, rash, intense itching, faintness soon after a dose (anaphylaxis). | Seek emergency treatment immediately. |
| **Common:** | |
| • Nausea, vomiting, abdominal cramps, nervousness, urgent urination, low blood sugar (hunger, anxiety, cold sweats, rapid pulse). | Discontinue. Call doctor right away. |
| • Ringing in ears, heartburn, indigestion, insomnia. | Continue. Call doctor when convenient. |
| **Infrequent:** | |
| • Weakness, headache, dizziness, drowsiness, agitation, tremor, confusion, irregular heartbeat. | Discontinue. Call doctor right away. |
| • Dry mouth, constipation. | Continue. Call doctor when convenient. |
| **Rare:** | |
| • Black or bloody vomit. | Discontinue. Seek emergency treatment. |
| • Change in vision; blurred vision; black, bloody or tarry stool; bloody urine; jaundice; dilated pupils. | Discontinue. Call doctor right away. |
| • Drowsiness. | Continue. Call doctor when convenient. |

## WARNINGS & PRECAUTIONS

**Don't take if:**
- You need to restrict sodium in your diet. Buffered effervescent tablets and sodium salicylate are high in sodium.

- Aspirin has a strong vinegar-like odor, which means it has decomposed.
- You have a peptic ulcer of stomach or duodenum, a bleeding disorder, heart disease.
- You are allergic to any stimulant or orphenadrine.

## Before you start, consult your doctor:
- If you have had stomach or duodenal ulcers, gout, heart disease or heart-rhythm disturbance, peptic ulcer.
- If you have asthma, nasal polyps, irregular heartbeat, hypoglycemia (low blood sugar), epilepsy, glaucoma, myasthenia gravis, difficulty emptying bladder.

## Over age 60:
- More likely to cause hidden bleeding in stomach or intestines. Watch for dark stools.
- Adverse reactions and side effects may be more frequent and severe than in younger persons.

## Pregnancy:
Risk to unborn child outweighs drug benefits. Don't use.

## Breast-feeding:
Drug passes into milk. Avoid drug or discontinue nursing until you finish medicine. Consult doctor for advice on maintaining milk supply.

## Infants & children:
- Overdose frequent and severe. Keep bottles out of children's reach.
- Consult doctor before giving to persons under age 18 who have fever and discomfort of viral illness, especially chicken pox and influenza. Probably increases risk of Reye's syndrome.
- Not recommended for children younger than 12.

## Prolonged use:
- Kidney damage. Periodic kidney-function test recommended.
- Stomach ulcers more likely.
- Increased internal-eye pressure.

## Skin & sunlight:
Aspirin combined with sunscreen may decrease sunburn.

## Driving, piloting or hazardous work:
Don't drive or pilot aircraft until you learn how medicine affects you. Don't work around dangerous machinery. Don't climb ladders or work in high places. Danger increases if you drink alcohol or take medicine affecting alertness and reflexes, such as antihistamines, tranquilizers, sedatives, pain medicine, narcotics and mind-altering drugs.

## Discontinuing:
- For chronic illness—Don't discontinue without doctor's advice until you complete prescribed dose, even though symptoms diminish or disappear.
- May be unnecessary to finish medicine if you take it for a short-term illness. Follow doctor's instructions.

## Others:
- Aspirin can complicate surgery, pregnancy, labor and delivery, and illness.
- For arthritis—Don't change dose without consulting doctor.
- Urine tests for blood sugar may be inaccurate.
- May produce or aggravate fibrocystic breast disease in women.

## POSSIBLE INTERACTION WITH OTHER DRUGS

| GENERIC NAME OR DRUG CLASS | COMBINED EFFECT |
|---|---|
| Acebutolol | Decreased antihypertensive effect of acebutolol. |
| Allopurinol | Decreased allopurinol effect. |
| Antacids | Decreased aspirin effect. |
| Anticholinergics | Increased anticholinergic effect. |
| Anticoagulants | Increased anticoagulant effect. Abnormal bleeding. |

*Continued page 969*

## POSSIBLE INTERACTION WITH OTHER SUBSTANCES

| INTERACTS WITH | COMBINED EFFECT |
|---|---|
| Alcohol: | Possible stomach irritation and bleeding, increased drowsiness. Avoid. |
| Beverages: Caffeine drinks. | Increased caffeine effect. |
| Cocaine: | Decreased orphenadrine effect. Overstimulation. Avoid. |
| Foods: | No proven problems. |
| Marijuana: | Increased effect of drugs. May lead to dangerous, rapid heartbeat. Increased dry mouth. Avoid. |
| Tobacco: | Increased heartbeat. Avoid. |

# OXACILLIN

## BRAND NAMES

Bactocill                    Prostaphlin

## BASIC INFORMATION

**Habit forming? No**
**Prescription needed? Yes**
**Available as generic? Yes**
**Drug class: Antibiotic (penicillin)**

## USES

Treatment of bacterial infections that are susceptible to oxacillin.

## DOSAGE & USAGE INFORMATION

**How to take:**
- Tablets or capsules—Swallow with liquid on an empty stomach 1 hour before or 2 hours after eating.
- Liquid—Take with cold beverage. Liquid form is perishable and effective for only 7 days at room temperature. Effective for 14 days if stored in refrigerator. Don't freeze.

**When to take:**
Follow instructions on prescription label or side of package. Doses should be evenly spaced. For example, 4 times a day means every 6 hours.

**If you forget a dose:**
Take as soon as you remember. Continue regular schedule.

**What drug does:**
Destroys susceptible bacteria. Does not kill viruses.

**Time lapse before drug works:**
May be several days before medicine affects infection.

**Don't take with:**
See Interaction column and consult doctor.

## OVERDOSE

**SYMPTOMS:**
**Severe diarrhea, nausea or vomiting.**
**WHAT TO DO:**
**Overdose unlikely to threaten life. If person takes much larger amount than prescribed, call doctor, poison-control center or hospital emergency room for instructions.**

## POSSIBLE ADVERSE REACTIONS OR SIDE EFFECTS

| SYMPTOMS | WHAT TO DO |
|---|---|
| **Life-threatening:** Hives, rash, intense itching, faintness soon after a dose (anaphylaxis). | Seek emergency treatment immediately. |
| **Common:** Dark or discolored tongue. | Continue. Tell doctor at next visit. |
| **Infrequent:** Mild nausea, vomiting, diarrhea. | Continue. Call doctor when convenient. |
| **Rare:** Unexplained bleeding. | Discontinue. Call doctor right away. |

## WARNINGS & PRECAUTIONS

**Don't take if:**
You are allergic to oxacillin, cephalosporin antibiotics, other penicillins or penicillamine. Life-threatening reaction may occur.

**Before you start, consult your doctor:**
If you are allergic to any substance or drug.

**Over age 60:**
You may have skin reactions, particularly around genitals and anus.

**Pregnancy:**
Studies inconclusive on harm to unborn child. Animal studies show fetal abnormalities. Decide with your doctor whether drug benefits justify risk to unborn child.

**Breast-feeding:**
Drug passes into milk. Child may become sensitive to penicillins and have allergic reactions to penicillin drugs. Avoid oxacillin or discontinue nursing until you finish medicine. Consult doctor for advice on maintaining milk supply.

**Infants & children:**
No problems expected.

**Prolonged use:**
You may become more susceptible to infections caused by germs not responsive to oxacillin.

**Skin & sunlight:**
No problems expected.

**Driving, piloting or hazardous work:**
Usually not dangerous. Most hazardous reactions likely to occur a few minutes after taking oxacillin.

**Discontinuing:**
Don't discontinue without doctor's advice until you complete prescribed dose, even though symptoms diminish or disappear.

**Others:**
No problems expected.

## POSSIBLE INTERACTION WITH OTHER DRUGS

| GENERIC NAME OR DRUG CLASS | COMBINED EFFECT |
|---|---|
| Beta-adrenergic blockers | Increased chance of anaphylaxis (see emergency information on inside front cover). |
| Chloramphenicol | Decreased effect of both drugs. |
| Erythromycins | Decreased effect of both drugs. |
| Loperamide | Decreased oxacillin effect. |
| Paromomycin | Decreased effect of both drugs. |
| Tetracyclines | Decreased effect of both drugs. |
| Troleandomycin | Decreased effect of both drugs. |

## POSSIBLE INTERACTION WITH OTHER SUBSTANCES

| INTERACTS WITH | COMBINED EFFECT |
|---|---|
| Alcohol: | Occasional stomach irritation. |
| Beverages: | None expected. |
| Cocaine: | No proven problems. |
| Foods: | None expected. |
| Marijuana: | No proven problems. |
| Tobacco: | None expected. |

# OXAZEPAM

## BRAND NAMES

| | |
|---|---|
| Apo-Oxazepam | Serax |
| Ox-Pam | Zapex |

## BASIC INFORMATION

**Habit forming? Yes**
**Prescription needed? Yes**
**Available as generic? No**
**Drug class: Tranquilizer (benzodiazepine)**

 USES

Treatment for nervousness or tension.

 DOSAGE & USAGE INFORMATION

**How to take:**
Tablet or capsule—Swallow with liquid. If you
can't swallow whole, crumble tablet or open
capsule and take with liquid or food.

**When to take:**
At the same time each day, according to
instructions on prescription label.

**If you forget a dose:**
Take as soon as you remember up to 2 hours
late. If more than 2 hours, wait for next
scheduled dose (don't double this dose).

**What drug does:**
Affects limbic system of brain—part that
controls emotions.

**Time lapse before drug works:**
2 hours. May take 6 weeks for full benefit.

**Don't take with:**
See Interaction column and consult doctor.

 OVERDOSE

**SYMPTOMS:**
**Drowsiness, weakness, tremor, stupor,**
**coma.**
**WHAT TO DO:**
- **Dial 0 (operator) or 911 (emergency) for an**
  **ambulance or medical help. Then give first**
  **aid immediately.**
- **If patient is unconscious and not**
  **breathing, give mouth-to-mouth breathing.**
  **If there is no heartbeat, use cardiac**
  **massage and mouth-to-mouth breathing**
  **(CPR). Don't try to make patient vomit. If**
  **you can't get help quickly, take patient to**
  **nearest emergency facility.**
- **See emergency information on inside**
  **covers.**

 POSSIBLE ADVERSE REACTIONS OR SIDE EFFECTS

| SYMPTOMS | WHAT TO DO |
|---|---|
| **Life-threatening:** None expected. | |
| **Common:** Clumsiness, drowsiness, dizziness. | Continue. Call doctor when convenient. |
| **Infrequent:** | |
| • Hallucinations, confusion, depression, irritability, rash, itchy skin, change in vision. | Discontinue. Call doctor right away. |
| • Constipation or diarrhea, nausea, vomiting, difficult urination. | Continue. Call doctor when convenient. |
| **Rare:** | |
| • Slow heartbeat, difficult breathing. | Discontinue. Seek emergency treatment. |
| • Mouth, throat ulcers; jaundice. | Discontinue. Call doctor right away. |

## WARNINGS & PRECAUTIONS

### Don't take if:
- You are allergic to any benzodiazepine.
- You have myasthenia gravis.
- You are active or recovering alcoholic.
- Patient is younger than 6 months.

### Before you start, consult your doctor:
- If you have liver, kidney or lung disease.
- If you have diabetes, epilepsy or porphyria.

### Over age 60:
Adverse reactions and side effects may be more frequent and severe than in younger persons. You need smaller doses for shorter periods of time. May develop agitation, rage or "hangover" effect.

### Pregnancy:
Risk to unborn child outweighs drug benefits. Don't use.

### Breast-feeding:
Drug passes into milk. Avoid drug or discontinue nursing until you finish medicine. Consult doctor for advice on maintaining milk supply.

### Infants & children:
Use only under medical supervision for children older than 6 months.

### Prolonged use:
May impair liver function.

### Skin & sunlight:
No problems expected.

### Driving, piloting or hazardous work:
Don't drive or pilot aircraft until you learn how medicine affects you. Don't work around dangerous machinery. Don't climb ladders or work in high places. Danger increases if you drink alcohol or take medicine affecting alertness and reflexes.

### Discontinuing:
Don't discontinue without consulting doctor. Dose may require gradual reduction if you have taken drug for a long time. Doses of other drugs may also require adjustment.

### Others:
- Hot weather, heavy exercise and profuse sweat may reduce excretion and cause overdose.
- Blood sugar may rise in diabetics, requiring insulin adjustment.

## POSSIBLE INTERACTION WITH OTHER DRUGS

| GENERIC NAME OR DRUG CLASS | COMBINED EFFECT |
| --- | --- |
| Anticonvulsants | Change in seizure frequency or severity. |
| Antidepressants | Increased sedative effect of both drugs. |
| Antihistamines | Increased sedative effect of both drugs. |
| Antihypertensives | Excessively low blood pressure. |
| Cimetidine | Excess sedation. |
| Disulfiram | Increased oxazepam effect. |
| Dronabinol | Increased effects of both drugs. Avoid. |
| MAO inhibitors | Convulsions, deep sedation, rage. |
| Molindone | Increased tranquilizer effect. |
| Narcotics | Increased sedative effect of both drugs. |
| Sedatives | Increased sedative effect of both drugs. |
| Sleep inducers | Increased sedative effect of both drugs. |
| Terfenadine | Possible oversedation. |
| Tranquilizers | Increased sedative effect of both drugs. |

## POSSIBLE INTERACTION WITH OTHER SUBSTANCES

| INTERACTS WITH | COMBINED EFFECT |
| --- | --- |
| Alcohol: | Heavy sedation. Avoid. |
| Beverages: | None expected. |
| Cocaine: | Decreased oxazepam effect. |
| Foods: | None expected. |
| Marijuana: | Heavy sedation. Avoid. |
| Tobacco: | Decreased oxazepam effect. |

# OXPRENOLOL

## BRAND NAMES

Slow-trasicor          Trasicor

## BASIC INFORMATION

Habit forming? No
Prescription needed? Yes
Available as generic? No
Drug class: Beta-adrenergic blocker

## USES

- Reduces frequency and severity of angina attacks.
- Stabilizes irregular heartbeat.
- Lowers blood pressure.
- Reduces frequency of migraine headaches. (Does not relieve headache pain.)

## DOSAGE & USAGE INFORMATION

**How to take:**
Tablet or capsule—Swallow with liquid. If you can't swallow whole, crumble tablet or open capsule and take with liquid or food.

**When to take:**
With meals or immediately after.

**If you forget a dose:**
Take as soon as you remember. Return to regular schedule, but allow 3 hours between doses.

**What drug does:**
- Blocks actions of sympathetic nervous system.
- Lowers heart's oxygen requirements.
- Slows nerve impulses through heart.
- Reduces blood-vessel contraction in several major organs and glands.

**Time lapse before drug works:**
1 to 4 hours.

*Continued next column*

## OVERDOSE

**SYMPTOMS:**
**Weakness, slow or weak pulse, blood-pressure drop, fainting, convulsions, cold and sweaty skin.**
**WHAT TO DO:**
- **Dial 0 (operator) or 911 (emergency) for an ambulance or medical help. Then give first aid immediately.**
- **See emergency information on inside covers.**

**Don't take with:**
Non-prescription drugs or drugs in interaction column without consulting doctor.

## POSSIBLE ADVERSE REACTIONS OR SIDE EFFECTS

| SYMPTOMS | WHAT TO DO |
|---|---|
| **Life-threatening:**<br>None expected. | |
| **Common:** | |
| • Pulse slower than 50 beats per minute. | Discontinue. Call doctor right away. |
| • Drowsiness, numbness or tingling of fingers or toes, dizziness, diarrhea, nausea, fatigue, weakness. | Continue. Call doctor when convenient. |
| • Dry skin, eyes or mouth; cold hands, feet. | Continue. Tell doctor at next visit. |
| **Infrequent:** | |
| • Hallucinations, nightmares, insomnia, headache, difficult breathing. | Discontinue. Call doctor right away. |
| • Confusion, depression, reduced alertness. | Continue. Call doctor when convenient. |
| • Constipation. | Continue. Tell doctor at next visit. |
| **Rare:** | |
| • Rash, sore throat, fever. | Discontinue. Call doctor right away. |
| • Unexplained bleeding or bruising. | Continue. Call doctor when convenient. |

## WARNINGS & PRECAUTIONS

**Don't take if:**
- You are allergic to any beta-adrenergic blocker.
- You have asthma.
- You have hay-fever symptoms.
- You have taken MAO inhibitors in past 2 weeks.

**Before you start, consult your doctor:**
- If you have heart disease or poor circulation to extremities.
- If you have hay fever, asthma, chronic bronchitis or emphysema.
- If you have overactive thyroid function.
- If you have impaired liver or kidney function.
- If you will have surgery within 2 months, including dental surgery, requiring general or spinal anesthesia.
- If you have diabetes or hypoglycemia.

**Over age 60:**
Adverse reactions and side effects may be more frequent and severe than in younger persons.

**Pregnancy:**
Risk to unborn child outweighs drug benefits. Don't use.

**Breast-feeding:**
Drug passes into milk. Avoid drug or discontinue nursing until you finish medicine. Consult doctor for advice on maintaining milk supply.

**Infants & children:**
Not recommended. Safety and dosage have not been established.

**Prolonged use:**
Weakens heart-muscle contractions.

**Skin & sunlight:**
No problems expected.

**Driving, piloting or hazardous work:**
Don't drive or pilot aircraft until you learn how medicine affects you. Don't work around dangerous machinery. Don't climb ladders or work in high places. Danger increases if you drink alcohol or take medicine affecting alertness and reflexes.

**Discontinuing:**
Don't discontinue without consulting doctor. Dose may require gradual reduction if you have taken drug for a long time. Doses of other drugs may also require adjustment.

**Others:**
May mask hypoglycemia.

## POSSIBLE INTERACTION WITH OTHER DRUGS

| GENERIC NAME OR DRUG CLASS | COMBINED EFFECT |
|---|---|
| Albuterol | Decreased albuterol effect and beta-adrenergic blocking effect. |
| Anesthetics used in surgery | Increased antihypertensive effect. |
| Antidiabetics | May make blood-sugar levels difficult to control. |
| Antihypertensives | Increased antihypertensive effect. |
| Anti-inflammatory drugs | Decreased antihypertensive effect of oxprenolol. |
| Calcium-channel blockers | May worsen congestive heart failure. |
| Clonidine | Possible blood-pressure rise once clonidine is discontinued. |
| Digitalis preparations | Increased **or** decreased heart rate. Improves irregular heartbeat. |
| Diuretics | Increased antihypertensive effect. |
| Ketoprofen | Decreased antihypertensive effect of oxprenolol |
| MAO inhibitors | Possible excessive blood-pressure rise once MAO inhibitor is discontinued. |
| Molindone | Increased tranquilizer effect. |
| Pentoxifylline | Increased antihypertensive effect. |
| Reserpine | Possible excessively low blood pressure and slow heartbeat. |
| Suprofen | Decreased antihypertensive effect of oxprenolol. |
| Sympathomimetics | Decreased effects of both drugs. |
| Timolol cyedrops | Possible increased oxprenolol effect. |
| Xanthine bronchodilators | Decreased effects of both drugs. |

## POSSIBLE INTERACTION WITH OTHER SUBSTANCES

| INTERACTS WITH | COMBINED EFFECT |
|---|---|
| Alcohol: | Excessive blood pressure drop. Avoid. |
| Beverages: | None expected. |
| Cocaine: | Irregular heartbeat. Avoid. |
| Foods: | None expected. |
| Marijuana: | Daily use—Impaired circulation to hands and feet. |
| Tobacco: | Possible irregular heartbeat. |

# OXTRIPHYLLINE & GUAIFENESIN

## BRAND NAMES

Brondecon          Brondelate

## BASIC INFORMATION

**Habit forming? No**
**Prescription needed? Yes**
**Available as generic? No**
**Drug class: Bronchodilator (xanthine),**
**          cough/cold preparation**

## USES

- Treatment for bronchial asthma symptoms.
- Loosens mucus in respiratory passages from allergies and infections.

## DOSAGE & USAGE INFORMATION

**How to take:**
Tablet or capsule—Swallow with liquid. If you can't swallow whole, crumble tablet or open capsule and take with liquid or food.

**When to take:**
Most effective taken on empty stomach 1 hour before or 2 hours after eating. However, may take with food to lessen stomach upset.

**If you forget a dose:**
Take as soon as you remember up to 2 hours late. If more than 2 hours, wait for next scheduled dose (don't double this dose).

**What drug does:**
- Relaxes and expands bronchial tubes.
- Increases production of watery fluids to thin mucus so it can be coughed out or absorbed.

**Time lapse before drug works:**
15 to 30 minutes.

**Don't take with:**
- Any stimulant.
- See Interaction column and consult doctor.

## OVERDOSE

**SYMPTOMS:**
**Restlessness, irritability, confusion, delirium, convulsions, rapid pulse, nausea, vomiting, coma.**
**WHAT TO DO:**
- **Dial 0 (operator) or 911 (emergency) for an ambulance or medical help. Then give first aid immediately.**
- **See emergency information on inside covers.**

## POSSIBLE ADVERSE REACTIONS OR SIDE EFFECTS

| SYMPTOMS | WHAT TO DO |
|---|---|
| **Life-threatening:** Difficult breathing, irregular or fast heartbeat. | Discontinue. Seek emergency treatment. |
| **Common:** Headache, irritability, nervousness, restlessness, insomnia, nausea, vomiting, abdominal pain, drowsiness. | Continue. Call doctor when convenient. |
| **Infrequent:** <br>• Hives, rash, red or flushed face, diarrhea. | Discontinue. Call doctor right away. |
| • Dizziness, lightheadedness, appetite loss. | Continue. Call doctor when convenient. |
| **Rare:** None expected. | |

## WARNINGS & PRECAUTIONS

**Don't take if:**
- You are allergic to any cough or cold preparation containing guaifenesin or any bronchodilator.
- You have an active peptic ulcer.

**Before you start, consult your doctor:**
- If you have had impaired kidney or liver function.
- If you gastritis, peptic ulcer, high blood pressure or heart disease.
- If you take medication for gout.

**Over age 60:**
Adverse reactions and side effects may be more frequent and severe than in younger persons. For drug to work, you must drink 8 to 10 glasses of fluid per day.

**Pregnancy:**
Risk to unborn child outweighs drug benefits. Don't use.

**Breast-feeding:**
Drug passes into milk. Avoid drug or discontinue nursing until you finish medicine. Consult doctor for advice on maintaining milk supply.

**Infants & children:**
Use only under medical supervision.

**Prolonged use:**
Stomach irritation.

**Skin & sunlight:**
No problems expected.

**Driving, piloting or hazardous work:**
Avoid if lightheaded or dizzy. Otherwise, no problems expected.

**Discontinuing:**
May be unnecessary to finish medicine. Follow doctor's instructions.

**Others:**
No problems expected.

## POSSIBLE INTERACTION WITH OTHER DRUGS

| GENERIC NAME OR DRUG CLASS | COMBINED EFFECT |
| --- | --- |
| Allopurinol | Decreased allopurinol effect. |
| Anticoagulants | Risk of bleeding. |
| Ephedrine | Increased effect of both drugs. |
| Epinephrine | Increased effect of both drugs. |
| Erythromycin | Increased bronchodilator effect. |
| Furosemide | Increased furosemide effect. |
| Lincomycins | Increased bronchodilator effect. |
| Lithium | Decreased lithium effect. |
| Probenecid | Decreased effect of both drugs. |
| Propranolol | Decreased bronchodilator effect. |
| Rauwolfia alkaloids | Rapid heartbeat. |
| Sulfinpyrazone | Decreased sulfinpyrazone effect. |
| Troleandomycin | Increased bronchodilator effect. |

## POSSIBLE INTERACTION WITH OTHER SUBSTANCES

| INTERACTS WITH | COMBINED EFFECT |
| --- | --- |
| Alcohol: | None expected. |
| Beverages: Caffeine drinks. | Nervousness and insomnia. You must drink 8 to 10 glasses of fluid per day for drug to work. |
| Cocaine: | Excess stimulation. Avoid. |
| Foods: | None expected. |
| Marijuana: | Slightly increased antiasthmatic effect of bronchodilator. |
| Tobacco: | Decreased bronchodilator effect and harmful for all conditions requiring bronchodilator treatment. Avoid. |

# OXYMETAZOLINE

## BRAND NAMES

See complete list of brand names in the *Brand Name Directory,* page 953.

## BASIC INFORMATION

**Habit forming? No**
**Prescription needed? No**
**Available as generic? Yes**
**Drug class: Sympathomimetic**

## USES

Relieves congestion of nose, sinuses and throat from allergies and infections.

## DOSAGE & USAGE INFORMATION

**How to take:**
Nasal solution, nasal spray—Use as directed on label. Avoid contamination. Don't use same container for more than 1 person.

**When to take:**
When needed, no more often than every 4 hours.

**If you forget a dose:**
Take as soon as you remember. Wait 4 hours for next dose.

**What drug does:**
Constricts walls of small arteries in nose, sinuses and eustachian tubes.

**Time lapse before drug works:**
5 to 30 minutes.

*Continued next column*

## OVERDOSE

**SYMPTOMS:**
**Headache, sweating, anxiety, agitation, rapid and irregular heartbeat.**
**WHAT TO DO:**
- **Dial 0 (operator) or 911 (emergency) for an ambulance or medical help. Then give first aid immediately.**
- **If patient is unconscious and not breathing, give mouth-to-mouth breathing. If there is no heartbeat, use cardiac massage and mouth-to-mouth breathing (CPR). If you can't get help quickly, take patient to nearest emergency facility.**
- **See emergency information on inside covers.**

**Don't take with:**
- Non-prescription drugs for allergy, cough or cold without consulting doctor.
- See Interaction column and consult doctor.

## POSSIBLE ADVERSE REACTIONS OR SIDE EFFECTS

| SYMPTOMS | WHAT TO DO |
|---|---|
| **Life-threatening:**<br>None expected. | |
| **Common:**<br>Runny, stuffy, burning, dry or stinging nose; sneezing; fast, irregular or pounding heartbeat. | Continue. Call doctor when convenient. |
| **Infrequent:**<br>Headache or lightheadedness, insomnia, nervousness. | Continue. Call doctor when convenient. |
| **Rare:**<br>None expected. | |

## WARNINGS & PRECAUTIONS

**Don't take if:**
You are allergic to any sympathomimetic nasal spray.

**Before you start, consult your doctor:**
- If you have heart disease or high blood pressure.
- If you have diabetes.
- If you have overactive thyroid.
- If you have taken MAO inhibitors in past 2 weeks.

**Over age 60:**
Adverse reactions and side effects may be more frequent and severe than in younger persons.

**Pregnancy:**
No proven harm to unborn child. Avoid if possible.

**Breast-feeding:**
No proven problems. Consult doctor.

**Infants & children:**
Don't give to children younger than 2.

**Prolonged use:**
Drug may lose effectiveness, cause increased congestion ("rebound effect," see Glossary) and irritate nasal membranes.

**Skin & sunlight:**
No problems expected.

**Driving, piloting or hazardous work:**
No problems expected.

**Discontinuing:**
May be unnecessary to finish medicine. Follow doctor's instructions.

**Others:**
No problems expected.

## POSSIBLE INTERACTION WITH OTHER DRUGS

| GENERIC NAME OR DRUG CLASS | COMBINED EFFECT |
|---|---|
| Acebutolol | Decreased effects of both drugs. |
| Antidepressants (tricyclics) | Increased oxymetazoline effect. |
| MAO inhibitors | Dangerous blood-pressure rise. |
| Minoxidil | Decreased minoxidil effect. |
| Nitrates | Possible decreased effects of both drugs. |
| Oxprenolol | Decreased effects of both drugs. |
| Sympathomimetics | Increased effect of both drugs, especially harmful side effects. |

## POSSIBLE INTERACTION WITH OTHER SUBSTANCES

| INTERACTS WITH | COMBINED EFFECT |
|---|---|
| Alcohol: | None expected. |
| Beverages: Caffeine drinks. | Nervousness or insomnia. |
| Cocaine: | Overstimulation. Avoid. |
| Foods: | None expected. |
| Marijuana: | Overstimulation. Avoid. |
| Tobacco: | None expected. |

# OXYPHENBUTAZONE

## BRAND NAMES

Oxalid          Tandearil
Oxybutazone

## BASIC INFORMATION

**Habit forming? No**
**Prescription needed? Yes**
**Available as generic? Yes**
**Drug class: Anti-inflammatory (non-steroid)**

## USES

- Treatment for joint pain, stiffness, inflammation and swelling of arthritis and gout.
- Pain reliever.
- Treatment for dysmenorrhea (painful or difficult menstruation).

## DOSAGE & USAGE INFORMATION

**How to take:**
Tablet or capsule—Swallow with liquid or food to lessen stomach irritation. If you can't swallow whole, crumble tablet or open capsule and take with liquid or food.

**When to take:**
At the same times each day.

**If you forget a dose:**
Take as soon as you remember up to 2 hours late. If more than 2 hours, wait for next scheduled dose (don't double this dose).

**What drug does:**
Reduces tissue concentration of prostaglandins (hormones which produce inflammation and pain).

**Time lapse before drug works:**
Begins in 4 to 24 hours. May require 3 weeks regular use for maximum benefit.

*Continued next column*

## OVERDOSE

**SYMPTOMS:**
**Confusion, agitation, incoherence, convulsions, possible hemorrhage from stomach or intestine, coma.**
**WHAT TO DO:**
- **Dial 0 (operator) or 911 (emergency) for an ambulance or medical help. Then give first aid immediately.**
- **See emergency information on inside covers.**

**Don't take with:**
See Interaction column and consult doctor.

## POSSIBLE ADVERSE REACTIONS OR SIDE EFFECTS

| SYMPTOMS | WHAT TO DO |
|---|---|
| **Life-threatening:** None expected. | |
| **Common:** | |
| • Dizziness, stomach upset. | Continue. Call doctor when convenient. |
| • Headache. | Continue. Tell doctor at next visit. |
| **Infrequent:** Depression, drowsiness, ringing in ears, constipation or diarrhea, vomiting, swollen feet or legs. | Continue. Call doctor when convenient. |
| **Rare:** | |
| • Convulsions; confusion; rash, hives or itchy skin; blurred vision; sore throat, fever, mouth ulcers; black stools; vomiting blood; difficult breathing; tightness in chest; unusual bleeding or bruising; blood in urine. | Discontinue. Call doctor right away. |
| • Urgent, frequent, painful or difficult urination; fatigue, weakness; weight gain. | Continue. Call doctor when convenient. |

## WARNINGS & PRECAUTIONS

**Don't take if:**
- You are allergic to aspirin or any non-steroid, anti-inflammatory drug.
- You have gastritis, peptic ulcer, enteritis, ileitis, ulcerative colitis.
- Patient is younger than 15.

**Before you start, consult your doctor:**
- If you have epilepsy.
- If you have Parkinson's disease.
- If you have been mentally ill.
- If you have had kidney disease or impaired kidney function, asthma, high blood pressure, heart failure, temporal arthritis, or polymyalgia rheumatica.

**Over age 60:**
Adverse reactions and side effects may be more frequent and severe than in younger persons.

**Pregnancy:**
Studies inconclusive on harm to unborn child. Animal studies show fetal abnormalities. Decide with your doctor whether drug benefits justify risk to unborn child.

**Breast-feeding:**
Drug filters into milk. May harm child. Avoid.

**Infants & children:**
Not recommended for those younger than 15. Use only under medical supervision.

**Prolonged use:**
- Eye damage.
- May cause rare bone-marrow damage, jaundice, reduced hearing.
- Periodic blood counts recommended if you use a long time.

**Skin & sunlight:**
No problems expected.

**Driving, piloting or hazardous work:**
Don't drive or pilot aircraft until you learn how medicine affects you. Don't work around dangerous machinery. Don't climb ladders or work in high places. Danger increases if you drink alcohol or take medicine affecting alertness and reflexes, such as antihistamines, tranquilizers, sedatives, pain medicine, narcotics and mind-altering drugs.

**Discontinuing:**
Don't discontinue without consulting doctor. Dose may require gradual reduction if you have taken drug for a long time. Doses of other drugs may also require adjustment.

**Others:**
No problems expected.

## POSSIBLE INTERACTION WITH OTHER DRUGS

| GENERIC NAME OR DRUG CLASS | COMBINED EFFECT |
|---|---|
| Acebutolol | Decreased antihypertensive effect of acebutolol. |
| Anticoagulants (oral) | Increased anticoagulant effect. |
| Antidiabetics (oral) | Increased antidiabetic effect. |
| Aspirin | Possible stomach ulcer. |
| Chloroquine | Possible skin toxicity. |
| Digitoxin | Decreased digitoxin effect. |
| Gold compounds | Possible increased likelihood of kidney damage. |
| Hydroxychloroquine | Possible skin toxicity. |
| Ketoprofen | Increased possibility of internal bleeding. |
| Methotrexate | Increased toxicity of both drugs to bone marrow. |
| Minoxidil | Decreased minoxidil effect. |
| Oxprenolol | Decreased antihypertensive effect of oxprenolol. |
| Penicillamine | Possible toxicity. |
| Phenytoin | Possible toxic phenytoin effect. |
| Trimethoprim | Possible bone-marrow toxicity. |

## POSSIBLE INTERACTION WITH OTHER SUBSTANCES

| INTERACTS WITH | COMBINED EFFECT |
|---|---|
| Alcohol: | Possible stomach ulcer or bleeding. |
| Beverages: | None expected. |
| Cocaine: | None expected. |
| Foods: | None expected. |
| Marijuana: | Increased pain relief from oxyphenbutazone. |
| Tobacco: | None expected. |

# PANCREATIN, PEPSIN, BILE SALTS, HYOSCYAMINE, ATROPINE, SCOPOLAMINE & PHENOBARBITAL

## BRAND NAMES

**Donnazyme**

## BASIC INFORMATION

**Habit forming? Yes**
**Prescription needed? Yes**
**Available as generic? No**
**Drug class: Digestant, sedative,**
        **anticholinergic**

## USES

- Replaces deficient digestive enzymes.
- Sometimes used to relieve indigestion.

## DOSAGE & USAGE INFORMATION

**How to take:**
Tablet—Swallow with liquid or food to lessen stomach irritation. If you can't swallow whole, crumble tablet and take with food or liquid.

**When to take:**
With or after meals.

**If you forget a dose:**
Skip it and resume schedule. Don't double-dose.

**What drug does:**
Blocks nerve impulses at parasympathetic nerve endings, preventing smooth muscle contraction and gland secretions.

**Time lapse before drug works:**
30 to 60 minutes.

**Don't take with:**
- Any medicine that will decrease mental alertness or reflexes, such as alcohol, other mind-altering drugs, cough/cold medicines,

*Continued next column*

## OVERDOSE

**SYMPTOMS:**
**Hallucinations, excitement, irregular heartbeat (too fast or too slow), fainting, collapse, coma.**
**WHAT TO DO:**
- **Dial 0 (operator) or 911 (emergency) for an ambulance or medical help. Then give first aid immediately.**
- **See emergency information on inside covers.**

antihistamines, allergy medicine, sedatives, tranquilizers (sleeping pills or "downers") barbiturates, seizure medicine, narcotics, other prescription medicine for pain, muscle relaxants, anesthetics.
- See Interaction column and consult doctor.

## POSSIBLE ADVERSE REACTIONS OR SIDE EFFECTS

| SYMPTOMS | WHAT TO DO |
|---|---|
| **Life-threatening:** None expected. | |
| **Common:** | |
| • Constipation, decreased sweating, headache. | Discontinue. Call doctor right away. |
| • Drowsiness, dry mouth, frequent urination. | Continue. Call doctor when convenient. |
| **Infrequent:** | |
| • Blurred vision. | Discontinue. Call doctor right away. |
| • Diminished sex drive, swallowing difficulty, sensitivity to light, insomnia. | Continue. Call doctor when convenient. |
| **Rare:** | |
| • Jaundice; unusual bleeding or bruising; swollen feet and ankles; abdominal pain; sore throat, fever, mouth sores; rash; hives; vomiting; joint pain; eye pain; diarrhea; blood in urine. | Discontinue. Call doctor right away. |
| • Unusual tiredness. | Continue. Call doctor when convenient. |

## WARNINGS & PRECAUTIONS

**Don't take if:**
- You are allergic to any of the drugs in this combination.
- You have trouble with stomach bloating, difficulty emptying your bladder completely, narrow-angle glaucoma, severe ulcerative colitis, porphyria.

**Before you start, consult your doctor:**
- If you have open-angle glaucoma, angina, chronic bronchitis or asthma, liver disease, hiatal hernia, enlarged prostate, myasthenia gravis, epilepsy, kidney or liver damage, anemia, chronic pain.

- If you will have surgery within 2 months, including dental surgery, requiring general or spinal anesthesia.

### Over age 60:
Adverse reactions and side effects may be more frequent and severe than in younger persons

### Pregnancy:
Risk to unborn child outweighs drug benefits. Don't use.

### Breast-feeding:
Drug passes into milk. Avoid drug or discontinue nursing until you finish medicine. Consult doctor for advice on maintaining milk supply.

### Infants & children:
Use only under medical supervision.

### Prolonged use:
- Chronic constipation, possible fecal impaction.
- May cause addiction, anemia, chronic intoxication.
- May lower body temperature, making exposure to cold temperatures hazardous.

### Skin & sunlight:
May cause rash or intensify sunburn in areas exposed to sun or sunlamp.

### Driving, piloting or hazardous work:
Don't drive or pilot aircraft until you learn how medicine affects you. Don't work around dangerous machinery. Don't climb ladders or work in high places. Danger increases if you drink alcohol or take medicine affecting alertness and reflexes, such as antihistamines, tranquilizers, sedatives, pain medicine, narcotics and mind-altering drugs.

### Discontinuing:
- May be unnecessary to finish medicine. Follow doctor's instructions.
- If you develop withdrawal symptoms of hallucinations, agitation or sleeplessness after discontinuing, call doctor right away.

### Others:
- Potential for abuse.
- Enzyme deficiencies probably better treated with identified separate substances rather than a mixture of components.

## POSSIBLE INTERACTION WITH OTHER DRUGS

| GENERIC NAME OR DRUG CLASS | COMBINED EFFECT |
|---|---|
| Amantadine | Increased atropine effect. |

| | |
|---|---|
| Anticholinergics (other) | Increased anticholinergic effect. |
| Anticoagulants (oral) | Decreased anticoagulant effect. |
| Antidepressants (tricyclic) | Decreased antidepressant effect. Possible dangerous oversedation. |
| Antidiabetics (oral) | Increased phenobartital effect. |
| Antihistamines | Increased atropine effect. |
| Anti-inflammatory drugs (non-steroidal) | Decreased anti-inflammatory effect. |
| Aspirin | Decreased aspirin effect. |
| Beta-adrenergic blockers | Decreased effect of beta-adrenergic blocker. |
| Contraceptives (oral) | Decreased contraceptive effect. |
| Cortisone drugs | Decreased cortisone effect. |
| Dronabinol | Increased phenobarbital effect. |
| Griseofulvin | Decreased griseofulvin effect. |
| Haloperidol | Increased internal-eye pressure. |

*Continued page 970*

## POSSIBLE INTERACTION WITH OTHER SUBSTANCES

| INTERACTS WITH | COMBINED EFFECT |
|---|---|
| Alcohol: | Possible fatal oversedation. Avoid. |
| Beverages: | None expected. |
| Cocaine: | Excessively rapid heartbeat. Avoid. |
| Foods: | None expected. |
| Marijuana: | Excessive sedation, drowsiness and dry mouth. |
| Tobacco: | May increase stomach acidity, decreasing the effectiveness of Donnazyme. Avoid. |

# PANCRELIPASE

## BRAND NAMES

| | |
|---|---|
| Cotazym | Ku-Zyme HP |
| Cotazym-S | Lipancreatin |
| Festal II | Pancrease |
| Ilozyme | Viokase |

## BASIC INFORMATION

**Habit forming? No**
**Prescription needed? Yes**
**Available as generic? No**
**Drug class: Enzyme (pancreatic)**

 **USES**

- Replaces pancreatic enzyme deficiency caused by surgery or disease.
- Treats fatty stools (steatorrhea).

 **DOSAGE & USAGE INFORMATION**

**How to take:**
- Capsules—Swallow whole. Do not take with milk or milk products.
- Powder—Sprinkle on liquid or soft food.

**When to take:**
Before meals.

**If you forget a dose:**
Take as soon as you remember up to 2 hours late. If more than 2 hours, wait for next scheduled dose (don't double this dose).

**What drug does:**
Enhances digestion of proteins, carbohydrates and fats.

**Time lapse before drug works:**
30 minutes.

**Don't take with:**
See Interaction column and consult doctor.

 **OVERDOSE**

**SYMPTOMS:**
Shortness of breath, wheezing, diarrhea.
**WHAT TO DO:**
Overdose unlikely to threaten life. If person takes much larger amount than prescribed, call doctor, poison-control center or hospital emergency room for instructions.

 **POSSIBLE ADVERSE REACTIONS OR SIDE EFFECTS**

| SYMPTOMS | WHAT TO DO |
|---|---|
| **Life-threatening:**<br>None expected. | |
| **Common:**<br>None expected. | |
| **Infrequent:**<br>None expected. | |
| **Rare:**<br>• Rash, hives, blood in urine, swollen feet or legs. | Discontinue. Call doctor right away. |
| • Nausea, joint pain. | Continue. Call doctor when convenient. |

# PANCRELIPASE

## WARNINGS & PRECAUTIONS

**Don't take if:**
You are allergic to pancreatin, pancrelipase, or pork.

**Before you start, consult your doctor:**
If you take any other medicines.

**Over age 60:**
Adverse reactions and side effects may be more frequent and severe than in younger persons.

**Pregnancy:**
Risk to unborn child outweighs drug benefits. Don't use.

**Breast-feeding:**
Drug passes into milk. Avoid drug or discontinue nursing until you finish medicine. Consult doctor for advice on maintaining milk supply.

**Infants & children:**
Under close medical supervision only.

**Prolonged use:**
No additional problems expected.

**Skin & sunlight:**
No problems expected.

**Driving, piloting or hazardous work:**
No problems expected.

**Discontinuing:**
Don't discontinue without consulting doctor. Dose may require gradual reduction if you have taken drug for a long time. Doses of other drugs may also require adjustment.

**Others:**
If you take powder form, avoid inhaling.

## POSSIBLE INTERACTION WITH OTHER DRUGS

| GENERIC NAME OR DRUG CLASS | COMBINED EFFECT |
|---|---|
| Calcium carbonate antacids. | Decreased effect of pancrelipase. |
| Iron preparations | Decreased iron absorption. |
| Magnesium hydroxide antacids | Decreased effect of pancrelipase. |

## POSSIBLE INTERACTION WITH OTHER SUBSTANCES

| INTERACTS WITH | COMBINED EFFECT |
|---|---|
| Alcohol: | Unknown. |
| Beverages: Milk. | Decreased effect of pancrelipase. |
| Cocaine: | Unknown. |
| Foods: Ice cream, milk products | Decreased effect of pancrelipase. |
| Marijuana: | Decreased absorption of pancrelipase. |
| Tobacco: | Decreased absorption of pancrelipase. |

# PANTOTHENIC ACID (VITAMIN B-5)

## BRAND AND GENERIC NAMES

CALCIUM
   PATOTHENATE
Dexol T.D.
Durasil

Pantholin
PANTOTHENIC ACID

**Ingredients in numerous multiple vitamin-mineral supplements.**

## BASIC INFORMATION

**Habit forming? No**
**Prescription needed? No**
**Available as generic? Yes**
**Drug class: Vitamin supplement**

## USES

Prevents and treats vitamin B-5 deficiency.

## DOSAGE & USAGE INFORMATION

**How to take:**
- Tablet or capsule—Swallow with liquid.
- Extended-release tablets—Swallow each dose whole with liquid.

**When to take:**
At the same times each day.

**If you forget a dose:**
Take as soon as you remember, then resume regular schedule.

**What drug does:**
Acts as co-enzyme in carbohydrate, protein and fat metabolism.

**Time lapse before drug works:**
15 to 20 minutes.

**Don't take with:**
- Levodopa—Small amounts of pantothenic acid will nullify levodopa effect. Carbidopa-levodopa combination not affected by this interaction.
- See Interaction column and consult doctor.

## OVERDOSE

**SYMPTOMS:**
**None expected.**
**WHAT TO DO:**
**Overdose unlikely to threaten life.**

## POSSIBLE ADVERSE REACTIONS OR SIDE EFFECTS

| SYMPTOMS | WHAT TO DO |
|---|---|
| **Life-threatening:** None expected. | |
| **Common:** None expected. | |
| **Infrequent:** None expected. | |
| **Rare:** None expected. | |

# PANTOTHENIC ACID (VITAMIN B-5)

 **WARNINGS & PRECAUTIONS**

**Don't take if:**
You are allergic to pantothenic acid.

**Before you start, consult your doctor:**
If you have hemophilia.

**Over age 60:**
No problems expected.

**Pregnancy:**
Don't exceed recommended dose.

**Breast-feeding:**
Don't exceed recommended dose.

**Infants & children:**
Don't exceed recommended dose.

**Prolonged use:**
Large doses for more than 1 month may cause toxicity.

**Skin & sunlight:**
No problems expected.

**Driving, piloting or hazardous work:**
No problems expected.

**Discontinuing:**
No problems expected.

**Others:**
Regular pantothenic acid supplements are recommended if you take chloramphenicol, cycloserine, ethionamide, hydralazine, immunosuppressants, isoniazid or penicillamine. These decrease pantothenic acid absorption and can cause anemia or tingling and numbness in hands and feet.

 **POSSIBLE INTERACTION WITH OTHER DRUGS**

| GENERIC NAME OR DRUG CLASS | COMBINED EFFECT |
|---|---|
| None expected. | |

 **POSSIBLE INTERACTION WITH OTHER SUBSTANCES**

| INTERACTS WITH | COMBINED EFFECT |
|---|---|
| Alcohol: | None expected. |
| Beverages: | None expected. |
| Cocaine: | None expected. |
| Foods: | None expected. |
| Marijuana: | None expected. |
| Tobacco: | May decrease pantothenic acid absorption. Decreased pantothenic acid effect. |

# PAPAVERINE

## BRAND NAMES

See complete list of brand names in the *Brand Name Directory,* page 954.

## BASIC INFORMATION

**Habit forming? No**
**Prescription needed? Yes**
**Available as generic? Yes**
**Drug class: Vasodilator**

 **USES**

Improves poor circulation in the extremities or brain.

 **DOSAGE & USAGE INFORMATION**

**How to take:**
- Tablet or capsule—Swallow with liquid or food to lessen stomach irritation. If you can't swallow whole, crumble tablet or open capsule and take with liquid or food.
- Extended-release tablets or capsules—Swallow whole with liquid.
- Liquid—Follow label instructions.

**When to take:**
At the same times each day.

**If you forget a dose:**
Take as soon as you remember up to 2 hours late. If more than 2 hours, wait for next scheduled dose (don't double this dose).

**What drug does:**
Relaxes and expands blood-vessel walls, allowing better distribution of oxygen and nutrients.

**Time lapse before drug works:**
30 to 60 minutes.

**Don't take with:**
- Non-prescription drugs without consulting doctor.
- See Interaction column and consult doctor.

 **OVERDOSE**

**SYMPTOMS:**
**Weakness, fainting, flush, sweating, stupor, irregular heartbeat.**
**WHAT TO DO:**
- **Dial 0 (operator) or 911 (emergency) for an ambulance or medical help. Then give first aid immediately.**
- **See emergency information on inside covers.**

 **POSSIBLE ADVERSE REACTIONS OR SIDE EFFECTS**

| SYMPTOMS | WHAT TO DO |
|---|---|
| **Life-threatening:** None expected. | |
| **Common:** | |
| • Drowsiness, dizziness, headache, flushed face, stomach irritation, indigestion, nausea, mild constipation, low blood pressure causing lethargy or dizziness (especially on change of position). | Continue. Call doctor when convenient. |
| • Dry mouth, throat. | Continue. Tell doctor at next visit. |
| **Infrequent:** | |
| • Rash, itchy skin, blurred or double vision, weakness. | Discontinue. Call doctor right away. |
| • Deep breathing, rapid heartbeat. | Continue. Call doctor when convenient. |
| **Rare:** Jaundice. | Discontinue. Call doctor right away. |

646

## WARNINGS & PRECAUTIONS

**Don't take if:**
You are allergic to any narcotic.

**Before you start, consult your doctor:**
- If you plan to become pregnant within medication period.
- If you have had a heart attack, heart disease, angina or stroke.
- If you have Parkinson's disease.

**Over age 60:**
Adverse reactions and side effects may be more frequent and severe than in younger persons.

**Pregnancy:**
No proven harm to unborn child. Avoid if possible.

**Breast-feeding:**
Drug filters into milk. May harm child. Avoid.

**Infants & children:**
Not recommended.

**Prolonged use:**
No problems expected.

**Skin & sunlight:**
No problems expected.

**Driving, piloting or hazardous work:**
Don't drive or pilot aircraft until you learn how medicine affects you. Don't work around dangerous machinery. Don't climb ladders or work in high places. Danger increases if you drink alcohol or take medicine affecting alertness and reflexes, such as antihistamines, tranquilizers, sedatives, pain medicine, narcotics and mind-altering drugs.

**Discontinuing:**
May be unnecessary to finish medicine. If drug does not help in 1 to 2 weeks, consult doctor about discontinuing.

**Others:**
- Periodic liver-function tests recommended.
- Internal eye-pressure measurements recommended if you have glaucoma.

## POSSIBLE INTERACTION WITH OTHER DRUGS

| GENERIC NAME OR DRUG CLASS | COMBINED EFFECT |
|---|---|
| Levodopa | Decreased levodopa effect. |
| Narcotics | Increased papaverine effect. |
| Pain relievers | Increased papaverine effect. |
| Sedatives | Increased papaverine effect. |
| Tranquilizers | Increased papaverine effect. |

## POSSIBLE INTERACTION WITH OTHER SUBSTANCES

| INTERACTS WITH | COMBINED EFFECT |
|---|---|
| Alcohol: | None expected. |
| Beverages: | None expected. |
| Cocaine: | Decreased papaverine effect. |
| Foods: | None expected. |
| Marijuana: | None expected. |
| Tobacco: | Decrease in papaverine's dilation of blood vessels. |

# PARA-AMINOSALICYLIC ACID (PAS)

## BRAND NAMES

Nemasol
Parasal
P.A.S.

P.A.S. Acid
Pasna
Teebacin

## BASIC INFORMATION

**Habit forming? No**
**Prescription needed? Yes**
**Available as generic? Yes**
**Drug class: Antitubercular**

## USES

Treatment for tuberculosis.

## DOSAGE & USAGE INFORMATION

**How to take:**
- Tablet—Swallow with liquid or food to lessen stomach irritation.
- Powder—Dissolve dose in water. Stir well and drink all liquid.

**When to take:**
At the same times each day.

**If you forget a dose:**
Take as soon as you remember up to 2 hours late. If more than 2 hours, wait for next scheduled dose (don't double this dose).

**What drug does:**
- Prevents growth of TB germs.
- Makes TB germs more susceptible to other antituberculosis drugs.

**Time lapse before drug works:**
6 months.

**Don't take with:**
See Interaction column and consult doctor.

## OVERDOSE

**SYMPTOMS:**
**Nausea, vomiting, diarrhea; rapid breathing; convulsions.**
**WHAT TO DO:**
- **Dial 0 (operator) or 911 (emergency) for an ambulance or medical help. Then give first aid immediately.**
- **See emergency information on inside covers.**

## POSSIBLE ADVERSE REACTIONS OR SIDE EFFECTS

| SYMPTOMS | WHAT TO DO |
|---|---|
| **Life-threatening:** None expected. | |
| **Common:** | |
| • Painful urination, chills, low back pain. | Discontinue. Call doctor right away. |
| • Diarrhea or stomach pain. | Continue. Call doctor when convenient. |
| **Infrequent:** | |
| • Confusion, blood in urine. | Discontinue. Call doctor right away. |
| • Headache; itchy, dry, puffy skin; light sensitivity; sore throat; fever; constipation or vomiting; swelling in front of neck; decreased sex drive in men; fatigue; weakness. | Continue. Call doctor when convenient. |
| • Menstrual irregularities. | Continue. Tell doctor at next visit. |
| **Rare:** Jaundice. | Discontinue. Call doctor right away. |

# PARA-AMINOSALICYLIC ACID (PAS)

## WARNINGS & PRECAUTIONS

**Don't take if:**
- You are allergic to PAS, aspirin or other salicylates.
- Tablets have turned brownish or purplish.

**Before you start, consult your doctor:**
- If you have ulcers in stomach or duodenum.
- If you have liver or kidney disease.
- If you have epilepsy.
- If you have adrenal insufficiency.
- If you have heart disease or congestive heart failure.
- If you have cancer.
- If you have overactive thyroid.

**Over age 60:**
Adverse reactions and side effects may be more frequent and severe than in younger persons.

**Pregnancy:**
Risk to unborn child outweighs drug benefits. Don't use.

**Breast-feeding:**
No proven problems. Consult doctor.

**Infants & children:**
Use only under medical supervision.

**Prolonged use:**
Enlarged thyroid gland and decreased function.

**Skin & sunlight:**
No problems expected.

**Driving, piloting or hazardous work:**
No problems expected.

**Discontinuing:**
No problems expected.

**Others:**
- Treatment may need to continue for several years or indefinitely.
- Periodic blood tests and liver- and kidney-function studies recommended.

## POSSIBLE INTERACTION WITH OTHER DRUGS

| GENERIC NAME OR DRUG CLASS | COMBINED EFFECT |
|---|---|
| Aminobenzoic acid (PABA) | Decreased effect of PAS. |
| Anticoagulants (oral) | Increased anticoagulant effect. |
| Anticonvulsants (hydantoin) | Increased anticonvulsant effect. |
| Aspirin | Stomach irritation. |
| Barbiturates | Oversedation. |
| Folic acid | Decreased effect of folic acid. |
| Probenecid | Increased PAS effect. Possible toxicity. |
| Rifampin | Decreased rifampin effect. |
| Sulfa drugs | Decreased effect of sulfa drugs. |
| Sulfinpyrazone | Increased PAS effect. Possible toxicity. |
| Tetracyclines | Reduced absorption of PAS. Space doses 3 hours apart. |

## POSSIBLE INTERACTION WITH OTHER SUBSTANCES

| INTERACTS WITH | COMBINED EFFECT |
|---|---|
| Alcohol: | Possible liver disease. |
| Beverages: | None expected |
| Cocaine: | None expected. |
| Foods: | None expected. |
| Marijuana: | None expected. |
| Tobacco: | None expected, but tobacco smoking may slow recovery. Avoid. |

# PARAMETHASONE

## BRAND NAMES

Haldrone

## BASIC INFORMATION

Habit forming? No
Prescription needed? Yes
Available as generic? No
Drug class: Cortisone drug (adrenal corticosteroid)

## USES

- Reduces inflammation caused by many different medical problems.
- Treatment for some allergic diseases, blood disorders, kidney diseases, asthma and emphysema.
- Replaces corticosteroid deficiencies.

## DOSAGE & USAGE INFORMATION

**How to take:**
Tablet—Swallow with liquid or food to lessen stomach irritation. If you can't swallow whole, crumble tablet and take with liquid or food.

**When to take:**
At the same times each day. Take once-a-day or once-every-other-day doses in mornings.

**If you forget a dose:**
- Several-doses-per-day prescription—Take as soon as you remember up to 2 hours late. If more than 2 hours, wait for next scheduled dose (don't double this dose).
- Once-a-day dose or less—Wait for next dose. Double this dose.

**What drug does:**
Decreases inflammatory responses.

**Time lapse before drug works:**
2 to 4 days.

**Don't take with:**
See Interaction column and consult doctor.

## OVERDOSE

**SYMPTOMS:**
Headache, convulsions, heart failure.

**WHAT TO DO:**
- **Dial 0 (operator) or 911 (emergency) for an ambulance or medical help. Then give first aid immediately.**
- **Additional emergency information on inside covers.**

## POSSIBLE ADVERSE REACTIONS OR SIDE EFFECTS

| SYMPTOMS | WHAT TO DO |
|---|---|
| **Life-threatening:** None expected. | |
| **Common:** | |
| • Acne, poor wound healing, indigestion, nausea, vomiting, thirst. | Continue. Call doctor when convenient. |
| **Infrequent:** | |
| • Black, bloody or tarry stool. | Discontinue. Seek emergency treatment. |
| • Blurred vision, halos around lights, sore throat, fever, muscle cramps. | Discontinue. Call doctor right away. |
| • Mood change, insomnia, restlessness, frequent urination, weight gain, round face, fatigue, weakness, TB recurrence, irregular menstrual periods. | Continue. Call doctor when convenient. |
| **Rare:** | |
| • Irregular heartbeat. | Discontinue. Seek emergency treatment. |
| • Rash. | Discontinue. Call doctor right away. |

## WARNINGS & PRECAUTIONS

**Don't take if:**
- You are allergic to any cortisone drug.
- You have tuberculosis or fungus infection.
- You have herpes infection of eyes, lips or genitals.

**Before you start, consult your doctor:**
- If you have had tuberculosis.
- If you have congestive heart failure.
- If you have diabetes.
- If you have peptic ulcer.
- If you have glaucoma.
- If you have underactive thyroid.
- If you have high blood pressure.
- If you have myasthenia gravis.
- If you have blood clots in legs or lungs.

**Over age 60:**
Adverse reactions and side effects may be more frequent and severe than in younger persons. Likely to aggravate edema, diabetes or ulcers. Likely to cause cataracts and osteoporosis (softening of the bones).

**Pregnancy:**
Risk to unborn child outweighs drug benefits. Don't use.

**Breast-feeding:**
Drug passes into milk. Avoid drug or discontinue nursing until you finish medicine. Consult doctor for advice on maintaining milk supply.

**Infants & children:**
Use only under medical supervision.

**Prolonged use:**
- Retards growth in children.
- Possible glaucoma, cataracts, diabetes, fragile bones and thin skin.
- Functional dependence.

**Skin & sunlight:**
No problems expected.

**Driving, piloting or hazardous work:**
No problems expected.

**Discontinuing:**
- Don't discontinue without doctor's advice until you complete prescribed dose, even though symptoms diminish or disappear.
- Drug affects your response to surgery, illness, injury or stress for 2 years after discontinuing. Tell anyone who takes medical care of you within 2 years about drug.

**Others:**
Avoid immunizations if possible.

## POSSIBLE INTERACTION WITH OTHER DRUGS

| GENERIC NAME OR DRUG CLASS | COMBINED EFFECT |
|---|---|
| Amphoterecin B | Potassium depletion. |
| Anticholinergics | Possible glaucoma. |
| Anticoagulants (oral) | Decreased anticoagulant effect. |
| Anticonvulsants (hydantoin) | Decreased paramethasone effect. |
| Antidiabetics (oral) | Decreased antidiabetic effect. |
| Antihistamines | Decreased paramethasone effect. |
| Aspirin | Increased paramethasone effect. |
| Barbiturates | Decreased paramethasone effect. Oversedation. |
| Beta-adrenergic blockers | Decreased paramethasone effect. |
| Chloral hydrate | Decreased paramethasone effect. |
| Chlorthalidone | Potassium depletion. |
| Cholinergics | Decreased cholinergic effect. |
| Contraceptives (oral) | Increased paramethasone effect. |
| Digitalis preparations | Dangerous potassium depletion. Possible digitalis toxicity. |
| Diuretics (thiazide) | Potassium depletion. |
| Ephedrine | Decreased paramethasone effect. |
| Estrogens | Increased paramethasone effect. |
| Ethacrynic acid | Potassium depletion. |
| Furosemide | Potassium depletion. |
| Glutethimide | Decreased paramethasone effect. |
| Indapamide | Possible excessive potassium loss, causing dangerous heartbeat irregularity. |
| Indomethacin | Increased paramethasone effect. |
| Insulin | Decreased insulin effect. |
| Isoniazid | Decreased isoniazid effect. |
| Oxyphenbutazone | Possible ulcers. |
| Phenylbutazone | Possible ulcers. |
| Potassium supplements | Decreased potassium effect. |
| Rifampin | Decreased paramethasone effect. |
| Sympathomimetics | Possible glaucoma. |

## POSSIBLE INTERACTION WITH OTHER SUBSTANCES

| INTERACTS WITH | COMBINED EFFECT |
|---|---|
| Alcohol: | Risk of stomach ulcers. |
| Beverages: | No proven problems. |
| Cocaine: | Overstimulation. Avoid. |
| Foods: | No proven problems. |
| Marijuana: | Decreased immunity. |
| Tobacco: | Increased paramethasone effect. Possible toxicity. |

# PAREGORIC

## BRAND NAMES

Brown Mixture
CM with Paregoric
Diban
Donnagel-PG

Kaoparin
Opium Tincture
Parepectolin
Pomalin

## BASIC INFORMATION

**Habit forming?** Yes
**Prescription needed?** Yes
**Available as generic?** Yes
**Drug class:** Narcotic, antidiarrheal

## USES

Reduces intestinal cramps and diarrhea.

## DOSAGE & USAGE INFORMATION

**How to take:**
Drops or liquid—Dilute dose in beverage before swallowing.

**When to take:**
As needed for diarrhea, no more often than every 4 hours.

**If you forget a dose:**
Take as soon as you remember. Wait 4 hours for next dose.

**What drug does:**
Anesthetizes surface membranes of intestines and blocks nerve impulses.

**Time lapse before drug works:**
2 to 6 hours.

**Don't take with:**
See Interaction column and consult doctor.

## OVERDOSE

**SYMPTOMS:**
Deep sleep; slow breathing; slow pulse; flushed, warm skin; constricted pupils.
**WHAT TO DO:**
- Dial 0 (operator) or 911 (emergency) for an ambulance or medical help. Then give first aid immediately.
- If patient is unconscious and not breathing, give mouth-to-mouth breathing. If there is no heartbeat, use cardiac massage and mouth-to-mouth breathing (CPR). Don't try to make patient vomit. If you can't get help quickly, take patient to nearest emergency facility.
- See emergency information on inside covers.

## POSSIBLE ADVERSE REACTIONS OR SIDE EFFECTS

| SYMPTOMS | WHAT TO DO |
|---|---|
| **Life-threatening:**<br>None expected. | |
| **Common:**<br>Dizziness, flushed face, unusual tiredness, difficult urination. | Continue. Call doctor when convenient. |
| **Infrequent:**<br>Severe constipation, abdominal pain, vomiting. | Discontinue. Call doctor right away. |
| **Rare:**<br>• Hives, rash, itchy skin, slow heartbeat, irregular breathing. | Discontinue. Call doctor right away. |
| • Depression. | Continue. Call doctor when convenient. |

## WARNINGS & PRECAUTIONS

**Don't take if:**
You are allergic to any narcotic.

**Before you start, consult your doctor:**
If you have impaired liver or kidney function.

**Over age 60:**
More likely to be drowsy, dizzy, unsteady or constipated.

**Pregnancy:**
No proven harm to unborn child. Avoid if possible.

**Breast-feeding:**
Drug filters into milk. May depress infant. Avoid.

**Infants & children:**
Use only under medical supervision.

**Prolonged use:**
Causes psychological and physical dependence.

**Skin & sunlight:**
No problems expected.

**Driving, piloting or hazardous work:**
Don't drive or pilot aircraft until you learn how medicine affects you. Don't work around dangerous machinery. Don't climb ladders or work in high places. Danger increases if you drink alcohol or take medicine affecting alertness and reflexes, such as antihistamines, tranquilizers, sedatives, pain medicine, narcotics and mind-altering drugs.

**Discontinuing:**
May be unnecessary to finish medicine. Follow doctor's instructions.

**Others:**
Great potential for abuse.

## POSSIBLE INTERACTION WITH OTHER DRUGS

| GENERIC NAME OR DRUG CLASS | COMBINED EFFECT |
|---|---|
| Analgesics | Increased analgesic effect. |
| Antidepressants | Increased sedative effect. |
| Antihistamines | Increased sedative effect. |
| Mind-altering drugs | Increased sedative effect. |
| Narcotics (other) | Increased narcotic effect. |
| Phenothiazines | Increased sedative effect of paregoric. |
| Sedatives | Excessive sedation. |
| Sleep inducers | Increased effect of sleep inducers. |
| Tranquilizers | Increased tranquilizer effect. |

## POSSIBLE INTERACTION WITH OTHER SUBSTANCES

| INTERACTS WITH | COMBINED EFFECT |
|---|---|
| Alcohol: | Increases alcohol's intoxicating effect. Avoid. |
| Beverages: | None expected. |
| Cocaine: | None expected. |
| Foods: | None expected. |
| Marijuana: | Impairs physical and mental performance. |
| Tobacco: | None expected. |

# PARGYLINE & METHYCLOTHIAZIDE

## BRAND NAMES

Eutron

## BASIC INFORMATION

**Habit forming?** No
**Prescription needed?** Yes
**Available as generic?** No
**Drug class:** Antihypertensive, MAO inhibitor

## USES

- Controls, but doesn't cure, high blood pressure.
- Reduces fluid retention (edema) caused by conditions such as heart disorders and liver disease.

## DOSAGE & USAGE INFORMATION

**How to take:**
Tablet or capsule—Swallow with liquid. If you can't swallow whole, crumble tablet or open capsule and take with liquid or food. Don't exceed dose.

**When to take:**
At the same times each day.

**If you forget a dose:**
Take as soon as you remember up to 2 hours late. If more than 2 hours, wait for next scheduled dose (don't double this dose).

**What drug does:**
- Forces sodium and water excretion, reducing body fluid.
- Relaxes muscle cells of small arteries.
- Reduced body fluid and relaxed arteries lower blood pressure.
- Inhibits nerve transmissions in brain that may cause hypertension.

**Time lapse before drug works:**
4 to 6 weeks for maximum effect.

*Continued next column*

## OVERDOSE

**SYMPTOMS:**
Cramps, weakness, drowsiness, weak pulse, restlessness, agitation, fever, convulsions, coma.
**WHAT TO DO:**
- **Dial 0 (operator) or 911 (emergency) for an ambulance or medical help. Then give first aid immediately.**
- **See emergency information on inside covers.**

**Don't take with:**
- Non-prescription drugs without consulting doctor.
- Non-prescription diet pills, nose drops, medicine for asthma, cough, cold or allergy, or medicine containing caffeine or alcohol.
- See Interaction column and consult doctor.

## POSSIBLE ADVERSE REACTIONS OR SIDE EFFECTS

| SYMPTOMS | WHAT TO DO |
|---|---|
| **Life-threatening:** | |
| Irregular heartbeat, weak pulse, chest pain, fast heartbeat. | Discontinue. Seek emergency treatment. |
| **Common:** | |
| • Constipation, frequent urination. | Discontinue. Call doctor right away. |
| • Dry mouth, increased thirst, muscle cramps, muscle pain. | Continue. Call doctor when convenient. |
| **Infrequent:** | |
| • Fainting. | Discontinue. Seek emergency treatment. |
| • Blurred vision, abdominal pain, nausea, vomiting, swollen feet and ankles, chills. | Discontinue. Call doctor right away. |
| • Dizziness, mood change, headache, muscle cramps, weakness, tiredness, weight gain or loss, nightmares, restlessness, shakiness. | Continue. Call doctor when convenient. |
| **Rare:** | |
| Sore throat; jaundice; headache; nausea; vomiting; fever; hallucinations; joint pain; rash; hives; sore throat, fever, mouth sores; unusual bruising; stiff or sore neck. | Discontinue. Call doctor right away. |

## WARNINGS & PRECAUTIONS

**Don't take if:**
- You are allergic to any MAO inhibitor.
- You are allergic to any thiazide diuretic drug.

**Before you start, consult your doctor:**
- If you are alcoholic or allergic to any sulfa drug.

- If you have asthma, diabetes, epilepsy, overactive thyroid, schizophrenia, Parkinson's disease, adrenal-gland tumor, gout, liver, pancreas or kidney disorder.
- If you have had a stroke.
- If you will have surgery within 2 months, including dental surgery, requiring general or spinal anesthesia.

**Over age 60:**
Not recommended.

**Pregnancy:**
Risk to unborn child outweighs drug benefits. Don't use.

**Breast-feeding:**
Drug passes into milk. Avoid drug or discontinue nursing until you finish medicine. Consult doctor for advice on maintaining milk supply.

**Infants & children:**
Not recommended.

**Prolonged use:**
May be toxic to liver.

**Skin & sunlight:**
May cause rash or intensify sunburn in areas exposed to sun or sunlamp.

**Driving, piloting or hazardous work:**
Don't drive or pilot aircraft until you learn how medicine affects you. Don't work around dangerous machinery. Don't climb ladders or work in high places. Danger increases if you drink alcohol or take medicine affecting alertness and reflexes, such as antihistamines, tranquilizers, sedatives, pain medicine, narcotics and mind-altering drugs.

**Discontinuing:**
- Don't discontinue without doctor's advice until you complete prescribed dose, even though symptoms diminish or disappear.
- Follow precautions regarding foods, drinks and other medicines for 2 weeks after discontinuing.

**Others:**
- May affect blood-sugar levels in patients with diabetes.
- Hot weather and fever may cause dehydration and drop in blood pressure. Dose may require temporary adjustment. Weigh daily and report any unexpected weight decreases to your doctor.
- May cause rise in uric acid, leading to gout.

## POSSIBLE INTERACTION WITH OTHER DRUGS

| GENERIC NAME OR DRUG CLASS | COMBINED EFFECT |
|---|---|
| Acebutolol | Increased antihypertensive effect. Dosages of both drugs may require adjustments. |
| Allopurinol | Decreased allopurinol effect. |
| Amphetamines | Blood-pressure rise to life-threatening level. |
| Anticholinergics | Increased anticholinergic effect. |
| Anticonvulsants | Changed seizure pattern. |
| Antidepressants (tricyclic) | Blood-pressure rise to life-threatening level. Possible fever, convulsions, delirium. |
| Antidiabetics (oral and insulin) | Excessively low blood sugar. |

*Continued page 970*

## POSSIBLE INTERACTION WITH OTHER SUBSTANCES

| INTERACTS WITH | COMBINED EFFECT |
|---|---|
| Alcohol: | Dangerous blood-pressure drop, increased sedation to dangerous level. |
| Beverages: Caffeine drinks. | Irregular heartbeat or high blood pressure. |
| Drinks containing tyramine (see Glossary). | Blood-pressure rise to life-threatening level. |
| Cocaine: | Overstimulation. Possibly fatal. |
| Foods: Foods containing tyramine (see Glossary). | Blood-pressure rise to life-threatening level. |
| Licorice. | Excessive potassium loss that causes dangerous heart rhythms. |
| Marijuana: | Overstimulation. May increase blood pressure. Avoid. |
| Tobacco: | No proven problems. |

# PEMOLINE

## BRAND NAMES

Cylert

## BASIC INFORMATION

**Habit forming? Yes**
**Prescription needed? Yes**
**Available as generic? No**
**Drug class: Central nervous system**
                    **stimulant**

## USES

- Decreases overactivity and lengthens attention span in hyperactive children.
- Treatment of minimal brain dysfunction.

## DOSAGE & USAGE INFORMATION

**How to take:**
Tablet or capsule—Swallow with liquid or food to lessen stomach irritation. If you can't swallow whole, crumble tablet or open capsule and take with liquid or food.

**When to take:**
At the same times each day.

**If you forget a dose:**
Take as soon as you remember up to 2 hours late. If more than 2 hours, wait for next scheduled dose (don't double this dose).

**What drug does:**
Stimulates brain to improve alertness, concentration and attention span. Calms the hyperactive child.

*Continued next column*

## OVERDOSE

**SYMPTOMS:**
**Rapid heartbeat, hallucinations, fever,**
**confusion, convulsions, coma.**
**WHAT TO DO:**
- **Dial 0 (operator) or 911 (emergency) for an ambulance or medical help. Then give first aid immediately.**
- **If patient is unconscious and not breathing, give mouth-to-mouth breathing. If there is no heartbeat, use cardiac massage and mouth-to-mouth breathing (CPR). Don't try to make patient vomit. If you can't get help quickly, take patient to nearest emergency facility.**
- **See emergency information on inside covers.**

**Time lapse before drug works:**
- 1 month or more for maximum effect on child.
- 30 minutes to stimulate adults.

**Don't take with:**
See Interaction column and consult doctor.

## POSSIBLE ADVERSE REACTIONS OR SIDE EFFECTS

| SYMPTOMS | WHAT TO DO |
|---|---|
| **Life-threatening:** None expected. | |
| **Common:** Insomnia. | Continue. Call doctor when convenient. |
| **Infrequent:** | |
| • Irritability, depression dizziness, headache, drowsiness, unusual movement of eyes, rapid heartbeat. | Discontinue. Call doctor right away. |
| • Rash, unusual movements of tongue, appetite loss, abdominal pain, nausea, weight loss. | Continue. Call doctor when convenient. |
| **Rare:** Jaundice. | Discontinue. Call doctor right away. |

## WARNINGS & PRECAUTIONS

**Don't take if:**
You are allergic to pemoline.

**Before you start, consult your doctor:**
- If you have liver disease.
- If you have kidney disease.
- If patient younger than 6 years.
- If there is marked emotional instability.

**Over age 60:**
Adverse reactions and side effects may be more frequent and severe than in younger persons.

**Pregnancy:**
No proven harm to unborn child. Avoid if possible.

**Breast-feeding:**
No problems expected. Consult doctor.

**Infants & children:**
Use only under close medical supervision for children 6 or older.

**Prolonged use:**
Rare possibility of physical growth retardation.

**Skin & sunlight:**
No problems expected.

**Driving, piloting or hazardous work:**
Don't drive or pilot aircraft until you learn how medicine affects you. Don't work around dangerous machinery. Don't climb ladders or work in high places. Danger increases if you drink alcohol or take medicine affecting alertness and reflexes, such as antihistamines, tranquilizers, sedatives, pain medicine, narcotics and mind-altering drugs.

**Discontinuing:**
Don't discontinue without consulting doctor. Dose may require gradual reduction if you have taken drug for a long time. Doses of other drugs may also require adjustment.

**Others:**
Dose must be carefully adjusted by doctor.

## POSSIBLE INTERACTION WITH OTHER DRUGS

| GENERIC NAME OR DRUG CLASS | COMBINED EFFECT |
| --- | --- |
| None identified. | |

## POSSIBLE INTERACTION WITH OTHER SUBSTANCES

| INTERACTS WITH | COMBINED EFFECT |
| --- | --- |
| Alcohol: | More chance of depression. Avoid. |
| Beverages: Caffeine drinks. | May raise blood pressure. Avoid. |
| Cocaine: | Overstimulation. Avoid. |
| Foods: | No problems expected. |
| Marijuana: | Unknown. |
| Tobacco: | Unknown. |

# PENICILLAMINE

## BRAND NAMES

| | |
|---|---|
| Cuprimine | Distamine |
| Depen | Pendramine |

## BASIC INFORMATION

**Habit forming? No**
**Prescription needed? Yes**
**Available as generic? Yes**
**Drug class: Chelating agent, antirheumatic, antidote (heavy-metal)**

## USES

- Treatment for rheumatoid arthritis.
- Prevention of kidney stones.
- Treatment for heavy-metal poisoning.

## DOSAGE & USAGE INFORMATION

**How to take:**
Tablets or capsules—With liquid on an empty stomach 1 hour before or 2 hours after eating.

**When to take:**
At the same times each day.

**If you forget a dose:**
- 1 dose a day—Take as soon as you remember up to 12 hours late. If more than 12 hours, wait for next scheduled dose (don't double this dose).
- More than 1 dose a day—Take as soon as you remember up to 2 hours late. If more than 2 hours, wait for next scheduled dose (don't double this dose).

**What drug does:**
- Combines with heavy metals so kidney can excrete them.
- Combines with cysteine (amino acid found in many foods) to prevent cysteine kidney stones.
- May improve protective function of some white-blood cells against rheumatoid arthritis.

*Continued next column*

## OVERDOSE

**SYMPTOMS:**
**Ulcers, sores, convulsions, coughing up blood, coma.**
**WHAT TO DO:**
- **Dial 0 (operator) or 911 (emergency) for an ambulance or medical help. Then give first aid immediately.**
- **See emergency information on inside covers.**

**Time lapse before drug works:**
2 to 3 months.

**Don't take with:**
See Interaction column and consult doctor.

## POSSIBLE ADVERSE REACTIONS OR SIDE EFFECTS

| SYMPTOMS | WHAT TO DO |
|---|---|
| **Life-threatening:**<br>None expected. | |
| **Common:**<br>Rash, itchy skin, joint pain, fever, swollen lymph glands. | Discontinue. Call doctor right away. |
| **Infrequent:**<br>• Sore throat, fever, unusual bruising, swollen feet or legs, bloody or cloudy urine, weight gain, fatigue, weakness. | Discontinue. Call doctor right away. |
| • Appetite loss, nausea, diarrhea, vomiting. | Continue. Call doctor when convenient. |
| **Rare:**<br>Double or blurred vision, pain, ringing in ears, ulcers, sores, white spots in mouth, difficult breathing, coughing up blood, jaundice. | Discontinue. Call doctor right away. |

## WARNINGS & PRECAUTIONS

**Don't take if:**
- You are allergic to penicillamine.
- You have severe anemia.

**Before you start, consult your doctor:**
- If you have kidney disease.
- If you are allergic to any penicillin antibiotic.

**Over age 60:**
More likely to damage blood cells and kidneys.

**Pregnancy:**
Risk to unborn child outweighs drug benefits.
Don't use.

**Breast-feeding:**
Drug filters into milk. May harm child. Avoid.

**Infants & children:**
Use only under medical supervision.

**Prolonged use:**
May damage blood cells, kidney, liver.

**Skin & sunlight:**
No problems expected.

**Driving, piloting or hazardous work:**
No problems expected.

**Discontinuing:**
No problems expected.

**Others:**
Request laboratory studies on blood and urine every 2 weeks. Kidney- and liver-function studies recommended every 6 months.

## POSSIBLE INTERACTION WITH OTHER DRUGS

| GENERIC NAME OR DRUG CLASS | COMBINED EFFECT |
| --- | --- |
| Flecainide | Possible decreased blood-cell production in bone marrow. |
| Gold compounds | Damage to blood cells and kidney. |
| Immunosuppressants | Damage to blood cells and kidney. |
| Iron supplements | Decreased effect of penicillamine. Wait 2 hours between doses. |
| Oxyphenbutazone | Damage to blood cells and kidney. |
| Phenylbutazone | Damage to blood cells and kidney. |
| Quinine | Damage to blood cells and kidney. |
| Tocainide | Possible decreased blood-cell production in bone marrow. |

## POSSIBLE INTERACTION WITH OTHER SUBSTANCES

| INTERACTS WITH | COMBINED EFFECT |
| --- | --- |
| Alcohol: | Increased side effects of penicillamine. |
| Beverages: | None expected. |
| Cocaine: | Increased side effects of penicillamine. |
| Foods: | None expected. |
| Marijuana: | Increased side effects of penicillamine. |
| Tobacco: | None expected. |

# PENICILLIN G

## BRAND NAMES

| | |
|---|---|
| Ayercillin | Penioral |
| Bicillin | Pentids |
| Bicillin L.A. | Permapen |
| Crystapen | Pfizerpen |
| Crysticillin | Pfizerpen-AS |
| Duracillin | Pfizerpen G |
| Duracillin A.S. | SK-Penicillin G |
| Megacillin | Wycillin |
| Novopen-G | |

## BASIC INFORMATION

Habit forming? No
Prescription needed? Yes
Available as generic? Yes
Drug class: Antibiotic (penicillin)

 USES

Treatment of bacterial infections that are susceptible to penicillin G.

 DOSAGE & USAGE INFORMATION

**How to take:**
- Tablets or capsules—Swallow with liquid on an empty stomach 1 hour before or 2 hours after eating.
- Liquid—Take with cold beverage. Liquid form is perishable and effective for only 7 days at room temperature. Effective for 14 days if stored in refrigerator. Don't freeze.

**When to take:**
Follow instructions on prescription label or side of package. Doses should be evenly spaced. For example, 4 times a day means every 6 hours.

**If you forget a dose:**
Take as soon as you remember. Continue regular schedule.

**What drug does:**
Destroys susceptible bacteria. Does not kill viruses.

*Continued next column*

 OVERDOSE

**SYMPTOMS:**
Severe diarrhea, nausea or vomiting.
**WHAT TO DO:**
Overdose unlikely to threaten life. If person takes much larger amount than prescribed, call doctor, poison-control center or hospital emergency room for instructions.

**Time lapse before drug works:**
May be several days before medicine affects infection.

**Don't take with:**
See Interaction column and consult doctor.

 POSSIBLE ADVERSE REACTIONS OR SIDE EFFECTS

| SYMPTOMS | WHAT TO DO |
|---|---|
| **Life-threatening:** | |
| Hives, rash, intense itching, faintness soon after a dose (anaphylaxis). | Seek emergency treatment immediately. |
| **Common:** | |
| Dark or discolored tongue. | Continue. Tell doctor at next visit. |
| **Infrequent:** | |
| Mild nausea, vomiting, diarrhea. | Continue. Call doctor when convenient. |
| **Rare:** | |
| Unexplained bleeding. | Discontinue. Call doctor right away. |

## WARNINGS & PRECAUTIONS

**Don't take if:**
You are allergic to penicillin G, cephalosporin antibiotics, other penicillins or penicillamine. Life-threatening reaction may occur.

**Before you start, consult your doctor:**
If you are allergic to any substance or drug.

**Over age 60:**
You may have skin reactions, particularly around genitals and anus.

**Pregnancy:**
Studies inconclusive on harm to unborn child. Animal studies show fetal abnormalities. Decide with your doctor whether drug benefits justify risk to unborn child.

**Breast-feeding:**
Drug passes into milk. Child may become sensitive to penicillins and have allergic reactions to penicillin drugs. Avoid penicillin G or discontinue nursing until you finish medicine. Consult doctor for advice on maintaining milk supply.

**Infants & children:**
No problems expected.

**Prolonged use:**
You may become more susceptible to infections caused by germs not responsive to penicillin G.

**Skin & sunlight:**
No problems expected.

**Driving, piloting or hazardous work:**
Usually not dangerous. Most hazardous reactions likely to occur a few minutes after taking penicillin G.

**Discontinuing:**
Don't discontinue without doctor's advice until you complete prescribed dose, even though symptoms diminish or disappear.

**Others:**
Urine sugar test for diabetes may show false positive result.

## POSSIBLE INTERACTION WITH OTHER DRUGS

| GENERIC NAME OR DRUG CLASS | COMBINED EFFECT |
|---|---|
| Beta-adrenergic blockers | Increased chance of anaphylaxis (see emergency information on inside front cover). |
| Calcium supplements | Decreased penicillin effect. |
| Chloramphenicol | Decreased effect of both drugs. |
| Erythromycins | Decreased effect of both drugs. |
| Loperamide | Decreased penicillin effect. |
| Paromomycin | Decreased effect of both drugs. |
| Tetracyclines | Decreased effect of both drugs. |
| Troleandomycin | Decreased effect of both drugs. |

## POSSIBLE INTERACTION WITH OTHER SUBSTANCES

| INTERACTS WITH | COMBINED EFFECT |
|---|---|
| Alcohol: | Occasional stomach irritation. |
| Beverages: | None expected. |
| Cocaine: | No proven problems. |
| Foods: | Decreased effect of penicillin G. |
| Marijuana: | No proven problems. |
| Tobacco: | None expected. |

# PENICILLIN V

## BRAND NAMES

| | |
|---|---|
| Beepen-VK | Penapar VK |
| Betapen-VK | Pfizerpen VK |
| Compocillin VK | Robicillin VK |
| Ledercillin VK | SK-Penicillin VK |
| Nadopen-V | Uticillin VK |
| Novapen V | V-Cillin |
| Novopen-VK | V-Cillin K |
| Pen-Vee K | Veetids |

## BASIC INFORMATION

**Habit forming? No**
**Prescription needed? Yes**
**Available as generic? Yes**
**Drug class: Antibiotic (penicillin)**

## USES

- Treatment of bacterial infections that are susceptible to penicillin V.
- Prevention of streptococcal infections in susceptible persons such as those with heart valves damaged by rheumatic fever.

## DOSAGE & USAGE INFORMATION

**How to take:**
- Tablets or capsules—Swallow with liquid on an empty stomach 1 hour before meals or 2 hours after eating.
- Liquid—Take with cold beverage. Liquid form is perishable and effective for only 7 days at room temperature. Effective for 14 days if stored in refrigerator. Don't freeze.

**When to take:**
Follow instructions on prescription label or side of package. Doses should be evenly spaced. For example, 4 times a day means every 6 hours.

**If you forget a dose:**
Take as soon as you remember. Continue regular schedule.

*Continued next column*

## OVERDOSE

**SYMPTOMS:**
**Severe diarrhea, nausea or vomiting.**
**WHAT TO DO:**
**Overdose unlikely to threaten life. If person takes much larger amount than prescribed, call doctor, poison-control center or hospital emergency room for instructions.**

**What drug does:**
Destroys susceptible bacteria. Does not kill viruses.

**Time lapse before drug works:**
May be several days before penicillin V affects infection.

**Don't take with:**
See Interaction column and consult doctor.

## POSSIBLE ADVERSE REACTIONS OR SIDE EFFECTS

| SYMPTOMS | WHAT TO DO |
|---|---|
| **Life-threatening:**<br>Hives, rash, intense itching, faintness soon after a dose (anaphylaxis). | Seek emergency treatment immediately. |
| **Common:**<br>Dark or discolored tongue. | Continue. Tell doctor at next visit. |
| **Infrequent:**<br>Mild nausea, vomiting, diarrhea. | Continue. Call doctor when convenient. |
| **Rare:**<br>Unexplained bleeding. | Discontinue. Call doctor right away. |

## WARNINGS & PRECAUTIONS

**Don't take if:**
You are allergic to penicillin V, cephalosporin antibiotics, other penicillins or penicillamine. Life-threatening reaction may occur.

**Before you start, consult your doctor:**
If you are allergic to any substance or drug.

**Over age 60:**
You may have skin reactions, particularly around genitals and anus.

**Pregnancy:**
Studies inconclusive on danger to unborn child. Decide with your doctor whether drug benefits justify risk to unborn child.

**Breast-feeding:**
Drug passes into milk. Child may become sensitive to penicillin. Child more likely to have future allergic reactions to penicillin. Avoid penicillin V or discontinue nursing until you finish medicine. Consult doctor for advice on maintaining milk supply.

**Infants & children:**
No problems expected.

**Prolonged use:**
You may become more susceptible to infections caused by germs not responsive to penicillin V.

**Skin & sunlight:**
No problems expected.

**Driving, piloting or hazardous work:**
Usually not dangerous. Most hazardous reactions likely to occur a few minutes after taking penicillin V.

**Discontinuing:**
Don't discontinue without doctor's advice until you have finished prescribed dose, even if symptoms diminish or disappear.

**Others:**
No problems expected.

## POSSIBLE INTERACTION WITH OTHER DRUGS

| GENERIC NAME OR DRUG CLASS | COMBINED EFFECT |
| --- | --- |
| Beta-adrenergic blockers | Increased chance of anaphylaxis (see emergency information on inside front cover). |
| Calcium supplements | Decreased penicillin effect. |
| Chloramphenicol | Decreased effect of both drugs. |
| Erythromycins | Decreased effect of both drugs. |
| Loperamide | Decreased penicillin effect. |
| Paromomycin | Decreased effect of both drugs. |
| Tetracyclines | Decreased effect of both drugs. |
| Troleandomycin | Decreased effect of both drugs. |

## POSSIBLE INTERACTION WITH OTHER SUBSTANCES

| INTERACTS WITH | COMBINED EFFECT |
| --- | --- |
| Alcohol: | Occasional stomach irritation. |
| Beverages: | None expected. |
| Cocaine: | No proven problems. |
| Foods: | Decreased effect of penicillin V. |
| Marijuana: | No proven problems. |
| Tobacco: | None expected. |

# PENTOBARBITAL

## BRAND NAMES

| | |
|---|---|
| Carbrital | Pentogen |
| Nembutal | Quless |
| Nova-Rectal | Wigraine-PB |
| Novopentobarb | |

## BASIC INFORMATION

**Habit forming? Yes**
**Prescription needed? Yes**
**Available as generic? Yes**
**Drug class: Sedative, hypnotic (barbiturate)**

## USES

- Reduces anxiety or nervous tension (low dose).
- Relieves insomnia (higher bedtime dose).

## DOSAGE & USAGE INFORMATION

**How to take:**
- Tablet, capsule or liquid—Swallow with food or liquid to lessen stomach irritation. If you can't swallow whole, crumble tablet or open capsule and take with liquid or food.
- Suppositories—Remove wrapper and moisten suppository with water. Gently insert larger end into rectum. Push well into rectum with finger.

**When to take:**
At the same times each day.

**If you forget a dose:**
Take as soon as you remember up to 2 hours late. If more than 2 hours, wait for next scheduled dose (don't double this dose).

**What drug does:**
May partially block nerve impulses at nerve-cell connections.

**Time lapse before drug works:**
60 minutes.

*Continued next column*

## OVERDOSE

**SYMPTOMS:**
Deep sleep, weak pulse, coma.
**WHAT TO DO:**
- Dial 0 (operator) or 911 (emergency) for an ambulance or medical help. Then give first aid immediately.
- See emergency information on inside covers.

**Don't take with:**
- Non-prescription drugs without consulting doctor.
- See Interaction column and consult doctor.

## POSSIBLE ADVERSE REACTIONS OR SIDE EFFECTS

| SYMPTOMS | WHAT TO DO |
|---|---|
| **Life-threatening:**<br>None expected. | |
| **Common:**<br>Dizziness, drowsiness, "hangover" effect. | Continue. Call doctor when convenient. |
| **Infrequent:** | |
| • Rash or hives; face, lip swelling; swollen eyelids; sore throat, fever. | Discontinue. Call doctor right away. |
| • Depression, confusion, slurred speech, diarrhea, nausea, vomiting, joint or muscle pain. | Continue. Call doctor when convenient. |
| **Rare:** | |
| • Agitation, slow heartbeat, difficult breathing, jaundice. | Discontinue. Call doctor right away. |
| • Unexplained bleeding or bruising. | Continue. Call doctor when convenient. |

## WARNINGS & PRECAUTIONS

**Don't take if:**
- You are allergic to any barbiturate.
- You have porphyria.

**Before you start, consult your doctor:**
- If you have epilepsy.
- If you have kidney or liver damage.
- If you have asthma.
- If you have anemia.
- If you have chronic pain.
- If you will have surgery within 2 months, including dental surgery, requiring general or spinal anesthesia.

**Over age 60:**
Adverse reactions and side effects may be more frequent and severe than in younger persons. Use small doses.

**Pregnancy:**
Risk to unborn child outweighs drug benefits. Don't use.

**Breast-feeding:**
Drug passes into milk. Avoid drug or discontinue nursing until you finish medicine. Consult doctor for advice on maintaining milk supply.

### Infants & children:
Use only under doctor's supervision.

### Prolonged use:
- May cause addiction, anemia, chronic intoxication.
- May lower body temperature, making exposure to cold temperatures hazardous.

### Skin & sunlight:
May cause rash or intensify sunburn in areas exposed to sun or sunlamp.

### Driving, piloting or hazardous work:
Don't drive or pilot aircraft until you learn how medicine affects you. Don't work around dangerous machinery. Don't climb ladders or work in high places. Danger increases if you drink alcohol or take medicine affecting alertness and reflexes.

### Discontinuing:
May be unnecessary to finish medicine. Follow doctor's instructions. If you develop withdrawal symptoms of hallucinations, agitation or sleeplessness after discontinuing, call doctor right away.

### Others:
Great potential for abuse.

## POSSIBLE INTERACTION WITH OTHER DRUGS

| GENERIC NAME OR DRUG CLASS | COMBINED EFFECT |
|---|---|
| Anticoagulants (oral) | Decreased anticoagulant effect. |
| Anticonvulsants | Changed seizure patterns. |
| Antidepressants (tricyclics) | Decreased antidepressant effect. Possible dangerous oversedation. |
| Antidiabetics (oral) | Increased pentobarbital effect. |
| Antihistamines | Dangerous sedation. Avoid. |
| Anti-inflammatory drugs (non-steroidal) | Decreased anti-inflammatory effect. |
| Aspirin | Decreased aspirin effect. |
| Beta-adrenergic blockers | Decreased effect of beta-adrenergic blocker. |
| Contraceptives (oral) | Decreased contraceptive effect. |
| Cortisone drugs | Decreased cortisone effect. |

| Digitoxin | Decreased digitoxin effect. |
|---|---|
| Doxycycline | Decreased doxycycline effect. |
| Dronabinol | Increased effects of both drugs. Avoid. |
| Griseofulvin | Decreased griseofulvin effect. |
| Indapamide | Increased indapamide effect. |
| MAO inhibitors | Increased pentobarbital effect. |
| Mind-altering drugs | Dangerous sedation. Avoid. |
| Molindone | Increased sedative effect. |
| Narcotics | Dangerous sedation. Avoid. |
| Pain relievers | Dangerous sedation. Avoid. |
| Sedatives | Dangerous sedation. Avoid. |
| Sleep inducers | Dangerous sedation. Avoid. |
| Tranquilizers | Dangerous sedation. Avoid. |
| Valproic acid | Increased pentobarbital effect. |

## POSSIBLE INTERACTION WITH OTHER SUBSTANCES

| INTERACTS WITH | COMBINED EFFECT |
|---|---|
| Alcohol: | Possible fatal oversedation. Avoid. |
| Beverages: | None expected. |
| Cocaine: | Decreased pentobarbital effect. |
| Foods: | None expected. |
| Marijuana: | Excessive sedation. Avoid. |
| Tobacco: | None expected. |

# PENTOXIFYLLINE

## BRAND NAMES

**Trental**

## BASIC INFORMATION

**Habit forming? No**
**Prescription needed? Yes**
**Available as generic? No**
**Drug class: Hemorrheologic agent**

 ## USES

Reduces pain in legs caused by poor circulation.

 ## DOSAGE & USAGE INFORMATION

**How to take:**
Extended-release tablets—Swallow whole with water and food.

**When to take:**
At mealtimes. Taking with food decreases the likelihood of irritating the stomach to cause nausea.

**If you forget a dose:**
Take as soon as you remember up to 3 hours late. If more than 3 hours, wait for next scheduled dose (don't double this dose).

**What drug does:**
● Reduces "stickiness" of red blood cells and improves flexibility of the red cells.
● Improves blood flow through blood vessels.

**Time lapse before drug works:**
1 hour. Several weeks for full effect on circulation.

**Don't take with:**
● Tobacco or medicines to treat hypertension.
● See Interaction column and consult doctor.

 ## OVERDOSE

**SYMPTOMS:**
**Drowsiness, flushed face, fainting, nervousness, convulsions, coma.**
**WHAT TO DO:**
● **Dial 0 (operator) or 911 (emergency) for an ambulance or medical help. Then give first aid immediately.**
● **See emergency information on inside covers.**

 ## POSSIBLE ADVERSE REACTIONS OR SIDE EFFECTS

| SYMPTOMS | WHAT TO DO |
|---|---|
| **Life-threatening:** | |
| Chest pain, irregular heartbeat. | Discontinue. Seek emergency treatment. |
| **Common:** | |
| None expected. | |
| **Infrequent:** | |
| Dizziness, headache, nausea, vomiting. | Discontinue. Call doctor right away. |
| **Rare:** | |
| None expected. | |

## WARNINGS & PRECAUTIONS

**Don't take if:**
You are allergic to pentoxifylline.

**Before you start, consult your doctor:**
If you are allergic to caffeine, theophylline, theobromine, aminophyllin, dyphyllin, oxtriphylline, theobromine.

**Over age 60:**
Adverse reactions and side effects may be more frequent and severe than in younger persons. Ask doctor about smaller doses.

**Pregnancy:**
Safety to unborn child unestablished. Avoid if possible.

**Breast-feeding:**
No problems expected, but ask doctor.

**Infants & children:**
Not recommended.

**Prolonged use:**
No problems expected.

**Skin & sunlight:**
No problems expected.

**Driving, piloting or hazardous work:**
Wait to see if drug causes drowsiness or dizziness. If none, no problems expected.

**Discontinuing:**
No problems expected.

**Others:**
Don't smoke.

## POSSIBLE INTERACTION WITH OTHER DRUGS

| GENERIC NAME OR DRUG CLASS | COMBINED EFFECT |
|---|---|
| Anithypertensives (high blood pressure medicine such as Acebutolol, Alseroxylen, Amiloride, Atenolol, Butmetanide, Captopril, Chlorothiazide, Chlorthalidone, Clonidine, Cyclothiazide, Guanethidine, Hydralazine, Methyldopa, Metoprolol, Spironolactone, Verapamil, Nadolol, Oxprenolol, Pindolol, Propranolol, Timolol) | Increased effect of hypertensive medication. |

## POSSIBLE INTERACTION WITH OTHER SUBSTANCES

| INTERACTS WITH | COMBINED EFFECT |
|---|---|
| Alcohol: | Unknown. Best to avoid. |
| Beverages: Coffee, tea or other caffeine-containing beverages. | May decrease effectiveness of pentoxifylline. |
| Cocaine: | Reduces pentoxifylline effect. |
| Foods: | None expected. |
| Marijuana: | Decreased effect of pentoxifylline. |
| Tobacco: | Decreased effect of pentoxifylline. |

# PERPHENAZINE

## BRAND NAMES

| | |
|---|---|
| Apo-Perphenazine | Phenazine |
| Etrafon | Triavil |
| PMS Levazine | Trilafon |

## BASIC INFORMATION

**Habit forming? No**
**Prescription needed? Yes**
**Available as generic? Yes**
**Drug class: Tranquilizer, antiemetic
 (phenothiazine)**

## USES

- Stops nausea, vomiting.
- Reduces anxiety, agitation.

## DOSAGE & USAGE INFORMATION

**How to take:**
- Tablet or capsule—Swallow with liquid or food to lessen stomach irritation.
- Suppositories—Remove wrapper and moisten suppository with water. Gently insert into rectum, large end first.
- Drops or liquid—Dilute dose in beverage.

**When to take:**
- Nervous and mental disorders—Take at the same times each day.
- Nausea and vomiting—Take as needed, no more often than every 4 hours.

**If you forget a dose:**
- Nervous and mental disorders—Take up to 2 hours late. If more than 2 hours, wait for next scheduled dose (don't double this dose).
- Nausea and vomiting—Take as soon as you remember. Wait 4 hours for next dose.

**What drug does:**
- Suppresses brain's vomiting center.
- Suppresses brain centers that control abnormal emotions and behavior.

*Continued next column*

## OVERDOSE

**SYMPTOMS:**
**Stupor, convulsions, coma.**
**WHAT TO DO:**
- **Dial 0 (operator) or 911 (emergency) for an ambulance or medical help. Then give first aid immediately.**
- **See emergency information on inside covers.**

**Time lapse before drug works:**
- Nausea and vomiting—1 hour or less.
- Nervous and mental disorders—4-6 weeks.

**Don't take with:**
- Antacid or medicine for diarrhea.
- Non-prescription drug for cough, cold or allergy.
- See Interaction column and consult doctor.

## POSSIBLE ADVERSE REACTIONS OR SIDE EFFECTS

| SYMPTOMS | WHAT TO DO |
|---|---|
| **Life-threatening:**<br>None expected. | |
| **Common:** | |
| • Muscle spasms of face and neck, unsteady gait. | Discontinue. Seek emergency treatment. |
| • Restlessness, tremor, drowsiness. | Discontinue. Call doctor right away. |
| • Decreased sweating, dry mouth, runny nose, constipation. | Continue. Call doctor when convenient. |
| **Infrequent:** | |
| • Fainting. | Discontinue. Seek emergency treatment. |
| • Rash. | Discontinue. Call doctor right away. |
| • Difficult urination, diminished sex drive, swollen breasts, menstrual irregularities. | Continue. Call doctor when convenient. |
| **Rare:**<br>Change in vision, jaundice, sore throat, fever. | Discontinue. Call doctor right away. |

# PERPHENAZINE

## WARNINGS & PRECAUTIONS

**Don't take if:**
- You are allergic to any phenothiazine.
- You have a blood or bone-marrow disease.

**Before you start, consult your doctor:**
- If you will have surgery within 2 months, including dental surgery, requiring general or spinal anesthesia.
- If you have asthma, emphysema or other lung disorder.
- If you take non-prescription ulcer medicine, asthma medicine or amphetamines.

**Over age 60:**
Adverse reactions and side effects may be more frequent and severe than in younger persons. More likely to develop involuntary movement of jaws, lips, tongue, chewing. Report this to your doctor immediately. Early treatment can help.

**Pregnancy:**
Risk to unborn child outweighs drug benefits. Don't use.

**Breast-feeding:**
Drug passes into milk. Avoid drug or discontinue nursing until you finish medicine. Consult doctor for advice on maintaining milk supply.

**Infants & children:**
Don't give to children younger than 2.

**Prolonged use:**
May lead to tardive dyskinesia (involuntary movement of jaws, lips, tongue, chewing).

**Skin & sunlight:**
May cause rash or intensify sunburn in areas exposed to sun or sunlamp. Skin may remain sensitive for 3 months after discontinuing.

**Driving, piloting or hazardous work:**
Don't drive or pilot aircraft until you learn how medicine affects you. Don't work around dangerous machinery. Don't climb ladders or work in high places. Danger increases if you drink alcohol or take medicine affecting alertness and reflexes.

**Discontinuing:**
- Nervous and mental disorders—Don't discontinue without doctor's advice until you complete prescribed dose, even though symptoms diminish or disappear.
- Nausea and vomiting—May be unnecessary to finish medicine. Follow doctor's instructions.

**Others:**
No problems expected.

## POSSIBLE INTERACTION WITH OTHER DRUGS

| GENERIC NAME OR DRUG CLASS | COMBINED EFFECT |
|---|---|
| Anticholinergics | Increased anticholinergic effect. |
| Antidepressants (tricyclic) | Increased perphenazine effect. |
| Antihistamines | Increased antihistamine effect. |
| Appetite suppressants | Decreased suppressant effect. |
| Dronabinol | Increased effects of both drugs. Avoid. |
| Levodopa | Decreased levodopa effect. |
| Mind-altering drugs | Increased effect of mind-altering drugs. |
| Molindone | Increased tranquilizer effect. |
| Narcotics | Increased narcotic effect. |
| Phenytoin | Increased phenytoin effect. |
| Quinidine | Impaired heart function. Dangerous mixture. |
| Sedatives | Increased sedative effect. |
| Tranquilizers (other) | Increased tranquilizer effect. |

## POSSIBLE INTERACTION WITH OTHER SUBSTANCES

| INTERACTS WITH | COMBINED EFFECT |
|---|---|
| Alcohol: | Dangerous oversedation. |
| Beverages: | None expected. |
| Cocaine: | Decreased perphenazine effect. Avoid. |
| Foods: | None expected. |
| Marijuana: | Drowsiness. May increase antinausea effect. |
| Tobacco: | None expected. |

## BRAND NAMES

Etrafon                    Triavil

## BASIC INFORMATION

**Habit forming? No**
**Prescription needed? Yes**
**Available as generic? Yes**
**Drug class: Tranquilizer (phenothiazine),**
            **antidepressant**

## USES

- Decreases nausea, vomiting.
- Gradually relieves, but doesn't cure, symptoms of depression, anxiety, agitation.

## DOSAGE & USAGE INFORMATION

**How to take:**
Tablet or capsule—Swallow with liquid.

**When to take:**
At the same time each day.

**If you forget a dose:**
Bedtime dose—If you forget your once-a-day bedtime dose, don't take it more than 3 hours late. If more than 3 hours, wait for next scheduled dose (don't double this dose).

**What drug does:**
- Suppresses brain's vomiting center.
- Suppresses brain centers that control abnormal emotions and behavior.
- Probably affects part of brain that controls messages between nerve cells.

*Continued next column*

## OVERDOSE

**SYMPTOMS:**
**Stupor, convulsions, hallucinations, coma.**
**WHAT TO DO:**
- **Dial 0 (operator) or 911 (emergency) for an ambulance or medical help. Then give first aid immediately.**
- **If patient is unconscious and not breathing, give mouth-to-mouth breathing. If there is no heartbeat, use cardiac massage and mouth-to-mouth breathing (CPR). Don't try to make patient vomit. If you can't get help quickly, take patient to nearest emergency facility.**
- **See emergency information on inside covers.**

**Time lapse before drug works:**
- Nausea and vomiting—1 hour or less.
- Nervous and mental disorders—4-6 weeks.
- Begins in 1 to 2 weeks. May require 4 to 6 weeks for maximum benefit.

**Don't take with:**
- Antacid or medicine for diarrhea.
- Non-prescription drug for cough, cold or allergy.
- Non-prescription drugs without consulting doctor.
- See Interaction column and consult doctor.

## POSSIBLE ADVERSE REACTIONS OR SIDE EFFECTS

| SYMPTOMS | WHAT TO DO |
|---|---|
| **Life-threatening:** | |
| Seizures, irregular heartbeat, weak pulse, fainting, muscle spasms. | Discontinue. Seek emergency treatment. |
| **Common:** | |
| • Headache, constipation, nausea, vomiting, irregular heartbeat, drowsiness. | Discontinue. Call doctor right away. |
| • Insomnia, dry mouth, "sweet tooth," decreased sweating, runny nose, constipation. | Continue. Call doctor when convenient. |
| **Infrequent:** | |
| • Hallucinations, dizziness, tremor, blurred vision, eye pain, vomiting. | Discontinue. Call doctor right away. |
| • Frequent urination, diminished sex drive, breast swelling, menstrual irregularities. | Continue. Call doctor when convenient. |
| **Rare:** | |
| • Rash; itchy skin; sore throat; jaundice; fever; change in vision; sore throat, fever, mouth sores. | Discontinue. Call doctor right away. |
| • Fatigue, weakness. | Continue. Call doctor when convenient. |

## WARNINGS & PRECAUTIONS

### Don't take if:
- You are allergic to any phenothiazine, tricyclic antidepressant.
- You have a blood or bone-marrow disease or glaucoma.
- You drink alcohol.
- You have had a heart attack within 6 weeks.
- You have taken MAO inhibitors within 2 weeks.
- Patient is younger than 12.

### Before you start, consult your doctor:
- If you have asthma, emphysema or other lung disorder.
- If you have an enlarged prostate, heart disease, high blood pressure, stomach or intestinal problems, overactive thyroid, liver disease.
- If you take non-prescription ulcer medicine, asthma medicine or amphetamines.
- If you will have surgery within 2 months, including dental surgery, requiring general or spinal anesthesia.

### Over age 60:
Adverse reactions and side effects may be more frequent and severe than in younger persons. More likely to develop involuntary movement of jaws, lips, tongue, chewing, difficult urination. Report this to your doctor immediately. Early treatment can help.

### Pregnancy:
Risk to unborn child outweighs drug benefits. Don't use.

### Breast-feeding:
Drug passes into milk. Avoid drug or discontinue nursing until you finish medicine. Consult doctor for advice on maintaining milk supply.

### Infants & children:
Don't give to children younger than 12.

### Prolonged use:
May lead to tardive dyskinesia (involuntary movement of jaws, lips, tongue, chewing).

### Skin & sunlight:
May cause rash or intensify sunburn in areas exposed to sun or sunlamp. Skin may remain sensitive for 3 months after discontinuing.

### Driving, piloting or hazardous work:
Don't drive or pilot aircraft until you learn how medicine affects you. Don't work around dangerous machinery. Don't climb ladders or work in high places. Danger increases if you drink alcohol or take medicine affecting alertness and reflexes, such as antihistamines, tranquilizers, sedatives, pain medicine, narcotics and mind-altering drugs.

### Discontinuing:
- Nervous and mental disorders—Don't discontinue without doctor's advice until you complete prescribed dose, even though symptoms diminish or disappear.
- Dose may require gradual reduction if you have taken drug for a long time. Doses of other drugs may also require adjustment.

### Others:
No problems expected.

## POSSIBLE INTERACTION WITH OTHER DRUGS

| GENERIC NAME OR DRUG CLASS | COMBINED EFFECT |
| --- | --- |
| Anticholinergics | Increased anticholinergic effect, increased sedation. |
| Anticoagulants (oral) | Increased anticoagulant effect. |
| Antihistamines | Increased antihistamine effect. |
| Appetite suppressants | Decreased suppressant effect. |
| Barbiturates | Decreased antidepressant effect. |
| Clonidine | Decreased clonidine effect. |
| Diuretics (thiazide) | Increased antidepressant effect. |
| Dronabinol | Increased effect of both drugs. |
| Ethchlorvynol | Delirium. |

*Continued page 971*

## POSSIBLE INTERACTION WITH OTHER SUBSTANCES

| INTERACTS WITH | COMBINED EFFECT |
| --- | --- |
| **Alcohol:** Beverages or medicines with alcohol. | Excessive intoxication. Avoid. |
| **Beverages:** Coffee. | Reduces effectiveness. |
| **Cocaine:** | Excessive intoxication. Avoid. |
| **Foods:** | None expected. |
| **Marijuana:** | Excessive drowsiness. Avoid. |
| **Tobacco:** | None expected. |

# PHENACETIN

## BRAND NAMES

A.P.C. Tablets
Aspirin Compound
   with Codeine
Emprazil
Fiorinal
P.A.C. Compound
Percodan

Propoxyphene
   Compound 65
Sinubid
SK-65 Compound
Soma Compound
Tabloid APC with
   Codeine

## BASIC INFORMATION

**Habit forming?** No
**Prescription needed?** Yes
**Available as generic?** Yes
**Drug class:** Analgesic, fever reducer

## USES

- Relieves pain.
- Reduces fever.

## DOSAGE & USAGE INFORMATION

**How to take:**
- Tablet or capsule—Swallow with liquid or food to lessen stomach irritation. You may chew or crush tablets.
- Extended-release tablets or capsules— Swallow each dose whole with liquid.

**When to take:**
At the same times each day.

**If you forget a dose:**
Take as soon as you remember up to 2 hours late. If more than 2 hours, wait for next scheduled dose (don't double this dose).

**What drug does:**
Reduces level of prostaglandins, a chemical involved in producing inflammation, fever, pain.

**Time lapse before drug works:**
15 minutes.

**Don't take with:**
See Interaction column and consult doctor.

## OVERDOSE

**SYMPTOMS:**
Sweating, bloody urine, convulsions, coma.
**WHAT TO DO:**
- Dial 0 (operator) or 911 (emergency) for an ambulance or medical help. Then give first aid immediately.
- See emergency information on inside covers.

## POSSIBLE ADVERSE REACTIONS OR SIDE EFFECTS

| SYMPTOMS | WHAT TO DO |
|---|---|
| **Life-threatening:** None expected. | |
| **Common:** None expected. | |
| **Infrequent:** | |
| • Rash; itchy skin; hives; sore throat, fever, mouth sores. | Discontinue. Call doctor right away. |
| • Confusion, drowsiness, nausea. | Continue. Call doctor when convenient. |
| **Rare:** | |
| • Black, bloody or tarry stools. | Discontinue. Seek emergency treatment. |
| • Easy bruising, swollen feet or legs, blood in urine, anemia, blue fingernails, fatigue, weakness. | Discontinue. Call doctor right away. |

## WARNINGS & PRECAUTIONS

**Don't take if:**
You are allergic to phenacetin, aspirin or any of the many mixtures which contain either.

**Before you start, consult your doctor:**
- If you have kidney or liver disease.
- If you have G6PD deficiency.

**Over age 60:**
Adverse reactions and side effects may be more frequent and severe than in younger persons.

**Pregnancy:**
May cause anemia in newborn. Avoid if possible.

**Breast-feeding:**
Drug passes into milk. Avoid drug or discontinue nursing until you finish medicine. Consult doctor for advice on maintaining milk supply.

**Infants & children:**
Not recommended.

**Prolonged use:**
Kidney damage. Don't take regularly without medical advice.

**Skin & sunlight:**
No problems expected.

**Driving, piloting or hazardous work:**
No problems expected.

**Discontinuing:**
May be unnecessary to finish medicine. Follow doctor's instructions.

**Others:**
No problems expected.

 ## POSSIBLE INTERACTION WITH OTHER DRUGS

| GENERIC NAME OR DRUG CLASS | COMBINED EFFECT |
| --- | --- |
| Phenobarbital | Decreased phenacetin effect. |

 ## POSSIBLE INTERACTION WITH OTHER SUBSTANCES

| INTERACTS WITH | COMBINED EFFECT |
| --- | --- |
| Alcohol: | None expected. |
| Beverages: | None expected. |
| Cocaine: | None expected. |
| Foods: | None expected. |
| Marijuana: | Increased pain relief. |
| Tobacco: | None expected. |

# PHENAZOPYRIDINE

## BRAND NAMES

| | |
|---|---|
| Azo-100 | Phen-Azo |
| Azodine | Phenazodine |
| Azo-Gantanol | Pyridiate |
| Azo-Gantrisin | Pyridium |
| Azo-Mandelamine | Pyridium Plus |
| Azo-Standard | Pyrodine |
| Azotrex | Pyronium |
| Baridium | Thiosulfil-A |
| Di-Azo | Urobiotic |

## BASIC INFORMATION

**Habit forming? No**
**Prescription needed? Yes**
**Available as generic? Yes**
**Drug class: Analgesic (urinary)**

## USES

Relieves pain of lower urinary-tract irritation, as in cystitis, urethritis or prostatitis. Relieves symptoms only. Phenazopyridine alone does not cure infections.

## DOSAGE & USAGE INFORMATION

**How to take:**
Tablet or capsule—Swallow with liquid or food to lessen stomach irritation.

**When to take:**
At the same times each day.

**If you forget a dose:**
Take as soon as you remember up to 2 hours late. If more than 2 hours, wait for next scheduled dose (don't double this dose).

**What drug does:**
Anesthetizes lower urinary tract. Relieves pain, burning, pressure and urgency to urinate.

**Time lapse before drug works:**
1 to 2 hours.

**Don't take with:**
No restrictions.

## OVERDOSE

**SYMPTOMS:**
Shortness of breath, weakness.
**WHAT TO DO:**
Overdose unlikely to threaten life. If person takes much larger amount than prescribed, call doctor, poison-control center or hospital emergency room for instructions.

## POSSIBLE ADVERSE REACTIONS OR SIDE EFFECTS

| SYMPTOMS | WHAT TO DO |
|---|---|
| **Life-threatening:** None expected. | |
| **Common:** Red-orange urine. | No action necessary. |
| **Infrequent:** Indigestion, fatigue, weakness. | Continue. Call doctor when convenient. |
| **Rare:** | |
| • Rash, jaundice. | Discontinue. Call doctor right away. |
| • Headache, anemia. | Continue. Call doctor when convenient. |

## WARNINGS & PRECAUTIONS

**Don't take if:**
- You have hepatitis.
- You are allergic to any urinary analgesic.

**Before you start, consult your doctor:**
If you have kidney or liver disease.

**Over age 60:**
Adverse reactions and side effects may be more frequent and severe than in younger persons.

**Pregnancy:**
No proven harm to unborn child. Avoid if possible.

**Breast-feeding:**
No problems expected.

**Infants & children:**
Not recommended.

**Prolonged use:**
- Orange or yellow skin.
- Anemia. Occasional blood studies recommended.

**Skin & sunlight:**
No problems expected.

**Driving, piloting or hazardous work:**
No problems expected.

**Discontinuing:**
May be unnecessary to finish medicine. Follow doctor's instructions.

**Others:**
No problems expected.

## POSSIBLE INTERACTION WITH OTHER DRUGS

| GENERIC NAME OR DRUG CLASS | COMBINED EFFECT |
|---|---|
| None | |

## POSSIBLE INTERACTION WITH OTHER SUBSTANCES

| INTERACTS WITH | COMBINED EFFECT |
|---|---|
| Alcohol: | None expected. |
| Beverages: | None expected. |
| Cocaine: | None expected. |
| Foods: | None expected. |
| Marijuana: | None expected. |
| Tobacco: | None expected. |

# PHENIRAMINE

## BRAND NAMES

| | |
|---|---|
| Citra Capsules | S-T Forte |
| Citra Forte | Symptrol |
| Dri-Hist No. 2 Meta | Triaminic |
| Caps | Triaminicin |
| Dristan Nasal Spray | Triaminicol |
| Fiogesic | Tussagesic |
| Inhistor | Tussaminic |
| Poly-Histine D | Tussirex Sugar-Free |
| Robitussin-AC | Ursinus |
| Ru-Tuss | |

## BASIC INFORMATION

**Habit forming? No**
**Prescription needed?**
  **High strength: Yes**
  **Low strength: No**
**Available as generic? Yes**
**Drug class: Antihistamine**

## USES

Reduces allergic symptoms such as hay fever, hives, rash or itching.

## DOSAGE & USAGE INFORMATION

**How to take:**
- Tablet, syrup or capsule—Swallow with liquid or food to lessen stomach irritation.
- Extended-release tablets or capsules—Swallow each dose whole.

**When to take:**
Varies with form. Follow label directions.

**If you forget a dose:**
Take as soon as you remember up to 2 hours late. If more than 2 hours, wait for next scheduled dose (don't double this dose).

*Continued next column*

## OVERDOSE

**SYMPTOMS:**
Convulsions, red face, hallucinations, coma.
**WHAT TO DO:**
- Dial 0 (operator) or 911 (emergency) for an ambulance or medical help. Then give first aid immediately.
- See emergency information on inside covers.

**What drug does:**
Blocks action of histamine after an allergic response triggers histamine release in sensitive cells.

**Time lapse before drug works:**
30 minutes.

**Don't take with:**
See Interaction column and consult doctor.

## POSSIBLE ADVERSE REACTIONS OR SIDE EFFECTS

| SYMPTOMS | WHAT TO DO |
|---|---|
| **Life-threatening:**<br>None expected. | |
| **Common:**<br>Drowsiness, dizziness, dry mouth, nose, throat, nausea. | Continue. Tell doctor at next visit. |
| **Infrequent:**<br>• Change in vision. | Discontinue. Call doctor right away. |
| • Less tolerance for contact lenses, difficult urination. | Continue. Call doctor when convenient. |
| • Appetite loss. | Continue. Tell doctor at next visit. |
| **Rare:**<br>Nightmares, agitation, irritability, sore throat, fever, rapid heartbeat, unusual bleeding or bruising, fatigue, weakness. | Discontinue. Call doctor right away. |

## WARNINGS & PRECAUTIONS

**Don't take if:**
You are allergic to any antihistamine.

**Before you start, consult your doctor:**
- If you have glaucoma.
- If you have enlarged prostate.
- If you have asthma.
- If you have kidney disease.
- If you have peptic ulcer.
- If you will have surgery within 2 months, including dental surgery, requiring general or spinal anesthesia.

**Over age 60:**
Don't exceed recommended dose. Adverse reactions and side effects may be more frequent and severe than in younger persons, especially urination difficulty, diminished alertness and other brain and nervous-system symptoms.

**Pregnancy:**
No proven harm to unborn child. Avoid if possible.

**Breast-feeding:**
Drug passes into milk. Avoid drug or discontinue nursing until you finish medicine. Consult doctor for advice on maintaining milk supply.

**Infants & children:**
Not recommended for premature or newborn infants. Otherwise, no problems expected.

**Prolonged use:**
Avoid. May damage bone-marrow and nerve cells.

**Skin & sunlight:**
May cause rash or intensify sunburn in areas exposed to sun or sunlamp.

**Driving, piloting or hazardous work:**
Don't drive or pilot aircraft until you learn how medicine affects you. Don't work around dangerous machinery. Don't climb ladders or work in high places. Danger increases if you drink alcohol or take medicine affecting alertness and reflexes, such as antihistamines, tranquilizers, sedatives, pain medicine, narcotics and mind-altering drugs.

**Discontinuing:**
No problems expected.

**Others:**
May mask symptoms of hearing damage from aspirin, other salicylates, cisplatin, paromomycin, vancomycin or anticonvulsants. Consult doctor if you use these.

 ## POSSIBLE INTERACTION WITH OTHER DRUGS

| GENERIC NAME OR DRUG CLASS | COMBINED EFFECT |
|---|---|
| Anticholinergics | Increased anticholinergic effect. |
| Antidepressants (tricyclic) | Increased pheniramine effect. |
| Antihistamines (other) | Excess sedation. Avoid. |
| Dronabinol | Increased effects of both drugs. Avoid. |
| Hypnotics | Excess sedation. Avoid. |
| MAO inhibitors | Increased pheniramine effect. |
| Mind-altering drugs | Excess sedation. Avoid. |
| Narcotics | Excess sedation. Avoid. |
| Sedatives | Excess sedation. Avoid. |
| Sleep inducers | Excess sedation. Avoid. |
| Tranquilizers | Excess sedation. Avoid. |

 ## POSSIBLE INTERACTION WITH OTHER SUBSTANCES

| INTERACTS WITH | COMBINED EFFECT |
|---|---|
| Alcohol: | Excess sedation. Avoid. |
| Beverages: Caffeine drinks. | Less pheniramine sedation. |
| Cocaine: | Decreased pheniramine effect. Avoid. |
| Foods: | None expected. |
| Marijuana: | Excess sedation. Avoid. |
| Tobacco: | None expected. |

# PHENOBARBITAL

## BRAND NAMES

See complete list of brand names in the *Brand Name Directory,* page 953.

## BASIC INFORMATION

**Habit forming? Yes**
**Prescription needed? Yes**
**Available as generic? Yes**
**Drug class: Sedative, hypnotic (barbiturate), anticonvulsant**

## USES

- Reduces anxiety or nervous tension (low dose).
- Relieves insomnia (higher bedtime dose).
- Prevents convulsions or seizures, such as epilepsy.

## DOSAGE & USAGE INFORMATION

**How to take:**
- Tablet, liquid or capsule—Swallow with liquid or food to lessen stomach irritation. If you can't swallow whole, crumble tablet or open capsule and take with liquid or food.
- Extended-release tablets or capsules—Swallow each dose whole.
- Drops—Dilute dose in beverage before swallowing.

**When to take:**
At the same times each day.

**If you forget a dose:**
Take as soon as you remember up to 2 hours late. If more than 2 hours, wait for next scheduled dose (don't double this dose).

**What drug does:**
May partially block nerve impulses at nerve-cell connections.

*Continued next column*

## OVERDOSE

**SYMPTOMS:**
**Deep sleep, weak pulse, coma.**
**WHAT TO DO:**
- **Dial 0 (operator) or 911 (emergency) for an ambulance or medical help. Then give first aid immediately.**
- **See emergency information on inside covers.**

**Time lapse before drug works:**
60 minutes.

**Don't take with:**
- Non-prescription drugs without consulting doctor.
- See Interaction column and consult doctor.

## POSSIBLE ADVERSE REACTIONS OR SIDE EFFECTS

| SYMPTOMS | WHAT TO DO |
|---|---|
| **Life-threatening:**<br>None expected. | |
| **Common:**<br>Dizziness, drowsiness, "hangover" effect. | Continue. Call doctor when convenient. |
| **Infrequent:**<br>• Rash or hives, face or lip swelling, swollen eyelids, sore throat, fever. | Discontinue. Call doctor right away. |
| • Depression, confusion, slurred speech, diarrhea, nausea, vomiting, joint or muscle pain. | Continue. Call doctor when convenient. |
| **Rare:**<br>• Agitation, slow heartbeat, difficult breathing, jaundice. | Discontinue. Call doctor right away. |
| • Unexplained bleeding or bruising. | Continue. Call doctor when convenient. |

## WARNINGS & PRECAUTIONS

**Don't take if:**
- You are allergic to any barbiturate.
- You have porphyria.

**Before you start, consult your doctor:**
- If you have epilepsy.
- If you have kidney or liver damage.
- If you have asthma.
- If you have anemia.
- If you have chronic pain.
- If you will have surgery within 2 months, including dental surgery, requiring general or spinal anesthesia.

**Over age 60:**
Adverse reactions and side effects may be more frequent and severe than in younger persons. Use small doses.

**Pregnancy:**
Risk to unborn child outweighs drug benefits. Don't use.

**Breast-feeding:**
Drug passes into milk. Avoid drug or discontinue nursing until you finish medicine. Consult doctor for advice on maintaining milk supply.

**Infants & children:**
Use only under doctor's supervision.

**Prolonged use:**
- May cause addiction, anemia, chronic intoxication.
- May lower body temperature, making exposure to cold temperatures hazardous.

**Skin & sunlight:**
May cause rash or intensify sunburn in areas exposed to sun or sunlamp.

**Driving, piloting or hazardous work:**
Don't drive or pilot aircraft until you learn how medicine affects you. Don't work around dangerous machinery. Don't climb ladders or work in high places. Danger increases if you drink alcohol or take medicine affecting alertness and reflexes.

**Discontinuing:**
May be unnecessary to finish medicine. Follow doctor's instructions. If you develop withdrawal symptoms of hallucinations, agitation or sleeplessness after discontinuing, call doctor right away.

**Others:**
Great potential for abuse.

## POSSIBLE INTERACTION WITH OTHER DRUGS

| GENERIC NAME OR DRUG CLASS | COMBINED EFFECT |
|---|---|
| Anticoagulants (oral) | Decreased anticoagulant effect. |
| Anticonvulsants | Changed seizure patterns. |
| Antidepressants (tricyclics) | Decreased antidepressant effect. Possible dangerous oversedation. |
| Antidiabetics (oral) | Increased phenobarbital effect. |
| Antihistamines | Dangerous sedation. Avoid. |
| Anti-inflammatory drugs (non-steroidal) | Decreased anti-inflammatory effect. |
| Aspirin | Decreased aspirin effect. |
| Beta-adrenergic blockers | Decreased effect of beta-adrenergic blocker. |

| | |
|---|---|
| Contraceptives (oral) | Decreased contraceptive effect. |
| Cortisone drugs | Decreased cortisone effect. |
| Digitoxin | Decreased digitoxin effect. |
| Doxycycline | Decreased doxycycline effect. |
| Dronabinol | Increased effects of both drugs. Avoid. |
| Griseofulvin | Decreased griseofulvin effect. |
| Indapamide | Increased indapamide effect. |
| MAO inhibitors | Increased phenobarbital effect. |
| Mind-altering drugs | Dangerous sedation. Avoid. |
| Molindone | Increased sedative effect. |
| Narcotics | Dangerous sedation. Avoid. |
| Pain relievers | Dangerous sedation. Avoid. |
| Sedatives | Dangerous sedation. Avoid. |
| Sleep inducers | Dangerous sedation. Avoid. |
| Tranquilizers | Dangerous sedation. Avoid. |
| Valproic acid | Increased phenobarbital effect. |

## POSSIBLE INTERACTION WITH OTHER SUBSTANCES

| INTERACTS WITH | COMBINED EFFECT |
|---|---|
| Alcohol: | Possible fatal oversedation. Avoid. |
| Beverages: | None expected. |
| Cocaine: | Decreased phenobarbital effect. |
| Foods: | None expected. |
| Marijuana: | Excessive sedation. Avoid. |
| Tobacco: | None expected. |

# PHENOLPHTHALEIN

## BRAND NAMES

| | |
|---|---|
| Agoral | Evac-U-Lax |
| Alophen | Ex-Lax |
| Correctol | Feen-A-Mint |
| Espotabs | Fructines-Vichy |
| Evac-Q-Kit | Phenolax |
| Evac-Q-Kwik | Prulet |
| Evac-U-Gen | Trilax |

## BASIC INFORMATION

**Habit forming? No**
**Prescription needed? No**
**Available as generic? Yes**
**Drug class: Laxative (stimulant)**

 ## USES

Constipation relief.

 ## DOSAGE & USAGE INFORMATION

**How to take:**
- Tablet or wafer—Swallow with liquid. If you can't swallow whole, chew or crumble and take with liquid or food.
- Liquid—Drink 6 to 8 glasses of water each day, in addition to one taken with each dose.
- Chewable tablets—Chew thoroughly before swallowing.

**When to take:**
Usually at bedtime with a snack, unless directed otherwise.

**If you forget a dose:**
Take as soon as you remember.

**What drug does:**
Acts on smooth muscles of intestine wall to cause vigorous bowel movement.

**Time lapse before drug works:**
6 to 10 hours.

*Continued next column*

 ## OVERDOSE

**SYMPTOMS:**
Vomiting, electrolyte depletion.
**WHAT TO DO:**
Overdose unlikely to threaten life. If person takes much larger amount than prescribed, call doctor, poison-control center or hospital emergency room for instructions.

**Don't take with:**
- See Interaction column and consult doctor.
- Don't take within 2 hours of taking another medicine. Laxative interferes with medicine absorption.

 ## POSSIBLE ADVERSE REACTIONS OR SIDE EFFECTS

| SYMPTOMS | WHAT TO DO |
|---|---|
| **Life-threatening:** | |
| None expected. | |
| **Common:** | |
| • Rectal irritation. | Continue. Call doctor when convenient. |
| • Pink to orange urine. | No action necessary. |
| **Infrequent:** | |
| • Dangerous potassium loss. | Discontinue. Call doctor right away. |
| • Belching, cramps, nausea. | Continue. Call doctor when convenient. |
| **Rare:** | |
| Irritability, confusion, headache, rash, difficult breathing, irregular heartbeat, muscle cramps, unusual tiredness or weakness, burning on urination. | Discontinue. Call doctor right away. |

## WARNINGS & PRECAUTIONS

### Don't take if:
- You have symptoms of appendicitis, inflamed bowel or intestinal blockage.
- You are allergic to a stimulant laxative.
- You have missed a bowel movement for only 1 or 2 days.

### Before you start, consult your doctor:
- If you have a colostomy or ileostomy.
- If you have congestive heart disease.
- If you have diabetes.
- If you have high blood pressure.
- If you have a laxative habit.
- If you have rectal bleeding.
- If you take other laxatives.

### Over age 60:
Adverse reactions and side effects may be more frequent and severe than in younger persons.

### Pregnancy:
Risk to mother and unborn child outweighs drug benefits. Don't use.

### Breast-feeding:
Drug passes into milk. Avoid drug or discontinue nursing until you finish medicine. Consult doctor for advice on maintaining milk supply.

### Infants & children:
Use only under medical supervision.

### Prolonged use:
Don't take for more than 1 week unless under a doctor's supervision. May cause laxative dependence.

### Skin & sunlight:
No problems expected.

### Driving, piloting or hazardous work:
No problems expected.

### Discontinuing:
May be unnecessary to finish medicine. Follow doctor's instructions.

### Others:
Don't take to "flush out" your system or as a "tonic."

## POSSIBLE INTERACTION WITH OTHER DRUGS

| GENERIC NAME OR DRUG CLASS | COMBINED EFFECT |
|---|---|
| Antacids | Tablet coating may dissolve too rapidly, irritating stomach or bowel. |
| Antihypertensives | May cause dangerous low potassium level. |
| Diuretics | May cause dangerous low potassium level. |

## POSSIBLE INTERACTION WITH OTHER SUBSTANCES

| INTERACTS WITH | COMBINED EFFECT |
|---|---|
| Alcohol: | None expected. |
| Beverages: Milk. | Tablet coating may dissolve too rapidly, irritating stomach or bowel. |
| Cocaine: | None expected. |
| Foods: | None expected. |
| Marijuana: | None expected. |
| Tobacco: | None expected. |

# PHENPROCOUMON

## BRAND NAMES

Liquamar                    Marcumar

## BASIC INFORMATION

**Habit forming? No**
**Prescription needed? Yes**
**Available as generic? Yes**
**Drug class: Anticoagulant**

## USES

Reduces blood clots. Used for abnormal clotting inside blood vessels.

## DOSAGE & USAGE INFORMATION

**How to take:**
Tablet—Swallow with liquid. If you can't swallow whole, crumble tablet and take with liquid or food.

**When to take:**
At the same time each day.

**If you forget a dose:**
Take as soon as you remember up to 12 hours late. If more than 12 hours, wait for next scheduled dose (don't double this dose). Inform your doctor of any missed doses.

**What drug does:**
Blocks action of vitamin K necessary for blood clotting.

**Time lapse before drug works:**
36 to 48 hours.

**Don't take with:**
See Interaction column and consult doctor.

## OVERDOSE

**SYMPTOMS:**
**Bloody vomit and bloody or black stools, red urine.**
**WHAT TO DO:**
- **Dial 0 (operator) or 911 (emergency) for an ambulance or medical help. Then give first aid immediately.**
- **See emergency information on inside covers.**

## POSSIBLE ADVERSE REACTIONS OR SIDE EFFECTS

| SYMPTOMS | WHAT TO DO |
|---|---|
| **Life-threatening:**<br>None expected. | |
| **Common:**<br>Bloating, gaseousness. | Continue. Tell doctor at next visit. |
| **Infrequent:**<br>● Black stools or bloody vomit, coughing up blood. | Discontinue. Seek emergency treatment. |
| ● Rash, hives, itchy skin, blurred vision, sore throat, easy bruising or bleeding, cloudy or red urine, back pain, jaundice, fever, chills, fatigue, weakness. | Discontinue. Call doctor right away. |
| ● Diarrhea, cramps, nausea, vomiting, swollen feet or legs, hair loss. | Continue. Call doctor when convenient. |
| **Rare:**<br>Dizziness, headache, mouth sores. | Discontinue. Call doctor right away. |

## WARNINGS & PRECAUTIONS

**Don't take if:**
- You have been allergic to any oral anticoagulant.
- You have a bleeding disorder.
- You have an active peptic ulcer.
- You have ulcerative colitis.

**Before you start, consult your doctor:**
- If you take any other drugs, including non-prescription drugs.
- If you have high blood pressure.
- If you have heavy or prolonged menstrual periods.
- If you have diabetes.
- If you have a bladder catheter.
- If you have serious liver or kidney disease.
- If you will have surgery within 2 months, including dental surgery, requiring general or spinal anesthesia.

**Over age 60:**
Adverse reactions and side effects may be more frequent and severe than in younger persons.

**Pregnancy:**
Risk to unborn child outweighs drug benefits. Don't use.

**Breast-feeding:**
Drug filters into milk. May harm child. Avoid.

**Infants & children:**
Use only under doctor's supervision.

**Prolonged use:**
No problems expected.

**Skin & sunlight:**
No problems expected.

**Driving, piloting or hazardous work:**
- Avoid hazardous activities that could cause injury.
- Don't drive if you feel dizzy or have blurred vision.

**Discontinuing:**
Don't discontinue without consulting doctor. Dose may require gradual reduction if you have taken drug for a long time. Doses of other drugs may also require adjustment.

**Others:**
Carry identification to state you take anticoagulants.

## POSSIBLE INTERACTION WITH OTHER DRUGS

| GENERIC NAME OR DRUG CLASS | COMBINED EFFECT |
| --- | --- |
| Acetaminophen | Increased phenprocoumon effect. |
| Allopurinol | Increased phenprocoumon effect. |
| Androgens | Increased phenprocoumon effect. |
| Antacids (large doses) | Decreased phenprocoumon effect. |
| Antibiotics | Increased phenprocoumon effect. |
| Anticonvulsants (hydantoin) | Increased effect of both drugs. |
| Antidepressants (tricyclic) | Increased phenprocoumon effect. |
| Antidiabetics (oral) | Increased phenprocoumon effect. |
| Antihistamines | Unpredictable increased or decreased anticoagulant effect |
| Barbiturates | Decreased phenprocoumon effect. |
| Benzodiazepines | Unpredictable increased or decreased anticoagulant effect. |
| Carbamazepine | Decreased phenprocoumon effect. |
| Chloral hydrate | Unpredictable increased or decreased anticoagulant effect. |

*Continued page 971*

## POSSIBLE INTERACTION WITH OTHER SUBSTANCES

| INTERACTS WITH | COMBINED EFFECT |
| --- | --- |
| Alcohol: | Can increase or decrease effect of anticoagulant. Use with caution. |
| Beverages: | None expected. |
| Cocaine: | None expected. |
| Foods: High in vitamin K such as fish, liver, spinach, cabbage. | May decrease anticoagulant effect. |
| Marijuana: | None expected. |
| Tobacco: | None expected. |

# PHENSUXIMIDE

## BRAND NAMES

Milontin

## BASIC INFORMATION

**Habit forming?** No
**Prescription needed?** Yes
**Available as generic?** No
**Drug class:** Anticonvulsant (succinimide)

## USES

Controls seizures in treatment of epilepsy.

## DOSAGE & USAGE INFORMATION

**How to take:**
Capsule or syrup—Swallow with liquid or food to lessen stomach irritation.

**When to take:**
Every day in regularly-spaced doses, according to prescription.

**If you forget a dose:**
Take as soon as you remember up to 2 hours late. If more than 2 hours, wait for next scheduled dose (don't double this dose).

**What drug does:**
Depresses nerve transmissions in part of brain that controls muscles.

**Time lapse before drug works:**
3 hours.

**Don't take with:**
See Interaction column and consult doctor.

## OVERDOSE

**SYMPTOMS:**
Coma
**WHAT TO DO:**
- Dial 0 (operator) or 911 (emergency) for an ambulance or medical help. Then give first aid immediately.
- If patient is unconscious and not breathing, give mouth-to-mouth breathing. If there is no heartbeat, use cardiac massage and mouth-to-mouth breathing (CPR). Don't try to make patient vomit. If you can't get help quickly, take patient to nearest emergency facility.
- See emergency information on inside covers.

## POSSIBLE ADVERSE REACTIONS OR SIDE EFFECTS

| SYMPTOMS | WHAT TO DO |
|---|---|
| **Life-threatening:** None expected. | |
| **Common:** Nausea, vomiting, stomach cramps, appetite loss. | Continue. Call doctor when convenient. |
| **Infrequent:** Dizziness, drowsiness, headache, irritability, mood change. | Continue. Call doctor when convenient. |
| **Rare:** • Rash, sore throat, fever, unusual bleeding or bruising. | Discontinue. Call doctor right away. |
| • Swollen lymph glands. | Continue. Call doctor when convenient. |

## WARNINGS & PRECAUTIONS

**Don't take if:**
You are allergic to any succinimide anticonvulsant.

**Before you start, consult your doctor:**
- If you plan to become pregnant within medication period.
- If you take other anticonvulsants.
- If you have blood disease.
- If you have kidney or liver disease.

**Over age 60:**
Adverse reactions and side effects may be more frequent and severe than in younger persons.

**Pregnancy:**
Risk to unborn child outweighs drug benefits. Don't use.

**Breast-feeding:**
Drug passes into milk. Avold drug or discontinue nursing.

**Infants & children:**
Use only under medical supervision.

**Prolonged use:**
No problems expected.

**Skin & sunlight:**
No problems expected.

**Driving, piloting or hazardous work:**
Don't drive or pilot aircraft until you learn how medicine affects you. Don't work around dangerous machinery. Don't climb ladders or work in high places. Danger increases if you drink alcohol or take medicine affecting alertness and reflexes, such as antihistamines, tranquilizers, sedatives, pain medicine, narcotics and mind-altering drugs.

**Discontinuing:**
Don't discontinue without doctor's advice until you complete prescribed dose, even though symptoms diminish or disappear.

**Others:**
- Your response to medicine should be checked regularly by your doctor. Dose and schedule may have to be altered frequently to fit individual needs.
- Periodic blood-cell counts, kidney- and liver-function studies recommended.

## POSSIBLE INTERACTION WITH OTHER DRUGS

| GENERIC NAME OR DRUG CLASS | COMBINED EFFECT |
|---|---|
| Anticonvulsants (other) | Increased effect of both drugs. |
| Antidepressants (tricyclic) | May provoke seizures. |
| Antipsychotics | May provoke seizures. |

## POSSIBLE INTERACTION WITH OTHER SUBSTANCES

| INTERACTS WITH | COMBINED EFFECT |
|---|---|
| Alcohol: | May provoke seizures. |
| Beverages: | None expected. |
| Cocaine: | May provoke seizures. |
| Foods: | None expected. |
| Marijuana: | May provoke seizures. |
| Tobacco: | None expected. |

# PHENYLBUTAZONE

## BRAND NAMES

Algoverine
Apo-Phenylbutazone
Azolid
Buffazone
Butagesic
Butazolidin
Intrabutazone

Malgesic
Nadozone
Neo-Zoline
Novobutazone
Phenbuff
Phenbutazone
Sterazolidin

## BASIC INFORMATION

Habit forming? No
Available as generic? Yes
Prescription needed? Yes
Drug class: Anti-inflammatory (non-steroid)

 ## USES

- Treatment for joint pain, stiffness, inflammation and swelling of arthritis and gout.
- Pain reliever.
- Treatment for dysmenorrhea (painful or difficult menstruation).

 ## DOSAGE & USAGE INFORMATION

**How to take:**
Tablet or capsule—Swallow with liquid or food to lessen stomach irritation. If you can't swallow whole, crumble tablet or open capsule and take with liquid or food.

**When to take:**
At the same times each day.

**If you forget a dose:**
Take as soon as you remember up to 2 hours late. If more than 2 hours, wait for next scheduled dose (don't double this dose).

*Continued next column*

 ## OVERDOSE

**SYMPTOMS:**
Confusion, agitation, incoherence, convulsions, possible hemorrhage from stomach or intestine, coma.
**WHAT TO DO:**
- **Dial 0 (operator) or 911 (emergency) for an ambulance or medical help. Then give first aid immediately.**
- **See emergency information on inside covers.**

**What drug does:**
Reduces tissue concentration of prostaglandins (hormones which produce inflammation and pain).

**Time lapse before drug works:**
Begins in 4 to 24 hours. May require 3 weeks regular use for maximum benefit.

**Don't take with:**
See Interaction column and consult doctor.

 ## POSSIBLE ADVERSE REACTIONS OR SIDE EFFECTS

| SYMPTOMS | WHAT TO DO |
|---|---|
| **Life-threatening:**<br>None expected. | |
| **Common:**<br>• Dizziness, stomach upset. | Continue. Call doctor when convenient. |
| • Headache. | Continue. Tell doctor at next visit. |
| **Infrequent:**<br>Depression, drowsiness, ringing in ears, constipation or diarrhea, vomiting, swollen feet or legs. | Continue. Call doctor when convenient. |
| **Rare:**<br>• Convulsions; confusion; rash, hives or itchy skin; blurred vision; sore throat, fever, mouth ulcers; black stools; vomiting blood; difficult breathing; tightness in chest; unusual bleeding or bruising; blood in urine. | Discontinue. Call doctor right away. |
| • Frequent, painful or difficult urination; fatigue; weakness; weight gain. | Continue. Call doctor when convenient. |

 ## WARNINGS & PRECAUTIONS

**Don't take if:**
- You are allergic to aspirin or any non-steroid, anti-inflammatory drug.
- You have gastritis, peptic ulcer, enteritis, ileitis, ulcerative colitis.
- Patient is younger than 15.

**Before you start, consult your doctor:**
- If you have epilepsy.
- If you have Parkinson's disease.
- If you have been mentally ill.
- If you have had kidney disease or impaired kidney function, asthma, high blood pressure, heart failure, temporal arthritis, or polymyalgia rheumatica.

**Over age 60:**
Adverse reactions and side effects may be more frequent and severe than in younger persons.

**Pregnancy:**
Studies inconclusive on harm to unborn child. Animal studies show fetal abnormalities. Decide with your doctor whether drug benefits justify risk to unborn child.

**Breast-feeding:**
Drug filters into milk. May harm child. Avoid.

**Infants & children:**
Not recommended for those younger than 15. Use only under medical supervision.

**Prolonged use:**
- Eye damage.
- May cause rare bone-marrow damage, jaundice (yellow skin and eyes), reduced hearing.
- Periodic blood counts recommended if you use a long time.

**Skin & sunlight:**
No problems expected.

**Driving, piloting or hazardous work:**
Don't drive or pilot aircraft until you learn how medicine affects you. Don't work around dangerous machinery. Don't climb ladders or work in high places. Danger increases if you drink alcohol or take medicine affecting alertness and reflexes, such as antihistamines, tranquilizers, sedatives, pain medicine, narcotics and mind-altering drugs.

**Discontinuing:**
Don't discontinue without consulting doctor. Dose may require gradual reduction if you have taken drug for a long time. Doses of other drugs may also require adjustment.

**Others:**
No problems expected.

## POSSIBLE INTERACTION WITH OTHER DRUGS

| GENERIC NAME OR DRUG CLASS | COMBINED EFFECT |
|---|---|
| Acebutolol | Decreased acebutolol effect. |
| Anticoagulants (oral) | Increased anticoagulant effect. |
| Aspirin | Possible stomach ulcer. |
| Antidiabetics (oral) | Increased antidiabetic effect. |
| Chloroquine | Possible skin toxicity. |
| Digitoxin | Decreased digitoxin effect. |
| Flecainide | Possible decreased blood-cell production in bone marrow. |
| Gold compounds | Possible increased likelihood of kidney damage. |
| Hydroxychloroquine | Possible skin toxicity. |
| Ketoprofen | Increased possibility of internal bleeding. |
| Methotrexate | Increased toxicity of both drugs to bone marrow. |
| Minoxidil | Decreased minoxidil effect. |
| Oxprenolol | Decreased antihypertensive effect of oxprenolol. |
| Penicillamine | Possible toxicity. |
| Phenytoin | Possible toxic phenytoin effect. |
| Tocainide | Possible decreased blood-cell production in bone marrow. |
| Trimethoprim | Possible bone-marrow toxicity. |

## POSSIBLE INTERACTION WITH OTHER SUBSTANCES

| INTERACTS WITH | COMBINED EFFECT |
|---|---|
| Alcohol: | Possible stomach ulcer or bleeding. |
| Beverages: | None expected. |
| Cocaine: | None expected. |
| Foods: | None expected. |
| Marijuana: | Increased pain relief from phenylbutazone. |
| Tobacco: | None expected. |

# PHENYLEPHRINE

## BRAND NAMES

See complete list of brand names in the *Brand Name Directory,* page 954.

## BASIC INFORMATION

**Habit forming? No**
**Prescription needed? No**
**Available as generic? Yes**
**Drug class: Sympathomimetic**

 ## USES

Temporary relief of congestion of nose, sinuses and throat caused by allergies, colds or sinusitis.

 ## DOSAGE & USAGE INFORMATION

**How to take:**
- Syrup, tablet or capsule—Swallow with liquid or food to lessen stomach irritation.
- Extended-release tablets or capsules—Swallow each dose whole.
- Nasal solution, nasal spray, nasal jelly—Take as directed on package.

**When to take:**
As needed, no more often than every 4 hours.

**If you forget a dose:**
Take when you remember. Wait 4 hours for next dose. Never double a dose.

**What drug does:**
Contracts blood-vessel walls of nose, sinus and throat tissues, enlarging airways.

**Time lapse before drug works:**
5 to 30 minutes.

**Don't take with:**
- Non-prescription drugs for asthma, cough, cold, allergy, appetite suppressants, sleeping pills or drugs containing caffeine without consulting doctor.
- See Interaction column and consult doctor.

 ## OVERDOSE

**SYMPTOMS:**
**Headache, heart palpitations, vomiting, blood-pressure rise, slow and forceful pulse.**
**WHAT TO DO:**
- **Dial 0 (operator) or 911 (emergency) for an ambulance or medical help. Then give first aid immediately.**
- **See emergency information on inside covers.**

 ## POSSIBLE ADVERSE REACTIONS OR SIDE EFFECTS

| SYMPTOMS | WHAT TO DO |
|---|---|
| **Life-threatening:** | |
| None expected. | |
| **Common:** | |
| • Fast or pounding heartbeat. | Discontinue. Call doctor right away. |
| • Headache or dizziness; shakiness; insomnia; nervousness; burning, dryness, stinging inside nose. | Continue. Call doctor when convenient. |
| **Infrequent:** | |
| Paleness. | Continue. Call doctor when convenient. |
| **Rare:** | |
| Unusual sweating. | Discontinue. Call doctor right away. |

## WARNINGS & PRECAUTIONS

**Don't take if:**
You are allergic to any sympathomimetic.

**Before you start, consult your doctor:**
- If you have high blood pressure.
- If you have heart disease.
- If you have diabetes.
- If you have overactive thyroid.
- If you have taken MAO inhibitors in past 2 weeks.

**Over age 60:**
Adverse reactions and side effects may be more frequent and severe than in younger persons.

**Pregnancy:**
Risk to unborn child outweighs drug benefits. Don't use.

**Breast-feeding:**
Drug passes into milk. Avoid drug or discontinue nursing until you finish medicine. Consult doctor for advice on maintaining milk supply.

**Infants & children:**
Use only under close supervision.

**Prolonged use:**
- "Rebound" congestion (see Glossary) and chemical irritation of nasal membranes.
- May cause functional dependence.

**Skin & sunlight:**
No problems expected.

**Driving, piloting or hazardous work:**
No problems expected.

**Discontinuing:**
May be unnecessary to finish medicine. Follow doctor's instructions.

**Others:**
No problems expected.

## POSSIBLE INTERACTION WITH OTHER DRUGS

| GENERIC NAME OR DRUG CLASS | COMBINED EFFECT |
|---|---|
| Acebutolol | Decreased effects of both drugs. |
| Amphetamines | Increased nervousness. |
| Antiasthmatics | Nervous stimulation. |
| Antidepressants (tricyclic) | Increased phenylephrine effect. |
| Antihypertensives | Decreased antihypertensive effect. |
| MAO inhibitors | Dangerous blood-pressure rise. |
| Nitrates | Possible decreased effects of both drugs. |
| Oxprenolol | Decreased effects of both drugs. |
| Sedatives | Decreased sedative effect. |
| Sympathomimetics (other) | Increased stimulant effect. |
| Tranquilizers | Decreased tranquilizer effect. |

## POSSIBLE INTERACTION WITH OTHER SUBSTANCES

| INTERACTS WITH | COMBINED EFFECT |
|---|---|
| Alcohol: | None expected. |
| Beverages: Caffeine drinks. | Excess brain stimulation. |
| Cocaine: | Excess brain stimulation. |
| Foods: | None expected. |
| Marijuana: | None expected. |
| Tobacco: | None expected. |

# PHENYLPROPANOLAMINE

## BRAND NAMES

See complete list of brand names in the *Brand Name Directory,* page 954.

## BASIC INFORMATION

**Habit forming? No**
**Prescription needed?**
   **High strength: Yes**
   **Low strength: No**
**Available as generic? Yes**
**Drug class: Sympathomimetic**

## USES

- Relieves bronchial asthma.
- Decreases congestion of breathing passages.
- Suppresses allergic reactions.
- Decreases appetite.

## DOSAGE & USAGE INFORMATION

**How to take:**
- Tablet or capsule—Swallow with liquid. You may chew or crush tablet.
- Extended-release tablets or capsules—Swallow each dose whole.
- Syrup—Take as directed on bottle.

**When to take:**
As needed, no more often than every 4 hours.

**If you forget a dose:**
Take up to 2 hours late. If more than 2 hours, wait for next dose (don't double this dose).

**What drug does:**
- Prevents cells from releasing allergy-causing chemicals (histamines).
- Relaxes muscles of bronchial tubes.
- Decreases blood-vessel size and blood flow, thus causing decongestion.

**Time lapse before drug works:**
30 to 60 minutes.

*Continued next column*

## OVERDOSE

**SYMPTOMS:**
**Severe anxiety, confusion, delirium, muscle tremors, rapid and irregular pulse.**
**WHAT TO DO:**
- **Dial 0 (operator) or 911 (emergency) for an ambulance or medical help. Then give first aid immediately.**
- **See emergency information on inside covers.**

**Don't take with:**
- Non-prescription drugs for cough, cold, allergy or asthma without consulting doctor.
- See Interaction column and consult doctor.

## POSSIBLE ADVERSE REACTIONS OR SIDE EFFECTS

| SYMPTOMS | WHAT TO DO |
|---|---|
| **Life-threatening:** | |
| None expected. | |
| **Common:** | |
| • Rapid heartbeat. | Discontinue. Call doctor right away. |
| • Nervousness, headache, paleness. | Continue. Call doctor when convenient. |
| • Insomnia. | Continue. Tell doctor at next visit. |
| **Infrequent:** | |
| • Irregular heartbeat. | Discontinue. Call doctor right away. |
| • Dizziness, appetite loss, nausea, vomiting, difficult urination. | Continue. Call doctor when convenient. |
| **Rare:** | |
| Tightness in chest. | Discontinue. Call doctor right away. |

## WARNINGS & PRECAUTIONS

**Don't take if:**
You are allergic to any sympathomimetic drug.

**Before you start, consult your doctor:**
- If you have high blood pressure.
- If you have diabetes.
- If you have overactive thyroid gland.
- If you have difficulty urinating.
- If you have taken any MAO inhibitors in past 2 weeks.
- If you have taken digitalis preparations in the last 7 days.
- If you will have surgery within 2 months, including dental surgery, requiring general or spinal anesthesia.

**Over age 60:**
More likely to develop high blood pressure, heart-rhythm disturbances, angina and to feel drug's stimulant effects.

**Pregnancy:**
No proven harm to unborn child. Avoid if possible.

**Breast-feeding:**
Drug passes into milk. Avoid drug or discontinue nursing until you finish medicine. Consult doctor for advice on maintaining milk supply.

**Infants & children:**
No special problems expected.

**Prolonged use:**
- Excessive doses—Rare toxic psychosis.
- Men with enlarged prostate gland may have more urination difficulty.

**Skin & sunlight:**
No known problems.

**Driving, piloting or hazardous work:**
No restrictions unless you feel dizzy.

**Discontinuing:**
May be unnecessary to finish medicine. Follow doctor's instructions.

**Others:**
No problems expected.

## POSSIBLE INTERACTION WITH OTHER DRUGS

| GENERIC NAME OR DRUG CLASS | COMBINED EFFECT |
|---|---|
| Acebutolol | Decreased effects of both drugs. |
| Anesthetics (general) | Increased phenylpropanolamine effect. |
| Antidepressants (tricyclic) | Increased effect of phenylpropanolamine. Excessive stimulation of heart and blood pressure. |
| Antihypertensives | Decreased antihypertensive effect. |
| Digitalis preparations | Serious heart-rhythm disturbances. |
| Epinephrine | Increased epinephrine effect. |
| Ergot preparations | Serious blood-pressure rise. |
| Guanethidine | Decreased effect of both drugs. |
| MAO inhibitors | Increased phenylpropanolamine effect. Dangerous blood-pressure rise. |
| Nitrates | Possible decreased effects of both drugs. |
| Oxprenolol | Decreased effects of both drugs. |

## POSSIBLE INTERACTION WITH OTHER SUBSTANCES

| INTERACTS WITH | COMBINED EFFECT |
|---|---|
| Alcohol: | None expected. |
| Beverages: Caffeine drinks. | Nervousness or insomnia. |
| Cocaine: | Rapid heartbeat. Avoid. |
| Foods: | None expected. |
| Marijuana: | Rapid heartbeat, possible heart-rhythm disturbance. Avoid. |
| Tobacco: | None expected. |

# PHENYLTOLOXAMINE

## BRAND NAMES

See complete list of brand names in the *Brand Name Directory,* page 955.

## BASIC INFORMATION

**Habit forming? No**
**Prescription needed? No**
**Available as generic? No**
**Drug class: Antihistamine**

## USES

Relieves symptoms of hay fever, allergic reactions and infections of nose and throat.

## DOSAGE & USAGE INFORMATION

**How to take:**
- Extended-release tablets or capsules—Swallow each dose whole with liquid.
- Syrup—Take as directed on label.
- Pediatric drops—Dilute dose in beverage before swallowing.

**When to take:**
As needed, no more often than every 3 hours.

**If you forget a dose:**
Take as soon as you remember. Wait 3 hours for next dose (don't double this dose).

**What drug does:**
Blocks histamine action in sensitized tissues.

**Time lapse before drug works:**
30 minutes.

**Don't take with:**
- Non-prescription drugs containing alcohol without consulting doctor.
- See Interaction column and consult doctor.

## OVERDOSE

**SYMPTOMS:**
- Adults—Drowsiness, confusion, incoordination, unsteadiness, muscle tremors, stupor, coma.
- Children—Excitement, hallucinations, overactivity, convulsions.

**WHAT TO DO:**
- Dial 0 (operator) or 911 (emergency) for an ambulance or medical help. Then give first aid immediately.
- See emergency information on inside covers.

## POSSIBLE ADVERSE REACTIONS OR SIDE EFFECTS

| SYMPTOMS | WHAT TO DO |
|---|---|
| **Life-threatening:** None expected. | |
| **Common:** Drowsiness, thick bronchial secretions. | Continue. Tell doctor at next visit. |
| **Infrequent:** | |
| • Stomach upset or pain, rapid heartbeat. | Discontinue. Call doctor right away. |
| • Confusion; dry mouth, nose, throat; ringing or buzzing in ears; painful or difficult urination, appetite loss. | Continue. Call doctor when convenient. |
| **Rare:** | |
| • Nightmares, agitation, irritability (especially children), change in vision, sore throat, fever, unusual bleeding or bruising, fatigue, weakness. | Discontinue. Call doctor right away. |
| • Unusual sweating. | Continue. Call doctor when convenient. |

## WARNINGS & PRECAUTIONS

**Don't take if:**
- You are allergic to any antihistamine.
- You have asthma attacks.
- You have glaucoma.
- You have urination difficulty.

**Before you start, consult your doctor:**
- If you have reacted badly to any antihistamine.
- If you have had peptic ulcer disease.
- If you will have surgery within 2 months, including dental surgery, requiring general or spinal anesthesia.

**Over age 60:**
Likely to be drowsy, dizzy or lethargic and have impaired thinking, judgment and memory. Increases urination problems from enlarged prostate gland.

**Pregnancy:**
No proven problems. Consult doctor.

**Breast-feeding:**
Drug passes into milk. Avoid drug or discontinue nursing until you finish medicine. Consult doctor for advice on maintaining milk supply.

**Infants & children:**
Use only under medical supervision.

**Prolonged use:**
No problems expected.

**Skin & sunlight:**
May cause rash or intensify sunburn in areas exposed to sun or sunlamp.

**Driving, piloting or hazardous work:**
Don't drive or pilot aircraft until you learn how medicine affects you. Don't work around dangerous machinery. Don't climb ladders or work in high places. Danger increases if you drink alcohol or take medicine affecting alertness and reflexes.

**Discontinuing:**
May be unnecessary to finish medicine. Follow doctor's instructions.

**Others:**
No problems expected.

## POSSIBLE INTERACTION WITH OTHER DRUGS

| GENERIC NAME OR DRUG CLASS | COMBINED EFFECT |
|---|---|
| Amphetamines | Decreased effect of phenyltoloxamine, especially drowsiness. |
| Anticholinergics | Increased anticholinergic effect. |
| Anticonvulsants (hydantoin) | Changed pattern of epileptic seizures. |
| Antidepressants (tricyclic) | Increased phenyltoloxamine effect. |
| Dronabinol | Increased effects of both drugs. Avoid. |
| Narcotics | Increased sedation. |
| Pain relievers | Increased sedation. |
| Sedatives | Increased sedation. |
| Sleep inducers | Increased sedation. |
| Tranquilizers | Increased sedation. |

## POSSIBLE INTERACTION WITH OTHER SUBSTANCES

| INTERACTS WITH | COMBINED EFFECT |
|---|---|
| Alcohol: | Rapid, excessive sedation. Use caution. |
| Beverages: | None expected. |
| Cocaine: | Decreased phenyltoloxamine effect. |
| Foods: | None expected. |
| Marijuana: | Excessive sedation. |
| Tobacco: | None expected. |

# PHENYTOIN

## BRAND NAMES

| | |
|---|---|
| Dantoin | Dilantin-30-Pediatric |
| Dilantin | Di-Phen |
| Dilantin Infatabs | Diphenylan |
| Dilantin Kapseals | Diphenylhydantoin |
| Dilantin-125 | Novophenytoin |

## BASIC INFORMATION

**Habit forming? No**
**Prescription needed? Yes**
**Available as generic? Yes**
**Drug class: Anticonvulsant (hydantoin)**

## USES

- Prevents epileptic seizures.
- Stabilizes irregular heartbeat.

## DOSAGE & USAGE INFORMATION

**How to take:**
- Tablet or capsule—Swallow with liquid.
- Extended-release tablets or capsules—Swallow each dose whole. If you take regular tablets, you may chew or crush them.

**When to take:**
At the same time each day.

**If you forget a dose:**
- If drug taken 1 time per day—Take as soon as you remember up to 12 hours late. If more than 12 hours, wait for next scheduled dose (don't double this dose).
- If taken several times per day—Take as soon as possible, then return to regular schedule.

**What drug does:**
Promotes sodium loss from nerve fibers. This lessens excitability and inhibits spread of nerve impulses.

*Continued next column*

## OVERDOSE

**SYMPTOMS:**
**Jerky eye movements; stagger; slurred speech; imbalance; drowsiness; blood-pressure drop; slow, shallow breathing; coma.**
**WHAT TO DO:**
- **Dial 0 (operator) or 911 (emergency) for an ambulance or medical help. Then give first aid immediately.**
- **See emergency information on inside covers.**

**Time lapse before drug works:**
7 to 10 days continual use.

**Don't take with:**
See Interaction column and consult doctor.

## POSSIBLE ADVERSE REACTIONS OR SIDE EFFECTS

| SYMPTOMS | WHAT TO DO |
|---|---|
| **Life-threatening:**<br>None expected. | |
| **Common:**<br>Enlarged, tender, receding gums with increased likelihood of bleeding; mild dizziness; sleeplessness; constipation; nausea, vomiting. | Continue. Call doctor when convenient. |
| **Infrequent:**<br>• Hallucinations, confusion, slurred speech, stagger, rash, change in vision. | Discontinue. Call doctor right away. |
| • Headache, drowsiness, diarrhea, muscle twitching. | Continue. Call doctor when convenient. |
| • Increased body and facial hair. | Continue. Tell doctor at next visit. |
| **Rare:**<br>Sore throat, fever, stomach pain, unusual bleeding or bruising, jaundice. | Discontinue. Call doctor right away. |

694

## WARNINGS & PRECAUTIONS

**Don't take if:**
You are allergic to any hydantoin anticonvulsant.

**Before you start, consult your doctor:**
- If you have had impaired liver function or disease.
- If you will have surgery within 2 months, including dental surgery, requiring general or spinal anesthesia.

**Over age 60:**
Adverse reactions and side effects may be more frequent and severe than in younger persons.

**Pregnancy:**
Risk to unborn child outweighs drug benefits. Don't use.

**Breast-feeding:**
Drug passes into milk. Avoid drug or discontinue nursing until you finish medicine. Consult doctor for advice on maintaining milk supply.

**Infants & children:**
Use only under medical supervision.

**Prolonged use:**
- Weakened bones.
- Lymph gland enlargement.
- Possible liver damage.
- Numbness and tingling of hands and feet.
- Continual back-and-forth eye movements.
- Bleeding, swollen or tender gums.

**Skin & sunlight:**
May cause rash or intensify sunburn in areas exposed to sun or sunlamp.

**Driving, piloting or hazardous work:**
Don't drive or pilot aircraft until you learn how medicine affects you. Don't work around dangerous machinery. Don't climb ladders or work in high places. Danger increases if you drink alcohol or take medicine affecting alertness and reflexes.

**Discontinuing:**
Don't discontinue without consulting doctor. Dose may require gradual reduction if you have taken drug for a long time. Doses of other drugs may also require adjustment.

**Others:**
No problems expected.

## POSSIBLE INTERACTION WITH OTHER DRUGS

| GENERIC NAME OR DRUG CLASS | COMBINED EFFECT |
|---|---|
| Amiodarone | Increased effect of phenytoin. |
| Anticoagulants | Increased effect of both drugs. |
| Antidepressants (tricyclic) | Decreased phenytoin effect. Phenytoin dose requires adjustment. |
| Antihypertensives | Increased effect of antihypertensive. |
| Aspirin | Increased phenytoin effect. |
| Barbiturates | Changed seizure pattern. |
| Carbonic anhydrase inhibitors | Increased chance of bone disease. |
| Chloramphenicol | Increased phenytoin effect. |
| Contraceptives (oral) | Increased seizures. Menstrual irregularities. |
| Cortisone drugs | Decreased cortisone effect. |
| Digitalis preparations | Decreased digitalis effect. |
| Disulfiram | Increased phenytoin effect. |
| Estrogens | Increased phenytoin effect. |
| Furosemide | Decreased furosemide effect. |

*Continued page 972*

## POSSIBLE INTERACTION WITH OTHER SUBSTANCES

| INTERACTS WITH | COMBINED EFFECT |
|---|---|
| Alcohol: | Possible decreased anticonvulsant effect. Use with caution. |
| Beverages: | None expected. |
| Cocaine: | Possible seizures. |
| Foods: | None expected. |
| Marijuana: | Drowsiness, unsteadiness, decreased anticonvulsant effect. |
| Tobacco: | None expected. |

# PILOCARPINE

## BRAND NAMES

Adsorbocarpine
Akarpine
Almocarpine
Isopto Carpine
Minims
Minims Pilocarpine
Miocarpine
Nova-Carpine
Ocusert Pilo

Pilocar
Pilocel
Pilokair
Pilomiotin
Pilopine HS
Piloptic
P.V. Carpine
P.V. Carpine Liquifilm

## BASIC INFORMATION

Habit forming? No
Prescription needed?
  U.S.: Yes
  Canada: No
Available as generic? Yes
Drug class: Antiglaucoma

 ## USES

Treatment for glaucoma.

 ## DOSAGE & USAGE INFORMATION

How to take:
- Drops—Apply to eyes. Close eyes for 1 or 2 minutes to absorb medicine.
- Eye system—Follow label directions.

When to take:
As directed on label.

*Continued next column*

 ## OVERDOSE

SYMPTOMS:
If swallowed—Nausea, vomiting, diarrhea, forceful urination, profuse sweating, rapid pulse, breathing difficulty, loss of consciousness.
WHAT TO DO:
- Dial 0 (operator) or 911 (emergency) for an ambulance or medical help. Then give first aid immediately.
- If patient is unconscious and not breathing, give mouth-to-mouth breathing. If there is no heartbeat, use cardiac massage and mouth-to-mouth breathing (CPR). Don't try to make patient vomit. If you can't get help quickly, take patient to nearest emergency facility.
- See emergency information on inside covers.

If you forget a dose:
Apply as soon as possible and return to prescribed schedule. Don't double dose.

What drug does:
Reduces internal-eye pressure.

Time lapse before drug works:
15 to 30 minutes.

Don't take with:
See Interaction column and consult doctor.

 ## POSSIBLE ADVERSE REACTIONS OR SIDE EFFECTS

| SYMPTOMS | WHAT TO DO |
|---|---|
| **Life-threatening:** None expected. | |
| **Common:** Pain, blurred or altered vision. | Continue. Call doctor when convenient. |
| **Infrequent:** <br> • Headache, eye irritation or twitching, nausea, vomiting, diarrhea, difficult breathing, muscle tremors. | Discontinue. Call doctor right away. |
| • Profuse sweating, unusual saliva flow. | Continue. Call doctor when convenient. |
| **Rare:** None expected. | |

## WARNINGS & PRECAUTIONS

**Don't take if:**
You are allergic to pilocarpine.

**Before you start, consult your doctor:**
- If you take sedatives, sleeping pills, tranquilizers, antidepressants, antihistamines, narcotics or mind-altering drugs.
- If you have asthma.
- If you have conjunctivitis (pink eye).

**Over age 60:**
Adverse reactions and side effects may be more frequent and severe than in younger persons.

**Pregnancy:**
No proven harm to unborn child. Avoid if possible.

**Breast-feeding:**
No proven problems. Consult doctor.

**Infants & children:**
Not recommended.

**Prolonged use:**
You may develop tolerance for drug, making it ineffective.

**Skin & sunlight:**
No problems expected.

**Driving, piloting or hazardous work:**
Don't drive or pilot aircraft until you learn how medicine affects you. Don't work around dangerous machinery. Don't climb ladders or work in high places. Danger increases if you drink alcohol or take medicine affecting alertness and reflexes, such as antihistamines, tranquilizers, sedatives, pain medicine, narcotics and mind-altering drugs.

**Discontinuing:**
Doctor may discontinue and substitute another drug to keep treatment effective.

**Others:**
- Can provoke asthma attack in susceptible individuals.
- Drops may impair vision for 2 to 3 hours.

## POSSIBLE INTERACTION WITH OTHER DRUGS

| GENERIC NAME OR DRUG CLASS | COMBINED EFFECT |
|---|---|
| Amphetamines | Decreased pilocarpine effect. |
| Anticholinergics | Decreased pilocarpine effect. |
| Appetite suppressants | Decreased pilocarpine effect. |
| Cortisone drugs | Decreased pilocarpine effect. |
| Glycopyrrolate | Increased glycopyrrolate effect. |
| Phenothiazines | Decreased pilocarpine effect. |

## POSSIBLE INTERACTION WITH OTHER SUBSTANCES

| INTERACTS WITH | COMBINED EFFECT |
|---|---|
| Alcohol: | May prolong alcohol's effect on brain. |
| Beverages: | None expected. |
| Cocaine: | Decreased pilocarpine effect. Avoid. |
| Foods: | None expected. |
| Marijuana: | Used once or twice weekly—May help lower internal eye pressure. |
| Tobacco: | None expected. |

# PINDOLOL

## BRAND NAMES

Pindolol        Visken

## BASIC INFORMATION

Habit forming? No
Prescription needed? Yes
Available as generic? No
Drug class: Beta-adrenergic blocker

 **USES**

- Reduces angina attacks.
- Stabilizes irregular heartbeat.
- Lowers blood pressure.
- Reduces frequency of migraine headaches. (Does not relieve headache pain.)
- Other uses prescribed by your doctor.

 **DOSAGE & USAGE INFORMATION**

**How to take:**
Tablet or capsule—Swallow with liquid. If you can't swallow whole, crumble tablet or open capsule and take with liquid or food.

**When to take:**
With meals or immediately after.

**If you forget a dose:**
Take as soon as you remember. Return to regular schedule, but allow 3 hours between doses.

**What drug does:**
- Blocks certain actions of sympathetic nervous system.
- Lowers heart's oxygen requirements.
- Slows nerve impulses through heart.
- Reduces blood vessel contraction in heart, scalp and other body parts.

*Continued next column*

 **OVERDOSE**

**SYMPTOMS:**
Weakness, slow or weak pulse, blood-pressure drop, fainting, convulsions, cold and sweaty skin.
**WHAT TO DO:**
- **Dial 0 (operator) or 911 (emergency) for an ambulance or medical help. Then give first aid immediately.**
- **See emergency information on inside covers.**

**Time lapse before drug works:**
1 to 4 hours.

**Don't take with:**
Non-prescription drugs or drugs in Interaction column without consulting doctor.

 **POSSIBLE ADVERSE REACTIONS OR SIDE EFFECTS**

| SYMPTOMS | WHAT TO DO |
|---|---|
| **Life-threatening:** None expected. | |
| **Common:** | |
| • Pulse slower than 50 beats per minute. | Discontinue. Call doctor right away. |
| • Drowsiness, numbness or tingling of fingers or toes, dizziness, diarrhea, nausea, fatigue, weakness. | Continue. Call doctor when convenient. |
| • Cold hands, feet; dry mouth, eyes, skin. | Continue. Tell doctor at next visit. |
| **Infrequent:** | |
| • Hallucinations, nightmares, insomnia, headache, difficult breathing, joint pain. | Discontinue. Call doctor right away. |
| • Confusion, depression, reduced alertness. | Continue. Call doctor when convenient. |
| • Constipation. | Continue. Tell doctor at next visit. |
| **Rare:** | |
| • Rash, sore throat, fever. | Discontinue. Call doctor right away. |
| • Unusual bleeding and bruising. | Continue. Call doctor when convenient. |

 **WARNINGS & PRECAUTIONS**

**Don't take if:**
- You are allergic to any beta-adrenergic blocker.
- You have asthma.
- You have hay fever symptoms.
- You have taken MAO inhibitors in past 2 weeks.

**Before you start, consult your doctor:**
- If you have heart disease or poor circulation to the extremities.
- If you have hay fever, asthma, chronic bronchitis, emphysema.
- If you have overactive thyroid function.
- If you have impaired liver or kidney function.
- If you will have surgery within 2 months, including dental surgery, requiring general or spinal anesthesia.
- If you have diabetes or hypoglycemia.

**Over age 60:**
Adverse reactions and side effects may be more frequent and severe than in younger persons.

**Pregnancy:**
Risk to unborn child outweighs drug benefits. Don't use.

**Breast-feeding:**
Drug passes into milk. Avoid drug or discontinue nursing until you finish medicine. Consult doctor for advice on maintaining milk supply.

**Infants & children:**
Not recommended.

**Prolonged use:**
Weakens heart muscle contractions.

**Skin & sunlight:**
No problems expected.

**Driving, piloting or hazardous work:**
Don't drive or pilot aircraft until you learn how medicine affects you. Don't work around dangerous machinery. Don't climb ladders or work in high places. Danger increases if you drink alcohol or take medicine affecting alertness and reflexes.

**Discontinuing:**
Don't discontinue without consulting doctor. Dose may require gradual reduction if you have taken drug for a long time. Doses of other drugs may also require adjustment.

**Others:**
May mask hypoglycemia.

## POSSIBLE INTERACTION WITH OTHER DRUGS

| GENERIC NAME OR DRUG CLASS | COMBINED EFFECT |
|---|---|
| Acebutolol | Increased antihypertensive effects of both drugs. Dosages may require adjustment. |
| Albuterol | Decreased albuterol effect and beta-adrenergic blocking effect |
| Antidiabetics | Increased antidiabetic effect. |
| Antihistamines | Decreased antihistamine effect. |
| Antihypertensives | Increased antihypertensive effect. |
| Anti-inflammatory drugs | Decreased anti-inflammatory effect. |

| | |
|---|---|
| Barbiturates | Increased barbiturate effect. Dangerous sedation. |
| Digitalis preparations | Can either increase or decrease heart rate. Improves irregular heartbeat. |
| Narcotics | Increased narcotic effect. Dangerous sedation. |
| Nitrates | Possible excessive blood-pressure drop. |
| Pentoxifylline | Increased antihypertensive effect. |
| Phenytoin | Increased pindolol effect. |
| Quinidine | Slows heart excessively. |
| Reserpine | Increased reserpine effect. Excessive sedation and depression. |
| Tocainide | May worsen congestive heart failure. |

## POSSIBLE INTERACTION WITH OTHER SUBSTANCES

| INTERACTS WITH | COMBINED EFFECT |
|---|---|
| Alcohol: | Excessive blood-pressure drop. Avoid. |
| Beverages: | None expected. |
| Cocaine: | Irregular heartbeat. Avoid. |
| Foods: | None expected. |
| Marijuana: | Daily use—Impaired circulation to hands and feet. |
| Tobacco: | Possible irregular heartbeat. |

# PIPERACETAZINE

## BRAND NAMES

Quide

## BASIC INFORMATION

**Habit forming? No**
**Prescription needed? Yes**
**Available as generic? Yes**
**Drug class: Tranquilizer, antiemetic
(phenothiazine)**

## USES

- Stops nausea, vomiting.
- Reduces anxiety, agitation.

## DOSAGE & USAGE INFORMATION

**How to take:**
- Tablet or capsule—Swallow with liquid or food to lessen stomach irritation.
- Suppositories—Remove wrapper and moisten suppository with water. Gently insert into rectum, large end first.
- Drops or liquid—Dilute dose in beverage.

**When to take:**
- Nervous and mental disorders—Take at the same times each day.
- Nausea and vomiting—Take as needed, no more often than every 4 hours.

**If you forget a dose:**
- Nervous and mental disorders—Take up to 2 hours late. If more than 2 hours, wait for next scheduled dose (don't double this dose).
- Nausea and vomiting—Take as soon as you remember. Wait 4 hours for next dose.

**What drug does:**
- Suppresses brain's vomiting center.
- Suppresses brain centers that control abnormal emotions and behavior.

**Time lapse before drug works:**
- Nausea and vomiting—1 hour or less.
- Nervous and mental disorders—4-6 weeks.

*Continued next column*

## OVERDOSE

**SYMPTOMS:**
**Stupor, convulsions, coma.**
**WHAT TO DO:**
- **Dial 0 (operator) or 911 (emergency) for an ambulance or medical help. Then give first aid immediately.**
- **See emergency information on inside covers.**

**Don't take with:**
- Antacid or medicine for diarrhea.
- Non-prescription drug for cough, cold or allergy.
- See Interaction column and consult doctor.

## POSSIBLE ADVERSE REACTIONS OR SIDE EFFECTS

| SYMPTOMS | WHAT TO DO |
|---|---|
| **Life-threatening:**<br>None expected. | |
| **Common:** | |
| • Muscle spasms of face and neck, unsteady gait. | Discontinue. Seek emergency treatment. |
| • Restlessness, tremor, drowsiness. | Discontinue. Call doctor right away. |
| • Decreased sweating, dry mouth, runny nose, constipation. | Continue. Call doctor when convenient. |
| **Infrequent:** | |
| • Fainting. | Discontinue. Seek emergency treatment. |
| • Rash. | Discontinue. Call doctor right away. |
| • Difficult urination, diminished sex drive, swollen breasts, menstrual irregularities. | Continue. Call doctor when convenient. |
| **Rare:** | |
| Change in vision, sore throat, fever, jaundice. | Discontinue. Call doctor right away. |

# PIPERACETAZINE

## WARNINGS & PRECAUTIONS

**Don't take if:**
- You are allergic to any phenothiazine.
- You have a blood or bone-marrow disease.

**Before you start, consult your doctor:**
- If you will have surgery within 2 months, including dental surgery, requiring general or spinal anesthesia.
- If you have asthma, emphysema or other lung disorder.
- If you take non-prescription ulcer medicine, asthma medicine or amphetamines.

**Over age 60:**
Adverse reactions and side effects may be more frequent and severe than in younger persons. More likely to develop involuntary movement of jaws, lips, tongue, chewing. Report this to your doctor immediately. Early treatment can help.

**Pregnancy:**
Risk to unborn child outweighs drug benefits. Don't use.

**Breast feeding:**
Drug passes into milk. Avoid drug or discontinue nursing until you finish medicine. Consult doctor for advice on maintaining milk supply.

**Infants & children:**
Don't give to children younger than 2.

**Prolonged use:**
May lead to tardive dyskinesia (involuntary movement of jaws, lips, tongue, chewing).

**Skin & sunlight:**
May cause rash or intensify sunburn in areas exposed to sun or sunlamp. Skin may remain sensitive for 3 months after discontinuing.

**Driving, piloting or hazardous work:**
Don't drive or pilot aircraft until you learn how medicine affects you. Don't work around dangerous machinery. Don't climb ladders or work in high places. Danger increases if you drink alcohol or take medicine affecting alertness and reflexes.

**Discontinuing:**
- Nervous and mental disorders—Don't discontinue without doctor's advice until you complete prescribed dose, even though symptoms diminish or disappear.
- Nausea and vomiting—May be unnecessary to finish medicine. Follow doctor's instructions.

**Others:**
No problems expected.

## POSSIBLE INTERACTION WITH OTHER DRUGS

| GENERIC NAME OR DRUG CLASS | COMBINED EFFECT |
|---|---|
| Anticholinergics | Increased anticholinergic effect. |
| Antidepressants (tricyclic) | Increased piperacetazine effect. |
| Antihistamines | Increased antihistamine effect. |
| Appetite suppressants | Decreased suppressant effect. |
| Dronabinol | Increased effects of both drugs. Avoid. |
| Levodopa | Decreased levodopa effect. |
| Mind-altering drugs | Increased effect of mind-altering drugs. |
| Narcotics | Increased narcotic effect. |
| Phenytoin | Increased phenytoin effect. |
| Quinidine | Impaired heart function. Dangerous mixture. |
| Sedatives | Increased sedative effect. |
| Tranquilizers (other) | Increased tranquilizer effect. |

## POSSIBLE INTERACTION WITH OTHER SUBSTANCES

| INTERACTS WITH | COMBINED EFFECT |
|---|---|
| Alcohol: | Dangerous oversedation. |
| Beverages: | None expected. |
| Cocaine: | Decreased piperacetazine effect. Avoid. |
| Foods: | None expected. |
| Marijuana: | Drowsiness. May increase antinausea effect. |
| Tobacco: | None expected. |

701

# PIROXICAM

## BRAND NAMES

Feldene

## BASIC INFORMATION

**Habit forming?** No
**Prescription needed?** Yes
**Available as generic?** No
**Drug class:** Anti-inflammatory (non-steroid)

 **USES**

- Relieves symptoms of rheumatoid arthritis, osteoarthritis and gout.
- Relieves symptoms of ankylosing spondylitis.

 **DOSAGE & USAGE INFORMATION**

**How to take:**
Tablet—Swallow with liquid or food to lessen stomach irritation. If you can't swallow whole, crumble tablet and take with liquid or food.

**When to take:**
At the same times each day.

**If you forget a dose:**
Take as soon as you remember up to 2 hours late. If more than 2 hours, wait for next scheduled dose (don't double this dose).

**What drug does:**
Reduces tissue concentration of prostaglandins (hormones that produce inflammation and pain).

**Time lapse before drug works:**
Begins in 4 to 24 hours. May require 3 weeks regular use for maximum benefit.

**Don't take with:**
See Interaction column and consult doctor.

 **OVERDOSE**

**SYMPTOMS:**
Confusion, agitation, incoherence, convulsions, possible hemorrhage from stomach or intestine, coma.
**WHAT TO DO:**
- Dial 0 (operator) or 911 (emergency) for an ambulance or medical help. Then give first aid immediately.
- See emergency information on inside covers.

 **POSSIBLE ADVERSE REACTIONS OR SIDE EFFECTS**

| SYMPTOMS | WHAT TO DO |
|---|---|
| **Life-threatening:** | |
| None expected. | |
| **Common:** | |
| • Dizziness, nausea, pain. | Continue. Call doctor when convenient. |
| • Headache. | Continue. Tell doctor at next visit. |
| **Infrequent:** | |
| Depression, drowsiness, ringing in ears, swollen feet or legs, constipation or diarrhea, vomiting. | Continue. Call doctor when convenient. |
| **Rare:** | |
| • Convulsions; confusion; rash, hives or itchy skin; blurred vision; black, bloody or tarry stool; difficult breathing; tightness in chest; rapid heartbeat; unusual bleeding or bruising; blood in urine; jaundice. | Discontinue. Call doctor right away. |
| • Painful or difficult urination, fatigue, weakness. | Continue. Call doctor when convenient. |

## WARNINGS & PRECAUTIONS

**Don't take if:**
- You are allergic to aspirin or any non-steroid, anti-inflammatory drug.
- You have gastritis, peptic ulcer, enteritis, ileitis, ulcerative colitis, asthma, heart failure, high blood pressure or bleeding problems.
- Patient is younger than 15.

**Before you start, consult your doctor:**
- If you have epilepsy.
- If you have Parkinson's disease.
- If you have been mentally ill.
- If you have had kidney disease or impaired kidney function.
- If you will have surgery within 2 months, including dental surgery, requiring general or spinal anesthesia.

**Over age 60:**
Adverse reactions and side effects may be more frequent and severe than in younger persons. Smaller than average doses may reduce unpleasant side effects.

**Pregnancy:**
Studies inconclusive on harm to unborn child. Animal studies show fetal abnormalities. Decide with your doctor whether drug benefits justify risk to unborn child.

**Breast-feeding:**
May harm child. Avoid.

**Infants & children:**
Not recommended for anyone younger than 15. Use only under medical supervision.

**Prolonged use:**
- Eye damage, reduced hearing, sore throat, fever.
- Weight gain.
- Request liver-function and bleeding time studies.

**Skin & sunlight:**
No problems expected.

**Driving, piloting or hazardous work:**
Don't drive or pilot aircraft until you learn how medicine affects you. Don't work around dangerous machinery. Don't climb ladders or work in high places. Danger increases if you drink alcohol or take medicine affecting alertness and reflexes.

**Discontinuing:**
Don't discontinue without consulting doctor. Dose may require gradual reduction if you have taken drug for a long time. Doses of other drugs may also require adjustment.

**Others:**
No problems expected.

## POSSIBLE INTERACTION WITH OTHER DRUGS

| GENERIC NAME OR DRUG CLASS | COMBINED EFFECT |
|---|---|
| Acebutolol | Decreased antihypertensive effect of acebutolol. |
| Anticoagulants (oral) | Increased risk of bleeding. |
| Aspirin | Increased risk of stomach ulcer. |
| Cortisone drugs | Increased risk of stomach ulcer. |
| Furosemide | Decreased diuretic effect of furosemide. |
| Gold compounds | Possible increased likelihood of kidney damage. |
| Minoxidil | Decreased minoxidil effect. |
| Oxprenolol | Decreased antihypertensive effect of oxprenolol. |
| Oxyphenbutazone | Possible stomach ulcer. |
| Phenylbutazone | Possible stomach ulcer. |
| Probenecid | Increased piroxicam effect. |
| Thyroid hormones | Rapid heartbeat, blood-pressure rise. |

## POSSIBLE INTERACTION WITH OTHER SUBSTANCES

| INTERACTS WITH | COMBINED EFFECT |
|---|---|
| Alcohol: | Possible stomach ulcer or bleeding. |
| Beverages: | None expected. |
| Cocaine: | Depression following cocaine use. Avoid. |
| Foods: | None expected. |
| Marijuana: | Increased pain relief from piroxicam, but may be depressing. |
| Tobacco: | Decreased absorption of piroxicam. Avoid tobacco. |

# POLOXAMER 188

## BRAND NAMES

Alaxin                    Poloxalkol

## BASIC INFORMATION

**Habit forming? No**
**Prescription needed? No**
**Available as generic? Yes**
**Drug class: Laxative (emollient)**

 ## USES

Constipation relief.

 ## DOSAGE & USAGE INFORMATION

**How to take:**
- Tablet or capsule—Swallow with liquid. Don't open capsules.
- Drops—Dilute dose in beverage before swallowing.
- Syrup—Take as directed on bottle.

**When to take:**
At the same time each day, preferably bedtime.

**If you forget a dose:**
Take as soon as you remember. Wait 12 hours for next dose. Return to regular schedule.

**What drug does:**
Makes stool hold fluid so it is easier to pass.

**Time lapse before drug works:**
2 to 3 days of continual use.

**Don't take with:**
- Other medicines at same time. Wait 2 hours.
- See Interaction column and consult doctor.

 ## OVERDOSE

**SYMPTOMS:**
**Appetite loss, nausea, vomiting, diarrhea.**
**WHAT TO DO:**
**Overdose unlikely to threaten life. If person takes much larger amount than prescribed, call doctor, poison-control center or hospital emergency room for instructions.**

 ## POSSIBLE ADVERSE REACTIONS OR SIDE EFFECTS

| SYMPTOMS | WHAT TO DO |
|---|---|
| **Life-threatening:** None expected. | |
| **Common:** None expected. | |
| **Infrequent:** Throat irritation (liquid only), intestinal and stomach cramps. | Continue. Call doctor when convenient. |
| **Rare:** Rash. | Discontinue. Call doctor right away. |

## WARNINGS & PRECAUTIONS

**Don't take if:**
- You are allergic to any emollient laxative.
- You have abdominal pain and fever that might be appendicitis.

**Before you start, consult your doctor:**
- If you are taking other laxatives.
- To be sure constipation isn't a sign of a serious disorder.

**Over age 60:**
You must drink 6 to 8 glasses of fluid every 24 hours for drug to work.

**Pregnancy:**
No problems expected. Consult doctor.

**Breast-feeding:**
No problems expected.

**Infants & children:**
No problems expected.

**Prolonged use:**
Avoid. Overuse of laxatives may damage intestine lining.

**Skin & sunlight:**
No problems expected.

**Driving, piloting or hazardous work:**
No problems expected.

**Discontinuing:**
May be unnecessary to finish medicine. Follow doctor's instructions.

**Others:**
No problems expected.

## POSSIBLE INTERACTION WITH OTHER DRUGS

| GENERIC NAME OR DRUG CLASS | COMBINED EFFECT |
|---|---|
| Danthron | Possible liver damage. |
| Digitalis preparations | Toxic absorption of digitalis. |
| Mineral oil | Increased mineral oil absorption into bloodstream. Avoid. |
| Phenolphthalein | Increased phenolphthalein absorption. Possible toxicity. |

## POSSIBLE INTERACTION WITH OTHER SUBSTANCES

| INTERACTS WITH | COMBINED EFFECT |
|---|---|
| Alcohol: | None expected. |
| Beverages: | None expected. |
| Cocaine: | None expected. |
| Foods: | None expected. |
| Marijuana: | None expected. |
| Tobacco: | None expected. |

## BRAND NAMES

Mitrolan

## BASIC INFORMATION

**Habit forming?** No
**Prescription needed?** No
**Available as generic?** No
**Drug class:** Laxative (bulk-forming),
antidiarrheal

## USES

- Relieves constipation and prevents straining for bowel movement.
- Stops diarrhea.

## DOSAGE & USAGE INFORMATION

**How to take:**
- Tablets (laxative)—Swallow with 8 oz. cold liquid. Drink 6 to 8 glasses of water each day in addition to the one with each dose.
- Tablets (diarrhea)—Take without water at half-hour intervals.

**When to take:**
At the same times each day.

**If you forget a dose:**
Take as soon as you remember. Resume regular schedule.

**What drug does:**
Absorbs water, stimulating the bowel to form a soft, bulky stool and decreasing watery diarrhea.

**Time lapse before drug works:**
May require 2 or 3 days to begin, then works in 12 to 24 hours.

**Don't take with:**
- See Interaction column and consult doctor.
- Don't take within 2 hours of taking another medicine.

## OVERDOSE

**SYMPTOMS:**
None expected.
**WHAT TO DO:**
Overdose unlikely to threaten life. If person takes much larger amount than prescribed, call doctor, poison-control center or hospital emergency room for instructions.

## POSSIBLE ADVERSE REACTIONS OR SIDE EFFECTS

| SYMPTOMS | WHAT TO DO |
|---|---|
| **Life-threatening:** None expected. | |
| **Common:** None expected. | |
| **Infrequent:** Swallowing difficulty, "lump in throat" sensation, nausea, vomiting, diarrhea. | Continue. Call doctor when convenient. |
| **Rare:** Itchy skin, rash, intestinal blockage, asthma. | Discontinue. Call doctor right away. |

## WARNINGS & PRECAUTIONS

**Don't take if:**
- You are allergic to any bulk-forming laxative.
- You have symptoms of appendicitis, inflamed bowel or intestinal blockage.
- You have missed a bowel movement for only 1 or 2 days.

**Before you start, consult your doctor:**
- If you have diabetes.
- If you have a laxative habit.
- If you have rectal bleeding.
- If you have difficulty swallowing.
- If you take other laxatives.

**Over age 60:**
Adverse reactions and side effects may be more frequent and severe than in younger persons.

**Pregnancy:**
Most bulk-forming laxatives contain sodium or sugars which may cause fluid retention. Avoid if possible.

**Breast-feeding:**
No problems expected.

**Infants & children:**
Use only under medical supervision.

**Prolonged use:**
Don't take for more than 1 week unless under a doctor's supervision. May cause laxative dependence.

**Skin & sunlight:**
No problems expected.

**Driving, piloting or hazardous work:**
No problems expected.

**Discontinuing:**
May be unnecessary to finish medicine. Follow doctor's instructions.

**Others:**
Don't take to "flush out" your system or as a "tonic."

## POSSIBLE INTERACTION WITH OTHER DRUGS

| GENERIC NAME OR DRUG CLASS | COMBINED EFFECT |
|---|---|
| Antibiotics | Decreased antibiotic effect. |
| Anticoagulants | Decreased anticoagulant effect. |
| Digitalis preparations | Decreased digitalis effect. |
| Salicylates (including aspirin) | Decreased salicylate effect. |

## POSSIBLE INTERACTION WITH OTHER SUBSTANCES

| INTERACTS WITH | COMBINED EFFECT |
|---|---|
| Alcohol: | None expected. |
| Beverages: | None expected. |
| Cocaine: | None expected. |
| Foods: | None expected. |
| Marijuana: | None expected. |
| Tobacco: | None expected. |

# POLYTHIAZIDE

## BRAND NAMES

Renese

## BASIC INFORMATION

**Habit forming?** No
**Prescription needed?** Yes
**Available as generic?** Yes
**Drug class:** Antihypertensive, diuretic
(thiazide)

## USES

- Controls, but doesn't cure, high blood pressure.
- Reduces fluid retention (edema) caused by conditions such as heart disorders and liver disease.

## DOSAGE & USAGE INFORMATION

**How to take:**
Tablet or capsule—Swallow with 8 oz. of liquid. If you can't swallow whole, crumble tablet or open capsule and take with liquid or food. Don't exceed dose.

**When to take:**
At the same time each day.

**If you forget a dose:**
Take as soon as you remember up to 2 hours late. If more than 2 hours, wait for next scheduled dose (don't double this dose).

**What drug does:**
- Forces sodium and water excretion, reducing body fluid.
- Relaxes muscle cells of small arteries.
- Reduced body fluid and relaxed arteries lower blood pressure.

**Time lapse before drug works:**
4 to 6 hours. May require several weeks to lower blood pressure.

*Continued next column*

## OVERDOSE

**SYMPTOMS:**
**Cramps, weakness, drowsiness, weak pulse, coma.**
**WHAT TO DO:**
- **Dial 0 (operator) or 911 (emergency) for an ambulance or medical help. Then give first aid immediately.**
- **See emergency information on inside covers.**

**Don't take with:**
- See Interaction column and consult doctor.
- Non-prescription drugs without consulting doctor.

## POSSIBLE ADVERSE REACTIONS OR SIDE EFFECTS

| SYMPTOMS | WHAT TO DO |
|---|---|
| **Life-threatening:** None expected. | |
| **Common:** None expected. | |
| **Infrequent:** | |
| • Blurred vision, severe abdominal pain, nausea, vomiting, irregular heartbeat, weak pulse. | Discontinue. Call doctor right away. |
| • Dizziness, mood change, headache, weakness, tiredness, weight changes. | Continue. Call doctor when convenient. |
| • Dry mouth, thirst. | Continue. Tell doctor at next visit. |
| **Rare:** | |
| • Rash or hives. | Discontinue. Seek emergency treatment. |
| • Jaundice, sore. throat, fever. | Discontinue. Call doctor right away. |

## WARNINGS & PRECAUTIONS

**Don't take if:**
You are allergic to any thiazide diuretic drug.

**Before you start, consult your doctor:**
- If you are allergic to any sulfa drug.
- If you have gout.
- If you have liver, pancreas or kidney disorder.

**Over age 60:**
Adverse reactions and side effects may be more frequent and severe than in younger persons, especially dizziness and excessive potassium loss.

**Pregnancy:**
Risk to unborn child outweighs drug benefits. Don't use.

**Breast-feeding:**
Drug passes into milk. Avoid drug or discontinue nursing.

**Infants & children:**
No problems expected.

**Prolonged use:**
You may need medicine to treat high blood pressure for the rest of your life.

**Skin & sunlight:**
May cause rash or intensify sunburn in areas exposed to sun or sunlamp.

**Driving, piloting or hazardous work:**
Don't drive or pilot aircraft until you learn how medicine affects you. Don't work around dangerous machinery. Don't climb ladders or work in high places. Danger increases if you drink alcohol or take medicine affecting alertness and reflexes, such as antihistamines, tranquilizers, sedatives, pain medicine, narcotics and mind-altering drugs.

**Discontinuing:**
Don't discontinue without medical advice.

**Others:**
- Hot weather and fever may cause dehydration and drop in blood pressure. Dose may require temporary adjustment. Weigh daily and report any unexpected weight decreases to your doctor.
- May cause rise in uric acid, leading to gout.
- May cause blood-sugar rise in diabetics.

## POSSIBLE INTERACTION WITH OTHER DRUGS

| GENERIC NAME OR DRUG CLASS | COMBINED EFFECT |
|---|---|
| Acebutolol | Increased antihypertensive effect. Dosages of both drugs may require adjustments. |
| Allopurinol | Decreased allopurinol effect. |
| Amiodarone | Increased risk of heartbeat irregularity due to low potassium. |
| Antidepressants (tricyclic) | Dangerous drop in blood pressure. Avoid combination unless under medical supervision. |
| Barbiturates | Increased polythiazide effect. |
| Calcium supplements | Increased calcium in blood. |
| Cholestyramine | Decreased polythiazide effect. |
| Cortisone drugs | Excessive potassium loss that causes dangerous heart rhythms. |
| Digitalis preparations | Excessive potassium loss that causes dangerous heart rhythms. |
| Diuretics (thiazide) | Increased effect of other thiazide diuretics. |
| Indapamide | Increased diuretic effect. |
| Labetolol | Increased antihypertensive effects. |
| Lithium | Increased effect of lithium. |
| MAO inhibitors | Increased polythiazide effect. |
| Nitrates | Excessive blood-pressure drop. |
| Oxprenolol | Increased antihypertensive effect. Dosages of both drugs may require adjustments. |
| Potassium supplements | Decreased potassium effect. |
| Probenecid | Decreased probenecid effect. |

## POSSIBLE INTERACTION WITH OTHER SUBSTANCES

| INTERACTS WITH | COMBINED EFFECT |
|---|---|
| Alcohol: | Dangerous blood-pressure drop. |
| Beverages: | None expected. |
| Cocaine: | None expected. |
| Foods: Licorice. | Excessive potassium loss that causes dangerous heart rhythms. |
| Marijuana: | May increase blood pressure. |
| Tobacco: | None expected. |

## BRAND NAMES

K-Phos Original          Neutra-Phos K

## BASIC INFORMATION

**Habit forming? No**
**Prescription needed? Yes**
**Available as generic? No**
**Drug class: Urinary acidifier, antiurolithic**
**(antikidney stones) electrolyte**
**replenisher**

## USES

- Provides supplement of phosphorous for people with diseases which decrease phosphorous absorption from food.
- Keeps uric acid to treat or prevent urinary tract infections and prevent stone formation.

## DOSAGE & USAGE INFORMATION

**How to take:**
- Tablets—Dissolve tablets in 3/4 to 1 glass of water. Let tablets soak 2 to 5 minutes, then stir to completely dissolve.
- Capsules—Swallow with food.

**When to take:**
After meals or with food to prevent or lessen stomach irritation or loose stools.

**If you forget a dose:**
Take within 1 hour then return to original schedule. If later than 1 hour, skip dose. Don't double-dose.

**What drug does:**
- Provides supplemental phosphates.
- Makes uric acid.

**Time lapse before drug works:**
30-60 minutes.

**Don't take with:**
See Interaction column and consult doctor.

## OVERDOSE

**SYMPTOMS:**
**Irregular heartbeat, blood-pressure drop with weakness, coma, cardiac arrest.**
**WHAT TO DO:**
- **Dial 0 (operator) or 911 (emergency) for an ambulance or medical help. Then give first aid immediately.**
- **See emergency information on inside covers.**

## POSSIBLE ADVERSE REACTIONS OR SIDE EFFECTS

| SYMPTOMS | WHAT TO DO |
|---|---|
| **Life-threatening:** | |
| Irregular heartbeat, shortness of breath. | Discontinue. Seek emergency treatment. |
| **Common:** | |
| Muscle cramps. | Discontinue. Call doctor right away. |
| **Infrequent:** | |
| Bone and joint pain, numbness or tingling in hands or feet, unusual tiredness, weakness, diarrhea, nausea, abdominal pain, vomiting. | Discontinue. Call doctor right away. |
| **Rare:** | |
| None expected. | |

## WARNINGS & PRECAUTIONS

**Don't take if:**
You have had allergic reaction to potassium, sodium or phosphates; severe kidney disease; severe burns.

**Before you start, consult your doctor:**
If you have heart problems, adrenal insufficiency, liver disease, high blood pressure, pregnancy, hypoparathyroidism, chronic kidney disease, osteomalacia, pancreatitis, rickets.

**Over age 60:**
Adverse reactions and side effects may be more frequent and severe than in younger persons. Ask doctor about smaller doses.

**Pregnancy:**
Risk to unborn child outweighs drug benefits. Don't use.

**Breast-feeding:**
No data available in humans.

**Infants & children:**
Use only under medical supervision.

**Prolonged use:**
Monitor ECG, serum calcium, phosphorous and potassium levels.

**Skin & sunlight:**
No problems expected.

**Driving, piloting or hazardous work:**
Avoid if medicine causes dizziness or confusion.

**Discontinuing:**
Don't discontinue without consulting doctor. Dose may require gradual reduction if you have taken drug for a long time. Doses of other drugs may also require adjustment.

**Others:**
Protect liquid medicine from freezing.

## POSSIBLE INTERACTION WITH OTHER DRUGS

| GENERIC NAME OR DRUG CLASS | COMBINED EFFECT |
|---|---|
| Cortisone drugs | Increased fluid retention. |
| Captopril | Level of potassium in blood too high. |
| Digitalis preparations | Level of potassium in blood too high. |
| Diuretics amiloride, triamterene, spironolactone | Level of potassium in blood too high. |
| Male hormones | Fluid retention. |
| Mexiletine | May decrease effectiveness of mexiletine. |
| Potassium supplements | Level of potassium in blood too high. |
| Quinidine | Increases quinidine effect. |
| Salicylates (including aspirin) | Level of salicylates in blood too high. |
| Vitamin D (calcifidiol and and calcitriol) | Level of phosphorous in blood too high. |

## POSSIBLE INTERACTION WITH OTHER SUBSTANCES

| INTERACTS WITH | COMBINED EFFECT |
|---|---|
| Alcohol: | None expected. |
| Beverages: Salty drinks such as tomato juice, commercial thirst quenchers, salt substitutes. | Increased fluid retention. |
| Cocaine: | May cause irregular heartbeat. |
| Foods: Salty foods such as canned soups, potato chips, TV dinners, hot dogs, pickles. | Increased fluid retention. |
| Marijuana: | May cause irregular heartbeat. |
| Tobacco: | May aggravate irregular heartbeat. |

# POTASSIUM & SODIUM PHOSPHATES

## BRAND AND GENERIC NAMES

DIBASIC POTASSIUM
& SODIUM
PHOSPHATES
K-Phos M.F.
K-Phos Neutral
K-Phos 2
MONOBASIC
POTASSIUM &
SODIUM
PHOSPHATES

Neutra-Phos
POTASSIUM &
SODIUM
PHOSPHATES
Uro-KP-Neutral

## BASIC INFORMATION

Habit forming? No
Prescription needed? Yes
Available as generic? Yes
Drug class: Urinary acidifier, antiurolithic
(antikidney stones) electrolyte
replenisher

## USES

- Provides supplement of phosphorous for people with diseases which decrease phosphorous absorption from food.
- Keeps uric acid to treat or prevent urinary tract infections and prevent stone formation.

## DOSAGE & USAGE INFORMATION

How to take:
Dissolve tablets in 3/4 to 1 glass of water. Let tablets soak 2 to 5 minutes, then stir to completely dissolve.

When to take:
After meals or with food to prevent or lessen stomach irritation or loose stools.

If you forget a dose:
Take within 1 hour then return to original schedule. If later than 1 hour, skip dose. Don't double-dose.

*Continued next column*

## OVERDOSE

SYMPTOMS:
Irregular heartbeat, blood-pressure drop with weakness, coma, cardiac arrest.
WHAT TO DO:
- Dial 0 (operator) or 911 (emergency) for an ambulance or medical help. Then give first aid immediately.
- See emergency information on inside covers.

What drug does:
- Provides supplemental phosphates.
- Makes uric acid.

Time lapse before drug works:
30-60 minutes.

Don't take with:
See Interaction column and consult doctor.

## POSSIBLE ADVERSE REACTIONS OR SIDE EFFECTS

| SYMPTOMS | WHAT TO DO |
|---|---|
| **Life-threatening:** Irregular heart-beat, difficult breathing, anxiety, weak legs. | Discontinue. Seek emergency treatment. |
| **Common:** None expected. | |
| **Infrequent:** Numbness or tingling in hands or feet, diarrhea, nausea, abdomnial pain, vomiting, headache, dizziness, muscle cramps, swollen feet and ankles, thirst, weakness. | Discontinue. Call doctor right away. |
| **Rare:** Confusion. | Discontinue. Call doctor right away. |

## WARNINGS & PRECAUTIONS

**Don't take if:**
You have had allergic reaction to potassium, sodium or phosphates; severe kidney disease; severe burns.

**Before you start, consult your doctor:**
If you have heart problems, adrenal insufficiency, liver disease, high blood pressure, pregnancy, hypoparathyroidism, chronic kidney disease, osteomalacia, pancreatitis, rickets.

**Over age 60:**
Adverse reactions and side effects may be more frequent and severe than in younger persons. Ask doctor about smaller doses.

**Pregnancy:**
Risk to unborn child outweighs drug benefits. Don't use.

**Breast-feeding:**
No data available in humans.

**Infants & children:**
Use only under medical supervision.

**Prolonged use:**
Monitor ECG, serum calcium, phosphorous and potassium levels.

**Skin & sunlight:**
No problems expected.

**Driving, piloting or hazardous work:**
Avoid if medicine causes dizziness or confusion.

**Discontinuing:**
Don't discontinue without consulting doctor. Dose may require gradual reduction if you have taken drug for a long time. Doses of other drugs may also require adjustment.

**Others:**
Protect liquid medicine from freezing.

## POSSIBLE INTERACTION WITH OTHER DRUGS

| GENERIC NAME OR DRUG CLASS | COMBINED EFFECT |
|---|---|
| Captopril | Level of potassium in blood too high. |
| Cortisone drugs | Increased fluid retention. |
| Digitalis preparations | Level of potassium in blood too high. |
| Diuretics such as: amiloride, triamterene, spironolactone | Level of potassium in blood too high. |
| Male hormones | Fluid retention. |
| Potassium supplements | Level of potassium in blood too high. |
| Quinidine | Increases quinidine effect. |
| Salicylates (including aspirin) | Level of salicylates in blood too high. |
| Vitamin D (calcifidiol and and calcitriol) | Level of phosphorous in blood too high. |

## POSSIBLE INTERACTION WITH OTHER SUBSTANCES

| INTERACTS WITH | COMBINED EFFECT |
|---|---|
| Alcohol: | None expected. |
| Beverages: Salty drinks such as tomato juice, commercial thirst quenchers, salt substitutes. | Increased fluid retention. |
| Cocaine: | May cause irregular heartbeat. |
| Foods: Salty foods such as canned soups, potato chips, TV dinners, hot dogs, pickles. | Increased fluid retention. |
| Marijuana: | May cause irregular heartbeat. |
| Tobacco: | May aggravate irregular heartbeat. |

# POTASSIUM SUPPLEMENTS

## BRAND NAMES

See complete list of brand names in the *Brand Name Directory,* page 955.

## BASIC INFORMATION

**Habit forming? No**
**Prescription needed? Yes**
**Available as generic? Yes**
**Drug class: Mineral supplement (potassium)**

## USES

- Treatment for potassium deficiency from diuretics, cortisone or digitalis medicines.
- Treatment for low potassium associated with some illnesses.

## DOSAGE & USAGE INFORMATION

**How to take:**
- Tablet or capsule—Swallow with liquid or food to lessen stomach irritation. You may chew or crush tablet.
- Extended-release tablets or capsules—Swallow each dose whole with liquid.
- Effervescent tablets, granules, powder or liquid—Dilute dose in water.

**When to take:**
At the same time each day, preferably with food or immediately after meals.

**If you forget a dose:**
Take as soon as you remember. Don't double next dose.

**What drug does:**
Preserves or restores normal function of nerve cells, heart and skeletal-muscle cells, kidneys, and stomach-juice secretions.

*Continued next column*

## OVERDOSE

**SYMPTOMS:**
**Paralysis of arms and legs, irregular heartbeat, blood-pressure drop, convulsions, coma, cardiac arrest.**
**WHAT TO DO:**
- **Dial 0 (operator) or 911 (emergency) for an ambulance or medical help. Then give first aid immediately.**
- **See emergency information on inside covers.**

**Time lapse before drug works:**
1 to 2 hours. Full benefit may require 12 to 24 hours.

**Don't take with:**
See Interaction column and consult doctor.

## POSSIBLE ADVERSE REACTIONS OR SIDE EFFECTS

| SYMPTOMS | WHAT TO DO |
|---|---|
| **Life-threatening:** None expected. | |
| **Common:** None expected. | |
| **Infrequent:** Diarrhea, nausea, vomiting, stomach discomfort. | Continue. Call doctor when convenient. |
| **Rare:** | |
| • Confusion, irregular heartbeat, difficult breathing, unusual fatigue, weakness, heaviness of legs. | Discontinue. Call doctor right away. |
| • Numbness or tingling in hands or feet. | Continue. Call doctor when convenient. |

## WARNINGS & PRECAUTIONS

**Don't take if:**
- You are allergic to any potassium supplement.
- You have acute or chronic kidney disease.

**Before you start, consult your doctor:**
- If you have Addison's disease or familial periodic paralysis.
- If you have heart disease.
- If you have intestinal blockage.
- If you have a stomach ulcer.
- If you use diuretics.
- If you use heart medicine.
- If you use laxatives or have chronic diarrhea.
- If you use salt substitutes or low-salt milk.

**Over age 60:**
Observe dose schedule strictly. Potassium balance is critical. Deviation above or below normal can have serious results.

**Pregnancy:**
No problems expected if you adhere strictly to prescribed dose.

**Breast-feeding:**
Studies inconclusive on harm to infant. Consult doctor.

**Infants & children:**
Use only under doctor's supervision.

**Prolonged use:**
- Slows absorption of vitamin B-12. May cause anemia.
- Request frequent lab tests to monitor potassium levels in blood, especially if you take digitalis preparations.

**Skin & sunlight:**
No problems expected.

**Driving, piloting or hazardous work:**
No problems expected.

**Discontinuing:**
Don't discontinue without consulting doctor. Dose may require gradual reduction if you have taken drug for a long time. Doses of other drugs may also require adjustment.

**Others:**
- Overdose or underdose serious. Frequent EKGs and laboratory blood studies to measure serum electrolytes and kidney function recommended.
- Prolonged diarrhea may call for increased dosage of potassium.
- Serious injury may necessitate temporary *decrease* in potassium.

## POSSIBLE INTERACTION WITH OTHER DRUGS

| GENERIC NAME OR DRUG CLASS | COMBINED EFFECT |
|---|---|
| Amiloride | Dangerous rise in blood potassium. |
| Atropine | Increased possibility of intestinal ulcers, which sometimes occur with oral potassium tablets. |
| Belladonna | Increased possibility of intestinal ulcers, which sometimes occur with oral potassium tablets. |
| Captopril | Possible increased potassium effect. |
| Cortisone medicines | Decreased effect of potassium. |
| Digitalis preparations | Possible irregular heartbeat. |
| Diuretics (thiazide) | Decreased potassium effect. |
| Laxatives | Possible decreased potassium effect. |
| Spironolactone | Dangerous rise in blood potassium. |
| Triamterene | Dangerous rise in blood potassium. |
| Vitamin B-12 | Extended-release tablets may decrease vitamin B-12 absorption and increase vitamin B-12 requirements. |

## POSSIBLE INTERACTION WITH OTHER SUBSTANCES

| INTERACTS WITH | COMBINED EFFECT |
|---|---|
| Alcohol: | None expected. |
| Beverages: Salty drinks such as tomato juice, commercial thirst quenchers. | Increased fluid retention. |
| Cocaine: | May cause irregular heartbeat. |
| Foods: Salty foods. | Increased fluid retention. |
| Marijuana: | May cause irregular heartbeat. |
| Tobacco: | None expected. |

# PRAZEPAM

## BRAND NAMES

Centrax

## BASIC INFORMATION

**Habit forming? Yes**
**Prescription needed? Yes**
**Available as generic? No**
**Drug class: Tranquilizer (benzodiazepine)**

 ## USES

Treatment for nervousness or tension.

 ## DOSAGE & USAGE INFORMATION

**How to take:**
Tablet or capsule—Swallow with liquid. If you can't swallow whole, crumble tablet or open capsule and take with liquid or food.

**When to take:**
At the same time each day, according to instructions on prescription label.

**If you forget a dose:**
Take as soon as you remember up to 2 hours late. If more than 2 hours, wait for next scheduled dose (don't double this dose).

**What drug does:**
Affects limbic system, the part of the brain that controls emotions.

**Time lapse before drug works:**
2 hours. May take 6 weeks for full benefit.

**Don't take with:**
See Interaction column and consult doctor.

 ## OVERDOSE

**SYMPTOMS:**
Drowsiness, weakness, tremor, stupor, coma.
**WHAT TO DO:**
- Dial 0 (operator) or 911 (emergency) for an ambulance or medical help. Then give first aid immediately.
- If patient is unconscious and not breathing, give mouth-to-mouth breathing. If there is no heartbeat, use cardiac massage and mouth-to-mouth breathing (CPR). Don't try to make patient vomit. If you can't get help quickly, take patient to nearest emergency facility.
- See emergency information on inside covers.

 ## POSSIBLE ADVERSE REACTIONS OR SIDE EFFECTS

| SYMPTOMS | WHAT TO DO |
|---|---|
| **Life-threatening:** | |
| None expected. | |
| **Common:** | |
| Clumsiness, drowsiness, dizziness. | Continue. Call doctor when convenient. |
| **Infrequent:** | |
| • Hallucinations, confusion, depression, irritability, rash, itchy skin, change in vision. | Discontinue. Call doctor right away. |
| • Constipation or diarrhea, nausea, vomiting, difficult urination. | Continue. Call doctor when convenient. |
| **Rare:** | |
| • Slow heartbeat, difficult breathing. | Discontinue. Seek emergency treatment. |
| • Mouth and throat ulcers, jaundice. | Discontinue. Call doctor right away. |

**WARNINGS & PRECAUTIONS**

**Don't take if:**
- You are allergic to any benzodiazepine.
- You have myasthenia gravis.
- You have glaucoma.
- You are active or recovering alcoholic.
- Patient is younger than 6 months.

**Before you start, consult your doctor:**
- If you have liver, kidney or lung disease.
- If you have diabetes, epilepsy or porphyria.

**Over age 60:**
Adverse reactions and side effects may be more frequent and severe than in younger persons. You need smaller doses for shorter periods of time. May develop agitation, rage or "hangover" effect.

**Pregnancy:**
Risk to unborn child outweighs drug benefits. Don't use.

**Breast-feeding:**
Drug passes into milk. Avoid drug or discontinue nursing until you finish medicine. Consult doctor for advice on maintaining milk supply.

**Infants & children:**
Use only under medical supervision for children older than 6 months.

**Prolonged use:**
May impair liver function.

**Skin & sunlight:**
No problems expected.

**Driving, piloting or hazardous work:**
Don't drive or pilot aircraft until you learn how medicine affects you. Don't work around dangerous machinery. Don't climb ladders or work in high places. Danger increases if you drink alcohol or take medicine affecting alertness and reflexes.

**Discontinuing:**
Don't discontinue without consulting doctor. Dose may require gradual reduction if you have taken drug for a long time. Doses of other drugs may also require adjustment.

**Others:**
- Hot weather, heavy exercise and profuse sweat may reduce excretion and cause overdose.
- Blood sugar may rise in diabetics, requiring insulin adjustment.

 **POSSIBLE INTERACTION WITH OTHER DRUGS**

| GENERIC NAME OR DRUG CLASS | COMBINED EFFECT |
|---|---|
| Anticonvulsants | Change in seizure frequency or severity. |
| Antidepressants | Increased sedative effect of both drugs. |
| Antihistamines | Increased sedative effect of both drugs. |
| Antihypertensives | Excessively low blood pressure. |
| Cimetidine | Excess sedation. |
| Disulfiram | Increased prazepam effect. |
| Dronabinol | Increased effects of both drugs. Avoid. |
| MAO inhibitors | Convulsions, deep sedation, rage. |
| Molindone | Increased tranquilizer effect. |
| Narcotics | Increased sedative effect of both drugs. |
| Sedatives | Increased sedative effect of both drugs. |
| Sleep inducers | Increased sedative effect of both drugs. |
| Tranquilizers | Increased sedative effect of both drugs. |

 **POSSIBLE INTERACTION WITH OTHER SUBSTANCES**

| INTERACTS WITH | COMBINED EFFECT |
|---|---|
| Alcohol: | Heavy sedation. Avoid. |
| Beverages: | None expected. |
| Cocaine: | Decreased prazepam effect. |
| Foods: | None expected. |
| Marijuana: | Heavy sedation. Avoid. |
| Tobacco: | Decreased prazepam effect. |

# PRAZOSIN

## BRAND NAMES

Minipress

## BASIC INFORMATION

Habit forming? No
Prescription needed? Yes
Available as generic? No
Drug class: Antihypertensive

## USES

- Treatment for high blood pressure.
- Improves congestive heart failure.

## DOSAGE & USAGE INFORMATION

**How to take:**
Tablet or capsule—Swallow with liquid. If you can't swallow whole, crumble tablet or open capsule and take with liquid or food.

**When to take:**
At the same times each day.

**If you forget a dose:**
Take as soon as you remember up to 2 hours late. If more than 2 hours, wait for next scheduled dose (don't double this dose).

**What drug does:**
Expands and relaxes blood-vessel walls to lower blood pressure.

**Time lapse before drug works:**
30 minutes.

**Don't take with:**
See Interaction column and consult doctor.

## OVERDOSE

**SYMPTOMS:**
Extreme weakness; loss of consciousness; cold, sweaty skin; weak, rapid pulse; coma.
**WHAT TO DO:**
- Dial 0 (operator) or 911 (emergency) for an ambulance or medical help. Then give first aid immediately.
- If patient is unconscious and not breathing, give mouth-to-mouth breathing. If there is no heartbeat, use cardiac massage and mouth-to-mouth breathing (CPR). Don't try to make patient vomit. If you can't get help quickly, take patient to nearest emergency facility.
- See emergency information on inside covers.

## POSSIBLE ADVERSE REACTIONS OR SIDE EFFECTS

| SYMPTOMS | WHAT TO DO |
|---|---|
| **Life-threatening:** | |
| None expected. | |
| **Common:** | |
| • Rapid heartbeat. | Discontinue. Call doctor right away. |
| • Vivid dreams, drowsiness, dizziness. | Continue. Call doctor when convenient. |
| **Infrequent:** | |
| • Rash or itchy skin, blurred vision, shortness of breath, chest pain. | Discontinue. Call doctor right away. |
| • Appetite loss, constipation or diarrhea, stomach pain, nausea, vomiting, fluid retention, joint or muscle aches. | Continue. Call doctor when convenient. |
| • Headache, irritability, depression, dry mouth, stuffy nose, increased urination. | Continue. Tell doctor at next visit. |
| **Rare:** | |
| Decreased sexual function. | Continue. Call doctor when convenient. |

## WARNINGS & PRECAUTIONS

**Don't take if:**
- You are allergic to prazosin.
- You are depressed.
- You will have surgery within 2 months, including dental surgery, requiring general or spinal anesthesia.

**Before you start, consult your doctor:**
- If you experience lightheadedness or fainting with other antihypertensive drugs.
- If you are easily depressed.
- If you have impaired brain circulation or have had a stroke.
- If you have coronary heart disease (with or without angina).
- If you have kidney disease or impaired liver function.

**Over age 60:**
Begin with no more than 1 mg. per day for first 3 days. Increases should be gradual and supervised by your doctor. Don't stand while taking. Sudden changes in position may cause falls. Sit or lie down promptly if you feel dizzy. If you have impaired brain circulation or coronary heart disease, excessive lowering of blood pressure should be avoided. Report problems to your doctor immediately.

**Pregnancy:**
Studies inconclusive on harm to unborn child. Animal studies show fetal abnormalities. Decide with your doctor whether drug benefits justify risk to child.

**Breast-feeding:**
No proven problems. Consult doctor.

**Infants & children:**
Not recommended.

**Prolonged use:**
No problems expected.

**Skin & sunlight:**
No problems expected.

**Driving, piloting or hazardous work:**
Don't drive or pilot aircraft until you learn how medicine affects you. Don't work around dangerous machinery. Don't climb ladders or work in high places.

**Discontinuing:**
Don't discontinue without doctor's advice until you complete prescribed dose, even though symptoms diminish or disappear.

**Others:**
First dose likely to cause fainting. Take it at night and get out of bed slowly next morning.

 ## POSSIBLE INTERACTION WITH OTHER DRUGS

| GENERIC NAME OR DRUG CLASS | COMBINED EFFECT |
|---|---|
| Acebutolol | Increased antihypertensive effect. Dosages may require adjustments. |
| Amitriptyline | Acute agitation. |
| Amphetamines | Decreased prazosin effect. |
| Antihypertensives (other) | Increased effect of other drugs. |
| Chlorpromazine | Acute agitation. |
| Enalapril | Possible excessive potassium in blood. |
| MAO inhibitors | Blood-pressure drop. |
| Nitrates | Possible excessive blood-pressure drop. |
| Nitroglycerin | Prolonged effect of prazosin. |
| Oxprenolol | Increased antihypertensive effect. Dosages may require adjustments. |

 ## POSSIBLE INTERACTION WITH OTHER SUBSTANCES

| INTERACTS WITH | COMBINED EFFECT |
|---|---|
| Alcohol: | Excessive blood-pressure drop. |
| Beverages: | None expected. |
| Cocaine: | Decreased prazosin effect. Avoid. |
| Foods: | None expected. |
| Marijuana: | Possible fainting. Avoid. |
| Tobacco: | Possible spasm of coronary arteries. Avoid. |

# PRAZOSIN & POLYTHIAZIDE

## BRAND NAMES

**Minizide**

## BASIC INFORMATION

**Habit forming? No**
**Prescription needed? Yes**
**Available as generic? No**
**Drug class: Antihypertensive, thiazide**
**diuretic**

## USES

- Controls, but doesn't cure, high blood pressure.
- Reduces fluid retention (edema) caused by conditions such as heart disorders and liver disease.

## DOSAGE & USAGE INFORMATION

**How to take:**
Tablet or capsule—Swallow with 8 oz. of liquid. If you can't swallow whole, crumble tablet or open capsule and take with liquid or food. Don't exceed dose.

**When to take:**
At the same times each day.

**If you forget a dose:**
Take as soon as you remember up to 2 hours late. If more than 2 hours, wait for next scheduled dose (don't double this dose).

*Continued next column*

## OVERDOSE

**SYMPTOMS:**
**Extreme weakness; loss of consciousness; cold, sweaty skin; weak, rapid pulse; cramps; weakness; drowsiness; coma.**
**WHAT TO DO:**
- **Dial 0 (operator) or 911 (emergency) for an ambulance or medical help. Then give first aid immediately.**
- **If patient is unconscious and not breathing, give mouth-to-mouth breathing. If there is no heartbeat, use cardiac massage and mouth-to-mouth breathing (CPR). Don't try to make patient vomit. If you can't get help quickly, take patient to nearest emergency facility.**
- **See emergency information on inside covers.**

**What drug does:**
- Expands and relaxes blood-vessel walls to lower blood pressure.
- Forces sodium and water excretion, reducing body fluid.
- Relaxes muscle cells of small arteries.
- Reduced body fluid and relaxed arteries lower blood pressure.

**Time lapse before drug works:**
4 to 6 hours. May require several weeks to lower blood pressure.

**Don't take with:**
- Non-prescription drugs without consulting doctor.
- See Interaction column and consult doctor.

## POSSIBLE ADVERSE REACTIONS OR SIDE EFFECTS

| SYMPTOMS | WHAT TO DO |
|---|---|
| **Life-threatening:** | |
| Irregular heartbeat, weak pulse, fast heartbeat, difficult breathing, chest pain. | Discontinue. Seek emergency treatment. |
| **Common:** | |
| Nightmares, vivid dreams, drowsiness, dizziness, dry mouth, stuffy nose. | Continue. Call doctor when convenient. |
| **Infrequent:** | |
| • Blurred vision, abdominal pain, nausea, vomiting. | Discontinue. Call doctor right away. |
| • Dizziness, mood change, headache, dry mouth, muscle pain, urgent urination, weakness, tiredness, weight gain or loss, runny nose, joint or muscle pain, agitation, depression, rash, appetite loss, constipation. | Continue. Call doctor when convenient. |
| **Rare:** | |
| • Sore throat, fever, mouth sores; jaundice. | Discontinue. Call doctor right away. |
| • Diminished sex drive. | Continue. Call doctor when convenient. |

## WARNINGS & PRECAUTIONS

**Don't take if:**
- You are allergic to any thiazide diuretic drug or prazosin.
- You are depressed.
- You will have surgery within 2 months, including dental surgery, requiring general or spinal anesthesia.

**Before you start, consult your doctor:**
- If you are allergic to any sulfa drug.
- If you have gout, impaired brain circulation or have had a stroke, coronary heart disease (with or without angina), kidney disease or impaired liver function.
- If you experience lightheadedness or fainting with other antihypertensive drugs.
- If you are easily depressed.

**Over age 60:**
- Adverse reactions and side effects may be more frequent and severe than in younger persons, especially dizziness and excessive potassium loss.
- Don't stand while taking. Sudden changes in position may cause falls. Sit or lie down promptly if you feel dizzy. If you have impaired brain circulation or coronary heart disease, excessive lowering of blood pressure should be avoided. Report problems to your doctor immediately.

**Pregnancy:**
Risk to unborn child outweighs drug benefits. Don't use.

**Breast-feeding:**
Drug passes into milk. Avoid drug or discontinue nursing until you finish medicine. Consult doctor for advice on maintaining milk supply.

**Infants & children:**
Not recommended.

**Prolonged use:**
You may need medicine to treat high blood pressure for the rest of your life.

**Skin & sunlight:**
May cause rash or intensify sunburn in areas exposed to sun or sunlamp.

**Driving, piloting or hazardous work:**
Don't drive or pilot aircraft until you learn how medicine affects you. Don't work around dangerous machinery. Don't climb ladders or work in high places. Danger increases if you drink alcohol or take medicine affecting alertness and reflexes, such as antihistamines, tranquilizers, sedatives, pain medicine, narcotics and mind-altering drugs.

**Discontinuing:**
Don't discontinue without consulting doctor.

**Others:**
- First dose likely to cause fainting. Take it at night and get out of bed slowly next morning.
- Hot weather and fever may cause dehydration and drop in blood pressure. Dose may require temporary adjustment. Weigh daily and report any unexpected weight decreases to your doctor.
- May cause rise in uric acid, leading to gout.
- May cause blood-sugar rise in diabetics.

## POSSIBLE INTERACTION WITH OTHER DRUGS

| GENERIC NAME OR DRUG CLASS | COMBINED EFFECT |
|---|---|
| Acebutolol | Increased antihypertensive effect. Dosages may require adjustments. |
| Allopurinol | Decreased allopurinol effect. |
| Amitriptyline | Acute agitation. |
| Amphetamines | Decreased prazosin effect. |
| Antidepressants (tricyclic) | Dangerous drop in blood pressure. Avoid combination unless under medical supervision. |
| Barbiturates | Increased polythiazide effect. |

*Continued page 973*

## POSSIBLE INTERACTION WITH OTHER SUBSTANCES

| INTERACTS WITH | COMBINED EFFECT |
|---|---|
| Alcohol: | Dangerous blood-pressure drop. Avoid. |
| Beverages: | None expected. |
| Cocaine: | Decreased prazosin effect. Avoid. |
| Foods: Licorice. | Excessive potassium loss that causes dangerous heart rhythms. |
| Marijuana: | Possible fainting, may increase blood pressure. Avoid. |
| Tobacco: | Possible spasm of coronary arteries. Avoid. |

# PREDNISOLONE

## BRAND NAMES

See complete list of brand names in the *Brand Name Directory,* page 955.

## BASIC INFORMATION

**Habit forming? No**
**Prescription needed? Yes**
**Available as generic? Yes**
**Drug class: Cortisone drug (adrenal corticosteroid)**

 USES

- Reduces inflammation caused by many different medical problems.
- Treatment for some allergic diseases, blood disorders, kidney diseases, asthma and emphysema.
- Replaces corticosteroid deficiencies.

 DOSAGE & USAGE INFORMATION

**How to take:**
Tablet—Swallow with liquid or food to lessen stomach irritation. If you can't swallow whole, crumble tablet and take with liquid or food.

**When to take:**
At the same times each day. Take once-a-day or once-every-other-day doses in mornings.

**If you forget a dose:**
- Several-doses-per-day prescription—Take as soon as you remember up to 2 hours late. If more than 2 hours, wait for next scheduled dose (don't double this dose).
- Once-a-day dose or less—Wait for next dose. Double this dose.

**What drug does:**
Decreases inflammatory responses.

**Time lapse before drug works:**
2 to 4 days.

**Don't take with:**
See Interaction column and consult doctor.

 OVERDOSE

**SYMPTOMS:**
**Headache, convulsions, heart failure.**
**WHAT TO DO:**
- **Dial 0 (operator) or 911 (emergency) for an ambulance or medical help. Then give first aid immediately.**
- **See emergency information on inside covers.**

 POSSIBLE ADVERSE REACTIONS OR SIDE EFFECTS

| SYMPTOMS | WHAT TO DO |
|---|---|
| **Life-threatening:**<br>None expected. | |
| **Common:**<br>Acne, poor wound healing, thirst, indigestion, nausea, vomiting. | Continue. Call doctor when convenient. |
| **Infrequent:**<br>• Black, bloody or tarry stool. | Discontinue. Seek emergency treatment. |
| • Blurred vision, halos around lights, sore throat, fever, muscle cramps, swollen legs or feet. | Discontinue. Call doctor right away. |
| • Mood change, insomnia, restlessness, frequent urination, weight gain, round face, fatigue, weakness, TB recurrence, irregular menstrual periods. | Continue. Call doctor when convenient. |
| **Rare:**<br>• Irregular heartbeat. | Discontinue. Seek emergency treatment. |
| • Rash. | Discontinue. Call doctor right away. |

 WARNINGS & PRECAUTIONS

**Don't take if:**
- You are allergic to any cortisone drug.
- You have tuberculosis or fungus infection.
- You have herpes infection of eyes, lips or genitals.

**Before you start, consult your doctor:**
- If you have had tuberculosis.
- If you have congestive heart failure.
- If you have diabetes.
- If you have peptic ulcer.
- If you have glaucoma.
- If you have underactive thyroid.
- If you have high blood pressure.
- If you have myasthenia gravis.
- If you have blood clots in legs or lungs.

**Over age 60:**
Adverse reactions and side effects may be more frequent and severe than in younger persons. Likely to aggravate edema, diabetes or ulcers. Likely to cause cataracts and osteoporosis (softening of the bones).

**Prolonged use:**
You may need medicine to treat high blood pressure for the rest of your life.

**Skin & sunlight:**
May cause rash or intensify sunburn in areas exposed to sun or sunlamp.

**Driving, piloting or hazardous work:**
Don't drive or pilot aircraft until you learn how medicine affects you. Don't work around dangerous machinery. Don't climb ladders or work in high places. Danger increases if you drink alcohol or take medicine affecting alertness and reflexes, such as antihistamines, tranquilizers, sedatives, pain medicine, narcotics and mind-altering drugs.

**Discontinuing:**
Don't discontinue without medical advice.

**Others:**
- Hot weather and fever may cause dehydration and drop in blood pressure. Dose may require temporary adjustment. Weigh daily and report any unexpected weight decreases to your doctor.
- May cause rise in uric acid, leading to gout.
- May cause blood-sugar rise in diabetics.

## POSSIBLE INTERACTION WITH OTHER DRUGS

| GENERIC NAME OR DRUG CLASS | COMBINED EFFECT |
| --- | --- |
| Acebutolol | Increased antihypertensive effect. Dosages of both drugs may require adjustments. |
| Allopurinol | Decreased allopurinol effect. |
| Amiodarone | Increased risk of heartbeat irregularity due to low potassium. |
| Antidepressants (tricyclic) | Dangerous drop in blood pressure. Avoid combination unless under medical supervision. |
| Barbiturates | Increased polythiazide effect. |
| Calcium supplements | Increased calcium in blood. |
| Chlorthalidone | Potassium depletion. |
| Cholinergics | Decreased cholinergic effect. |
| Contraceptives (oral) | Increased prednisolone effect. |
| Digitalis preparations | Dangerous potassium depletion. Possible digitalis toxicity. |
| Diuretics (thiazide) | Potassium depletion. |
| Ephedrine | Decreased prednisolone effect. |
| Estrogens | Increased prednisolone effect. |
| Ethacrynic acid | Potassium depletion. |
| Furosemide | Potassium depletion. |
| Glutethimide | Decreased prednisolone effect. |
| Indapamide | Possible excessive potassium loss, causing dangerous heartbeat irregularity. |
| Indomethacin | Increased prednisolone effect. |
| Insulin | Decreased insulin effect. |
| Isoniazid | Decreased isoniazid effect. |
| Oxyphenbutazone | Possible ulcers. |
| Phenylbutazone | Possible ulcers. |
| Potassium supplements | Decreased potassium effect. |
| Rifampin | Decreased prednisolone effect. |
| Sympathomimetics | Possible glaucoma. |

## POSSIBLE INTERACTION WITH OTHER SUBSTANCES

| INTERACTS WITH | COMBINED EFFECT |
| --- | --- |
| Alcohol: | Risk of stomach ulcers. |
| Beverages: | No proven problems. |
| Cocaine: | Overstimulation. Avoid. |
| Foods: | No proven problems. |
| Marijuana: | Decreased immunity. |
| Tobacco: | Increased prednisolone effect. Possible toxicity. |

# PREDNISONE

## BRAND NAMES

| | |
|---|---|
| Apo-Prednisone | Panasol |
| Colisone | Paracort |
| Cortan | Prednicen-M |
| Deltasone | SK-Prednisone |
| Liquid-Pred | Sterapred |
| Meticorten | Sterazolidin |
| Novoprednisone | Winpred |
| Orasone | |

## BASIC INFORMATION

**Habit forming?** No
**Prescription needed?** Yes
**Available as generic?** Yes
**Drug class:** Cortisone drug (adrenal corticosteroid)

 ## USES

- Reduces inflammation caused by many different medical problems.
- Treatment for some allergic diseases, blood disorders, kidney diseases, asthma and emphysema.
- Replaces corticosteroid deficiencies.

 ## DOSAGE & USAGE INFORMATION

**How to take:**
Tablet or syrup—Swallow with liquid or food to lessen stomach irritation. If you can't swallow whole, crumble tablet.

**When to take:**
At the same times each day. Take once-a-day or once-every-other-day doses in mornings.

**If you forget a dose:**
- Several-doses-per-day prescription—Take as soon as you remember up to 2 hours late. If more than 2 hours, wait for next scheduled dose (don't double this dose).
- Once-a-day dose or less—Wait for next dose. Double this dose.

*Continued next column*

 ## OVERDOSE

**SYMPTOMS:**
Headache, convulsions, heart failure.
**WHAT TO DO:**
- **Dial 0 (operator) or 911 (emergency) for an ambulance or medical help. Then give first aid immediately.**
- **See emergency information on inside covers.**

**What drug does:**
Decreases inflammatory responses.

**Time lapse before drug works:**
2 to 4 days.

**Don't take with:**
See Interaction column and consult doctor.

 ## POSSIBLE ADVERSE REACTIONS OR SIDE EFFECTS

| SYMPTOMS | WHAT TO DO |
|---|---|
| **Life-threatening:**<br>None expected. | |
| **Common:**<br>Acne, poor wound healing, thirst, indigestion, nausea, vomiting. | Continue. Call doctor when convenient. |
| **Infrequent:** | |
| • Black, bloody or tarry stool. | Discontinue. Seek emergency treatment. |
| • Blurred vision, halos around lights, sore throat, fever, muscle cramps, swollen legs or feet. | Discontinue. Call doctor right away. |
| • Mood change, insomnia, restlessness, frequent urination, weight gain, round face, fatigue, weakness, TB recurrence, irregular menstrual periods. | Continue. Call doctor when convenient. |
| **Rare:** | |
| • Irregular heartbeat. | Discontinue. Seek emergency treatment. |
| • Rash. | Discontinue. Call doctor right away. |

## WARNINGS & PRECAUTIONS

**Don't take if:**
- You are allergic to any cortisone drug.
- You have tuberculosis or fungus infection.
- You have herpes infection of eyes, lips or genitals.

**Before you start, consult your doctor:**
- If you have had tuberculosis.
- If you have congestive heart failure.
- If you have diabetes.
- If you have peptic ulcer.
- If you have glaucoma.
- If you have underactive thyroid.
- If you have high blood pressure.
- If you have myasthenia gravis.
- If you have blood clots in legs or lungs.

**Over age 60:**
Adverse reactions and side effects may be more frequent and severe than in younger persons. Likely to aggravate edema, diabetes or ulcers. Likely to cause cataracts and osteoporosis (softening of the bones).

**Pregnancy:**
Risk to unborn child outweighs drug benefits. Don't use.

**Breast-feeding:**
Drug passes into milk. Avoid drug or discontinue nursing until you finish medicine. Consult doctor for advice on maintaining milk supply.

**Infants & children:**
Use only under medical supervision.

**Prolonged use:**
- Retards growth in children.
- Possible glaucoma, cataracts, diabetes, fragile bones and thin skin.
- Functional dependence.

**Skin & sunlight:**
No problems expected.

**Driving, piloting or hazardous work:**
No problems expected.

**Discontinuing:**
- Don't discontinue without doctor's advice until you complete prescribed dose, even though symptoms diminish or disappear.
- Drug affects your response to surgery, illness, injury or stress for 2 years after discontinuing. Tell anyone who takes medical care of you within 2 years about drug.

**Others:**
Avoid immunizations if possible.

## POSSIBLE INTERACTION WITH OTHER DRUGS

| GENERIC NAME OR DRUG CLASS | COMBINED EFFECT |
|---|---|
| Amphoterecin B | Potassium depletion. |
| Anticholinergics | Possible glaucoma. |
| Anticoagulants (oral) | Decreased anticoagulant effect. |
| Anticonvulsants (hydantoin) | Decreased prednisone effect. |
| Antidiabetics (oral) | Decreased antidiabetic effect. |
| Antihistamines | Decreased prednisone effect. |
| Aspirin | Increased prednisone effect. |
| Barbiturates | Decreased prednisone effect. Oversedation. |
| Beta-adrenergic blockers | Decreased prednisone effect. |
| Chloral hydrate | Decreased prednisone effect. |
| Chlorthalidone | Potassium depletion. |
| Cholinergics | Decreased cholinergic effect. |
| Contraceptives (oral) | Increased prednisone effect. |
| Digitalis preparations | Dangerous potassium depletion. Possible digitalis toxicity. |
| Diuretics (thiazide) | Potassium depletion. |
| Ephedrine | Decreased prednisone effect. |
| Estrogens | Increased prednisone effect. |

*Continued page 973*

## POSSIBLE INTERACTION WITH OTHER SUBSTANCES

| INTERACTS WITH | COMBINED EFFECT |
|---|---|
| Alcohol: | Risk of stomach ulcers. |
| Beverages: | No proven problems. |
| Cocaine: | Overstimulation. Avoid. |
| Foods: | No proven problems. |
| Marijuana: | Decreased immunity. |
| Tobacco: | Increased prednisone effect. Possible toxicity. |

# PRIMIDONE

## BRAND NAMES

Apo-Primidone     Mysoline
Myidone          Sertan

## BASIC INFORMATION

Habit forming? No
Prescription needed? Yes
Available as generic? Yes
Drug class: Anticonvulsant

## USES

Prevents epileptic seizures.

## DOSAGE & USAGE INFORMATION

**How to take:**
- Tablet or capsule—Swallow with liquid. If you can't swallow whole, crumble tablet or open capsule and take with liquid or food.
- Liquid—If desired, dilute dose in beverage before swallowing.

**When to take:**
Daily in regularly spaced doses, according to doctor's prescription.

**If you forget a dose:**
Take as soon as you remember up to 2 hours late. If more than 2 hours, wait for next scheduled dose (don't double this dose).

**What drug does:**
Probably inhibits repetitious spread of impulses along nerve pathways.

*Continued next column*

## OVERDOSE

**SYMPTOMS:**
Slow, shallow breathing; weak, rapid pulse; confusion, deep sleep, coma.
**WHAT TO DO:**
- Dial 0 (operator) or 911 (emergency) for an ambulance or medical help. Then give first aid immediately.
- If patient is unconscious and not breathing, give mouth-to-mouth breathing. If there is no heartbeat, use cardiac massage and mouth-to-mouth breathing (CPR). Don't try to make patient vomit. If you can't get help quickly, take patient to nearest emergency facility.
- See emergency information on inside covers.

**Time lapse before drug works:**
2 to 3 weeks.

**Don't take with:**
See Interaction column and consult doctor.

## POSSIBLE ADVERSE REACTIONS OR SIDE EFFECTS

| SYMPTOMS | WHAT TO DO |
|---|---|
| **Life-threatening:** | |
| None expected. | |
| **Common:** | |
| • Difficult breathing. | Discontinue. Call doctor right away. |
| • Confusion, change in vision. | Continue. Call doctor when convenient. |
| • Clumsiness, dizziness, drowsiness. | Continue. Tell doctor at next visit. |
| **Infrequent:** | |
| • Unusual excitement, particularly in children. | Discontinue. Call doctor right away. |
| • Headache, fatigue, weakness. | Continue. Call doctor when convenient. |
| **Rare:** | |
| • Rash or hives, nausea, vomiting, appetite loss. | Discontinue. Call doctor right away. |
| • Swollen eyelids. | Continue. Call doctor when convenient. |
| • Decreased sexual ability. | Continue. Tell doctor at next visit. |

## WARNINGS & PRECAUTIONS

**Don't take if:**
- You are allergic to any barbiturate.
- You have had porphyria.

**Before you start, consult your doctor:**
- If you have had liver, kidney or lung disease or asthma.
- If you have lupus.

**Over age 60:**
Adverse reactions and side effects may be more frequent and severe than in younger persons.

**Pregnancy:**
Studies inconclusive on harm to unborn child. Animal studies show fetal abnormalities. Decide with your doctor whether drug benefits justify risk to unborn child.

**Breast-feeding:**
Drug filters into milk. May harm child. Avoid.

**Infants & children:**
Use only under medical supervision.

**Prolonged use:**
- Enlarged lymph and thyroid glands.
- Anemia.
- Rickets in children and osteomalacia (insufficient calcium to bones) in adults.

**Skin & sunlight:**
None expected.

**Driving, piloting or hazardous work:**
Don't drive or pilot aircraft until you learn how medicine affects you. Don't work around dangerous machinery. Don't climb ladders or work in high places. Danger increases if you drink alcohol or take medicine affecting alertness and reflexes.

**Discontinuing:**
Don't discontinue abruptly or without doctor's advice until you complete prescribed dose, even though symptoms diminish or disappear.

**Others:**
- Tell doctor if you become ill or injured and must interrupt dose schedule.
- Periodic laboratory blood tests of drug level recommended.

 **POSSIBLE INTERACTION WITH OTHER DRUGS**

| GENERIC NAME OR DRUG CLASS | COMBINED EFFECT |
|---|---|
| Anticoagulants (oral) | Decreased primidone effect. |
| Anticonvulsants (other) | Changed seizure pattern. |
| Antidepressants | Increased antidepressant effect. |
| Antidiabetics | Increased effect of primidone sedation. |
| Antihistamines | Increased effect of primidone sedation. |
| Aspirin | Decreased aspirin effect. |
| Contraceptives (oral) | Decreased contraceptive effect. |
| Cortisone drugs | Decreased cortisone effect. |

| | |
|---|---|
| Digitalis preparations | Decreased digitalis effect. |
| Griseofulvin | Decreased griseofulvin effect. |
| Isoniazid | Increased isoniazid effect. |
| MAO inhibitors | Increased effect of primidone sedation. |
| Mind-altering drugs | Increased effect of mind-altering drugs. |
| Narcotics | Increased narcotic effect. |
| Oxyphenbutazone | Decreased oxyphenbutazone effect. |
| Phenylbutazone | Decreased phenylbutazone effect. |
| Sedatives | Increased sedative effect. |
| Sleep inducers | Increased effect of sleep inducer. |
| Tranquilizers | Increased tranquilizer effect. |

 **POSSIBLE INTERACTION WITH OTHER SUBSTANCES**

| INTERACTS WITH | COMBINED EFFECT |
|---|---|
| Alcohol: | Dangerous sedative effect. Avoid. |
| Beverages: | None expected. |
| Cocaine: | Decreased primidone effect. |
| Foods: | Possible need for more vitamin D. |
| Marijuana: | Decreased anticonvulsant effect of primidone. Drowsiness, unsteadiness. |
| Tobacco: | None expected. |

# PROBENECID

## BRAND NAMES

Benacen
Benemid
Benuryl
ColBENEMID

Col-Probenecid
Polycillin-PRB
Probalan
SK-Probenecid

## BASIC INFORMATION

**Habit forming?** No
**Prescription needed?** Yes
**Available as generic?** Yes
**Drug class:** Antigout (uricosuric)

## USES

- Treatment for chronic gout.
- Increases blood levels of penicillins and cephalosporins.

## DOSAGE & USAGE INFORMATION

**How to take:**
Tablet or capsule—Swallow with liquid or food to lessen stomach irritation. If you can't swallow whole, crumble tablet or open capsule and take with liquid or food.

**When to take:**
At the same time each day.

**If you forget a dose:**
Take as soon as you remember up to 12 hours late. If more than 12 hours, wait for next scheduled dose (don't double this dose).

**What drug does:**
- Forces kidneys to excrete uric acid.
- Reduces amount of penicillin excreted in urine.

**Time lapse before drug works:**
May require several months of regular use to prevent acute gout.

*Continued next column*

## OVERDOSE

**SYMPTOMS:**
Breathing difficulty, severe nervous agitation, convulsions, delirium, coma.
**WHAT TO DO:**
- Dial 0 (operator) or 911 (emergency) for an ambulance or medical help. Then give first aid immediately.
- See emergency information on inside covers.

---

**Don't take with:**
- Non-prescription drugs containing aspirin or caffeine.
- See Interaction column and consult doctor.

## POSSIBLE ADVERSE REACTIONS OR SIDE EFFECTS

| SYMPTOMS | WHAT TO DO |
|---|---|
| **Life-threatening:** None expected. | |
| **Common:** Headache, appetite loss, nausea, vomiting. | Continue. Call doctor when convenient. |
| **Infrequent:** | |
| • Blood in urine, low back pain. | Discontinue. Call doctor right away. |
| • Dizziness, flushed face, itchy skin. | Continue. Call doctor when convenient. |
| • Painful or frequent urination. | Continue. Tell doctor at next visit. |
| **Rare:** Sore throat; difficult breathing; unusual bleeding or bruising; red, painful joint; jaundice; fever. | Discontinue. Call doctor right away. |

## WARNINGS & PRECAUTIONS

### Don't take if:
- You are allergic to any uricosuric.
- You have acute gout.
- Patient is younger than 2.

### Before you start, consult your doctor:
- If you have had kidney stones or kidney disease.
- If you have a peptic ulcer.
- If you have bone-marrow or blood-cell disease.

### Over age 60:
Adverse reactions and side effects may be more frequent and severe than in younger persons.

### Pregnancy:
Studies inconclusive on harm to unborn child. Animal studies show fetal abnormalities. Decide with your doctor whether drug benefits justify risk to unborn child.

### Breast-feeding:
No proven problems.

### Infants & children:
Not recommended.

### Prolonged use:
Possible kidney damage.

### Skin & sunlight:
No problems expected.

### Driving, piloting or hazardous work:
Avoid if you feel dizzy. Otherwise, no problems expected.

### Discontinuing:
Don't discontinue without consulting doctor. Dose may require gradual reduction if you have taken drug for a long time. Doses of other drugs may also require adjustment.

### Others:
If signs of gout attack develop while taking medicine, consult doctor.

## POSSIBLE INTERACTION WITH OTHER DRUGS

| GENERIC NAME OR DRUG CLASS | COMBINED EFFECT |
| --- | --- |
| Acetohexamide | Increased acetohexamide effect. |
| Anticoagulants (oral) | Increased anticoagulant effect. |
| Aspirin | Decreased probenecid effect. |
| Cephalosporins | Increased cephalosporin effect. |
| Dapsone | Increased dapsone effect. Increased toxicity. |
| Diuretics (thiazide) | Decreased probenecid effect. |
| Indapamide | Decreased probenecid effect. |
| Indomethacin | Increased adverse effects of indomethacin. |
| Methotrexate | Increased methotrexate toxicity. |
| Nitrofurantoin | Increased effect of nitrofurantoin. |
| Para-aminosalicylic acid (PAS) | Increased effect of para-aminosalicylic acid. |
| Penicillins | Enhanced penicillin effect. |
| Pyrazinamide | Decreased probenecid effect. |
| Salicylates | Decreased probenecid effect. |
| Sulfa drugs | Slows elimination. May cause harmful accumulation of sulfa. |

## POSSIBLE INTERACTION WITH OTHER SUBSTANCES

| INTERACTS WITH | COMBINED EFFECT |
| --- | --- |
| Alcohol: | Decreased probenecid effect. |
| Beverages: Caffeine drinks. | Loss of probenecid effectiveness. |
| Cocaine: | None expected. |
| Foods: | None expected. |
| Marijuana: | Daily use—Decreased probenecid effect. |
| Tobacco: | None expected. |

## BRAND NAMES

Colabid  Proben-C
Col Benemid

## BASIC INFORMATION

Habit forming? No
Prescription needed? Yes
Available as generic? Yes
Drug class: Antigout (uricosuric)

## USES

- Increases blood levels of penicillins and cephalosporins.
- Relieves joint pain, inflammation, swelling from gout.

## DOSAGE & USAGE INFORMATION

**How to take:**
Tablet or capsule—Swallow with liquid or food to lessen stomach irritation. If you can't swallow whole, crumble tablet or open capsule and take with liquid or food.

**When to take:**
At the same time each day.

**If you forget a dose:**
Take as soon as you remember up to 12 hours late. If more than 12 hours, wait for next scheduled dose (don't double this dose).

**What drug does:**
- Forces kidneys to excrete uric acid.
- Reduces amount of penicillin excreted in urine.
- Decreases acidity of joint tissues and prevents deposits of uric-acid crystals.

*Continued next column*

## OVERDOSE

**SYMPTOMS:**
**Breathing difficulty, severe nervous agitation, convulsions, bloody urine, diarrhea, muscle weakness, fever, stupor, delirium, coma.**
**WHAT TO DO:**
- **Dial 0 (operator) or 911 (emergency) for an ambulance or medical help. Then give first aid immediately.**
- **See emergency information on inside covers.**

**Time lapse before drug works:**
12 to 48 hours.

**Don't take with:**
- Non-prescription drugs containing aspirin or caffeine.
- See Interaction column and consult doctor.

## POSSIBLE ADVERSE REACTIONS OR SIDE EFFECTS

| SYMPTOMS | WHAT TO DO |
|---|---|
| **Life-threatening:**<br>Blood in urine; convulsions; severe muscle weakness; difficult breathing; burning feeling of stomach, throat or skin. | Discontinue. Seek emergency treatment. |
| **Common:**<br>Diarrhea, headache, abdominal pain. | Discontinue. Call doctor right away. |
| **Infrequent:**<br>• Back pain; painful, difficult urination. | Discontinue. Call doctor right away. |
| • Dizziness, red or flushed face, urgent urination, sore gums, hair loss. | Continue. Call doctor when convenient. |
| **Rare:**<br>Sudden decrease in urine output; nausea; vomiting; mood change; fever; diarrhea; jaundice; numbness or tingling in hands or feet; rash; sore throat, fever, mouth sores; swollen feet and ankles; unexplained bleeding or bruising; weight gain or loss. | Discontinue. Call doctor right away. |

## WARNINGS & PRECAUTIONS

**Don't take if:**
You are allergic to any uricosuric or colchicine.

**Before you start, consult your doctor:**
- If you have had kidney stones, kidney disease, heart or liver disease, peptic ulcers or ulcerative colitis.
- If you have bone-marrow or blood-cell disease.
- If you will have surgery within 2 months, including dental surgery, requiring general or spinal anesthesia.

**Over age 60:**
Adverse reactions and side effects may be more frequent and severe than in younger persons. Colchicine has a narrow margin of safety for people in this age group.

**Pregnancy:**
Risk to unborn child outweighs drug benefits. Don't use.

**Breast-feeding:**
No problems expected, but consult doctor.

**Infants & children:**
Not recommended.

**Prolonged use:**
- Possible kidney damage.
- Permanent hair loss.
- Anemia. Request blood counts.
- Numbness or tingling in hands and feet.

**Skin & sunlight:**
No problems expected.

**Driving, piloting or hazardous work:**
Don't drive or pilot aircraft until you learn how medicine affects you. Don't work around dangerous machinery. Don't climb ladders or work in high places. Danger increases if you drink alcohol or take medicine affecting alertness and reflexes, such as antihistamines, tranquilizers, sedatives, pain medicine, narcotics and mind-altering drugs.

**Discontinuing:**
- May be unnecessary to finish medicine. Follow doctor's instructions.
- Stop taking if severe digestive upsets occur before symptoms are relieved.

**Others:**
- If signs of gout attack develop while taking medicine, consult doctor.
- Limit each course of treatment to 8 mg. Don't exceed 3 mg. per 24 hours.
- Possible sperm damage. May cause birth defects if child conceived while father taking colchicine.

 **POSSIBLE INTERACTION WITH OTHER DRUGS**

| GENERIC NAME OR DRUG CLASS | COMBINED EFFECT |
|---|---|
| Acetohexamide | Increased acetohexamide effect. |
| Amphetamines | Increased amphetamine effect. |

| | |
|---|---|
| Anticoagulants | Irregular effect on anticoagulation, sometimes increased, sometimes decreased. Follow prothrombin times. |
| Antidepressants | Oversedation. |
| Antihistamines | Oversedation. |
| Antihypertensives | Decreased antihypertensive effect. |
| Appetite suppressants | Increased suppressant effect. |
| Cephalosporins | Increased cephalosporin effect. |
| Dapsone | Increased dapsone effect. Increased toxicity. |
| Diuretics (thiazide) | Decreased probenecid effect. |
| Indapamide | Increased probenecid effect. |
| Indomethacin | Increased adverse effects of indomethacin. |
| Methotrexate | Increased methotrexate effect. |
| Mind-altering drugs | Oversedation. |
| Narcotics | Oversedation. |
| Nitrofurantoin | Increased nitrofurantoin effect. |
| Para-aminosalicylic acid (PAS) | Increased effect of para-aminosalicylic acid. |
| Penicillins | Enhanced penicillin effect. |

*Continued page 974*

 **POSSIBLE INTERACTION WITH OTHER SUBSTANCES**

| INTERACTS WITH | COMBINED EFFECT |
|---|---|
| Alcohol: | Decreased probenecid effect. |
| **Beverages:** Caffeine drinks. | Loss of probenecid effectiveness. |
| Herbal teas. | Increased colchicine effect. Avoid. |
| Cocaine: | Overstimulation. Avoid. |
| Foods: | No proven problems. |
| Marijuana: | Decreased colchicine and probenecid effect. |
| Tobacco: | No proven problems. |

# PROBUCOL

## BRAND NAMES

Lorelco

## BASIC INFORMATION

**Habit forming?** No
**Prescription needed?** Yes
**Available as generic?** No
**Drug class:** Antihyperlipidemic

## USES

Lowers cholesterol level in blood in persons with type IIa hyperlipoproteinemia.

## DOSAGE & USAGE INFORMATION

**How to take:**
Tablet or capsule—Swallow with liquid. If you can't swallow whole, crumble tablet or open capsule and take with liquid or food.

**When to take:**
With morning and evening meals.

**If you forget a dose:**
Take as soon as you remember up to 2 hours late. If more than 2 hours, wait for next scheduled dose (don't double this dose).

**What drug does:**
Reduces serum cholesterol without reducing liver cholesterol.

**Time lapse before drug works:**
3 to 4 months.

**Don't take with:**
Other medicines or vitamins. Separate by 1 to 2 hours.

## OVERDOSE

**SYMPTOMS:**
None reported.
**WHAT TO DO:**
**Overdose unlikely to threaten life. If person takes much larger amount than prescribed, call doctor, poison-control center or hospital emergency room for instructions.**

## POSSIBLE ADVERSE REACTIONS OR SIDE EFFECTS

| SYMPTOMS | WHAT TO DO |
|---|---|
| **Life-threatening:** None expected. | |
| **Common:** Bloating, diarrhea, nausea, vomiting, stomach pain. | Discontinue. Call doctor right away. |
| **Infrequent:** | |
| • Dizziness, headache. | Discontinue. Call doctor right away. |
| • Numbness or tingling in feet, toes, fingers, face. | Continue. Call doctor when convenient. |
| **Rare:** | |
| • Swelling of hands, face, feet, mouth. | Discontinue. Seek emergency treatment. |
| • Rash. | Discontinue. Call doctor right away. |
| • Insomnia, blurred vision, diminished taste. | Continue. Call doctor when convenient. |

## WARNINGS & PRECAUTIONS

**Don't take if:**
You are allergic to probucol.

**Before you start, consult your doctor:**
- If you have liver disease such as cirrhosis.
- If you have heartbeat irregularity.
- If you have congestive heart failure that is not under control.
- If you have gallstones.

**Over age 60:**
Adverse reactions and side effects may be more frequent and severe than in younger persons.

**Pregnancy:**
No proven problems. Avoid if possible. Continue using birth-control methods for 6 months after discontinuing medicine.

**Breast-feeding:**
Not recommended. Animal studies show drug passes into milk. Studies not available for human beings.

**Infants & children:**
Not recommended. Safety and dosage have not been established.

**Prolonged use:**
Request serum cholesterol and serum triglyceride laboratory studies every 2 to 4 months.

**Skin & sunlight:**
No problems expected.

**Driving, piloting or hazardous work:**
If medicine does not cause dizziness, no problems expected.

**Discontinuing:**
Don't discontinue without consulting doctor. Dose may require gradual reduction if you have taken drug for a long time. Doses of other drugs may also require adjustment.

**Others:**
Medicine works best in conjunction with low-fat, low-cholesterol diet and an active, regular exercise program.

## POSSIBLE INTERACTION WITH OTHER DRUGS

| GENERIC NAME OR DRUG CLASS | COMBINED EFFECT |
| --- | --- |
| Clofibrate | Combination no more effective than one drug only, so don't take both. |

## POSSIBLE INTERACTION WITH OTHER SUBSTANCES

| INTERACTS WITH | COMBINED EFFECT |
| --- | --- |
| Alcohol: | May aggravate liver problems. Avoid. |
| Beverages: | None expected. |
| Cocaine: | None expected. |
| Foods: | None expected. |
| Marijuana: | None expected. |
| Tobacco: | None expected. |

# PROCAINAMIDE

## BRAND NAMES

| | |
|---|---|
| Procan | Pronestyl |
| Procan SR | Pronestyl SR |
| Procamide | Rhythmin |
| Procapan | Sub-Quin |
| Promine | |

## BASIC INFORMATION

**Habit forming? No**
**Prescription needed? Yes**
**Available as generic? Yes**
**Drug class: Antiarrhythmic**

 ## USES

Stabilizes irregular heartbeat.

 ## DOSAGE & USAGE INFORMATION

**How to take:**
- Tablet or capsule—Swallow with liquid.
- Extended-release tablets or capsules—Swallow each dose whole. If you take regular tablets, you may chew or crush them.

**When to take:**
Best taken on empty stomach, 1 hour before or 2 hours after meals. If necessary, may be taken with food or milk to lessen stomach upset.

**If you forget a dose:**
Take as soon as you remember up to 2 hours late. If more than 2 hours, wait for next scheduled dose (don't double this dose).

**What drug does:**
Slows activity of pacemaker (rhythm-control center of heart) and delays transmission of electrical impulses.

**Time lapse before drug works:**
30 to 60 minutes.

**Don't take with:**
See Interaction column and consult doctor.

 ## OVERDOSE

**SYMPTOMS:**
Fast and irregular heartbeat, stupor, fainting, cardiac arrest.
**WHAT TO DO:**
- Dial 0 (operator) or 911 (emergency) for an ambulance or medical help. Then give first aid immediately.
- See emergency information on inside covers.

 ## POSSIBLE ADVERSE REACTIONS OR SIDE EFFECTS

| SYMPTOMS | WHAT TO DO |
|---|---|
| **Life-threatening:**<br>None expected. | |
| **Common:**<br>Diarrhea, appetite loss, nausea, vomiting. | Continue. Call doctor when convenient. |
| **Infrequent:**<br>• Joint pain, painful breathing. | Discontinue. Call doctor right away. |
| • Dizziness. | Continue. Call doctor when convenient. |
| **Rare:**<br>• Hallucinations, confusion, depression, itchy skin, rash, sore throat, fever. | Discontinue. Call doctor right away. |
| • Fatigue. | Continue. Call doctor when convenient. |

## WARNINGS & PRECAUTIONS

**Don't take if:**
- You are allergic to procainamide.
- You have myasthenia gravis.

**Before you start, consult your doctor:**
- If you are allergic to local anesthetics that end in "caine."
- If you have had liver or kidney disease or impaired kidney function.
- If you have had lupus.
- If you take digitalis preparations.
- If you will have surgery within 2 months, including dental surgery, requiring general or spinal anesthesia.

**Over age 60:**
Adverse reactions and side effects may be more frequent and severe than in younger persons.

**Pregnancy:**
No proven harm to unborn child. Avoid if possible.

**Breast-feeding:**
No proven problems. Consult doctor.

**Infants & children:**
Not recommended.

**Prolonged use:**
May cause lupus-like illness.

**Skin & sunlight:**
No problems expected.

**Driving, piloting or hazardous work:**
Use caution if you feel dizzy or weak. Otherwise, no problems expected.

**Discontinuing:**
Don't discontinue without doctor's advice until you complete prescribed dose, even though symptoms diminish or disappear.

**Others:**
No problems expected.

## POSSIBLE INTERACTION WITH OTHER DRUGS

| GENERIC NAME OR DRUG CLASS | COMBINED EFFECT |
| --- | --- |
| Acetazolamide | Increased procainamide effect. |
| Ambenonium | Decreased ambenonium effect. |
| Antihypertensives | Increased antihypertensive effect. |
| Antimyasthenics | Decreased antimyasthenic effect. |
| Anticholinergics | Increased anticholinergic effect. |
| Flecainide | Possible irregular heartbeat. |
| Kanamycin | Severe muscle weakness, impaired breathing. |
| Neomycin | Severe muscle weakness, impaired breathing. |
| Tocainide | Increased likelihood of adverse reactions with either drug. |

## POSSIBLE INTERACTION WITH OTHER SUBSTANCES

| INTERACTS WITH | COMBINED EFFECT |
| --- | --- |
| Alcohol: | None expected. |
| Beverages: Caffeine drinks, iced drinks. | Irregular heartbeat. |
| Cocaine: | Decreased procainamide effect. |
| Foods: | None expected. |
| Marijuana: | None expected. |
| Tobacco: | Decreased procainamide effect. |

# PROCARBAZINE

## BRAND NAMES

Matulane                    Natulan

## BASIC INFORMATION

**Habit forming? No**
**Prescription needed? Yes**
**Available as generic? No**
**Drug class: Antineoplastic**

 **USES**

Treatment for some kinds of cancer.

 **DOSAGE & USAGE INFORMATION**

**How to take:**
Tablet or capsule—Swallow with liquid after light meal. Don't drink fluids with meals. Drink extra fluids between meals. Avoid sweet or fatty foods.

**When to take:**
At the same time each day.

**If you forget a dose:**
Take as soon as you remember. Don't double dose ever.

**What drug does:**
Inhibits abnormal cell reproduction. Procarbazine is an alkylating agent and a MAO inhibitor.

**Time lapse before drug works:**
Up to 6 weeks for full effect.

**Don't take with:**
See Interaction column and consult doctor.

 **OVERDOSE**

**SYMPTOMS:**
**Restlessness, agitation, fever, convulsions, bleeding.**
**WHAT TO DO:**
● **Dial 0 (operator) or 911 (emergency) for an ambulance or medical help. Then give first aid immediately.**
● **If patient is unconscious and not breathing, give mouth-to-mouth breathing. If there is no heartbeat, use cardiac massage and mouth-to-mouth breathing (CPR). Don't try to make patient vomit. If you can't get help quickly, take patient to nearest emergency facility.**
● **See emergency information on inside covers.**

 **POSSIBLE ADVERSE REACTIONS OR SIDE EFFECTS**

| SYMPTOMS | WHAT TO DO |
|---|---|
| **Life-threatening:** | |
| None expected. | |
| **Common:** | |
| ● Fatigue, weakness. | Continue. Call doctor when convenient. |
| ● Dizziness when changing position, dry mouth, constipation, difficult urination. | Continue. Tell doctor at next visit. |
| **Infrequent:** | |
| ● Fainting. | Discontinue. Seek emergency treatment. |
| ● Severe headache, abnormal bleeding or bruising, chest pain. | Discontinue. Call doctor right away. |
| ● Hallucinations, insomnia, nightmares, diarrhea, rapid or pounding heartbeat, swollen feet or legs. | Continue. Call doctor when convenient. |
| ● Diminished sex drive. | Continue. Tell doctor at next visit. |
| **Rare:** | |
| Rash, nausea, vomiting, stiff neck, jaundice, fever. | Discontinue. Call doctor right away. |

## WARNINGS & PRECAUTIONS

**Don't take if:**
- You are allergic to any MAO inhibitor.
- You have heart disease, congestive heart failure, heart-rhythm irregularities or high blood pressure.
- You have liver or kidney disease.

**Before you start, consult your doctor:**
- If you are alcoholic.
- If you have asthma.
- If you have had a stroke.
- If you have diabetes or epilepsy.
- If you have overactive thyroid.
- If you have schizophrenia.
- If you have Parkinson's disease.
- If you have adrenal-gland tumor.
- If you will have surgery within 2 months, including dental surgery, requiring general or spinal anesthesia.

**Over age 60:**
Not recommended.

**Pregnancy:**
Avoid if possible.

**Breast-feeding:**
Safety not established. Consult doctor.

**Infants & children:**
Not recommended.

**Prolonged use:**
May be toxic to liver.

**Skin & sunlight:**
May cause rash or intensify sunburn in areas exposed to sun or sunlamp.

**Driving, piloting or hazardous work:**
Don't drive or pilot aircraft until you learn how medicine affects you. Don't work around dangerous machinery. Don't climb ladders or work in high places. Danger increases if you drink alcohol or take medicine affecting alertness and reflexes.

**Discontinuing:**
- Don't discontinue without doctor's advice until you complete prescribed dose, even though symptoms diminish or disappear.
- Follow precautions regarding foods, drinks and other medicines for 2 weeks after discontinuing.

**Others:**
- May affect blood-sugar levels in patients with diabetes.
- Fever may indicate that MAO inhibitor dose requires adjustment.

## POSSIBLE INTERACTION WITH OTHER DRUGS

| GENERIC NAME OR DRUG CLASS | COMBINED EFFECT |
|---|---|
| Amphetamines | Blood-pressure rise to life-threatening level. |
| Anticonvulsants | Changed seizure pattern. |
| Antidepressants (tricyclic) | Blood-pressure rise to life-threatening level. |
| Antidiabetics (oral and insulin) | Excessively low blood sugar. |
| Caffeine | Irregular heartbeat or high blood pressure. |
| Carbamazepine | Fever, seizures. Avoid. |
| Cyclobenzaprine | Fever, seizures. Avoid. |
| Diuretics | Excessively low blood pressure. |
| Guanethidine | Blood-pressure rise to life-threatening level. |
| Levodopa | Sudden, severe blood-pressure rise. |
| MAO inhibitors (other) | High fever, convulsions, death. |

## POSSIBLE INTERACTION WITH OTHER SUBSTANCES

| INTERACTS WITH | COMBINED EFFECT |
|---|---|
| Alcohol: | Increased sedation to dangerous level. |
| Beverages: Caffeine drinks. | Irregular heartbeat or high blood pressure. |
| Drinks containing tyramine (see Glossary). | Blood-pressure rise to life-threatening level. |
| Cocaine: | Overstimulation. Possibly fatal. |
| Foods: Foods containing tyramine (see Glossary). | Blood-pressure rise to life-threatening level. |
| Marijuana: | Overstimulation. Avoid. |
| Tobacco: | No proven problems. |

# PROCHLORPERAZINE

## BRAND NAMES

| | |
|---|---|
| Chlorazine | Prochlor-Iso |
| Combid | Pro-Iso |
| Compazine | Stemetil |
| Eskatrol | |

## BASIC INFORMATION

**Habit forming?** No
**Prescription needed?** Yes
**Available as generic?** Yes
**Drug class:** Tranquilizer, antiemetic (phenothiazine)

 ## USES

- Stops nausea, vomiting.
- Reduces anxiety, agitation.

 ## DOSAGE & USAGE INFORMATION

**How to take:**
- Tablet or capsule—Swallow with liquid or food to lessen stomach irritation.
- Suppositories—Remove wrapper and moisten suppository with water. Gently insert into rectum, large end first.
- Drops or liquid—Dilute dose in beverage.

**When to take:**
- Nervous and mental disorders—Take at the same times each day.
- Nausea and vomiting—Take as needed, no more often than every 4 hours.

**If you forget a dose:**
- Nervous and mental disorders—Take up to 2 hours late. If more than 2 hours, wait for next scheduled dose (don't double this dose).
- Nausea and vomiting—Take as soon as you remember. Wait 4 hours for next dose.

*Continued next column*

 ## OVERDOSE

**SYMPTOMS:**
Stupor, convulsions, coma.
**WHAT TO DO:**
- **Dial 0 (operator) or 911 (emergency) for an ambulance or medical help. Then give first aid immediately.**
- **See emergency information on inside covers.**

**What drug does:**
- Suppresses brain's vomiting center.
- Suppresses brain centers that control abnormal emotions and behavior.

**Time lapse before drug works:**
- Nausea and vomiting—1 hour or less.
- Nervous and mental disorders—4-6 weeks.

**Don't take with:**
- Antacid or medicine for diarrhea.
- Non-prescription drug for cough, cold or allergy.
- See Interaction column and consult doctor.

 ## POSSIBLE ADVERSE REACTIONS OR SIDE EFFECTS

| SYMPTOMS | WHAT TO DO |
|---|---|
| **Life-threatening:** | |
| None expected. | |
| **Common:** | |
| • Muscle spasms of face and neck, unsteady gait. | Discontinue. Seek emergency treatment. |
| • Restlessness, tremor, drowsiness. | Discontinue. Call doctor right away. |
| • Decreased sweating, dry mouth, runny nose, constipation. | Continue. Call doctor when convenient. |
| **Infrequent:** | |
| • Fainting. | Discontinue. Seek emergency treatment. |
| • Rash. | Discontinue. Call doctor right away. |
| • Difficult urination, diminished sex drive, swollen breasts, menstrual irregularities. | Continue. Call doctor when convenient. |
| **Rare:** | |
| Change in vision, sore throat, fever, jaundice. | Discontinue. Call doctor right away. |

## WARNINGS & PRECAUTIONS

**Don't take if:**
- You are allergic to any phenothiazine.
- You have a blood or bone-marrow disease.

**Before you start, consult your doctor:**
- If you will have surgery within 2 months, including dental surgery, requiring general or spinal anesthesia.
- If you have asthma, emphysema or other lung disorder.
- If you take non-prescription ulcer medicine, asthma medicine or amphetamines.

**Over age 60:**
Adverse reactions and side effects may be more frequent and severe than in younger persons. More likely to develop involuntary movement of jaws, lips, tongue, chewing. Report this to your doctor immediately. Early treatment can help.

**Pregnancy:**
Risk to unborn child outweighs drug benefits. Don't use.

**Breast-feeding:**
Drug passes into milk. Avoid drug or discontinue nursing until you finish medicine. Consult doctor for advice on maintaining milk supply.

**Infants & children:**
Don't give to children younger than 2.

**Prolonged use:**
May lead to tardive dyskinesia (involuntary movement of jaws, lips, tongue, chewing).

**Skin & sunlight:**
May cause rash or intensify sunburn in areas exposed to sun or sunlamp. Skin may remain sensitive for 3 months after discontinuing.

**Driving, piloting or hazardous work:**
Don't drive or pilot aircraft until you learn how medicine affects you. Don't work around dangerous machinery. Don't climb ladders or work in high places. Danger increases if you drink alcohol or take medicine affecting alertness and reflexes.

**Discontinuing:**
- Nervous and mental disorders—Don't discontinue without doctor's advice until you complete prescribed dose, even though symptoms diminish or disappear.
- Nausea and vomiting—May be unnecessary to finish medicine. Follow doctor's instructions.

## POSSIBLE INTERACTION WITH OTHER DRUGS

| GENERIC NAME OR DRUG CLASS | COMBINED EFFECT |
|---|---|
| Anticholinergics | Increased anticholinergic effect. |
| Antidepressants (tricyclic) | Increased prochlorperazine effect. |
| Antihistamines | Increased antihistamine effect. |
| Appetite suppressants | Decreased suppressant effect. |
| Dronabinol | Increased effects of both drugs. Avoid. |
| Levodopa | Decreased levodopa effect. |
| Mind-altering drugs | Increased effect of mind-altering drugs. |
| Molindone | Increased tranquilizer effect. |
| Narcotics | Increased narcotic effect. |
| Phenytoin | Increased phenytoin effect. |
| Quinidine | Impaired heart function. Dangerous mixture. |
| Sedatives | Increased sedative effect. |
| Tranquilizers (other) | Increased tranquilizer effect. |

## POSSIBLE INTERACTION WITH OTHER SUBSTANCES

| INTERACTS WITH | COMBINED EFFECT |
|---|---|
| Alcohol: | Dangerous oversedation. |
| Beverages: | None expected. |
| Cocaine: | Decreased prochlorperazine effect. Avoid. |
| Foods: | None expected. |
| Marijuana: | Drowsiness. May increase antinausea effect. |
| Tobacco: | None expected. |

# PROCHLORPERAZINE & ISOPROPAMIDE

## BRAND NAMES

**Combid Spansules**

## BASIC INFORMATION

**Habit forming? No**
**Prescription needed? Yes**
**Available as generic? No**
**Drug class: Antispasmodic, antiemetic,**
            **tranquilizer (phenothiazine)**

## USES

- Stops nausea, vomiting.
- Reduces anxiety, agitation.
- Reduces spasms of digestive system.

## DOSAGE & USAGE INFORMATION

**How to take:**
- Tablet or capsule—Swallow with liquid or food to lessen stomach irritation.
- Extended-release tablets or capsules—Swallow each dose whole. If you take regular tablets, you may chew or crush them.

**When to take:**
30 minutes before meals (unless directed otherwise by doctor).

**If you forget a dose:**
Take as soon as you remember up to 2 hours late. If more than 2 hours, wait for next scheduled dose (don't double this dose).

*Continued next column*

## OVERDOSE

**SYMPTOMS:**
**Dilated pupils, rapid pulse and breathing, dizziness, fever, hallucinations, confusion, slurred speech, agitation, flushed face, convulsions, stupor, coma.**
**WHAT TO DO:**
- **Dial 0 (operator) or 911 (emergency) for an ambulance or medical help. Then give first aid immediately.**
- **See emergency information on inside covers.**

**What drug does:**
- Suppresses brain's vomiting center.
- Suppresses brain centers that control abnormal emotions and behavior.
- Blocks nerve impulses at parasympathetic nerve endings, preventing muscle contractions and gland secretions of organs involved.

**Time lapse before drug works:**
15 to 30 minutes.

**Don't take with:**
- Antacid or medicine for diarrhea.
- Non-prescription drugs for cough, cold or allergy.
- See Interaction column and consult doctor.

## POSSIBLE ADVERSE REACTIONS OR SIDE EFFECTS

| SYMPTOMS | WHAT TO DO |
|---|---|
| **Life-threatening:**<br>Fainting, dilated pupils, rapid pulse, hallucinations, muscle spasms, unsteady gait. | Discontinue. Seek emergency treatment. |
| **Common:** | |
| • Restlessness, tremor, confusion, drowsiness, rash. | Discontinue. Call doctor right away. |
| • Decreased sweating, dry mouth, runny nose, constipation, nausea. | Continue. Call doctor when convenient. |
| **Infrequent:** | |
| • Painful, difficult urination; vomiting. | Discontinue. Call doctor right away. |
| • Headache, diminished sex drive, swollen breasts, menstrual irregularities. | Continue. Call doctor when convenient. |
| **Rare:** | |
| Hives; change in vision; eye pain; sore throat, fever, mouth sores. | Discontinue. Call doctor right away. |

## WARNINGS & PRECAUTIONS

**Don't take if:**
- You are allergic to any anticholinergic or phenothiazine.
- You have trouble with stomach bloating, difficulty emptying your bladder completely, narrow-angle glaucoma, severe ulcerative colitis, a blood or bone-marrow disease.

## Before you start, consult your doctor:

- If you have open-angle glaucoma, angina, chronic bronchitis or asthma, hiatal hernia, liver disease, enlarged prostate, myasthenia gravis, peptic ulcer, emphysema or other lung disorder.
- If you take non-prescription ulcer medicine, asthma medicine or amphetamines.
- If you will have surgery within 2 months, including dental surgery, requiring general or spinal anesthesia.

## Over age 60:

Adverse reactions and side effects may be more frequent and severe than in younger persons. More likely to develop involuntary movement of jaws, lips, tongue, chewing. Report this to your doctor immediately. Early treatment can help.

## Pregnancy:

Risk to unborn child outweighs drug benefits. Don't use.

## Breast-feeding:

Drug passes into milk. Avoid drug or discontinue nursing until you finish medicine. Consult doctor for advice on maintaining milk supply.

## Infants & children:

Use only under medical supervision.

## Prolonged use:

- Chronic constipation, possible fecal impaction.
- May lead to tardive dyskinesia (involuntary movement of jaws, lips, tongue, chewing).

## Skin & sunlight:

May cause rash or intensify sunburn in areas exposed to sun or sunlamp. Skin may remain sensitive for 3 months after discontinuing.

## Driving, piloting or hazardous work:

Don't drive or pilot aircraft until you learn how medicine affects you. Don't work around dangerous machinery. Don't climb ladders or work in high places. Danger increases if you drink alcohol or take medicine affecting alertness and reflexes, such as antihistamines, tranquilizers, sedatives, pain medicine, narcotics and mind-altering drugs.

## Discontinuing:

- May be unnecessary to finish medicine. Follow doctor's instructions.
- If you develop withdrawal symptoms of hallucinations, agitation or sleeplessness after discontinuing, call doctor right away.

## Others:

No problems expected.

## POSSIBLE INTERACTION WITH OTHER DRUGS

| GENERIC NAME OR DRUG CLASS | COMBINED EFFECT |
|---|---|
| Amantadine | Increased isopropamide effect. |
| Anticholinergics | Increased anticholingeric effect. |
| Antidepressants (tricyclic) | Increased atropine effect. Increased sedation. |
| Antihistamlnes | Increased isopropamide effect. |
| Appetite suppressants | Decreased suppressant effect. |
| Cortisone drugs | Increased internal-eye pressure. |
| Dronabinol | Increased effect of both drugs. Avoid. |
| Haloperidol | Increased internal-eye pressure. |
| Levodopa | Decreased levodopa effect. |
| MAO inhibitors | Increased isopropamide effect. |
| Meperidine | Increased isopropamide effect. |
| Methylphenidate | Increased isopropamide effect. |
| Mind-altering drugs | Increased effect of mind-altering drugs. |
| Narcotics | Increased narcotic effect. |

*Continued page 974*

## POSSIBLE INTERACTION WITH OTHER SUBSTANCES

| INTERACTS WITH | COMBINED EFFECT |
|---|---|
| Alcohol: | Dangerous oversedation. |
| Beverages: | None expected. |
| Cocaine: | Excessively rapid heartbeat. Avoid. |
| Foods: | None expected. |
| Marijuana: | Drowsiness and dry mouth. May increase antinausea effect. |
| Tobacco: | None expected. |

# PROCYCLIDINE

## BRAND NAMES

Kemadrin         Procyclid
PMS Procyclidine

## BASIC INFORMATION

Habit forming? No
Prescription needed? Yes
Available as generic? No
Drug class: Antidyskinetic, antiparkinsonism

## USES

- Treatment of Parkinson's disease.
- Treatment of adverse effects of phenothiazines.

## DOSAGE & USAGE INFORMATION

**How to take:**
Tablets or capsules—Take with food to lessen stomach irritation.

**When to take:**
At the same times each day.

**If you forget a dose:**
Take as soon as you remember up to 2 hours late. If more than 2 hours, wait for next scheduled dose (don't double this dose).

**What drug does:**
- Balances chemical reactions necessary to send nerve impulses within base of brain.
- Improves muscle control and reduces stiffness.

*Continued next column*

## OVERDOSE

**SYMPTOMS:**
Agitation, dilated pupils, hallucinations, dry mouth, rapid heartbeat, sleepiness.
**WHAT TO DO:**
- Dial 0 (operator) or 911 (emergency) for an ambulance or medical help. Then give first aid immediately.
- If patient is unconscious and not breathing, give mouth-to-mouth breathing. If there is no heartbeat, use cardiac massage and mouth-to-mouth breathing (CPR). Don't try to make patient vomit. If you can't get help quickly, take patient to nearest emergency facility.
- See emergency information on inside covers.

**Time lapse before drug works:**
1 to 2 hours.

**Don't take with:**
- Non-prescription drugs for colds, cough or allergy.
- See Interaction column and consult doctor.

## POSSIBLE ADVERSE REACTIONS OR SIDE EFFECTS

| SYMPTOMS | WHAT TO DO |
|---|---|
| **Life-threatening:** None expected. | |
| **Common:** | |
| • Blurred vision, light sensitivity, constipation, nausea, vomiting. | Continue. Call doctor when convenient. |
| • Frequent, painful or difficult urination. | Continue. Tell doctor at next visit. |
| **Infrequent:** None expected. | |
| **Rare:** | |
| • Rash, eye pain. | Discontinue. Call doctor right away. |
| • Confusion, dizziness, sore mouth or tongue, muscle cramps, numbness or weakness in hands or feet. | Continue. Call doctor when convenient. |

# PROCYCLIDINE

## WARNINGS & PRECAUTIONS

**Don't take if:**
You are allergic to any antidyskinetic.

**Before you start, consult your doctor:**
- If you have had glaucoma.
- If you have had high blood pressure or heart disease.
- If you have had impaired liver function.
- If you have had kidney disease or urination difficulty.

**Over age 60:**
More sensitive to drug. Aggravates symptoms of enlarged prostate. Causes impaired thinking, hallucinations, nightmares. Consult doctor about any of these.

**Pregnancy:**
Studies inconclusive on harm to unborn child. Animal studies show fetal abnormalities. Decide with your doctor whether drug benefits justify risk to unborn child.

**Breast-feeding:**
No problems expected.

**Infants & children:**
Not recommended for children 3 and younger. Use for older children only under doctor's supervision.

**Prolonged use:**
Possible glaucoma.

**Skin & sunlight:**
No problems expected.

**Driving, piloting or hazardous work:**
Don't drive or pilot aircraft until you learn how medicine affects you. Don't work around dangerous machinery. Don't climb ladders or work in high places. Danger increases if you drink alcohol or take medicine affecting alertness and reflexes, such as antihistamines, tranquilizers, sedatives, pain medicine, narcotics and mind-altering drugs.

**Discontinuing:**
Don't discontinue without consulting doctor. Dose may require gradual reduction if you have taken drug for a long time. Doses of other drugs may also require adjustment.

**Others:**
- Internal eye pressure should be measured regularly.
- Avoid becoming overheated.

## POSSIBLE INTERACTION WITH OTHER DRUGS

| GENERIC NAME OR DRUG CLASS | COMBINED EFFECT |
|---|---|
| Amantadine | Increased amantadine effect. |
| Antidepressants (tricyclic) | Increased procyclidine effect. May cause glaucoma. |
| Antihistamines | Increased procyclidine effect. |
| Levodopa | Increased levodopa effect. Improved results in treating Parkinson's disease. |
| Meperidine | Increased procyclidine effect. |
| MAO inhibitors | Increased procyclidine effect. |
| Orphenadrine | Increased procyclidine effect. |
| Phenothiazines | Behavior changes. |
| Primidone | Excessive sedation. |
| Procainamide | Increased procainamide effect. |
| Quinidine | Increased procyclidine effect. |
| Tranquilizers | Excessive sedation. |

## POSSIBLE INTERACTION WITH OTHER SUBSTANCES

| INTERACTS WITH | COMBINED EFFECT |
|---|---|
| Alcohol: | None expected. |
| Beverages: | None expected. |
| Cocaine: | Decreased procyclidine effect. Avoid. |
| Foods: | None expected. |
| Marijuana: | None expected. |
| Tobacco: | None expected. |

743

# PROMAZINE

## BRAND NAMES

Norzine
Promanyl

Prozine
Sparine

## BASIC INFORMATION

Habit forming? No
Prescription needed? Yes
Available as generic? Yes
Drug class: Tranquilizer, antiemetic
(phenothiazine)

 USES

- Stops nausea, vomiting.
- Reduces anxiety, agitation.

 DOSAGE & USAGE INFORMATION

### How to take:

- Tablet or capsule—Swallow with liquid or food to lessen stomach irritation.
- Suppositories—Remove wrapper and moisten suppository with water. Gently insert into rectum, large end first.
- Drops or liquid—Dilute dose in beverage.

### When to take:

- Nervous and mental disorders—Take at the same times each day.
- Nausea and vomiting—Take as needed, no more often than every 4 hours.

### If you forget a dose:

- Nervous and mental disorders—Take up to 2 hours late. If more than 2 hours, wait for next scheduled dose (don't double this dose).
- Nausea and vomiting—Take as soon as you remember. Wait 4 hours for next dose.

### What drug does:

- Suppresses brain's vomiting center.
- Suppresses brain centers that control abnormal emotions and behavior.

*Continued next column*

 OVERDOSE

SYMPTOMS:
Stupor, convulsions, coma.
WHAT TO DO:
- Dial 0 (operator) or 911 (emergency) for an ambulance or medical help. Then give first aid immediately.
- See emergency information on inside covers.

## Time lapse before drug works:

- Nausea and vomiting—1 hour or less.
- Nervous and mental disorders—4-6 weeks.

### Don't take with:

- Antacid or medicine for diarrhea.
- Non-prescription drug for cough, cold or allergy.
- See Interaction column and consult doctor.

 POSSIBLE ADVERSE REACTIONS OR SIDE EFFECTS

| SYMPTOMS | WHAT TO DO |
|---|---|
| **Life-threatening:**<br>None expected. | |
| **Common:** | |
| • Muscle spasms of face and neck, unsteady gait. | Discontinue. Seek emergency treatment. |
| • Restlessness, tremor, drowsiness. | Discontinue. Call doctor right away. |
| • Decreased sweating, dry mouth, runny nose, constipation. | Continue. Call doctor when convenient. |
| **Infrequent:** | |
| • Fainting. | Discontinue. Seek emergency treatment. |
| • Rash. | Discontinue. Call doctor right away. |
| • Difficult urination, diminished sex drive, swollen breasts, menstrual irregularities. | Continue. Call doctor when convenient. |
| **Rare:**<br>Change in vision, sore throat, fever, jaundice. | Discontinue. Call doctor right away. |

## WARNINGS & PRECAUTIONS

### Don't take if:
- You are allergic to any phenothiazine.
- You have a blood or bone-marrow disease.

### Before you start, consult your doctor:
- If you will have surgery within 2 months, including dental surgery, requiring general or spinal anesthesia.
- If you have asthma, emphysema or other lung disorder.
- If you take non-prescription ulcer medicine, asthma medicine or amphetamines.

### Over age 60:
Adverse reactions and side effects may be more frequent and severe than in younger persons. More likely to develop involuntary movement of jaws, lips, tongue, chewing. Report this to your doctor immediately. Early treatment can help.

### Pregnancy:
Risk to unborn child outweighs drug benefits. Don't use.

### Breast-feeding:
Drug passes into milk. Avoid drug or discontinue nursing until you finish medicine. Consult doctor for advice on maintaining milk supply.

### Infants & children:
Don't give to children younger than 2.

### Prolonged use:
May lead to tardive dyskinesia (involuntary movement of jaws, lips, tongue, chewing).

### Skin & sunlight:
May cause rash or intensify sunburn in areas exposed to sun or sunlamp. Skin may remain sensitive for 3 months after discontinuing.

### Driving, piloting or hazardous work:
Don't drive or pilot aircraft until you learn how medicine affects you. Don't work around dangerous machinery. Don't climb ladders or work in high places. Danger increases if you drink alcohol or take medicine affecting alertness and reflexes.

### Discontinuing:
- Nervous and mental disorders—Don't discontinue without doctor's advice until you complete prescribed dose, even though symptoms diminish or disappear.
- Nausea and vomiting—May be unnecessary to finish medicine. Follow doctor's instructions.

## POSSIBLE INTERACTION WITH OTHER DRUGS

| GENERIC NAME OR DRUG CLASS | COMBINED EFFECT |
| --- | --- |
| Anticholinergics | Increased anticholinergic effect. |
| Antidepressants (tricyclic) | Increased promazine effect. |
| Antihistamines | Increased antihistamine effect. |
| Appetite suppressants | Decreased suppressant effect. |
| Dronabinol | Increased effects of both drugs. Avoid. |
| Levodopa | Decreased levodopa effect. |
| Mind-altering drugs | Increased effect of mind-altering drugs. |
| Molindone | Increased tranquilizer effect. |
| Narcotics | Increased narcotic effect. |
| Phenytoin | Increased phenytoin effect. |
| Quinidine | Impaired heart function. Dangerous mixture. |
| Sedatives | Increased sedative effect. |
| Tranquilizers (other) | Increased tranquilizer effect. |

## POSSIBLE INTERACTION WITH OTHER SUBSTANCES

| INTERACTS WITH | COMBINED EFFECT |
| --- | --- |
| Alcohol: | Dangerous oversedation. |
| Beverages: | None expected. |
| Cocaine: | Decreased promazine effect. Avoid. |
| Foods: | None expected. |
| Marijuana: | Drowsiness. May increase antinausea effect. |
| Tobacco: | None expected. |

# PROMETHAZINE

## BRAND NAMES

See complete list of brand names in the *Brand Name Directory,* page 955.

## BASIC INFORMATION

**Habit forming? No**
**Prescription needed? Yes**
**Available as generic? Yes**
**Drug class: Antihistamine, tranquilizer
(phenothiazine)**

 ## USES

- Stops nausea, vomiting and dizziness of motion sickness.
- Produces mild sedation and light sleep.
- Reduces allergic symptoms of hay fever and hives.

 ## DOSAGE & USAGE INFORMATION

**How to take:**
- Tablets or liquid—Swallow with water.
- Suppositories—Remove wrapper and moisten suppository with water. Gently insert larger end into rectum. Push well into rectum with finger.

**When to take:**
Take as needed, no more often than every 12 hours.

**If you forget a dose:**
Take as soon as you remember. Wait 12 hours for next dose.

**What drug does:**
- Blocks stimulation of brain's vomiting center.
- Suppresses brain centers that control abnormal emotions and behavior.
- Blocks histamine action in sensitized cells.

**Time lapse before drug works:**
1 to 2 hours.

*Continued next column*

 ## OVERDOSE

**SYMPTOMS:**
**Stupor, convulsions, coma.**
**WHAT TO DO:**
- **Dial 0 (operator) or 911 (emergency) for an ambulance or medical help. Then give first aid immediately.**
- **See emergency information on inside covers.**

**Don't take with:**
- Antacid or medicine for diarrhea.
- Non-prescription drug for cough, cold or allergy.
- See Interaction column and consult doctor.

 ## POSSIBLE ADVERSE REACTIONS OR SIDE EFFECTS

| SYMPTOMS | WHAT TO DO |
|---|---|
| **Life-threatening:** | |
| None expected. | |
| **Common:** | |
| • Restlessness, tremor, drowsiness. | Discontinue. Call doctor right away. |
| • Decreased sweating, dry mouth, runny nose, constipation. | Continue. Call doctor when convenient. |
| **Infrequent:** | |
| • Fainting. | Discontinue. Seek emergency treatment. |
| • Rash, muscle spasms of face and neck, unsteady gait. | Discontinue. Call doctor right away. |
| • Difficult urination, diminished sex drive, swollen breasts, menstrual irregularities. | Continue. Call doctor when convenient. |
| **Rare:** | |
| Change in vision, sore throat, fever, jaundice. | Discontinue. Call doctor right away. |

 ## WARNINGS & PRECAUTIONS

**Don't take if:**
- You are allergic to any phenothiazine.
- You have a blood or bone-marrow disease.

**Before you start, consult your doctor:**
- If you will have surgery within 2 months, including dental surgery, requiring general or spinal anesthesia.
- If you have asthma, emphysema or other lung disorder.
- If you take non-prescription ulcer medicine, asthma medicine or amphetamines.

**Over age 60:**
Adverse reactions and side effects may be more frequent and severe than in younger persons. More likely to develop tardive dyskinesia (involuntary movement of jaws, lips, tongue, chewing). Report this to your doctor immediately. Early treatment can help.

**Pregnancy:**
Risk to unborn child outweighs drug benefits. Don't use.

**Breast-feeding:**
Drug passes into milk. Avoid drug or discontinue nursing until you finish medicine. Consult doctor for advice on maintaining milk supply.

**Infants & children:**
Don't give to children younger than 2.

**Prolonged use:**
May lead to tardive dyskinesia (involuntary movement of jaws, lips, tongue, chewing).

**Skin & sunlight:**
May cause rash or intensify sunburn in areas exposed to sun or sunlamp. Skin may remain sensitive for 3 months after discontinuing.

**Driving, piloting or hazardous work:**
Don't drive or pilot aircraft until you learn how medicine affects you. Don't work around dangerous machinery. Don't climb ladders or work in high places. Danger increases if you drink alcohol or take medicine affecting alertness and reflexes.

**Discontinuing:**
- Nervous and mental disorders—Don't discontinue without doctor's advice until you complete prescribed dose, even though symptoms diminish or disappear.
- Nausea, vomiting or allergy—May be unnecessary to finish medicine. Follow doctor's instructions.

**Others:**
No problems expected.

## POSSIBLE INTERACTION WITH OTHER DRUGS

| GENERIC NAME OR DRUG CLASS | COMBINED EFFECT |
|---|---|
| Antacids | Decreased promethazine effect. |
| Anticholinergics | Increased anticholinergic effect. |
| Anticonvulsants (hydantoin) | Increased anticonvulsant effect. |

| | |
|---|---|
| Antidepressants (tricyclic) | Increased promethazine effect. |
| Antihistamines (other) | Increased antihistamine effect. |
| Appetite suppressants | Decreased suppressant effect. |
| Barbiturates | Oversedation. |
| Dronabinol | Increased effects of both drugs. Avoid. |
| Glycopyrrolate | Possible increased glycopyrrolate effect. |
| Guanethidine | Decreased guanethidine effect. |
| Levodopa | Decreased levodopa effect. |
| MAO inhibitors | Increased promethazine effect. |
| Mind-altering drugs | Increased effect of mind-altering drugs. |
| Molindone | Increased sedative and antihistamine effect. |
| Narcotics | Increased narcotic effect. |
| Sedatives | Increased sedative effect. |
| Terfenadine | Possible oversedation. |
| Tranquilizers (other) | Increased tranquilizer effect. |

## POSSIBLE INTERACTION WITH OTHER SUBSTANCES

| INTERACTS WITH | COMBINED EFFECT |
|---|---|
| Alcohol: | Dangerous sedation. |
| Beverages: | None expected. |
| Cocaine: | Decreased effect of promethazine. Avoid. |
| Foods: | None expected. |
| Marijuana: | Drowsiness. May increase antinausea effect. |
| Tobacco: | None expected. |

# PROPANTHELINE

## BRAND NAMES

Banlin
Norpanth
Novopropanthil
Pro-Banthine
Pro-Banthine with
  Phenobarbital

Propanthel
Ropanth
SK-Propantheline

## BASIC INFORMATION

**Habit forming? No**
**Prescription needed?**
  **High strength: Yes**
  **Low strength: No**
**Available as generic? Yes**
**Drug class: Antispasmodic, anticholinergic**

 **USES**

Reduces spasms of digestive system, bladder
and urethra.

 **DOSAGE & USAGE INFORMATION**

**How to take:**
Tablet—Swallow with liquid or food to lessen
stomach irritation.

**When to take:**
30 minutes before meals (unless directed
otherwise by doctor).

**If you forget a dose:**
Take as soon as you remember up to 2 hours
late. If more than 2 hours, wait for next
scheduled dose (don't double this dose).

**What drug does:**
Blocks nerve impulses at parasympathetic nerve
endings, preventing muscle contractions and
gland secretions of organs involved.

**Time lapse before drug works:**
15 to 30 minutes.

**Don't take with:**
See Interaction column and consult doctor.

 **OVERDOSE**

**SYMPTOMS:**
**Dilated pupils, rapid pulse and breathing,
dizziness, fever, hallucinations, confusion,
slurred speech, agitation, flushed face,
convulsions, coma.**
**WHAT TO DO:**
- **Dial 0 (operator) or 911 (emergency) for an
  ambulance or medical help. Then give first
  aid immediately.**
- **See emergency information on inside
  covers.**

 **POSSIBLE ADVERSE REACTIONS OR SIDE EFFECTS**

| SYMPTOMS | WHAT TO DO |
|---|---|
| **Life-threatening:** | |
| None expected. | |
| **Common:** | |
| ● Confusion, delirium, rapid heartbeat. | Discontinue. Call doctor right away. |
| ● Nausea, vomiting, decreased sweating. | Continue. Call doctor when convenient. |
| ● Constipation. | Continue. Tell doctor at next visit. |
| ● Dry ears, nose, throat. | No action necessary. |
| **Infrequent:** | |
| Headache, difficult urination. | Continue. Call doctor when convenient. |
| **Rare:** | |
| Rash or hives, pain, blurred vision. | Discontinue. Call doctor right away. |

 **WARNINGS & PRECAUTIONS**

**Don't take if:**
- You are allergic to any anticholinergic.
- You have trouble with stomach bloating.
- You have difficulty emptying your bladder
  completely.
- You have narrow-angle glaucoma.
- You have severe ulcerative colitis.

**Before you start, consult your doctor:**
- If you have open-angle glaucoma.
- If you have angina.
- If you have chronic bronchitis or asthma.
- If you have hiatal hernia.
- If you have liver disease.
- If you have enlarged prostate.
- If you have myasthenia gravis.
- If you have peptic ulcer.
- If you will have surgery within 2 months,
  including dental surgery, requiring general or
  spinal anesthesia.

**Over age 60:**
Adverse reactions and side effects may be
more frequent and severe than in younger
persons.

**Pregnancy:**
Studies inconclusive on harm to unborn child.
Animal studies show fetal abnormalities. Decide
with your doctor whether drug benefits justify
risk to unborn child.

# PROPANTHELINE

**Breast-feeding:**
Drug passes into milk and decreases milk flow. Avoid drug or discontinue nursing until you finish medicine. Consult doctor for advice on maintaining milk supply.

**Infants & children:**
Use only under medical supervision.

**Prolonged use:**
Chronic constipation, possible fecal impaction. Consult doctor immediately.

**Skin & sunlight:**
No problems expected.

**Driving, piloting or hazardous work:**
Use disqualifies you for piloting aircraft. Otherwise, no problems expected.

**Discontinuing:**
May be unnecessary to finish medicine. Follow doctor's instructions.

**Others:**
No problems expected.

 **POSSIBLE INTERACTION WITH OTHER DRUGS**

| GENERIC NAME OR DRUG CLASS | COMBINED EFFECT |
| --- | --- |
| Amantadine | Increased propantheline effect. |
| Anticholinergics (other) | Increased propantheline effect. |
| Antidepressants (tricyclic) | Increased propantheline effect. Increased sedation. |
| Antihistamines | Increased propantheline effect. |
| Cortisone drugs | Increased internal eye pressure. |
| Haloperidol | Increased internal eye pressure. |
| MAO inhibitors | Increased propantheline effect. |
| Meperidine | Increased propantheline effect. |
| Methylphenidate | Increased propantheline effect. |
| Molindone | Increased anticholinergic effect. |
| Nitrates | Increased internal-eye pressure. |
| Orphenadrine | Increased propantheline effect. |
| Phenothiazines | Increased propantheline effect. |
| Pilocarpine | Loss of pilocarpine effect in glaucoma treatment. |
| Potassium supplements | Increased possibility of intestinal ulcers with oral potassium tablets. |
| Terfenadine | Possible increased propantheline effect. |
| Vitamin C | Decreased propantheline effect. Avoid large doses of vitamin C. |

 **POSSIBLE INTERACTION WITH OTHER SUBSTANCES**

| INTERACTS WITH | COMBINED EFFECT |
| --- | --- |
| Alcohol: | None expected. |
| Beverages: | None expected. |
| Cocaine: | Excessively rapid heartbeat. Avoid. |
| Foods: | None expected. |
| Marijuana: | Drowsiness and dry mouth. |
| Tobacco: | None expected. |

# PROPRANOLOL

## BRAND NAMES

| | |
|---|---|
| Apo-Propranolol | Inderide |
| Detensol | Novopranol |
| Inderal | Panolol |
| Inderal LA | pms-Propranolol |

## BASIC INFORMATION

**Habit forming? No**
**Prescription needed? Yes**
**Available as generic? Yes**
**Drug class: Beta-adrenergic blocker**

## USES

- Reduces angina attacks.
- Stabilizes irregular heartbeat.
- Lowers blood pressure.
- Reduces frequency of migraine headaches. (Does not relieve headache pain.)
- Other uses prescribed by your doctor.

## DOSAGE & USAGE INFORMATION

**How to take:**
Tablet or capsule—Swallow with liquid. If you can't swallow whole, crumble tablet or open capsule and take with liquid or food.

**When to take:**
With meals or immediately after.

**If you forget a dose:**
Take as soon as you remember. Return to regular schedule, but allow 3 hours between doses.

**What drug does:**
- Blocks certain actions of sympathetic nervous system.
- Lowers heart's oxygen requirements.
- Slows nerve impulses through heart.
- Reduces blood vessel contraction in heart, scalp and other body parts.

*Continued next column*

## OVERDOSE

**SYMPTOMS:**
**Weakness, slow or weak pulse, blood-pressure drop, fainting, convulsions, cold and sweaty skin.**
**WHAT TO DO:**
- **Dial 0 (operator) or 911 (emergency) for an ambulance or medical help. Then give first aid immediately.**
- **See emergency information on inside covers.**

**Time lapse before drug works:**
1 to 4 hours.

**Don't take with:**
Non-prescription drugs or drugs in Interaction column without consulting doctor.

## POSSIBLE ADVERSE REACTIONS OR SIDE EFFECTS

| SYMPTOMS | WHAT TO DO |
|---|---|
| **Life-threatening:** | |
| None expected. | |
| **Common:** | |
| • Pulse slower than 50 beats per minute. | Discontinue. Call doctor right away. |
| • Drowsiness, numbness or tingling of fingers or toes, dizziness, diarrhea, nausea, fatigue, weakness. | Continue. Call doctor when convenient. |
| • Cold hands or feet; dry mouth, eyes and skin. | Continue. Tell doctor at next visit. |
| **Infrequent:** | |
| • Hallucinations, nightmares, insomnia, headache, difficult breathing, joint pain. | Discontinue. Call doctor right away. |
| • Confusion, depression, reduced alertness, impotence. | Continue. Call doctor when convenient. |
| • Constipation. | Continue. Tell doctor at next visit. |
| **Rare:** | |
| • Rash, sore throat, fever. | Discontinue. Call doctor right away. |
| • Unusual bleeding and bruising. | Continue. Call doctor when convenient. |

## WARNINGS & PRECAUTIONS

**Don't take if:**
- You are allergic to any beta-adrenergic blocker.
- You have asthma.
- You have hay fever symptoms.
- You have taken MAO inhibitors in past 2 weeks.

**Before you start, consult your doctor:**
- If you have heart disease or poor circulation to the extremities.
- If you have hay fever, asthma, chronic bronchitis, emphysema.
- If you have overactive thyroid function.
- If you have impaired liver or kidney function.
- If you will have surgery within 2 months, including dental surgery, requiring general or spinal anesthesia.
- If you have diabetes or hypoglycemia.

**Over age 60:**
Adverse reactions and side effects may be more frequent and severe than in younger persons.

**Pregnancy:**
Risk to unborn child outweighs drug benefits. Don't use.

**Breast-feeding:**
Drug passes into milk. Avoid drug or discontinue nursing until you finish medicine. Consult doctor for advice on maintaining milk supply.

**Infants & children:**
Not recommended.

**Prolonged use:**
Weakens heart muscle contractions.

**Skin & sunlight:**
No problems expected.

**Driving, piloting or hazardous work:**
Don't drive or pilot aircraft until you learn how medicine affects you. Don't work around dangerous machinery. Don't climb ladders or work in high places. Danger increases if you drink alcohol or take medicine affecting alertness and reflexes.

**Discontinuing:**
Don't discontinue without consulting doctor. Dose may require gradual reduction if you have taken drug for a long time. Doses of other drugs may also require adjustment.

**Others:**
May mask hypoglycemia.

## POSSIBLE INTERACTION WITH OTHER DRUGS

| GENERIC NAME OR DRUG CLASS | COMBINED EFFECT |
| --- | --- |
| Acebutolol | Increased antihypertensive effects of both drugs. Dosages may require adjustment. |
| Albuterol | Decreased Albuterol effect and Beta-adrenergic blocking effect |
| Antidiabetics | Increased antidiabetic effect. |
| Antihistamines | Decreased antihistamine effect. |
| Antihypertensives | Increased antihypertensive effect. |
| Anti-inflammatory drugs | Decreased anti-inflammatory effect. |
| Barbiturates | Increased barbiturate effect. Dangerous sedation. |
| Digitalis preparations | Can either increase or decrease heart rate. Improves irregular heartbeat. |
| Molindone | Increased tranquilizer effect. |
| Narcotics | Increased narcotic effect. Dangerous sedation. |
| Nitrates | Possible excessive blood-pressure drop. |
| Pentoxifylline | Increased antihypertensive effect. |
| Phenytoin | Increased propranolol effect. |
| Quinidine | Slows heart excessively. |
| Reserpine | Increased reserpine effect. Excessive sedation and depression. |
| Tocainide | May worsen congestive heart failure. |

## POSSIBLE INTERACTION WITH OTHER SUBSTANCES

| INTERACTS WITH | COMBINED EFFECT |
| --- | --- |
| Alcohol: | Excessive blood-pressure drop. Avoid. |
| Beverages: | None expected. |
| Cocaine: | Irregular heartbeat. Avoid. |
| Foods: | None expected. |
| Marijuana: | Daily use—Impaired circulation to hands and feet. |
| Tobacco: | Possible irregular heartbeat. |

# PSEUDOEPHEDRINE

## BRAND NAMES

See complete list of brand names in the *Brand Name Directory,* page 955.

## BASIC INFORMATION

**Habit forming? No**
**Prescription needed?**
  **U.S.: High strength—Yes**
          **Low strength—No**
  **Canada: No**
**Available as generic? Yes**
**Drug class: Sympathomimetic**

 USES

Reduces congestion of nose, sinuses and throat from allergies and infections.

 DOSAGE & USAGE INFORMATION

**How to take:**
- Tablet or capsule—Swallow with liquid. You may chew or crush tablet.
- Extended-release tablets or capsules—Swallow each dose whole.
- Syrup—Take as directed on label.

**When to take:**
- At the same times each day.
- To prevent insomnia, take last dose of day a few hours before bedtime.

**If you forget a dose:**
Take up to 2 hours late. If more than 2 hours, wait for next dose (don't double this dose).

**What drug does:**
Decreases blood volume in nasal tissues, shrinking tissues and enlarging airways.

*Continued next column*

 OVERDOSE

**SYMPTOMS:**
**Nervousness, restlessness, headache, rapid or irregular heartbeat, sweating, nausea, vomiting, anxiety, confusion, delirium, muscle tremors.**
**WHAT TO DO:**
- **Dial 0 (operator) or 911 (emergency) for an ambulance or medical help. Then give first aid immediately.**
- **See emergency information on inside covers.**

**Time lapse before drug works:**
15 to 20 minutes.

**Don't take with:**
- See Interaction column and consult doctor.
- Non-prescription drugs with caffeine without consulting doctor.

 POSSIBLE ADVERSE REACTIONS OR SIDE EFFECTS

| SYMPTOMS | WHAT TO DO |
|---|---|
| **Life-threatening:**<br>None expected. | |
| **Common:**<br>Agitation, insomnia. | Continue. Tell doctor at next visit. |
| **Infrequent:**<br>• Nausea or vomiting, irregular or slow heartbeat, difficult breathing, unusually fast or pounding heartbeat, painful or difficult urination, increased sweating. | Discontinue. Call doctor right away. |
| • Dizziness, headache, shakiness, weakness. | Continue. Call doctor when convenient. |
| • Paleness. | Continue. Tell doctor at next visit. |
| **Rare:**<br>Hallucinations, seizures. | Discontinue. Seek emergency treatment. |

## WARNINGS & PRECAUTIONS

**Don't take if:**
You are allergic to any sympathomimetic drug.

**Before you start, consult your doctor:**
- If you have overactive thyroid or diabetes.
- If you have taken any MAO inhibitors in past 2 weeks.
- If you take digitalis preparations or have high blood pressure or heart disease.
- If you will have surgery within 2 months, including dental surgery, requiring general or spinal anesthesia.
- If you have urination difficulty.

**Over age 60:**
Adverse reactions and side effects may be more frequent and severe than in younger persons.

**Pregnancy:**
No proven harm to unborn child. Avoid if possible.

**Breast-feeding:**
Drug passes into milk. Avoid drug or discontinue nursing until you finish medicine. Consult doctor for advice on maintaining milk supply.

**Infants & children:**
Keep dose low or avoid.

**Prolonged use:**
No proven problems.

**Skin & sunlight:**
No problems expected.

**Driving, piloting or hazardous work:**
Avoid if you feel dizzy. Otherwise, no problems expected..

**Discontinuing:**
May be unnecessary to finish medicine. Follow doctor's instructions.

**Others:**
No problems expected.

## POSSIBLE INTERACTION WITH OTHER DRUGS

| GENERIC NAME OR DRUG CLASS | COMBINED EFFECT |
|---|---|
| Antidepressants (tricyclic) | Increased pseudoephedrine effect. |
| Antihypertensives | Decreased antihypertensive effect. |
| Beta-adrenergic blockers | Decreased effects of both drugs. |
| Calcium supplements | Increased pseudoephedrine effect. |
| Digitalis preparations | Irregular heartbeat. |
| Epinephrine | Increased epinephrine effect. Excessive heart stimulation and blood-pressure increase. |
| Ergot preparations | Serious blood-pressure rise. |
| Guanethidine | Decreased effect of both drugs. |
| MAO inhibitors | Increased pseudoephedrine effect. |
| Nitrates | Possible decreased effects of both drugs. |

## POSSIBLE INTERACTION WITH OTHER SUBSTANCES

| INTERACTS WITH | COMBINED EFFECT |
|---|---|
| Alcohol: | None expected. |
| Beverages: Caffeine drinks. | Nervousness or insomnia. |
| Cocaine: | Dangerous stimulation. Avoid. |
| Foods: | None expected. |
| Marijuana: | Rapid heartbeat. |
| Tobacco: | None expected. |

# PSORALENS

## BRAND AND GENERIC NAMES

METHOXSALEN
Methoxsalen Lotion
 (Topical)
Oxsoralen

Oxsoralen (Topical)
TRIOXSALEN
Trisoralen

## BASIC INFORMATION

**Habit forming? No**
**Prescription needed? Yes**
**Available as generic? No**
**Drug class: Repigmenting agent (psoralen)**

 USES

- Repigmenting skin affected with vitiligo (absence of skin pigment).
- Treatment for psoriasis, when other treatments haven't helped.
- Treatment for mycosis fungoides.

 DOSAGE & USAGE INFORMATION

**How to take or apply:**
- Tablet or capsule—Swallow with liquid or food to lessen stomach irritation.
- Topical—As directed by doctor.

**When to take or apply:**
2 to 4 hours before exposure to sunlight or sunlamp.

**If you forget a dose:**
Take as soon as you remember. Delay sun exposure for at least 2 hours after taking.

**What drug does:**
Helps pigment cells when used in conjunction with ultraviolet light.

**Time lapse before drug works:**
- For vitiligo, up to 6 months.
- For psoriasis, 10 weeks or longer.
- For tanning, 3 to 4 days.

**Don't take with:**
Any other medicine which causes skin sensitivity to sun. Ask pharmacist.

 OVERDOSE

**SYMPTOMS:**
Blistering skin, swelling feet and legs.
**WHAT TO DO:**
Overdose unlikely to threaten life. If person takes much larger amount than prescribed, call doctor, poison-control center or hospital emergency room for instructions.

 POSSIBLE ADVERSE REACTIONS OR SIDE EFFECTS

| SYMPTOMS | WHAT TO DO |
|---|---|
| **Life-threatening:** None expected. | |
| **Always:** | |
| • Increased skin sensitivity to sun. | Always protect from overexposure. |
| • Increased eye sensitivity to sunlight. | Always protect with wrap-around sunglasses. |
| **Infrequent:** None expected. | |
| **Rare:** Hepatitis with jaundice, blistering and peeling. | Discontinue. Call doctor right away. |

 WARNINGS & PRECAUTIONS

**Don't take if:**
- You are allergic to any other psoralen.
- You are unwilling or unable to remain under close medical supervision.

**Before you start, consult your doctor:**
- If you have heart or liver disease.
- If you have allergy to sunlight.
- If you have cataracts.
- If you have albinism.
- If you have lupus erythematosis, porphyria, chronic infection, skin cancer or peptic ulcer.
- If you will have surgery within 2 months, including dental surgery, requiring general or spinal anesthesia.

**Over age 60:**
Adverse reactions and side effects may be more frequent and severe than in younger persons.

**Pregnancy:**
Risk to unborn child outweighs drug benefits. Don't use.

**Breast-feeding:**
Drug passes into milk. Avoid drug or discontinue nursing until you finish medicine. Consult doctor for advice on maintaining milk supply.

**Infants & children:**
Not recommended.

**Prolonged use:**
Increased chance of toxic effects.

**Skin & sunlight:**
Too much can burn skin. Cover skin for 24 hours before and 8 hours following treatments.

**Driving, piloting or hazardous work:**
No problems expected. Protect eyes and skin from bright light.

**Discontinuing:**
Skin may remain sensitive for some time after treatment stops. Use extra protection from sun.

**Others:**
- Use sunblock on lips.
- Don't use just to make skin tan.

 ## POSSIBLE INTERACTION WITH OTHER DRUGS

| GENERIC NAME OR DRUG CLASS | COMBINED EFFECT |
|---|---|
| **Any medicine causing sensitization to sunlight, such as: acetohexamide, amitriptyline, anthralin, barbiturates, bendroflumethiazide, carbamazepine, chlordiazepoxide, chloroqulne, chlorothiazide, chloropromazine, chloropropamide, chlortetracycline, chlorthalidone, clindamycin, coal tar derivatives, cyproheptadine, demeclocycline, desipramine, diethylstllbrestrol, diphenhydramine, doxepin, doxycycline, estrogen, fluphenazine, gold preparations, glyburide, griseofulvin, hydrochlorothiazide, hydroflumethiazide, imipramine, lincomycin, mesoridazine, methacycline, nalidixic acid, nortriptyline, oral contraceptives, oxyphenbutazone, oxytetracycline,** | Greatly increased likelihood of extreme sensitivity to sunlight. |

**perphenazine, phenobarbital, phenylbutazone, phenytoin, prochlorperazine, promazine, promethazine, protriptyline, pyrazinamide, sulfonamides, tetracycline, thioridazine, thiazide diuretics, tolazamide, tolbutamide, tranylcypromine, triamterene, trifluoperazine, trimeprazine, trimipramine, triprolidine.**

 ## POSSIBLE INTERACTION WITH OTHER SUBSTANCES

| INTERACTS WITH | COMBINED EFFECT |
|---|---|
| **Alcohol:** | May increase chance of liver toxicity. |
| **Beverages:** Lime drinks. | Avoid—toxic. |
| **Cocaine:** | Increased chance of toxicity. Avoid. |
| **Foods:** Those containing furocoumarin (limes, parsley, figs, parsnips, carrots, celery, mustard). | May cause toxic effects to psoralens. |
| **Marijuana:** | Increased chance of toxicity. Avoid. |
| **Tobacco:** | May cause uneven absorption of medicine. Avoid. |

755

# PSYLLIUM

## BRAND NAMES

See complete list of brand names in the *Brand Name Directory,* page 956.

## BASIC INFORMATION

**Habit forming? No**
**Prescription needed? No**
**Available as generic? Yes**
**Drug class: Laxative (bulk-forming)**

 **USES**

Relieves constipation and prevents straining for bowel movement.

 **DOSAGE & USAGE INFORMATION**

**How to take:**
Powder, flakes or granules—Dilute dose in 8 oz. cold water or fruit juice.

**When to take:**
At the same time each day, preferably morning.

**If you forget a dose:**
Take as soon as you remember. Resume regular schedule.

**What drug does:**
Absorbs water, stimulating the bowel to form a soft, bulky stool.

**Time lapse before drug works:**
May require 2 or 3 days to begin, then works in 12 to 24 hours.

**Don't take with:**
- See Interaction column and consult doctor.
- Don't take within 2 hours of taking another medicine.

 **OVERDOSE**

**SYMPTOMS:**
**None expected.**
**WHAT TO DO:**
**Overdose unlikely to threaten life. If person takes much larger amount than prescribed, call doctor, poison-control center or hospital emergency room for instructions.**

 **POSSIBLE ADVERSE REACTIONS OR SIDE EFFECTS**

| SYMPTOMS | WHAT TO DO |
|---|---|
| **Life-threatening**<br>None expected. | |
| **Common:**<br>None expected. | |
| **Infrequent:**<br>Swallowing difficulty, "lump in throat" sensation. | Continue. Call doctor when convenient. |
| **Rare:**<br>Rash, itchy skin, intestinal blockage, asthma. | Discontinue. Call doctor right away. |

## WARNINGS & PRECAUTIONS

**Don't take if:**
- You are allergic to any bulk-forming laxative.
- You have symptoms of appendicitis, inflamed bowel or intestinal blockage.
- You have missed a bowel movement for only 1 or 2 days.

**Before you start, consult your doctor:**
- If you have diabetes.
- If you have kidney disease.
- If you have a laxative habit.
- If you have rectal bleeding.
- If you have difficulty swallowing.
- If you take other laxatives.

**Over age 60:**
Adverse reactions and side effects may be more frequent and severe than in younger persons.

**Pregnancy:**
Most bulk-forming laxatives contain sodium or sugars which may cause fluid retention. Avoid if possible.

**Breast-feeding:**
No problems expected.

**Infants & children:**
Use only under medical supervision.

**Prolonged use:**
Don't take for more than 1 week unless under a doctor's supervision. May cause laxative dependence.

**Skin & sunlight:**
No problems expected.

**Driving, piloting or hazardous work:**
No problems expected.

**Discontinuing:**
May be unnecessary to finish medicine. Follow doctor's instructions.

**Others:**
Don't take to "flush out" your system, or as a "tonic."

 ## POSSIBLE INTERACTION WITH OTHER DRUGS

| GENERIC NAME OR DRUG CLASS | COMBINED EFFECT |
|---|---|
| Antibiotics | Decreased antibiotic effect. |
| Anticoagulants | Decreased anticoagulant effect. |
| Digitalis preparations | Decreased digitalis effect. |
| Salicylates (including aspirin) | Decreased salicylate effect. |

 ## POSSIBLE INTERACTION WITH OTHER SUBSTANCES

| INTERACTS WITH | COMBINED EFFECT |
|---|---|
| Alcohol: | None expected. |
| Beverages: | None expected. |
| Cocaine: | None expected. |
| Foods: | None expected. |
| Marijuana: | None expected. |
| Tobacco: | None expected. |

# PYRIDOSTIGMINE

## BRAND NAMES

Mestinon             Regonol
Mestinon Timespans

## BASIC INFORMATION

Habit forming? No
Prescription needed? Yes
Available as generic? Yes
Drug class: Cholinergic (anticholinesterase)

 ## USES

- Treatment of myasthenia gravis.
- Treatment of urinary retention and abdominal distention.
- Antidote to adverse effects of muscle relaxants used in surgery.

 ## DOSAGE & USAGE INFORMATION

**How to take:**
- Tablet or syrup—Swallow with liquid or food to lessen stomach irritation.
- Extended-release tablets or capsules—Swallow each dose whole. If you take regular tablets, you may chew or crush them.

**When to take:**
As directed, usually 3 or 4 times a day.

**If you forget a dose:**
Take as soon as you remember up to 2 hours late. If more than 2 hours, wait for next scheduled dose (don't double this dose).

*Continued next column*

 ## OVERDOSE

**SYMPTOMS:**
Muscle weakness, cramps, twitching or clumsiness; severe diarrhea, nausea, vomiting, stomach cramps or pain; breathing difficulty; confusion, irritability, nervousness, restlessness, fear; unusually slow heartbeat; seizures.
**WHAT TO DO:**
- Dial 0 (operator) or 911 (emergency) for an ambulance or medical help. Then give first aid immediately.
- See emergency information on inside covers.

**What drug does:**
Inhibits the chemical activity of an enzyme (cholinesterase) so nerve impulses can cross the junction of nerves and muscles.

**Time lapse before drug works:**
3 hours.

**Don't take with:**
See Interaction column and consult doctor.

 ## POSSIBLE ADVERSE REACTIONS OR SIDE EFFECTS

| SYMPTOMS | WHAT TO DO |
|---|---|
| **Life-threatening:** | |
| None expected. | |
| **Common:** | |
| • Mild diarrhea, nausea, vomiting, stomach cramps or pain. | Discontinue. Call doctor right away. |
| • Excess saliva, unusual sweating. | Continue. Call doctor when convenient. |
| **Infrequent:** | |
| • Confusion, irritability. | Discontinue. Seek emergency treatment. |
| • Constricted pupils, watery eyes, lung congestion, frequent urge to urinate. | Continue. Call doctor when convenient. |
| **Rare:** | |
| None expected. | |

## WARNINGS & PRECAUTIONS

**Don't take if:**
- You are allergic to any cholinergic or bromide.
- You take mecamylamine.

**Before you start, consult your doctor:**
- If you plan to become pregnant within medication period.
- If you have bronchial asthma.
- If you have heartbeat irregularities.
- If you have urinary obstruction or urinary-tract infection.

**Over age 60:**
Adverse reactions and side effects may be more frequent and severe than in younger persons.

**Pregnancy:**
No proven harm to unborn child. Avoid if possible. May increase uterus contractions close to delivery.

**Breast-feeding:**
No problems expected, but consult doctor.

**Infants & children:**
Not recommended.

**Prolonged use:**
Medication may lose effectiveness. Discontinuing for a few days may restore effect.

**Skin & sunlight:**
No problems expected.

**Driving, piloting or hazardous work:**
Don't drive or pilot aircraft until you learn how medicine affects you. Don't work around dangerous machinery. Don't climb ladders or work in high places. Danger increases if you drink alcohol or take medicine affecting alertness and reflexes, such as antihistamines, tranquilizers, sedatives, pain medicine, narcotics and mind-altering drugs.

**Discontinuing:**
Don't discontinue without doctor's advice until you complete prescribed dose, even though symptoms diminish or disappear.

**Others:**
No problems expected.

## POSSIBLE INTERACTION WITH OTHER DRUGS

| GENERIC NAME OR DRUG CLASS | COMBINED EFFECT |
|---|---|
| Anesthetics (local or general) | Decreased pyridostigmine effect. |
| Antiarrhythmics | Decreased pyridostigmine effect. |
| Antibiotics | Decreased pyridostigmine effect. |
| Anticholinergics | Decreased pyridostigmine effect. May mask severe side effects. |
| Cholinergics (other) | Reduced intestinal-tract function. Possible brain and nervous-system toxicity. |
| Mecamylamine | Decreased pyridostigmine effect. |
| Nitrates | Decreased pyridostigmine effect. |
| Quinidine | Decreased pyridostigmine effect. |

## POSSIBLE INTERACTION WITH OTHER SUBSTANCES

| INTERACTS WITH | COMBINED EFFECT |
|---|---|
| Alcohol: | No proven problems with small doses. |
| Beverages: | None expected. |
| Cocaine: | Decreased pyridostigmine effect. Avoid. |
| Foods: | None expected. |
| Marijuana: | No proven problems. |
| Tobacco: | No proven problems. |

# PYRIDOXINE (VITAMIN B-6)

## BRAND NAMES

| | |
|---|---|
| Alba-Lybe | Hexa-Betalin |
| Al-Vite | Hexacrest |
| Beelith | Hexavibex |
| Beesix | Mega-B |
| Bendectin | Nu-Iron-V |
| Eldertonic | Pyroxine |
| Glutofac | Rodex |
| Hemo-vite | Tex Six T.R. |
| Herpecin-L | Vicon |

## BASIC INFORMATION

**Habit forming? No**
**Prescription needed?**
  **High strength: Yes**
  **Low strength: No**
**Available as generic? Yes**
**Drug class: Vitamin supplement**

## USES

- Prevention and treatment of pyridoxine deficiency.
- Treatment of some forms of anemia.

## DOSAGE & USAGE INFORMATION

**How to take:**
- Tablets—Swallow with liquid.
- Extended-release tablets—Swallow each dose whole with liquid.

**When to take:**
At the same times each day.

**If you forget a dose:**
Take as soon as you remember, then resume regular schedule.

**What drug does:**
Acts as co-enzyme in carbohydrate, protein and fat metabolism.

**Time lapse before drug works:**
15 to 20 minutes.

**Don't take with:**
- Levodopa—Small amounts of pyridoxine will nullify levodopa effect. Carbidopa-levodopa combination not affected by this interaction.
- See Interaction column and consult doctor.

## OVERDOSE

**SYMPTOMS:**
**None expected.**
**WHAT TO DO:**
**Overdose unlikely to threaten life.**

## POSSIBLE ADVERSE REACTIONS OR SIDE EFFECTS

| SYMPTOMS | WHAT TO DO |
|---|---|

**Life-threatening:**
None expected.

**Common:**
None expected.

**Infrequent:**
None expected.

**Rare:**
None expected.

## WARNINGS & PRECAUTIONS

**Don't take if:**
You are allergic to pyridoxine.

**Before you start, consult your doctor:**
If you are pregnant or breast-feeding.

**Over age 60:**
No problems expected.

**Pregnancy:**
Don't exceed recommended dose.

**Breast-feeding:**
Don't exceed recommended dose.

**Infants & children:**
Don't exceed recommended dose.

**Prolonged use:**
Large doses for more than 1 month may cause toxicity.

**Skin & sunlight:**
No problems expected.

**Driving, piloting or hazardous work:**
No problems expected.

**Discontinuing:**
No problems expected.

**Others:**
Regular pyridoxine supplements recommended if you take chloramphenicol, cycloserine, ethionamide, hydralazine, immunosuppressants, isoniazid or penicillamine. These decrease pyridoxine absorption and can cause anemia or tingling and numbness in hands and feet.

## POSSIBLE INTERACTION WITH OTHER DRUGS

| GENERIC NAME OR DRUG CLASS | COMBINED EFFECT |
|---|---|
| Chloramphenicol | Decreased pyridoxine effect. |
| Contraceptives (oral) | Decreased pyridoxine effect. |
| Cycloserine | Decreased pyridoxine effect. |
| Ethionamide | Decreased pyridoxine effect. |
| Hydralazine | Decreased pyridoxine effect. |
| Hypnotics (barbiturates) | Decreased hypnotic effect. |
| Immunosuppressants | Decreased pyridoxine effect. |
| Isoniazid | Decreased pyridoxine effect. |
| Levodopa | Decreased levodopa effect. |
| Penicillamine | Decreased pyridoxine effect. |
| Phenytoin | Decreased phenytoin effect. |

## POSSIBLE INTERACTION WITH OTHER SUBSTANCES

| INTERACTS WITH | COMBINED EFFECT |
|---|---|
| Alcohol: | None expected. |
| Beverages: | None expected. |
| Cocaine: | None expected. |
| Foods: | None expected. |
| Marijuana: | None expected. |
| Tobacco: | May decrease pyridoxine absorption. Decreased pyridoxine effect. |

# PYRILAMINE

## BRAND NAMES

See complete list of brand names in the *Brand Name Directory,* page 956.

## BASIC INFORMATION

**Habit forming? No**
**Prescription needed? No**
**Available as generic? Yes**
**Drug class: Antihistamine**

## USES

- Reduces allergic symptoms such as hay fever, hives, rash or itching.
- Prevents motion sickness, nausea, vomiting.
- Induces sleep.

## DOSAGE & USAGE INFORMATION

**How to take:**
Tablet or capsule—Swallow with liquid or food to lessen stomach irritation.

**When to take:**
Varies with form. Follow label directions.

**If you forget a dose:**
Take as soon as you remember up to 2 hours late. If more than 2 hours, wait for next scheduled dose (don't double this dose).

**What drug does:**
Blocks action of histamine after an allergic response triggers histamine release in sensitive cells.

*Continued next column*

## OVERDOSE

**SYMPTOMS:**
Convulsions, red face, hallucinations, coma.
**WHAT TO DO:**
- **Dial 0 (operator) or 911 (emergency) for an ambulance or medical help. Then give first aid immediately.**
- **If patient is unconscious and not breathing, give mouth-to-mouth breathing. If there is no heartbeat, use cardiac massage and mouth-to-mouth breathing (CPR). Don't try to make patient vomit. If you can't get help quickly, take patient to nearest emergency facility.**
- **See emergency information on inside covers.**

**Time lapse before drug works:**
30 minutes.

**Don't take with:**
See Interaction column and consult doctor.

## POSSIBLE ADVERSE REACTIONS OR SIDE EFFECTS

| SYMPTOMS | WHAT TO DO |
|---|---|
| **Life-threatening:** None expected. | |
| **Common:** Drowsiness; dizziness; dry mouth, nose and throat; nausea. | Continue. Tell doctor at next visit. |
| **Infrequent:** | |
| • Change in vision. | Discontinue. Call doctor right away. |
| • Less tolerance for contact lenses, urination difficulty. | Continue. Call doctor when convenient. |
| • Appetite loss. | Continue. Tell doctor at next visit. |
| **Rare:** Nightmares, agitation, irritability, sore throat, fever, rapid heartbeat, unusual bleeding or bruising, fatigue, weakness. | Discontinue. Call doctor right away. |

## WARNINGS & PRECAUTIONS

**Don't take if:**
You are allergic to any antihistamine.

**Before you start, consult your doctor:**
- If you have glaucoma.
- If you have enlarged prostate.
- If you have asthma.
- If you have kidney disease.
- If you have peptic ulcer.
- If you will have surgery within 2 months, including dental surgery, requiring general or spinal anesthesia.

**Over age 60:**
Don't exceed recommended dose. Adverse reactions and side effects may be more frequent and severe than in younger persons, especially urination difficulty, diminished alertness and other brain and nervous-system symptoms.

**Pregnancy:**
No proven harm to unborn child. Avoid if possible.

**Breast-feeding:**
Drug passes into milk. Avoid drug or discontinue nursing until you finish medicine. Consult doctor for advice on maintaining milk supply.

**Infants & children:**
Not recommended for premature or newborn infants. Otherwise, no problems expected.

**Prolonged use:**
Avoid. May damage bone marrow and nerve cells.

**Skin & sunlight:**
May cause rash or intensify sunburn in areas exposed to sun or sunlamp.

**Driving, piloting or hazardous work:**
Don't drive or pilot aircraft until you learn how medicine affects you. Don't work around dangerous machinery. Don't climb ladders or work in high places. Danger increases if you drink alcohol or take medicine affecting alertness and reflexes, such as antihistamines, tranquilizers, sedatives, pain medicine, narcotics and mind-altering drugs.

**Discontinuing:**
No problems expected.

**Others:**
May mask symptoms of hearing damage from aspirin, other salicylates, cisplatin, paromomycin, vancomycin or anticonvulsants. Consult doctor if you use these.

## POSSIBLE INTERACTION WITH OTHER DRUGS

| GENERIC NAME OR DRUG CLASS | COMBINED EFFECT |
| --- | --- |
| Anticholinergics | Increased anticholinergic effect. |
| Antidepressants (tricyclic) | Increased pyrilamine effect. Excess sedation. |
| Antihistamines (other) | Excess sedation. Avoid. |
| Dronabinol | Increased effects of both drugs. Avoid. |
| Hypnotics | Excess sedation. Avoid. |
| MAO inhibitors | Increased pyrilamine effect. |
| Mind-altering drugs | Excess sedation. Avoid. |
| Molindone | Increased sedative and antihistamine effect. |
| Narcotics | Excess sedation. Avoid. |
| Sedatives | Excess sedation. Avoid. |
| Sleep inducers | Excess sedation. Avoid. |
| Tranquilizers | Excess sedation. Avoid. |

## POSSIBLE INTERACTION WITH OTHER SUBSTANCES

| INTERACTS WITH | COMBINED EFFECT |
| --- | --- |
| Alcohol: | Excess sedation. Avoid. |
| Beverages: Caffeine drinks. | Less pyrilamine sedation. |
| Cocaine: | Decreased pyrilamine effect. Avoid. |
| Foods: | None expected. |
| Marijuana: | Excess sedation. Avoid. |
| Tobacco: | None expected. |

# PYRILAMINE & PENTOBARBITAL

## BRAND NAMES

Wans

## BASIC INFORMATION

Habit forming? Yes
Prescription needed? Yes
Available as generic? No
Drug class: Antihistamine, sedative
(barbiturate)

 ## USES

- Prevents and relieves motion sickness, nausea, vomiting.
- Induces sleep.

 ## DOSAGE & USAGE INFORMATION

**How to take:**
Suppositories—Remove wrapper and moisten suppository with water. Gently insert larger end into rectum. Push well into rectum with finger.

**When to take:**
As directed when needed.

**If you forget a dose:**
Take as soon as you remember up to 2 hours late. If more than 2 hours, wait for next scheduled dose (don't double this dose).

*Continued next column*

 ## OVERDOSE

**SYMPTOMS:**
Deep sleep, weak pulse, convulsions, red face, hallucinations, coma.
**WHAT TO DO:**
- Dial 0 (operator) or 911 (emergency) for an ambulance or medical help. Then give first aid immediately.
- If patient is unconscious and not breathing, give mouth-to-mouth breathing. If there is no heartbeat, use cardiac massage and mouth-to-mouth breathing (CPR). Don't try to make patient vomit. If you can't get help quickly, take patient to nearest emergency facility.
- See emergency information on inside covers.

**What drug does:**
- May partially block nerve impulses at nerve-cell connections in nausea center of brain.
- Blocks action of histamine after an allergic response triggers histamine release in sensitive cells.

**Time lapse before drug works:**
30 minutes.

**Don't take with:**
- Non-prescription drugs without consulting doctor.
- See Interaction column and consult doctor.

 ## POSSIBLE ADVERSE REACTIONS OR SIDE EFFECTS

| SYMPTOMS | WHAT TO DO |
|---|---|
| **Life-threatening:** | |
| Slow or fast heartbeat, difficult breathing. | Discontinue. Seek emergency treatment. |
| **Common:** | |
| • Drowsiness, agitation. | Discontinue. Call doctor right away. |
| • Dizziness, "hangover" effect, dry mouth. | Continue. Call doctor when convenient. |
| **Infrequent:** | |
| • Rash; swelling of face, lip or eyelid; change in vision; nausea; vomiting; diarrhea; appetite loss. | Discontinue. Call doctor right away. |
| • Less tolerance for contact lens, joint or muscle pain, frequent urination. | Continue. Call doctor when convenient. |
| **Rare:** | |
| Sore throat, fever, mouth sores; urgent urination; jaundice. | Discontinue. Call doctor right away. |

 ## WARNINGS & PRECAUTIONS

**Don't take if:**
- You are allergic to any antihistamine or barbiturate.
- You have porphyria.

**Before you start, consult your doctor:**
- If you have glaucoma, enlarged prostate, peptic ulcer, epilepsy, kidney or liver damage, asthma, anemia, chronic pain.
- If you will have surgery within 2 months, including dental surgery, requiring general or spinal anesthesia.

**Over age 60:**
Don't exceed recommended dose. Adverse reactions and side effects may be more frequent and severe than in younger persons, especially urination difficulty, diminished alertness and other brain and nervous-system symptoms.

**Pregnancy:**
Risk to unborn child outweighs drug benefits. Don't use.

**Breast-feeding:**
Drug passes into milk. Avoid drug or discontinue nursing until you finish medicine. Consult doctor for advice on maintaining milk supply.

**Infants & children:**
Not recommended for premature or newborn infants. Use only under doctor's supervision.

**Prolonged use:**
- May damage bone marrow and nerve cells. Avoid.
- May cause addiction, anemia, chronic intoxication.
- May lower body temperature, making exposure to cold temperatures hazardous.

**Skin & sunlight:**
May cause rash or intensify sunburn in areas exposed to sun or sunlamp.

**Driving, piloting or hazardous work:**
Don't drive or pilot aircraft until you learn how medicine affects you. Don't work around dangerous machinery. Don't climb ladders or work in high places. Danger increases if you drink alcohol or take medicine affecting alertness and reflexes, such as antihistamines, tranquilizers, sedatives, pain medicine, narcotics and mind-altering drugs.

**Discontinuing:**
- May be unnecessary to finish medicine. Follow doctor's instructions.
- If you develop withdrawal symptoms of hallucinations, agitation or sleeplessness after discontinuing, call doctor right away.

**Others:**
- May mask symptoms of hearing damage from aspirin, other salicylates, cisplatin, paromomycin, vancomycin or anticonvulsants. Consult your doctor if you use these.
- Great potential for abuse.

## POSSIBLE INTERACTION WITH OTHER DRUGS

| GENERIC NAME OR DRUG CLASS | COMBINED EFFECT |
|---|---|
| Anticholinergics | Increased anticholinergics effect. |
| Anticoagulants | Decreased anticoagulant effect. |
| Anticonvulsants | Changed seizure patterns. |
| Antidepressants (tricyclics) | Possible dangerous oversedation. Increased pyrilamine effect. |
| Antidiabetics | Increased pentobarbital effect. |
| Antihistamines | Dangerous sedation. Avoid. |
| Anti-inflammatory drugs (non-steroidal) | Decreased anti-inflammatory effect. |
| Aspirin | Decreased aspirin effect. |
| Beta-adrenergic blockers | Decreased effect of beta-adrenergic blocker. |
| Contraceptives (oral) | Decreased contraceptive effect. |
| Cortisone drugs | Decreased cortisone effect. |
| Digitoxin | Decreased digitoxin effect. |
| Doxycycline | Decreased doxycycline effect. |
| Dronabinol | Increased effect of both drugs. |

*Continued page 974*

## POSSIBLE INTERACTION WITH OTHER SUBSTANCES

| INTERACTS WITH | COMBINED EFFECT |
|---|---|
| Alcohol: | Possible fatal oversedation. Avoid. |
| Beverages: Caffeine drinks. | Less pyrilamine sedation. |
| Cocaine: | Decreased Wans effect. Avoid. |
| Foods: | None expected. |
| Marijuana: | Excessive sedation. Avoid. |
| Tobacco: | None expected. |

# PYRVINIUM

## BRAND NAMES

Pamovin      Vanquin
Povan        Viprynium
Pyr-pam

## BASIC INFORMATION

**Habit forming?** No
**Prescription needed?** Yes
**Available as generic?** No
**Drug class:** Antihelminthic (antiworm
            medication)

## USES

Treatment for pinworm infestation.

## DOSAGE & USAGE INFORMATION

**How to take:**
* Tablet—Swallow whole with food or liquid.
  Don't crush or chew tablet.
* Liquid—Take with food or liquid.

**When to take:**
According to label instructions. Usually a single
dose, which may be repeated in 2 or 3 weeks.

**If you forget a dose:**
Take when remembered.

**What drug does:**
Interferes with a metabolic process in the
infecting parasite and kills it.

**Time lapse before drug works:**
12 hours.

**Don't take with:**
Non-prescription drugs for pinworms.

## OVERDOSE

**SYMPTOMS:**
**Increased severity of adverse reactions and
side effects.**
**WHAT TO DO:**
**Overdose unlikely to threaten life. If person
takes much larger amount than prescribed,
call doctor, poison-control center or hospital
emergency room for instructions.**

## POSSIBLE ADVERSE REACTIONS OR SIDE EFFECTS

| SYMPTOMS | WHAT TO DO |
|---|---|
| **Life-threatening:** None expected. | |
| **Common:** None expected. | |
| **Infrequent:** None expected. | |
| **Rare:** | |
| • Rash. | Discontinue. Call doctor right away. |
| • Dizziness, stomach cramps, nausea, vomiting. | Continue. Call doctor when convenient. |

## WARNINGS & PRECAUTIONS

**Don't take if:**
You are allergic to any antihelminthic drug.

**Before you start, consult your doctor:**
- If you have kidney or liver disease.
- If you have a bowel disease or inflammation.

**Over age 60:**
Adverse reactions and side effects may be more frequent and severe than in younger persons.

**Pregnancy:**
No proven harm to unborn child. Avoid if possible.

**Breast-feeding:**
No problems expected, but consult doctor.

**Infants & children:**
No problems expected.

**Prolonged use:**
Not recommended.

**Skin & sunlight:**
May cause rash or intensify sunburn in areas exposed to sun or sunlamp.

**Driving, piloting or hazardous work:**
Avoid if you feel dizzy. Otherwise, no problems expected.

**Discontinuing:**
Don't discontinue without doctor's advice until you complete prescribed dose, even though symptoms diminish or disappear.

**Others:**
- This medicine is a dye that permanently stains most materials. Teeth will be stained a few days. Stool and vomit may be red.
- Pinworm infestations are highly contagious. All family members should be treated at the same time.

 ## POSSIBLE INTERACTION WITH OTHER DRUGS

| GENERIC NAME OR DRUG CLASS | COMBINED EFFECT |
|---|---|
| None | |

 ## POSSIBLE INTERACTION WITH OTHER SUBSTANCES

| INTERACTS WITH | COMBINED EFFECT |
|---|---|
| Alcohol: | None expected. |
| Beverages: | None expected. |
| Cocaine: | None expected. |
| Foods: | None expected. |
| Marijuana: | None expected. |
| Tobacco: | None expected. |

# QUINESTROL

## BRAND NAMES

Estrovis

## BASIC INFORMATION

**Habit forming?** No
**Prescription needed?** Yes
**Available as generic?** Yes
**Drug class:** Female sex hormone (estrogen)

## USES

- Treatment for symptoms of menopause and menstrual-cycle irregularity.
- Replacement for female hormone deficiency.

## DOSAGE & USAGE INFORMATION

**How to take:**
Tablet—Swallow with liquid. If you can't swallow whole, crumble tablet and take with liquid or food.

**When to take:**
At the same time each day.

**If you forget a dose:**
Take as soon as you remember up to 12 hours late. If more than 12 hours, wait for next scheduled dose (don't double this dose).

**What drug does:**
Restores normal estrogen level in tissues.

**Time lapse before drug works:**
10 to 20 days.

**Don't take with:**
See Interaction column and consult doctor.

## OVERDOSE

**SYMPTOMS:**
**Nausea, vomiting, fluid retention, breast enlargement and discomfort, abnormal vaginal bleeding.**
**WHAT TO DO:**
**Overdose unlikely to threaten life. If person takes much larger amount than prescribed, call doctor, poison-control center or hospital emergency room for instructions.**

## POSSIBLE ADVERSE REACTIONS OR SIDE EFFECTS

| SYMPTOMS | WHAT TO DO |
|---|---|
| **Life-threatening:** | |
| None expected. | |
| **Common:** | |
| ● Stomach cramps. | Discontinue. Call doctor right away. |
| ● Appetite loss. | Continue. Call doctor when convenient. |
| ● Nausea; diarrhea; swollen ankles, feet; swollen, tender breasts. | Continue. Tell doctor at next visit. |
| **Infrequent:** | |
| ● Rash, stomach or side pain. | Discontinue. Call doctor right away. |
| ● Depression, dizziness, irritability, vomiting, breast lumps. | Continue. Call doctor when convenient. |
| ● Brown blotches, hair loss, vaginal discharge or bleeding, changes in sex drive. | Continue. Tell doctor at next visit. |
| **Rare:** | |
| Jaundice. | Discontinue. Call doctor right away. |

## WARNINGS & PRECAUTIONS

**Don't take if:**
- You are allergic to any estrogen-containing drugs.
- You have impaired liver function.
- You have had blood clots, stroke or heart attack.
- You have unexplained vaginal bleeding.

**Before you start, consult your doctor:**
- If you have had cancer of breast or reproductive organs, fibrocystic breast disease, fibroid tumors of the uterus or endometriosis.
- If you have had migraine headaches, epilepsy or porphyria.
- If you have diabetes, high blood pressure, asthma, congestive heart failure, kidney disease or gallstones.
- If you plan to become pregnant within 3 months.

**Over age 60:**
Controversial. You and your doctor must decide if drug risks outweigh benefits.

**Pregnancy:**
Risk to unborn child outweighs drug benefits. Don't use.

**Breast-feeding:**
Drug filters into milk. May harm child. Avoid.

**Infants & children:**
Not recommended.

**Prolonged use:**
Increased growth of fibroid tumors of uterus. Possible association with cancer of uterus.

**Skin & sunlight:**
May cause rash or intensify sunburn in areas exposed to sun or sunlamp.

**Driving, piloting or hazardous work:**
No problems expected.

**Discontinuing:**
You may need to discontinue quinestrol periodically. Consult your doctor.

**Others:**
In rare instances, may cause blood clot in lung, brain or leg. Symptoms are *sudden* severe headache, coordination loss, vision change, chest pain, breathing difficulty, slurred speech, pain in legs or groin. Seek emergency treatment immediately.

## POSSIBLE INTERACTION WITH OTHER DRUGS

| GENERIC NAME OR DRUG CLASS | COMBINED EFFECT |
|---|---|
| Anticoagulants (oral) | Decreased anticoagulant effect. |
| Anticonvulsants (hydantoin) | Increased seizures. |
| Antidiabetics (oral) | Unpredictable increase or decrease in blood sugar. |
| Carbamazepine | Increased seizures. |
| Clofibrate | Decreased clofibrate effect. |
| Meprobamate | Increased quinestrol effect. |
| Phenobarbital | Decreased quinestrol effect. |
| Primidone | Decreased quinestrol effect. |
| Rifampin | Decreased quinestrol effect. |
| Thyroid hormones | Decreased thyroid effect. |

## POSSIBLE INTERACTION WITH OTHER SUBSTANCES

| INTERACTS WITH | COMBINED EFFECT |
|---|---|
| Alcohol: | None expected. |
| Beverages: | None expected. |
| Cocaine: | No proven problems. |
| Foods: | None expected. |
| Marijuana: | Possible menstrual irregularities and bleeding between periods. |
| Tobacco: | Increased risk of blood clots leading to stroke or heart attack. |

# QUINETHAZONE

## BRAND NAMES

**Aquamox**          **Hydromox**

## BASIC INFORMATION

**Habit forming?** No
**Prescription needed?** Yes
**Available as generic?** Yes
**Drug class:** Antihypertensive, diuretic
(thiazide)

## USES

- Controls, but doesn't cure, high blood pressure.
- Reduces fluid retention (edema) caused by conditions such as heart disorders and liver disease.

## DOSAGE & USAGE INFORMATION

**How to take:**
Tablet or capsule—Swallow with liquid. If you can't swallow whole, crumble tablet or open capsule and take with liquid or food. Don't exceed dose.

**When to take:**
At the same time each day.

**If you forget a dose:**
Take as soon as you remember up to 2 hours late. If more than 2 hours, wait for next scheduled dose (don't double this dose).

**What drug does:**
- Forces sodium and water excretion, reducing body fluid.
- Relaxes muscle cells of small arteries.
- Reduced body fluid and relaxed arteries lower blood pressure.

*Continued next column*

## OVERDOSE

**SYMPTOMS:**
**Cramps, weakness, drowsiness, weak pulse, coma.**
**WHAT TO DO:**
- **Dial 0 (operator) or 911 (emergency) for an ambulance or medical help. Then give first aid immediately.**
- **See emergency information on inside covers.**

**Time lapse before drug works:**
4 to 6 hours. May require several weeks to lower blood pressure.

**Don't take with:**
- See Interaction column and consult doctor.
- Non-prescription drugs without consulting doctor.

## POSSIBLE ADVERSE REACTIONS OR SIDE EFFECTS

| SYMPTOMS | WHAT TO DO |
|---|---|
| **Life-threatening:**<br>None expected. | |
| **Common:**<br>None expected. | |
| **Infrequent:** | |
| • Blurred vision, severe abdominal pain, nausea, vomiting, irregular heartbeat, weak pulse. | Discontinue. Call doctor right away. |
| • Dizziness, mood change, headache, weakness, tiredness, weight changes. | Continue. Call doctor when convenient. |
| • Dry mouth, thirst. | Continue. Tell doctor at next visit. |
| **Rare:** | |
| • Rash or hives. | Discontinue. Seek emergency treatment. |
| • Sore throat, fever, jaundice. | Discontinue. Call doctor right away. |

## WARNINGS & PRECAUTIONS

**Don't take if:**
You are allergic to any thiazide diuretic drug.

**Before you start, consult your doctor:**
- If you are allergic to any sulfa drug.
- If you have gout.
- If you have liver, pancreas or liver disorder.

**Over age 60:**
Adverse reactions and side effects may be more frequent and severe than in younger persons, especially dizziness and excessive potassium loss.

**Pregnancy:**
Risk to unborn child outweighs drug benefits. Don't use.

**Breast-feeding:**
Drug passes into milk. Avoid drug or discontinue nursing.

**Infants & children:**
No problems expected.

**Prolonged use:**
You may need medicine to treat high blood pressure for the rest of your life.

**Skin & sunlight:**
May cause rash or intensify sunburn in areas exposed to sun or sunlamp.

**Driving, piloting or hazardous work:**
Don't drive or pilot aircraft until you learn how medicine affects you. Don't work around dangerous machinery. Don't climb ladders or work in high places. Danger increases if you drink alcohol or take medicine affecting alertness and reflexes, such as antihistamines, tranquilizers, sedatives, pain medicine, narcotics and mind-altering drugs.

**Discontinuing:**
Don't discontinue without medical advice.

**Others:**
- Hot weather and fever may cause dehydration and drop in blood pressure. Dose may require temporary adjustment. Weigh daily and report any unexpected weight decreases to your doctor.
- May cause rise in uric acid, leading to gout.
- May cause blood-sugar rise in diabetics.

 **POSSIBLE INTERACTION WITH OTHER DRUGS**

| GENERIC NAME OR DRUG CLASS | COMBINED EFFECT |
|---|---|
| Acebutolol | Increased antihypertensive effect. Dosages of both drugs may require adjustments. |
| Allopurinol | Decreased allopurinol effect. |
| Amiodarone | Increased risk of heartbeat irregularity due to low potassium. |
| Antidepressants (tricyclic) | Dangerous drop in blood pressure. Avoid combination unless under medical supervision. |
| Barbiturates | Increased quinethazone effect. |
| Calcium supplements | Increased calcium in blood. |
| Cholestyramine | Decreased quinethazone effect. |

| | |
|---|---|
| Cortisone drugs | Excessive potassium loss that causes dangerous heart rhythms. |
| Digitalis preparations | Excessive potassium loss that causes dangerous heart rhythms. |
| Diuretics (thiazide) | Increased effect of other thiazide diuretics. |
| Enalapril | Possible excessive potassium in blood. |
| Indapamide | Increased diuretic effect. |
| Labetolol | Increased antihypertensive effects. |
| Lithium | Increased effect of lithium. |
| MAO inhibitors | Increased quinethazone effect. |
| Nitrates | Excessive blood-pressure drop. |
| Oxprenolol | Increased antihypertensive effect. Dosages of both drugs may require adjustments. |
| Potassium supplements | Decreased potassium effect. |
| Probenecid | Decreased probenecid effect. |

 **POSSIBLE INTERACTION WITH OTHER SUBSTANCES**

| INTERACTS WITH | COMBINED EFFECT |
|---|---|
| Alcohol: | Dangerous blood-pressure drop. |
| Beverages: | None expected. |
| Cocaine: | None expected. |
| Foods: Licorice. | Excessive potassium loss that causes dangerous heart rhythms. |
| Marijuana: | May increase blood pressure. |
| Tobacco: | None expected. |

# QUINIDINE

## BRAND NAMES

| | |
|---|---|
| Apo-Quinidine | Quinalan |
| Biquin Durules | Quinate |
| Cardioquin | Quinidex Extentabs |
| Cin-Quin | Quinobarb |
| Duraquin | Quinora |
| Novoquinidin | SK-Quinidine Sulfate |
| Quinaglute Dura-Tabs | |

## BASIC INFORMATION

Habit forming? No
Prescription needed?
 U.S.: Yes
  Canada: No
Available as generic? Yes
Drug class: Antiarrhythmic

 USES

Corrects heart-rhythm disorders.

 DOSAGE & USAGE INFORMATION

How to take:
- Tablet or capsule—Swallow with liquid or food to lessen stomach irritation.
- Extended-release tablets or capsules—Swallow each dose whole. If you take regular tablets, you may chew or crush them.

When to take:
At the same times each day.

If you forget a dose:
Take as soon as you remember up to 2 hours late. If more than 2 hours, wait for next scheduled dose (don't double this dose).

*Continued next column*

 OVERDOSE

SYMPTOMS:
Confusion, severe blood-pressure drop, breathing difficulty, fainting.
WHAT TO DO:
- Dial 0 (operator) or 911 (emergency) for an ambulance or medical help. Then give first aid immediately.
- If patient is unconscious and not breathing, give mouth-to-mouth breathing. If there is no heartbeat, use cardiac massage and mouth-to-mouth breathing (CPR). Don't try to make patient vomit. If you can't get help quickly, take patient to nearest emergency facility.
- See emergency information on inside covers.

What drug does:
Delays nerve impulses to the heart to regulate heartbeat.

Time lapse before drug works:
2 to 4 hours.

Don't take with:
See Interaction column and consult doctor.

 POSSIBLE ADVERSE REACTIONS OR SIDE EFFECTS

| SYMPTOMS | WHAT TO DO |
|---|---|
| **Life-threatening:** None expected. | |
| **Common:** Bitter taste, diarrhea, nausea, vomiting. | Discontinue. Call doctor right away. |
| **Infrequent:** • Dizziness, lightheadedness, fainting, headache, confusion, rash, change in vision, difficult breathing, rapid heartbeat. | Discontinue. Call doctor right away. |
| • Ringing in ears. | Continue. Call doctor when convenient. |
| **Rare:** • Unusual bleeding or bruising. | Discontinue. Call doctor right away. |
| • Weakness. | Continue. Call doctor when convenient. |

## WARNINGS & PRECAUTIONS

**Don't take if:**
- You are allergic to quinidine.
- You have an active infection.

**Before you start, consult your doctor:**
About any drug you take, including non-prescription drugs.

**Over age 60:**
Adverse reactions and side effects may be more frequent and severe than in younger persons.

**Pregnancy:**
Risk to unborn child outweighs drug benefits. Don't use.

**Breast-feeding:**
Drug filters into milk. May harm child. Avoid.

**Infants & children:**
No problems expected.

**Prolonged use:**
No problems expected.

**Skin & sunlight:**
No problems expected.

**Driving, piloting or hazardous work:**
Don't drive or pilot aircraft until you learn how medicine affects you. Don't work around dangerous machinery. Don't climb ladders or work in high places. Danger increases if you drink alcohol or take medicine affecting alertness and reflexes, such as antihistamines, tranquilizers, sedatives, pain medicine, narcotics and mind-altering drugs.

**Discontinuing:**
Don't discontinue without doctor's advice until you complete prescribed dose, even though symptoms diminish or disappear.

**Others:**
No problems expected.

## POSSIBLE INTERACTION WITH OTHER DRUGS

| GENERIC NAME OR DRUG CLASS | COMBINED EFFECT |
|---|---|
| Anticholinergics | Increased anticholinergic effect. |
| Anticoagulants | Increased anticoagulant effect. |
| Antidepressants (tricyclic) | Irregular heartbeat. |
| Antihypertensives | Increased antihypertensive effect. |
| Calcium supplements | Increased quinidine effect. |
| Cholinergics | Decreased cholinergic effect. |
| Citrates | Prolongs citrate effect. |
| Digitalis preparations | Slows heartbeat excessively. |
| Flecainide | Possible irregular heartbeat. |
| Molindone | Impaired heart function. Dangerous mixture. |
| Phenytoin | Increased quinidine effect. |
| Propranolol | Slows heartbeat excessively. |
| Pyrimethamine | Increased quinidine effect. |
| Rauwolfia alkaloids | Seriously disturbs heart rhythms. |
| Tocainide | Increased possibility of adverse reactions from either drug. |

## POSSIBLE INTERACTION WITH OTHER SUBSTANCES

| INTERACTS WITH | COMBINED EFFECT |
|---|---|
| Alcohol: | None expected. |
| Beverages: Caffeine drinks. | Causes rapid heartbeat. Use sparingly. |
| Cocaine: | Irregular heartbeat. Avoid. |
| Foods: | None expected. |
| Marijuana: | Can cause fainting. |
| Tobacco: | Irregular heartbeat. Avoid. |

# QUININE

## BRAND NAMES

| | |
|---|---|
| Coco-Quinine | Quindan |
| Kinine | Quine |
| NovoQuinie | Quinite |
| Quinamm | Strema |

## BASIC INFORMATION

**Habit forming? No**
**Prescription needed?**
  **High strength: Yes**
  **Low strength: No**
**Available as generic? Yes**
**Drug class: Antiprotozoal**

## USES

- Treatment or prevention of malaria.
- Relief of muscle cramps.

## DOSAGE & USAGE INFORMATION

**How to take:**
Liquid, tablet or capsule—Swallow with liquid or food to lessen stomach irritation.

**When to take:**
- Prevention—At the same time each day, usually at bedtime.
- Treatment—At the same times each day in evenly spaced doses.

**If you forget a dose:**
- Prevention—Take as soon as you remember up to 12 hours late. If more than 12 hours, wait for next scheduled dose (don't double this dose).
- Treatment—Take as soon as you remember up to 2 hours late. If more than 2 hours, wait for next scheduled dose (don't double this dose).

*Continued next column*

## OVERDOSE

**SYMPTOMS:**
Severe impairment of vision and hearing; severe nausea, vomiting, diarrhea; shallow breathing, fast heartbeat; apprehension, confusion, delirium.
**WHAT TO DO:**
Dial 0 (operator) or 911 (emergency) for an ambulance or medical help. Then give first aid immediately.

**What drug does:**
- Reduces contractions of skeletal muscles.
- Increases blood flow.
- Interferes with genes in malaria micro-organisms.

**Time lapse before drug works:**
May require several days or weeks for maximum effect.

**Don't take with:**
See Interaction column and consult doctor.

## POSSIBLE ADVERSE REACTIONS OR SIDE EFFECTS

| SYMPTOMS | WHAT TO DO |
|---|---|
| **Life-threatening:** | |
| None expected. | |
| **Common:** | |
| • Blurred vision or change in vision. | Discontinue. Call doctor right away. |
| • Dizziness, headache, stomach discomfort, mild nausea, vomiting, diarrhea. | Continue. Call doctor when convenient. |
| • Ringing or buzzing in ears, impaired hearing. | Continue. Tell doctor at next visit. |
| **Infrequent:** | |
| Rash, hives, itchy skin, difficult breathing. | Discontinue. Call doctor right away. |
| **Rare:** | |
| Sore throat, fever, unusual bleeding or bruising, unusual tiredness or weakness. | Discontinue. Call doctor right away. |

# WARNINGS & PRECAUTIONS

**Don't take if:**
You are allergic to quinine or quinidine.

**Before you start, consult your doctor:**
- If you plan to become pregnant within medication period.
- If you have asthma.
- If you have eye disease, hearing problems or ringing in the ears.
- If you have heart disease.
- If you have myasthenia gravis.

**Over age 60:**
Adverse reactions and side effects may be more frequent and severe than in younger persons.

**Pregnancy:**
Risk to unborn child outweighs drug benefits. Don't use.

**Breast-feeding:**
Drug filters into milk. May harm child. Avoid.

**Infants & children:**
Use only under medical supervision.

**Prolonged use:**
May develop headache, blurred vision, nausea, temporary hearing loss, but seldom need to discontinue because of these symptoms.

**Skin & sunlight:**
No problems expected.

**Driving, piloting or hazardous work:**
Avoid if you feel dizzy or have blurred vision. Otherwise, no problems expected.

**Discontinuing:**
Don't discontinue without doctor's advice until you complete prescribed dose, even though symptoms diminish or disappear.

**Others:**
Don't confuse with quinidine, a medicine for heart-rhythm problems.

# POSSIBLE INTERACTION WITH OTHER DRUGS

| GENERIC NAME OR DRUG CLASS | COMBINED EFFECT |
| --- | --- |
| Antacids (with aluminum hydroxide) | Decreased quinine effect. |
| Anticoagulants | Increased anticoagulant effect. |
| Quinidine | Possible toxic effects of quinine. |
| Sodium bicarbonate | Possible toxic effects of quinine. |

# POSSIBLE INTERACTION WITH OTHER SUBSTANCES

| INTERACTS WITH | COMBINED EFFECT |
| --- | --- |
| Alcohol: | No proven problems. |
| Beverages: | None expected. |
| Cocaine: | No proven problems. |
| Foods: | None expected. |
| Marijuana: | No proven problems. |
| Tobacco: | None expected. |

# RADIO-PHARMACEUTICALS

## BRAND NAMES

See complete list of brand names in the *Brand Name Directory,* page 956.

## BASIC INFORMATION

**Habit forming? No**
**Prescription needed? Yes**
**Available as generic? Yes**
**Drug class: Radio-pharmaceuticals**

 USES

To help establish an accurate diagnosis for many medical problems, such as pernicious anemia, malabsorption, iron metabolism, cancer, abscess, infection, cerebrospinal fluid flow, blood volume, kidney diseases, lung diseases, pancreas diseases, red blood cell disorders, spleen diseases, thyroid diseases, thyroid cancer, brain diseases or tumor, bladder diseases, eye tumors, liver diseases, heart diseases, bone diseases, bone marrow diseases.

 DOSAGE & USAGE INFORMATION

**How to take:**
- As directed by nuclear medicine specialist. Most are given intravenously by the doctor, some are taken by mouth.
- Drink lots of liquids and urinate often after test to decrease possible radiation effect on the urinary bladder.

**When to take:**
According to individual instructions.

**If you forget a dose:**
Take as soon as you remember.

**What drug does:**
Very small quantities of radioactive substances concentrate in various organs of the body and become measurable. Pictures or readings of the organ or system under study become possible.

**Time lapse before drug works:**
Varies between products.

**Don't take with:**
Any other medicine without consulting doctor.

 OVERDOSE

**SYMPTOMS:**
**None expected.**
**WHAT TO DO:**
**None expected.**

 POSSIBLE ADVERSE REACTIONS OR SIDE EFFECTS

| SYMPTOMS | WHAT TO DO |
|---|---|
| **Life-threatening:**<br>None expected. | |
| **Common:**<br>None expected. | |
| **Infrequent:**<br>Drowsiness; fast heartbeat; swollen feet, ankles, hands or throat; abdominal pain; rash; hives; nausea; vomiting, headache; red or flushed face; fever; fainting. | Discontinue. Call doctor right away. |
| **Rare:**<br>None expected. | |

## WARNINGS & PRECAUTIONS

**Don't take if:**
You are allergic to the prescribed drug.

**Before you start, consult your doctor:**
- If you have had allergic reactions to human serum albumin.
- If you are allergic to anything.

**Over age 60:**
Adverse reactions and side effects may be more frequent and severe than in younger persons. Ask doctor about smaller doses.

**Pregnancy:**
Avoid during pregnancy if possible.

**Breast-feeding:**
Drug passes into milk. Avoid drug or discontinue nursing until you finish medicine. Consult doctor for advice on maintaining milk supply.

**Infants & children:**
No problems expected.

**Prolonged use:**
Not intended for prolonged use.

**Skin & sunlight:**
No problems expected.

**Driving, piloting or hazardous work:**
No problems expected.

**Discontinuing:**
No problems expected.

**Others:**
Some of these agents may accumulate in the urinary bladder. To decrease chance of excessive radiation, drink 8 oz. of fluid every 1 hour for 10-12 hours following the test, unless otherwise specified by your doctor.

## POSSIBLE INTERACTION WITH OTHER DRUGS

| GENERIC NAME OR DRUG CLASS | COMBINED EFFECT |
|---|---|
| None expected. | |

## POSSIBLE INTERACTION WITH OTHER SUBSTANCES

| INTERACTS WITH | COMBINED EFFECT |
|---|---|
| Alcohol: | None expected. |
| Beverages: | None expected. |
| Cocaine: | None expected. |
| Foods: | None expected. |
| Marijuana: | None expected. |
| Tobacco: | None expected. |

# RANITIDINE

## BRAND NAMES

Zantac

## BASIC INFORMATION

**Habit forming? No**
**Prescription needed? Yes**
**Available as generic? No**
**Drug class: Histamine H2 antagonist**

## USES

- Treatment for duodenal ulcer.
- Decreases acid in stomach.

## DOSAGE & USAGE INFORMATION

**How to take:**
Tablets—Swallow with liquid.

**When to take:**
At same times each day.

**If you forget a dose:**
Take as soon as you remember up to 2 hours late. If more than 2 hours, wait for next scheduled dose (don't double this dose).

**What drug does:**
Decreases stomach-acid production.

**Time lapse before drug works:**
2 to 3 hours.

**Don't take with:**
- Alcohol.
- See Interaction column and consult doctor.

## OVERDOSE

**SYMPTOMS:**
**Muscular tremors, vomiting, rapid breathing, coma.**
**WHAT TO DO:**
- **Dial 0 (operator) or 911 (emergency) for an ambulance or medical help. Then give first aid immediately.**
- **If patient is unconscious and not breathing, give mouth-to-mouth breathing. If there is no heartbeat, use cardiac massage and mouth-to-mouth breathing (CPR). Don't try to make patient vomit. If you can't get help quickly, take patient to nearest emergency facility.**
- **See emergency information on inside covers.**

## POSSIBLE ADVERSE REACTIONS OR SIDE EFFECTS

| SYMPTOMS | WHAT TO DO |
|---|---|
| **Life-threatening:**<br>None expected. | |
| **Common:**<br>None expected. | |
| **Infrequent:** | |
| • Rash. | Discontinue. Call doctor right away. |
| • Headache, dizziness, constipation, abdominal pain, nausea. | Continue. Call doctor when convenient. |
| **Rare:**<br>Jaundice. | Discontinue. Call doctor right away. |

## WARNINGS & PRECAUTIONS

**Don't take if:**
You are allergic to any histamine H2 antagonist.

**Before you start, consult your doctor:**
If you have kidney disease.

**Over age 60:**
Adverse reactions and side effects may be more frequent and severe than in younger persons.

**Pregnancy:**
No proven harm to unborn child. Avoid if possible.

**Breast-feeding:**
Drug passes into milk. Avoid drug or discontinue nursing until you finish medicine. Consult doctor for advice on maintaining milk supply.

**Infants & children:**
Not recommended.

**Prolonged use:**
Not recommended. Use for short term only.

**Skin & sunlight:**
No problems expected.

**Driving, piloting or hazardous work:**
Avoid if you feel dizzy. Otherwise, no problems expected.

**Discontinuing:**
Don't discontinue without consulting doctor until you finish prescribed dose, even though symptoms diminish or disappear.

**Others:**
No problems expected.

## POSSIBLE INTERACTION WITH OTHER DRUGS

| GENERIC NAME OR DRUG CLASS | COMBINED EFFECT |
|---|---|
| Antacids | Decreased absorption of ranitidine if taken simultaneously. |
| Ketoconazole | Decreased absorption of ranitidine. |

## POSSIBLE INTERACTION WITH OTHER SUBSTANCES

| INTERACTS WITH | COMBINED EFFECT |
|---|---|
| Alcohol: | Decreased ranitidine effect. |
| Beverages: | None expected. |
| Cocaine: | No proven problems. |
| Foods: | None expected. |
| Marijuana: | No proven problems. |
| Tobacco: | Decreased ranitidine effect. |

# RAUWOLFIA ALKALOIDS

## BRAND AND GENERIC NAMES

See complete list of brand and generic names in the *Brand Name Directory,* page 956.

## BASIC INFORMATION

**Habit forming?** No
**Prescription needed?** Yes
**Available as generic?** Yes
**Drug class:** Antihypertensive, tranquilizer (rauwolfia alkaloid)

## USES

- Treatment for high blood pressure.
- Tranquilizer for mental and emotional disturbances.

## DOSAGE & USAGE INFORMATION

**How to take:**
Tablet—Swallow with liquid or food to lessen stomach irritation. If you can't swallow whole, crumble tablet and take with liquid or food.

**When to take:**
At the same times each day.

**If you forget a dose:**
Take as soon as you remember up to 2 hours late. If more than 2 hours, wait for next scheduled dose (don't double this dose).

**What drug does:**
- Interferes with nerve impulses and relaxes blood-vessel muscles, reducing blood pressure.
- Suppresses brain centers that control emotions.

**Time lapse before drug works:**
3 weeks continual use required to determine effectiveness.

**Don't take with:**
See Interaction column and consult doctor.

## OVERDOSE

**SYMPTOMS:**
**Drowsiness; slow, weak pulse; slow, shallow breathing; diarrhea; coma; flush; low body temperature.**
**WHAT TO DO:**
- **Dial 0 (operator) or 911 (emergency) for an ambulance or medical help. Then give first aid immediately.**
- **See emergency information on inside covers.**

## POSSIBLE ADVERSE REACTIONS OR SIDE EFFECTS

| SYMPTOMS | WHAT TO DO |
|---|---|
| **Life-threatening:** None expected. | |
| **Common:** | |
| • Depression. | Continue. Call doctor when convenient. |
| • Headache, drowsiness or faintness, lethargy, eye redness, stuffy nose, impotence, diminished sex drive. | Continue. Tell doctor at next visit. |
| **Infrequent:** | |
| • Black stool; bloody vomit; chest pain; shortness of breath; irregular or slow heartbeat; stiffness in muscles, bones, joints. | Discontinue. Call doctor right away. |
| • Trembling hands. | Continue. Call doctor when convenient. |
| **Rare:** | |
| • Rash or itchy skin, sore throat, fever, stomach pain, nausea, vomiting, unusual bleeding or bruising, jaundice. | Discontinue. Call doctor right away. |
| • Painful urination. | Continue. Call doctor when convenient. |

## WARNINGS & PRECAUTIONS

**Don't take if:**
- You are allergic to any rauwolfia alkaloid.
- You are depressed.
- You have active peptic ulcer.
- You have ulcerative colitis.

**Before you start, consult your doctor:**
- If you have been depressed.
- If you have had peptic ulcer, ulcerative colitis or gallstones.
- If you have epilepsy.
- If you will have surgery within 2 months, including dental surgery, requiring general or spinal anesthesia.

**Over age 60:**
Adverse reactions and side effects may be more frequent and severe than in younger persons.

**Pregnancy:**
Studies inconclusive on harm to unborn child. Animal studies show fetal abnormalities. Decide with your doctor whether drug benefits justify risk to unborn child.

**Breast-feeding:**
Drug passes into milk. Avoid drug or discontinue nursing until you finish medicine. Consult doctor for advice on maintaining milk supply.

**Infants & children:**
Not recommended.

**Prolonged use:**
Causes cancer in laboratory animals. Consult your doctor if you have family or personal history of cancer.

**Skin & sunlight:**
No problems expected.

**Driving, piloting or hazardous work:**
Avoid if you feel drowsy, dizzy or faint. Otherwise, no problems expected.

**Discontinuing:**
Don't discontinue without consulting doctor. Dose may require gradual reduction if you have taken drug for a long time. Doses of other drugs may also require adjustment.

**Others:**
Consult your doctor if you do isometric exercises. These raise blood pressure. Drug may intensify blood-pressure rise.

## POSSIBLE INTERACTION WITH OTHER DRUGS

| GENERIC NAME OR DRUG CLASS | COMBINED EFFECT |
|---|---|
| Acebutolol | Possible increased effects of both drugs, causing excessively low blood pressure and slow heartbeat. |
| Anticoagulants (oral) | Unpredictable increased or decreased effect of anticoagulant. |
| Anticonvulsants | Serious change in seizure pattern. |
| Antidepressants | Increased antidepressant effect. |
| Antihistamines | Increased antihistamine effect. |
| Aspirin | Decreased aspirin effect. |

| Beta-adrenergic blockers | Increased effect of rauwolfia alkaloids. Excessive sedation. |
|---|---|
| Digitalis preparations | Irregular heartbeat. |
| Dronabinol | Increased effects of both drugs. Avoid. |
| Levodopa | Decreased levodopa effect. |
| MAO inhibitors | Severe depression. |
| Mind-altering drugs | Excessive sedation. |
| Pentoxifylline | Increased antihypertensive effect. |

## POSSIBLE INTERACTION WITH OTHER SUBSTANCES

| INTERACTS WITH | COMBINED EFFECT |
|---|---|
| Alcohol: | Increased intoxication. Use with extreme caution. |
| Beverages: Carbonated drinks. | Decreased rauwolfia alkaloids effect. |
| Cocaine: | Decreased rauwolfia alkaloids effect. |
| Foods: Spicy foods. | Possible digestive upset. |
| Marijuana: | Occasional use—Mild drowsiness. Daily use—Moderate drowsiness, low blood pressure, depression. |
| Tobacco: | No problems expected. |

781

# RAUWOLFIA & THIAZIDE DIURETICS

## BRAND NAMES

See complete list of brand names in the *Brand Name Directory,* page 957.

## BASIC INFORMATION

**Habit forming? No**
**Prescription needed? Yes**
**Available as generic? Yes**
**Drug class: Antihypertensive, diuretic, tranquilizer**

 ## USES

- Controls, but doesn't cure, high blood pressure.
- Reduces fluid retention (edema).

 ## DOSAGE & USAGE INFORMATION

**How to take:**
Tablet or capsule—Swallow with liquid. If you can't swallow whole, crumble tablet or open capsule and take with liquid or food.

**When to take:**
At the same time each day.

**If you forget a dose:**
Take as soon as you remember up to 2 hours late. If more than 2 hours, wait for next scheduled dose (don't double this dose).

**What drug does:**
- Forces sodium and water excretion, reducing body fluid.
- Reduced body fluid and relaxed arteries lower blood pressure.
- Interferes with nerve impulses and relaxes blood-vessel muscles, reducing blood pressure.
- Suppresses brain centers that control emotion.

*Continued next column*

 ## OVERDOSE

**SYMPTOMS:**
**Cramps; weakness; drowsiness; slow, weak pulse; slow, shallow breathing; diarrhea; flush; low body temperature; coma.**
**WHAT TO DO:**
- **Dial 0 (operator) or 911 (emergency) for an ambulance or medical help. Then give first aid immediately.**
- **See emergency information on inside covers.**

**Time lapse before drug works:**
3 weeks continual use required to determine effectiveness.

**Don't take with:**
- Non-prescription drugs without consulting doctor.
- See Interaction column and consult doctor.

 ## POSSIBLE ADVERSE REACTIONS OR SIDE EFFECTS

| SYMPTOMS | WHAT TO DO |
|---|---|
| **Life-threatening:** | |
| Irregular heart-beat, weak pulse, hives, black stool, bloody vomit. | Discontinue. Seek emergency treatment. |
| **Common:** | |
| Lethargy, drowsiness, tremor, depression, red eyes, runny nose. | Continue. Call doctor when convenient. |
| **Infrequent:** | |
| • Blurred vision, abdominal pain, nausea, vomiting, irregular heartbeat, joint pain. | Discontinue. Call doctor right away. |
| • Dizziness, mood change, headache, dry mouth, weakness, tiredness, weight gain or loss. | Continue. Call doctor when convenient. |
| **Rare:** | |
| • Sore throat, fever, mouth sores; jaundice; unexplained bleeding or bruising. | Discontinue. Call doctor right away. |
| • Rash, painful or difficult urination, tremor, impotence. | Continue. Call doctor when convenient. |

 ## WARNINGS & PRECAUTIONS

**Don't take if:**
- You are allergic to any thiazide diuretic drug or any rauwolfia alkaloid.
- You are depressed.
- You have active peptic ulcer or ulcerative colitis.

## Before you start, consult your doctor:

- If you are allergic to any sulfa drug.
- If you have gout, liver, pancreas or kidney disorder, epilepsy.
- If you have had peptic ulcer, ulcerative colitis or gallstones.
- If you have been depressed.
- If you will have surgery within 2 months, including dental surgery, requiring general or spinal anesthesia.

## Over age 60:

Adverse reactions and side effects may be more frequent and severe than in younger persons, especially dizziness and excessive potassium loss.

## Pregnancy:

Risk to unborn child outweighs drug benefits. Don't use.

## Breast-feeding:

Drug passes into milk. Avoid drug or discontinue nursing until you finish medicine. Consult doctor for advice on maintaining milk supply.

## Infants & children:

Not recommended.

## Prolonged use:

- You may need medicine to treat high blood pressure for the rest of your life.
- Causes cancer in laboratory animals. Consult your doctor if you have family or personal history of cancer.

## Skin & sunlight:

May cause rash or intensify sunburn in areas exposed to sun or sunlamp.

## Driving, piloting or hazardous work:

Don't drive or pilot aircraft until you learn how medicine affects you. Don't work around dangerous machinery. Don't climb ladders or work in high places. Danger increases if you drink alcohol or take medicine affecting alertness and reflexes, such as antihistamines, tranquilizers, sedatives, pain medicine, narcotics and mind-altering drugs.

## Discontinuing:

Don't discontinue without consulting doctor. Dose may require gradual reduction if you have taken drug for a long time. Doses of other drugs may also require adjustment.

## Others:

- Hot weather and fever may cause dehydration and drop in blood pressure. Dose may require temporary adjustment. Weigh daily and report any unexpected weight decreases to your doctor.
- May cause rise in uric acid, leading to gout.
- May cause blood-sugar rise in diabetics.
- Consult your doctor if you do isometric exercises. These raise blood pressure. Drug may intensify blood-pressure rise.

## POSSIBLE INTERACTION WITH OTHER DRUGS

| GENERIC NAME OR DRUG CLASS | COMBINED EFFECT |
|---|---|
| Acebutolol | Possible increased effect of both drugs, causing excessively low blood pressure and slow heartbeat. |
| Anticoagulants (oral) | Unpredictable increased or decreased effect of anticoagulant. |
| Anticonvulsants | Serious change in seizure pattern. |
| Antidepressants (tricyclic) | Dangerous drop in blood pressure. Avoid combination unless under medical supervision. |
| Antihistamines | Increased antihistamine effect. |
| Aspirin | Decreased aspirin effect. |
| Barbiturates | Increased hydrochlorothiazide effect. |

*Continued page 974*

## POSSIBLE INTERACTION WITH OTHER SUBSTANCES

| INTERACTS WITH | COMBINED EFFECT |
|---|---|
| Alcohol: | Increased intoxication. Dangerous blood-pressure drop. Avoid. |
| Beverages: Carbonated drinks. | Decreased rauwolfia effect. |
| Cocaine: | Decreased rauwolfia effect. |
| Foods: Spicy foods. | Possible digestive upset. |
| Licorice. | Excessive potassium loss that causes dangerous heart rhythms. |
| Marijuana: | Occasional use—Mild drowsiness. Daily use—Moderate drowsiness, low blood pressure, depression. |
| Tobacco: | No proven problems. |

# RESERPINE & HYDRALAZINE

## BRAND NAMES

**Serpasil-Apresoline**

## BASIC INFORMATION

**Habit forming? No**
**Prescription needed? Yes**
**Available as generic? No**
**Drug class: Antihypertensive, tranquilizer**
**(rauwolfia alkaloid)**

 **USES**

Treatment for high blood pressure and congestive heart failure.

 **DOSAGE & USAGE INFORMATION**

**How to take:**
Tablet—Swallow with liquid or food to lessen stomach irritation. If you can't swallow whole, crumble tablet and take with liquid or food.

**When to take:**
At the same times each day.

**If you forget a dose:**
Take as soon as you remember up to 2 hours late. If more than 2 hours, wait for next scheduled dose (don't double this dose).

*Continued next column*

 **OVERDOSE**

**SYMPTOMS:**
**Drowsiness, slow, shallow breathing; diarrhea; flush; low body temperature; rapid, weak heartbeat; fainting; extreme weakness; cold, sweaty skin; coma.**
**WHAT TO DO:**
- **Dial 0 (operator) or 911 (emergency) for an ambulance or medical help. Then give first aid immediately.**
- **If patient is unconscious and not breathing, give mouth-to-mouth breathing. If there is no heartbeat, use cardiac massage and mouth-to-mouth breathing (CPR). Don't try to make patient vomit. If you can't get help quickly, take patient to nearest emergency facility.**
- **See emergency information on inside covers.**

## What drug does:
- Interferes with nerve impulses and relaxes blood-vessel muscles, reducing blood pressure.
- Suppresses brain centers that control emotions.

## Time lapse before drug works:
Regular use for several weeks may be necessary to determine drug's effectiveness.

## Don't take with:
- Non-prescription drugs containing alcohol without consulting doctor.
- See Interaction column and consult doctor.

 **POSSIBLE ADVERSE REACTIONS OR SIDE EFFECTS**

| SYMPTOMS | WHAT TO DO |
|---|---|
| **Life-threatening:** | |
| Fainting, black stool, black vomit, chest pain, rapid or irregular heartbeat. | Discontinue. Seek emergency treatment. |
| **Common:** | |
| • Nausea, vomiting. | Discontinue. Call doctor right away. |
| • Headache, drowsiness, runny nose, diarrhea, appetite loss. | Continue. Call doctor when convenient. |
| **Infrequent:** | |
| • Rash, hives, joint pain. | Discontinue. Call doctor right away. |
| • Confusion; dizziness; red or flushed face; irritated, red, watery eyes; constipation; joint stiffness; weakness. | Continue. Call doctor when convenient. |
| **Rare:** | |
| Unexplained bleeding or bruising, sore throat, abdominal pain, jaundice, swollen lymph glands. | Discontinue. Call doctor right away. |

## WARNINGS & PRECAUTIONS

**Don't take if:**
- If you are allergic to any rauwolfia alkaloid or hydralazine.
- You are depressed.
- You have active peptic ulcer, ulcerative colitis, or history of coronary-artery disease or rheumatic heart disease.

**Before you start, consult your doctor:**
- If you have been depressed.
- If you have had peptic ulcer, ulcerative colitis, gallstones, lupus, a stroke, kidney disease or impaired kidney function.
- If you have epilepsy.
- If you will have surgery within 2 months, including dental surgery, requiring general or spinal anesthesia.

**Over age 60:**
Adverse reactions and side effects may be more frequent and severe than in younger persons.

**Pregnancy:**
Risk to unborn child outweighs drug benefits. Don't use.

**Breast-feeding:**
Drug passes into milk. Avoid drug or discontinue nursing until you finish medicine. Consult doctor for advice on maintaining milk supply.

**Infants & children:**
Not recommended.

**Prolonged use:**
- Causes cancer in laboratory animals. Consult your doctor if you have family or personal history of cancer.
- May cause lupus (a connective tissue illness with arthritis, anemia and kidney malfunction).
- Possible psychosis.
- May cause numbness, tingling in hands or feet.

**Skin & sunlight:**
No problems expected.

**Driving, piloting or hazardous work:**
Don't drive or pilot aircraft until you learn how medicine affects you. Don't work around dangerous machinery. Don't climb ladders or work in high places. Danger increases if you drink alcohol or take medicine affecting alertness and reflexes, such as antihistamines, tranquilizers, sedatives, pain medicine, narcotics and mind-altering drugs.

**Discontinuing:**
Don't discontinue without consulting doctor. Dose may require gradual reduction if you have taken drug for a long time. Doses of other drugs may also require adjustment.

**Others:**
- Consult your doctor if you do isometric exercises. These raise blood pressure. Drug may intensify blood-pressure rise.
- Vitamin B-6 diet supplement may be advisable. Consult doctor.

## POSSIBLE INTERACTION WITH OTHER DRUGS

| GENERIC NAME OR DRUG CLASS | COMBINED EFFECT |
|---|---|
| Acebutolol | Possible increased effect of both drugs, causing excessively low blood pressure and slow heartbeat. |
| Amphetamines | Decreased hydralazine effect. |
| Anticoagulants (oral) | Unpredictable increased or decreased effect of anticoagulant. |
| Anticonvulsants | Serious change in seizure pattern. |
| Antidepressants | Increased antidepressant effect. |
| Antihistamines | Increased antihistamine effect. |
| Antihypertensives (other) | Increased antihypertensive effect. |

*Continued page 975*

## POSSIBLE INTERACTION WITH OTHER SUBSTANCES

| INTERACTS WITH | COMBINED EFFECT |
|---|---|
| Alcohol: | Increased intoxication. Avoid. |
| Beverages: Carbonated drinks. | Decreased rauwolfia alkaloids effect. |
| Cocaine: | Dangerous blood-pressure rise. Avoid. |
| Foods: Spicy foods. | Possible digestive upset. |
| Marijuana: | Occasional use—Mild drowsiness. Daily use—Moderate drowsiness, low blood pressure, depression. |
| Tobacco: | Possible angina attacks. |

# RESERPINE, HYDRALAZINE & HYDROCHLOROTHIAZIDE

## BRAND NAMES

Hydrap-Es
Hyserp
R-HCTZ-H

Ser-Ap-Es
Tri-Hydroserpine
Unipres

## BASIC INFORMATION

**Habit forming?** No
**Prescription needed?** Yes
**Available as generic?** No
**Drug class:** Antihypertensive

 USES

- Treatment for high blood pressure and congestive heart failure.
- Reduces fluid retention (edema).

 DOSAGE & USAGE INFORMATION

**How to take:**
Tablet or capsule—Swallow with liquid. If you can't swallow whole, crumble tablet or open capsule and take with liquid or food.

**When to take:**
At the same times each day.

**If you forget a dose:**
Take as soon as you remember up to 2 hours late. If more than 2 hours, wait for next scheduled dose (don't double this dose).

*Continued next column*

 OVERDOSE

**SYMPTOMS:**
Drowsiness; slow, shallow breathing; diarrhea; flush; low body temperature; rapid, weak heartbeat; fainting; extreme weakness; cold, sweaty skin; cramps, coma.
**WHAT TO DO:**
- **Dial 0 (operator) or 911 (emergency) for an ambulance or medical help. Then give first aid immediately.**
- **If patient is unconscious and not breathing, give mouth-to-mouth breathing. If there is no heartbeat, use cardiac massage and mouth-to-mouth breathing (CPR). Don't try to make patient vomit. If you can't get help quickly, take patient to nearest emergency facility.**
- **See emergency information on inside covers.**

**What drug does:**
- Interferes with nerve impulses and relaxes blood-vessel muscles, reducing blood pressure.
- Suppresses brain centers that control emotions.
- Forces sodium and water excretion, reducing body fluid.
- Reduced body fluid and relaxed arteries lower blood pressure.

**Time lapse before drug works:**
Regular use for several weeks may be necessary to determine drug's effectiveness.

**Don't take with:**
- Non-prescription drugs containing alcohol without consulting doctor.
- See Interaction column and consult doctor.

 POSSIBLE ADVERSE REACTIONS OR SIDE EFFECTS

| SYMPTOMS | WHAT TO DO |
|---|---|
| **Life-threatening:** | |
| Rapid or irregular heartbeat, weak pulse, fainting, black stool, black or bloody vomit, chest pain. | Discontinue. Seek emergency treatment. |
| **Common:** | |
| • Nausea, vomiting. | Discontinue. Call doctor right away. |
| • Headache, drowsiness, runny nose, diarrhea, appetite loss. | Continue. Call doctor when convenient. |
| **Infrequent:** | |
| • Blurred vision, abdominal pain, rash, hives, joint pain. | Discontinue. Call doctor right away. |
| • Dizziness; mood change; headache; dry mouth; weakness; tiredness; weight gain or loss; eyes red, watery, irritated; confusion; constipation; red or flushed face; joint stiffness. | Continue. Call doctor when convenient. |
| **Rare:** | |
| Sore throat; jaundice; unexplained bleeding or bruising; sore throat, fever, mouth sores. | Discontinue. Call doctor right away. |

# RESERPINE, HYDRALAZINE & HYDROCHLOROTHIAZIDE

## WARNINGS & PRECAUTIONS

### Don't take if:
- You are allergic to any rauwolfia alkaloid, hydralazine, or any thiazide diuretic drug.
- You are depressed.
- You have active peptic ulcer, ulcerative colitis, history of coronary-artery disease or rheumatic heart disease.

### Before you start, consult your doctor:
- If you have been depressed.
- If you have had peptic ulcer, ulcerative colitis, gallstones, kidney disease or impaired kidney function, lupus or a stroke.
- If you have epilepsy, gout, liver, pancreas or kidney disorder.
- If you feel pain in chest, neck or arms on physical exertion.
- If you are allergic to any sulfa drug.
- If you will have surgery within 2 months, including dental surgery, requiring general or spinal anesthesia.

### Over age 60:
Adverse reactions and side effects may be more frequent and severe than in younger persons, especially dizziness and excessive potassium loss.

### Pregnancy:
Risk to unborn child outweighs drug benefits. Don't use.

### Breast-feeding:
Drug passes into milk. Avoid drug or discontinue nursing until you finish medicine.

### Infants & children:
Not recommended.

### Prolonged use:
- Causes cancer in laboratory animals. Consult your doctor if you have family or personal history of cancer.
- May cause lupus.
- Possible psychosis.
- May cause numbness, tingling in hands or feet.

### Skin & sunlight:
May cause rash or intensify sunburn in areas exposed to sun or sunlamp.

### Driving, piloting or hazardous work:
Don't drive or pilot aircraft until you learn how medicine affects you. Don't work around dangerous machinery. Don't climb ladders or work in high places. Danger increases if you drink alcohol or take medicine affecting alertness and reflexes.

### Discontinuing:
Don't discontinue without consulting doctor. Dose may require gradual reduction if you have taken drug for a long time. Doses of other drugs may also require adjustment.

### Others:
- Consult your doctor if you do isometric exercises. These raise blood pressure. Drug may intensify blood-pressure rise.
- Vitamin B-6 supplement may be advisable. Consult doctor.
- Hot weather and fever may cause dehydration and drop in blood pressure. Dose may require temporary adjustment. Weigh daily and report any unexpected weight decreases to your doctor.
- May cause rise in uric acid, leading to gout.
- May cause blood-sugar rise in diabetics.

## POSSIBLE INTERACTION WITH OTHER DRUGS

| GENERIC NAME OR DRUG CLASS | COMBINED EFFECT |
| --- | --- |
| Acebutolol | Possible increased effects of drugs. |

*Continued page 975*

## POSSIBLE INTERACTION WITH OTHER SUBSTANCES

| INTERACTS WITH | COMBINED EFFECT |
| --- | --- |
| Alcohol: | Increased intoxication. Avoid. |
| Beverages: Carbonated drinks. | Decreased rauwolfia alkaloids effect. |
| Cocaine: | Dangerous blood-pressure rise. Avoid. |
| Foods: Spicy foods. | Possible digestive upset. |
| Licorice. | Excessive potassium loss that causes dangerous heart rhythms. |
| Marijuana: | Weakness on standing. May increase blood pressure. Occasional use—Mild drowsiness. Daily use—Moderate drowsiness, low blood pressure, depression. |
| Tobacco: | Possible angina attacks. |

# RIBAVIRIN

## BRAND NAMES

Tribavirin      Viramid
Vilona         Virazole

## BASIC INFORMATION

**Habit forming? No**
**Prescription needed? Yes**
**Available as generic? No**
**Drug class: Antiviral**

## USES

- Treats severe viral pneumonia.
- Treats influenza A and B.
- It does *not* treat other viruses such as the common cold.

## DOSAGE & USAGE INFORMATION

**How to take:**
By inhalation of a fine mist through mouth. Requires a special sprayer attached to oxygen mask, face mask for infants or hood.

**When to take:**
As ordered by your doctor.

**If you forget a dose:**
Use as soon as you remember.

**What drug does:**
Kills virus or prevents its growth.

**Time lapse before drug works:**
Begins working in 1 hour. May require treatment for 12 to 18 hours per day for 3 to 7 days.

**Don't take with:**
See Interaction column and consult doctor.

## OVERDOSE

**SYMPTOMS:**
**None expected.**
**WHAT TO DO:**
**Overdose unlikely to threaten life. If person takes much larger amount than prescribed, call doctor, poison-control center or hospital emergency room for instructions.**

## POSSIBLE ADVERSE REACTIONS OR SIDE EFFECTS

| SYMPTOMS | WHAT TO DO |
|---|---|
| **Life-threatening:** None expected. | |
| **Common:** None expected. | |
| **Infrequent:** Blurred vision; dizziness; fainting; eye irritation; eyes more sensitive to light; red, swollen or itchy eyes. | Discontinue. Call doctor right away. |
| **Rare:** None expected. | |

## WARNINGS & PRECAUTIONS

**Don't take if:**
You are allergic to ribavirin.

**Before you start, consult your doctor:**
If you are now on low-salt, low-sugar or any special diet.

**Over age 60:**
Adverse reactions and side effects may be more frequent and severe than in younger persons. Ask doctor about smaller doses.

**Pregnancy:**
Risk to unborn child outweighs drug benefits. Don't use.

**Breast-feeding:**
Drug passes into milk. Avoid drug or discontinue nursing until you finish medicine. Consult doctor for advice on maintaining milk supply.

**Infants & children:**
Use only under close medical supervision.

**Prolonged use:**
No problems expected.

**Skin & sunlight:**
No problems expected.

**Driving, piloting or hazardous work:**
Don't drive or pilot aircraft until you learn how medicine affects you. Don't work around dangerous machinery. Don't climb ladders or work in high places. Danger increases if you drink alcohol or take medicine affecting alertness and reflexes, such as antihistamines, tranquilizers, sedatives, pain medicine, narcotics and mind-altering drugs.

**Discontinuing:**
Don't discontinue without consulting doctor. Dose may require gradual reduction if you have taken drug for a long time. Doses of other drugs may also require adjustment.

**Others:**
No problems expected.

## POSSIBLE INTERACTION WITH OTHER DRUGS

| GENERIC NAME OR DRUG CLASS | COMBINED EFFECT |
| --- | --- |
| None expected. | |

## POSSIBLE INTERACTION WITH OTHER SUBSTANCES

| INTERACTS WITH | COMBINED EFFECT |
| --- | --- |
| Alcohol: | None expected. |
| Beverages: | None expected. |
| Cocaine: | None expected. |
| Foods: | None expected. |
| Marijuana: | None expected. |
| Tobacco: | None expected. |

## BRAND NAMES

Riobin-50        Many multivitamin
                 preparations.

## BASIC INFORMATION

Habit forming? No
Prescription needed? No
Available as generic? Yes
Drug class: Vitamin supplement

 ## USES

- Dietary supplement to ensure normal growth and health.
- Dietary supplement to treat symptoms caused by deficiency of B-2: sores in mouth, eyes sensitive to light, itching and peeling skin.
- Infections, stomach problems, burns, alcoholism, liver disease.
- Overactive thyroid may cause need for extra Vitamin B-2.

 ## DOSAGE & USAGE INFORMATION

How to take:
Tablet or capsule—Swallow with liquid or food to lessen stomach irritation. If you can't swallow whole, crumble tablet or open capsule and take with liquid or food.

When to take:
At the same times each day.

If you forget a dose:
Take as soon as you remember. Resume regular schedule. Don't double dose.

What drug does:
Promotes normal growth and health.

Time lapse before drug works:
Requires continual intake.

Don't take with:
See Interaction column and consult doctor.

 ## OVERDOSE

SYMPTOMS:
Dark urine, nausea, vomiting.
WHAT TO DO:
Overdose unlikely to threaten life. If person takes much larger amount than prescribed, call doctor, poison-control center or hospital emergency room for instructions.

 ## POSSIBLE ADVERSE REACTIONS OR SIDE EFFECTS

| SYMPTOMS | WHAT TO DO |
|---|---|
| **Life-threatening:** None expected. | |
| **Common:** Urine yellow in color. | No action necessary. |
| **Infrequent:** None expected. | |
| **Rare:** None expected. | |

## WARNINGS & PRECAUTIONS

**Don't take if:**
- You are allergic to any B vitamin.
- You have chronic kidney failure.

**Before you start, consult your doctor:**
If you are pregnant or plan pregnancy.

**Over age 60:**
No problems expected.

**Pregnancy:**
Recommended. Consult doctor.

**Breast-feeding:**
Recommended. Consult doctor.

**Infants & children:**
Consult doctor.

**Prolonged use:**
No problems expected.

**Skin & sunlight:**
No problems expected.

**Driving, piloting or hazardous work:**
No problems expected.

**Discontinuing:**
No problems expected.

**Others:**
A balanced diet should provide all the vitamin B-2 a healthy person needs and make supplements unnecessary during periods of good health. Best sources are milk, meats and green leafy vegetables.

## POSSIBLE INTERACTION WITH OTHER DRUGS

| GENERIC NAME OR DRUG CLASS | COMBINED EFFECT |
|---|---|
| Antidepressants (tricyclic) | Decreased riboflavin effect. |
| Phenothiazines | Decreased riboflavin effect. |
| Probenecid | Decreased riboflavin effect. |

## POSSIBLE INTERACTION WITH OTHER SUBSTANCES

| INTERACTS WITH | COMBINED EFFECT |
|---|---|
| Alcohol: | Prevents uptake and absorption of vitamin B-2. |
| Beverages: | No problems expected. |
| Cocaine: | No problems expected. |
| Foods: | No problems expected. |
| Marijuana: | No problems expected. |
| Tobacco: | Prevents absorption of vitamin B-2 and other vitamins and nutrients. |

# RIFAMPIN

## BRAND NAMES

Rifadin
Rifamate
Rifampicin

Rifomycin
Rimactane
Rofact

## BASIC INFORMATION

**Habit forming? No**
**Prescription needed? Yes**
**Available as generic? No**
**Drug class: Antibiotic (rifamycin)**

## USES

Treatment for tuberculosis and other infections.
Requires daily use for 1 to 2 years.

## DOSAGE & USAGE INFORMATION

**How to take:**
Capsule—Swallow with liquid. If you can't
swallow whole, open capsule and take with
liquid or small amount of food. For child, mix
with small amount of applesauce or jelly.

**When to take:**
1 hour before or 2 hours after a meal.

**If you forget a dose:**
Take as soon as you remember up to 2 hours
late. If more than 2 hours, wait for next
scheduled dose (don't double this dose).

**What drug does:**
Prevents multiplication of tuberculosis germs.

*Continued next column*

## OVERDOSE

**SYMPTOMS:**
**Slow, shallow breathing; weak, rapid pulse;**
**cold, sweaty skin; coma.**
**WHAT TO DO:**
- **Dial 0 (operator) or 911 (emergency) for an**
  **ambulance or medical help. Then give first**
  **aid immediately.**
- **If patient is unconscious and not**
  **breathing, give mouth-to-mouth breathing.**
  **If there is no heartbeat, use cardiac**
  **massage and mouth-to-mouth breathing**
  **(CPR). Don't try to make patient vomit. If**
  **you can't get help quickly, take patient to**
  **nearest emergency facility.**
- **See emergency information on inside**
  **covers.**

**Time lapse before drug works:**
Usually 2 weeks. May require 1 to 2 years
without missed doses for maximum benefit.

**Don't take with:**
See Interaction column and consult doctor.

## POSSIBLE ADVERSE REACTIONS OR SIDE EFFECTS

| SYMPTOMS | WHAT TO DO |
|---|---|
| **Life-threatening:**<br>None expected. | |
| **Common:**<br>Diarrhea; reddish urine, stool, saliva, sweat and tears. | Continue. Call doctor when convenient. |
| **Infrequent:** | |
| • Rash, itchy skin, blurred vision, difficult breathing. | Discontinue. Call doctor right away. |
| • Dizziness, unsteady gait, confusion, muscle or bone pain. | Continue. Call doctor when convenient. |
| • Headache. | Continue. Tell doctor at next visit. |
| **Rare:** | |
| • Sore throat, mouth or tongue; jaundice. | Discontinue. Call doctor right away. |
| • Appetite loss, vomiting, less urination. | Continue. Call doctor when convenient. |

## WARNINGS & PRECAUTIONS

**Don't take if:**
- You are allergic to rifampin.
- You wear soft contact lenses.

**Before you start, consult your doctor:**
If you are alcoholic or have liver disease.

**Over age 60:**
Adverse reactions and side effects may be more frequent and severe than in younger persons.

**Pregnancy:**
Studies inconclusive on harm to unborn child. Animal studies show fetal abnormalities. Decide with your doctor whether drug benefits justify risk to unborn child.

**Breast-feeding:**
No proven problems. Consult doctor.

**Infants & children:**
Use only under medical supervision.

**Prolonged use:**
You may become more susceptible to infections caused by germs not responsive to rifampin.

**Skin & sunlight:**
No problems expected.

**Driving, piloting or hazardous work:**
Don't drive or pilot aircraft until you learn how medicine affects you. Don't work around dangerous machinery. Don't climb ladders or work in high places. Danger increases if you drink alcohol or take medicine affecting alertness and reflexes, such as antihistamines, tranquilizers, sedatives, pain medicine, narcotics and mind-altering drugs.

**Discontinuing:**
Don't discontinue without doctor's advice until you complete prescribed dose, even though symptoms diminish or disappear.

**Others:**
No problems expected.

## POSSIBLE INTERACTION WITH OTHER DRUGS

| GENERIC NAME OR DRUG CLASS | COMBINED EFFECT |
|---|---|
| Anticoagulants (oral) | Decreased anticoagulant effect. |
| Barbiturates | Decreased barbiturate effect. |
| Contraceptives (oral) | Decreased contraceptive effect. * |
| Cortisone drugs | Decreased effect of cortisone drugs. |
| Dapsone | Decreased dapsone effect. |
| Digitoxin | Decreased digitoxin effect. |
| Flecainide | Possible decreased blood-cell production in bone marrow. |
| Isoniazid | Possible toxicity to liver. |
| Methadone | Decreased methadone effect. |
| Para-aminosalicylic acid (PAS) | Decreased rifampin effect. |
| Probenecid | Possible toxicity to liver. |
| Tocainide | Possible decreased blood-cell production in bone marrow. |
| Tolbutamide | Decreased tolbutamide effect. |
| Trimethoprim | Decreased trimethoprim effect. |

## POSSIBLE INTERACTION WITH OTHER SUBSTANCES

| INTERACTS WITH | COMBINED EFFECT |
|---|---|
| Alcohol: | Possible toxicity to liver. |
| Beverages: | None expected. |
| Cocaine: | No proven problems. |
| Foods: | None expected. |
| Marijuana: | No proven problems. |
| Tobacco: | None expected. |

# RITODRINE

## BRAND NAMES

Yutopar

## BASIC INFORMATION

**Habit forming?** No
**Prescription needed?** Yes
**Available as generic?** No
**Drug class:** Labor inhibitor; Beta-adrenergic
stimulator

## USES

Halts premature labor in pregnancies of 20 or
more weeks.

## DOSAGE & USAGE INFORMATION

**How to take:**
Tablet or capsule—Swallow with liquid or food
to lessen stomach irritation. If you can't swallow
whole, crumble tablet or open capsule and take
with liquid or food.

**When to take:**
Every 4 to 6 hours until term.

**If you forget a dose:**
Take as soon as you remember up to 2 hours
late. If more than 2 hours, wait for next
scheduled dose (don't double this dose).

**What drug does:**
Inhibits contractions of uterus (womb).

*Continued next column*

## OVERDOSE

**SYMPTOMS:**
**Rapid, irregular heartbeat to 120 or more;
shortness of breath.**
**WHAT TO DO:**
- **Dial 0 (operator) or 911 (emergency) for an
  ambulance or medical help. Then give first
  aid immediately.**
- **If patient is unconscious and not
  breathing, give mouth-to-mouth breathing.
  If there is no heartbeat, use cardiac
  massage and mouth-to-mouth breathing
  (CPR). Don't try to make patient vomit. If
  you can't get help quickly, take patient to
  nearest emergency facility.**
- **See emergency information on inside
  covers.**

**Time lapse before drug works:**
30 to 60 minutes (oral form). Faster
intravenously.

**Don't take with:**
See Interaction column and consult doctor.

## POSSIBLE ADVERSE REACTIONS OR SIDE EFFECTS

| SYMPTOMS | WHAT TO DO |
|---|---|
| **Life-threatening:**<br>None expected. | |
| **Always:**<br>Increased heart rate. | Continue. Call doctor when convenient. |
| **Common:**<br>• Irregular heartbeat. | Discontinue. Call doctor right away. |
| • Increased systolic blood pressure. | Continue. Tell doctor at next visit. |
| **Infrequent:**<br>• Shortness of breath. | Discontinue. Call doctor right away. |
| • Nervousness, trembling, headache, nausea, vomiting. | Continue. Call doctor when convenient. |
| **Rare:**<br>Rash. | Discontinue. Call doctor right away. |

## WARNINGS & PRECAUTIONS

**Don't take if:**
- You have heart disease.
- You have eclampsia.
- You have lung congestion.
- You have infection in the uterus.
- You have an overactive thyroid.
- You have a bleeding disorder.

**Before you start, consult your doctor:**
- If you have asthma.
- If you have diabetes.
- If you have high blood pressure.
- If you have pre-eclampsia.

**Over age 60:**
Not used.

**Pregnancy:**
Ritodrine crosses placenta, but animal studies show that it causes no effects on fetuses. Benefits versus risks must be assessed by you and your doctor.

**Breast-feeding:**
Not applicable.

**Infants & children:**
Not used.

**Prolonged use:**
Request blood sugar and electrolytes measurements.

**Skin & sunlight:**
No problems expected.

**Driving, piloting or hazardous work:**
Don't drive or pilot aircraft until you learn how medicine affects you. Don't work around dangerous machinery. Don't climb ladders or work in high places. Danger increases if you drink alcohol or take medicine affecting alertness and reflexes, such as antihistamines, tranquilizers, sedatives, pain medicine, narcotics and mind-altering drugs.

**Discontinuing:**
Don't discontinue without consulting doctor. Dose may require gradual reduction if you have taken drug for a long time. Doses of other drugs may also require adjustment.

**Others:**
No problems expected.

## POSSIBLE INTERACTION WITH OTHER DRUGS

| GENERIC NAME OR DRUG CLASS | COMBINED EFFECT |
|---|---|
| Adrenal corticosteroids | Increased chance of fluid in lungs of mother. Avoid. |
| Beta-adrenergic blockers | Decreased effect of ritodrine. |
| Sympathomimetics | Increased side effects of both. |

## POSSIBLE INTERACTION WITH OTHER SUBSTANCES

| INTERACTS WITH | COMBINED EFFECT |
|---|---|
| Alcohol: | Increased adverse effects. Avoid. |
| Beverages: | No problems expected. |
| Cocaine: | Injury to fetus. Avoid. |
| Foods: | No problems expected. |
| Marijuana: | Injury to fetus. Avoid. |
| Tobacco: | Injury to fetus. Avoid. |

# SALICYLATES

## BRAND AND GENERIC NAMES

See complete list of brand and generic names in the *Brand Name Directory*, page 957.

## BASIC INFORMATION

**Habit forming? No**
**Prescription needed? No**
**Available as generic? Yes**
**Drug class: Analgesic, anti-inflammatory**
      **(salicylate)**

## USES

- Reduces pain, fever, inflammation.
- Relieves swelling, stiffness, joint pain of arthritis or rheumatism.

## DOSAGE & USAGE INFORMATION

**How to take:**
- Tablet or capsule—Swallow with liquid.
- Extended-release tablets or capsules—Swallow each dose whole.
- Suppositories—Remove wrapper and moisten suppository with water. Gently insert into rectum, large end first.

**When to take:**
Pain, fever, inflammation—As needed, no more often than every 4 hours.

**If you forget a dose:**
- Pain, fever—Take as soon as you remember. Wait 4 hours for next dose.
- Arthritis—Take as soon as you remember up to 2 hours late. Return to regular schedule.

*Continued next column*

## OVERDOSE

**SYMPTOMS:**
Ringing in ears; nausea; vomiting; dizziness; fever; deep, rapid breathing; hallucinations; convulsions; coma.
**WHAT TO DO:**
- Dial 0 (operator) or 911 (emergency) for an ambulance or medical help. Then give first aid immediately.
- See emergency information on inside covers.

**What drug does:**
- Affects hypothalamus, the part of the brain that regulates temperature by dilating small blood vessels in skin.
- Prevents clumping of platelets (small blood cells) so blood vessels remain open.
- Decreases prostaglandin effect.
- Suppresses body's pain messages.

**Time lapse before drug works:**
30 minutes for pain, fever, arthritis.

**Don't take with:**
- Tetracyclines. Space doses 1 hour apart.
- See Interaction column and consult doctor.

## POSSIBLE ADVERSE REACTIONS OR SIDE EFFECTS

| SYMPTOMS | WHAT TO DO |
|---|---|
| **Life-threatening:** | |
| Hives, rash, intense itching, faintness soon after a dose (anaphylaxis); black or bloody vomit; blood in urine. | Seek emergency treatment immediately. |
| **Common:** | |
| • Nausea, vomiting, abdominal pain. | Discontinue. Seek emergency treatment. |
| • Heartburn, indigestion. | Continue. Call doctor when convenient. |
| • Ringing in ears. | Continue. Tell doctor at next visit. |
| **Infrequent:** | |
| None expected. | |
| **Rare:** | |
| • Black stools, unexplained fever. | Discontinue. Seek emergency treatment. |
| • Rash, hives, itchy skin, diminished vision, shortness of breath, wheezing, jaundice. | Discontinue. Call doctor right away. |
| • Drowsiness. | Continue. Call doctor when convenient. |

## WARNINGS & PRECAUTIONS

**Don't take if:**
- You need to restrict sodium in your diet. Buffered effervescent tablets and sodium salicylate are high in sodium.
- Salicylates have a strong vinegar-like odor, which means it has decomposed.
- You have a peptic ulcer of stomach or duodenum.
- You have a bleeding disorder.

**Before you start, consult your doctor:**
- If you have had stomach or duodenal ulcers.
- If you have had gout.
- If you have asthma or nasal polyps.

**Over age 60:**
More likely to cause hidden bleeding in stomach or intestines. Watch for dark stools.

**Pregnancy:**
Risk to unborn child outweighs drug benefits. Don't use.

**Breast-feeding:**
Drug passes into milk. Avoid drug or discontinue nursing until you finish medicine. Consult doctor for advice on maintaining milk supply.

**Infants & children:**
Overdose frequent and severe. Keep bottles out of children's reach.

**Prolonged use:**
Kidney damage. Periodic kidney-function test recommended.

**Skin & sunlight:**
Aspirin combined with sunscreen may decrease sunburn.

**Driving, piloting or hazardous work:**
No restrictions unless you feel drowsy.

**Discontinuing:**
For chronic illness—Don't discontinue without doctor's advice until you complete prescribed dose, even though symptoms diminish or disappear.

**Others:**
- Salicylates can complicate surgery, pregnancy, labor and delivery, and illness.
- For arthritis—Don't change dose without consulting doctor.
- Urine tests for blood sugar may be inaccurate.

## POSSIBLE INTERACTION WITH OTHER DRUGS

| GENERIC NAME OR DRUG CLASS | COMBINED EFFECT |
|---|---|
| Acebutolol | Decreased antihypertensive effect of acebutolol. |
| Allopurinol | Decreased allopurinol effect. |
| Antacids | Decreased salicylate effect. |
| Anticoagulants | Increased anticoagulant effect. Abnormal bleeding. |
| Antidiabetics (oral) | Low blood sugar. |

| | |
|---|---|
| Anti-inflammatory drugs (non-steroid) | Risk of stomach bleeding and ulcers. |
| Aspirin (other) | Likely salicylate toxicity. |
| Calcium supplements | Increased salicylate effect. |
| Cortisone drugs | Increased cortisone effect. Risk of ulcers and stomach bleeding. |
| Furosemide | Possible salicylate toxicity. |
| Gold compounds | Increased likelihood of kidney damage. |
| Indomethacin | Risk of stomach bleeding and ulcers. |
| Ketoprofen | Increased possibility of internal bleeding. |
| Methotrexate | Increased methotrexate effect. |
| Minoxidil | Decreased minoxidil effect. |
| Oxprenolol | Decreased antihypertensive effect of oxprenolol. |
| Para-aminosalicylic acid (PAS) | Possible salicylate toxicity. |
| Penicillins | Increased effect of both drugs. |
| Phenobarbital | Decreased salicylate effect. |
| Phenytoin | Increased phenytoin effect. |
| Probenecid | Decreased probenecid effect. |

*Continued page 976*

## POSSIBLE INTERACTION WITH OTHER SUBSTANCES

| INTERACTS WITH | COMBINED EFFECT |
|---|---|
| Alcohol: | Possible stomach irritation and bleeding. Avoid. |
| Beverages: | None expected. |
| Cocaine: | None expected. |
| Foods: | None expected. |
| Marijuana: | Possible increased pain relief, but marijuana may slow body's recovery. Avoid. |
| Tobacco: | None expected. |

# SCOPOLAMINE (HYOSCINE)

## BRAND NAMES

See complete list of brand names in the *Brand Name Directory,* page 957.

## BASIC INFORMATION

**Habit forming? No**
**Prescription needed?**
  **High strength: Yes**
  **Low strength: No**
**Available as generic? Yes**
**Drug class: Antispasmodic, anticholinergic**

## USES

- Reduces spasms of digestive system, bladder and urethra.
- Relieves painful menstruation.
- Prevents motion sickness.

## DOSAGE & USAGE INFORMATION

**How to take:**
- Tablet or capsule—Swallow with liquid or food to lessen stomach irritation.
- Extended-release tablets or capsules—Swallow each dose whole.
- Drops—Dilute dose in beverage.
- Skin discs—Clean application site. Change application sites with each dose.

**When to take:**
- Motion sickness—Apply disc 30 minutes before departure.
- Other uses—Take 30 minutes before meals (unless directed otherwise by doctor).

**If you forget a dose:**
Take up to 2 hours late. If more than 2 hours, wait for next dose (don't double this dose).

*Continued next column*

## OVERDOSE

**SYMPTOMS:**
**Dilated pupils, rapid pulse and breathing, dizziness, fever, hallucinations, confusion, slurred speech, agitation, flushed face, convulsions, coma.**
**WHAT TO DO:**
- **Dial 0 (operator) or 911 (emergency) for an ambulance or medical help. Then give first aid immediately.**
- **See emergency information on inside covers.**

**What drug does:**
Blocks nerve impulses at parasympathetic nerve endings, preventing muscle contractions and gland secretions of organs involved.

**Time lapse before drug works:**
15 to 30 minutes.

**Don't take with:**
See Interaction column and consult doctor.

## POSSIBLE ADVERSE REACTIONS OR SIDE EFFECTS

| SYMPTOMS | WHAT TO DO |
|---|---|
| **Life-threatening:** | |
| None expected. | |
| **Common:** | |
| • Confusion, delirium, rapid heartbeat. | Discontinue. Call doctor right away. |
| • Nausea, vomiting, decreased sweating. | Continue. Call doctor when convenient. |
| • Constipation. | Continue. Tell doctor at next visit. |
| • Dryness in ears, nose, throat. | No action necessary. |
| **Infrequent:** | |
| Headache, difficult urination. | Continue. Call doctor when convenient. |
| **Rare:** | |
| Rash or hives, pain, blurred vision. | Discontinue. Call doctor right away. |

## WARNINGS & PRECAUTIONS

**Don't take if:**
- You are allergic to any anticholinergic.
- You have trouble with stomach bloating.
- You have difficulty emptying your bladder completely.
- You have narrow-angle glaucoma.
- You have severe ulcerative colitis.

**Before you start, consult your doctor:**
- If you have open-angle glaucoma.
- If you have angina.
- If you have chronic bronchitis or asthma.
- If you have hiatal hernia.
- If you have liver disease.
- If you have enlarged prostate.
- If you have myasthenia gravis.
- If you have peptic ulcer.
- If you will have surgery within 2 months, including dental surgery, requiring general or spinal anesthesia.

**Over age 60:**
Adverse reactions and side effects may be more frequent and severe than in younger persons.

**Pregnancy:**
Studies inconclusive on harm to unborn child. Animal studies show fetal abnormalities. Decide with your doctor whether drug benefits justify risk to unborn child.

**Breast-feeding:**
Drug passes into milk and decreases milk flow. Avoid drug or discontinue nursing until you finish medicine. Consult doctor for advice on maintaining milk supply.

**Infants & children:**
Use only under medical supervision.

**Prolonged use:**
Chronic constipation, possible fecal impaction. Consult doctor immediately.

**Skin & sunlight:**
No problems expected.

**Driving, piloting or hazardous work:**
Use disqualifies you for piloting aircraft. Otherwise, no problems expected.

**Discontinuing:**
May be unnecessary to finish medicine. Follow doctor's instructions.

**Others:**
No problems expected.

## POSSIBLE INTERACTION WITH OTHER DRUGS

| GENERIC NAME OR DRUG CLASS | COMBINED EFFECT |
|---|---|
| Amantadine | Increased scopolamine effect. |
| Anticholinergics (other) | Increased scopolamine effect. |
| Antidepressants (tricyclic) | Increased scopolamine effect. Increased sedation. |

| | COMBINED EFFECT |
|---|---|
| Antihistamines | Increased scopolamine effect. |
| Cortisone drugs | Increased internal-eye pressure. |
| Haloperidol | Increased internal-eye pressure. |
| MAO inhibitors | Increased scopolamine effect. |
| Meperidine | Increased scopolamine effect. |
| Methylphenidate | Increased scopolamine effect. |
| Molindone | Increased anticholinergic effect. |
| Nitrates | Increased internal-eye pressure. |
| Orphenadrine | Increased scopolamine effect. |
| Phenothiazines | Increased scopolamine effect. |
| Pilocarpine | Loss of pilocarpine effect in glaucoma treatment. |
| Potassium supplements | Possible intestinal ulcers with oral potassium tablets. |
| Vitamin C | Decreased scopolamine effect. Avoid large doses of vitamin C. |

## POSSIBLE INTERACTION WITH OTHER SUBSTANCES

| INTERACTS WITH | COMBINED EFFECT |
|---|---|
| Alcohol: | None expected. |
| Beverages: | None expected. |
| Cocaine: | Excessively rapid heartbeat. Avoid. |
| Foods: | None expected. |
| Marijuana: | Drowsiness, dry mouth. |
| Tobacco: | None expected. |

# SECOBARBITAL

## BRAND NAMES

Novo Secobarb       Seral
Secogen             Tuinal
Seconal

## BASIC INFORMATION

**Habit forming? Yes**
**Prescription needed? Yes**
**Available as generic? Yes**
**Drug class: Sedative, hypnotic (barbiturate)**

 USES

- Reduces anxiety or nervous tension (low dose).
- Relieves insomnia (higher bedtime dose).

 DOSAGE & USAGE INFORMATION

**How to take:**
- Tablet, capsule or liquid—Swallow with food or liquid to lessen stomach irritation. If you can't swallow whole, crumble tablet or open capsule and take with liquid or food.
- Suppositories—Remove wrapper and moisten suppository with water. Gently insert larger end into rectum. Push well into rectum with finger.

**When to take:**
At the same times each day.

**If you forget a dose:**
Take as soon as you remember up to 2 hours late. If more than 2 hours, wait for next scheduled dose (don't double this dose).

**What drug does:**
May partially block nerve impulses at nerve-cell connections.

**Time lapse before drug works:**
60 minutes.

**Don't take with:**
- Non-prescription drugs without consulting doctor.
- See Interaction column and consult doctor.

 OVERDOSE

**SYMPTOMS:**
**Deep sleep, weak pulse, coma.**
**WHAT TO DO:**
- **Dial 0 (operator) or 911 (emergency) for an ambulance or medical help. Then give first aid immediately.**
- **See emergency information on inside covers.**

 POSSIBLE ADVERSE REACTIONS OR SIDE EFFECTS

| SYMPTOMS | WHAT TO DO |
|---|---|
| **Life-threatening:** None expected. | |
| **Common:** Dizziness, drowsiness, "hangover" effect. | Continue. Call doctor when convenient. |
| **Infrequent:** | |
| • Rash or hives; swollen face, lip or eyelids; sore throat, fever. | Discontinue. Call doctor right away. |
| • Depression, confusion, slurred speech, diarrhea, nausea, vomiting, joint or muscle pain. | Continue. Call doctor when convenient. |
| **Rare:** | |
| • Agitation, slow heartbeat, difficult breathing, jaundice. | Discontinue. Call doctor right away. |
| • Unexplained bleeding or bruising. | Continue. Call doctor when convenient. |

 WARNINGS & PRECAUTIONS

**Don't take if:**
- You are allergic to any barbiturate.
- You have porphyria.

**Before you start, consult your doctor:**
- If you have epilepsy.
- If you have kidney or liver damage.
- If you have asthma.
- If you have anemia.
- If you have chronic pain.
- If you will have surgery within 2 months, including dental surgery, requiring general or spinal anesthesia.

**Over age 60:**
Adverse reactions and side effects may be more frequent and severe than in younger persons. Use small doses.

**Pregnancy:**
Risk to unborn child outweighs drug benefits. Don't use.

**Breast-feeding:**
Drug passes into milk. Avoid drug or discontinue nursing until you finish medicine. Consult doctor for advice on maintaining milk supply.

**Infants & children:**
Use only under doctor's supervision.

# SECOBARBITAL

**Prolonged use:**
- May cause addiction, anemia, chronic intoxication.
- May lower body temperature, making exposure to cold temperatures hazardous.

**Skin & sunlight:**
May cause rash or intensify sunburn in areas exposed to sun or sunlamp.

**Driving, piloting or hazardous work:**
Don't drive or pilot aircraft until you learn how medicine affects you. Don't work around dangerous machinery. Don't climb ladders or work in high places. Danger increases if you drink alcohol or take medicine affecting alertness and reflexes.

**Discontinuing:**
May be unnecessary to finish medicine. Follow doctor's instructions. If you develop withdrawal symptoms of hallucinations, agitation or sleeplessness after discontinuing, call doctor right away.

**Others:**
Great potential for abuse.

 ## POSSIBLE INTERACTION WITH OTHER DRUGS

| GENERIC NAME OR DRUG CLASS | COMBINED EFFECT |
|---|---|
| Anticoagulants (oral) | Decreased anticoagulant effect. |
| Anticonvulsants | Changed seizure patterns. |
| Antidepressants (tricyclics) | Decreased antidepressant effect. Increased sedation. |
| Antidiabetics (oral) | Increased secobarbital effect. |
| Antihistamines | Dangerous sedation. Avoid. |
| Anti-inflammatory drugs (non-steroidal) | Decreased anti-inflammatory effect. |
| Aspirin | Decreased aspirin effect. |
| Beta-adrenergic blockers | Decreased effect of beta-adrenergic blocker. |
| Contraceptives (oral) | Decreased contraceptive effect. |

| | |
|---|---|
| Cortisone drugs | Decreased cortisone effect. |
| Digitoxin | Decreased digitoxin effect. |
| Doxycycline | Decreased doxycycline effect. |
| Dronabinol | Increased effects of both drugs. Avoid. |
| Griseofulvin | Decreased griseofulvin effect. |
| Indapamide | Increased indapamide effect. |
| MAO inhibitors | Increased secobarbital effect. |
| Mind-altering drugs | Dangerous sedation. Avoid. |
| Molindone | Increased sedative effect. |
| Narcotics | Dangerous sedation. Avoid. |
| Pain relievers | Dangerous sedation. Avoid. |
| Sedatives | Dangerous sedation. Avoid. |
| Sleep inducers | Dangerous sedation. Avoid. |
| Tranquilizers | Dangerous sedation. Avoid. |
| Valproic acid | Increased secobarbital effect. |

 ## POSSIBLE INTERACTION WITH OTHER SUBSTANCES

| INTERACTS WITH | COMBINED EFFECT |
|---|---|
| Alcohol: | Possible fatal oversedation. Avoid. |
| Beverages: | None expected. |
| Cocaine: | Decreased secobarbital effect. |
| Foods: | None expected. |
| Marijuana: | Excessive sedation. Avoid. |
| Tobacco: | None expected. |

# SENNA

## BRAND NAMES

Black Draught
Black-Draught Lax
  Senna
Casa-Fru
Dr. Caldwell's Senna
  Laxative

Fletcher's Castoria
Senexon
Senokot
Senolax
Swiss Kriss
X-Prep

## BASIC INFORMATION

**Habit forming? No**
**Prescription needed? No**
**Available as generic? Yes**
**Drug class: Laxative (stimulant)**

## USES

Constipation relief.

## DOSAGE & USAGE INFORMATION

**How to take:**
- Tablet—Swallow with liquid. If you can't swallow whole, chew or crumble tablet and take with liquid or food.
- Liquid, granules—Drink 6 to 8 glasses of water each day, in addition to one taken with each dose.

**When to take:**
Usually at bedtime with a snack, unless directed otherwise.

**If you forget a dose:**
Take as soon as you remember.

**What drug does:**
Acts on smooth muscles of intestine wall to cause vigorous bowel movement.

**Time lapse before drug works:**
6 to 10 hours.

**Don't take with:**
- See Interaction column and consult doctor.
- Don't take within 2 hours of taking another medicine. Laxative interferes with medicine absorption.

## OVERDOSE

**SYMPTOMS:**
**Vomiting, electrolyte depletion.**
**WHAT TO DO:**
**Overdose unlikely to threaten life. If person takes much larger amount than prescribed, call doctor, poison-control center or hospital emergency room for instructions.**

## POSSIBLE ADVERSE REACTIONS OR SIDE EFFECTS

| SYMPTOMS | WHAT TO DO |
|---|---|
| **Life-threatening:** | |
| None expected. | |
| **Common:** | |
| • Rectal irritation. | Continue. Call doctor when convenient. |
| • Yellow-brown or red-violet urine. | No action necessary. |
| **Infrequent:** | |
| • Dangerous potassium loss. | Discontinue. Call doctor right away. |
| • Belching, cramps, nausea. | Continue. Call doctor when convenient. |
| **Rare:** | |
| • Irritability, confusion, headache, rash, difficult breathing, irregular heartbeat, muscle cramps, unusual tiredness or weakness. | Discontinue. Call doctor right away. |
| • Burning on urination. | Continue. Call doctor when convenient. |

## WARNINGS & PRECAUTIONS

**Don't take if:**
- You have symptoms of appendicitis, inflamed bowel or intestinal blockage.
- You are allergic to a stimulant laxative.
- You have missed a bowel movement for only 1 or 2 days.

**Before you start, consult your doctor:**
- If you have a colostomy or ileostomy.
- If you have congestive heart disease.
- If you have diabetes.
- If you have high blood pressure.
- If you have a laxative habit.
- If you have rectal bleeding.
- If you take other laxatives.

**Over age 60:**
Adverse reactions and side effects may be more frequent and severe than in younger persons.

**Pregnancy:**
Risk to mother and unborn child outweighs drug benefits. Don't use.

**Breast-feeding:**
Drug passes into milk. Avoid drug or discontinue nursing until you finish medicine. Consult doctor for advice on maintaining milk supply.

**Infants & children:**
Use only under medical supervision.

**Prolonged use:**
Don't take for more than 1 week unless under a doctor's supervision. May cause laxative dependence.

**Skin & sunlight:**
No problems expected.

**Driving, piloting or hazardous work:**
No problems expected.

**Discontinuing:**
May be unnecessary to finish medicine. Follow doctor's instructions.

**Others:**
Don't take to "flush out" your system or as a "tonic."

## POSSIBLE INTERACTION WITH OTHER DRUGS

| GENERIC NAME OR DRUG CLASS | COMBINED EFFECT |
| --- | --- |
| Antihypertensives | May cause dangerous low potassium level. |
| Diuretics | May cause dangerous low potassium level. |

## POSSIBLE INTERACTION WITH OTHER SUBSTANCES

| INTERACTS WITH | COMBINED EFFECT |
| --- | --- |
| Alcohol: | None expected. |
| Beverages: | None expected. |
| Cocaine: | None expected. |
| Foods: | None expected. |
| Marijuana: | None expected. |
| Tobacco: | None expected. |

## BRAND NAMES

| | |
|---|---|
| Glysennid | Senokot |
| Nytilax | X-Prep |

## BASIC INFORMATION

**Habit forming?** No
**Prescription needed?** No
**Available as generic?** Yes
**Drug class:** Laxative (stimulant)

## USES

Constipation relief.

## DOSAGE & USAGE INFORMATION

**How to take:**
- Tablet—Swallow with liquid. If you can't swallow whole, chew or crumble tablet and take with liquid or food.
- Liquid, granules—Drink 6 to 8 glasses of water each day, in addition to one taken with each dose.

**When to take:**
Usually at bedtime with a snack, unless directed otherwise.

**If you forget a dose:**
Take as soon as you remember.

**What drug does:**
Acts on smooth muscles of intestine wall to cause vigorous bowel movement.

**Time lapse before drug works:**
6 to 10 hours.

**Don't take with:**
- See Interaction column and consult doctor.
- Don't take within 2 hours of taking another medicine. Laxative interferes with medicine absorption.

## OVERDOSE

**SYMPTOMS:**
**Vomiting, electrolyte depletion.**
**WHAT TO DO:**
**Overdose unlikely to threaten life. If person takes much larger amount than prescribed, call doctor, poison-control center or hospital emergency room for instructions.**

## POSSIBLE ADVERSE REACTIONS OR SIDE EFFECTS

| SYMPTOMS | WHAT TO DO |
|---|---|
| **Life-threatening:** | |
| None expected. | |
| **Common:** | |
| • Rectal irritation. | Continue. Call doctor when convenient. |
| • Yellow-brown or red-violet urine. | No action necessary. |
| **Infrequent:** | |
| • Dangerous potassium loss. | Discontinue. Call doctor right away. |
| • Belching, cramps, nausea. | Continue. Call doctor when convenient. |
| **Rare:** | |
| • Irritability, confusion, headache, rash, difficult breathing, irregular heartbeat, muscle cramps, unusual tiredness or weakness. | Discontinue. Call doctor right away. |
| • Burning on urination. | Continue. Call doctor when convenient. |

## WARNINGS & PRECAUTIONS

**Don't take if:**
- You have symptoms of appendicitis, inflamed bowel or intestinal blockage.
- You are allergic to a stimulant laxative.
- You have missed a bowel movement for only 1 or 2 days.

**Before you start, consult your doctor:**
- If you have a colostomy or ileostomy.
- If you have congestive heart disease.
- If you have diabetes.
- If you have high blood pressure.
- If you have a laxative habit.
- If you have rectal bleeding.
- If you take other laxatives.

**Over age 60:**
Adverse reactions and side effects may be more frequent and severe than in younger persons.

**Pregnancy:**
Risk to mother and unborn child outweighs drug benefits. Don't use.

**Breast-feeding:**
Drug passes into milk. Avoid drug or discontinue nursing until you finish medicine. Consult doctor for advice on maintaining milk supply.

**Infants & children:**
Use only under medical supervision.

**Prolonged use:**
Don't take for more than 1 week unless under a doctor's supervision. May cause laxative dependence.

**Skin & sunlight:**
No problems expected.

**Driving, piloting or hazardous work:**
No problems expected.

**Discontinuing:**
May be unnecessary to finish medicine. Follow doctor's instructions.

**Others:**
Don't take to "flush out" your system or as a "tonic."

## POSSIBLE INTERACTION WITH OTHER DRUGS

| GENERIC NAME OR DRUG CLASS | COMBINED EFFECT |
|---|---|
| Antihypertensives | May cause dangerous low potassium level. |
| Diuretics | May cause dangerous low potassium level. |

## POSSIBLE INTERACTION WITH OTHER SUBSTANCES

| INTERACTS WITH | COMBINED EFFECT |
|---|---|
| Alcohol: | None expected. |
| Beverages: | None expected. |
| Cocaine: | None expected. |
| Foods: | None expected. |
| Marijuana: | None expected. |
| Tobacco: | None expected. |

# SIMETHICONE

## BRAND NAMES

| | |
|---|---|
| Barriere | Ovol |
| Celluzyme | Phazyme |
| Di-Gel | Phazyme 125 |
| Gas-X | Riopan Plus |
| Gelusil | Simeco |
| Mygel | Silain |
| Mylanta | Tri-Cone |
| Mylicon | |

## BASIC INFORMATION

Habit forming? No
Prescription needed? No
Available as generic? Yes
Drug class: Antiflatulent

## USES

- Treatment for retention of abdominal gas.
- Used prior to x-ray of abdomen to reduce gas shadows.

## DOSAGE & USAGE INFORMATION

**How to take:**
- Tablet—Swallow with liquid.
- Liquid—Dissolve in water. Drink complete dose.
- Chewable tablets—Chew completely. Don't swallow whole.

**When to take:**
After meals and at bedtime.

**If you forget a dose:**
Take when remembered if needed.

**What drug does:**
Reduces surface tension of gas bubbles in stomach.

**Time lapse before drug works:**
10 minutes.

**Don't take with:**
No restrictions.

## OVERDOSE

**SYMPTOMS:**
None expected.
**WHAT TO DO:**
Overdose unlikely to threaten life.

## POSSIBLE ADVERSE REACTIONS OR SIDE EFFECTS

| SYMPTOMS | WHAT TO DO |
|---|---|
| **Life-threatening:** None expected. | |
| **Common:** None expected. | |
| **Infrequent:** None expected. | |
| **Rare:** None expected. | |

## WARNINGS & PRECAUTIONS

**Don't take if:**
You are allergic to simethicone.

**Before you start, consult your doctor:**
No problems expected.

**Over age 60:**
No problems expected.

**Pregnancy:**
No proven harm to unborn child. Avoid if possible.

**Breast-feeding:**
No problems expected.

**Infants & children:**
Not recommended.

**Prolonged use:**
No problems expected.

**Skin & sunlight:**
No problems expected.

**Driving, piloting or hazardous work:**
No problems expected.

**Discontinuing:**
May be unnecessary to finish medicine. Discontinue when symptoms disappear.

**Others:**
No problems expected.

## POSSIBLE INTERACTION WITH OTHER DRUGS

| GENERIC NAME OR DRUG CLASS | COMBINED EFFECT |
|---|---|
| None | |

## POSSIBLE INTERACTION WITH OTHER SUBSTANCES

| INTERACTS WITH | COMBINED EFFECT |
|---|---|
| Alcohol: | None expected. |
| Beverages: | None expected. |
| Cocaine: | None expected. |
| Foods: | None expected. |
| Marijuana: | None expected. |
| Tobacco: | None expected. |

# SODIUM BICARBONATE

## BRAND NAMES

Alka-Citrate
  Compound
Alka-Seltzer Antacid
Arm and Hammer
  Baking Soda
Bell/ans
Bisodol
Bisodol Powder
Brioschi
Bromo Seltzer

Ceo-Two
Chembicarb
Citrocarbonate
Eno
Fizrin
Infalyte
Neut
Seidlitz Powder
Soda Mint

## BASIC INFORMATION

Habit forming? No
Prescription needed? No
Available as generic? Yes
Drug class: Antacid

 USES

Treatment for hyperacidity in upper gastrointestinal tract, including stomach and esophagus. Symptoms may be heartburn or acid indigestion. Diseases include peptic ulcer, gastritis, esophagitis, hiatal hernia.

 DOSAGE & USAGE INFORMATION

**How to take:**
- Tablet—Swallow with liquid.
- Chewable tablets or wafers—Chew well before swallowing.
- Powder—Dilute dose in beverage before swallowing.

**When to take:**
1 to 3 hours after meals unless directed otherwise by your doctor.

**If you forget a dose:**
Take as soon as you remember.

**What drug does:**
- Neutralizes some of the hydrochloric acid in the stomach.
- Reduces action of pepsin, a digestive enzyme.

*Continued next column*

 OVERDOSE

**SYMPTOMS:**
Weakness, fatigue, dizziness.
**WHAT TO DO:**
Overdose unlikely to threaten life. If person takes much larger amount than prescribed, call doctor, poison-control center or hospital emergency room for instructions.

**Time lapse before drug works:**
15 minutes.

**Don't take with:**
Other medicines at the same time. Decreases absorption of other drugs.

 POSSIBLE ADVERSE REACTIONS OR SIDE EFFECTS

| SYMPTOMS | WHAT TO DO |
|---|---|
| **Life-threatening:** | |
| None expected. | |
| **Common:** | |
| • Constipation, appetite loss, weight gain. | Continue. Call doctor when convenient. |
| • Belching. | Continue. Tell doctor at next visit. |
| **Infrequent:** | |
| • Lower abdominal pain and swelling, bone pain, muscle weakness, swollen wrists or ankles. | Discontinue. Call doctor right away. |
| • Mood change, nausea, vomiting, weight loss. | Continue. Call doctor when convenient. |
| **Rare:** | |
| None expected. | |

## WARNINGS & PRECAUTIONS

**Don't take if:**
You are allergic to any antacid.

**Before you start, consult your doctor:**
- If you have kidney disease, liver disease, high blood pressure or congestive heart failure.
- If you have chronic constipation or diarrhea.
- If you have symptoms of appendicitis.
- If you have stomach or intestinal bleeding.

**Over age 60:**
Adverse reactions and side effects may be more frequent and severe than in younger persons. Diarrhea or constipation particularly likely.

**Pregnancy:**
Risk to unborn child outweighs drug benefits. Don't use.

**Breast-feeding:**
Drug passes into milk. Avoid drug or discontinue nursing until you finish medicine. Consult doctor for advice on maintaining milk supply.

**Infants & children:**
Use only under medical supervision.

**Prolonged use:**
Prolonged use with calcium supplements or milk leads to too much calcium in blood.

**Skin & sunlight:**
No problems expected.

**Driving, piloting or hazardous work:**
No problems expected.

**Discontinuing:**
May be unnecessary to finish medicine. Follow doctor's instructions.

**Others:**
Don't take longer than 2 weeks unless under medical supervision.

## POSSIBLE INTERACTION WITH OTHER DRUGS

| GENERIC NAME OR DRUG CLASS | COMBINED EFFECT |
|---|---|
| Amphetamine | Increased amphetamine effect. |
| Anticoagulants | Decreased anticoagulant effect. |
| Iron supplements | Decreased iron effect. |
| Meperidine | Increased meperidine effect. |
| Mexiletine | May slow elimination of mexiletine and cause need to adjust dosage. |
| Nalidixic acid | Decreased effect of nalidixic acid. |
| Oxyphenbutazone | Decreased oxyphenbutazone effect. |
| Para-aminosalicylic acid (PAS) | Decreased PAS effect. |
| Penicillins | Decreased penicillin effect. |
| Pentobarbital | Decreased pentobarbital effect. |
| Phenylbutazone | Decreased phenylbutazone effect. |
| Pseudoephedrine | Increased pseudoephedrine effect. |
| Quinidine | Increased quinidine effect. |
| Salicylates | Decreased salicylate effect. |
| Sulfa drugs | Decreased sulfa effect. |
| Tetracyclines | Decreased tetracycline effect. |

## POSSIBLE INTERACTION WITH OTHER SUBSTANCES

| INTERACTS WITH | COMBINED EFFECT |
|---|---|
| Alcohol: | Decreased antacid effect. |
| Beverages: | No proven problems. |
| Cocaine: | No proven problems. |
| Foods: | Decreased antacid effect. Wait 1 hour after eating. |
| Marijuana: | No proven problems. |
| Tobacco: | Decreased antacid effect. |

# SODIUM CARBONATE

## BRAND NAMES

Rolaids

## BASIC INFORMATION

**Habit forming?** No
**Prescription needed?** No
**Available as generic?** Yes
**Drug class:** Antacid

 ## USES

Treatment for hyperacidity in upper gastrointestinal tract, including stomach and esophagus. Symptoms may be heartburn or acid indigestion. Diseases include peptic ulcer, gastritis, esophagitis, hiatal hernia.

 ## DOSAGE & USAGE INFORMATION

**How to take:**
Chewable tablets or wafers—Chew well before swallowing.

**When to take:**
1 to 3 hours after meals unless directed otherwise by your doctor.

**If you forget a dose:**
Take as soon as you remember.

**What drug does:**
- Neutralizes some of the hydrochloric acid in the stomach.
- Reduces action of pepsin, a digestive enzyme.

**Time lapse before drug works:**
15 minutes.

**Don't take with:**
Other medicines at the same time. Decreases absorption of other drugs.

 ## OVERDOSE

**SYMPTOMS:**
Weakness, fatigue, dizziness.
**WHAT TO DO:**
Overdose unlikely to threaten life. If person takes much larger amount than prescribed, call doctor, poison-control center or hospital emergency room for instructions.

 ## POSSIBLE ADVERSE REACTIONS OR SIDE EFFECTS

| SYMPTOMS | WHAT TO DO |
|---|---|
| **Life-threatening:**<br>None expected. | |
| **Common:**<br>Constipation, appetite loss. | Continue. Call doctor when convenient. |
| **Infrequent:**<br>• Lower abdominal pain and swelling, bone pain, muscle weakness, swollen wrists or ankles. | Discontinue. Call doctor right away. |
| • Mood change, nausea, vomiting, weight loss. | Continue. Call doctor when convenient. |
| **Rare:**<br>None expected. | |

# SODIUM CARBONATE

## WARNINGS & PRECAUTIONS

**Don't take if:**
You are allergic to any antacid.

**Before you start, consult your doctor:**
- If you have kidney disease, liver disease, high blood pressure or congestive heart failure.
- If you have chronic constipation or diarrhea.
- If you have symptoms of appendicitis.
- If you have stomach or intestinal bleeding.

**Over age 60:**
Adverse reactions and side effects may be more frequent and severe than in younger persons. Diarrhea or constipation particularly likely.

**Pregnancy:**
Risk to unborn child outweighs drug benefits. Don't use.

**Breast-feeding:**
Drug passes into milk. Avoid drug or discontinue nursing until you finish medicine. Consult doctor for advice on maintaining milk supply.

**Infants & children:**
Use only under medical supervision.

**Prolonged use:**
Fluid retention.

**Skin & sunlight:**
No problems expected.

**Driving, piloting or hazardous work:**
No problems expected.

**Discontinuing:**
May be unnecessary to finish medicine. Follow doctor's instructions.

**Others:**
Don't take longer than 2 weeks unless under medical supervision.

## POSSIBLE INTERACTION WITH OTHER DRUGS

| GENERIC NAME OR DRUG CLASS | COMBINED EFFECT |
|---|---|
| Anticoagulants | Decreased anticoagulant effect. |
| Chlorpromazine | Decreased chlorpromazine effect. |
| Digitalis preparations | Decreased digitalis effect. |
| Iron supplements | Decreased iron effect. |
| Meperidine | Increased meperidine effect. |
| Nalidixic acid | Decreased effect of nalidixic acid. |
| Oxyphenbutazone | Decreased oxyphenbutazone effect. |
| Para-aminosalicylic acid (PAS) | Decreased PAS effect. |
| Penicillins | Decreased penicillin effect. |
| Pentobarbital | Decreased pentobarbital effect. |
| Phenylbutazone | Decreased phenylbutazone effect. |
| Pseudoephedrine | Increased pseudoephedrine effect. |
| Sulfa drugs | Decreased sulfa effect. |
| Tetracyclines | Decreased tetracycline effect. |
| Vitamins A and C | Decreased vitamin effect. |

## POSSIBLE INTERACTION WITH OTHER SUBSTANCES

| INTERACTS WITH | COMBINED EFFECT |
|---|---|
| Alcohol: | Decreased antacid effect. |
| Beverages: | No proven problems. |
| Cocaine: | No proven problems. |
| Foods: | Decreased antacid effect. Wait 1 hour after eating. |
| Marijuana: | No proven problems. |
| Tobacco: | Decreased antacid effect. |

# SODIUM FLUORIDE

## BRAND NAMES

| | |
|---|---|
| Denta-Fl | Luride-SF |
| Flo-Tab | Nafeen |
| Fluor-A-Day | Pediaflor |
| Fluorident | Pedi-Dent |
| Fluoritab | Solu-Flur |
| Fluorodex | Stay-Flo |
| Flura | Studaflor |
| Karidium | Thera-Flur |
| Luride | |

Numerous other multiple vitamin-mineral supplements.

## BASIC INFORMATION

**Habit forming? No**
**Prescription needed? Yes**
**Available as generic? Yes**
**Drug class: Mineral supplement (fluoride)**

## USES

Reduces tooth cavities.

## DOSAGE & USAGE INFORMATION

**How to take:**
- Tablet—Swallow with liquid or crumble tablet and take with liquid (*not* milk) or food.
- Liquid—Measure with dropper and take directly or with liquid.
- Chewable tablets—Chew slowly and thoroughly before swallowing.

**When to take:**
Usually at bedtime after teeth are thoroughly brushed.

**If you forget a dose:**
Take as soon as you remember. Don't double a forgotten dose. Return to schedule.

*Continued next column*

## OVERDOSE

**SYMPTOMS:**
**Stomach cramps or pain, nausea, faintness, vomiting (possibly bloody), diarrhea, black stools, shallow breathing.**
**WHAT TO DO:**
- **Dial 0 (operator) or 911 (emergency) for an ambulance or medical help. Then give first aid immediately.**
- **See emergency information on inside covers.**

**What drug does:**
Provides supplemental fluoride to combat tooth decay.

**Time lapse before drug works:**
8 weeks to provide maximum effect.

**Don't take with:**
- Other medicine simultaneously.
- See Interaction column.

## POSSIBLE ADVERSE REACTIONS OR SIDE EFFECTS

| SYMPTOMS | WHAT TO DO |
|---|---|
| **Life-threatening:**<br>None expected. | |
| **Common:**<br>None expected. | |
| **Infrequent:**<br>Rash. | Discontinue. Call doctor right away. |
| **Rare:**<br>• Severe upsets (digestive) only with overdose. | Discontinue. Seek emergency treatment. |
| • Sores in mouth and lips. | Discontinue. Call doctor right away. |

## WARNINGS & PRECAUTIONS

**Don't take if:**
- Your water supply contains 0.7 parts fluoride per million. Too much fluoride stains teeth permanently.
- You are allergic to any fluoride-containing product.
- You have underactive thyroid.

**Before you start, consult your doctor:**
Not necessary.

**Over age 60:**
No problems expected.

**Pregnancy:**
No problems expected.

**Breast-feeding:**
No problems expected.

**Infants & children:**
No problems expected except accidental overdose. Keep vitamin-mineral supplements out of children's reach.

**Prolonged use:**
Excess may cause discolored teeth and decreased calcium in blood.

**Skin & sunlight:**
No problems expected.

**Driving, piloting or hazardous work:**
No problems expected.

**Discontinuing:**
No problems expected.

**Others:**
Store in original plastic container. Fluoride decomposes glass.

## POSSIBLE INTERACTION WITH OTHER DRUGS

| GENERIC NAME OR DRUG CLASS | COMBINED EFFECT |
|---|---|
| None | |

## POSSIBLE INTERACTION WITH OTHER SUBSTANCES

| INTERACTS WITH | COMBINED EFFECT |
|---|---|
| Alcohol: | None expected. |
| Beverages: Milk. | Prevents absorption of fluoride. Space dose 2 hours before or after milk. |
| Cocaine: | None expected. |
| Foods: | None expected. |
| Marijuana: | None expected. |
| Tobacco: | None expected. |

# SODIUM PHOSPHATE

## BRAND NAMES

**Fleet Phospho-Soda**  **Sal Hepatica**
**Phospho-Soda**

## BASIC INFORMATION

**Habit forming? No**
**Prescription needed? No**
**Available as generic? Yes**
**Drug class: Laxative (hyperosmotic)**

 ## USES

Constipation relief.

 ## DOSAGE & USAGE INFORMATION

**How to take:**
Liquid, effervescent tablet or powder—Dilute
dose in beverage before swallowing.

**When to take:**
Usually once a day, preferably in the morning.

**If you forget a dose:**
Take as soon as you remember up to 8 hours
before bedtime. If later, wait for next scheduled
dose (don't double this dose). Don't take at
bedtime.

**What drug does:**
Draws water into bowel from other body tissues.
Causes distention through fluid accumulation,
which promotes soft stool and accelerates
bowel motion.

**Time lapse before drug works:**
30 minutes to 3 hours.

**Don't take with:**
See Interaction column and consult doctor.

 ## OVERDOSE

**SYMPTOMS:**
**Fluid depletion, weakness, vomiting,**
**fainting.**
**WHAT TO DO:**
**Overdose unlikely to threaten life. If person**
**takes much larger amount than prescribed,**
**call doctor, poison-control center or hospital**
**emergency room for instructions.**

 ## POSSIBLE ADVERSE REACTIONS OR SIDE EFFECTS

| SYMPTOMS | WHAT TO DO |
|---|---|
| **Life-threatening:** | |
| None expected. | |
| **Common:** | |
| None expected. | |
| **Infrequent:** | |
| • Irregular heartbeat. | Discontinue. Call doctor right away. |
| • Increased thirst, cramps, nausea, diarrhea, gaseousness. | Continue. Tell doctor at next visit. |
| **Rare:** | |
| Dizziness, confusion, tiredness or weakness. | Continue. Call doctor when convenient. |

## WARNINGS & PRECAUTIONS

**Don't take if:**
- You are allergic to any hyperosmotic laxative.
- You have symptoms of appendicitis, inflamed bowel or intestinal blockage.
- You have missed a bowel movement for only 1 or 2 days.

**Before you start, consult your doctor:**
- If you have congestive heart disease.
- If you have diabetes.
- If you have high blood pressure.
- If you have a colostomy or ileostomy.
- If you have kidney disease.
- If you have a laxative habit.
- If you have rectal bleeding.
- If you take another laxative.

**Over age 60:**
Adverse reactions and side effects may be more frequent and severe than in younger persons.

**Pregnancy:**
Salt content may cause fluid retention and swelling. Avoid if possible.

**Breast-feeding:**
No problems expected.

**Infants & children:**
Use only under medical supervision.

**Prolonged use:**
Don't take for more than 1 week unless under a doctor's supervision. May cause laxative dependence.

**Skin & sunlight:**
No problems expected.

**Driving, piloting or hazardous work:**
No problems expected.

**Discontinuing:**
May be unnecessary to finish medicine. Follow doctor's instructions.

**Others:**
- Don't take to "flush out" your system or as a "tonic."
- Don't take within 2 hours of taking another medicine.

## POSSIBLE INTERACTION WITH OTHER DRUGS

| GENERIC NAME OR DRUG CLASS | COMBINED EFFECT |
|---|---|
| Chlordiazepoxide | Decreased chlordiazepoxide effect. |
| Chlorpromazine | Decreased chlorpromazine effect. |
| Dicumarol | Decreased dicumarol effect. |
| Digoxin | Decreased digoxin effect. |
| Isoniazid | Decreased isoniazid effect. |
| Mexiletine | May decrease effectiveness of mexiletine. |
| Tetracyclines | Possible intestinal blockage. |

## POSSIBLE INTERACTION WITH OTHER SUBSTANCES

| INTERACTS WITH | COMBINED EFFECT |
|---|---|
| Alcohol: | None expected. |
| Beverages: | None expected. |
| Cocaine: | None expected. |
| Foods: | None expected. |
| Marijuana: | None expected. |
| Tobacco: | None expected. |

# SPIRONOLACTONE

## BRAND NAMES

| | |
|---|---|
| Aldactazide | Sincomen |
| Aldactone | Spironazide |
| Novospiroton | |

## BASIC INFORMATION

**Habit forming?** No
**Prescription needed?** Yes
**Available as generic?** Yes
**Drug class:** Antihypertensive, diuretic

## USES

- Reduces high blood pressure.
- Prevents fluid retention.

## DOSAGE & USAGE INFORMATION

**How to take:**
Tablet—Swallow with liquid or food to lessen stomach irritation. If you can't swallow whole, crumble tablet and take with liquid or food.

**When to take:**
- 1 dose a day—Take after breakfast.
- More than 1 dose a day—Take last dose no later than 6 p.m.

**If you forget a dose:**
- 1 dose a day—Take as soon as you remember up to 12 hours late. If more than 12 hours, wait for next scheduled dose (don't double this dose).
- More than 1 dose a day—Take as soon as you remember. Wait 6 hours for next dose.

**What drug does:**
- Increases sodium and water excretion through increased urine production, decreasing body fluid and blood pressure.
- Retains potassium.

*Continued next column*

## OVERDOSE

**SYMPTOMS:**
Thirst, drowsiness, confusion, fatigue, weakness, nausea, vomiting, irregular heartbeat, excessive blood-pressure drop.
**WHAT TO DO:**
- Dial 0 (operator) or 911 (emergency) for an ambulance or medical help. Then give first aid immediately.
- See emergency information on inside covers.

**Time lapse before drug works:**
3 to 5 days.

**Don't take with:**
See Interaction column and consult doctor.

## POSSIBLE ADVERSE REACTIONS OR SIDE EFFECTS

| SYMPTOMS | WHAT TO DO |
|---|---|
| **Life-threatening:**<br>None expected. | |
| **Common:**<br>Drowsiness or headache, thirst, nausea, vomiting, diarrhea. | Continue. Call doctor when convenient. |
| **Infrequent:**<br>• Confusion, irregular heartbeat, shortness of breath, unusual sweating. | Discontinue. Call doctor right away. |
| • Numbness, tingling in hands or feet; menstrual irregularities; tender breasts; change in sex drive. | Continue. Call doctor when convenient. |
| **Rare:**<br>• Rash or itchy skin. | Discontinue. Call doctor right away. |
| • Deep voice in women. | Continue. Tell doctor at next visit. |

## WARNINGS & PRECAUTIONS

**Don't take if:**
- You are allergic to spironolactone.
- You have impaired kidney function.
- Your serum potassium level is high.

**Before you start, consult your doctor:**
- If you have had kidney or liver disease.
- If you will have surgery within 2 months, including dental surgery, requiring general or spinal anesthesia.

**Over age 60:**
- Limit use to 2 to 3 weeks if possible.
- Adverse reactions and side effects may be more frequent and severe than in younger persons.
- Heat or fever can reduce blood pressure. May require dose adjustment.
- Overdose and extended use may cause blood clots.

**Pregnancy:**
No proven harm to unborn child. Avoid if possible.

**Breast-feeding:**
No proven problems. Consult doctor.

**Infants & children:**
Use only under medical supervision.

**Prolonged use:**
Potassium retention with irregular heartbeat, unusual weakness and confusion.

**Skin & sunlight:**
No problems expected.

**Driving, piloting or hazardous work:**
Avoid if you feel drowsy. Otherwise, no problems expected.

**Discontinuing:**
Consult doctor about adjusting doses of other drugs.

**Others:**
No problems expected.

## POSSIBLE INTERACTION WITH OTHER DRUGS

| GENERIC NAME OR DRUG CLASS | COMBINED EFFECT |
|---|---|
| Acebutolol | Increased antihypertensive effect. Dosages of both drugs may require adjustment. |
| Amiodarone | Increased risk of heartbeat irregularity due to low potassium. |
| Anticoagulants (oral) | Decreased anticoagulant effect. |
| Antihypertensives (other) | Increased antihypertensive effect. |
| Aspirin | Decreased spironolactone effect. |
| Calcium supplements | Increased calcium in blood. |
| Digitalis preparations | Decreased digitalis effect. |
| Diuretics (other) | Increased effect of both drugs. Beneficial if needed and dose is correct. |
| Enalapril | Possible excessive potassium in blood. |
| Labetolol | Increased antihypertensive effects. |
| Laxatives | Reduced potassium levels. |
| Lithium | Likely lithium toxicity. |
| Nitrates | Excessive blood-pressure drop. |
| Oxprenolol | Increased antihypertensive effect. Dosages of both drugs may require adjustment. |
| Pentoxifylline | Increased antihypertensive effect. |
| Potassium supplements | Dangerous potassium retention, causing possible heartbeat irregularity. |
| Sodium bicarbonate | Reduces high potassium levels. |
| Triamterene | Dangerous potassium retention. |

## POSSIBLE INTERACTION WITH OTHER SUBSTANCES

| INTERACTS WITH | COMBINED EFFECT |
|---|---|
| Alcohol: | None expected. |
| Beverages: Low-salt milk. | Possible potassium toxicity. |
| Cocaine: | Decreased spironolactone effect. |
| Foods: Salt. | Don't restrict unless directed by doctor. |
| Salt substitutes. | Possible potassium toxicity. |
| Marijuana: | Increased thirst, fainting. |
| Tobacco: | None expected. |

## BRAND NAMES

**Aldactazide**

## BASIC INFORMATION

**Habit forming? Yes**
**Prescription needed? Yes**
**Available as generic? No**
**Drug class: Antihypertensive, diuretic**
**        (thiazide)**

 ## USES

- Controls, but doesn't cure, high blood pressure.
- Reduces fluid retention (edema).

 ## DOSAGE & USAGE INFORMATION

**How to take:**
Tablet or capsule—Swallow with liquid. If you can't swallow whole, crumble tablet or open capsule and take with liquid or food.

**When to take:**
- 1 dose a day—Take after breakfast.
- More than 1 dose a day—Take last dose no later than 6 p.m.

**If you forget a dose:**
- 1 dose a day—Take as soon as you remember up to 12 hours late. If more than 12 hours, wait for next scheduled dose (don't double this dose).
- More than 1 dose a day—Take as soon as you remember. Wait 6 hours for next dose.

*Continued next column*

 ## OVERDOSE

**SYMPTOMS:**
**Thirst, drowsiness, confusion, fatigue, weakness, nausea, vomiting, cramps, irregular heartbeat, weak pulse, excessive blood-pressure drop, coma.**
**WHAT TO DO:**
- **Dial 0 (operator) or 911 (emergency) for an ambulance or medical help. Then give first aid immediately.**
- **See emergency information on inside covers.**

**What drug does:**
- Increases sodium and water excretion through increased urine production.
- Retains potassium.
- Relaxes muscle cells of small arteries.
- Reduced body fluid and relaxed arteries lower blood pressure.

**Time lapse before drug works:**
4 to 6 hours. May require several weeks to lower blood pressure.

**Don't take with:**
- See Interaction column and consult doctor.
- Non-prescription drugs without consulting doctor.

 ## POSSIBLE ADVERSE REACTIONS OR SIDE EFFECTS

| SYMPTOMS | WHAT TO DO |
|---|---|
| **Life-threatening:** | |
| Irregular heartbeat, weak pulse, shortness of breath. | Discontinue. Seek emergency treatment. |
| **Common:** | |
| Drowsiness, headache, thirst. | Continue. Call doctor when convenient. |
| **Infrequent:** | |
| • Blurred vision, abdominal pain, nausea, vomiting. | Discontinue. Call doctor right away. |
| • Dizziness, mood change, headache, dry mouth, menstrual irregularities, tender breasts, diminished sex drive, increased sweating, weakness, tiredness, weight gain or loss, confusion, numbness or tingling in hands or feet, diarrhea. | Continue. Call doctor when convenient. |
| **Rare:** | |
| • Sore throat, jaundice, rash. | Discontinue. Call doctor right away. |
| • Deepening of voice in women. | Continue. Call doctor when convenient. |

# SPIRONOLACTONE & HYDROCHLOROTHIAZIDE

## WARNINGS & PRECAUTIONS

**Don't take if:**
You are allergic to any thiazide diuretic drug.

**Before you start, consult your doctor:**
- If you are allergic to any sulfa drug.
- If you have gout, liver, pancreas or kidney disorder.
- If you have had kidney or liver disease.
- If you will have surgery within 2 months, including dental surgery, requiring general or spinal anesthesia.

**Over age 60:**
- Adverse reactions and side effects may be more frequent and severe than in younger persons, especially dizziness and excessive potassium loss.
- Limit use to 2 to 3 weeks if possible.
- Heat or fever can reduce blood pressure. May require dose adjustment.
- Overdose and extended use may cause blood clots.

**Pregnancy:**
Risk to unborn child outweighs drug benefits. Don't use.

**Breast-feeding:**
Drug passes into milk. Avoid drug or discontinue nursing until you finish medicine.

**Infants & children:**
Use only under medical supervision.

**Prolonged use:**
- You may need medicine to treat high blood pressure for the rest of your life.
- Potassium retention with irregular heartbeat, unusual weakness and confusion.

**Skin & sunlight:**
May cause rash or intensify sunburn in areas exposed to sun or sunlamp.

**Driving, piloting or hazardous work:**
Don't drive or pilot aircraft until you learn how medicine affects you. Don't work around dangerous machinery. Don't climb ladders or work in high places. Danger increases if you drink alcohol or take medicine affecting alertness and reflexes.

**Discontinuing:**
- Don't discontinue without medical advice.
- Consult doctor about adjusting doses of other drugs.

**Others:**
- Hot weather and fever may cause dehydration and drop in blood pressure. Dose may require temporary adjustment. Weigh daily and report any unexpected weight decreases to your doctor.
- May cause rise in uric acid, leading to gout.
- May cause blood-sugar rise in diabetics.

## POSSIBLE INTERACTION WITH OTHER DRUGS

| GENERIC NAME OR DRUG CLASS | COMBINED EFFECT |
|---|---|
| Acebutolol | Increased antihypertensive effect. Dosages of both drugs may require adjustment. |
| Allopurinol | Decreased allopurinol effect. |
| Anticoagulants (oral) | Decreased anticoagulant effect. |
| Antidepressants (tricyclic) | Dangerous drop in blood pressure. Avoid combination unless under medical supervision. |

*Continued page 976*

## POSSIBLE INTERACTION WITH OTHER SUBSTANCES

| INTERACTS WITH | COMBINED EFFECT |
|---|---|
| Alcohol: | Dangerous blood-pressure drop. |
| Beverages: Low-salt milk. | Possible potassium toxicity. |
| Cocaine: | Decreased spironolactone effect. |
| Foods: Salt. | Don't restrict unless directed by doctor. |
| Salt substitutes. | Possible potassium toxicity. |
| Marijuana: | May increase blood pressure. Increased thirst, fainting. |
| Tobacco: | None expected. |

# SUCRALFATE

## BRAND NAMES

Carafate                    Sulcrate

## BASIC INFORMATION

**Habit forming? No**
**Prescription needed? Yes**
**Available as generic? No**
**Drug class: Anti-ulcer**

## USES

Treatment of duodenal ulcer.

## DOSAGE & USAGE INFORMATION

**How to take:**
Tablet or capsule—Swallow with liquid or food
to lessen stomach irritation. If you can't swallow
whole, crumble tablet or open capsule and take
with liquid or food.

**When to take:**
1 hour before meals and at bedtime. Allow 2
hours to elapse before taking other prescription
medicines.

**If you forget a dose:**
Take as soon as you remember up to 2 hours
late. If more than 2 hours, wait for next
scheduled dose (don't double this dose).

**What drug does:**
Covers ulcer site and protects from acid,
enzymes and bile salts.

**Time lapse before drug works:**
Begins in 30 minutes. May require several days
to relieve pain.

**Don't take with:**
See Interaction column and consult doctor.

## OVERDOSE

**SYMPTOMS:**
**No data available yet for this new drug.**
**WHAT TO DO:**
**Overdose unlikely to threaten life. If person
takes much larger amount than prescribed,
call doctor, poison-control center or hospital
emergency room for instructions.**

## POSSIBLE ADVERSE REACTIONS OR SIDE EFFECTS

| SYMPTOMS | WHAT TO DO |
|---|---|
| **Life-threatening:**<br>None expected. | |
| **Common:**<br>Constipation. | Continue. Call doctor when convenient. |
| **Infrequent:**<br>Dizziness, sleepiness, rash, itchy skin, abdominal pain, nausea, vomiting, indigestion, back pain. | Continue. Call doctor when convenient. |
| **Rare:**<br>None expected. | |

## WARNINGS & PRECAUTIONS

**Don't take if:**
You are allergic to sucralfate.

**Before you start, consult your doctor:**
If you will have surgery within 2 months, including dental surgery, requiring general or spinal anesthesia.

**Over age 60:**
Adverse reactions and side effects may be more frequent and severe than in younger persons.

**Pregnancy:**
No proven harm to unborn child. Avoid if possible.

**Breast-feeding:**
Unknown effects.

**Infants & children:**
Safety not established.

**Prolonged use:**
Request blood counts if medicine needed longer than 8 weeks.

**Skin & sunlight:**
No problems expected.

**Driving, piloting or hazardous work:**
Don't drive or pilot aircraft until you learn how medicine affects you. Don't work around dangerous machinery. Don't climb ladders or work in high places. Danger increases if you drink alcohol or take medicine affecting alertness and reflexes, such as antihistamines, tranquilizers, sedatives, pain medicine, narcotics and mind-altering drugs.

**Discontinuing:**
Don't discontinue without consulting doctor. Dose may require gradual reduction if you have taken drug for a long time. Doses of other drugs may also require adjustment.

**Others:**
No problems expected.

## POSSIBLE INTERACTION WITH OTHER DRUGS

| GENERIC NAME OR DRUG CLASS | COMBINED EFFECT |
|---|---|
| Cimetidine | Decreased absorption of cimetidine if taken simultaneously. |
| Phenytoin | Decreased absorption of phenytoin if taken simultaneously. |
| Tetracyclines | Decreased absorption of tetracycline if taken simultaneously. |

## POSSIBLE INTERACTION WITH OTHER SUBSTANCES

| INTERACTS WITH | COMBINED EFFECT |
|---|---|
| Alcohol: | Irritates ulcer. Avoid. |
| Beverages: Caffeine. | Irritates ulcer. Avoid. |
| Cocaine: | May make ulcer worse. Avoid. |
| Foods: | No problems expected. |
| Marijuana: | May make ulcer worse. Avoid. |
| Tobacco: | May make ulcer worse. Avoid. |

# SULFACYTINE

## BRAND NAMES

Renoquid

## BASIC INFORMATION

**Habit forming? No**
**Prescription needed? Yes**
**Available as generic? Yes**
**Drug class: Sulfa (sulfonamide)**

## USES

Treatment for infections responsive to this drug.

## DOSAGE & USAGE INFORMATION

**How to take:**
Tablet—Swallow with liquid. Instructions to take on empty stomach mean 1 hour before or 2 hours after eating.

**When to take:**
At the same times each day, evenly spaced.

**If you forget a dose:**
Take as soon as you remember up to 2 hours late. If more than 2 hours, wait for next scheduled dose (don't double this dose).

**What drug does:**
Interferes with a nutrient (folic acid) necessary for growth and reproduction of bacteria. Will not attack viruses.

**Time lapse before drug works:**
2 to 5 days to affect infection.

**Don't take with:**
See Interaction column and consult doctor.

## OVERDOSE

**SYMPTOMS:**
Less urine, bloody urine, coma.
**WHAT TO DO:**
- Dial 0 (operator) or 911 (emergency) for an ambulance or medical help. Then give first aid immediately.
- See emergency information on inside covers.

## POSSIBLE ADVERSE REACTIONS OR SIDE EFFECTS

| SYMPTOMS | WHAT TO DO |
|---|---|
| **Life-threatening:**<br>None expected. | |
| **Common:**<br>• Itchy skin, rash. | Discontinue. Call doctor right away. |
| • Headache, dizziness, appetite loss, nausea, vomiting, diarrhea. | Continue. Call doctor when convenient. |
| **Infrequent:**<br>Red, peeling or blistering skin; sore throat; fever; swallowing difficulty; unusual bruising; aching joints or muscles; jaundice. | Discontinue. Call doctor right away. |
| **Rare:**<br>Painful urination, low back pain. | Discontinue. Call doctor right away. |

## WARNINGS & PRECAUTIONS

**Don't take if:**
You are allergic to any sulfa drug.

**Before you start, consult your doctor:**
- If you are allergic to carbonic anhydrase inhibitors, oral antidiabetics or thiazide diuretics.
- If you are allergic by nature.
- If you have liver or kidney disease.
- If you have porphyria.
- If you have developed anemia from use of any drug.

**Over age 60:**
Adverse reactions and side effects may be more frequent and severe than in younger persons.

**Pregnancy:**
Risk to unborn child outweighs drug benefits. Don't use.

**Breast-feeding:**
Drug passes into milk. Avoid drug or discontinue nursing until you finish medicine. Consult doctor for advice on maintaining milk supply.

**Infants & children:**
Don't give to infants younger than 1 month.

**Prolonged use:**
- May enlarge thyroid gland.
- You may become more susceptible to infections caused by germs not responsive to this drug.
- Request frequent blood counts, liver- and kidney-function studies.

**Skin & sunlight:**
May cause rash or intensify sunburn in areas exposed to sun or sunlamp.

**Driving, piloting or hazardous work:**
Avoid if you feel dizzy. Otherwise, no problems expected.

**Discontinuing:**
Don't discontinue without doctor's advice until you complete prescribed dose, even though symptoms diminish or disappear.

**Others:**
- Drink 2 quarts of liquid each day to prevent adverse reactions.
- If you require surgery, tell anesthetist you take sulfa. Pentothal anesthesia should not be used.

## POSSIBLE INTERACTION WITH OTHER DRUGS

| GENERIC NAME OR DRUG CLASS | COMBINED EFFECT |
|---|---|
| Aminobenzoate potassium | Possible decreased sulfa effect. |
| Anticoagulants (oral) | Increased anticoagulant effect. |
| Anticonvulsants (hydantoin) | Toxic effect on brain. |
| Aspirin | Increased sulfa effect. |
| Calcium supplements | Decreased sulfa effect. |
| Isoniazid | Possible anemia. |
| Methenamine | Possible kidney blockage. |
| Methotrexate | Increased methotrexate effect. |
| Oxyphenbutazone | Increased sulfa effect. |
| Para-aminosalicylic acid (PAS) | Decreased sulfa effect. |
| Penicillins | Decreased penicillin effect. |
| Phenylbutazone | Increased sulfa effect. |
| Probenecid | Increased sulfa effect. |
| Sulfinpyrazone | Increased sulfa effect. |
| Trimethoprim | Increased sulfa effect. |

## POSSIBLE INTERACTION WITH OTHER SUBSTANCES

| INTERACTS WITH | COMBINED EFFECT |
|---|---|
| Alcohol: | Increased alcohol effect. |
| Beverages: Less than 2 quarts of fluid daily. | Kidney damage. |
| Cocaine: | None expected. |
| Foods: | None expected. |
| Marijuana: | None expected. |
| Tobacco: | None expected. |

# SULFAMETHOXAZOLE

## BRAND NAMES

| | |
|---|---|
| Apo-Sulfamethoxazole | Gantrisin |
| Apo-Sulfatrim | Methoxanol |
| Azo Gantanol | Novotrimel |
| Bactrim | Protrin |
| Cetamide | Roubac |
| Cotrim | Septra |
| Cotrim D.S. | SMZ-TMP |
| Co-trimoxazole | Sulfamethoprim |
| Gantanol | |

## BASIC INFORMATION

**Habit forming? No**
**Prescription needed? Yes**
**Available as generic? Yes**
**Drug class: Sulfa (sulfonamide)**

## USES

Treatment for infections responsive to this drug.

## DOSAGE & USAGE INFORMATION

**How to take:**
- Tablet—Swallow with liquid. Instructions to take on empty stomach mean 1 hour before or 2 hours after eating.
- Liquid—Shake carefully before measuring.

**When to take:**
At the same times each day, evenly spaced.

**If you forget a dose:**
Take as soon as you remember up to 2 hours late. If more than 2 hours, wait for next scheduled dose (don't double this dose).

**What drug does:**
Interferes with a nutrient (folic acid) necessary for growth and reproduction of bacteria. Will not attack viruses.

*Continued next column*

## OVERDOSE

**SYMPTOMS:**
Less urine, bloody urine, coma.
**WHAT TO DO:**
- Dial 0 (operator) or 911 (emergency) for an ambulance or medical help. Then give first aid immediately.
- See emergency information on inside covers.

**Time lapse before drug works:**
2 to 5 days to affect infection.

**Don't take with:**
See Interaction column and consult doctor.

## POSSIBLE ADVERSE REACTIONS OR SIDE EFFECTS

| SYMPTOMS | WHAT TO DO |
|---|---|
| **Life-threatening:**<br>None expected. | |
| **Common:**<br>• Itchy skin, rash. | Discontinue. Call doctor right away. |
| • Headache, dizziness, appetite loss, nausea, vomiting, diarrhea. | Continue. Call doctor when convenient. |
| **Infrequent:**<br>Red, peeling or blistering skin; sore throat; fever; swallowing difficulty; unusual bruising; aching joints or muscles; jaundice. | Discontinue. Call doctor right away. |
| **Rare:**<br>Painful urination, low back pain. | Discontinue. Call doctor right away. |

## WARNINGS & PRECAUTIONS

**Don't take if:**
You are allergic to any sulfa drug.

**Before you start, consult your doctor:**
- If you are allergic to carbonic anhydrase inhibitors, oral antidiabetics or thiazide diuretics.
- If you are allergic by nature.
- If you have liver or kidney disease.
- If you have porphyria.
- If you have developed anemia from use of any drug.

**Over age 60:**
Adverse reactions and side effects may be more frequent and severe than in younger persons.

**Pregnancy:**
Risk to unborn child outweighs drug benefits. Don't use.

**Breast-feeding:**
Drug passes into milk. Avoid drug or discontinue nursing until you finish medicine. Consult doctor for advice on maintaining milk supply.

**Infants & children:**
Don't give to infants younger than 1 month.

**Prolonged use:**
- May enlarge thyroid gland.
- You may become more susceptible to infections caused by germs not responsive to this drug.
- Request frequent blood counts, liver- and kidney-function studies.

**Skin & sunlight:**
May cause rash or intensify sunburn in areas exposed to sun or sunlamp.

**Driving, piloting or hazardous work:**
Avoid if you feel dizzy. Otherwise, no problems expected.

**Discontinuing:**
Don't discontinue without doctor's advice until you complete prescribed dose, even though symptoms diminish or disappear.

**Others:**
- Drink 2 quarts of liquid each day to prevent adverse reactions.
- If you require surgery, tell anesthetist you take sulfa. Pentothal anesthesia should not be used.

## POSSIBLE INTERACTION WITH OTHER DRUGS

| GENERIC NAME OR DRUG CLASS | COMBINED EFFECT |
|---|---|
| Aminobenzoate potassium | Possible decreased sulfa effect. |
| Anticoagulants (oral) | Increased anticoagulant effect. |
| Anticonvulsants (hydantoin) | Toxic effect on brain. |
| Aspirin | Increased sulfa effect. |
| Calcium supplements | Decreased sulfa effect. |
| Isoniazid | Possible anemia. |
| Methenamine | Possible kidney blockage. |
| Methotrexate | Increased methotrexate effect. |
| Oxyphenbutazone | Increased sulfa effect. |
| Para-aminosalicylic acid (PAS) | Decreased sulfa effect. |
| Penicillins | Decreased penicillin effect. |
| Phenylbutazone | Increased sulfa effect. |
| Probenecid | Increased sulfa effect. |
| Sulfinpyrazone | Increased sulfa effect. |
| Trimethoprim | Increased sulfa effect. |

## POSSIBLE INTERACTION WITH OTHER SUBSTANCES

| INTERACTS WITH | COMBINED EFFECT |
|---|---|
| Alcohol: | Increased alcohol effect. |
| Beverages: Less than 2 quarts of fluid daily. | Kidney damage. |
| Cocaine: | None expected. |
| Foods: | None expected. |
| Marijuana: | None expected. |
| Tobacco: | None expected. |

# SULFASALAZINE

## BRAND NAMES

Azulfidine
Azulfidine En-Tabs

Salazopyrin
SAS-500

## BASIC INFORMATION

**Habit forming? No**
**Prescription needed? Yes**
**Available as generic? Yes**
**Drug class: Sulfa (sulfonamide)**

 **USES**

Treatment for ulceration and bleeding during active phase of ulcerative colitis.

 **DOSAGE & USAGE INFORMATION**

**How to take:**
- Tablet—Swallow with liquid. Instructions to take on empty stomach mean 1 hour before or 2 hours after eating.
- Liquid—Shake carefully before measuring.

**When to take:**
At the same times each day, evenly spaced.

**If you forget a dose:**
Take as soon as you remember up to 2 hours late. If more than 2 hours, wait for next scheduled dose (don't double this dose).

**What drug does:**
Anti-inflammatory action reduces tissue destruction in colon.

**Time lapse before drug works:**
2 to 5 days.

**Don't take with:**
See Interaction column and consult doctor.

 **OVERDOSE**

**SYMPTOMS:**
**Less urine, bloody urine, coma.**
**WHAT TO DO:**
- **Dial 0 (operator) or 911 (emergency) for an ambulance or medical help. Then give first aid immediately.**
- **See emergency information on inside covers.**

 **POSSIBLE ADVERSE REACTIONS OR SIDE EFFECTS**

| SYMPTOMS | WHAT TO DO |
|---|---|
| **Life-threatening:**<br>None expected. | |
| **Common:** | |
| • Itchy skin, rash. | Discontinue. Call doctor right away. |
| • Headache, dizziness, appetite loss, nausea, vomiting, diarrhea. | Continue. Call doctor when convenient. |
| • Orange urine. | Continue. Tell doctor at next visit. |
| **Infrequent:**<br>Red, peeling or blistering skin; sore throat; fever; swallowing difficulty; unusual bruising; aching joints or muscles; jaundice. | Discontinue. Call doctor right away. |
| **Rare:**<br>Painful urination, low back pain. | Discontinue. Call doctor right away. |

## WARNINGS & PRECAUTIONS

**Don't take if:**
You are allergic to any sulfa drug.

**Before you start, consult your doctor:**
- If you are allergic to carbonic anhydrase inhibitors, oral antidiabetics or thiazide diuretics.
- If you are allergic by nature.
- If you have liver or kidney disease.
- If you have porphyria.
- If you have developed anemia from use of any drug.

**Over age 60:**
Adverse reactions and side effects may be more frequent and severe than in younger persons.

**Pregnancy:**
Risk to unborn child outweighs drug benefits. Don't use.

**Breast-feeding:**
Drug passes into milk. Avoid drug or discontinue nursing until you finish medicine. Consult doctor for advice on maintaining milk supply.

**Infants & children:**
Don't give to infants younger than 1 month.

**Prolonged use:**
- May enlarge thyroid gland.
- You may become more susceptible to infections caused by germs not responsive to this drug.
- Request frequent blood counts, liver- and kidney-function studies.

**Skin & sunlight:**
May cause rash or intensify sunburn in areas exposed to sun or sunlamp.

**Driving, piloting or hazardous work:**
Avoid if you feel dizzy. Otherwise, no problems expected.

**Discontinuing:**
Don't discontinue without doctor's advice until you complete prescribed dose, even though symptoms diminish or disappear.

**Others:**
- Drink 2 quarts of liquid each day to prevent adverse reactions.
- If you require surgery, tell anesthetist you take sulfa. Pentothal anesthesia should not be used.

## POSSIBLE INTERACTION WITH OTHER DRUGS

| GENERIC NAME OR DRUG CLASS | COMBINED EFFECT |
|---|---|
| Aminobenzoate potassium | Possible decreased sulfa effect. |
| Antibiotics | Decreased sulfa effect. |
| Anticoagulants (oral) | Increased anticoagulant effect. |
| Anticonvulsants (hydantoin) | Toxic effect on brain. |
| Aspirin | Increased sulfa effect. |
| Calcium supplements | Decreased sulfa efffect. |
| Digoxin | Decreased digoxin effect. |
| Iron supplements | Decreased sulfa effect. |
| Isoniazid | Possible anemia. |
| Methenamine | Possible kidney blockage. |
| Methotrexate | Increased methotrexate effect. |
| Oxyphenbutazone | Increased sulfa effect. |
| Para-aminosalicylic acid (PAS) | Decreased sulfa effect. |
| Penicillins | Decreased penicillin effect. |
| Phenylbutazone | Increased sulfa effect. |
| Probenecid | Increased sulfa effect. |
| Sulfinpyrazone | Increased sulfa effect. |
| Trimethoprim | Increased sulfa effect. |
| Vitamin C | Possible kidney damage. Avoid large doses of vitamin C. |

## POSSIBLE INTERACTION WITH OTHER SUBSTANCES

| INTERACTS WITH | COMBINED EFFECT |
|---|---|
| Alcohol: | Increased alcohol effect. |
| Beverages: Less than 2 quarts of fluid daily. | Kidney damage. |
| Cocaine: | None expected. |
| Foods: | None expected. |
| Marijuana: | None expected. |
| Tobacco: | None expected. |

# SULFINPYRAZONE

## BRAND NAMES

Antazone
Anturan
Anturane
Apo-Sulfinpyrazone
Aprazone
Novopyrazone
Zynol

## BASIC INFORMATION

Habit forming? No
Prescription needed? Yes
Available as generic? Yes
Drug class: Antigout (uricosuric)

 **USES**

- Treatment for chronic gout.
- Reduces severity of recurrent heart attack. (This use is experimental and not yet approved by F.D.A.)

 **DOSAGE & USAGE INFORMATION**

**How to take:**
Tablet or capsule—Swallow with liquid or food to lessen stomach irritation. If you can't swallow whole, crumble tablet or open capsule and take with liquid or food.

**When to take:**
At the same times each day.

**If you forget a dose:**
Take as soon as you remember up to 2 hours late. If more than 2 hours, wait for next scheduled dose (don't double this dose).

*Continued next column*

 **OVERDOSE**

**SYMPTOMS:**
Breathing difficulty, imbalance, convulsions, coma.
**WHAT TO DO:**
- Dial 0 (operator) or 911 (emergency) for an ambulance or medical help. Then give first aid immediately.
- If patient is unconscious and not breathing, give mouth-to-mouth breathing. If there is no heartbeat, use cardiac massage and mouth-to-mouth breathing (CPR). Don't try to make patient vomit. If you can't get help quickly, take patient to nearest emergency facility.
- See emergency information on inside covers.

**What drug does:**
Reduces uric-acid level in blood and tissues by increasing amount of uric acid secreted in urine by kidneys.

**Time lapse before drug works:**
May require 6 months to prevent gout attacks.

**Don't take with:**
See Interaction column and consult doctor.

 **POSSIBLE ADVERSE REACTIONS OR SIDE EFFECTS**

| SYMPTOMS | WHAT TO DO |
|---|---|
| **Life-threatening:** None expected. | |
| **Common:** None expected. | |
| **Infrequent:** | |
| • Painful or difficult urination. | Discontinue. Call doctor right away. |
| • Rash, nausea, vomiting, stomach pain, low back pain. | Continue. Call doctor when convenient. |
| **Rare:** | |
| • Black, bloody or tarry stools. | Discontinue. Seek emergency treatment. |
| • Sore throat; fever; unusual bleeding or bruising; red, painful joints; blood in urine; fatigue or weakness. | Discontinue. Call doctor right away. |

## WARNINGS & PRECAUTIONS

**Don't take if:**
- You are allergic to any uricosuric.
- You have acute gout.
- You have active ulcers (stomach or duodenal), enteritis or ulcerative colitis.
- You have blood-cell disorders.
- You are allergic to oxyphenbutazone or phenylbutazone.

**Before you start, consult your doctor:**
If you have kidney or blood disease.

**Over age 60:**
Adverse reactions and side effects may be more frequent and severe than in younger persons. You require lower dose because of decreased kidney function.

**Pregnancy:**
Studies inconclusive on harm to unborn child. Animal studies show fetal abnormalities. Decide with your doctor whether drug benefits justify risk to unborn child.

**Breast-feeding:**
No proven problems. Consult doctor.

**Infants & children:**
Not recommended.

**Prolonged use:**
Possible kidney damage.

**Skin & sunlight:**
No problems expected.

**Driving, piloting or hazardous work:**
No problems expected.

**Discontinuing:**
Don't discontinue without consulting doctor. Dose may require gradual reduction if you have taken drug for a long time. Doses of other drugs may also require adjustment.

**Others:**
- Drink 10 to 12 glasses of water each day you take this medicine.
- Periodic blood and urine laboratory tests recommended.

## POSSIBLE INTERACTION WITH OTHER DRUGS

| GENERIC NAME OR DRUG CLASS | COMBINED EFFECT |
|---|---|
| Anticoagulants (oral) | Increased anticoagulant effect. |
| Antidiabetics (oral) | Increased antidiabetic effect. |
| Aspirin | Bleeding tendency. Decreased sulfinpyrazone effect. |
| Cephalexin | Increased effect of cephalexin. |
| Cephradine | Increased effect of cephradine. |
| Contraceptives (oral) | Increased bleeding between menstrual periods. |
| Diuretics | Decreased sulfinpyrazone effect. |
| Flecainide | Possible decreased blood-cell production in bone marrow. |
| Insulin | Increased insulin effect. |
| Penicillins | Increased penicillin effect. |
| Probenecid | Possible increased sulfinpyrazone effect. |
| Salicylates | Bleeding tendency. Decreased sulfinpyrazone effect. |
| Sulfa drugs | Increased effect of sulfa drugs |
| Tocainide | Possible decreased blood-cell production in bone marrow. |

## POSSIBLE INTERACTION WITH OTHER SUBSTANCES

| INTERACTS WITH | COMBINED EFFECT |
|---|---|
| Alcohol: | Decreased sulfinpyrazone effect. |
| Beverages: Caffeine drinks. | Decreased sulfinpyrazone effect. |
| Cocaine: | None expected. |
| Foods: | None expected. |
| Marijuana: | Occasional use—None expected. Daily use—May increase blood level of uric acid. |
| Tobacco: | None expected. |

# SULFISOXAZOLE

## BRAND NAMES

See complete list of brand names in the *Brand Name Directory,* page 957.

## BASIC INFORMATION

**Habit forming? No**
**Prescription needed? Yes**
**Available as generic? Yes**
**Drug class: Sulfa (sulfonamide)**

## USES

Treatment for infections responsive to this drug.

## DOSAGE & USAGE INFORMATION

**How to take:**
- Tablet—Swallow with liquid. Instructions to take on empty stomach mean 1 hour before or 2 hours after eating.
- Liquid—Shake carefully before measuring.

**When to take:**
At the same times each day, evenly spaced.

**If you forget a dose:**
Take as soon as you remember up to 2 hours late. If more than 2 hours, wait for next scheduled dose (don't double this dose).

**What drug does:**
Interferes with a nutrient (folic acid) necessary for growth and reproduction of bacteria. Will not attack viruses.

**Time lapse before drug works:**
2 to 5 days to affect infection.

**Don't take with:**
See Interaction column and consult doctor.

## OVERDOSE

**SYMPTOMS:**
**Less urine, bloody urine, coma.**
**WHAT TO DO:**
- Dial 0 (operator) or 911 (emergency) for an ambulance or medical help. Then give first aid immediately.
- See emergency information on inside covers.

## POSSIBLE ADVERSE REACTIONS OR SIDE EFFECTS

| SYMPTOMS | WHAT TO DO |
|---|---|
| **Life-threatening:** | |
| None expected. | |
| **Common:** | |
| • Itchy skin, rash. | Discontinue. Call doctor right away. |
| • Headache, dizziness, appetite loss, nausea, vomiting, diarrhea. | Continue. Call doctor when convenient. |
| **Infrequent:** | |
| Red, peeling or blistering skin; sore throat; fever; swallowing difficulty; unusual bruising; aching joints or muscles; jaundice. | Discontinue. Call doctor right away. |
| **Rare:** | |
| Painful urination, low back pain. | Discontinue. Call doctor right away. |

## WARNINGS & PRECAUTIONS

**Don't take if:**
You are allergic to any sulfa drug.

**Before you start, consult your doctor:**
- If you are allergic to carbonic anhydrase inhibitors, oral antidiabetics or thiazide diuretics.
- If you are allergic by nature.
- If you have liver or kidney disease.
- If you have porphyria.
- If you have developed anemia from use of any drug.

**Over age 60:**
Adverse reactions and side effects may be more frequent and severe than in younger persons.

**Pregnancy:**
Risk to unborn child outweighs drug benefits. Don't use.

**Breast-feeding:**
Drug passes into milk. Avoid drug or discontinue nursing until you finish medicine. Consult doctor for advice on maintaining milk supply.

**Infants & children:**
Don't give to infants younger than 1 month.

**Prolonged use:**
- May enlarge thyroid gland.
- You may become more susceptible to infections caused by germs not responsive to this drug.
- Request frequent blood counts, liver- and kidney-function studies.

**Skin & sunlight:**
May cause rash or intensify sunburn in areas exposed to sun or sunlamp.

**Driving, piloting or hazardous work:**
Avoid if you feel dizzy. Otherwise, no problems expected.

**Discontinuing:**
Don't discontinue without doctor's advice until you complete prescribed dose, even though symptoms diminish or disappear.

**Others:**
- Drink 2 quarts of liquid each day to prevent adverse reactions.
- If you require surgery, tell anesthetist you take sulfa.

## POSSIBLE INTERACTION WITH OTHER DRUGS

| GENERIC NAME OR DRUG CLASS | COMBINED EFFECT |
|---|---|
| Aminobenzoate potassium | Possible decreased sulfisoxazole effect. |
| Anticoagulants (oral) | Increased anticoagulant effect. |
| Anticonvulsants (hydantoin) | Toxic effect on brain. |
| Aspirin | Increased sulfa effect. |
| Calcium supplements | Decreased sulfa effect. |
| Flecainide | Possible decreased blood-cell production in bone marrow. |
| Isoniazid | Possible anemia. |
| Methenamine | Possible kidney blockage. |
| Methotrexate | Increased possibility of toxic side effects from methotrexate. |
| Oxyphenbutazone | Increased sulfa effect. |
| Para-aminosalicylic acid (PAS) | Decreased sulfa effect. |
| Penicillins | Decreased penicillin effect. |
| Phenylbutazone | Increased sulfa effect. |
| Probenecid | Increased sulfa effect. |
| Sulfinpyrazone | Increased sulfa effect. |
| Tocainide | Possible decreased blood-cell production in bone marrow. |
| Trimethoprim | Increased sulfa effect. |

## POSSIBLE INTERACTION WITH OTHER SUBSTANCES

| INTERACTS WITH | COMBINED EFFECT |
|---|---|
| Alcohol: | Increased alcohol effect. |
| Beverages: Less than 2 quarts of fluid daily. | Kidney damage. |
| Cocaine: | None expected. |
| Foods: | None expected. |
| Marijuana: | None expected. |
| Tobacco: | None expected. |

# SULFONAMIDES & PHENAZOPYRIDINE

## BRAND AND GENERIC NAMES

Azo Gantanol
Azo Gantrisin
Azo-Soxazole
Azo-Sulfamethoxazole
Azo-Sulfisoxazole
Suldiazo

Sulfafurazole &
  Phenazopyridine
SULFAMETHOXAZOLE
  & PHENAZOPYRIDINE
SULFISOXAZOLE &
  PHENAZOPYRIDINE

## BASIC INFORMATION

**Habit forming?** No
**Prescription needed?** Yes
**Available as generic?** Yes
**Drug class:** Analgesic (urinary) sulfonamide

## USES

- Treatment for infections responsive to this drug.
- Relieves pain of lower urinary-tract irritation, as in cystitis, urethritis or prostatitis.

## DOSAGE & USAGE INFORMATION

**How to take:**
Tablet—Swallow with liquid. Instructions to take on empty stomach mean 1 hour before or 2 hours after eating.

**When to take:**
At the same times each day, evenly spaced.

**If you forget a dose:**
Take as soon as you remember up to 2 hours late. If more than 2 hours, wait for next scheduled dose (don't double this dose).

*Continued next column*

## OVERDOSE

**SYMPTOMS:**
Less urine, bloody urine, shortness of breath, weakness, coma.
**WHAT TO DO:**
- Dial 0 (operator) or 911 (emergency) for an ambulance or medical help. Then give first aid immediately.
- See emergency information on inside covers.

**What drug does:**
- Interferes with a nutrient (folic acid) necessary for growth and reproduction of bacteria. Will not attack viruses.
- Anesthetizes lower urinary tract. Relieves pain, burning, pressure and urgency to urinate.

**Time lapse before drug works:**
2 to 5 days to affect infection.

**Don't take with:**
See Interaction column and consult doctor.

## POSSIBLE ADVERSE REACTIONS OR SIDE EFFECTS

| SYMPTOMS | WHAT TO DO |
|---|---|
| **Life-threatening:**<br>None expected. | |
| **Common:** | |
| • Rash, itchy skin. | Discontinue. Call doctor right away. |
| • Dizziness, diarrhea, headache, appetite loss, nausea, vomiting. | Continue. Call doctor when convenient. |
| **Infrequent:** | |
| • Joint pain; swallowing difficulty; pale skin; blistering; peeling of skin; sore throat, fever, mouth sores; unexplained bleeding or bruising; weakness; jaundice; increased sun sensitivity. | Discontinue. Call doctor right away. |
| • Abdominal pain, indigestion. | Continue. Call doctor when convenient. |
| **Rare:**<br>Back pain, neck swelling. | Discontinue. Call doctor right away. |

## WARNINGS & PRECAUTIONS

**Don't take if:**
- You are allergic to any sulfa drug or urinary analgesic.
- You have hepatitis.

**Before you start, consult your doctor:**
- If you are allergic to carbonic anhydrase inhibitors, oral antidiabetics or thiazide diuretics.
- If you are allergic by nature.
- If you have liver or kidney disease, porphyria.
- If you have developed anemia from use of any drug.

**Over age 60:**
Adverse reactions and side effects may be more frequent and severe than in younger persons.

**Pregnancy:**
Risk to unborn child outweighs drug benefits. Don't use.

**Breast-feeding:**
Drug passes into milk. Avoid drug or discontinue nursing until you finish medicine. Consult doctor for advice on maintaining milk supply.

**Infants & children:**
Don't give to infants younger than 1 month.

**Prolonged use:**
- May enlarge thyroid gland.
- You may become more susceptible to infections caused by germs not responsive to this drug.
- Request frequent blood counts, liver- and kidney-function studies.
- Orange or yellow skin.
- Anemia. Occasional blood studies recommended.

**Skin & sunlight:**
May cause rash or intensify sunburn in areas exposed to sun or sunlamp.

**Driving, piloting or hazardous work:**
Avoid if you feel dizzy. Otherwise, no problems expected.

**Discontinuing:**
Don't discontinue without doctor's advice until you complete prescribed dose, even though symptoms diminish or disappear.

**Others:**
- Drink 2 quarts of liquid each day to prevent adverse reactions.
- If you require surgery, tell anesthetist you take sulfa.
- Will probably cause urine to be reddish orange. Requires no action.

## POSSIBLE INTERACTION WITH OTHER DRUGS

| GENERIC NAME OR DRUG CLASS | COMBINED EFFECT |
|---|---|
| Aminobenzoate potassium | Possible decreased sulfa effect. |
| Anticoagulants (oral) | Increased anticoagulant effect. |
| Anticonvulsants (hydantoin) | Toxic effect on brain. |
| Aspirin | Increased sulfa effect. |
| Isoniazid | Possible anemia. |
| Methenamine | Possible kidney blockage. |
| Methotrexate | Increased methotrexate effect. |
| Oxyphenbutazone | Increased sulfa effect. |
| Para-aminosalicylic acid (PAS) | Decreased sulfa effect. |
| Penicillins | Decreased penicillin effect. |
| Phenylbutazone | Increased sulfa effect. |
| Probenecid | Increased sulfa effect. |
| Sulfinpyrazone | Increased sulfa effect. |
| Trimethoprim | Increased sulfa effect. |

## POSSIBLE INTERACTION WITH OTHER SUBSTANCES

| INTERACTS WITH | COMBINED EFFECT |
|---|---|
| Alcohol: | Increased alcohol effect. |
| Beverages: Less than 2 quarts of fluid daily. | Kidney damage. |
| Cocaine: | None expected. |
| Foods: | None expected. |
| Marijuana: | None expected. |
| Tobacco: | None expected. |

# SULINDAC

## BRAND NAMES

Clinoril

## BASIC INFORMATION

**Habit forming? No**
**Available as generic? Yes**
**Prescription needed? Yes**
**Drug class: Anti-inflammatory (non-steroid)**

 **USES**

- Treatment for joint pain, stiffness, inflammation and swelling of arthritis and gout.
- Pain reliever.

 **DOSAGE & USAGE INFORMATION**

**How to take:**
Tablet—Swallow with liquid or food to lessen stomach irritation. If you can't swallow whole, crumble tablet and take with liquid or food.

**When to take:**
At the same times each day.

**If you forget a dose:**
Take as soon as you remember up to 2 hours late. If more than 2 hours, wait for next scheduled dose (don't double this dose).

**What drug does:**
Reduces tissue concentration of prostaglandins (hormones which produce inflammation and pain).

**Time lapse before drug works:**
Begins in 4 to 24 hours. May require 3 weeks regular use for maximum benefit.

**Don't take with:**
See Interaction column and consult doctor.

 **OVERDOSE**

**SYMPTOMS:**
**Confusion, agitation, incoherence, convulsions, possible hemorrhage from stomach or intestine, coma.**
**WHAT TO DO:**
- **Dial 0 (operator) or 911 (emergency) for an ambulance or medical help. Then give first aid immediately.**
- **See emergency information on inside covers.**

 **POSSIBLE ADVERSE REACTIONS OR SIDE EFFECTS**

| SYMPTOMS | WHAT TO DO |
|---|---|
| **Life-threatening:** None expected. | |
| **Common:** | |
| • Dizziness, nausea, pain. | Continue. Call doctor when convenient. |
| • Headache. | Continue. Tell doctor at next visit. |
| **Infrequent:** Depression, drowsiness, ringing in ears, constipation or diarrhea, vomiting, swollen feet or legs. | Continue. Call doctor when convenient. |
| **Rare:** | |
| • Convulsions; confusion; rash, hives or itchy skin; blurred vision; black, bloody or tarry stool; difficult breathing; tightness in chest; rapid heartbeat; unusual bleeding or bruising; blood in urine; jaundice. | Discontinue. Call doctor right away. |
| • Frequent, painful or difficult urination; fatigue; weakness. | Continue. Call doctor when convenient. |

# SULINDAC

## WARNINGS & PRECAUTIONS

### Don't take if:
- You are allergic to aspirin or any non-steroid, anti-inflammatory drug.
- You have gastritis, peptic ulcer, enteritis, ileitis, ulcerative colitis, asthma, heart failure, high blood pressure or bleeding problems.
- You have had recent rectal bleeding and suppository form has been prescribed.
- Patient is younger than 15.

### Before you start, consult your doctor:
- If you have epilepsy.
- If you have Parkinson's disease.
- If you have been mentally ill.
- If you have had kidney disease or impaired kidney function.

### Over age 60:
Adverse reactions and side effects may be more frequent and severe than in younger persons.

### Pregnancy:
Studies inconclusive on harm to unborn child. Decide with your doctor whether drug benefits justify risk to unborn child.

### Breast-feeding:
May harm child. Avoid.

### Infants & children:
Not recommended for those younger than 15. Use only under medical supervision.

### Prolonged use:
- Eye damage.
- Reduced hearing.
- Sore throat, fever.
- Weight gain.

### Skin & sunlight:
No problems expected.

### Driving, piloting or hazardous work:
Don't drive or pilot aircraft until you learn how medicine affects you. Don't work around dangerous machinery. Don't climb ladders or work in high places. Danger increases if you drink alcohol or take medicine affecting alertness and reflexes, such as antihistamines, tranquilizers, sedatives, pain medicine, narcotics and mind-altering drugs.

### Discontinuing:
Don't discontinue without consulting doctor. Dose may require gradual reduction if you have taken drug for a long time. Doses of other drugs may also require adjustment.

### Others:
No problems expected.

## POSSIBLE INTERACTION WITH OTHER DRUGS

| GENERIC NAME OR DRUG CLASS | COMBINED EFFECT |
|---|---|
| Acebutolol | Decreased antihypertensive effect of acebutolol. |
| Anticoagulants (oral) | Increased risk of bleeding. |
| Aspirin | Increased risk of stomach ulcer. |
| Cortisone drugs | Increased risk of stomach ulcer. |
| Furosemide | Decreased diuretic effect of furosemide. |
| Gold compounds | Possible increased likelihood of kidney damage. |
| Ketoprofen | Increased possibility of internal bleeding. |
| Minoxidil | Decreased minoxidil effect. |
| Oxprenolol | Decreased antihypertensive effect of oxprenolol. |
| Oxyphenbutazone | Possible stomach ulcer. |
| Phenylbutazone | Possible stomach ulcer. |
| Probenecid | Increased sulindac effect. |
| Thyroid hormones | Rapid heartbeat, blood-pressure rise. |

## POSSIBLE INTERACTION WITH OTHER SUBSTANCES

| INTERACTS WITH | COMBINED EFFECT |
|---|---|
| Alcohol: | Possible stomach ulcer or bleeding. |
| Beverages: | None expected. |
| Cocaine: | None expected. |
| Foods: | None expected. |
| Marijuana: | Increased pain relief from sulindac. |
| Tobacco: | None expected. |

835

# SUPROFEN

## BRAND NAMES

Suprol

## BASIC INFORMATION

Habit forming? No
Prescription needed? Yes
Available as generic? No
Drug class: Analgesic, antidysmenorreal
(non-steroidal anti-inflammatory
analgesic [NSAIA])

## USES

- Treatment of pain.
- Treatment of soft-tissue athletic injuries.
- Treats dysmenorrhea.

## DOSAGE & USAGE INFORMATION

**How to take:**
Capsules—Take with full glass of water while
sitting or standing upright. Take on an empty
stomach, either 1/2 hour before or 2 hours after
meals. If stomach irritation occurs, may take
with food or aluminum hydroxide or magnesium
hydroxide antacids.

**When to take:**
At the same times each day.

**If you forget a dose:**
Take as soon as you remember up to 2 hours
late. If more than 2 hours, wait for next
scheduled dose (don't double this dose).

**What drug does:**
Reduces tissue concentration of prostaglandins
(hormones which produce inflammation and
pain).

**Time lapse before drug works:**
Begins in 4 to 24 hours. May require 3 weeks
regular use for maximum benefit.

*Continued next column*

## OVERDOSE

**SYMPTOMS:**
Confusion, agitation, incoherence,
convulsions, possible hemorrhage from
stomach or intestine, coma.
**WHAT TO DO:**
- **Dial 0 (operator) or 911 (emergency) for an
  ambulance or medical help. Then give first
  aid immediately.**
- **See emergency information on inside
  covers.**

---

**Don't take with:**
- Large doses of acetaminophen. Combination
  increases possibility of kidney damage.
- See Interaction column and consult doctor.

## POSSIBLE ADVERSE REACTIONS OR SIDE EFFECTS

| SYMPTOMS | WHAT TO DO |
|---|---|
| **Life-threatening:** | |
| Hives, rash, intense itching, faintness soon after a dose (anaphylaxis); breathing difficulty; tightness in chest; rapid heartbeat. | Discontinue. Seek emergency treatment. |
| **Common:** | |
| Dizziness, headache, nausea, pain, depression, drowsiness, ringing in ears. | Continue. Call doctor when convenient. |
| **Infrequent:** | |
| • Flank pain. | Discontinue. Call doctor right away. |
| • Constipation or diarrhea, vomiting. | Continue. Call doctor when convenient. |
| **Rare:** | |
| • Bloody or black, tarry stools; convulsions; confusion; rash, hives or itch; blurred vision; unusual bleeding or bruising; jaundice; blood in urine; difficult, painful or frequent urination. | Discontinue. Call doctor right away. |
| • Fatigue, weakness. | Continue. Call doctor when convenient. |

## WARNINGS & PRECAUTIONS

**Don't take if:**
- You are allergic to suprofen, aspirin or any
  non-steroid, anti-inflammatory drug.
- You have gastritis, peptic ulcer, enteritis,
  ileitis, ulcerative colitis, asthma, heart failure,
  high blood pressure or bleeding problems.
- Patient is younger than 15.

**Before you start, consult your doctor:**
- If you have epilepsy or Parkinson's disease.
- If you have been mentally ill.
- If you have had kidney disease or impaired
  kidney function.

**Over age 60:**
Adverse reactions and side effects may be more frequent and severe than in younger persons.

**Pregnancy:**
Studies inconclusive on harm to unborn child. Decide with your doctor whether drug benefits justify risk to unborn child.

**Breast-feeding:**
May harm child. Avoid.

**Infants & children:**
Not recommended for anyone younger than 15. Use only under medical supervision.

**Prolonged use:**
- Eye damage.
- Reduced hearing.
- Sore throat, fever.
- Weight gain.

**Skin & sunlight:**
No problems expected.

**Driving, piloting or hazardous work:**
Don't drive or pilot aircraft until you learn how medicine affects you. Don't work around dangerous machinery. Don't climb ladders or work in high places. Danger increases if you drink alcohol or take medicine affecting alertness and reflexes, such as antihistamines, tranquilizers, sedatives, pain medicine, narcotics and mind-altering drugs.

**Discontinuing:**
Don't discontinue without consulting doctor. Dose may require gradual reduction if you have taken drug for a long time. Doses of other drugs may also require adjustment.

**Others:**
No problems expected.

 **POSSIBLE INTERACTION WITH OTHER DRUGS**

| GENERIC NAME OR DRUG CLASS | COMBINED EFFECT |
|---|---|
| Acebutolol | Decreased antihypertensive effect of acebutolol. |
| Anticoagulants (oral) | Increased risk of bleeding. |
| Any other non-steroidal anti-inflammatory analgesic, such as oxyphenbutazone, phenylbutazone, fenoprofen, ibuprofen, indomethacin, meclofenamate, naproxen, salicylates, sulindac, tolmetin | Increased possibility of internal bleeding. |
| Aspirin | Increased risk of stomach ulcer. |
| Cortisone drugs | Increased risk of stomach ulcer and bleeding. |
| Furosemide | Decreased diuretic effect of furosemide. |
| Gold compounds | Possible increased likelihood of kidney damage. |
| Lithium | May increase lithium in blood. |
| Minoxidil | Decreased minoxidil effect. |
| Nifedipine | Increases chance of nifedipine toxicity |
| Oxprenolol | Increased antihypertensive effect of oxprenolol. |
| Oxyphenbutazone | Possible stomach ulcer. |
| Phenylbutazone | Possible stomach ulcer. |
| Probenecid | Increased suprofen effect. |
| Thyroid hormones | Rapid heartbeat, blood-pressure rise. |
| Verapamil | Increases chance of verapamil toxicity. |

 **POSSIBLE INTERACTION WITH OTHER SUBSTANCES**

| INTERACTS WITH | COMBINED EFFECT |
|---|---|
| Alcohol: | Possible stomach ulcer or bleeding. Avoid. |
| Beverages: | None expected. |
| Cocaine: | None expected. |
| Foods: | None expected. |
| Marijuana: | Increased pain relief from suprofen. |
| Tobacco: | None expected. |

## BRAND NAMES

| | |
|---|---|
| Axotal | Lotusate |
| Buff-A-Comp | Marnal |
| Butal Compound | Plexonal |
| Fiorinal | Protensin |
| Isollyl | Sandoptal |
| Lanorinal | Tenstan |

## BASIC INFORMATION

**Habit forming? Yes**
**Prescription needed? Yes**
**Available as generic? Yes**
**Drug class: Sedative, hypnotic (barbiturate)**

 ## USES

- Reduces anxiety or nervous tension (low dose).
- Relieves insomnia (higher bedtime dose).

 ## DOSAGE & USAGE INFORMATION

**How to take:**
Tablet or capsule—Swallow with liquid or food to lessen stomach irritation. If you can't swallow whole, crumble tablet or open capsule and take with liquid or food.

**When to take:**
At the same times each day.

**If you forget a dose:**
Take as soon as you remember up to 2 hours late. If more than 2 hours, wait for next scheduled dose (don't double this dose).

**What drug does:**
May partially block nerve impulses at nerve-cell connections.

**Time lapse before drug works:**
60 minutes.

**Don't take with:**
- Non-prescription drugs without consulting doctor.
- See Interaction column and consult doctor.

 ## OVERDOSE

**SYMPTOMS:**
Deep sleep, weak pulse, coma.
**WHAT TO DO:**
- Dial 0 (operator) or 911 (emergency) for an ambulance or medical help. Then give first aid immediately.
- See emergency information on inside covers.

 ## POSSIBLE ADVERSE REACTIONS OR SIDE EFFECTS

| SYMPTOMS | WHAT TO DO |
|---|---|
| **Life-threatening:** None expected. | |
| **Common:** Dizziness, drowsiness, "hangover" effect. | Continue. Call doctor when convenient. |
| **Infrequent:** | |
| • Rash or hives; swollen face, lip, eyelids; sore throat; fever. | Discontinue. Call doctor right away. |
| • Depression, confusion, slurred speech, diarrhea, nausea, vomiting, joint or muscle pain. | Continue. Call doctor when convenient. |
| **Rare:** | |
| • Agitation, slow heartbeat, difficult breathing, jaundice. | Discontinue. Call doctor right away. |
| • Unexplained bleeding or bruising. | Continue. Call doctor when convenient. |

 ## WARNINGS & PRECAUTIONS

**Don't take if:**
- You are allergic to any barbiturate.
- You have porphyria.

**Before you start, consult your doctor:**
- If you have epilepsy, kidney or liver damage, asthma, anemia, or chronic pain.
- If you will have surgery within 2 months, including dental surgery, requiring general or spinal anesthesia.

**Over age 60:**
Adverse reactions and side effects may be more frequent and severe than in younger persons. Use small doses.

**Pregnancy:**
Risk to unborn child outweighs drug benefits. Don't use.

**Breast-feeding:**
Drug passes into milk. Avoid drug or discontinue nursing until you finish medicine. Consult doctor for advice on maintaining milk supply.

**Infants & children:**
Use only under doctor's supervision.

**Prolonged use:**
- May cause addiction, anemia, chronic intoxication.
- May lower body temperature, making exposure to cold temperatures hazardous.

**Skin & sunlight:**
May cause rash or intensify sunburn in areas exposed to sun or sunlamp.

**Driving, piloting or hazardous work:**
Don't drive or pilot aircraft until you learn how medicine affects you. Don't work around dangerous machinery. Don't climb ladders or work in high places. Danger increases if you drink alcohol or take medicine affecting alertness and reflexes.

**Discontinuing:**
May be unnecessary to finish medicine. Follow doctor's instructions. If you develop withdrawal symptoms of hallucinations, agitation or sleeplessness after discontinuing, call doctor right away.

**Others:**
No problems expected.

 ## POSSIBLE INTERACTION WITH OTHER DRUGS

| GENERIC NAME OR DRUG CLASS | COMBINED EFFECT |
|---|---|
| Anticoagulants (oral) | Decreased anticoagulant effect. |
| Anticonvulsants | Changed seizure patterns. |
| Antidepressants (tricyclics) | Decreased antidepressant effect. Possible dangerous oversedation. |
| Antidiabetics (oral) | Increased talbutal (butalbital) effect. |
| Antihistamines | Dangerous sedation. Avoid. |
| Anti-inflammatory drugs (non-steroidal) | Decreased anti-inflammatory effect. |
| Aspirin | Decreased aspirin effect. |
| Beta-adrenergic blockers | Decreased effect of beta-adrenergic blocker. |
| Contraceptives (oral) | Decreased contraceptive effect. |
| Cortisone drugs | Decreased cortisone effect. |
| Digitoxin | Decreased digitoxin effect. |
| Doxycycline | Decreased doxycycline effect. |
| Dronabinol | Increased effects of both drugs. Avoid. |
| Griseofulvin | Decreased griseofulvin effect. |
| Indapamide | Increased indapamide effect. |
| MAO inhibitors | Increased talbutal (butalbital) effect. |
| Mind-altering drugs | Dangerous sedation. Avoid. |
| Molindone | Increased sedative effect. |
| Narcotics | Dangerous sedation. Avoid. |
| Pain relievers | Dangerous sedation. Avoid. |
| Sedatives | Dangerous sedation. Avoid. |
| Sleep inducers | Dangerous sedation. Avoid. |
| Tranquilizers | Dangerous sedation. Avoid. |
| Valproic acid | Increased talbutal (butalbital) effect. |

 ## POSSIBLE INTERACTION WITH OTHER SUBSTANCES

| INTERACTS WITH | COMBINED EFFECT |
|---|---|
| Alcohol: | Possible fatal oversedation. Avoid. |
| Beverages: | None expected. |
| Cocaine: | Decreased talbutal (butalbital) effect. |
| Foods: | None expected. |
| Marijuana: | Excessive sedation. Avoid. |
| Tobacco: | None expected. |

# TEMAZEPAM

## BRAND NAMES

Restoril

## BASIC INFORMATION

Habit forming? Yes
Prescription needed? Yes
Available as generic? Yes
Drug class: Tranquilizer (benzodiazepine)

 **USES**

Treatment for insomnia.

 **DOSAGE & USAGE INFORMATION**

**How to take:**
Tablet or capsule—Swallow with liquid. If you can't swallow whole, crumble tablet or open capsule and take with liquid or food.

**When to take:**
At the same time each day, according to instructions on prescription label.

**If you forget a dose:**
Take as soon as you remember up to 2 hours late. If more than 2 hours, wait for next scheduled dose (don't double this dose).

**What drug does:**
Affects limbic system of brain—part that controls emotions. Induces near-normal sleep pattern.

**Time lapse before drug works:**
30 minutes.

**Don't take with:**
See Interaction column and consult doctor.

 **OVERDOSE**

**SYMPTOMS:**
**Drowsiness, weakness, tremor, stupor, coma.**
**WHAT TO DO:**
- **Dial 0 (operator) or 911 (emergency) for an ambulance or medical help. Then give first aid immediately.**
- **If patient is unconscious and not breathing, give mouth-to-mouth breathing. If there is no heartbeat, use cardiac massage and mouth-to-mouth breathing (CPR). Don't try to make patient vomit. If you can't get help quickly, take patient to nearest emergency facility.**
- **See emergency information on inside covers.**

 **POSSIBLE ADVERSE REACTIONS OR SIDE EFFECTS**

| SYMPTOMS | WHAT TO DO |
|---|---|
| **Life-threatening:** | |
| None expected. | |
| **Common:** | |
| Clumsiness, drowsiness, dizziness. | Continue. Call doctor when convenient. |
| **Infrequent:** | |
| • Hallucinations, confusion, depression, irritability, rash, itchy skin, change in vision. | Discontinue. Call doctor right away. |
| • Constipation or diarrhea, nausea, vomiting, difficult urination. | Continue. Call doctor when convenient. |
| **Rare:** | |
| • Slow heartbeat, difficult breathing. | Discontinue. Seek emergency treatment. |
| • Mouth or throat ulcers, jaundice. | Discontinue. Call doctor right away. |

## WARNINGS & PRECAUTIONS

**Don't take if:**
- You are allergic to any benzodiazepine.
- You have myasthenia gravis.
- You are active or recovering alcoholic.
- Patient is younger than 6 months.

**Before you start, consult your doctor:**
- If you have liver, kidney or lung disease.
- If you have diabetes, epilepsy or porphyria.

**Over age 60:**
Adverse reactions and side effects may be more frequent and severe than in younger persons. May develop agitation, rage or "hangover" effect.

**Pregnancy:**
Risk to unborn child outweighs drug benefits. Don't use.

**Breast-feeding:**
Drug passes into milk. Avoid drug or discontinue nursing until you finish medicine. Consult doctor for advice on maintaining milk supply.

**Infants & children:**
Use only under medical supervision for children older than 6 months.

**Prolonged use:**
May impair liver function.

**Skin & sunlight:**
No problems expected.

**Driving, piloting or hazardous work:**
Don't drive or pilot aircraft until you learn how medicine affects you. Don't work around dangerous machinery. Don't climb ladders or work in high places. Danger increases if you drink alcohol or take medicine affecting alertness and reflexes.

**Discontinuing:**
Don't discontinue without doctor's advice until you complete prescribed dose, even though symptoms diminish or disappear.

**Others:**
- Hot weather, heavy exercise and profuse sweat may reduce excretion and cause overdose.
- Blood sugar may rise in diabetics, requiring insulin adjustment.

## POSSIBLE INTERACTION WITH OTHER DRUGS

| GENERIC NAME OR DRUG CLASS | COMBINED EFFECT |
|---|---|
| Anticonvulsants | Change in seizure frequency or severity. |
| Antidepressants | Increased sedative effect of both drugs. |
| Antihistamines | Increased sedative effect of both drugs. |
| Antihypertensives | Excessively low blood pressure. |
| Cimetidine | Excess sedation. |
| Disulfiram | Increased temazepam effect. |
| Dronabinol | Increased effects of both drugs. Avoid. |
| MAO inhibitors | Convulsions, deep sedation, rage. |
| Molindone | Increased sedative effect. |
| Narcotics | Increased sedative effect of both drugs. |
| Sedatives | Increased sedative effect of both drugs. |
| Tranquilizers | Increased sedative effect of both drugs. |

## POSSIBLE INTERACTION WITH OTHER SUBSTANCES

| INTERACTS WITH | COMBINED EFFECT |
|---|---|
| Alcohol: | Heavy sedation. Avoid. |
| Beverages: | None expected. |
| Cocaine: | Decreased temazepam effect. |
| Foods: | None expected. |
| Marijuana: | Heavy sedation. Avoid. |
| Tobacco: | Decreased temazepam effect. |

# TERBUTALINE

## BRAND NAMES

Brethaire          Bricanyl
Brethine

## BASIC INFORMATION

**Habit forming?** No
**Prescription needed?** Yes
**Available as generic?** No
**Drug class:** Sympathomimetic

## USES

Treatment of bronchial asthma, bronchitis and emphysema.

## DOSAGE & USAGE INFORMATION

**How to take:**
Tablet or capsule—Swallow with liquid or food to lessen stomach irritation.

**When to take:**
At the same times each day.

**If you forget a dose:**
Take as soon as you remember up to 2 hours late. If more than 2 hours, wait for next scheduled dose (don't double this dose).

**What drug does:**
Dilates constricted bronchial tubes.

**Time lapse before drug works:**
30 minutes.

**Don't take with:**
See Interaction column and consult doctor.

## OVERDOSE

**SYMPTOMS:**
**Rapid heartbeat, chest pain, tremors.**
**WHAT TO DO:**
- **Dial 0 (operator) or 911 (emergency) for an ambulance or medical help. Then give first aid immediately.**
- **If patient is unconscious and not breathing, give mouth-to-mouth breathing. If there is no heartbeat, use cardiac massage and mouth-to-mouth breathing (CPR). Don't try to make patient vomit. If you can't get help quickly, take patient to nearest emergency facility.**
- **See emergency information on inside covers.**

## POSSIBLE ADVERSE REACTIONS OR SIDE EFFECTS

| SYMPTOMS | WHAT TO DO |
|---|---|
| **Life-threatening:** None expected. | |
| **Common:** Headache, nervousness, restlessness, trembling. | Continue. Call doctor when convenient. |
| **Infrequent:** • Drowsiness, nausea, vomiting, fast or pounding heartbeat, cramps, weakness. | Discontinue. Call doctor right away. |
| • Unusual sweating. | Continue. Call doctor when convenient. |
| **Rare:** None expected. | |

## WARNINGS & PRECAUTIONS

**Don't take if:**
You are allergic to any sympathomimetic.

**Before you start, consult your doctor:**
- If you have diabetes.
- If you have heart disease or high blood pressure.
- If you have overactive thyroid.
- If you have had seizures.
- If you take non-prescription amphetamines or other asthma medicines.

**Over age 60:**
Adverse reactions and side effects may be more frequent and severe than in younger persons.

**Pregnancy:**
No proven harm to unborn child. Avoid if possible. May prolong labor and delivery.

**Breast-feeding:**
No proven problems. Avoid if possible.

**Infants & children:**
Use only under medical supervision.

**Prolonged use:**
No problems expected.

**Skin & sunlight:**
No problems expected.

**Driving, piloting or hazardous work:**
Avoid if you feel drowsy. Otherwise, no problems expected.

**Discontinuing:**
May be unnecessary to finish medicine. Follow doctor's instructions.

**Others:**
If troubled breathing does not improve or worsens after using medicine, don't increase dose. Consult doctor.

## POSSIBLE INTERACTION WITH OTHER DRUGS

| GENERIC NAME OR DRUG CLASS | COMBINED EFFECT |
|---|---|
| Albuterol | Increased effect of both drugs, especially harmful side effects. |
| Antidepressants (tricyclics) | Increased terbutaline effect. |
| Beta-adrenergic blockers | Decreased effects of both drugs. |
| Ephedrine | Increased terbutaline effect. Excess heart stimulation. |
| Epinephrine | Increased terbutaline effect. Excess heart stimulation. |
| MAO inhibitors | Increased terbutaline effect. Dangerous. Avoid. |
| Minoxidil | Decreased minoxidil effect. |
| Nitrates | Possible decreased effects of both drugs. |
| Sympathomimetics | Increased terbutaline effect. |

## POSSIBLE INTERACTION WITH OTHER SUBSTANCES

| INTERACTS WITH | COMBINED EFFECT |
|---|---|
| Alcohol: | None expected. |
| Beverages: | None expected. |
| Cocaine: | Overstimulation. |
| Foods: | None expected. |
| Marijuana: | Possible increased therapeutic effect of terbutaline. May cause lung disorders to worsen. |
| Tobacco: | No interactions expected, but smoking may slow body's recovery. Avoid. |

# TERFENADINE

## BRAND NAMES

Seldane    Vantac

## BASIC INFORMATION

**Habit forming? No**
**Prescription needed? No**
**Available as generic? No**
**Drug class: Antihistamine**

## USES

Reduces allergic symptoms such as hay fever, hives, rash or itching. Less likely to cause drowsiness than most other antihistamines.

## DOSAGE & USAGE INFORMATION

**How to take:**
Tablet—Swallow with water or food to lessen stomach irritation.

**When to take:**
Follow prescription instructions.

**If you forget a dose:**
Take as soon as you remember up to 2 hours late. If more than 2 hours, wait for next scheduled dose (don't double this dose).

**What drug does:**
Blocks effects of histamine, a chemical produced by the body as a result of contact with an allergen.

**Time lapse before drug works:**
1 to 2 hours; maximum effect at 3 to 4 hours.

**Don't take with:**
See Interaction column and consult doctor.

## OVERDOSE

**SYMPTOMS:**
Flushed face, hallucinations.
**WHAT TO DO:**
- Dial 0 (operator) or 911 (emergency) for an ambulance or medical help. Then give first aid immediately.
- See emergency information on inside covers.

## POSSIBLE ADVERSE REACTIONS OR SIDE EFFECTS

| SYMPTOMS | WHAT TO DO |
|---|---|
| **Life-threatening:** None expected. | |
| **Common:** None expected. | |
| **Infrequent:** None expected. | |
| **Rare:** | |
| • Swollen lips. | Discontinue. Seek emergency treatment. |
| • Rapid heart rate. | Discontinue. Call doctor right away. |
| • Nightmares, mild visual disturbances, nausea, vomiting, change in bowel habits, hair loss. | Continue. Call doctor when convenient. |
| • Depression, difficulty in falling asleep, sore throat, irregular heartbeat, frequent urination, mildly painful menstruation. | Continue. Tell doctor at next visit. |

## WARNINGS & PRECAUTIONS

**Don't take if:**
- You are allergic to terfenadine.
- You have urinary-tract blockage.

**Before you start, consult your doctor:**
- If you are allergic to other antihistamines.
- If you are under age 12.
- If you are allergic to any substance or any medicine.
- If you are pregnant or expect to become pregnant.
- If you have asthma.
- If you will have surgery within 2 months, including dental surgery, requiring general or spinal anesthesia.
- If you plan to have skin tests for allergies.

**Over age 60:**
Don't exceed recommended dose. Adverse reactions and side effects may be more frequent and severe than in younger persons, especially urination difficulty, diminished alertness and other brain and nervous-system symptoms.

**Pregnancy:**
No proven harm to unborn child. Avoid if possible.

**Breast-feeding:**
Drug passes into milk. Avoid drug or discontinue nursing until you finish medicine. Consult doctor for advice on maintaining milk supply.

**Infants & children:**
Not recommended for premature or newborn infants. Otherwise, no problems expected.

**Prolonged use:**
Avoid. May damage bone marrow and nerve cells.

**Skin & sunlight:**
May cause rash or intensify sunburn in areas exposed to sun or sunlamp.

**Driving, piloting or hazardous work:**
Don't drive or pilot aircraft until you learn how medicine affects you. Sedation and dizziness are less likely to occur with terfenadine than with other antihistamines.

**Discontinuing:**
No problems expected.

**Others:**
May mask symptoms of hearing damage from aspirin, other salicylates, cisplatin, paramomycin, vancomycin or anticonvulsants. Consult doctor if you use these.

## POSSIBLE INTERACTION WITH OTHER DRUGS

| GENERIC NAME OR DRUG CLASS | COMBINED EFFECT |
|---|---|
| Aspirin in large doses regularly | Terfenadine may conceal overdose of aspirin, such as ringing in the ears. |
| Anticholinergics | Possible increased anticholinergic effect. |
| Antidepressants | Possible increased side effects of antidepressants. |
| Antihistamines (other) | Possible oversedation. Avoid. |
| Hypnotics | Possible oversedation. |
| MAO inhibitors | Increased side effects of MAO inhibitors. |
| Molindone | Increased antihistamine effect. |
| Narcotics | Possible oversedation. |
| Sedatives | Possible oversedation. |
| Sleep Inducers | Possible oversedation. |
| Tranquilizers | Possible oversedation. |

## POSSIBLE INTERACTION WITH OTHER SUBSTANCES

| INTERACTS WITH | COMBINED EFFECT |
|---|---|
| Alcohol: | Possible oversedation. |
| Beverages: | None expected. |
| Cocaine: | Decreased terfenadine effect. |
| Foods: | None expected. |
| Marijuana: | None expected. |
| Tobacco: | None expected. |

# TERPIN HYDRATE

## BRAND NAMES

Cotussis
Prunicodeine
SK-Terpin Hydrate
  w/Codeine

Terpin Hydrate and
  Codeine Syrup
Terpin Hydrate Elixir

## BASIC INFORMATION

**Habit forming? Yes**
**Prescription needed? No**
**Available as generic? Yes**
**Drug class: Expectorant**

## USES

Decreases cough due to simple bronchial irritation.

## DOSAGE & USAGE INFORMATION

**How to take:**
Follow each dose with 8 oz. water. Works better in combination with a cool-air vaporizer.

**When to take:**
3 to 4 times each day, spaced at least 4 hours apart.

**If you forget a dose:**
Take as soon as you remember. Wait 4 hours for next dose.

**What drug does:**
Loosens mucus in bronchial tubes to make mucus easier to cough up.

**Time lapse before drug works:**
10 to 15 minutes.

**Don't take with:**
See Interaction column and consult doctor.

## OVERDOSE

**SYMPTOMS:**
**Nausea, drowsiness.**
**WHAT TO DO:**
**Overdose unlikely to threaten life. If person takes much larger amount than prescribed, call doctor, poison-control center or hospital emergency room for instructions.**

## POSSIBLE ADVERSE REACTIONS OR SIDE EFFECTS

| SYMPTOMS | WHAT TO DO |
|---|---|
| **Life-threatening:** None expected. | |
| **Common:** None expected. | |
| **Infrequent:** Nausea, vomiting, stomach pain. | Continue. Call doctor when convenient. |
| **Rare:** Symptoms of alcohol intoxication, especially in children. | Discontinue. Call doctor right away. |

## WARNINGS & PRECAUTIONS

**Don't take if:**
- You are allergic to terpin hydrate.
- You are a recovering or active alcoholic.

**Before you start, consult your doctor:**
If you plan to become pregnant within medication period.

**Over age 60:**
No problems expected.

**Pregnancy:**
Risk to unborn child outweighs drug benefits. Don't use.

**Breast-feeding:**
Drug filters into milk. May harm child. Avoid.

**Infants & children:**
Use only under medical supervision.

**Prolonged use:**
Habit forming.

**Skin & sunlight:**
No problems expected.

**Driving, piloting or hazardous work:**
Don't drive or pilot aircraft until you learn how medicine affects you. Don't work around dangerous machinery. Don't climb ladders or work in high places. Danger increases if you drink alcohol or take medicine affecting alertness and reflexes, such as antihistamines, tranquilizers, sedatives, pain medicine, narcotics and mind-altering drugs.

**Discontinuing:**
May be unnecessary to finish medicine. Follow doctor's instructions.

**Others:**
- Exceeding recommended doses may cause intoxication; drug is 42.5% alcohol.
- Frequently combined with codeine, which increases hazards.

## POSSIBLE INTERACTION WITH OTHER DRUGS

| GENERIC NAME OR DRUG CLASS | COMBINED EFFECT |
|---|---|
| Antidepressants | Increased effect of terpin hydrate. |
| Antihistamines | Increased effect of terpin hydrate. |
| Muscle relaxants | Increased effect of terpin hydrate. |
| Narcotics | Increased effect of terpin hydrate. |
| Sedatives | Increased effect of terpin hydrate. |
| Sleep inducers | Increased effect of terpin hydrate. |
| Tranquilizers | Increased effect of terpin hydrate. |

## POSSIBLE INTERACTION WITH OTHER SUBSTANCES

| INTERACTS WITH | COMBINED EFFECT |
|---|---|
| Alcohol: | Increased sedative effect of both drugs. Avoid. |
| Beverages: | None expected. |
| Cocaine: | Unpredictable effect on nervous system. Avoid. |
| Foods: | None expected. |
| Marijuana: | Unpredictable effect on nervous system. Avoid. |
| Tobacco: | None expected. |

# TESTOSTERONE & ESTRADIOL

## BRAND NAMES

See complete list of brand names in the *Brand Name Directory,* page 957.

## BASIC INFORMATION

**Habit forming? No**
**Prescription needed? Yes**
**Available as generic? No**
**Drug class: Androgens-estrogens**

## USES

- Prevents breast fullness in new mothers after childbirth.
- Relieves menopause symptoms such as unnecessary sweating, hot flashes, chills, faintness and dizziness.

## DOSAGE & USAGE INFORMATION

**How to take:**
Given by injection, deeply intramuscular.

**When to take:**
When directed.

**If you forget a dose:**
Check with your doctor.

**What drug does:**
- Restores normal estrogen level in tissues.
- Stimulates cells that produce male sex characteristics.
- Replaces hormone deficiencies.
- Stimulates red-blood-cell production.
- Suppresses production of estrogen.

**Time lapse before drug works:**
10 to 20 days.

**Don't take with:**
See Interaction column and consult doctor.

## OVERDOSE

**SYMPTOMS:**
**Nausea, vomiting, fluid retention, breast enlargement and discomfort, abnormal vaginal bleeding.**
**WHAT TO DO:**
**Overdose unlikely to threaten life. If person takes much larger amount than prescribed, call doctor, poison-control center or hospital emergency room for instructions.**

## POSSIBLE ADVERSE REACTIONS OR SIDE EFFECTS

| SYMPTOMS | WHAT TO DO |
|---|---|
| **Life-threatening:**<br>Hives, black stool, black or bloody vomit, intense itching, weakness, loss of consciousness. | Discontinue. Seek emergency treatment. |
| **Common:** | |
| • Red or flushed face; rash; swollen, tender breasts. | Discontinue. Call doctor right away. |
| • Depression, confusion, dizziness, irritability, acne or oily skin (females), enlarged clitoris, deepened voice, appetite loss, increased sex drive. | Continue. Call doctor when convenient. |
| **Infrequent:** | |
| • Nausea, vomiting, diarrhea, unusual vaginal bleeding or discharge. | Discontinue. Call doctor right away. |
| • Swollen feet and ankles, increased libido in some women. | Continue. Call doctor when convenient. |
| **Rare:** | |
| • Jaundice, abdominal pain. | Discontinue. Call doctor right away. |
| • Brown blotches on skin; hair loss; sore throat, fever, mouth sores. | Continue. Call doctor when convenient. |

## WARNINGS & PRECAUTIONS

**Don't take if:**
- You are allergic to any male hormone or any estrogen-containing drugs.
- You have impaired liver function.
- You have had blood clots, stroke or heart attack.
- You have unexplained vaginal bleeding.

**Before you start, consult your doctor:**
- If you might be pregnant or plan to become pregnant within 3 months.
- If you have heart disease, arteriosclerosis, diabetes, liver disease, high blood pressure, asthma, congestive heart failure, kidney disease or gallstones.
- If you have high level of blood calcium.
- If you have had migraine headaches, epilepsy or porphyria.
- If you have had cancer of breast or reproductive organs, fibrocystic breast disease, fibroid tumors of the uterus or endometriosis.

**Over age 60:**
- May stimulate sexual activity.
- Can make high blood pressure or heart disease worse.
- Controversial. You and your doctor must decide if drug risks outweigh benefits.

**Pregnancy:**
Risk to unborn child outweighs drug benefits. Don't use.

**Breast-feeding:**
Drug passes into milk. Avoid drug or discontinue nursing until you finish medicine. Consult doctor for advice on maintaining milk supply.

**Infants & children:**
Not recommended.

**Prolonged use:**
- Increased growth of fibroid tumors of uterus.
- Possible kidney stones.
- Unnatural hair growth and deep voice in women.

**Skin & sunlight:**
May cause rash or intensify sunburn in areas exposed to sun or sunlamp.

**Driving, piloting or hazardous work:**
No problems expected.

**Discontinuing:**
You may need to discontinue estrogens periodically. Consult your doctor.

**Others:**
- In rare instances, may cause blood clot in lung, brain or leg. Symptoms are *sudden* severe headache, coordination loss, vision change, chest pain, breathing difficulty, slurred speech, pain in legs or groin. Seek emergency treatment immediately.
- Will not increase strength in athletes.
- Read carefully the paper delivered with your prescription called "Information for the Patient."

## POSSIBLE INTERACTION WITH OTHER DRUGS

| GENERIC NAME OR DRUG CLASS | COMBINED EFFECT |
|---|---|
| Anticonvulsants (hydantoin) | Increased seizures. |
| Antidiabetics (oral) | Unpredictable increase or decrease in blood sugar. |
| Carbamazepine | Increased seizures. |
| Chlorzoxazone | Decreased androgen effect. |
| Clofibrate | Decreased clofibrate effect. |
| Meprobamate | Increased estrogen effect. |
| Oxyphenbutazone | Decreased androgen effect. |
| Phenobarbital | Decreased androgen and estrogen effect. |
| Phenylbutazone | Decreased androgen effect. |
| Primidone | Decreased estrogen effect. |
| Rifampin | Decreased estrogen effect. |
| Thyroid hormones | Decreased thyroid effect. |

## POSSIBLE INTERACTION WITH OTHER SUBSTANCES

| INTERACTS WITH | COMBINED EFFECT |
|---|---|
| Alcohol: | None expected. |
| Beverages: | None expected. |
| Cocaine: | No proven problems. |
| Foods: Salt. | Excessive fluid retention (edema). Decrease salt intake while taking male hormones. |
| Marijuana: | Decreased blood levels of androgens. Possible menstrual irregularities and bleeding between periods. |
| Tobacco: | Increased risk of blood clots leading to stroke or heart attack. |

## BRAND AND GENERIC NAMES

See complete list of brand and generic names in the *Brand Name Directory,* page 958.

## BASIC INFORMATION

**Habit forming? No**
**Prescription needed? Yes**
**Available as generic? Yes**
**Drug class: Antibiotic (tetracycline)**

## USES

- Treatment for infections susceptible to any tetracycline. Will not cure virus infections such as colds or flu.
- Treatment for acne.

## DOSAGE & USAGE INFORMATION

**How to take:**
- Tablet or capsule—Take on empty stomach 1 hour before or 2 hours after eating. If you can't swallow whole, crumble tablet or open capsule and take with liquid or food.
- Liquid—Shake well. Take with measuring spoon.

**When to take:**
At the same times each day, evenly spaced.

**If you forget a dose:**
Take as soon as you remember up to 2 hours late. If more than 2 hours, wait for next scheduled dose (don't double this dose).

**What drug does:**
Prevents germ growth and reproduction.

**Time lapse before drug works:**
- Infections—May require 5 days to affect infection.
- Acne—May require 4 weeks to affect acne.

**Don't take with:**
- Non-prescription drugs without consulting doctor.
- See Interaction column and consult doctor.

## OVERDOSE

**SYMPTOMS:**
**Severe nausea, vomiting, diarrhea.**
**WHAT TO DO:**
**Overdose unlikely to threaten life. If person takes much larger amount than prescribed, call doctor, poison-control center or hospital emergency room for instructions.**

## POSSIBLE ADVERSE REACTIONS OR SIDE EFFECTS

| SYMPTOMS | WHAT TO DO |
|---|---|
| **Life-threatening:** | |
| None expected. | |
| **Common:** | |
| • Sore mouth or tongue, nausea, vomiting, diarrhea, abdominal burning. | Discontinue. Seek emergency treatment. |
| • Itching around rectum and genitals. | Discontinue. Call doctor right away. |
| • Dark tongue. | Continue. Tell doctor at next visit. |
| **Infrequent:** | |
| • Headache, rash. | Discontinue. Call doctor right away. |
| • Excessive thirst, increased urination. | Continue. Call doctor when convenient. |
| **Rare:** | |
| Blurred vision, jaundice. | Discontinue. Call doctor right away. |

## WARNINGS & PRECAUTIONS

**Don't take if:**
You are allergic to any tetracycline antibiotic.

**Before you start, consult your doctor:**
● If you have kidney or liver disease.
● If you have lupus.
● If you have myasthenia gravis.

**Over age 60:**
Dosage usually less than in younger adults.
More likely to cause itching around rectum. Ask your doctor how to prevent it.

**Pregnancy:**
Risk to unborn child outweighs drug benefits.
Don't use.

**Breast-feeding:**
Drug passes into milk. Avoid drug or discontinue nursing until you finish medicine.
Consult doctor for advice on maintaining milk supply.

**Infants & children:**
May cause permanent teeth malformation or discoloration in children less than 8 years old.
Don't use.

**Prolonged use:**
● You may become more susceptible to infections caused by germs not responsive to tetracycline.
● May cause rare problems in liver, kidney or bone marrow. Periodic laboratory blood studies, liver- and kidney-function tests recommended if you use drug a long time.

**Skin & sunlight:**
May cause rash or intensify sunburn in areas exposed to sun or sunlamp.

**Driving, piloting or hazardous work:**
No problems expected.

**Discontinuing:**
Don't discontinue without doctor's advice until you complete prescribed dose, even though symptoms diminish or disappear.

**Others:**
No problems expected.

## POSSIBLE INTERACTION WITH OTHER DRUGS

| GENERIC NAME OR DRUG CLASS | COMBINED EFFECT |
|---|---|
| Antacids | Decreased tetracycline effect. |
| Anticoagulants (oral) | Increased anticoagulant effect. |
| Calcium supplements | Decreased tetracycline effect. |
| Contraceptives (oral) | Decreased contraceptive effect. |
| Digitalis preparations | Increased digitalis effect. |
| Lithium | Increased lithium effect. |
| Mineral supplements (iron, calcium, magnesium, zinc) | Decreased tetracycline absorption. Separate doses by 1 to 2 hours. |
| Penicillins | Decreased penicillin effect. |
| Sodium bicarbonate | Decreased tetracycline effect. |

## POSSIBLE INTERACTION WITH OTHER SUBSTANCES

| INTERACTS WITH | COMBINED EFFECT |
|---|---|
| Alcohol: | Possible liver damage. Avoid. |
| Beverages: Milk. | Decreased tetracycline absorption. Take dose 2 hours after or 1 hour before drinking. |
| Cocaine: | No proven problems. |
| Foods: Dairy products. | Decreased tetracycline absorption. Take dose 2 hours after or 1 hour before eating. |
| Marijuana: | No interactions expected, but marijuana may slow body's recovery. Avoid. |
| Tobacco: | None expected. |

# THEOPHYLLINE, EPHEDRINE & BARBITURATES

## BRAND NAMES

| | |
|---|---|
| Azma Aid | T.E.P. |
| Ephenyllin | Thalfed |
| Lardet | Theocord |
| Primatene "P" | Theodrine |
| Formula | Theofedral |
| Tedral | Theophenyllin |
| Tedral SA | Theoral |

## BASIC INFORMATION

**Habit forming? Yes**
**Prescription needed? Some yes, others no**
**Available as generic? Some yes, others no**
**Drug class: Bronchodilator,**
**sympathomimetic, barbiturate,**
**sedative**

## USES

- Treatment for bronchial asthma symptoms.
- Decreases congestion of breathing passages.
- Suppresses allergic reactions.
- Reduces anxiety or nervous tension (low dose).

## DOSAGE & USAGE INFORMATION

**How to take:**
- Tablet or capsule—Swallow with liquid.
- Extended-release tablets or capsules—Swallow each dose whole. If you take regular tablets, you may chew or crush them

**When to take:**
Most effective taken on empty stomach 1 hour before or 2 hours after eating. However, may take with food to lessen stomach upset.

*Continued next column*

## OVERDOSE

**SYMPTOMS:**
**Restlessness, irritability, anxiety, confusion, delirium, muscle tremors, convulsions, rapid and irregular pulse, coma.**
**WHAT TO DO:**
- **Dial 0 (operator) or 911 (emergency) for an ambulance or medical help. Then give first aid immediately.**
- **See emergency information on inside covers.**

## If you forget a dose:
Take as soon as you remember up to 2 hours late. If more than 2 hours, wait for next scheduled dose (don't double this dose).

## What drug does:
- Relaxes and expands bronchial tubes.
- Prevents cells from releasing allergy-causing chemicals (histamines).
- Decreases blood-vessel size and blood flow, thus causing decongestion.
- May partially block nerve impulses at nerve-cell connections.

## Time lapse before drug works:
15 to 30 minutes.

## Don't take with:
- See Interaction column and consult doctor.
- Non-prescription drugs with ephedrine, pseudoephedrine or epinephrine.
- Non-prescription drugs for cough, cold, allergy or asthma without consulting doctor.

## POSSIBLE ADVERSE REACTIONS OR SIDE EFFECTS

| SYMPTOMS | WHAT TO DO |
|---|---|
| **Life-threatening:**<br>Difficult breathing, uncontrollable rapid heart rate, loss of consciousness. | Discontinue. Seek emergency treatment. |
| **Common:** | |
| • Headache, irritability, nervousness, restlessness, insomnia, nausea, vomiting, abdominal pain, "hangover" effect. | Discontinue. Call doctor right away. |
| • Dizziness, lightheadedness, paleness, irregular heartbeat. | Continue. Call doctor when convenient. |
| **Infrequent:** | |
| • Rash; hives; red or flushed face; appetite loss; diarrhea; cough; confusion; slurred speech; eyelid, face, lip swelling; joint pain. | Discontinue. Call doctor right away. |
| • Frequent urination. | Continue. Call doctor when convenient. |
| **Rare:**<br>Agitation; sore throat, fever, mouth sores; jaundice. | Discontinue. Call doctor right away. |

# THEOPHYLLINE, EPHEDRINE & BARBITURATES

## WARNINGS & PRECAUTIONS

### Don't take if:
- You are allergic to any bronchodilator or barbiturate.
- You are allergic to ephedrine or any sympathomimetic drug.
- You have an active peptic ulcer or porphyria.

### Before you start, consult your doctor:
- If you have gastritis, peptic ulcer, high blood pressure or heart disease, diabetes, overactive thyroid gland, difficulty urinating, epilepsy, kidney or liver damage, asthma, anemia, chronic pain, taken any MAO inhibitor in past 2 weeks, taken digitalis preparations in the last 7 days.
- If you have had impaired kidney or liver function.
- If you take medication for gout.
- If you will have surgery within 2 months, including dental surgery, requiring general or spinal anesthesia.

### Over age 60:
- Adverse reactions and side effects may be more frequent and severe than in younger persons. Use small doses.
- More likely to develop high blood pressure, heart-rhythm disturbances, angina and to feel drug's stimulant effects.

### Pregnancy:
Risk to unborn child outweighs drug benefits. Don't use.

### Breast-feeding:
Drug passes into milk. Avoid drug or discontinue nursing until you finish medicine.

### Infants & children:
Use only under medical supervision.

### Prolonged use:
- Stomach irritation.
- Excessive doses—Rare toxic psychosis.
- Men with enlarged prostate gland may have more urination difficulty.
- May cause addiction, anemia, chronic intoxication.
- May lower body temperature, making exposure to cold temperatures hazardous.

### Skin & sunlight:
May cause rash or intensify sunburn in areas exposed to sun or sunlamp.

### Driving, piloting or hazardous work:
Don't drive or pilot aircraft until you learn how medicine affects you. Don't work around dangerous machinery. Don't climb ladders or work in high places. Danger increases if you drink alcohol or take medicine affecting alertness and reflexes.

### Discontinuing:
- May be unnecessary to finish medicine. Follow doctor's instructions.
- If you develop withdrawal symptoms of hallucinations, agitation or sleeplessness after discontinuing, call doctor right away.

### Others:
Potential for abuse.

## POSSIBLE INTERACTION WITH OTHER DRUGS

| GENERIC NAME OR DRUG CLASS | COMBINED EFFECT |
|---|---|
| Allopurinol | Decreased allopurinol effect. |
| Anticoagulants (oral) | Decreased anticoagulant effect. |
| Anticonvulsants | Changed seizure patterns. |
| Antidepressants (tricyclics) | Decreased antidepressant effect. Possible dangerous oversedation. |
| Antidiabetics (oral) | Increased phenobarbital effect. |
| Antihistamines | Dangerous sedation. Avoid. |

*Continued page 976*

## POSSIBLE INTERACTION WITH OTHER SUBSTANCES

| INTERACTS WITH | COMBINED EFFECT |
|---|---|
| Alcohol: | Possible fatal oversedation. Avoid. |
| Beverages: Caffeine drinks. | Nervousness or insomnia. |
| Cocaine: | Rapid heartbeat. Avoid. |
| Foods: | None expected. |
| Marijuana: | Rapid heartbeat, possible heart-rhythm disturbance. |
| Tobacco: | Decreased bronchodilator effect. |

# THEOPHYLLINE, EPHEDRINE, GUAIFENESIN & BARBITURATES

## BRAND NAMES

Bronkolixir
Bronkotabr
Guaiaphed

Lardet Expectorant
Mudrane GG
Quibron Plus

## BASIC INFORMATION

**Habit forming?** Yes (barbiturates)
**Prescription needed?** Yes
**Available as generic?** No
**Drug class:** Bronchodilator (xanthine), cough/cold preparation, sympathomimetic, sedative

 **USES**

- Treatment for symptoms of bronchial asthma, emphysema, chronic bronchitis.
- Relieves wheezing, coughing and shortness of breath.

 **DOSAGE & USAGE INFORMATION**

**How to take:**
- Tablet or capsule—Swallow with liquid.
- Extended-release tablets or capsules—Swallow each dose whole. If you take regular tablets, you may chew or crush them.

**When to take:**
Most effective taken on empty stomach 1 hour before or 2 hours after eating. However, may take with food to lessen stomach upset.

*Continued next column*

 **OVERDOSE**

**SYMPTOMS:**
**Restlessness, irritability, confusion, muscle tremors, severe anxiety, rapid and irregular pulse, mild weakness, nausea, vomiting, delirium, coma.**
**WHAT TO DO:**
- **Overdose unlikely to threaten life. Depending on severity of symptoms and amount taken, call doctor, poison-control center or hospital emergency room for instructions.**
- **Dial 0 (operator) or 911 (emergency) for an ambulance or medical help. Then give first aid immediately.**
- **See emergency information on inside covers.**

**If you forget a dose:**
Take as soon as you remember up to 2 hours late. If more than 2 hours, wait for next scheduled dose (don't double this dose).

**What drug does:**
- Relaxes and expands bronchial tubes.
- Prevents cells from releasing allergy-causing chemicals (histamines).
- Relaxes muscles of bronchial tubes.
- Decreases blood-vessel size and blood flow, thus causing decongestion.
- Increases production of watery fluids to thin mucus so it can be coughed out or absorbed.
- May partially block nerve impulses at nerve-cell connections.

**Time lapse before drug works:**
30 to 60 minutes.

**Don't take with:**
- Non-prescription drugs with ephedrine, pseudoephedrine or epinephrine.
- Non-prescription drugs for cough, cold, allergy or asthma without consulting doctor.
- See Interaction column and consult doctor.

 **POSSIBLE ADVERSE REACTIONS OR SIDE EFFECTS**

| SYMPTOMS | WHAT TO DO |
|---|---|
| **Life-threatening:** | |
| Difficult breathing, uncontrollable rapid heart rate, loss of consciousness. | Discontinue. Seek emergency treatment. |
| **Common:** | |
| • Headache, irritability, nervousness, restlessness, insomnia, nausea, vomiting, abdominal pain. | Discontinue. Call doctor right away. |
| • Dizziness, lightheadedness, paleness, irregular heartbeat. | Continue. Call doctor when convenient. |
| **Infrequent:** | |
| • Skin rash or hives, red or flushed face, appetite loss, diarrhea, abdominal pain. | Discontinue. Call doctor right away. |
| • Frequent urination. | Continue. Call doctor when convenient. |
| **Rare:** | |
| None expected. | |

# THEOPHYLLINE, EPHEDRINE, GUAIFENESIN & BARBITURATES

## WARNINGS & PRECAUTIONS

**Don't take if:**
- You are allergic to any bronchodilator, ephedrine, any sympathomimetic drug, cough or cold preparation containing guaifenesin.
- You have an active peptic ulcer.

**Before you start, consult your doctor:**
- If you have had impaired kidney or liver function.
- If you have gastritis, peptic ulcer, high blood pressure, heart disease, diabetes, overactive thyroid gland, difficulty urinating, epilepsy, anemia, chronic pain, taken any MAO inhibitor in past 2 weeks, taken digitalis preparations in the last 7 days.
- If you take medication for gout.
- If you will have surgery within 2 months, including dental surgery, requiring general or spinal anesthesia.

**Over age 60:**
- Adverse reactions and side effects may be more frequent and severe than in younger persons. Use small doses. For drug to work, you must drink 8 to 10 glasses of fluid per day.
- More likely to develop high blood pressure, heart-rhythm disturbances, angina and to feel drug's stimulant effects.

**Pregnancy:**
Risk to unborn child outweighs drug benefits. Don't use.

**Breast-feeding:**
Drug passes into milk. Avoid drug or discontinue nursing until you finish medicine. Consult doctor for advice on maintaining milk supply.

**Infants & children:**
Use only under medical supervision.

**Prolonged use:**
- Stomach irritation.
- Excessive doses—Rare toxic psychosis.
- Men with enlarged prostate gland may have more urination difficulty.
- May cause addiction, anemia, chronic intoxication.
- May lower body temperature, making exposure to cold temperature hazardous.

**Skin & sunlight:**
May cause rash or intensify sunburn in areas exposed to sun or sunlamp.

**Driving, piloting or hazardous work:**
Don't drive or pilot aircraft until you learn how medicine affects you. Don't work around dangerous machinery. Don't climb ladders or work in high places. Danger increases if you drink alcohol or take medicine affecting alertness and reflexes, such as antihistamines, tranquilizers, sedatives, pain medicine, narcotics and mind-altering drugs.

**Discontinuing:**
- May be unnecessary to finish medicine. Follow doctor's instructions.
- If you develop withdrawal symptoms of hallucinations, agitation or sleeplessness after discontinuing, call doctor right away.

**Others:**
Great potential for abuse.

## POSSIBLE INTERACTION WITH OTHER DRUGS

| GENERIC NAME OR DRUG CLASS | COMBINED EFFECT |
|---|---|
| Allopurinol | Decreased allopurinol effect. |
| Anticonvulsants | Changed seizure patterns. |

*Continued page 977*

## POSSIBLE INTERACTION WITH OTHER SUBSTANCES

| INTERACTS WITH | COMBINED EFFECT |
|---|---|
| Alcohol: | Possible fatal oversedation. Avoid. |
| Beverages:<br><br>Caffeine drinks. | You must drink 8 to 10 glasses of fluid per day for drug to work. Nervousness and insomnia. |
| Cocaine: | Rapid heartbeat. Excess stimulation. Avoid. |
| Foods: | None expected. |
| Marijuana: | Excessive sedation, rapid heartbeat, possible heart-rhythm disturbance. Avoid. |
| Tobacco: | Decreased bronchodilator effect. Smoking is damaging to all problems this medicine treats. Avoid. |

# THEOPHYLLINE, EPHEDRINE & HYDROXYZINE

## BRAND NAMES

| | |
|---|---|
| Brophed | Marax D.F. |
| Hydromax | Moxy Compound |
| Hydrophed | T.E.H. Compound |
| Marax | Theozine |

## BASIC INFORMATION

**Habit forming? No**
**Prescription needed? Yes**
**Available as generic? No**
**Drug class: Bronchodilator (xanthine), sympathomimetic, antihistamine, tranquilizer**

## USES

- Treatment for symptoms of bronchial asthma, emphysema, chronic bronchitis.
- Relieves wheezing, coughing and shortness of breath.

## DOSAGE & USAGE INFORMATION

**How to take:**
- Tablet or capsule—Swallow with liquid.
- Extended-release tablets or capsules—Swallow each dose whole. If you take regular tablets, you may chew or crush them.

**When to take:**
Most effective taken on empty stomach 1 hour before or 2 hours after eating. However, may take with food to lessen stomach upset.

**If you forget a dose:**
Take as soon as you remember up to 2 hours late. If more than 2 hours, wait for next scheduled dose (don't double this dose).

*Continued next column*

## OVERDOSE

**SYMPTOMS:**
**Restlessness, irritability, confusion, severe anxiety, muscle tremors, rapid and irregular pulse, agitation, purposeless movements, delirium, convulsions, coma.**
**WHAT TO DO:**
- **Dial 0 (operator) or 911 (emergency) for an ambulance or medical help. Then give first aid immediately.**
- **See emergency information on inside covers.**

## What drug does:
- Relaxes and expands bronchial tubes.
- Prevents cells from releasing allergy-causing chemicals (histamines).
- Relaxes muscles of bronchial tubes.
- Decreases blood-vessel size and blood flow, thus causing decongestion.
- May reduce activity in areas of the brain that influence emotional stability.

## Time lapse before drug works:
15 to 60 minutes.

## Don't take with:
- Non-prescription drugs with ephedrine, pseudoephedrine or epinephrine.
- Non-prescription drugs for cough, cold, allergy or asthma without consulting doctor.
- See Interaction column and consult doctor.

## POSSIBLE ADVERSE REACTIONS OR SIDE EFFECTS

| SYMPTOMS | WHAT TO DO |
|---|---|
| **Life-threatening:** | |
| Difficult breathing, uncontrollable rapid heart rate, loss of consciousness. | Discontinue. Seek emergency treatment. |
| **Common:** | |
| • Headache, irritability, nervousness, restlessness, insomnia, nausea, vomiting, abdominal pain. | Discontinue. Call doctor right away. |
| • Dizziness, lightheadedness, paleness, irregular heartbeat. | Continue. Call doctor when convenient. |
| **Infrequent:** | |
| • Skin rash or hives, red or flushed face, appetite loss, diarrhea, abdominal pain. | Discontinue. Call doctor right away. |
| • Frequent urination. | Continue. Call doctor when convenient. |
| **Rare:** | |
| Tremor. | Discontinue. Call doctor right away. |

## WARNINGS & PRECAUTIONS

**Don't take if:**
- You are allergic to any bronchodilator, ephedrine, any sympathomimetic drug, or antihistamine.
- You have an active peptic ulcer.

**Before you start, consult your doctor:**
- If you have had impaired kidney or liver function.
- If you have gastritis, peptic ulcer, high blood pressure, heart disease, diabetes, overactive thyroid gland, difficulty urinating, epilepsy, taken any MAO inhibitor in past 2 weeks, taken digitalis preparations in the last 7 days.
- If you take medication for gout.
- If you will have surgery within 2 months, including dental surgery, requiring general or spinal anesthesia.

**Over age 60:**
- Adverse reactions and side effects may be more frequent and severe than in younger persons.
- More likely to develop increased urination difficulty, high blood pressure, heart-rhythm disturbances, angina and to feel drug's stimulant effects.

**Pregnancy:**
Risk to unborn child outweighs drug benefits. Don't use.

**Breast-feeding:**
Drug passes into milk. Avoid drug or discontinue nursing until you finish medicine. Consult doctor for advice on maintaining milk supply.

**Infants & children:**
Use only under medical supervision.

**Prolonged use:**
- Stomach irritation.
- Excessive doses—Rare toxic psychosis.
- Men with enlarged prostate gland may have more urination difficulty.
- Tolerance develops and reduces effectiveness.

**Skin & sunlight:**
No problems expected.

**Driving, piloting or hazardous work:**
Don't drive or pilot aircraft until you learn how medicine affects you. Don't work around dangerous machinery. Don't climb ladders or work in high places. Danger increases if you drink alcohol or take medicine affecting alertness and reflexes, such as antihistamines, tranquilizers, sedatives, pain medicine, narcotics and mind-altering drugs.

**Discontinuing:**
Don't discontinue without consulting doctor. Dose may require gradual reduction if you have taken drug for a long time. Doses of other drugs may also require adjustment.

**Others:**
No problems expected.

## POSSIBLE INTERACTION WITH OTHER DRUGS

| GENERIC NAME OR DRUG CLASS | COMBINED EFFECT |
|---|---|
| Allopurinol | Decreased allopurinol effect. |
| Anticoagulants (oral) | Increased anticoagulant effect. |
| Anticonvulsants (hydantoin) | Decreased anticonvulsant effect. |
| Antidepressants (tricyclics) | Increased effect of ephedrine. Excess stimulation of heart and blood pressure. |
| Antihistamines | Increased hydroxyzine effect. |
| Antihypertensives | Decreased antihypertensive effect. |

*Continued page 978*

## POSSIBLE INTERACTION WITH OTHER SUBSTANCES

| INTERACTS WITH | COMBINED EFFECT |
|---|---|
| Alcohol: | Increased sedation and intoxication. Avoid. |
| Beverages: Caffeine drinks. | Nervousness and insomnia. |
| Cocaine: | Excess stimulation and rapid heartbeat. Avoid. |
| Foods: | None expected. |
| Marijuana: | Slightly increased antiasthmatic effect of bronchodilator. Rapid heartbeat, possible heart-rhythm disturbance. |
| Tobacco: | Decreased bronchodilator effect. Smoking is damaging to all problems this medicine treats. Avoid. |

# THEOPHYLLINE & GUAIFENESIN

## BRAND NAMES

| | |
|---|---|
| Asbcon G Inlay Tabs | Slo-Phyllin GG |
| Bronchial | Syncophylate-GG |
| Elixophyllin-GG | Theocolate |
| Glycery T | Theolair-Plus |
| Lanophyllin-GG | Theolate |
| Quibron | |

## BASIC INFORMATION

**Habit forming? No**
**Prescription needed? Yes**
**Available as generic? No**
**Drug class: Bronchodilator, expectorant**

 ## USES

- Treatment for bronchial asthma symptoms.
- Loosens mucus in respiratory passages.
- Relieves coughing, wheezing, shortness of breath.

 ## DOSAGE & USAGE INFORMATION

**How to take:**
- Tablet or capsule—Swallow with liquid.
- Extended-release tablets or capsules—Swallow each dose whole. If you take regular tablets, you may chew or crush them.

**When to take:**
Most effective taken on empty stomach 1 hour before or 2 hours after eating. However, may take with food to lessen stomach upset.

**If you forget a dose:**
Take as soon as you remember up to 2 hours late. If more than 2 hours, wait for next scheduled dose (don't double this dose).

*Continued next column*

 ## OVERDOSE

**SYMPTOMS:**
**Restlessness, irritability, confusion, drowsiness, mild weakness, nausea, vomiting, delirium, convulsions, rapid pulse, coma.**
**WHAT TO DO:**
- **Dial 0 (operator) or 911 (emergency) for an ambulance or medical help. Then give first aid immediately.**
- **See emergency information on inside covers.**

**What drug does:**
- Relaxes and expands bronchial tubes.
- Increases production of watery fluids to thin mucus so it can be coughed out or absorbed.

**Time lapse before drug works:**
15 to 30 minutes.

**Don't take with:**
See Interaction column and consult doctor.

 ## POSSIBLE ADVERSE REACTIONS OR SIDE EFFECTS

| SYMPTOMS | WHAT TO DO |
|---|---|
| **Life-threatening:**<br>Difficult breathing, uncontrollable heart rate, loss of consciousness. | Discontinue. Seek emergency treatment. |
| **Common:**<br>• Headache, irritability, nervousness, restlessness, insomnia, drowsiness, nausea, vomiting, abdominal pain. | Discontinue. Call doctor right away. |
| • Dizziness, lightheadedness, diarrhea, abdominal pain. | Continue. Call doctor when convenient. |
| **Infrequent:**<br>Skin rash or hives, red or flushed face, appetite loss, diarrhea. | Discontinue. Call doctor right away. |
| **Rare:**<br>None expected. | |

## WARNINGS & PRECAUTIONS

**Don't take if:**
- You are allergic to any bronchodilator or cough or cold preparation containing guaifenesin.
- You have an active peptic ulcer.

**Before you start, consult your doctor:**
- If you have had impaired kidney or liver function.
- If you have gastritis, peptic ulcer, high blood pressure or heart disease.
- If you take medication for gout.

**Over age 60:**
Adverse reactions and side effects may be more frequent and severe than in younger persons. For drug to work, you must drink 8 to 10 glasses of fluid per day.

**Pregnancy:**
Risk to unborn child outweighs drug benefits. Don't use.

**Breast-feeding:**
Drug passes into milk. Avoid drug or discontinue nursing until you finish medicine. Consult doctor for advice on maintaining milk supply.

**Infants & children:**
Use only under medical supervision.

**Prolonged use:**
Stomach irritation.

**Skin & sunlight:**
No problems expected.

**Driving, piloting or hazardous work:**
Avoid if lightheaded, drowsy or dizzy. Otherwise, no problems expected.

**Discontinuing:**
May be unnecessary to finish medicine. Follow doctor's instructions.

**Others:**
No problems expected.

## POSSIBLE INTERACTION WITH OTHER DRUGS

| GENERIC NAME OR DRUG CLASS | COMBINED EFFECT |
|---|---|
| Allopurinol | Decreased allopurinol effect. |
| Anticoagulants | Risk of bleeding. |
| Ephedrine | Increased effect of both drugs. |
| Epinephrine | Increased effect of both drugs. |
| Erythromycin | Increased bronchodilator effect. |
| Furosemide | Increased furosemide effect. |
| Lincomycins | Increased bronchodilator effect. |
| Lithium | Decreased lithium effect. |
| Probenecid | Decreased effect of both drugs. |
| Propranolol | Decreased bronchodilator effect. |
| Rauwolfia alkaloids | Rapid heartbeat. |
| Sulfinpyrazone | Decreased sulfinpyrazone effect. |
| Troleandomycin | Increased bronchodilator effect. |

## POSSIBLE INTERACTION WITH OTHER SUBSTANCES

| INTERACTS WITH | COMBINED EFFECT |
|---|---|
| Alcohol: | No proven problems. |
| Beverages: | You must drink 8 to 10 glasses of fluid per day for drug to work. |
| Caffeine drinks. | Nervousness and insomnia. |
| Cocaine: | Excess stimulation. Avoid. |
| Foods: | None expected. |
| Marijuana: | Slightly increased antiasthmatic effect of bronchodilator. |
| Tobacco: | Decreased bronchodilator effect. Cigarette smoking makes worse all problems that this medicine treats. Avoid. |

# THIABENDAZOLE

## BRAND NAMES

Foldan
Mintezol
Mintezol (Topical)

Minzolum
Triasox

## BASIC INFORMATION

**Habit forming?** No
**Prescription needed?** Yes
**Available as generic?** No
**Drug class:** Antihelminthic (antiworm medication)

## USES

Treatment of parasite infestations.

## DOSAGE & USAGE INFORMATION

**How to take or apply:**
- Tablet or capsule—Swallow with liquid or food to lessen stomach irritation.
- Topical suspension—Apply to end of each tunnel or burrow made by worm.

**When to take or apply:**
- Tablet or capsule—According to instructions on prescription, after meals.
- Topical—2 to 4 times daily up to 14 days.

**If you forget a dose:**
Take as soon as you remember up to 2 hours late. If more than 2 hours, wait for next scheduled dose (don't double this dose).

**What drug does:**
Kills larvae and adult worms.

*Continued next column*

## OVERDOSE

**SYMPTOMS:**
Aching, fever, blistered skin, seizures.
**WHAT TO DO:**
- Dial 0 (operator) or 911 (emergency) for an ambulance or medical help. Then give first aid immediately.
- If patient is unconscious and not breathing, give mouth-to-mouth breathing. If there is no heartbeat, use cardiac massage and mouth-to-mouth breathing (CPR). Don't try to make patient vomit. If you can't get help quickly, take patient to nearest emergency facility.
- See emergency information on inside covers.

**Time lapse before drug works:**
Varies according to degree of infestation.

**Don't take with:**
See Interaction column and consult doctor.

## POSSIBLE ADVERSE REACTIONS OR SIDE EFFECTS

| SYMPTOMS | WHAT TO DO |
|---|---|
| **Life-threatening:** | |
| None expected. | |
| **Common:** | |
| • Nausea, vomiting, abdominal pain. | Discontinue. Call doctor right away. |
| • Dizziness, drowsiness, head-ache, nausea, appetite loss, bedwetting. | Continue. Call doctor when convenient. |
| • Asparagus-like odor of urine. | Continue. Tell doctor at next visit. |
| **Infrequent:** | |
| • Redness, blistering with fever, rash with itchy skin, aching joints and muscles. | Discontinue. Call doctor right away. |
| • Ringing or buzzing in ears, numbness or tingling in hands and feet. | Continue. Call doctor when convenient. |
| **Rare:** | |
| Blurred or yellow vision. | Discontinue. Call doctor right away. |

## WARNINGS & PRECAUTIONS

**Don't take if:**
You are allergic to thiabendazole.

**Before you start, consult your doctor:**
- If you have kidney disease.
- If you have liver disease.

**Over age 60:**
Adverse reactions and side effects may be more frequent and severe than in younger persons.

**Pregnancy:**
Risk to unborn child outweighs drug benefits. Don't use.

**Breast-feeding:**
Unknown effect. Consult doctor.

**Infants & children:**
Use only under medical supervision.

**Prolonged use:**
Request follow-up stool exams 2 to 3 weeks following treatment.

**Skin & sunlight:**
No problems expected.

**Driving, piloting or hazardous work:**
Don't drive or pilot aircraft until you learn how medicine affects you. Don't work around dangerous machinery. Don't climb ladders or work in high places. Danger increases if you drink alcohol or take medicine affecting alertness and reflexes, such as antihistamines, tranquilizers, sedatives, pain medicine, narcotics and mind-altering drugs.

**Discontinuing:**
May be unnecessary to finish medicine. Follow doctor's instructions.

**Others:**
To prevent reinfection: Deworm household pets regularly. Cover sand boxes. Cook all pork until well done.

## POSSIBLE INTERACTION WITH OTHER DRUGS

| GENERIC NAME OR DRUG CLASS | COMBINED EFFECT |
|---|---|
| None expected. | |

## POSSIBLE INTERACTION WITH OTHER SUBSTANCES

| INTERACTS WITH | COMBINED EFFECT |
|---|---|
| Alcohol: | Decreased thiabendazole effect. |
| Beverages: | No problems expected. |
| Cocaine: | Decreased thiabendazole effect. |
| Foods: | Take with foods to decrease nausea. |
| Marijuana: | Decreased thiabendazole effect. |
| Tobacco: | May decrease absorption of medicine. |

# THIAMINE (VITAMIN B-1)

## BRAND NAMES

Betalin S      Biamine
Betaxin      Pan-B-1
Bewon
**Numerous other multiple vitamin-mineral supplements.**

## BASIC INFORMATION

**Habit forming? No**
**Prescription needed? No**
**Available as generic? Yes**
**Drug class: Vitamin supplement**

## USES

- Dietary supplement to promote normal growth, development and health.
- Treatment for beri-beri (a thiamine-deficiency disease).
- Dietary supplement for alcoholism, cirrhosis, overactive thyroid, infection, breast-feeding, absorption diseases, pregnancy, prolonged diarrhea, burns.

## DOSAGE & USAGE INFORMATION

**How to take:**
Tablet or liquid—Swallow with beverage or food to lessen stomach irritation.

**When to take:**
At the same time each day.

**If you forget a dose:**
Take when remembered. Return to regular schedule.

**What drug does:**
- Promotes normal growth and development.
- Combines with an enzyme to metabolize carbohydrates.

**Time lapse before drug works:**
15 minutes.

**Don't take with:**
See Interaction column and consult doctor.

## OVERDOSE

**SYMPTOMS:**
**Increased severity of adverse reactions and side effects.**
**WHAT TO DO:**
**Overdose unlikely to threaten life. If person takes much larger amount than prescribed, call doctor, poison-control center or hospital emergency room for instructions.**

## POSSIBLE ADVERSE REACTIONS OR SIDE EFFECTS

| SYMPTOMS | WHAT TO DO |
|---|---|
| **Life-threatening:** | |
| Hives, rash, intense itching, faintness soon after a dose (anaphylaxis). | Seek emergency treatment immediately. |
| **Common:** | |
| None expected. | |
| **Infrequent:** | |
| None expected. | |
| **Rare:** | |
| • Wheezing. | Discontinue. Seek emergency treatment. |
| • Rash or itchy skin. | Discontinue. Call doctor right away. |

# THIAMINE (VITAMIN B-1)

## WARNINGS & PRECAUTIONS

**Don't take if:**
You are allergic to any B vitamin.

**Before you start, consult your doctor:**
If you have liver or kidney disease.

**Over age 60:**
No problems expected.

**Pregnancy:**
No problems expected.

**Breast-feeding:**
No problems expected.

**Infants & children:**
No problems expected.

**Prolonged use:**
No problems expected.

**Skin & sunlight:**
No problems expected.

**Driving, piloting or hazardous work:**
No problems expected.

**Discontinuing:**
No problems expected.

**Others:**
A balanced diet should provide enough thiamine for healthy people to make supplement unnecessary. Best dietary sources of thiamine are whole-grain cereals and meats.

## POSSIBLE INTERACTION WITH OTHER DRUGS

| GENERIC NAME OR DRUG CLASS | COMBINED EFFECT |
|---|---|
| Barbiturates | Decreased thiamine effect. |

## POSSIBLE INTERACTION WITH OTHER SUBSTANCES

| INTERACTS WITH | COMBINED EFFECT |
|---|---|
| **Alcohol:** | None expected. |
| **Beverages:** Carbonates, citrates (additives listed on many beverage labels). | Decreased thiamine effect. |
| **Cocaine:** | None expected. |
| **Foods:** Carbonates, citrates (additives listed on many food labels). | Decreased thiamine effect. |
| **Marijuana:** | None expected. |
| **Tobacco:** | None expected. |

# THIORIDAZINE

## BRAND NAMES

Apo-Thioridazine
Mellaril
Mellaril S
Millazine
Novoridazine

PMS Thioridazine
SK-Thioridazine
  Hydrochloride
Thioril

## BASIC INFORMATION

**Habit forming? No**
**Prescription needed? Yes**
**Available as generic? Yes**
**Drug class: Tranquilizer, antiemetic**
      **(phenothiazine)**

## USES

- Stops nausea, vomiting.
- Reduces anxiety, agitation.

## DOSAGE & USAGE INFORMATION

**How to take:**
- Tablet or capsule—Swallow with liquid or food to lessen stomach irritation.
- Suppositories—Remove wrapper and moisten suppository with water. Gently insert into rectum, large end first.
- Drops or liquid—Dilute dose in beverage.

**When to take:**
- Nervous and mental disorders—Take at the same times each day.
- Nausea and vomiting—Take as needed, no more often than every 4 hours.

**If you forget a dose:**
- Nervous and mental disorders—Take up to 2 hours late. If more than 2 hours, wait for next scheduled dose (don't double this dose).
- Nausea and vomiting—Take as soon as you remember. Wait 4 hours for next dose.

*Continued next column*

## OVERDOSE

**SYMPTOMS:**
**Stupor, convulsions, coma.**
**WHAT TO DO:**
- **Dial 0 (operator) or 911 (emergency) for an ambulance or medical help. Then give first aid immediately.**
- **See emergency information on inside covers.**

## What drug does:
- Suppresses brain's vomiting center.
- Suppresses brain centers that control abnormal emotions and behavior.

## Time lapse before drug works:
- Nausea and vomiting—1 hour or less.
- Nervous and mental disorders—4-6 weeks.

## Don't take with:
- Antacid or medicine for diarrhea.
- Non-prescription drug for cough, cold or allergy.
- See Interaction column and consult doctor.

## POSSIBLE ADVERSE REACTIONS OR SIDE EFFECTS

| SYMPTOMS | WHAT TO DO |
|---|---|
| **Life-threatening:**<br>None expected. | |
| **Common:** | |
| • Muscle spasms of face and neck, unsteady gait. | Discontinue. Seek emergency treatment. |
| • Restlessness, tremor, drowsiness. | Discontinue. Call doctor right away. |
| • Decreased sweating, dry mouth, nasal congestion, constipation. | Continue. Call doctor when convenient. |
| **Infrequent:** | |
| • Fainting. | Discontinue. Seek emergency treatment. |
| • Rash. | Discontinue. Call doctor right away. |
| • Difficult urination, less interest in sex, swollen breasts, menstrual irregularities. | Continue. Call doctor when convenient. |
| **Rare:**<br>Change in vision, jaundice, sore throat, fever. | Discontinue. Call doctor right away. |

## WARNINGS & PRECAUTIONS

**Don't take if:**
- You are allergic to any phenothiazine.
- You have a blood or bone-marrow disease.

**Before you start, consult your doctor:**
- If you will have surgery within 2 months, including dental surgery, requiring general or spinal anesthesia.
- If you have asthma, emphysema or other lung disorder.
- If you take non-prescription ulcer medicine, asthma medicine or amphetamines.

**Over age 60:**
Adverse reactions and side effects may be more frequent and severe than in younger persons. More likely to develop involuntary movement of jaws, lips, tongue, chewing. Report this to your doctor immediately. Early treatment can help.

**Pregnancy:**
Risk to unborn child outweighs drug benefits. Don't use.

**Breast-feeding:**
Drug passes into milk. Avoid drug or discontinue nursing until you finish medicine. Consult doctor for advice on maintaining milk supply.

**Infants & children:**
Don't give to children younger than 2.

**Prolonged use:**
May lead to tardive dyskinesia (involuntary movement of jaws, lips, tongue, chewing).

**Skin & sunlight:**
May cause rash or intensify sunburn in areas exposed to sun or sunlamp. Skin may remain sensitive for 3 months after discontinuing.

**Driving, piloting or hazardous work:**
Don't drive or pilot aircraft until you learn how medicine affects you. Don't work around dangerous machinery. Don't climb ladders or work in high places. Danger increases if you drink alcohol or take medicine affecting alertness and reflexes.

**Discontinuing:**
- Nervous and mental disorders—Don't discontinue without doctor's advice until you complete prescribed dose, even though symptoms diminish or disappear.
- Nausea and vomiting—May be unnecessary to finish medicine. Follow doctor's instructions.

**Others:**
No problems expected.

## POSSIBLE INTERACTION WITH OTHER DRUGS

| GENERIC NAME OR DRUG CLASS | COMBINED EFFECT |
|---|---|
| Anticholinergics | Increased anticholinergic effect. |
| Antidepressants (tricyclic) | Increased thioridazine effect. |
| Antihistamines | Increased antihistamine effect. |
| Appetite suppressants | Decreased suppressant effect. |
| Dronabinol | Increased effects of both drugs. Avoid. |
| Levodopa | Decreased levodopa effect. |
| Mind-altering drugs | Increased effect of mind-altering drugs. |
| Molindone | Increased tranquilizer effect. |
| Narcotics | Increased narcotic effect. |
| Phenytoin | Increased phenytoin effect. |
| Quinidine | Impaired heart function. Dangerous mixture. |
| Sedatives | Increased sedative effect. |
| Tranquilizers (other) | Increased tranquilizer effect. |

## POSSIBLE INTERACTION WITH OTHER SUBSTANCES

| INTERACTS WITH | COMBINED EFFECT |
|---|---|
| Alcohol: | Dangerous oversedation. |
| Beverages: | None expected. |
| Cocaine: | Decreased thioridazine effect. Avoid. |
| Foods: | None expected. |
| Marijuana: | Drowsiness. May increase antinausea effect. |
| Tobacco: | None expected. |

# THIOTHIXENE

## BRAND NAMES

Navane

## BASIC INFORMATION

**Habit forming?** No
**Prescription needed?** Yes
**Available as generic?** No
**Drug class:** Tranquilizer (thioxanthine), antiemetic

## USES

- Reduces anxiety, agitation, psychosis.
- Stops vomiting.

## DOSAGE & USAGE INFORMATION

**How to take:**
- Capsule—Swallow with liquid. If you can't swallow whole, open capsule and take with liquid or food.
- Syrup—Dilute dose in beverage before swallowing.

**When to take:**
At the same time each day.

**If you forget a dose:**
Take as soon as you remember up to 2 hours late. If more than 2 hours, wait for next scheduled dose (don't double this dose).

**What drug does:**
Corrects imbalance of nerve impulses.

*Continued next column*

## OVERDOSE

**SYMPTOMS:**
**Drowsiness, dizziness, weakness, muscle rigidity, twitching, tremors, confusion, dry mouth, blurred vision, rapid pulse, shallow breathing, low blood pressure, convulsions, coma.**
**WHAT TO DO:**
- **Dial 0 (operator) or 911 (emergency) for an ambulance or medical help. Then give first aid immediately.**
- **If patient is unconscious and not breathing, give mouth-to-mouth breathing. If there is no heartbeat, use cardiac massage and mouth-to-mouth breathing (CPR). Don't try to make patient vomit. If you can't get help quickly, take patient to nearest emergency facility.**
- **See emergency information on inside covers.**

---

**Time lapse before drug works:**
3 weeks.

**Don't take with:**
See Interaction column and consult doctor.

## POSSIBLE ADVERSE REACTIONS OR SIDE EFFECTS

| SYMPTOMS | WHAT TO DO |
|---|---|
| **Life-threatening:** None expected. | |
| **Common:** | |
| • Fainting, restlessness, jerky and involuntary movements, blurred vision, rapid heartbeat. | Discontinue. Call doctor right away. |
| • Dizziness, drowsiness, constipation, muscle spasms, shuffling walk, decreased sweating. | Continue. Call doctor when convenient. |
| • Dry mouth, nasal congestion. | Continue. Tell doctor at next visit. |
| **Infrequent:** | |
| • Rash. | Discontinue. Call doctor right away. |
| • Less sexual ability, difficult urination. | Continue. Call doctor when convenient. |
| • Menstrual irregularities, swollen breasts. | Continue. Tell doctor at next visit. |
| **Rare:** | |
| Sore throat, fever, jaundice. | Discontinue. Call doctor right away. |

## WARNINGS & PRECAUTIONS

**Don't take if:**
- You are allergic to any thioxanthine or phenothiazine tranquilizer.
- You have serious blood disorder.
- You have Parkinson's disease.
- Patient is younger than 12.

**Before you start, consult your doctor:**
- If you have had liver or kidney disease.
- If you have epilepsy or glaucoma.
- If you have high blood pressure or heart disease (especially angina).
- If you use alcohol daily.
- If you will have surgery within 2 months, including dental surgery, requiring general or spinal anesthesia.

**Over age 60:**
Adverse reactions and side effects may be more frequent and severe than in younger persons.

**Pregnancy:**
No proven harm to unborn child. Avoid if possible.

**Breast-feeding:**
Studies inconclusive. Consult your doctor.

**Infants & children:**
Not recommended.

**Prolonged use:**
- Pigment deposits in lens and retina of eye.
- Involuntary movements of jaws, lips, tongue (tardive dyskinesia).

**Skin & sunlight:**
May cause rash or intensify sunburn in areas exposed to sun or sunlamp.

**Driving, piloting or hazardous work:**
Don't drive or pilot aircraft until you learn how medicine affects you. Don't work around dangerous machinery. Don't climb ladders or work in high places. Danger increases if you drink alcohol or take medicine affecting alertness and reflexes.

**Discontinuing:**
Don't discontinue without consulting doctor. Dose may require gradual reduction if you have taken drug for a long time. Doses of other drugs may also require adjustment.

**Others:**
Hot temperatures increase chance of heat stroke.

## POSSIBLE INTERACTION WITH OTHER DRUGS

| GENERIC NAME OR DRUG CLASS | COMBINED EFFECT |
|---|---|
| Anticholinergics | Increased anticholinergic effect. |
| Anticonvulsants | Change in seizure pattern. |
| Antidepressants (tricyclic) | Increased thiothixene effect. Excessive sedation. |
| Antihistamines | Increased thiothixene effect. Excessive sedation. |
| Antihypertensives | Excessively low blood pressure. |

| | |
|---|---|
| Barbiturates | Increased thiothixene effect. Excessive sedation. |
| Bethanechol | Decreased bethanechol effect. |
| Dronabinol | Increased effects of both drugs. Avoid. |
| Guanethidine | Decreased guanethidine effect. |
| Levodopa | Decreased levodopa effect. |
| MAO inhibitors | Excessive sedation. |
| Mind-altering drugs | Increased thiothixene effect. Excessive sedation. |
| Narcotics | Increased thiothixene effect. Excessive sedation. |
| Sedatives | Increased thiothixene effect. Excessive sedation. |
| Sleep inducers | Increased thiothixene effect. Excessive sedation. |
| Tranquilizers | Increased thiothixene effect. Excessive sedation. |

## POSSIBLE INTERACTION WITH OTHER SUBSTANCES

| INTERACTS WITH | COMBINED EFFECT |
|---|---|
| Alcohol: | Excessive brain depression. Avoid. |
| Beverages: | None expected. |
| Cocaine: | Decreased thiothixene effect. Avoid. |
| Foods: | None expected. |
| Marijuana: | Daily use—Fainting likely, possible psychosis. |
| Tobacco: | None expected. |

# THYROGLOBULIN

## BRAND NAMES

Proloid

## BASIC INFORMATION

Habit forming? No
Prescription needed? Yes
Available as generic? Yes
Drug class: Thyroid hormone

## USES

Replacement for thyroid hormone deficiency.

## DOSAGE & USAGE INFORMATION

**How to take:**
- Tablet or capsule—Swallow with liquid.
- Extended-release tablets or capsules—Swallow each dose whole. If you take regular tablets, you may chew or crush them.

**When to take:**
At the same time each day before a meal or on awakening.

**If you forget a dose:**
Take as soon as you remember up to 12 hours late. If more than 12 hours, wait for next scheduled dose (don't double this dose).

**What drug does:**
Increases cell metabolism rate.

**Time lapse before drug works:**
48 hours.

**Don't take with:**
See Interaction column and consult doctor.

## OVERDOSE

**SYMPTOMS:**
"Hot" feeling, heart palpitations, nervousness, sweating, hand tremors, insomnia, rapid and irregular pulse, headache, irritability, diarrhea, weight loss, muscle cramps.
**WHAT TO DO:**
Overdose unlikely to threaten life. If person takes much larger amount than prescribed, call doctor, poison-control center or hospital emergency room for instructions.

## POSSIBLE ADVERSE REACTIONS OR SIDE EFFECTS

| SYMPTOMS | WHAT TO DO |
|---|---|
| **Life-threatening:** None expected. | |
| **Common:** | |
| • Tremor, headache, irritability, insomnia. | Discontinue. Call doctor right away. |
| • Appetite change, diarrhea, leg cramps, menstrual irregularities, fever, heat sensitivity, unusual sweating, weight loss. | Continue. Call doctor when convenient. |
| **Infrequent:** Hives, rash, vomiting, chest pain, rapid and irregular heartbeat, shortness of breath. | Discontinue. Call doctor right away. |
| **Rare:** None expected. | |

## WARNINGS & PRECAUTIONS

**Don't take if:**
- You have had a heart attack within 6 weeks.
- You have no thyroid deficiency, but use this to lose weight.

**Before you start, consult your doctor:**
- If you have heart disease or high blood pressure.
- If you have diabetes.
- If you have Addison's disease, have had adrenal gland deficiency or use epinephrine, ephedrine or isoproterenol for asthma.

**Over age 60:**
More sensitive to thyroid hormone. May need smaller doses.

**Pregnancy:**
Considered safe if for thyroid deficiency only.

**Breast-feeding:**
Present in milk. Considered safe if dose is correct.

**Infants & children:**
Use only under medical supervision.

**Prolonged use:**
No problems expected, if dose is correct.

**Skin & sunlight:**
No problems expected.

**Driving, piloting or hazardous work:**
No problems expected.

**Discontinuing:**
Don't discontinue without consulting doctor. Dose may require gradual reduction if you have taken drug for a long time. Doses of other drugs may also require adjustment.

**Others:**
Digestive upsets, tremors, cramps, nervousness, insomnia or diarrhea may indicate need for dose adjustment.

## POSSIBLE INTERACTION WITH OTHER DRUGS

| GENERIC NAME OR DRUG CLASS | COMBINED EFFECT |
|---|---|
| Amphetamines | Increased amphetamine effect. |
| Anticoagulants (oral) | Increased anticoagulant effect. |
| Antidepressants (tricyclic) | Increased antidepressant effect. Irregular heartbeat. |
| Antidiabetics | Antidiabetic may require adjustment. |
| Aspirin (large doses, continuous use) | Increased thyroglobulin effect. |
| Barbiturates | Decreased barbiturate effect. |
| Cholestyramine | Decreased thyroglobulin effect. |
| Contraceptives (oral) | Decreased thyroglobulin effect. |
| Cortisone drugs | Requires dose adjustment to prevent cortisone deficiency. |
| Digitalis preparations | Increased digitalis effect. |
| Ephedrine | Increased ephedrine effect. |
| Epinephrine | Increased epinephrine effect. |
| Methylphenidate | Increased methylphenidate effect. |
| Phenytoin | Increased thyroglobulin effect. |

## POSSIBLE INTERACTION WITH OTHER SUBSTANCES

| INTERACTS WITH | COMBINED EFFECT |
|---|---|
| Alcohol: | None expected. |
| Beverages: | None expected. |
| Cocaine: | Excess stimulation. Avoid. |
| Foods: Soybeans. | Heavy consumption interferes with thyroid function. |
| Marijuana: | None expected. |
| Tobacco: | None expected. |

# THYROID

## BRAND NAMES

| | |
|---|---|
| Armour | S-P-T |
| Cytomel | Synthroid |
| Euthroid | Thyrar |
| Levothroid | Thyrocrine |
| Proloid | |

## BASIC INFORMATION

**Habit forming? No**
**Prescription needed? Yes**
**Available as generic? Yes**
**Drug class: Thyroid hormone**

## USES

Replacement for thyroid hormone deficiency.

## DOSAGE & USAGE INFORMATION

**How to take:**
- Tablet or capsule—Swallow with liquid.
- Extended-release tablets or capsules—Swallow each dose whole. If you take regular tablets, you may chew or crush them.

**When to take:**
At the same time each day before a meal or on awakening.

**If you forget a dose:**
Take as soon as you remember up to 12 hours late. If more than 12 hours, wait for next scheduled dose (don't double this dose).

**What drug does:**
Increases cell metabolism rate.

**Time lapse before drug works:**
48 hours.

**Don't take with:**
See Interaction column and consult doctor.

## OVERDOSE

**SYMPTOMS:**
"Hot" feeling, heart palpitations, nervousness, sweating, hand tremors, insomnia, rapid and irregular pulse, headache, irritability, diarrhea, weight loss, muscle cramps.
**WHAT TO DO:**
Overdose unlikely to threaten life. If person takes much larger amount than prescribed, call doctor, poison-control center or hospital emergency room for instructions.

## POSSIBLE ADVERSE REACTIONS OR SIDE EFFECTS

| SYMPTOMS | WHAT TO DO |
|---|---|
| **Life-threatening:**<br>None expected. | |
| **Common:** | |
| • Tremor, headache, irritability, insomnia. | Discontinue. Call doctor right away. |
| • Appetite change, diarrhea, leg cramps, menstrual irregularities, fever, heat sensitivity, unusual sweating, weight loss. | Continue. Call doctor when convenient. |
| **Infrequent:**<br>Hives, rash, vomiting, chest pain, rapid and irregular heartbeat, shortness of breath. | Discontinue. Call doctor right away. |
| **Rare:**<br>None expected. | |

## WARNINGS & PRECAUTIONS

**Don't take if:**
- You have had a heart attack within 6 weeks.
- You have no thyroid deficiency, but use this to lose weight.

**Before you start, consult your doctor:**
- If you have heart disease or high blood pressure.
- If you have diabetes.
- If you have Addison's disease, have had adrenal gland deficiency or use epinephrine, ephedrine or isoproterenol for asthma.

**Over age 60:**
More sensitive to thyroid hormone. May need smaller doses.

**Pregnancy:**
Considered safe if for thyroid deficiency only.

**Breast-feeding:**
Present in milk. Considered safe if dose is correct.

**Infants & children:**
Use only under medical supervision.

**Prolonged use:**
No problems expected, if dose is correct.

**Skin & sunlight:**
No problems expected.

**Driving, piloting or hazardous work:**
No problems expected.

**Discontinuing:**
Don't discontinue without consulting doctor. Dose may require gradual reduction if you have taken drug for a long time. Doses of other drugs may also require adjustment.

**Others:**
Digestive upsets, tremors, cramps, nervousness, insomnia or diarrhea may indicate need for dose adjustment.

## POSSIBLE INTERACTION WITH OTHER DRUGS

| GENERIC NAME OR DRUG CLASS | COMBINED EFFECT |
|---|---|
| Amphetamines | Increased amphetamine effect. |
| Anticoagulants (oral) | Increased anticoagulant effect. |
| Antidepressants (tricyclic) | Increased antidepressant effect. Irregular heartbeat. |
| Antidiabetics | Antidiabetic may require adjustment. |
| Aspirin (large doses, continuous use) | Increased thyroid effect. |
| Barbiturates | Decreased barbiturate effect. |
| Cholestyramine | Decreased thyroid effect. |
| Contraceptives (oral) | Decreased thyroid effect. |
| Cortisone drugs | Requires dose adjustment to prevent cortisone deficiency. |
| Digitalis preparations | Increased digitalis effect. |
| Ephedrine | Increased ephedrine effect. |
| Epinephrine | Increased epinephrine effect. |
| Methylphenidate | Increased methylphenidate effect. |
| Phenytoin | Increased thyroid effect. |

## POSSIBLE INTERACTION WITH OTHER SUBSTANCES

| INTERACTS WITH | COMBINED EFFECT |
|---|---|
| Alcohol: | None expected. |
| Beverages: | None expected. |
| Cocaine: | Excess stimulation. Avoid. |
| Foods: Soybeans. | Heavy consumption interferes with thyroid function. |
| Marijuana: | None expected. |
| Tobacco: | None expected. |

# THYROXINE (T-4, LEVOTHYROXINE)

## BRAND NAMES

| | |
|---|---|
| Choloxin | L-Thyroxine |
| Cytolen | L-T-S |
| Elthroxin | Noroxine |
| Euthroid | Ro-Thyroxine |
| Letter | Synthroid |
| Levoid | Thyrolar |
| Levothroid | |

## BASIC INFORMATION

**Habit forming? No**
**Prescription needed? Yes**
**Available as generic? Yes**
**Drug class: Thyroid hormone**

## USES

Replacement for thyroid hormone deficiency.

## DOSAGE & USAGE INFORMATION

**How to take:**
- Tablet or capsule—Swallow with liquid.
- Extended-release tablets or capsules—Swallow each dose whole. If you take regular tablets, you may chew or crush them.

**When to take:**
At the same time each day before a meal or on awakening.

**If you forget a dose:**
Take as soon as you remember up to 12 hours late. If more than 12 hours, wait for next scheduled dose (don't double this dose).

**What drug does:**
Increases cell metabolism rate.

**Time lapse before drug works:**
48 hours.

**Don't take with:**
See Interaction column and consult doctor.

## OVERDOSE

**SYMPTOMS:**
**"Hot" feeling, heart palpitations, nervousness, sweating, hand tremors, insomnia, rapid and irregular pulse, headache, irritability, diarrhea, weight loss, muscle cramps.**
**WHAT TO DO:**
**Overdose unlikely to threaten life. If person takes much larger amount than prescribed, call doctor, poison-control center or hospital emergency room for instructions.**

## POSSIBLE ADVERSE REACTIONS OR SIDE EFFECTS

| SYMPTOMS | WHAT TO DO |
|---|---|
| **Life-threatening:**<br>None expected. | |
| **Common:** | |
| • Tremor, headache, irritability, insomnia. | Discontinue. Call doctor right away. |
| • Appetite change, diarrhea, leg cramps, menstrual irregularities, fever, heat sensitivity, unusual sweating, weight loss. | Continue. Call doctor when convenient. |
| **Infrequent:** | |
| Hives, rash, vomiting, chest pain, rapid and irregular heartbeat, shortness of breath. | Discontinue. Call doctor right away. |
| **Rare:**<br>None expected. | |

## WARNINGS & PRECAUTIONS

**Don't take if:**
- You have had a heart attack within 6 weeks.
- You have no thyroid deficiency, but use this to lose weight.

**Before you start, consult your doctor:**
- If you have heart disease or high blood pressure.
- If you have diabetes.
- If you have Addison's disease, have had adrenal gland deficiency or use epinephrine, ephedrine or isoproterenol for asthma.

**Over age 60:**
More sensitive to thyroid hormone. May need smaller doses.

**Pregnancy:**
Considered safe if for thyroid deficiency only.

**Breast-feeding:**
Present in milk. Considered safe if dose is correct.

**Infants & children:**
Use only under medical supervision.

**Prolonged use:**
No problems expected, if dose is correct.

**Skin & sunlight:**
No problems expected.

**Driving, piloting or hazardous work:**
No problems expected.

**Discontinuing:**
Don't discontinue without consulting doctor. Dose may require gradual reduction if you have taken drug for a long time. Doses of other drugs may also require adjustment.

**Others:**
Digestive upsets, tremors, cramps, nervousness, insomnia or diarrhea may indicate need for dose adjustment.

## POSSIBLE INTERACTION WITH OTHER DRUGS

| GENERIC NAME OR DRUG CLASS | COMBINED EFFECT |
|---|---|
| Amphetamines | Increased amphetamine effect. |
| Anticoagulants (oral) | Increased anticoagulant effect. |
| Antidepressants (tricyclic) | Increased antidepressant effect. Irregular heartbeat. |
| Antidiabetics | Antidiabetic may require adjustment. |
| Aspirin (large doses, continuous use) | Increased thyroxine effect. |
| Barbiturates | Decreased barbiturate effect. |
| Cholestyramine | Decreased thyroxine effect. |
| Contraceptives (oral) | Decreased thyroxine effect. |
| Cortisone drugs | Requires dose adjustment to prevent cortisone deficiency. |
| Digitalis preparations | Increased digitalis effect. |
| Ephedrine | Increased ephedrine effect. |
| Epinephrine | Increased epinephrine effect. |
| Methylphenidate | Increased methylphenidate effect. |
| Phenytoin | Increased thyroxine effect. |

## POSSIBLE INTERACTION WITH OTHER SUBSTANCES

| INTERACTS WITH | COMBINED EFFECT |
|---|---|
| Alcohol: | None expected. |
| Beverages: | None expected. |
| Cocaine: | Excess stimulation. Avoid. |
| Foods: Soybeans. | Heavy consumption interferes with thyroid function. |
| Marijuana: | None expected. |
| Tobacco: | None expected. |

# TICARCILLIN

## BRAND NAMES

**Ticar**

## BASIC INFORMATION

**Habit forming? No**
**Prescription needed? Yes**
**Available as generic? Yes**
**Drug class: Antibiotic (penicillin)**

 ## USES

Treatment of bacterial infections that are susceptible to ticarcillin.

 ## DOSAGE & USAGE INFORMATION

**How to take:**
By injection only.

**When to take:**
Follow doctor's instructions.

**If you forget a dose:**
Consult doctor.

**What drug does:**
Destroys susceptible bacteria. Does not kill viruses.

**Time lapse before drug works:**
May be several days before medicine affects infection.

**Don't take with:**
See Interaction column and consult doctor.

 ## OVERDOSE

**SYMPTOMS:**
**Severe diarrhea, nausea, edema or vomiting.**
**WHAT TO DO:**
**Overdose unlikely to threaten life. If person takes much larger amount than prescribed, call doctor, poison-control center or hospital emergency room for instructions.**

 ## POSSIBLE ADVERSE REACTIONS OR SIDE EFFECTS

| SYMPTOMS | WHAT TO DO |
|---|---|
| **Life-threatening:** | |
| Hives, rash, intense itching, faintness soon after a dose (anaphylaxis). | Seek emergency treatment immediately. |
| **Common:** | |
| Dark or discolored tongue. | Continue. Tell doctor at next visit. |
| **Infrequent:** | |
| Mild nausea, vomiting, diarrhea. | Continue. Call doctor when convenient. |
| **Rare:** | |
| Unexplained bleeding. | Discontinue. Call doctor right away. |

## WARNINGS & PRECAUTIONS

**Don't take if:**
You are allergic to ticarcillin, cephalosporin antibiotics, other penicillins or penicillamine. Life-threatening reaction may occur.

**Before you start, consult your doctor:**
If you are allergic to any substance or drug.

**Over age 60:**
You may have skin reactions, particularly around genitals and anus.

**Pregnancy:**
Studies inconclusive on harm to unborn child. Animal studies show fetal abnormalities. Decide with your doctor whether drug benefits justify risk to unborn child.

**Breast-feeding:**
Drug passes into milk. Child may become sensitive to penicillins and have allergic reactions to penicillin drugs. Avoid ticarcillin or discontinue nursing until you finish medicine. Consult doctor for advice on maintaining milk supply.

**Infants & children:**
No problems expected.

**Prolonged use:**
You may become more susceptible to infections caused by germs not responsive to ticarcillin.

**Skin & sunlight:**
No problems expected.

**Driving, piloting or hazardous work:**
Usually not dangerous. Most hazardous reactions likely to occur a few minutes after taking ticarcillin.

**Discontinuing:**
Don't discontinue without doctor's advice until you complete prescribed dose, even though symptoms diminish or disappear.

**Others:**
No problems expected.

## POSSIBLE INTERACTION WITH OTHER DRUGS

| GENERIC NAME OR DRUG CLASS | COMBINED EFFECT |
|---|---|
| Beta-adrenergic blockers | Increased chance of anaphylaxis (see emergency information on inside front cover). |
| Chloramphenicol | Decreased effect of both drugs. |
| Erythromycins | Decreased effect of both drugs. |
| Loperamide | Decreased ticarcillin effect. |
| Paromomycin | Decreased effect of both drugs. |
| Tetracyclines | Decreased effect of both drugs. |
| Troleandomycin | Decreased effect of both drugs. |

## POSSIBLE INTERACTION WITH OTHER SUBSTANCES

| INTERACTS WITH | COMBINED EFFECT |
|---|---|
| Alcohol: | Occasional stomach irritation. |
| Beverages: | None expected. |
| Cocaine: | No proven problems. |
| Foods: | None expected. |
| Marijuana: | No proven problems. |
| Tobacco: | None expected. |

# TIMOLOL

## BRAND NAMES

Blocadren          Timoptic
Timolide

## BASIC INFORMATION

**Habit forming? No**
**Prescription needed? Yes**
**Available as generic? No**
**Drug class: Beta-adrenergic blocker,**
**antiglaucoma agent**

## USES

- Reduces angina attacks.
- Stabilizes irregular heartbeat.
- Lowers blood pressure.
- Reduces frequency of migraine headaches.
  (Does not relieve headache pain.)
- Decreases internal-eye pressure of glaucoma
  (ophthalmic drops).

## DOSAGE & USAGE INFORMATION

**How to take:**
- Eye drops—Wash hands. Apply slight
  pressure with finger to inside corner of eye.
  Pull lower eyelid down. Put drop just above
  lowered eyelid. Close eye gently for 2
  minutes. Don't blink.
- Tablet or capsule—Swallow with liquid or
  crumble and take with food.

**When to take:**
- Tablet or capsule—With meals or
  immediately after.
- Eye drops—Follow prescription directions.

**If you forget a dose:**
Take as soon as you remember. Return to
regular schedule, but allow 3 hours between
doses.

*Continued next column*

## OVERDOSE

**SYMPTOMS:**
**Weakness; slow or weak pulse;**
**blood-pressure drop; fainting; convulsions;**
**cold, sweaty skin.**
**WHAT TO DO:**
- **Dial 0 (operator) or 911 (emergency) for an**
  **ambulance or medical help. Then give first**
  **aid immediately.**
- **See emergency information on inside**
  **covers.**

## What drug does:

- Blocks certain actions of sympathetic nervous
  system.
- Lowers heart's oxygen requirements.
- Slows nerve impulses through heart.
- Reduces blood vessel contraction in heart,
  scalp and other body parts.
- Eye drops lower pressure inside eye.

## Time lapse before drug works:
1 to 4 hours.

## Don't take with:
Non-prescription drugs or drugs in Interaction
column without consulting doctor.

## POSSIBLE ADVERSE REACTIONS OR SIDE EFFECTS

| SYMPTOMS | WHAT TO DO |
|---|---|
| **Life-threatening:** | |
| None expected. | |
| **Common:** | |
| • Pulse slower than 50 beats per minute. | Discontinue. Call doctor right away. |
| • Drowsiness, numbness or tingling of fingers or toes, dizziness, diarrhea, nausea, fatigue, weakness. | Continue. Call doctor when convenient. |
| • Cold hands or feet; dry mouth, eyes and skin. | Continue. Tell doctor at next visit. |
| **Infrequent:** | |
| • Hallucinations, nightmares, insomnia, headache, difficult breathing. | Discontinue. Call doctor right away. |
| • Confusion, depression, reduced alertness, impotence. | Continue. Call doctor when convenient. |
| • Constipation. | Continue. Tell doctor at next visit. |
| **Rare:** | |
| • Rash, sore throat, fever. | Discontinue. Call doctor right away. |
| • Unusual bleeding or bruising. | Continue. Call doctor when convenient. |

## WARNINGS & PRECAUTIONS

**Don't take if:**
- You are allergic to any beta-adrenergic
  blocker.
- You have asthma.
- You have hay fever symptoms.
- You have taken MAO inhibitors in past 2
  weeks.

**Before you start, consult your doctor:**
- If you have heart disease or poor circulation to the extremities.
- If you have hay fever, asthma, chronic bronchitis, emphysema.
- If you have overactive thyroid function.
- If you have impaired liver or kidney function.
- If you will have surgery within 2 months, including dental surgery, requiring general or spinal anesthesia.
- If you have diabetes or hypoglycemia.

**Over age 60:**
Adverse reactions and side effects may be more frequent and severe than in younger persons.

**Pregnancy:**
Risk to unborn child outweighs drug benefits. Don't use.

**Breast-feeding:**
Drug passes into milk. Avoid drug or discontinue nursing until you finish medicine. Consult doctor about maintaining milk supply.

**Infants & children:**
Not recommended.

**Prolonged use:**
Weakens heart muscle contractions.

**Skin & sunlight:**
No problems expected.

**Driving, piloting or hazardous work:**
Don't drive or pilot aircraft until you learn how medicine affects you. Don't work around dangerous machinery. Don't climb ladders or work in high places. Danger increases if you drink alcohol or take medicine affecting alertness and reflexes.

**Discontinuing:**
Don't discontinue without consulting doctor. Dose may require gradual reduction if you have taken drug for a long time. Doses of other drugs may also require adjustment.

**Others:**
- May mask hypoglycemia.
- Side effects, such as burning or stinging of the eye, may also occur with timolol used as eye drops.

## POSSIBLE INTERACTION WITH OTHER DRUGS

| GENERIC NAME OR DRUG CLASS | COMBINED EFFECT |
|---|---|
| Acebutolol | Increased antihypertensive effects of both drugs. Dosages may require adjustment. |
| Albuterol | Decreased albuterol effect and beta-adrenergic blocking effect. |
| Antidiabetics | Increased antidiabetic effect. |
| Antihistamines | Decreased antihistamine effect. |
| Antihypertensives | Increased antihypertensive effect. |
| Anti-inflammatory drugs | Decreased effect of anti-inflammatory. |
| Barbiturates | Increased barbiturate effect. Dangerous sedation. |
| Digitalis preparations | Increased or decreased heart rate. Improves irregular heartbeat. |
| Narcotics | Increased narcotic effect. Dangerous sedation. |
| Nitrates | Possible excessive blood-pressure drop. |
| Pentoxifylline | Increased antihypertensive effect. |
| Phenytoin | Increased timolol effect. |
| Quinidine | Slows heart excessively. |
| Reserpine | Increased reserpine effect. Excessive sedation, depression. |
| Tocainide | May worsen congestive heart failure. |

## POSSIBLE INTERACTION WITH OTHER SUBSTANCES

| INTERACTS WITH | COMBINED EFFECT |
|---|---|
| Alcohol: | Excessive blood-pressure drop. Avoid. |
| Beverages: | None expected. |
| Cocaine: | Irregular heartbeat. Avoid. |
| Foods: | None expected. |
| Marijuana: | Daily use—Impaired circulation to hands and feet. |
| Tobacco: | Possible irregular heartbeat. |

# TOCAINIDE

## BRAND NAMES

Tonocard

## BASIC INFORMATION

**Habit forming? No**
**Prescription needed? Yes**
**Available as generic? No**
**Drug class: Antiarrhythmic**

## USES

Stabilizes irregular heartbeat, particularly irregular contractions of the ventricles of the heart or a too rapid heart rate.

## DOSAGE & USAGE INFORMATION

**How to take:**
Tablet—Swallow with food, water or milk. Dosage may need to be changed according to individual response.

**When to take:**
Take at regular times each day. For example, instructions to take 3 times a day means every 8 hours.

**If you forget a dose:**
Take as soon as you remember up to 4 hours late. If more than 4 hours, wait for next scheduled dose (don't double this dose).

**What drug does:**
Decreases excitability of cells of heart muscle.

**Time lapse before drug works:**
30 minutes to 2 hours.

**Don't take with:**
- See Interaction column and consult doctor.
- Wear identification information that states that you take this medicine so during an emergency a physician will know to avoid additional medicines that might be harmful or dangerous.

## OVERDOSE

**SYMPTOMS:**
**Convulsions, depressed breathing, cardiac arrest.**
**WHAT TO DO:**
- **Dial 0 (operator) or 911 (emergency) for an ambulance or medical help. Then give first aid immediately.**
- **See emergency information on inside covers.**

## POSSIBLE ADVERSE REACTIONS OR SIDE EFFECTS

| SYMPTOMS | WHAT TO DO |
|---|---|
| **Life-threatening:** | |
| None expected. | |
| **Common:** | |
| Nausea, vomiting. | Discontinue. Call doctor right away. |
| **Infrequent:** | |
| • Trembling. | Discontinue. Call doctor right away. |
| • Lightheadedness. | Continue. Call doctor when convenient. |
| **Rare:** | |
| • Sore throat, red tongue, mouth ulcers, unexplained bleeding or bruising, fever, chills. | Discontinue. Seek emergency treatment. |
| • Blurred vision, may accelerate heart rate or worsen irregular heartbeat, cough, difficult breathing, wheezing, may decrease white blood-cell count. | Discontinue. Call doctor right away. |
| • Numbness or tingling in hands or feet, rash, joint pain, swollen feet and ankles, unusual sweating. | Continue. Call doctor when convenient. |

## WARNINGS & PRECAUTIONS

**Don't take if:**
- You are allergic to tocainide or anesthetics whose names end in "caine."
- You have myasthenia gravis.

**Before you start, consult your doctor:**
- If you have congestive heart failure.
- If you are pregnant or plan to become pregnant.
- If you take anticancer drugs, trimethoprim, pyrimethamine, primaquine, phenylbutazone, penicillamine or oxyphenbutazone. These may affect blood-cell production in bone marrow.
- If you take any other heart medicine such as digitalis, flucystosine, colchicine, chloramphenicol, beta-adrenergic blockers or azathioprine. These can worsen heartbeat irregularity.
- If you will have surgery within 2 months, including dental surgery, requiring general, local or spinal anesthesia.
- If you have liver or kidney disease.

**Over age 60:**
Adverse reactions and side effects may be more frequent and severe than in younger persons.

**Pregnancy:**
No proven harm to unborn child. Nevertheless, avoid if possible.

**Breast-feeding:**
Avoid if possible.

**Infants & children:**
Not recommended. Safety and dosage have not been established.

**Prolonged use:**
Request periodic lab studies on blood, liver function, potassium levels.

**Skin & sunlight:**
No problems expected.

**Driving, piloting or hazardous work:**
Use caution if medicine causes you to feel dizzy or weak. Otherwise, no problems expected.

**Discontinuing:**
Don't discontinue without consulting doctor, even though symptoms diminish or disappear.

**Others:**
No problems expected.

## POSSIBLE INTERACTION WITH OTHER DRUGS

| GENERIC NAME OR DRUG CLASS | COMBINED EFFECT |
|---|---|
| Antiarrhythmics (others) | Increased possibility of adverse reactions from either drug. |
| Beta-adrenergic blockers | Possible irregular heartbeat. May worsen congestive heart failure. |
| Bone-marrow depressants, such as anticancer drugs, azathyoprine, chloramphenicol, colchicine, flucytosine, oxyphenbutazone, penicillamine, phenylbutazone, primaquine, pyrimethamine, trimethoprim. | Possible decreased production of blood cells in bone marrow. |

## POSSIBLE INTERACTION WITH OTHER SUBSTANCES

| INTERACTS WITH | COMBINED EFFECT |
|---|---|
| Alcohol: | Possible irregular heartbeat. Avoid. |
| Beverages: Caffeine drinks, iced drinks. | Possible irregular heartbeat. |
| Cocaine: | Possible lightheadedness, dizziness, quivering, convulsions. |
| Foods: | None expected. |
| Marijuana: | None expected. |
| Tobacco: | Possible irregular heartbeat. |

# TOLAZAMIDE

## BRAND NAMES

Ronase                    Tolinase

## BASIC INFORMATION

**Habit forming?** No
**Prescription needed?** Yes
**Available as generic?** Yes
**Drug class:** Antidiabetic (oral), sulfonurea

 **USES**

Treatment for diabetes in adults who can't control blood sugar by diet, weight loss and exercise.

 **DOSAGE & USAGE INFORMATION**

**How to take:**
Tablet—Swallow with liquid or food to lessen stomach irritation. If you can't swallow whole, crumble tablet and take with liquid or food.

**When to take:**
At the same times each day.

**If you forget a dose:**
Take as soon as you remember up to 2 hours late. If more than 2 hours, wait for next scheduled dose (don't double this dose).

**What drug does:**
Stimulates pancreas to produce more insulin. Insulin in blood forces cells to use sugar in blood.

**Time lapse before drug works:**
3 to 4 hours. May require 2 weeks for maximum benefit.

**Don't take with:**
See Interaction column and consult doctor.

 **OVERDOSE**

**SYMPTOMS:**
**Excessive hunger, nausea, anxiety, cool skin, cold sweats, drowsiness, rapid heartbeat, weakness, unconsciousness, coma.**
**WHAT TO DO:**
- **Dial 0 (operator) or 911 (emergency) for an ambulance or medical help. Then give first aid immediately.**
- **See emergency information on inside covers.**

 **POSSIBLE ADVERSE REACTIONS OR SIDE EFFECTS**

| SYMPTOMS | WHAT TO DO |
|---|---|
| **Life-threatening:** None expected. | |
| **Common:** | |
| • Dizziness. | Discontinue. Call doctor right away. |
| • Diarrhea, appetite loss, nausea, stomach pain, heartburn. | Continue. Call doctor when convenient. |
| **Infrequent:** Low blood sugar (hunger, anxiety, cold sweats, rapid pulse). | Discontinue. Seek emergency treatment. |
| **Rare:** Fatigue, itchy skin or rash, sore throat, fever, ringing in ears, unusual bleeding or bruising, jaundice. | Discontinue. Call doctor right away. |

 **WARNINGS & PRECAUTIONS**

**Don't take if:**
- You are allergic to any sulfonurea.
- You have impaired kidney or liver function.

**Before you start, consult your doctor:**
- If you have a severe infection.
- If you have thyroid disease.
- If you take insulin.
- If you have heart disease.

**Over age 60:**
Dose usually smaller than for younger adults. Avoid "low-blood-sugar" episodes because repeated ones can damage brain permanently.

**Pregnancy:**
No proven harm to unborn child. Avoid if possible.

**Breast-feeding:**
Drug filters into milk. May lower baby's blood sugar. Avoid.

**Infants & children:**
Don't give to infants or children.

**Prolonged use:**
None expected.

**Skin & sunlight:**
May cause rash or intensify sunburn in areas exposed to sun or sunlamp.

**Driving, piloting or hazardous work:**
No problems expected unless you develop hypoglycemia (low blood sugar). If so, avoid driving or hazardous activity.

**Discontinuing:**
Don't discontinue without consulting doctor. Dose may require gradual reduction if you have taken drug for a long time. Doses of other drugs may also require adjustment.

**Others:**
Don't exceed recommended dose. Hypoglycemia (low blood sugar) may occur, even with proper dose schedule. You must balance medicine, diet and exercise.

## POSSIBLE INTERACTION WITH OTHER DRUGS

| GENERIC NAME OR DRUG CLASS | COMBINED EFFECT |
|---|---|
| Androgens | Increased tolazamide effect. |
| Anticoagulants (oral) | Unpredictable prothrombin times. |
| Anticonvulsants (hydantoin) | Decreased tolazamide effect. |
| Anti-inflammatory drugs (non-steroidal) | Increased tolazamide effect. |
| Aspirin | Increased tolazamide effect. |
| Beta-adrenergic blockers | Increased tolazamide effect. Possible increased difficulty in regulating blood-sugar levels. |
| Chloramphenicol | Increased tolazamide effect. |
| Clofibrate | Increased tolazamide effect. |
| Contraceptives (oral) | Decreased tolazamide effect. |
| Cortisone drugs | Decreased tolazamide effect. |
| Diuretics (thiazide) | Decreased tolazamide effect. |
| Epinephrine | Decreased tolazamide effect. |
| Estrogens | Increased tolazamide effect. |
| Guanethidine | Unpredictable tolazamide effect. |
| Isoniazid | Decreased tolazamide effect. |
| Labetolol | Increased antidiabetic effect, may mask hypoglycemia. |
| MAO inhibitors | Increased tolazamide effect. |
| Oxyphenbutazone | Increased tolazamide effect. |
| Phenylbutazone | Increased tolazamide effect. |
| Phenyramidol | Increased tolazamide effect. |
| Probenecid | Increased tolazamide effect. |
| Pyrazinamide | Decreased tolazamide effect. |
| Sulfaphenazole | Increased tolazamide effect. |
| Sulfa drugs | Increased tolazamide effect. |
| Thyroid hormones | Decreased tolazamide effect. |

## POSSIBLE INTERACTION WITH OTHER SUBSTANCES

| INTERACTS WITH | COMBINED EFFECT |
|---|---|
| Alcohol: | Disulfiram reaction (see Glossary). Avoid. |
| Beverages: | None expected. |
| Cocaine: | No proven problems. |
| Foods: | None expected. |
| Marijuana: | Decreased tolazamide effect. Avoid. |
| Tobacco: | None expected. |

# TOLBUTAMIDE

## BRAND NAMES

Apo-Tolbutamide
Mobenol
Neo-Dibetic
Novobutamide

Oramide
Orinase
SK-Tolbutamide
Tolbutone

## BASIC INFORMATION

**Habit forming?** No
**Prescription needed?** Yes
**Available as generic?** Yes
**Drug class:** Antidiabetic (oral), sulfonurea

 USES

Treatment for diabetes in adults who can't control blood sugar by diet, weight loss and exercise.

 DOSAGE & USAGE INFORMATION

**How to take:**
Tablet—Swallow with liquid or food to lessen stomach irritation. If you can't swallow whole, crumble tablet and take with liquid or food.

**When to take:**
At the same times each day.

**If you forget a dose:**
Take as soon as you remember up to 2 hours late. If more than 2 hours, wait for next scheduled dose (don't double this dose).

**What drug does:**
Stimulates pancreas to produce more insulin. Insulin in blood forces cells to use sugar in blood.

**Time lapse before drug works:**
3 to 4 hours. May require 2 weeks for maximum benefit.

**Don't take with:**
See Interaction column and consult doctor.

 OVERDOSE

**SYMPTOMS:**
Excessive hunger, nausea, anxiety, cool skin, cold sweats, drowsiness, rapid heartbeat, weakness, unconsciousness, coma.
**WHAT TO DO:**
- **Dial 0 (operator) or 911 (emergency) for an ambulance or medical help. Then give first aid immediately.**
- **See emergency information on inside covers.**

 POSSIBLE ADVERSE REACTIONS OR SIDE EFFECTS

| SYMPTOMS | WHAT TO DO |
|---|---|
| **Life-threatening:**<br>None expected. | |
| **Common:**<br>• Dizziness. | Discontinue. Call doctor right away. |
| • Diarrhea, appetite loss, nausea, stomach pain, heartburn. | Continue. Call doctor when convenient. |
| **Infrequent:**<br>Low blood sugar (hunger, anxiety, cold sweats, rapid pulse). | Discontinue. Seek emergency treatment. |
| **Rare:**<br>Fatigue, itchy skin or rash, sore throat, fever, ringing in ears, unusual bleeding or bruising, jaundice. | Discontinue. Call doctor right away. |

 WARNINGS & PRECAUTIONS

**Don't take if:**
- You are allergic to any sulfonurea.
- You have impaired kidney or liver function.

**Before you start, consult your doctor:**
- If you have a severe infection.
- If you have thyroid disease.
- If you take insulin.
- If you have heart disease.

**Over age 60:**
Dose usually smaller than for younger adults. Avoid "low-blood-sugar" episodes because repeated ones can damage brain permanently.

**Pregnancy:**
No proven harm to unborn child. Avoid if possible.

**Breast-feeding:**
Drug filters into milk. May lower baby's blood sugar. Avoid.

**Infants & children:**
Don't give to infants or children.

**Prolonged use:**
None expected.

**Skin & sunlight:**
May cause rash or intensify sunburn in areas exposed to sun or sunlamp.

**Driving, piloting or hazardous work:**
No problems expected unless you develop hypoglycemia (low blood sugar). If so, avoid driving or hazardous activity.

**Discontinuing:**
Don't discontinue without consulting doctor. Dose may require gradual reduction if you have taken drug for a long time. Doses of other drugs may also require adjustment.

**Others:**
Don't exceed recommended dose. Hypoglycemia (low blood sugar) may occur, even with proper dose schedule. You must balance medicine, diet and exercise.

## POSSIBLE INTERACTION WITH OTHER DRUGS

| GENERIC NAME OR DRUG CLASS | COMBINED EFFECT |
|---|---|
| Androgens | Increased tolbutamide effect. |
| Anticoagulants (oral) | Unpredictable prothrombin times. |
| Anticonvulsants (hydantoin) | Decreased tolbutamide effect. |
| Anti-inflammatory drugs (non-steroidal) | Increased tolbutamide effect. |
| Aspirin | Increased tolbutamide effect. |
| Beta-adrenergic blockers | Increased tolbutamide effect. Possible increased difficulty in regulating blood-sugar levels. |
| Chloramphenicol | Increased tolbutamide effect. |
| Clofibrate | Increased tolbutamide effect. |
| Contraceptives (oral) | Decreased tolbutamide effect. |
| Cortisone drugs | Decreased tolbutamide effect. |
| Diuretics (thiazide) | Decreased tolbutamide effect. |
| Epinephrine | Decreased tolbutamide effect. |
| Estrogens | Increased tolbutamide effect. |
| Guanethidine | Unpredictable tolbutamide effect. |
| Isoniazid | Decreased tolbutamide effect. |
| Labetolol | Increased antidiabetic effect, may mask hypoglycemia. |
| MAO inhibitors | Increased tolbutamide effect. |
| Oxyphenbutazone | Increased tolbutamide effect. |
| Phenylbutazone | Increased tolbutamide effect. |
| Phenyramidol | Increased tolbutamide effect. |
| Probenecid | Increased tolbutamide effect. |
| Pyrazinamide | Decreased tolbutamide effect. |
| Sulfa drugs | Increased tolbutamide effect. |
| Sulfaphenazole | Increased tolbutamide effect. |
| Thyroid hormones | Decreased tolbutamide effect. |

## POSSIBLE INTERACTION WITH OTHER SUBSTANCES

| INTERACTS WITH | COMBINED EFFECT |
|---|---|
| Alcohol: | Disulfiram reaction (see Glossary). Avoid. |
| Beverages: | None expected. |
| Cocaine: | No proven problems. |
| Foods: | None expected. |
| Marijuana: | Decreased tolbutamide effect. Avoid. |
| Tobacco: | None expected. |

# TOLMETIN

## BRAND NAMES

Tolectin                    Tolectin DS

## BASIC INFORMATION

**Habit forming? No**
**Prescription needed? Yes**
**Available as generic? No**
**Drug class: Anti-inflammatory (non-steroid)**

## USES

- Treatment for joint pain, stiffness, inflammation and swelling of arthritis and gout.
- Pain reliever.

## DOSAGE & USAGE INFORMATION

**How to take:**
Tablet or capsule—Swallow with liquid or food to lessen stomach irritation. If you can't swallow whole, crumble tablet or open capsule and take with liquid or food.

**When to take:**
At the same times each day.

**If you forget a dose:**
Take as soon as you remember up to 2 hours late. If more than 2 hours, wait for next scheduled dose (don't double this dose).

**What drug does:**
Reduces tissue concentration of prostaglandins (hormones which produce inflammation and pain).

**Time lapse before drug works:**
Begins in 4 to 24 hours. May require 3 weeks regular use for maximum benefit.

**Don't take with:**
See Interaction column and consult doctor.

## OVERDOSE

**SYMPTOMS:**
**Confusion, agitation, incoherence, convulsions, possible hemorrhage from stomach or intestine, coma.**
**WHAT TO DO:**
- **Dial 0 (operator) or 911 (emergency) for an ambulance or medical help. Then give first aid immediately.**
- **See emergency information on inside covers.**

## POSSIBLE ADVERSE REACTIONS OR SIDE EFFECTS

| SYMPTOMS | WHAT TO DO |
|---|---|
| **Life-threatening:** None expected. | |
| **Common:** | |
| • Dizziness, nausea, pain. | Continue. Call doctor when convenient. |
| • Headache. | Continue. Tell doctor at next visit. |
| **Infrequent:** Depression, drowsiness, ringing in ears, swollen feet or legs, constipation or diarrhea, vomiting. | Continue. Call doctor when convenient. |
| **Rare:** | |
| • Convulsions; confusion; rash, hives or itchy skin; blurred vision; black, bloody or tarry stools; difficult breathing; tightness in chest; rapid heartbeat; unusual bleeding or bruising; blood in urine; jaundice. | Discontinue. Call doctor right away. |
| • Painful or difficult urination, fatigue, weakness. | Continue. Call doctor when convenient. |

## WARNINGS & PRECAUTIONS

**Don't take if:**
- You are allergic to aspirin or any non-steroid, anti-inflammatory drug.
- You have gastritis, peptic ulcer, enteritis, ileitis, ulcerative colitis, asthma, heart failure, high blood pressure or bleeding problems.
- Patient is younger than 15.

**Before you start, consult your doctor:**
- If you have epilepsy.
- If you have Parkinson's disease.
- If you have been mentally ill.
- If you have had kidney disease or impaired kidney function.

**Over age 60:**
Adverse reactions and side effects may be more frequent and severe than in younger persons.

**Pregnancy:**
Studies inconclusive on harm to unborn child. Decide with your doctor whether drug benefits justify risk to unborn child.

**Breast-feeding:**
May harm child. Avoid.

**Infants & children:**
Not recommended for anyone younger than 15. Use only under medical supervision.

**Prolonged use:**
- Eye damage.
- Reduced hearing.
- Sore throat, fever.
- Weight gain.

**Skin & sunlight:**
No problems expected.

**Driving, piloting or hazardous work:**
Don't drive or pilot aircraft until you learn how medicine affects you. Don't work around dangerous machinery. Don't climb ladders or work in high places. Danger increases if you drink alcohol or take medicine affecting alertness and reflexes, such as antihistamines, tranquilizers, sedatives, pain medicine, narcotics and mind-altering drugs.

**Discontinuing:**
Don't discontinue without consulting doctor. Dose may require gradual reduction if you have taken drug for a long time. Doses of other drugs may also require adjustment.

**Others:**
No problems expected.

## POSSIBLE INTERACTION WITH OTHER DRUGS

| GENERIC NAME OR DRUG CLASS | COMBINED EFFECT |
|---|---|
| Acebutolol | Decreased antihypertensive effect of acebutolol. |
| Anticoagulants (oral) | Increased risk of bleeding. |
| Aspirin | Increased risk of stomach ulcer. |
| Cortisone drugs | Increased risk of stomach ulcer. |
| Furosemide | Decreased diuretic effect of furosemide. |
| Gold compounds | Possible increased likelihood of kidney damage. |
| Ketoprofen | Increased possibility of internal bleeding. |
| Minoxidil | Decreased minoxidil effect. |
| Oxprenolol | Decreased antihypertensive effect of oxprenolol. |
| Oxyphenbutazone | Possible stomach ulcer. |
| Phenylbutazone | Possible stomach ulcer. |
| Probenecid | Increased tolmetin effect. |
| Thyroid hormones | Rapid heartbeat, blood-pressure rise. |

## POSSIBLE INTERACTION WITH OTHER SUBSTANCES

| INTERACTS WITH | COMBINED EFFECT |
|---|---|
| Alcohol: | Possible stomach ulcer or bleeding. |
| Beverages: | None expected. |
| Cocaine: | None expected. |
| Foods: | None expected. |
| Marijuana: | Increased pain relief from tolmetin. |
| Tobacco: | None expected. |

# TRAZODONE

## BRAND NAMES

**Desyrel**        **Desyrel Dividose**

## BASIC INFORMATION

**Habit forming? No**
**Prescription needed? Yes**
**Available as generic? No**
**Drug class: Antidepressant (non-tricyclic)**

 **USES**

- Treats mental depression.
- Treats anxiety.

 **DOSAGE & USAGE INFORMATION**

**How to take:**
Tablet or capsule—Swallow with liquid or food to lessen stomach irritation. If you can't swallow whole, crumble tablet or open capsule and take with liquid or food.

**When to take:**
According to prescription directions. Bedtime dose usually higher than other doses.

**If you forget a dose:**
Take as soon as you remember up to 2 hours late. If more than 2 hours, wait for next scheduled dose (don't double this dose).

**What drug does:**
Inhibits serotonin uptake in brain cells.

**Time lapse before drug works:**
2 to 4 weeks for full effect.

**Don't take with:**
See Interaction column and consult doctor.

 **OVERDOSE**

**SYMPTOMS:**
Fainting, irregular heartbeat, chest pain, seizures, coma.
**WHAT TO DO:**
- Dial 0 (operator) or 911 (emergency) for an ambulance or medical help. Then give first aid immediately.
- If patient is unconscious and not breathing, give mouth-to-mouth breathing. If there is no heartbeat, use cardiac massage and mouth-to-mouth breathing (CPR). Don't try to make patient vomit. If you can't get help quickly, take patient to nearest emergency facility.
- See emergency information on inside covers.

 **POSSIBLE ADVERSE REACTIONS OR SIDE EFFECTS**

| SYMPTOMS | WHAT TO DO |
|---|---|
| **Life-threatening:**<br>None expected. | |
| **Common:**<br>None expected. | |
| **Infrequent:** | |
| • Tremor, incoordination, blood pressue rise or drop, rapid heartbeat, shortness of breath, fainting. | Discontinue. Call doctor right away. |
| • Dizziness on standing, confusion, disorientation, drowsiness, excitement, fatigue, headache, nervousness, rash, itchy skin, blurred vision, ringing in ears, dry mouth, bad taste, diarrhea, nausea, vomiting, constipation, aching, prolonged penile erections, menstrual changes, diminished sex drive. | Continue. Call doctor when convenient. |
| **Rare:**<br>None expected. | |

## WARNINGS & PRECAUTIONS

**Don't take if:**
- You are allergic to trazodone.
- You are thinking about suicide.

**Before you start, consult your doctor:**
- If you have heart rhythm problem.
- If you have any heart disease.
- If you will have surgery within 2 months, including dental surgery, requiring general or spinal anesthesia.

**Over age 60:**
Adverse reactions and side effects may be more frequent and severe than in younger persons.

**Pregnancy:**
Risk to unborn child outweighs drug benefits. Don't use.

**Breast-feeding:**
Drug passes into milk. Avoid drug or discontinue nursing until you finish medicine. Consult doctor for advice on maintaining milk supply.

**Infants & children:**
Not recommended.

**Prolonged use:**
Occasional blood counts, especially if you have fever and sore throat.

**Skin & sunlight:**
No problems expected.

**Driving, piloting or hazardous work:**
Don't drive or pilot aircraft until you learn how medicine affects you. Don't work around dangerous machinery. Don't climb ladders or work in high places. Danger increases if you drink alcohol or take medicine affecting alertness and reflexes, such as antihistamines, tranquilizers, sedatives, pain medicine, narcotics and mind-altering drugs.

**Discontinuing:**
Don't discontinue without consulting doctor. Dose may require gradual reduction if you have taken drug for a long time. Doses of other drugs may also require adjustment.

**Others:**
Electroshock therapy should be avoided.

## POSSIBLE INTERACTION WITH OTHER DRUGS

| GENERIC NAME OR DRUG CLASS | COMBINED EFFECT |
|---|---|
| Antidepressants (other) | Excess drowsiness. |
| Antihistamines | Excess drowsiness. |
| Antihypertensives | Too low blood pressure. Avoid. |
| Barbiturates | Too low blood pressure. Avoid. |
| Digitalis preparations | Increased digitalis level in blood. |
| MAO inhibitors | May add to toxic effect of each. |
| Narcotics | Excess drowsiness. |
| Phenytoin | Increased phenytoin level in blood. |
| Sedatives | Excess drowsiness. |
| Tranquilizers | Excess drowsiness. |

## POSSIBLE INTERACTION WITH OTHER SUBSTANCES

| INTERACTS WITH | COMBINED EFFECT |
|---|---|
| Alcohol: | Excess sedation. Avoid. |
| Beverages: Caffeine. | May add to heartbeat irregularity. Avoid. |
| Cocaine: | May add to heartbeat irregularity. Avoid. |
| Foods: | No problems expected. |
| Marijuana: | May add to heartbeat irregularity. Avoid. |
| Tobacco: | May add to heartbeat irregularity. Avoid. |

# TRETINOIN

## BRAND NAMES

**Retin-A**          **StieVAA**
**Retinoic Acid**    **Vitamin A Acid**

## BASIC INFORMATION

**Habit forming? No**
**Prescription needed? Yes**
**Available as generic? Yes**
**Drug class: Antiacne (topical)**

 USES

Treatment for acne, psoriasis, ichthyosis, keratosis, folliculitis, flat warts.

 DOSAGE & USAGE INFORMATION

**How to use:**
Wash skin with non-medicated soap, pat dry, wait 20 minutes before applying.
- Cream or gel—Apply to affected areas with fingertips and rub in gently.
- Solution—Apply to affected areas with gauze pad or cotton swab. Avoid getting too wet so medicine doesn't drip into eyes, mouth, lips or inside nose.
- Follow manufacturer's directions on container.

**When to use:**
At the same time each day.

**If you forget an application:**
Use as soon as you remember.

**What drug does:**
Increases skin-cell turnover so skin layer peels off more easily.

**Time lapse before drug works:**
2 to 3 weeks. May require 6 weeks for maximum improvement.

**Don't use with:**
- Benzoyl peroxide. Apply 12 hours apart.
- See Interaction column and consult doctor.

 OVERDOSE

**SYMPTOMS:**
**None expected.**
**WHAT TO DO:**
**If person swallows drug, call doctor, poison-control center or hospital emergency room for instructions.**

 POSSIBLE ADVERSE REACTIONS OR SIDE EFFECTS

| SYMPTOMS | WHAT TO DO |
|---|---|
| **Life-threatening:**<br>None expected. | |
| **Common:** | |
| • Pigment change in treated area, warmth or stinging, peeling. | Continue. Tell doctor at next visit. |
| • Senstivity to wind or cold. | No action necessary. |
| **Infrequent:**<br>Blistering, crusting, severe burning, swelling. | Discontinue. Call doctor right away. |
| **Rare:**<br>None expected. | |

## WARNINGS & PRECAUTIONS

**Don't take if:**
- You are allergic to tretinoin.
- You are sunburned, windburned or have an open skin wound.

**Before you start, consult your doctor:**
If you have eczema.

**Over age 60:**
Not recommended.

**Pregnancy:**
No proven harm to unborn child. Avoid if possible.

**Breast-feeding:**
No problems expected.

**Infants & children:**
Not recommended.

**Prolonged use:**
No problems expected.

**Skin & sunlight:**
- May cause rash or intensify sunburn in areas exposed to sun or sunlamp.
- In some animal studies, tretinoin caused skin tumors to develop faster when treated area was exposed to ultraviolet light (sunlight or sunlamp). No proven similar effects in humans.

**Driving, piloting or hazardous work:**
No problems expected.

**Discontinuing:**
Don't discontinue without doctor's advice until you complete prescribed dose, even though symptoms diminish or disappear.

**Others:**
Acne may get worse before improvement starts in 2 or 3 weeks. Don't wash face more than 2 or 3 times daily.

## POSSIBLE INTERACTION WITH OTHER DRUGS

| GENERIC NAME OR DRUG CLASS | COMBINED EFFECT |
|---|---|
| Antiacne topical preparations (other) | Severe skin irritation. |
| Cosmetics (medicated) | Severe skin irritation. |
| Skin preparations with alcohol | Severe skin irritation. |
| Soaps or cleansers (abrasive) | Severe skin irritation. |

## POSSIBLE INTERACTION WITH OTHER SUBSTANCES

| INTERACTS WITH | COMBINED EFFECT |
|---|---|
| Alcohol: | None expected. |
| Beverages: | None expected. |
| Cocaine: | None expected. |
| Foods: | None expected. |
| Marijuana: | None expected. |
| Tobacco: | None expected. |

## BRAND NAMES

See complete list of brand names in the *Brand Name Directory,* page 958.

## BASIC INFORMATION

**Habit forming? No**
**Prescription needed? Yes**
**Available as generic? Yes**
**Drug class: Cortisone drug (adrenal**
**corticosteroid)**

## USES

- Reduces inflammation caused by many different medical problems.
- Treatment for some allergic diseases, blood disorders, kidney diseases, asthma and emphysema.
- Replaces corticosteroid deficiencies.

## DOSAGE & USAGE INFORMATION

**How to take:**
Tablet or syrup—Swallow with liquid or food to lessen stomach irritation. If you can't swallow whole, crumble tablet.

**When to take:**
At the same times each day. Take once-a-day or once-every-other-day doses in mornings.

**If you forget a dose:**
- Several-doses-per-day prescription—Take as soon as you remember up to 2 hours late. If more than 2 hours, wait for next scheduled dose (don't double this dose).
- Once-a-day dose or less—Wait for next dose. Double this dose.

**What drug does:**
Decreases inflammatory responses.

**Time lapse before drug works:**
2 to 4 days.

**Don't take with:**
See Interaction column and consult doctor.

## OVERDOSE

**SYMPTOMS:**
**Headache, convulsions, heart failure.**
**WHAT TO DO:**
- **Dial 0 (operator) or 911 (emergency) for an ambulance or medical help. Then give first aid immediately.**
- **See emergency information on inside covers.**

## POSSIBLE ADVERSE REACTIONS OR SIDE EFFECTS

| SYMPTOMS | WHAT TO DO |
|---|---|
| **Life-threatening:**<br>None expected. | |
| **Common:**<br>Acne, thirst, indigestion, nausea, vomiting, poor wound healing. | Continue. Call doctor when convenient. |
| **Infrequent:** | |
| • Black, bloody or tarry stool. | Discontinue. Seek emergency treatment. |
| • Blurred vision, halos around lights, muscle cramps, swollen legs and feet, sore throat, fever. | Discontinue. Call doctor right away. |
| • Mood change, insomnia, restlessness, frequent urination, weight gain, round face, fatigue, weakness, TB recurrence, menstrual irregularities. | Continue. Call doctor when convenient. |
| **Rare:** | |
| • Irregular heartbeat. | Discontinue. Seek emergency treatment. |
| • Rash. | Discontinue. Call doctor right away. |

## WARNINGS & PRECAUTIONS

**Don't take if:**
- You are allergic to any cortisone drug.
- You have tuberculosis or fungus infection.
- You have herpes infection of eyes, lips or genitals.

**Before you start, consult your doctor:**
- If you have had tuberculosis.
- If you have congestive heart failure.
- If you have diabetes.
- If you have peptic ulcer.
- If you have glaucoma.
- If you have underactive thyroid.
- If you have high blood pressure.
- If you have myasthenia gravis.
- If you have blood clots in legs or lungs.

**Over age 60:**
Adverse reactions and side effects may be more frequent and severe than in younger persons. Likely to aggravate edema, diabetes or ulcers. Likely to cause cataracts and osteoporosis (softening of the bones).

**Pregnancy:**
Risk to unborn child outweighs drug benefits. Don't use.

**Breast-feeding:**
Drug passes into milk. Avoid drug or discontinue nursing until you finish medicine. Consult doctor for advice on maintaining milk supply.

**Infants & children:**
Use only under medical supervision.

**Prolonged use:**
- Retards growth in children.
- Possible glaucoma, cataracts, diabetes, fragile bones and thin skin.
- Functional dependence.

**Skin & sunlight:**
No problems expected.

**Driving, piloting or hazardous work:**
No problems expected.

**Discontinuing:**
- Don't discontinue without doctor's advice until you complete prescribed dose, even though symptoms diminish or disappear.
- Drug affects your response to surgery, illness, injury or stress for 2 years after discontinuing. Tell anyone who takes medical care of you within 2 years about drug.

**Others:**
Avoid immunizations if possible.

## POSSIBLE INTERACTION WITH OTHER DRUGS

| GENERIC NAME OR DRUG CLASS | COMBINED EFFECT |
|---|---|
| Amphoterecin B | Potassium depletion. |
| Anticholinergics | Possible glaucoma. |
| Anticoagulants (oral) | Decreased anticoagulant effect. |
| Anticonvulsants (hydantoin) | Decreased triamcinolone effect. |
| Antidiabetics (oral) | Decreased antidiabetic effect. |
| Antihistamines | Decreased triamcinolone effect. |
| Aspirin | Increased triamcinolone effect. |
| Barbiturates | Decreased triamcinolone effect. Oversedation. |
| Beta-adrenergic blockers | Decreased triamcinolone effect. |
| Chloral hydrate | Decreased triamcinolone effect. |
| Chlorthalidone | Potassium depletion. |

| | |
|---|---|
| Cholinergics | Decreased cholinergic effect. |
| Contraceptives (oral) | Increased triamcinolone effect. |
| Digitalis preparations | Dangerous potassium depletion. Possible digitalis toxicity. |
| Diuretics (thiazide) | Potassium depletion. |
| Ephedrine | Decreased triamcinolone effect. |
| Estrogens | Increased triamcinolone effect. |
| Ethacrynic acid | Potassium depletion. |
| Furosemide | Potassium depletion. |
| Glutethimide | Decreased triamcinolone effect. |
| Indapamide | Possible excessive potassium loss, causing dangerous heartbeat irregularity. |
| Indomethacin | Increased triamcinolone effect. |
| Insulin | Decreased insulin effect. |
| Isoniazid | Decreased isoniazid effect. |
| Oxyphenbutazone | Possible ulcers. |
| Phenylbutazone | Possible ulcers. |
| Potassium supplements | Decreased potassium effect. |
| Rifampin | Decreased triamcinolone effect. |
| Sympathomimetics | Possible glaucoma. |

## POSSIBLE INTERACTION WITH OTHER SUBSTANCES

| INTERACTS WITH | COMBINED EFFECT |
|---|---|
| Alcohol: | Risk of stomach ulcers. |
| Beverages: | No proven problems. |
| Cocaine: | Overstimulation. Avoid. |
| Foods: | No proven problems. |
| Marijuana: | Decreased immunity. |
| Tobacco: | Increased triamcinolone effect. Possible toxicity. |

# TRIAMTERENE

## BRAND NAMES

Dyazide          Maxzide
Dyrenium

## BASIC INFORMATION

**Habit forming? No**
**Prescription needed? Yes**
**Available as generic? No**
**Drug class: Antihypertensive, diuretic**

## USES

- Reduces fluid retention (edema).
- Reduces potassium loss.

## DOSAGE & USAGE INFORMATION

**How to take:**
Tablet or capsule—Swallow with liquid or food to lessen stomach irritation. If you can't swallow whole, crumble tablet or open capsule and take with liquid or food.

**When to take:**
- 1 dose per day—Take after breakfast.
- More than 1 dose per day—Take last dose no later than 6 p.m.

**If you forget a dose:**
Take as soon as you remember up to 6 hours late. If more than 6 hours, wait for next scheduled dose (don't double this dose).

**What drug does:**
Increases urine production to eliminate sodium and water from body while conserving potassium.

*Continued next column*

## OVERDOSE

**SYMPTOMS:**
Lethargy, irregular heartbeat, coma.
**WHAT TO DO:**
- Dial 0 (operator) or 911 (emergency) for an ambulance or medical help. Then give first aid immediately.
- If patient is unconscious and not breathing, give mouth-to-mouth breathing. If there is no heartbeat, use cardiac massage and mouth-to-mouth breathing (CPR). Don't try to make patient vomit. If you can't get help quickly, take patient to nearest emergency facility.
- See emergency information on inside covers.

**Time lapse before drug works:**
2 hours. May require 2 to 3 days for maximum benefit.

**Don't take with:**
See Interaction column and consult doctor.

## POSSIBLE ADVERSE REACTIONS OR SIDE EFFECTS

| SYMPTOMS | WHAT TO DO |
|---|---|
| **Life-threatening:** None expected. | |
| **Common:** None expected. | |
| **Infrequent:** | |
| • Drowsiness, confusion, dry mouth, thirst, irregular heartbeat, shortness of breath, unusual tiredness, weakness. | Discontinue. Call doctor right away. |
| • Diarrhea. | Continue. Call doctor when convenient. |
| • Anxiety. | Continue. Tell doctor at next visit. |
| **Rare:** | |
| • Rash, sore throat, fever, red or inflamed tongue, unusual bleeding or bruising. | Discontinue. Call doctor right away. |
| • Headache. | Continue. Tell doctor at next visit. |

## WARNINGS & PRECAUTIONS

**Don't take if:**
- You are allergic to triamterene.
- You have had severe liver or kidney disease.

**Before you start, consult your doctor:**
- If you have gout.
- If you have diabetes.
- If you will have surgery within 2 months, including dental surgery, requiring general or spinal anesthesia.

**Over age 60:**
- Warm weather or fever can decrease blood pressure. Dose may require adjustment.
- Extended use can increase blood clots.

**Pregnancy:**
No proven harm to unborn child. Avoid if possible.

**Breast-feeding:**
Present in milk. Avoid

**Infants & children:**
Used infrequently. Use only under medical supervision.

**Prolonged use:**
Potassium retention which may lead to heart-rhythm problems.

**Skin & sunlight:**
May cause rash or intensify sunburn in areas exposed to sun or sunlamp.

**Driving, piloting or hazardous work:**
Avoid if you feel drowsy or confused. Otherwise, no problems expected.

**Discontinuing:**
Don't discontinue without consulting doctor. Dose may require gradual reduction if you have taken drug for a long time. Doses of other drugs may also require adjustment.

**Others:**
No problems expected.

## POSSIBLE INTERACTION WITH OTHER DRUGS

| GENERIC NAME OR DRUG CLASS | COMBINED EFFECT |
|---|---|
| Acebutolol | Increased antihypertensive effect. Dosages may require adjustment. |
| Amiodarone | Increased risk of heartbeat irregularity due to low potassium. |
| Antidiabetics (oral) | Decreased antidiabetic effect. |
| Antihypertensives (other) | Increased effect of other antihypertensives. |
| Calcium supplements | Increased calcium in blood. |
| Digitalis preparations | Decreased digitalis effect. |
| Enalapril | Possible excessive potassium in blood. |
| Labetolol | Increased antihypertensive effects. |
| Lithium | Increased lithium effect. |
| Nitrates | Excessive blood-pressure drop. |
| Oxprenolol | Increased antihypertensive effect. Dosages may require adjustment. |
| Potassium supplements | Possible excessive potassium retention. |
| Spironolactone | Dangerous retention of potassium. |

## POSSIBLE INTERACTION WITH OTHER SUBSTANCES

| INTERACTS WITH | COMBINED EFFECT |
|---|---|
| Alcohol: | None expected. |
| Beverages: | None expected. |
| Cocaine: | Decreased triamterene effect. |
| Foods: Salt. | Don't restrict unless directed by doctor. |
| Marijuana: | Daily use—Fainting likely. |
| Tobacco: | None expected. |

# TRIAMTERENE & HYDROCHLOROTHIAZIDE

## BRAND NAMES

Dyazide                    Maxzide

## BASIC INFORMATION

Habit forming? No
Prescription needed? Yes
Available as generic? No
Drug class: Diuretic

 **USES**

- Reduces fluid retention (edema).
- Reduces potassium loss.
- Controls, but doesn't cure, high blood pressure.

 **DOSAGE & USAGE INFORMATION**

**How to take:**
Tablet or capsule—Swallow with liquid. If you can't swallow whole, crumble tablet or open capsule and take with liquid or food.

**When to take:**
- 1 dose per day—Take after breakfast.
- More than 1 dose per day—Take last dose no later than 6 p.m.

**If you forget a dose:**
Take as soon as you remember up to 6 hours late. If more than 6 hours, wait for next scheduled dose (don't double this dose).

**What drug does:**
- Increases urine production to eliminate sodium and water from body while conserving potassium.

*Continued next column*

 **OVERDOSE**

**SYMPTOMS:**
**Lethargy, irregular heartbeat, cramps, weakness, drowsiness, weak pulse, coma.**
**WHAT TO DO:**
- **Dial 0 (operator) or 911 (emergency) for an ambulance or medical help. Then give first aid immediately.**
- **If patient is unconscious and not breathing, give mouth-to-mouth breathing. If there is no heartbeat, use cardiac massage and mouth-to-mouth breathing (CPR). Don't try to make patient vomit. If you can't get help quickly, take patient to nearest emergency facility.**
- **See emergency information on inside covers.**

- Forces sodium and water excretion, reducing body fluid.
- Relaxes muscle cells of small arteries.
- Reduced body fluid and relaxed arteries lower blood pressure.

**Time lapse before drug works:**
4 to 6 hours. May require several weeks to lower blood pressure.

**Don't take with:**
- Non-prescription drugs without consulting doctor.
- See Interaction column and consult doctor.

 **POSSIBLE ADVERSE REACTIONS OR SIDE EFFECTS**

| SYMPTOMS | WHAT TO DO |
|---|---|
| **Life-threatening:** | |
| Irregular heartbeat, weak pulse, shortness of breath. | Discontinue. Seek emergency treatment. |
| **Common:** | |
| • Mood change, muscle cramps. | Discontinue. Call doctor right away. |
| • Numbness or tingling in hands or feet. | Continue. Call doctor when convenient. |
| **Infrequent:** | |
| • Blurred vision, abdominal pain, nausea, vomiting. | Discontinue. Call doctor right away. |
| • Dizziness, mood change, headache, dry mouth, weakness, tiredness, weight gain or loss. | Continue. Call doctor when convenient. |
| **Rare:** | |
| • Sore throat, fever, mouth sores; jaundice; rash; joint or muscle pain; hives; unexplained bleeding or bruising. | Discontinue. Call doctor right away. |
| • Corners of mouth cracked, weakness. | Continue. Call doctor when convenient. |

 **WARNINGS & PRECAUTIONS**

**Don't take if:**
- If you are allergic to triamterene or any thiazide diuretic drug.
- If you have had severe liver or kidney disease.

**Before you start, consult your doctor:**
- If you have gout, diabetes, liver, pancreas or kidney disorder.
- You are allergic to any sulfa drug.
- If you will have surgery within 2 months, including dental surgery, requiring general or spinal anesthesia.

**Over age 60:**
- Adverse reactions and side effects may be more frequent and severe than in younger persons, especially dizziness and excessive potassium loss.
- Warm weather or fever can decrease blood pressure. Dose may require adjustment.
- Extended use can increase blood clots.

**Pregnancy:**
Risk to unborn child outweighs drug benefits. Don't use.

**Breast-feeding:**
Drug passes into milk. Avoid drug or discontinue nursing until you finish medicine. Consult doctor for advice on maintaining milk supply.

**Infants & children:**
Used infrequently. Use only under medical supervision.

**Prolonged use:**
Potassium retention which may lead to heart-rhythm problems.

**Skin & sunlight:**
May cause rash or intensify sunburn in areas exposed to sun or sunlamp.

**Driving, piloting or hazardous work:**
Don't drive or pilot aircraft until you learn how medicine affects you. Don't work around dangerous machinery. Don't climb ladders or work in high places. Danger increases if you drink alcohol or take medicine affecting alertness and reflexes, such as antihistamines, tranquilizers, sedatives, pain medicine, narcotics and mind-altering drugs.

**Discontinuing:**
Don't discontinue without consulting doctor. Dose may require gradual reduction if you have taken drug for a long time. Doses of other drugs may also require adjustment.

**Others:**
- Hot weather and fever may cause dehydration and drop in blood pressure. Dose may require temporary adjustment. Weigh daily and report any unexpected weight decreases to your doctor.
- May cause rise in uric acid, leading to gout.
- May cause blood-sugar rise in diabetics.

## POSSIBLE INTERACTION WITH OTHER DRUGS

| GENERIC NAME OR DRUG CLASS | COMBINED EFFECT |
|---|---|
| Acebutolol | Decreased antihypertensive effect of acebutolol. |
| Allopurinol | Decreased allopurinol effect. |
| Antidepressants | Dangerous drop in blood pressure. Avoid combination unless under medical supervision. |
| Antidiabetics (oral) | Decreased antidiabetic effect. |
| Barbiturates | Increased hydrochlorothiazide effect. |
| Cholestyramine | Decreased hydrochlorothiazide effect. |
| Cortisone drugs | Excessive potassium loss that causes dangerous heart rhythms. |
| Digitalis preparations | Excessive potassium loss that causes dangerous heart rhythms. |
| Diuretics (thiazide) | Increased effect of other thiazide diuretics. |
| Indapamide | Increased diuretic effect. |
| Lithium | Increased lithium effect. |
| MAO inhibitors | Increased hydrochlorothiazide effect. |
| Nitrates | Excessive blood-pressure drop. |

*Continued page 979*

## POSSIBLE INTERACTION WITH OTHER SUBSTANCES

| INTERACTS WITH | COMBINED EFFECT |
|---|---|
| Alcohol: | Dangerous blood-pressure drop. |
| Beverages: | None expected. |
| Cocaine: | Decreased triamterene effect. |
| Foods: Salt. | Don't restrict unless directed by doctor. |
| Marijuana: | Daily use—Fainting likely. |
| Tobacco: | Decreases drug's effectiveness. |

# TRIAZOLAM

## BRAND NAMES

Halcion

## BASIC INFORMATION

**Habit forming? Yes**
**Prescription needed? Yes**
**Available as generic? No**
**Drug class: Tranquilizer (benzodiazepine)**

## USES

Treatment of insomnia. Not recommended for more than 2 weeks maximum.

## DOSAGE & USAGE INFORMATION

**How to take:**
Tablet or capsule—Swallow with liquid. If you can't swallow whole, crumble tablet or open capsule and take with liquid or food.

**When to take:**
At the same time each day, according to instructions on prescription label.

**If you forget a dose:**
Take as soon as you remember up to 2 hours late. If more than 2 hours, wait for next scheduled dose (don't double this dose).

**What drug does:**
Affects limbic system, the part of the brain that controls emotions.

**Time lapse before drug works:**
2 hours. May take 6 weeks for full benefit.

**Don't take with:**
See Interaction column and consult doctor.

## OVERDOSE

**SYMPTOMS:**
**Drowsiness, weakness, tremor, stupor, coma.**
**WHAT TO DO:**
- **Dial 0 (operator) or 911 (emergency) for an ambulance or medical help. Then give first aid immediately.**
- **If patient is unconscious and not breathing, give mouth-to-mouth breathing. If there is no heartbeat, use cardiac massage and mouth-to-mouth breathing (CPR). Don't try to make patient vomit. If you can't get help quickly, take patient to nearest emergency facility.**
- **See emergency information on inside covers.**

## POSSIBLE ADVERSE REACTIONS OR SIDE EFFECTS

| SYMPTOMS | WHAT TO DO |
|---|---|
| **Life-threatening:** None expected. | |
| **Common:** Clumsiness, drowsiness, dizziness. | Continue. Call doctor when convenient. |
| **Infrequent:** | |
| • Hallucinations, confusion, depression, irritability, rash, itchy skin, change in vision. | Discontinue. Call doctor right away. |
| • Constipation or diarrhea, nausea, vomiting, difficult urination. | Continue. Call doctor when convenient. |
| **Rare:** | |
| • Slow heartbeat, difficult breathing. | Discontinue. Seek emergency treatment. |
| • Mouth or throat ulcers, jaundice. | Discontinue. Call doctor right away. |

## WARNINGS & PRECAUTIONS

**Don't take if:**
- You are allergic to any benzodiazepine.
- You have myasthenia gravis.
- You are active or recovering alcoholic.
- Patient is younger than 6 months.

**Before you start, consult your doctor:**
- If you have liver, kidney or lung disease.
- If you have diabetes, epilepsy or porphyria.
- If you will have surgery within 2 months, including dental surgery, requiring general or spinal anesthesia.

**Over age 60:**
Adverse reactions and side effects may be more frequent and severe than in younger persons. You need smaller doses for shorter periods of time. May develop agitation, rage or "hangover" effect.

**Pregnancy:**
Risk to unborn child outweighs drug benefits. Don't use.

**Breast-feeding:**
Drug passes into milk. Avoid drug or discontinue nursing until you finish medicine. Consult doctor for advice on maintaining milk supply.

**Infants & children:**
Use only under medical supervision for children older than 6 months.

**Prolonged use:**
May impair liver function.

**Skin & sunlight:**
No problems expected.

**Driving, piloting or hazardous work:**
Don't drive or pilot aircraft until you learn how medicine affects you. Don't work around dangerous machinery. Don't climb ladders or work in high places. Danger increases if you drink alcohol or take medicine affecting alertness and reflexes.

**Discontinuing:**
Don't discontinue without consulting doctor. Dose may require gradual reduction if you have taken drug for a long time. Doses of other drugs may also require adjustment.

**Others:**
- Hot weather, heavy exercise and profuse sweat may reduce excretion and cause overdose.
- Blood sugar may rise in diabetics, requiring insulin adjustment.

## POSSIBLE INTERACTION WITH OTHER DRUGS

| GENERIC NAME OR DRUG CLASS | COMBINED EFFECT |
|---|---|
| Anticonvulsants | Change in seizure frequency or severity. |
| Antidepressants | Increased sedative effect of both drugs. |
| Antihistamines | Increased sedative effect of both drugs. |
| Antihypertensives | Excessively low blood pressure. |
| Cimetidine | Excess sedation. |
| Disulfiram | Increased triazolam effect. |
| Dronabinol | Increased effects of both drugs. Avoid. |
| MAO inhibitors | Convulsions, deep sedation, rage. |
| Molindone | Increased sedative effect. |
| Narcotics | Increased sedative effect of both drugs. |
| Sedatives | Increased sedative effect of both drugs. |
| Sleep inducers | Increased sedative effect of both drugs. |
| Tranquilizers | Increased sedative effect of both drugs. |

## POSSIBLE INTERACTION WITH OTHER SUBSTANCES

| INTERACTS WITH | COMBINED EFFECT |
|---|---|
| Alcohol: | Heavy sedation. Avoid. |
| Beverages: | None expected. |
| Cocaine: | Decreased triazolam effect. |
| Foods: | None expected. |
| Marijuana: | Heavy sedation. Avoid. |
| Tobacco: | Decreased triazolam effect. |

# TRICHLORMETHIAZIDE

## BRAND NAMES

| | |
|---|---|
| Metahydrin | Naqua |
| Metatensin | Naquival |

## BASIC INFORMATION

**Habit forming?** No
**Prescription needed?** Yes
**Available as generic?** Yes
**Drug class:** Antihypertensive, diuretic
(thiazide)

## USES

- Controls, but doesn't cure, high blood pressure.
- Reduces fluid retention (edema) caused by conditions such as heart disorders and liver disease.

## DOSAGE & USAGE INFORMATION

**How to take:**
Tablet or capsule—Swallow with liquid. If you can't swallow whole, crumble tablet or open capsule and take with liquid or food. Don't exceed dose.

**When to take:**
At the same time each day.

**If you forget a dose:**
Take as soon as you remember up to 2 hours late. If more than 2 hours, wait for next scheduled dose (don't double this dose).

**What drug does:**
- Forces sodium and water excretion, reducing body fluid.
- Relaxes muscle cells of small arteries.
- Reduced body fluid and relaxed arteries lower blood pressure.

**Time lapse before drug works:**
4 to 6 hours. May require several weeks to lower blood pressure.

*Continued next column*

## OVERDOSE

**SYMPTOMS:**
**Cramps, weakness, drowsiness, weak pulse, coma.**
**WHAT TO DO:**
- **Dial 0 (operator) or 911 (emergency) for an ambulance or medical help. Then give first aid immediately.**
- **See emergency information on inside covers.**

**Don't take with:**
- See Interaction column and consult doctor.
- Non-prescription drugs without consulting doctor.

## POSSIBLE ADVERSE REACTIONS OR SIDE EFFECTS

| SYMPTOMS | WHAT TO DO |
|---|---|
| **Life-threatening:**<br>None expected. | |
| **Common:**<br>None expected. | |
| **Infrequent:** | |
| • Blurred vision, severe abdominal pain, nausea, vomiting, irregular heartbeat, weak pulse, sore throat, fever. | Discontinue. Call doctor right away. |
| • Dizziness, mood change, headache, weakness, tiredness, weight changes. | Continue. Call doctor when convenient. |
| • Dry mouth, thirst. | Continue. Tell doctor at next visit. |
| **Rare:** | |
| • Rash or hives. | Discontinue. Seek emergency treatment. |
| • Jaundice. | Discontinue. Call doctor right away. |

## WARNINGS & PRECAUTIONS

**Don't take if:**
You are allergic to any thiazide diuretic drug.

**Before you start, consult your doctor:**
- If you are allergic to any sulfa drug.
- If you have gout.
- If you have liver, pancreas or kidney disorder.

**Over age 60:**
Adverse reactions and side effects may be more frequent and severe than in younger persons, especially dizziness and excessive potassium loss.

**Pregnancy:**
Risk to unborn child outweighs drug benefits. Don't use.

**Breast-feeding:**
Drug passes into milk. Avoid drug or discontinue nursing.

**Infants & children:**
No problems expected.

**Prolonged use:**
You may need medicine to treat high blood pressure for the rest of your life.

**Skin & sunlight:**
May cause rash or intensify sunburn in areas exposed to sun or sunlamp.

**Driving, piloting or hazardous work:**
Don't drive or pilot aircraft until you learn how medicine affects you. Don't work around dangerous machinery. Don't climb ladders or work in high places. Danger increases if you drink alcohol or take medicine affecting alertness and reflexes, such as antihistamines, tranquilizers, sedatives, pain medicine, narcotics and mind-altering drugs.

**Discontinuing:**
Don't discontinue without medical advice.

**Others:**
- Hot weather and fever may cause dehydration and drop in blood pressure. Dose may require temporary adjustment. Weigh daily and report any unexpected weight decreases to your doctor.
- May cause rise in uric acid, leading to gout.
- May cause blood-sugar rise in diabetics.

 **POSSIBLE INTERACTION WITH OTHER DRUGS**

| GENERIC NAME OR DRUG CLASS | COMBINED EFFECT |
|---|---|
| Acebutolol | Increased antihypertensive effect. Dosages of both drugs may require adjustments. |
| Allopurinol | Decreased allopurinol effect. |
| Amiodarone | Increased risk of heartbeat irregularity due to low potassium. |
| Antidepressants (tricyclic) | Dangerous drop in blood pressure. Avoid combination unless under medical supervision. |
| Barbiturates | Increased trichlormethiazide effect. |
| Calcium supplements | Increased calcium in blood. |
| Cholestyramine | Decreased trichlormethiazide effect. |
| Cortisone drugs | Excessive potassium loss that causes dangerous heart rhythms. |

| | |
|---|---|
| Digitalis preparations | Excessive potassium loss that causes dangerous heart rhythms. |
| Diuretics (thiazide) | Increased effect of other thiazide diuretics. |
| Indapamide | Increased diuretic effect. |
| Labetolol | Increased antihypertensive effects. |
| Lithium | Increased effect of lithium. |
| MAO inhibitors | Increased trichlormethiazide effect. |
| Nitrates | Excessive blood-pressure drop. |
| Oxprenolol | Increased antihypertensive effect. Dosages of both drugs may require adjustments. |
| Potassium supplements | Decreased potassium effect. |
| Probenecid | Decreased probenecid effect. |

 **POSSIBLE INTERACTION WITH OTHER SUBSTANCES**

| INTERACTS WITH | COMBINED EFFECT |
|---|---|
| Alcohol: | Dangerous blood-pressure drop. |
| Beverages: | None expected. |
| Cocaine: | None expected. |
| Foods: Licorice. | Excessive potassium loss that causes dangerous heart rhythms. |
| Marijuana: | May increase blood pressure. |
| Tobacco: | None expected. |

# TRICYCLIC ANTIDEPRESSANTS

## BRAND NAMES

See complete list of brand names in the *Brand Name Directory,* page 958.

## BASIC INFORMATION

**Habit forming? No**
**Prescription needed? Yes**
**Available as generic? Yes**
**Drug class: Antidepressant (tricyclic)**

## USES

- Gradually relieves, but doesn't cure, symptoms of depression.
- Imipramine is also used to decrease bedwetting.

## DOSAGE & USAGE INFORMATION

**How to take:**
Tablet or capsule—Swallow with liquid.

**When to take:**
At the same time each day, usually at bedtime.

**If you forget a dose:**
Bedtime dose—If you forget your once-a-day bedtime dose, don't take it more than 3 hours late. If more than 3 hours, wait for next scheduled dose. Don't double this dose.

**What drug does:**
Probably affects part of brain that controls messages between nerve cells.

**Time lapse before drug works:**
Begins in 1 to 2 weeks. May require 4 to 6 weeks for maximum benefit.

*Continued next column*

## OVERDOSE

**SYMPTOMS:**
**Hallucinations, convulsions, coma.**
**WHAT TO DO:**
- **Dial 0 (operator) or 911 (emergency) for an ambulance or medical help. Then give first aid immediately.**
- **If patient is unconscious and not breathing, give mouth-to-mouth breathing. If there is no heartbeat, use cardiac massage and mouth-to-mouth breathing (CPR). Don't try to make patient vomit. If you can't get help quickly, take patient to nearest emergency facility.**
- **See emergency information on inside covers.**

**Don't take with:**
- Non-prescription drugs without consulting doctor.
- See Interaction column and consult doctor.

## POSSIBLE ADVERSE REACTIONS OR SIDE EFFECTS

| SYMPTOMS | WHAT TO DO |
|---|---|
| **Life-threatening:** | |
| Seizures. | Seek emergency treatment immediately. |
| **Common:** | |
| • Headache, dry mouth or unpleasant taste, constipation or diarrhea, nausea, indigestion, fatigue, weakness. | Continue. Call doctor when convenient. |
| • Insomnia, "sweet tooth." | Continue. Tell doctor at next visit. |
| **Infrequent:** | |
| • Hallucinations, shakiness, dizziness, fainting, blurred vision, eye pain, vomiting, irregular heartbeat or slow pulse. | Discontinue. Call doctor right away. |
| • Difficult urination. | Continue. Call doctor when convenient. |
| **Rare:** | |
| Rash, itchy skin, sore throat, jaundice, fever. | Discontinue. Call doctor right away. |

## WARNINGS & PRECAUTIONS

**Don't take if:**
- You are allergic to any tricyclic antidepressant.
- You drink alcohol.
- You have had a heart attack within 6 weeks.
- You have glaucoma.
- You have taken MAO inhibitors within 2 weeks.
- Patient is younger than 12.

**Before you start, consult your doctor:**
- If you will have surgery within 2 months, including dental surgery, requiring general or spinal anesthesia.
- If you have an enlarged prostate.
- If you have heart disease or high blood pressure.
- If you have stomach or intestinal problems.
- If you have an overactive thyroid.
- If you have asthma.
- If you have liver disease.

**Over age 60:**
More likely to develop urination difficulty and side effects such as seizures, hallucinations, shaking, dizziness, fainting, headache, insomnia.

**Pregnancy:**
Studies inconclusive on harm to unborn child. Animal studies show fetal abnormalities. Decide with your doctor whether drug benefits justify risk to unborn child.

**Breast-feeding:**
Drug passes into milk. Avoid drug or discontinue nursing until you finish medicine. Consult doctor about maintaining milk supply.

**Infants & children:**
Don't give to children younger than 12.

**Prolonged use:**
No problems expected.

**Skin & sunlight:**
May cause rash or intensify sunburn in areas exposed to sun or sunlamp.

**Driving, piloting or hazardous work:**
Don't drive or pilot aircraft until you learn how medicine affects you. Don't work around dangerous machinery. Don't climb ladders or work in high places. Danger increases if you drink alcohol or take medicine affecting alertness and reflexes.

**Discontinuing:**
Don't discontinue without consulting doctor. Dose may require gradual reduction if you have taken drug for a long time. Doses of other drugs may also require adjustment.

**Others:**
No problems expected.

 **POSSIBLE INTERACTION WITH OTHER DRUGS**

| GENERIC NAME OR DRUG CLASS | COMBINED EFFECT |
|---|---|
| Anticoagulants (oral) | Increased anticoagulant effect. |
| Anticholinergics | Increased sedation. |
| Antihistamines | Increased antihistamine effect. |
| Barbiturates | Decreased antidepressant effect. |
| Clonidine | Decreased clonidine effect. |
| Diuretics (thiazide) | Increased antidepressant effect. |
| Ethchlorvynol | Delirium. |
| Guanethidine | Decreased guanethidine effect. |
| MAO inhibitors | Fever, delirium, convulsions. |
| Methyldopa | Decreased methyldopa effect. |
| Molindone | Increased molindone effect. |
| Narcotics | Dangerous oversedation. |
| Phenytoin | Decreased phenytoin effect. |
| Quinidine | Irregular heartbeat. |
| Sedatives | Dangerous oversedation. |
| Sympathomimetics | Increased sympathomimetic effect. |
| Thyroid hormones | Irregular heartbeat. |

 **POSSIBLE INTERACTION WITH OTHER SUBSTANCES**

| INTERACTS WITH | COMBINED EFFECT |
|---|---|
| Alcohol: Beverages or medicines with alcohol. | Excessive intoxication. Avoid. |
| Beverages: | None expected. |
| Cocaine: | Excessive intoxication. Avoid. |
| Foods: | None expected. |
| Marijuana: | Excessive drowsiness. Avoid. |
| Tobacco: | None expected. |

# TRIDIHEXETHYL

## BRAND NAMES

Milpath        Pathilon
Pathibamate

## BASIC INFORMATION

**Habit forming?** No
**Prescription needed?**
  **Low strength:** No
  **High strength:** Yes
**Available as generic?** Yes
**Drug class:** Antispasmodic, anticholinergic

 **USES**

Reduces spasms of digestive system, bladder and urethra.

 **DOSAGE & USAGE INFORMATION**

**How to take:**
Tablet—Swallow with liquid or food to lessen stomach irritation.

**When to take:**
30 minutes before meals (unless directed otherwise by doctor).

**If you forget a dose:**
Take as soon as you remember up to 2 hours late. If more than 2 hours, wait for next scheduled dose (don't double this dose).

**What drug does:**
Blocks nerve impulses at parasympathetic nerve endings, preventing muscle contractions and gland secretions of organs involved.

**Time lapse before drug works:**
15 to 30 minutes.

**Don't take with:**
See Interaction column and consult doctor.

 **OVERDOSE**

**SYMPTOMS:**
**Dilated pupils, rapid pulse and breathing, dizziness, fever, hallucinations, confusion, slurred speech, agitation, flushed face, convulsions, coma.**
**WHAT TO DO:**
- **Dial 0 (operator) or 911 (emergency) for an ambulance or medical help. Then give first aid immediately.**
- **See emergency information on inside covers.**

 **POSSIBLE ADVERSE REACTIONS OR SIDE EFFECTS**

| SYMPTOMS | WHAT TO DO |
|---|---|
| **Life-threatening:** | |
| None expected. | |
| **Common:** | |
| • Confusion, delirium, rapid heartbeat. | Discontinue. Call doctor right away. |
| • Nausea, vomiting, decreased sweating. | Continue. Call doctor when convenient. |
| • Constipation. | Continue. Tell doctor at next visit. |
| • Dryness in ears, nose, throat. | No action necessary. |
| **Infrequent:** | |
| Difficult urination, headache. | Continue. Call doctor when convenient. |
| **Rare:** | |
| Rash or hives, pain, blurred vision. | Discontinue. Call doctor right away. |

 **WARNINGS & PRECAUTIONS**

**Don't take if:**
- You are allergic to any anticholinergic.
- You have trouble with stomach bloating.
- You have difficulty emptying your bladder completely.
- You have narrow-angle glaucoma.
- You have severe ulcerative colitis.

**Before you start, consult your doctor:**
- If you have open-angle glaucoma.
- If you have angina.
- If you have chronic bronchitis or asthma.
- If you have hiatal hernia.
- If you have liver disease.
- If you have enlarged prostate.
- If you have myasthenia gravis.
- If you have peptic ulcer.
- If you will have surgery within 2 months, including dental surgery, requiring general or spinal anesthesia.

**Over age 60:**
Adverse reactions and side effects may be more frequent and severe than in younger persons.

**Pregnancy:**
Studies inconclusive on harm to unborn child. Animal studies show fetal abnormalities. Decide with your doctor whether drug benefits justify risk to unborn child.

**Breast-feeding:**
Drug passes into milk and decreases milk flow. Avoid drug or discontinue nursing until you finish medicine. Consult doctor for advice on maintaining milk supply.

**Infants & children:**
Use only under medical supervision.

**Prolonged use:**
Chronic constipation, possible fecal impaction. Consult doctor immediately.

**Skin & sunlight:**
No problems expected.

**Driving, piloting or hazardous work:**
Use disqualifies you for piloting aircraft. Otherwise, no problems expected.

**Discontinuing:**
May be unnecessary to finish medicine. Follow doctor's instructions.

**Others:**
No problems expected.

## POSSIBLE INTERACTION WITH OTHER DRUGS

| GENERIC NAME OR DRUG CLASS | COMBINED EFFECT |
|---|---|
| Amantadine | Increased tridihexethyl effect. |
| Anticholinergics (other) | Increased tridihexethyl effect. |
| Antidepressants (tricyclic) | Increased tridihexethyl effect. Increased sedation. |
| Antihistamines | Increased tridihexethyl effect. |
| Cortisone drugs | Increased internal-eye pressure. |
| Haloperidol | Increased internal-eye pressure. |

| | |
|---|---|
| MAO inhibitors | Increased tridihexethyl effect. |
| Meperidine | Increased tridihexethyl effect. |
| Methylphenidate | Increased tridihexethyl effect. |
| Nitrates | Increased internal-eye pressure. |
| Orphenadrine | Increased tridihexethyl effect. |
| Phenothiazines | Increased tridihexethyl effect. |
| Pilocarpine | Loss of pilocarpine effect in glaucoma treatment. |
| Potassium supplements | Possible intestinal ulcers with oral potassium tablets. |
| Vitamin C | Decreased tridihexethyl effect. Avoid large doses of vitamin C. |

## POSSIBLE INTERACTION WITH OTHER SUBSTANCES

| INTERACTS WITH | COMBINED EFFECT |
|---|---|
| Alcohol: | None expected. |
| Beverages: | None expected. |
| Cocaine: | Excessively rapid heartbeat. Avoid. |
| Foods: | None expected. |
| Marijuana: | Drowsiness and dry mouth. |
| Tobacco: | None expected. |

# TRIFLUOPERAZINE

## BRAND NAMES

Apo-Trifluoperazine
Clinazine
Novoflurazine
Pentazine
Solazine
Stelazine
Suprazine
Terfluzine
Triflurin
Tripazine

## BASIC INFORMATION

**Habit forming? No**
**Prescription needed? Yes**
**Available as generic? Yes**
**Drug class: Tranquilizer, antiemetic**
**(phenothiazine)**

## USES

- Stops nausea, vomiting.
- Reduces anxiety, agitation.

## DOSAGE & USAGE INFORMATION

**How to take:**
- Tablet or capsule—Swallow with liquid or food to lessen stomach irritation.
- Suppositories—Remove wrapper and moisten suppository with water. Gently insert into rectum, large end first.
- Drops or liquid—Dilute dose in beverage.

**When to take:**
- Nervous and mental disorders—Take at the same times each day.
- Nausea and vomiting—Take as needed, no more often than every 4 hours.

**If you forget a dose:**
- Nervous and mental disorders—Take up to 2 hours late. If more than 2 hours, wait for next scheduled dose (don't double this dose).
- Nausea and vomiting—Take as soon as you remember. Wait 4 hours for next dose.

**What drug does:**
- Suppresses brain's vomiting center.
- Suppresses brain centers that control abnormal emotions and behavior.

*Continued next column*

## OVERDOSE

**SYMPTOMS:**
Stupor, convulsions, coma.
**WHAT TO DO:**
- Dial 0 (operator) or 911 (emergency) for an ambulance or medical help. Then give first aid immediately.
- See emergency information on inside covers.

**Time lapse before drug works:**
- Nausea and vomiting—1 hour or less.
- Nervous and mental disorders—4-6 weeks.

**Don't take with:**
- Antacid or medicine for diarrhea.
- Non-prescription drug for cough, cold or allergy.
- See Interaction column and consult doctor.

## POSSIBLE ADVERSE REACTIONS OR SIDE EFFECTS

| SYMPTOMS | WHAT TO DO |
|---|---|
| **Life-threatening:**<br>None expected. | |
| **Common:** | |
| • Muscle spasms of face and neck, unsteady gait. | Discontinue. Seek emergency treatment. |
| • Restlessness, tremor, drowsiness. | Discontinue. Call doctor right away. |
| • Decreased sweating, dry mouth, nasal congestion, constipation. | Continue. Call doctor when convenient. |
| **Infrequent:** | |
| • Fainting. | Discontinue. Seek emergency treatment. |
| • Rash. | Discontinue. Call doctor right away. |
| • Difficult urination, less interest in sex, swollen breasts, menstrual irregularities. | Continue. Call doctor when convenient. |
| **Rare:**<br>Change in vision, sore throat, fever, jaundice. | Discontinue. Call doctor right away. |

## WARNINGS & PRECAUTIONS

**Don't take if:**
- You are allergic to any phenothiazine.
- You have a blood or bone-marrow disease.

**Before you start, consult your doctor:**
- If you will have surgery within 2 months, including dental surgery, requiring general or spinal anesthesia.
- If you have asthma, emphysema or other lung disorder.
- If you take non-prescription ulcer medicine, asthma medicine or amphetamines.

**Over age 60:**
Adverse reactions and side effects may be more frequent and severe than in younger persons. More likely to develop involuntary movement of jaws, lips, tongue, chewing. Report this to your doctor immediately. Early treatment can help.

**Pregnancy:**
Risk to unborn child outweighs drug benefits. Don't use.

**Breast-feeding:**
Drug passes into milk. Avoid drug or discontinue nursing until you finish medicine. Consult doctor for advice on maintaining milk supply.

**Infants & children:**
Don't give to children younger than 2.

**Prolonged use:**
May lead to tardive dyskinesia (involuntary movement of jaws, lips, tongue, chewing).

**Skin & sunlight:**
May cause rash or intensify sunburn in areas exposed to sun or sunlamp. Skin may remain sensitive for 3 months after discontinuing.

**Driving, piloting or hazardous work:**
Don't drive or pilot aircraft until you learn how medicine affects you. Don't work around dangerous machinery. Don't climb ladders or work in high places. Danger increases if you drink alcohol or take medicine affecting alertness and reflexes.

**Discontinuing:**
- Nervous and mental disorders—Don't discontinue without doctor's advice until you complete prescribed dose, even though symptoms diminish or disappear.
- Nausea and vomiting—May be unnecessary to finish medicine. Follow doctor's instructions.

**Others:**
No problems expected.

## POSSIBLE INTERACTION WITH OTHER DRUGS

| GENERIC NAME OR DRUG CLASS | COMBINED EFFECT |
| --- | --- |
| Anticholinergics | Increased anticholinergic effect. |
| Antidepressants (tricyclic) | Increased trifluoperazine effect. |
| Antihistamines | Increased antihistamine effect. |
| Appetite suppressants | Decreased suppressant effect. |
| Dronabinol | Increased effects of both drugs. Avoid. |
| Levodopa | Decreased levodopa effect. |
| Mind-altering drugs | Increased effect of mind-altering drugs. |
| Molindone | Increased tranquilizer effect. |
| Narcotics | Increased narcotic effect. |
| Phenytoin | Increased phenytoin effect. |
| Quinidine | Impaired heart function. Dangerous mixture. |
| Sedatives | Increased sedative effect. |
| Tranquilizers (other) | Increased tranquilizer effect. |

## POSSIBLE INTERACTION WITH OTHER SUBSTANCES

| INTERACTS WITH | COMBINED EFFECT |
| --- | --- |
| Alcohol: | Dangerous oversedation. |
| Beverages: | None expected. |
| Cocaine: | Decreased trifluoperazine effect. Avoid. |
| Foods: | None expected. |
| Marijuana: | Drowsiness. May increase antinausea effect. |
| Tobacco: | None expected. |

# TRIFLUPROMAZINE

## BRAND NAMES

Psyquil          Vesprin

## BASIC INFORMATION

Habit forming? No
Prescription needed? Yes
Available as generic? Yes
Drug class: Tranquilizer, antiemetic
          (phenothiazine)

 **USES**

- Stops nausea, vomiting.
- Reduces anxiety, agitation.

 **DOSAGE & USAGE INFORMATION**

**How to take:**
- Tablet or capsule—Swallow with liquid or food to lessen stomach irritation.
- Suppositories—Remove wrapper and moisten suppository with water. Gently insert into rectum, large end first.
- Drops or liquid—Dilute dose in beverage.

**When to take:**
- Nervous and mental disorders—Take at the same times each day.
- Nausea and vomiting—Take as needed, no more often than every 4 hours.

**If you forget a dose:**
- Nervous and mental disorders—Take up to 2 hours late. If more than 2 hours, wait for next scheduled dose (don't double this dose).
- Nausea and vomiting—Take as soon as you remember. Wait 4 hours for next dose.

**What drug does:**
- Suppresses brain's vomiting center.
- Suppresses brain centers that control abnormal emotions and behavior.

**Time lapse before drug works:**
- Nausea and vomiting—1 hour or less.
- Nervous and mental disorders—4-6 weeks.

*Continued next column*

 **OVERDOSE**

**SYMPTOMS:**
Stupor, convulsions, coma.
**WHAT TO DO:**
- Dial 0 (operator) or 911 (emergency) for an ambulance or medical help. Then give first aid immediately.
- See emergency information on inside covers.

**Don't take with:**
- Antacid or medicine for diarrhea.
- Non-prescription drug for cough, cold or allergy.
- See Interaction column and consult doctor.

 **POSSIBLE ADVERSE REACTIONS OR SIDE EFFECTS**

| SYMPTOMS | WHAT TO DO |
|---|---|
| **Life-threatening:** | |
| None expected. | |
| **Common:** | |
| • Muscle spasms of face and neck, unsteady gait. | Discontinue. Seek emergency treatment. |
| • Restlessness, tremor, drowsiness. | Discontinue. Call doctor right away. |
| • Decreased sweating, dry mouth, nasal congestion, constipation. | Continue. Call doctor when convenient. |
| **Infrequent:** | |
| • Fainting. | Discontinue. Seek emergency treatment. |
| • Rash. | Discontinue. Call doctor right away. |
| • Difficult urination, less interest in sex, swollen breasts, menstrual irregularities. | Continue. Call doctor when convenient. |
| **Rare:** | |
| Change in vision, sore throat, fever, jaundice. | Discontinue. Call doctor right away. |

## WARNINGS & PRECAUTIONS

**Don't take if:**
- You are allergic to any phenothiazine.
- You have a blood or bone-marrow disease.

**Before you start, consult your doctor:**
- If you will have surgery within 2 months, including dental surgery, requiring general or spinal anesthesia.
- If you have asthma, emphysema or other lung disorder.
- If you take non-prescription ulcer medicine, asthma medicine or amphetamines.

**Over age 60:**
Adverse reactions and side effects may be more frequent and severe than in younger persons. More likely to develop involuntary movement of jaws, lips, tongue, chewing. Report this to your doctor immediately. Early treatment can help.

**Pregnancy:**
Risk to unborn child outweighs drug benefits. Don't use.

**Breast-feeding:**
Drug passes into milk. Avoid drug or discontinue nursing until you finish medicine. Consult doctor for advice on maintaining milk supply.

**Infants & children:**
Don't give to children younger than 2.

**Prolonged use:**
May lead to tardive dyskinesia (involuntary movement of jaws, lips, tongue, chewing).

**Skin & sunlight:**
May cause rash or intensify sunburn in areas exposed to sun or sunlamp. Skin may remain sensitive for 3 months after discontinuing.

**Driving, piloting or hazardous work:**
Don't drive or pilot aircraft until you learn how medicine affects you. Don't work around dangerous machinery. Don't climb ladders or work in high places. Danger increases if you drink alcohol or take medicine affecting alertness and reflexes.

**Discontinuing:**
- Nervous and mental disorders—Don't discontinue without doctor's advice until you complete prescribed dose, even though symptoms diminish or disappear.
- Nausea and vomiting—May be unnecessary to finish medicine. Follow doctor's instructions.

**Others:**
No problems expected.

## POSSIBLE INTERACTION WITH OTHER DRUGS

| GENERIC NAME OR DRUG CLASS | COMBINED EFFECT |
|---|---|
| Anticholinergics | Increased anticholinergic effect. |
| Antidepressants (tricyclic) | Increased triflupromazine effect. |
| Antihistamines | Increased antihistamine effect. |
| Appetite suppressants | Decreased suppressant effect. |
| Dronabinol | Increased effects of both drugs. Avoid. |
| Levodopa | Decreased levodopa effect. |
| Mind-altering drugs | Increased effect of mind-altering drugs. |
| Molindone | Increased tranquilizer effect. |
| Narcotics | Increased narcotic effect. |
| Phenytoin | Increased phenytoin effect. |
| Quinidine | Impaired heart function. Dangerous mixture. |
| Sedatives | Increased sedative effect. |
| Tranquilizers (other) | Increased tranquilizer effect. |

## POSSIBLE INTERACTION WITH OTHER SUBSTANCES

| INTERACTS WITH | COMBINED EFFECT |
|---|---|
| Alcohol: | Dangerous oversedation. |
| Beverages: | None expected. |
| Cocaine: | Decreased triflupromazine effect. Avoid. |
| Foods: | None expected. |
| Marijuana: | Drowsiness. May increase antinausea effect. |
| Tobacco: | None expected. |

# TRIHEXYPHENIDYL

## BRAND NAMES

| | |
|---|---|
| Aparkane | T.H.P. |
| Apo-Trihex | Tremin |
| Artane | Trihexane |
| Artane Sequels | Trihexidyl |
| Novohexidyl | Trihexy |

## BASIC INFORMATION

**Habit forming? No**
**Prescription needed? Yes**
**Available as generic? Yes**
**Drug class: Antidyskinetic, antiparkinsonism**

## USES

- Treatment of Parkinson's disease.
- Treatment of adverse effects of phenothiazines.

## DOSAGE & USAGE INFORMATION

**How to take:**
Tablets or capsules—Take with food to lessen stomach irritation.

**When to take:**
At the same times each day.

**If you forget a dose:**
Take as soon as you remember up to 2 hours late. If more than 2 hours, wait for next scheduled dose (don't double this dose).

**What drug does:**
- Balances chemical reactions necessary to send nerve impulses within base of brain.
- Improves muscle control and reduces stiffness.

*Continued next column*

## OVERDOSE

**SYMPTOMS:**
**Agitation, dilated pupils, hallucinations, dry mouth, rapid heartbeat, sleepiness.**
**WHAT TO DO:**
- **Dial 0 (operator) or 911 (emergency) for an ambulance or medical help. Then give first aid immediately.**
- **If patient is unconscious and not breathing, give mouth-to-mouth breathing. If there is no heartbeat, use cardiac massage and mouth-to-mouth breathing (CPR). Don't try to make patient vomit. If you can't get help quickly, take patient to nearest emergency facility.**
- **See emergency information on inside covers.**

**Time lapse before drug works:**
1 to 2 hours.

**Don't take with:**
- Non-prescription drugs for colds, cough or allergy.
- See Interaction column and consult doctor.

## POSSIBLE ADVERSE REACTIONS OR SIDE EFFECTS

| SYMPTOMS | WHAT TO DO |
|---|---|
| **Life-threatening:** | |
| None expected. | |
| **Common:** | |
| • Blurred vision, light sensitivity, constipation, nausea, vomiting. | Continue. Call doctor when convenient. |
| • Painful or difficult urination. | Continue. Tell doctor at next visit. |
| **Infrequent:** | |
| None expected. | |
| **Rare:** | |
| • Rash, eye pain. | Discontinue. Call doctor right away. |
| • Confusion, dizziness, sore mouth or tongue, muscle cramps, numbness or tingling in hands or feet. | Continue. Call doctor when convenient. |

## WARNINGS & PRECAUTIONS

**Don't take if:**
You are allergic to any antidyskinetic.

**Before you start, consult your doctor:**
- If you have had glaucoma.
- If you have had high blood pressure or heart disease.
- If you have had impaired liver function.
- If you have had kidney disease or urination difficulty.

**Over age 60:**
More sensitive to drug. Aggravates symptoms of enlarged prostate. Causes impaired thinking, hallucinations, nightmares. Consult doctor about any of these.

**Pregnancy:**
Studies inconclusive on harm to unborn child. Animal studies show fetal abnormalities. Decide with your doctor whether drug benefits justify risk to unborn child.

**Breast-feeding:**
No problems expected.

**Infants & children:**
Not recommended for children 3 and younger. Use for older children only under doctor's supervision.

**Prolonged use:**
Possible glaucoma.

**Skin & sunlight:**
No problems expected.

**Driving, piloting or hazardous work:**
Don't drive or pilot aircraft until you learn how medicine affects you. Don't work around dangerous machinery. Don't climb ladders or work in high places. Danger increases if you drink alcohol or take medicine affecting alertness and reflexes, such as antihistamines, tranquilizers, sedatives, pain medicine, narcotics and mind-altering drugs.

**Discontinuing:**
Don't discontinue without consulting doctor. Dose may require gradual reduction if you have taken drug for a long time. Doses of other drugs may also require adjustment.

**Others:**
- Internal eye pressure should be measured regularly.
- Avoid becoming overheated.

## POSSIBLE INTERACTION WITH OTHER DRUGS

| GENERIC NAME OR DRUG CLASS | COMBINED EFFECT |
| --- | --- |
| Amantadine | Increased amantadine effect. |
| Antidepressants (tricyclic) | Increased trihexyphenidyl effect. May cause glaucoma. |
| Antihistamines | Increased trihexyphenidyl effect. |
| Levodopa | Increased levodopa effect. Improved results in treating Parkinson's disease. |
| MAO inhibitors | Increased trihexyphenidyl effect. |
| Meperidine | Increased trihexyphenidyl effect. |
| Orphenadrine | Increased trihexyphenidyl effect. |
| Phenothiazines | Behavior changes. |
| Primidone | Excessive sedation. |
| Procainamide | Increased procainamide effect. |
| Quinidine | Increased trihexyphenidyl effect. |
| Tranquilizers | Excessive sedation. |

## POSSIBLE INTERACTION WITH OTHER SUBSTANCES

| INTERACTS WITH | COMBINED EFFECT |
| --- | --- |
| Alcohol: | None expected. |
| Beverages: | None expected. |
| Cocaine: | Decreased trihexyphenidyl effect. Avoid. |
| Foods: | None expected. |
| Marijuana: | None expected. |
| Tobacco: | None expected. |

# TRIMEPRAZINE

## BRAND NAMES

Panectyl                    Temaril

## BASIC INFORMATION

**Habit forming?** No
**Prescription needed?** Yes
**Available as generic?** Yes
**Drug class:** Tranquilizer (phenothiazine), antihistamine

 ## USES

Relieves itching of hives, skin allergies, chickenpox.

 ## DOSAGE & USAGE INFORMATION

**How to take:**
- Tablet or syrup—Swallow with liquid or food to lessen stomach irritation.
- Extended-release capsules—Swallow each dose whole. If you take regular tablets, you may chew or crush them.

**When to take:**
At the same times each day.

**If you forget a dose:**
Take as soon as you remember up to 2 hours late. If more than 2 hours, wait for next scheduled dose (don't double this dose).

**What drug does:**
Blocks histamine action in skin.

**Time lapse before drug works:**
1 to 2 hours.

**Don't take with:**
- Antacid or medicine for diarrhea.
- Non-prescription drug for cough, cold or allergy.
- See Interaction column and consult doctor.

 ## OVERDOSE

**SYMPTOMS:**
Stupor, convulsions, coma.
**WHAT TO DO:**
- Dial 0 (operator) or 911 (emergency) for an ambulance or medical help. Then give first aid immediately.
- See emergency information on inside covers.

 ## POSSIBLE ADVERSE REACTIONS OR SIDE EFFECTS

| SYMPTOMS | WHAT TO DO |
|---|---|
| **Life-threatening:** None expected. | |
| **Common:** | |
| • Restlessness, tremor, drowsiness. | Discontinue. Call doctor right away. |
| • Decreased sweating, dry mouth, nasal congestion, constipation. | Continue. Call doctor when convenient. |
| **Infrequent:** | |
| • Fainting. | Discontinue. Seek emergency treatment. |
| • Rash, muscle spasms of face and neck, unsteady gait. | Discontinue. Call doctor right away. |
| • Difficult urination, less interest in sex, swollen breasts, menstrual irregularities. | Continue. Call doctor when convenient. |
| **Rare:** | |
| Change in vision, sore throat, fever, jaundice. | Discontinue. Call doctor right away. |

## WARNINGS & PRECAUTIONS

**Don't take if:**
- You are allergic to any phenothiazine.
- You have a blood or bone-marrow disease.

**Before you start, consult your doctor:**
- If you will have surgery within 2 months, including dental surgery, requiring general or spinal anesthesia.
- If you have asthma, emphysema or other lung disorder.
- If you take non-prescription ulcer medicine, asthma medicine or amphetamines.

**Over age 60:**
Adverse reactions and side effects may be more frequent and severe than in younger persons. More likely to develop tardive dyskinesia (involuntary movement of jaws, lips, tongue, chewing). Report this to your doctor immediately. Early treatment can help.

**Pregnancy:**
Risk to unborn child outweighs drug benefits. Don't use.

**Breast-feeding:**
Drug passes into milk. Avoid drug or discontinue nursing until you finish medicine. Consult doctor for advice on maintaining milk supply.

**Infants & children:**
Don't give to children younger than 2.

**Prolonged use:**
May lead to tardive dyskinesia (involuntary movement of jaws, lips, tongue, chewing).

**Skin & sunlight:**
May cause rash or intensify sunburn in areas exposed to sun or sunlamp. Skin may remain sensitive for 3 months after discontinuing.

**Driving, piloting or hazardous work:**
Don't drive or pilot aircraft until you learn how medicine affects you. Don't work around dangerous machinery. Don't climb ladders or work in high places. Danger increases if you drink alcohol or take medicine affecting alertness and reflexes.

**Discontinuing:**
May be unnecessary to finish medicine. Follow doctor's instructions.

**Others:**
No problems expected.

## POSSIBLE INTERACTION WITH OTHER DRUGS

| GENERIC NAME OR DRUG CLASS | COMBINED EFFECT |
|---|---|
| Antacids | Decreased trimeprazine effect. |
| Anticholinergics | Increased anticholinergic effect. |
| Anticonvulsants (hydantoin) | Increased anticonvulsant effect. |
| Antidepressants (tricyclic) | Increased trimeprazine effect. |
| Antihistamines (other) | Increased antihistamine effect. |
| Appetite suppressants | Decreased suppressant effect. |
| Barbiturates | Oversedation. |
| Dronabinol | Increased effects of both drugs. Avoid. |
| Guanethidine | Decreased guanethidine effect. |
| Levodopa | Decreased levodopa effect |
| MAO inhibitors | Increased trimeprazine effect. |
| Mind-altering drugs | Increased effect of mind-altering drugs. |
| Molindone | Increased sedative and antihistamine effect. |
| Narcotics | Increased narcotic effect. |
| Sedatives | Increased sedative effect. |
| Tranquilizers | Increased tranquilizer effect. Avoid. |

## POSSIBLE INTERACTION WITH OTHER SUBSTANCES

| INTERACTS WITH | COMBINED EFFECT |
|---|---|
| Alcohol: | Dangerous oversedation. |
| Beverages: | None expected. |
| Cocaine: | Decreased effect of trimeprazine. Avoid. |
| Foods: | None expected. |
| Marijuana: | Drowsiness. |
| Tobacco: | None expected. |

# TRIMETHOBENZAMIDE

## BRAND NAMES

| | |
|---|---|
| Stemetic | Tigan |
| Tegamide | Tiject-20 |
| Ticon | |

## BASIC INFORMATION

**Habit forming? No**
**Prescription needed? Yes**
**Available as generic? Yes**
**Drug class: Antiemetic**

 ## USES

Reduces nausea and vomiting.

 ## DOSAGE & USAGE INFORMATION

**How to take:**
- Capsule—Swallow with liquid. If you can't swallow whole, open capsule and take with liquid or food.
- Suppositories—Remove wrapper and moisten suppository with water. Gently insert larger end into rectum. Push well into rectum with finger.

**When to take:**
When needed, no more often than label directs.

**If you forget a dose:**
Take when you remember. Wait as long as label directs for next dose.

**What drug does:**
Possibly blocks nerve impulses to brain's vomiting centers.

**Time lapse before drug works:**
20 to 40 minutes.

*Continued next column*

 ## OVERDOSE

**SYMPTOMS:**
Confusion, convulsions, coma.
**WHAT TO DO:**
- Dial 0 (operator) or 911 (emergency) for an ambulance or medical help. Then give first aid immediately.
- If patient is unconscious and not breathing, give mouth-to-mouth breathing. If there is no heartbeat, use cardiac massage and mouth-to-mouth breathing (CPR). Don't try to make patient vomit. If you can't get help quickly, take patient to nearest emergency facility.
- See emergency information on inside covers.

**Don't take with:**
Non-prescription drugs or drugs in Interaction column without consulting doctor.

 ## POSSIBLE ADVERSE REACTIONS OR SIDE EFFECTS

| SYMPTOMS | WHAT TO DO |
|---|---|
| **Life-threatening:**<br>None expected. | |
| **Common:**<br>None expected. | |
| **Infrequent:**<br>• Rash, blurred vision, low blood pressure. | Discontinue. Call doctor right away. |
| • Dizziness, drowsiness, headache, diarrhea, muscle cramps, unusual tiredness. | Continue. Call doctor when convenient. |
| **Rare:**<br>Seizures, tremor, depression, sore throat, fever, repeated vomiting, back pain, jaundice. | Discontinue. Call doctor right away. |

## WARNINGS & PRECAUTIONS

**Don't take if:**
- You are allergic to trimethobenzamide.
- You are allergic to local anesthetics and have suppository form.

**Before you start, consult your doctor:**
If you have reacted badly to antihistamines.

**Over age 60:**
More susceptible to low blood pressure and sedative effects of this drug.

**Pregnancy:**
No proven harm to unborn child. Avoid if possible.

**Breast-feeding:**
No proven problems. Avoid if possible.

**Infants & children:**
- Injectable form not recommended.
- Avoid during viral infections. Drug may contribute to Reyes' syndrome.

**Prolonged use:**
- Damages blood-cell production of bone marrow.
- Causes Parkinson-like symptoms of tremors, rigidity.

**Skin & sunlight:**
Possible sun sensitivity. Use caution.

**Driving, piloting or hazardous work:**
- Use disqualifies you for piloting aircraft.
- Don't drive until you learn how medicine affects you. Don't work around dangerous machinery. Don't climb ladders or work in high places. Danger increases if you drink alcohol or take medicine affecting alertness and reflexes, such as antihistamines, tranquilizers, sedatives, pain medicine, narcotics and mind-altering drugs.

**Discontinuing:**
May be unnecessary to finish medicine. Follow doctor's instructions.

**Others:**
No problems expected.

## POSSIBLE INTERACTION WITH OTHER DRUGS

| GENERIC NAME OR DRUG CLASS | COMBINED EFFECT |
|---|---|
| Antidepressants | Increased sedative effect. |
| Antihistamines | Increased sedative effect. |
| Barbiturates | Increased effect of both drugs. |
| Belladonna | Increased effect of both drugs. |
| Cholinergics | Increased effect of both drugs. |
| Mind-altering drugs | Increased effect of mind-altering drug. |
| Narcotics | Increased sedative effect. |
| Phenothiazines | Increased effect of both drugs. |
| Sedatives | Increased sedative effect. |
| Sleep inducers | Increased effect of sleep inducer. |
| Tranquilizers | Increased sedative effect. |

## POSSIBLE INTERACTION WITH OTHER SUBSTANCES

| INTERACTS WITH | COMBINED EFFECT |
|---|---|
| Alcohol: | Oversedation. Avoid. |
| Beverages: | None expected. |
| Cocaine: | None expected. |
| Foods: | None expected. |
| Marijuana: | Increased antinausea effect. |
| Tobacco: | None expected. |

# TRIMETHOPRIM

## BRAND NAMES

| | |
|---|---|
| Apo-Sulfatrim | Rovbac |
| Bactrim | Septra |
| Cotrim | SMZ-TMP |
| Novotrimel | Syraprim |
| Proloprim | Trimpex |
| Protrin | |

## BASIC INFORMATION

**Habit forming? No**
**Prescription needed? Yes**
**Available as generic? Yes**
**Drug class: Antimicrobial**

## USES

- Treatment for urinary-tract infections susceptible to trimethoprim.
- Helps prevent recurrent urinary-tract infections if taken once a day.

## DOSAGE & USAGE INFORMATION

**How to take:**
- Tablet or capsule—Swallow with liquid or food to lessen stomach irritation.
- Drops—Dilute dose in beverage before swallowing.

**When to take:**
Space doses evenly in 24 hours to keep constant amount in urine.

**If you forget a dose:**
Take as soon as possible. Wait 5 to 6 hours before next dose. Then return to regular schedule.

**What drug does:**
Stops harmful bacterial germs from multiplying. Will not kill viruses.

**Time lapse before drug works:**
2 to 5 days.

**Don't take with:**
See Interaction column and consult doctor.

## OVERDOSE

**SYMPTOMS:**
**Nausea, vomiting, diarrhea.**
**WHAT TO DO:**
**Overdose unlikely to threaten life. If person takes much larger amount than prescribed, call doctor, poison-control center or hospital emergency room for instructions.**

## POSSIBLE ADVERSE REACTIONS OR SIDE EFFECTS

| SYMPTOMS | WHAT TO DO |
|---|---|
| **Life-threatening:**<br>None expected. | |
| **Common:**<br>Rash, itchy skin. | Discontinue. Seek emergency treatment. |
| **Infrequent:**<br>• Diarrhea, nausea, vomiting, abdominal pain. | Discontinue. Call doctor right away. |
| • Headache. | Continue. Call doctor when convenient. |
| **Rare:**<br>• Blue fingernails, lips and skin; difficult breathing. | Discontinue. Seek emergency treatment. |
| • Sore throat, fever. | Discontinue. Call doctor right away. |

## WARNINGS & PRECAUTIONS

**Don't take if:**
You are allergic to trimethoprim or any sulfa drug.

**Before you start, consult your doctor:**
If you have had liver or kidney disease.

**Over age 60:**
- Reduced liver and kidney function may require reduced dose.
- More likely to have severe anal and genital itch.
- Increased susceptibility to anemia.

**Pregnancy:**
Studies inconclusive on harm to unborn child. Animal studies show fetal abnormalities. Decide with your doctor whether drug benefits justify risk to unborn child.

**Breast-feeding:**
No proven harm to unborn child. Avoid if possible.

**Infants & children:**
Use under medical supervision only.

**Prolonged use:**
Anemia.

**Skin & sunlight:**
May cause rash or intensify sunburn in areas exposed to sun or sunlamp.

**Driving, piloting or hazardous work:**
No problems expected.

**Discontinuing:**
Don't discontinue without doctor's advice until you complete prescribed dose, even though symptoms diminish or disappear.

**Others:**
No problems expected.

## POSSIBLE INTERACTION WITH OTHER DRUGS

| GENERIC NAME OR DRUG CLASS | COMBINED EFFECT |
|---|---|
| Diuretics (thiazide) | Unusual bleeding or bruising. |
| Flecainide | Possible decreased blood-cell production in bone marrow. |
| Sulfamethoxazole | Beneficial increase of sulfamethoxazole effect. |
| Tocainide | Possible decreased blood-cell production in bone marrow. |

## POSSIBLE INTERACTION WITH OTHER SUBSTANCES

| INTERACTS WITH | COMBINED EFFECT |
|---|---|
| Alcohol: | Increased alcohol effect with Bactrim or Septra. |
| Beverages: | None expected. |
| Cocaine: | No proven problems. |
| Foods: | None expected. |
| Marijuana: | None expected. |
| Tobacco: | None expected. |

# TRIPELENNAMINE

## BRAND NAMES

PBZ  
PBZ-SR  

Pyribenzamine  
Ro-Hist

## BASIC INFORMATION

Habit forming? No  
Prescription needed?  
  High strength: Yes  
  Low strength: No  
Available as generic? Yes  
Drug class: Antihistamine

## USES

- Reduces allergic symptoms such as hay fever, hives, rash or itching.
- Induces sleep.

## DOSAGE & USAGE INFORMATION

**How to take:**
- Tablet or liquid—Swallow with liquid or food to lessen stomach irritation.
- Extended-release tablets—Swallow each dose whole.

**When to take:**  
Varies with form. Follow label directions.

**If you forget a dose:**  
Take as soon as you remember up to 2 hours late. If more than 2 hours, wait for next scheduled dose (don't double this dose).

**What drug does:**  
Blocks action of histamine after an allergic response triggers histamine release in sensitive cells.

*Continued next column*

## OVERDOSE

**SYMPTOMS:**  
Convulsions, red face, hallucinations, coma.  
**WHAT TO DO:**
- **Dial 0 (operator) or 911 (emergency) for an ambulance or medical help. Then give first aid immediately.**
- **If patient is unconscious and not breathing, give mouth-to-mouth breathing. If there is no heartbeat, use cardiac massage and mouth-to-mouth breathing (CPR). Don't try to make patient vomit. If you can't get help quickly, take patient to nearest emergency facility.**
- **See emergency information on inside covers.**

**Time lapse before drug works:**  
30 minutes.

**Don't take with:**  
See Interaction column and consult doctor.

## POSSIBLE ADVERSE REACTIONS OR SIDE EFFECTS

| SYMPTOMS | WHAT TO DO |
|---|---|
| **Life-threatening:**<br>None expected. | |
| **Common:**<br>Drowsiness; dizziness; dry mouth, nose and throat; nausea. | Continue. Tell doctor at next visit. |
| **Infrequent:**<br>• Change in vision. | Discontinue. Call doctor right away. |
| • Less tolerance for contact lenses, difficult urination. | Continue. Call doctor when convenient. |
| • Appetite loss. | Continue. Tell doctor at next visit. |
| **Rare:**<br>Nightmares, agitation, irritability, sore throat, fever, rapid heartbeat, unusual bleeding or bruising, fatigue, weakness. | Discontinue. Call doctor right away. |

## WARNINGS & PRECAUTIONS

**Don't take if:**
You are allergic to any antihistamine.

**Before you start, consult your doctor:**
- If you have glaucoma.
- If you have enlarged prostate.
- If you have asthma.
- If you have kidney disease.
- If you have peptic ulcer.
- If you will have surgery within 2 months, including dental surgery, requiring general or spinal anesthesia.

**Over age 60:**
Don't exceed recommended dose. Adverse reactions and side effects may be more frequent and severe than in younger persons, especially urination difficulty, diminished alertness and other brain and nervous-system symptoms.

**Pregnancy:**
No proven harm to unborn child. Avoid if possible.

**Breast-feeding:**
Drug passes into milk. Avoid drug or discontinue nursing until you finish medicine. Consult doctor for advice on maintaining milk supply.

**Infants & children:**
Not recommended for premature or newborn infants. Otherwise, no problems expected.

**Prolonged use:**
Avoid. May damage bone marrow and nerve cells.

**Skin & sunlight:**
May cause rash or intensify sunburn in areas exposed to sun or sunlamp.

**Driving, piloting or hazardous work:**
Don't drive or pilot aircraft until you learn how medicine affects you. Don't work around dangerous machinery. Don't climb ladders or work in high places. Danger increases if you drink alcohol or take medicine affecting alertness and reflexes, such as antihistamines, tranquilizers, sedatives, pain medicine, narcotics and mind-altering drugs.

**Discontinuing:**
No problems expected.

**Others:**
May mask symptoms of hearing damage from aspirin, other salicylates, cisplatin, paromomycin, vancomycin or anticonvulsants. Consult doctor if you use these.

## POSSIBLE INTERACTION WITH OTHER DRUGS

| GENERIC NAME OR DRUG CLASS | COMBINED EFFECT |
|---|---|
| Anticholinergics | Increased anticholinergic effect. |
| Antidepressants (tricyclic) | Increased tripelennamine effect. Excess sedation. |
| Antihistamines (other) | Excess sedation. Avoid. |
| Dronabinol | Increased effects of both drugs. Avoid. |
| Hypnotics | Excess sedation. Avoid. |
| MAO inhibitors | Increased tripelennamine effect. |
| Mind-altering drugs | Excess sedation. Avoid. |
| Molindone | Increased antihistamine effect. |
| Narcotics | Excess sedation. Avoid. |
| Sedatives | Excess sedation. Avoid. |
| Sleep inducers | Excess sedation. Avoid. |
| Tranquilizers | Excess sedation. Avoid. |

## POSSIBLE INTERACTION WITH OTHER SUBSTANCES

| INTERACTS WITH | COMBINED EFFECT |
|---|---|
| Alcohol: | Excess sedation. Avoid. |
| Beverages: Caffeine drinks. | Less tripelennamine sedation. |
| Cocaine: | Decreased tripelennamine effect. Avoid. |
| Foods: | None expected. |
| Marijuana: | Excess sedation. Avoid. |
| Tobacco: | None expected. |

# TRIPROLIDINE

## BRAND NAMES

Actidil
Actifed
Bayidyl
Eldafed

Triafed-C
Trifed
Tripodrine

## BASIC INFORMATION

Habit forming? No
Prescription needed?
  High Strength: Yes
  Low strength: No
Available as generic? Yes
Drug class: Antihistamine

 **USES**

- Reduces allergic symptoms such as hay fever, hives, rash or itching.
- Induces sleep.

 **DOSAGE & USAGE INFORMATION**

**How to take:**
Tablet or syrup—Swallow with liquid or food to lessen stomach irritation.

**When to take:**
Varies with form. Follow label directions.

**If you forget a dose:**
Take as soon as you remember up to 2 hours late. If more than 2 hours, wait for next scheduled dose (don't double this dose).

**What drug does:**
Blocks action of histamine after an allergic response triggers histamine release in sensitive cells.

*Continued next column*

 **OVERDOSE**

**SYMPTOMS:**
Convulsions, red face, hallucinations, coma.
**WHAT TO DO:**
- Dial 0 (operator) or 911 (emergency) for an ambulance or medical help. Then give first aid immediately.
- If patient is unconscious and not breathing, give mouth-to-mouth breathing. If there is no heartbeat, use cardiac massage and mouth-to-mouth breathing (CPR). Don't try to make patient vomit. If you can't get help quickly, take patient to nearest emergency facility.
- See emergency information on inside covers.

**Time lapse before drug works:**
30 minutes.

**Don't take with:**
See Interaction column and consult doctor.

 **POSSIBLE ADVERSE REACTIONS OR SIDE EFFECTS**

| SYMPTOMS | WHAT TO DO |
|---|---|
| **Life-threatening:** None expected. | |
| **Common:** Drowsiness; dizziness; dry mouth, nose and throat; nausea. | Continue. Tell doctor at next visit. |
| **Infrequent:** • Change in vision. | Discontinue. Call doctor right away. |
| • Less tolerance for contact lenses, difficult urination. | Continue. Call doctor when convenient. |
| • Appetite loss. | Continue. Tell doctor at next visit. |
| **Rare:** Nightmares, agitation, irritability, sore throat, fever, rapid heartbeat, unusual bleeding or bruising, fatigue, weakness. | Discontinue. Call doctor right away. |

## WARNINGS & PRECAUTIONS

**Don't take if:**
You are allergic to any antihistamine.

**Before you start, consult your doctor:**
- If you have glaucoma.
- If you have enlarged prostate.
- If you have asthma.
- If you have kidney disease.
- If you have peptic ulcer.
- If you will have surgery within 2 months, including dental surgery, requiring general or spinal anesthesia.

**Over age 60:**
Don't exceed recommended dose. Adverse reactions and side effects may be more frequent and severe than in younger persons, especially urination difficulty, diminished alertness and other brain and nervous-system symptoms.

**Pregnancy:**
No proven harm to unborn child. Avoid if possible.

**Breast-feeding:**
Drug passes into milk. Avoid drug or discontinue nursing until you finish medicine. Consult doctor for advice on maintaining milk supply.

**Infants & children:**
Not recommended for premature or newborn infants. Otherwise, no problems expected.

**Prolonged use:**
Avoid. May damage bone marrow and nerve cells.

**Skin & sunlight:**
May cause rash or intensify sunburn in areas exposed to sun or sunlamp.

**Driving, piloting or hazardous work:**
Don't drive or pilot aircraft until you learn how medicine affects you. Don't work around dangerous machinery. Don't climb ladders or work in high places. Danger increases if you drink alcohol or take medicine affecting alertness and reflexes, such as antihistamines, tranquilizers, sedatives, pain medicine, narcotics and mind-altering drugs.

**Discontinuing:**
No problems expected.

**Others:**
May mask symptoms of hearing damage from aspirin, other salicylates, cisplatin, paromomycin, vancomycin or anticonvulsants. Consult doctor if you use these.

## POSSIBLE INTERACTION WITH OTHER DRUGS

| GENERIC NAME OR DRUG CLASS | COMBINED EFFECT |
|---|---|
| Anticholinergics | Increased anticholinergic effect. |
| Antidepressants (tricyclic) | Increased triprolidine effect. Excess sedation. |
| Antihistamines (other) | Excess sedation. Avoid. |
| Dronabinol | Increased effects of both drugs. Avoid. |
| Hypnotics | Excess sedation. Avoid. |
| MAO inhibitors | Increased triprolidine effect. |
| Mind-altering drugs | Excess sedation. Avoid. |
| Molindone | Increased antihistamine effect. |
| Narcotics | Excess sedation. Avoid. |
| Sedatives | Excess sedation. Avoid. |
| Sleep inducers | Excess sedation. Avoid. |
| Tranquilizers | Excess sedation. Avoid. |

## POSSIBLE INTERACTION WITH OTHER SUBSTANCES

| INTERACTS WITH | COMBINED EFFECT |
|---|---|
| Alcohol: | Excess sedation. Avoid. |
| Beverages: Caffeine drinks. | Less triprolidine sedation. |
| Cocaine: | Decreased triprolidine effect. Avoid. |
| Foods: | None expected. |
| Marijuana: | Excess sedation. Avoid. |
| Tobacco: | None expected. |

# VALPROIC ACID (DIPROPYLACETIC ACID)

## BRAND NAMES

Depakene          Epival
Depakote

## BASIC INFORMATION

**Habit forming?** No
**Prescription needed?** Yes
**Available as generic?** Yes
**Drug class:** Anticonvulsant

## USES

Controls petit mal (absence) seizures in treatment of epilepsy.

## DOSAGE & USAGE INFORMATION

**How to take:**
Tablet or capsule—Swallow with liquid or food to lessen stomach irritation.

**When to take:**
Once a day.

**If you forget a dose:**
Take as soon as you remember. Don't ever double dose.

**What drug does:**
Increases concentration of gamma aminobutyric acid, which inhibits nerve transmission in parts of brain.

**Time lapse before drug works:**
1 to 4 hours.

**Don't take with:**
See Interaction column and consult doctor.

## OVERDOSE

**SYMPTOMS:**
Coma
**WHAT TO DO:**
- Dial 0 (operator) or 911 (emergency) for an ambulance or medical help. Then give first aid immediately.
- If patient is unconscious and not breathing, give mouth-to-mouth breathing. If there is no heartbeat, use cardiac massage and mouth-to-mouth breathing (CPR). Don't try to make patient vomit. If you can't get help quickly, take patient to nearest emergency facility.
- See emergency information on inside covers.

## POSSIBLE ADVERSE REACTIONS OR SIDE EFFECTS

| SYMPTOMS | WHAT TO DO |
|---|---|
| **Life-threatening:** | |
| None expected. | |
| **Common:** | |
| Menstrual irregularities. | Continue. Call doctor when convenient. |
| **Infrequent:** | |
| • Rash, blood spots under skin, hair loss, bleeding (heart and lungs), easy bruising. | Discontinue. Call doctor right away. |
| • Sleepiness, weakness, easily upset emotionally, depression, psychic changes, headache, incoordination, nausea, vomiting, abdominal cramps, appetite change. | Continue. Call doctor when convenient. |
| **Rare:** | |
| • Double vision, unusual movements of eyes (nystagmus). | Discontinue. Call doctor right away. |
| • Anemia. | Continue. Call doctor when convenient. |

# VALPROIC ACID (DIPROPYLACETIC ACID)

## WARNINGS & PRECAUTIONS

**Don't take if:**
You are allergic to valproic acid.

**Before you start, consult your doctor:**
- If you have blood, kidney or liver disease.
- If you will have surgery within 2 months, including dental surgery, requiring general or spinal anesthesia.

**Over age 60:**
Adverse reactions and side effects may be more frequent and severe than in younger persons.

**Pregnancy:**
No proven harm to unborn child. Avoid if possible.

**Breast-feeding:**
Unknown effect.

**Infants & children:**
Under close medical supervision only.

**Prolonged use:**
Request periodic blood tests, liver and kidney function tests.

**Skin & sunlight:**
No problems expected.

**Driving, piloting or hazardous work:**
Don't drive or pilot aircraft until you learn how medicine affects you. Don't work around dangerous machinery. Don't climb ladders or work in high places. Danger increases if you drink alcohol or take medicine affecting alertness and reflexes, such as antihistamines, tranquilizers, sedatives, pain medicine, narcotics and mind-altering drugs.

**Discontinuing:**
Don't discontinue without consulting doctor. Dose may require gradual reduction if you have taken drug for a long time. Doses of other drugs may also require adjustment.

**Others:**
No problems expected.

## POSSIBLE INTERACTION WITH OTHER DRUGS

| GENERIC NAME OR DRUG CLASS | COMBINED EFFECT |
|---|---|
| Anticoagulants | Increased chance of bleeding. |
| Aspirin | Increased chance of bleeding. |
| Central nervous system depressants: Antidepressants, antihistamines, narcotics, sedatives, sleeping pills, tranquilizers, muscle relaxants | Increased sedative effect. |
| Clonazepam | May prolong seizure. |
| Dypiradamole | Increased chance of bleeding. |
| Flecainide | Possible decreased blood-cell production in bone marrow. |
| MAO inhibitors | Increased sedative effect. |
| Phenytoin | Unpredictable. Dose may require adjustment. |
| Primidone | Increased chance of toxicity. |
| Sulfinpyrazone | Increased chance of bleeding. |
| Tocainide | Possible decreased blood-cell production in bone marrow. |

## POSSIBLE INTERACTION WITH OTHER SUBSTANCES

| INTERACTS WITH | COMBINED EFFECT |
|---|---|
| Alcohol: | Deep sedation. Avoid. |
| Beverages: | No problems expected. |
| Cocaine: | Increased brain sensitivity. Avoid. |
| Foods: | No problems expected. |
| Marijuana: | Increased brain sensitivity. Avoid. |
| Tobacco: | Decreased valproic acid effect. |

# VERAPAMIL

## BRAND NAMES

Calan                    Isoptin

## BASIC INFORMATION

**Habit forming? No**
**Prescription needed? Yes**
**Available as generic? No**
**Drug class: Calcium-channel blocker,**
              **antiarrhythmic, antianginal**

## USES

- Prevents angina attacks.
- Stabilizes irregular heartbeat.

## DOSAGE & USAGE INFORMATION

**How to take:**
Tablet—Swallow with liquid.

**When to take:**
At the same times each day 1 hour before or 2 hours after eating.

**If you forget a dose:**
Take as soon as you remember up to 2 hours late. If more than 2 hours, wait for next scheduled dose (don't double this dose).

**What drug does:**
- Reduces work that heart must perform.
- Reduces normal artery pressure.
- Increases oxygen to heart muscle.

**Time lapse before drug works:**
1 to 2 hours.

**Don't take with:**
See Interaction column and consult doctor.

## OVERDOSE

**SYMPTOMS:**
**Unusually fast or unusually slow heartbeat, loss of consciousness, cardiac arrest.**
**WHAT TO DO:**
- **Dial 0 (operator) or 911 (emergency) for an ambulance or medical help. Then give first aid immediately.**
- **If patient is unconscious and not breathing, give mouth-to-mouth breathing. If there is no heartbeat, use cardiac massage and mouth-to-mouth breathing (CPR). Don't try to make patient vomit. If you can't get help quickly, take patient to nearest emergency facility.**
- **See emergency information on inside covers.**

## POSSIBLE ADVERSE REACTIONS OR SIDE EFFECTS

| SYMPTOMS | WHAT TO DO |
|---|---|
| **Life-threatening:** None expected. | |
| **Common:** Tiredness. | Continue. Tell doctor at next visit. |
| **Infrequent:** | |
| • Unusually fast or unusually slow heartbeat, wheezing, cough, shortness of breath. | Discontinue. Call doctor right away. |
| • Dizziness; numbness or tingling in hands and feet; swollen feet, ankles or legs; difficult urination. | Continue. Call doctor when convenient. |
| • Nausea, constipation. | Continue. Tell doctor at next visit. |
| **Rare:** | |
| • Fainting. | Discontinue. Call doctor right away. |
| • Headache. | Continue. Tell doctor at next visit. |

## WARNINGS & PRECAUTIONS

**Don't take if:**
- You are allergic to verapamil.
- You have very low blood pressure.

**Before you start, consult your doctor:**
- If you have kidney or liver disease.
- If you have high blood pressure.
- If you have heart disease other than coronary-artery disease.

**Over age 60:**
Adverse reactions and side effects may be more frequent and severe than in younger persons.

**Pregnancy:**
No proven harm to unborn child. Avoid if possible.

**Breast-feeding:**
Safety not established. Avoid if possible.

**Infants & children:**
Not recommended.

**Prolonged use:**
No problems expected.

**Skin & sunlight:**
No problems expected.

**Driving, piloting or hazardous work:**
Avoid if you feel dizzy. Otherwise, no problems expected.

**Discontinuing:**
Don't discontinue without doctor's advice until you complete prescribed dose, even though symptoms diminish or disappear.

**Others:**
Learn to check your own pulse rate. If it drops to 50 beats per minute or lower, don't take verapamil until your consult your doctor.

## POSSIBLE INTERACTION WITH OTHER DRUGS

| GENERIC NAME OR DRUG CLASS | COMBINED EFFECT |
|---|---|
| Amiodarone | Increased likelihood of slow heartbeat. |
| Anticoagulants (oral) | Increased anticoagulant effect. |
| Anticonvulsants (hydantoin) | Increased anticonvulsant effect. |
| Antihypertensives | Dangerous blood-pressure drop. |
| Beta-adrenergic blockers | Possible irregular heartbeat. |
| Calcium (large doses) | Decreased verapamil effect. |
| Digitalis preparations | Increased digitalis effect. May need to reduce dose. |
| Disopyramide | May cause dangerously slow, fast or irregular heartbeat. |
| Diuretics | Dangerous blood-pressure drop. |
| Enalapril | Possible excessive potassium in blood. |
| Flecainide | Possible irregular heartbeat. |
| Ketoprofen | Increased chance of toxicity of verapamil. |
| Nitrates | Reduced angina attacks. |
| Oxprenolol | Possible greater difficulty in treating patients with congestive heart failure. |
| Pentoxifylline | Increased antihypertensive effect. |
| Quinidine | Increased quinidine effect. |

| | |
|---|---|
| Suprofen | Increased chance of toxicity of verapamil. |
| Tocainide | Possible irregular heartbeat. |
| Vitamin D (large doses) | Decreased verapamil effect. |

## POSSIBLE INTERACTION WITH OTHER SUBSTANCES

| INTERACTS WITH | COMBINED EFFECT |
|---|---|
| Alcohol: | Dangerously low blood pressure. Avoid. |
| Beverages: | None expected. |
| Cocaine: | Possible irregular heartbeat. Avoid. |
| Foods: | None expected. |
| Marijuana: | Possible irregular heartbeat. Avoid. |
| Tobacco: | Possible rapid heartbeat. Avoid. |

# VITAMIN A

## BRAND NAMES

Acon
Afaxin
Alphalin

Aquasol A
Dispatabs
Sust-A

Numerous multiple vitamin-mineral
supplements.

## BASIC INFORMATION

**Habit forming? No**
**Prescription needed? No**
**Available as generic? Yes**
**Drug class: Vitamin supplement**

 ## USES

Dietary supplement to ensure normal growth
and health, especially eyes and skin.

 ## DOSAGE & USAGE INFORMATION

**How to take:**
Tablet or capsule—Swallow with liquid. If you
can't swallow whole, crumble tablet or open
capsule and take with liquid or food.

**When to take:**
At the same time each day.

**If you forget a dose:**
Take as soon as you remember. Resume
regular schedule.

**What drug does:**
- Prevents night blindness.
- Promotes normal growth and health.

**Time lapse before drug works:**
Requires continual intake.

**Don't take with:**
See Interaction column and consult doctor.

 ## OVERDOSE

**SYMPTOMS:**
Increased adverse reactions and side
effects. Jaundice (rare, but may occur with
large doses).
**WHAT TO DO:**
Overdose unlikely to threaten life. If person
takes much larger amount than prescribed,
call doctor, poison-control center or hospital
emergency room for instructions.

 ## POSSIBLE ADVERSE REACTIONS OR SIDE EFFECTS

| SYMPTOMS | WHAT TO DO |
|---|---|
| **Life-threatening:**<br>None expected. | |
| **Common:**<br>None expected. | |
| **Infrequent:**<br>Confusion, dizziness, drowsiness, headache, irritability, dry lips, peeling skin, hair loss. | Continue. Call doctor when convenient. |
| **Rare:** | |
| • Bulging soft spot on baby's head, double vision. | Discontinue. Call doctor right away. |
| • Diarrhea, appetite loss, nausea, vomiting. | Continue. Call doctor when convenient. |

## WARNINGS & PRECAUTIONS

**Don't take if:**
You have chronic kidney failure.

**Before you start, consult your doctor:**
If you have any kidney disorder.

**Over age 60:**
No problems expected.

**Pregnancy:**
Don't take more than 6,000 units daily.

**Breast-feeding:**
No problems expected.

**Infants & children:**
- Avoid large doses.
- Keep vitamin-mineral supplements out of children's reach.

**Prolonged use:**
No problems expected.

**Skin & sunlight:**
No problems expected.

**Driving, piloting or hazardous work:**
No problems expected.

**Discontinuing:**
Don't discontinue without doctor's advice until you complete prescribed dose, even though symptoms diminish or disappear.

**Others:**
- Don't exceed dose. Too much over a long time may be harmful.
- A balanced diet should provide all the vitamin A a healthy person needs and prevent need for supplements. Best sources are liver, yellow-orange fruits and vegetables, dark-green, leafy vegetables, milk, butter and margarine.

## POSSIBLE INTERACTION WITH OTHER DRUGS

| GENERIC NAME OR DRUG CLASS | COMBINED EFFECT |
|---|---|
| Anticoagulants | Increased anticoagulant effect with large doses (over 10,000 I.U.) of vitamin A. |
| Calcium supplements | Decreased vitamin effect. |
| Cholestyramine | Decreased vitamin A absorption. |
| Colestipol | Decreased vitamin absorption. |
| Mineral oil (long term) | Decreased vitamin A absorption. |
| Neomycin | Decreased vitamin absorption. |
| Vitamin E (excess dose) | Vitamin A depletion. |

## POSSIBLE INTERACTION WITH OTHER SUBSTANCES

| INTERACTS WITH | COMBINED EFFECT |
|---|---|
| Alcohol: | None expected. |
| Beverages: | None expected. |
| Cocaine: | None expected. |
| Foods: | None expected. |
| Marijuana: | None expected. |
| Tobacco: | None expected. |

# VITAMIN B-12 (CYANOCOBALAMIN)

## BRAND NAMES

See complete list of brand names in the *Brand Name Directory*, page 958.

## BASIC INFORMATION

**Habit forming? No**
**Prescription needed? No**
**Available as generic? Yes**
**Drug class: Vitamin supplement**

 ## USES

- Dietary supplement for normal growth, development and health.
- Treatment for nerve damage.
- Treatment for pernicious anemia.
- Treatment and prevention of vitamin B-12 deficiencies in people who have had stomach or intestines surgically removed.
- Prevention of vitamin B-12 deficiency in strict vegetarians and persons with absorption diseases.

 ## DOSAGE & USAGE INFORMATION

**How to take:**
- Tablets—Swallow with liquid.
- Injection—Follow doctor's directions.

**When to take:**
- Oral—At the same time each day.
- Injection—Follow doctor's directions.

**If you forget a dose:**
Take when remembered. Don't double next dose. Resume regular schedule.

**What drug does:**
Acts as enzyme to promote normal fat and carbohydrate metabolism and protein synthesis.

**Time lapse before drug works:**
15 minutes.

**Don't take with:**
See Interaction column and consult doctor.

 ## OVERDOSE

**SYMPTOMS:**
**Increased adverse reactions and side effects.**
**WHAT TO DO:**
**Overdose unlikely to threaten life. If person takes much larger amount than prescribed, call doctor, poison-control center or hospital emergency room for instructions.**

 ## POSSIBLE ADVERSE REACTIONS OR SIDE EFFECTS

| SYMPTOMS | WHAT TO DO |
|---|---|
| **Life-threatening:**<br>Hives, rash, intense itching, faintness soon after a dose (anaphylaxis). | Seek emergency treatment immediately. |
| **Common:**<br>None expected. | |
| **Infrequent:**<br>None expected. | |
| **Rare:** | |
| • Itchy skin, wheezing. | Discontinue. Call doctor right away. |
| • Diarrhea. | Continue. Call doctor when convenient. |

## WARNINGS & PRECAUTIONS

**Don't take if:**
You have Leber's disease (optic nerve atrophy).

**Before you start, consult your doctor:**
- If you have gout.
- If you have heart disease.

**Over age 60:**
Don't take more than 100mg per day unless prescribed by your doctor.

**Pregnancy:**
No problems expected.

**Breast-feeding:**
No problems expected.

**Infants & children:**
No problems expected.

**Prolonged use:**
No problems expected.

**Skin & sunlight:**
No problems expected.

**Driving, piloting or hazardous work:**
No problems expected.

**Discontinuing:**
Don't discontinue without doctor's advice until you complete prescribed dose, even though symptoms diminish or disappear.

**Others:**
- A balanced diet should provide all the vitamin B-12 a healthy person needs and make supplements unnecessary. Best sources are meat, fish, egg yolk and cheese.
- Tablets should be used only for diet supplements. All other uses of vitamin B-12 require injections.
- Don't take large doses of vitamin C (1,000mg or more per day) unless prescribed by your doctor.

## POSSIBLE INTERACTION WITH OTHER DRUGS

| GENERIC NAME OR DRUG CLASS | COMBINED EFFECT |
|---|---|
| Anticonvulsants | Decreased absorption of vitamin B-12. |
| Aspirin | Decreased absorption of vitamin B-12. |
| Chloramphenicol | Decreased vitamin B-12 effect. |
| Colchicine | Decreased absorption of vitamin B-12. |
| Neomycin | Decreased absorption of vitamin B-12. |
| Potassium (extended-release forms) | Decreased absorption of vitamin B-12. |
| Vitamin C (ascorbic acid) | Destroys vitamin B-12 if taken at same time. Take 2 hours apart. |

## POSSIBLE INTERACTION WITH OTHER SUBSTANCES

| INTERACTS WITH | COMBINED EFFECT |
|---|---|
| Alcohol: | Decreased absorption of vitamin B-12. |
| Beverages: | None expected. |
| Cocaine: | None expected. |
| Foods: | None expected. |
| Marijuana: | None expected. |
| Tobacco: | None expected. |

# VITAMIN C (ASCORBIC ACID)

## BRAND NAMES

See complete list of brand names in the *Brand Name Directory,* page 958.

## BASIC INFORMATION

**Habit forming? No**
**Prescription needed? No**
**Available as generic? Yes**
**Drug class: Vitamin supplement**

## USES

- Prevention and treatment of scurvy and other vitamin-C deficiencies.
- Treatment of anemia.
- Maintenance of acid urine.

## DOSAGE & USAGE INFORMATION

**How to take:**
- Tablets, capsules, liquid—Swallow with 8 oz. water.
- Extended-release tablets—Swallow whole.
- Drops—Squirt directly into mouth or mix with liquid or food.

**When to take:**
1, 2 or 3 times per day, as prescribed on label.

**If you forget a dose:**
Take as soon as you remember. Return to regular schedule.

**What drug does:**
- May help form collagen.
- Increases iron absorption from intestine.
- Contributes to hemoglobin and red-blood-cell production in bone marrow.

**Time lapse before drug works:**
1 week.

**Don't take with:**
See Interaction column and consult doctor.

## OVERDOSE

**SYMPTOMS:**
**Diarrhea, vomiting, dizziness.**
**WHAT TO DO:**
**Overdose unlikely to threaten life. If person takes much larger amount than prescribed, call doctor, poison-control center or hospital emergency room for instructions.**

## POSSIBLE ADVERSE REACTIONS OR SIDE EFFECTS

| SYMPTOMS | WHAT TO DO |
|---|---|
| **Life-threatening:** | |
| None expected. | |
| **Common:** | |
| None expected. | |
| **Infrequent:** | |
| • Mild diarrhea, nausea, vomiting. | Discontinue. Call doctor right away. |
| • Flushed face. | Continue. Call doctor when convenient. |
| **Rare:** | |
| • Kidney stones with high doses, anemia. | Discontinue. Call doctor right away. |
| • Headache. | Continue. Tell doctor at next visit. |

## WARNINGS & PRECAUTIONS

**Don't take if:**
You are allergic to vitamin C.

**Before you start, consult your doctor:**
- If you have sickle-cell or other anemia.
- If you have had kidney stones.
- If you have gout.

**Over age 60:**
Don't take more than 100mg per day unless prescribed by your doctor.

**Pregnancy:**
No proven harm to unborn child. Avoid large doses.

**Breast-feeding:**
Avoid large doses.

**Infants & children:**
- Avoid large doses.
- Keep vitamin-mineral supplements out of children's reach.

**Prolonged use:**
Large doses for longer than 2 months may cause kidney stones.

**Skin & sunlight:**
No problems expected.

**Driving, piloting or hazardous work:**
No problems expected.

**Discontinuing:**
No problems expected.

**Others:**
- Store in cool, dry place.
- May cause inaccurate tests for sugar in urine or blood in stool.
- May cause crisis in patients with sickle-cell anemia.
- A balanced diet should provide all the vitamin C a healthy person needs and make supplements unnecessary. Best sources are citrus, strawberries, cantaloupe and raw peppers.
- Don't take large doses of vitamin C (1,000mg or more per day) unless prescribed by your doctor.

## POSSIBLE INTERACTION WITH OTHER DRUGS

| GENERIC NAME OR DRUG CLASS | COMBINED EFFECT |
|---|---|
| Anticholinergics | Decreased anticholinergic effect. |
| Anticoagulants (oral) | Decreased anticoagulant effect. |
| Aspirin | Decreased vitamin C effect. |
| Barbiturates | Decreased vitamin C effect. Increased barbiturate effect. |
| Contraceptives (oral) | Decreased vitamin C effect. |
| Estrogens | Increased likelihood of adverse effects from estrogen with 1gm or more of vitamin C per day. |
| Iron supplements | Increased iron effect. |
| Mexiletine | May decrease effectiveness of mexiletine. |
| Mineral oil | Decreased vitamin C effect. |
| Quinidine | Decreased quinidine effect. |
| Salicylates | Decreased vitamin C effect. |
| Tetracyclines | Decreased vitamin C effect. |
| Tranquilizers (phenothiazine) | Decreased phenothiazine effect if no vitamin C deficiency exists. |

## POSSIBLE INTERACTION WITH OTHER SUBSTANCES

| INTERACTS WITH | COMBINED EFFECT |
|---|---|
| Alcohol: | None expected. |
| Beverages: | None expected. |
| Cocaine: | None expected. |
| Foods: | None expected. |
| Marijuana: | None expected. |
| Tobacco: | Increased requirement for vitamin C. |

# VITAMIN D

## BRAND NAMES

| | |
|---|---|
| Calciferol | Drisdol |
| Calcifidiol | Ergocalciferol |
| Calcitriol | Hytakerol |
| Calderol | Ostoforte |
| Deltalin | Radiostol |
| DHT | Radiostol Forte |
| Dihydrotachysterol | Rocaltrol |

Numerous other multiple vitamin-mineral supplements.

## BASIC INFORMATION

**Habit forming?** No
**Prescription needed?**
  Low strength: No
  High strength: Yes
**Available as generic?** Yes
**Drug class:** Vitamin supplement

 USES

- Dietary supplement.
- Prevention of rickets (bone disease).
- Treatment for hypocalcemia (low blood calcium) in kidney disease.
- Treatment for postoperative muscle contractions.

 DOSAGE & USAGE INFORMATION

**How to take:**
- Tablet or capsule—Swallow with liquid.
- Drops—Dilute dose in beverage.

**When to take:**
As directed, usually once a day at the same time each day.

**If you forget a dose:**
Take up to 12 hours late. If more than 12 hours, wait for next dose (don't double this dose).

*Continued next column*

 OVERDOSE

**SYMPTOMS:**
Severe stomach pain, nausea, vomiting, weight loss; bone and muscle pain; increased urination, cloudy urine; mood or mental changes (possible psychosis); high blood pressure, irregular heartbeat; eye irritation or light sensitivity; itchy skin.
**WHAT TO DO:**
Overdose unlikely to threaten life. If person takes much larger amount than prescribed, call doctor, poison-control center or hospital emergency room for instructions.

**What drug does:**
Maintains growth and health. Prevents rickets. Essential so body can use calcium and phosphate.

**Time lapse before drug works:**
2 hours. May require 2 to 3 weeks of continual use for maximum effect.

**Don't take with:**
Non-prescription drugs or drugs in Interaction column without consulting doctor.

 POSSIBLE ADVERSE REACTIONS OR SIDE EFFECTS

| SYMPTOMS | WHAT TO DO |
|---|---|
| **Life-threatening:** None expected. | |
| **Common:** None expected. | |
| **Infrequent:** Headache, metallic taste in mouth, thirst, dry mouth, constipation, appetite loss, nausea, vomiting. | Continue. Call doctor when convenient. |
| **Rare:** None expected. | |

## WARNINGS & PRECAUTIONS

**Don't take if:**
You are allergic to medicine containing vitamin D.

**Before you start, consult your doctor:**
- If you plan to become pregnant while taking vitamin D.
- If you have epilepsy.
- If you have heart or blood-vessel disease.
- If you have kidney disease.

**Over age 60:**
Adverse reactions and side effects may be more frequent and severe than in younger persons.

**Pregnancy:**
Risk to unborn child outweighs drug benefits. Don't use.

**Breast-feeding:**
No problems expected, but consult doctor.

**Infants & children:**
- Avoid large doses.
- Keep vitamins out of children's reach.

**Prolonged use:**
No problems expected.

**Skin & sunlight:**
No problems expected.

**Driving, piloting or hazardous work:**
No problems expected.

**Discontinuing:**
Don't discontinue without doctor's advice until you complete prescribed dose, even though symptoms diminish or disappear.

**Others:**
- Don't exceed dose. Too much over a long time may be harmful.
- A balanced diet should provide all the vitamin D a healthy person needs and make supplements unnecessary. Best sources are fish and vitamin-D fortified milk and bread.

## POSSIBLE INTERACTION WITH OTHER DRUGS

| GENERIC NAME OR DRUG CLASS | COMBINED EFFECT |
|---|---|
| Antacids (magnesium-containing) | Possible excess magnesium. |
| Anticonvulsants (hydantoin) | Decreased vitamin D effect. |
| Calcium (high doses) | Excess calcium in blood. |
| Calcium-channel blockers | Decreased effect of calcium-channel blockers. |
| Calcium supplements | Excessive absorption of vitamin D. |
| Cholestyramine | Decreased vitamin D effect. |
| Colestipol | Decreased vitamin D absorption. |
| Digitalis preparations | Heartbeat irregularities. |
| Mineral oil | Decreased vitamin D effect. |
| Neomycin | Decreased vitamin D absorption. |
| Phenobarbital | Decreased vitamin D effect. |
| Phosphorous preparations | Accumulation of excess phosphorous. |
| Vitamin D (other) | Possible toxicity. |

## POSSIBLE INTERACTION WITH OTHER SUBSTANCES

| INTERACTS WITH | COMBINED EFFECT |
|---|---|
| Alcohol: | None expected. |
| Beverages: | None expected. |
| Cocaine: | None expected. |
| Foods: | None expected. |
| Marijuana: | None expected. |
| Tobacco: | None expected. |

# VITAMIN E

## BRAND NAMES

| | |
|---|---|
| Aquasol E | Eprolin |
| Chew-E | Epsilan-M |
| Daltose | Pheryl-E |
| Eferol | Viterra E |

Numerous other multiple vitamin-mineral supplements.

## BASIC INFORMATION

Habit forming? No
Prescription needed? No
Available as generic? Yes
Drug class: Vitamin supplement

 **USES**

- Dietary supplement to promote normal growth, development and health.
- Treatment and prevention of vitamin-E deficiency, especially in premature or low birth-weight infants.
- Treatment for fibrocystic disease of the breast.
- Treatment for circulatory problems to the lower extremities.
- Treatment for sickle-cell anemia.
- Treatment for lung toxicity from air pollution.

 **DOSAGE & USAGE INFORMATION**

How to take:
- Tablet, capsule or chewable tablets—Swallow with liquid or food to lessen stomach irritation.
- Drops—Dilute dose in beverage before swallowing or squirt directly into mouth.

When to take:
At the same times each day.

If you forget a dose:
Take when you remember. Don't double next dose.

What drug does:
- Promotes normal growth and development.
- Prevents oxidation in body.

*Continued next column*

 **OVERDOSE**

SYMPTOMS:
Nausea, vomiting.
WHAT TO DO:
Overdose unlikely to threaten life. If person takes much larger amount than prescribed, call doctor, poison-control center or hospital emergency room for instructions.

Time lapse before drug works:
Not determined.

Don't take with:
See Interaction column and consult doctor.

 **POSSIBLE ADVERSE REACTIONS OR SIDE EFFECTS**

| SYMPTOMS | WHAT TO DO |
|---|---|
| **Life-threatening:**<br>None expected. | |
| **Common:**<br>None expected. | |
| **Infrequent:**<br>Nausea, stomach pain, muscle aches, pain in lower legs, fever, tiredness, weakness. | Continue. Call doctor when convenient. |
| **Rare:**<br>None expected. | |

## WARNINGS & PRECAUTIONS

**Don't take if:**
You are allergic to vitamin E.

**Before you start, consult your doctor:**
- If you have had blood clots in leg veins (thrombophlebitis).
- If you have liver disease.

**Over age 60:**
No problems expected. Avoid excessive doses.

**Pregnancy:**
No problems expected with normal daily requirements. Don't exceed prescribed dose.

**Breast-feeding:**
No problems expected.

**Infants & children:**
Use only under medical supervision.

**Prolonged use:**
Toxic accumulation of vitamin E. Don't exceed recommended dose.

**Skin & sunlight:**
No problems expected.

**Driving, piloting or hazardous work:**
No problems expected.

**Discontinuing:**
No problems expected.

**Others:**
A balanced diet should provide all the vitamin E a healthy person needs and make supplements unnecessary. Best sources are vegetable oils, whole-grain cereals, liver.

## POSSIBLE INTERACTION WITH OTHER DRUGS

| GENERIC NAME OR DRUG CLASS | COMBINED EFFECT |
|---|---|
| Anticoagulants (oral) | Increased anticoagulant effect. |
| Cholestyramine | Decreased vitamin E absorption. |
| Colestipol | Decreased vitamin E absorption. |
| Iron supplements | Decreased effect of iron supplement in patients with iron-deficiency anemia. Decreased vitamin E effect in healthy persons. |
| Neomycin | Decreased vitamin E absorption. |
| Vitamin A | Recommended dose of vitamin E— Increased benefit and decreased toxicity of vitamin A. Excess dose of vitamin E—Vitamin A depletion. |

## POSSIBLE INTERACTION WITH OTHER SUBSTANCES

| INTERACTS WITH | COMBINED EFFECT |
|---|---|
| Alcohol: | None expected. |
| Beverages: | None expected. |
| Cocaine: | None expected. |
| Foods: | None expected. |
| Marijuana: | None expected. |
| Tobacco: | None expected. |

# VITAMIN K

## BRAND NAMES

| | |
|---|---|
| Konakion | Mephyton |
| Menadione | Phytonadione |
| Menadiol | Synkayvite |

## BASIC INFORMATION

**Habit forming? No**
**Prescription needed? No**
**Available as generic? Yes**
**Drug class: Vitamin supplement**

 **USES**

- Dietary supplement.
- Treatment for bleeding disorders and malabsorption diseases due to vitamin K deficiency.
- Treatment for hemorrhagic disease of the newborn.
- Treatment for bleeding due to overdose of oral anticoagulants.

 **DOSAGE & USAGE INFORMATION**

**How to take:**
Tablet—Swallow with liquid. If you can't swallow whole, crumble tablet or open capsule and take with liquid or food.

**When to take:**
At the same time each day.

**If you forget a dose:**
Take as soon as you remember up to 12 hours late. If more than 12 hours, wait for next scheduled dose (don't double this dose).

**What drug does:**
- Promotes growth, development and good health.
- Supplies a necessary ingredient for blood clotting.

**Time lapse before drug works:**
15 to 30 minutes to support blood clotting.

**Don't take with:**
See Interaction column and consult doctor.

 **OVERDOSE**

**SYMPTOMS:**
**Nausea, vomiting.**
**WHAT TO DO:**
**Overdose unlikely to threaten life. If person takes much larger amount than prescribed, call doctor, poison-control center or hospital emergency room for instructions.**

 **POSSIBLE ADVERSE REACTIONS OR SIDE EFFECTS**

| SYMPTOMS | WHAT TO DO |
|---|---|
| **Life-threatening:** None expected. | |
| **Common:** None expected. | |
| **Infrequent:** Unusual taste. | Continue. Call doctor when convenient. |
| **Rare:** None expected. | |

## WARNINGS & PRECAUTIONS

**Don't take if:**
- You are allergic to vitamin K.
- You have G6PD deficiency.
- You have liver disease.

**Before you start, consult your doctor:**
If you are pregnant.

**Over age 60:**
No problems expected.

**Pregnancy:**
Don't exceed dose.

**Breast-feeding:**
No problems expected.

**Infants & children:**
Phytonadione is the preferred form for hemorrhagic disease of the newborn.

**Prolonged use:**
No problems expected.

**Skin & sunlight:**
No problems expected.

**Driving, piloting or hazardous work:**
No problems expected.

**Discontinuing:**
No problems expected.

**Others:**
- Tell all doctors and dentists you consult that you take this medicine.
- Don't exceed dose. Too much over a long time may be harmful.
- A balanced diet should provide all the vitamin K a healthy person needs and make supplements unnecessary. Best sources are green, leafy vegetables, meat or dairy products.

## POSSIBLE INTERACTION WITH OTHER DRUGS

| GENERIC NAME OR DRUG CLASS | COMBINED EFFECT |
|---|---|
| Anticoagulants (oral) | Decreased anticoagulant effect. |
| Cholestyramine | Decreased vitamin K effect. |
| Colestipol | Decreased vitamin K absorption. |
| Mineral oil (long term) | Vitamin K deficiency. |
| Neomycin | Decreased vitamin K absorption. |
| Sulfa drugs | Vitamin K deficiency. |

## POSSIBLE INTERACTION WITH OTHER SUBSTANCES

| INTERACTS WITH | COMBINED EFFECT |
|---|---|
| Alcohol: | None expected. |
| Beverages: | None expected. |
| Cocaine: | None expected. |
| Foods: | None expected. |
| Marijuana: | None expected. |
| Tobacco: | None expected. |

# VITAMINS & FLUORIDE

## BRAND AND GENERIC NAMES

Adeflor
Cari-Tab
Mulvidren-F
Poly-Vi-Flor
**MULTIPLE VITAMINS & FLUORIDE**
**VITAMINS A, D & C & FLUORIDE**

Tri-Vi-Flor
Vi-Daylin/F
Vi-Penta F

## BASIC INFORMATION

**Habit forming? No**
**Prescription needed? Yes**
**Available as generic? No**
**Drug class: Vitamins, minerals**

## USES

- Reduces incidence of tooth cavities (fluoride). Children who need supplements should take until age 16.
- Prevents deficiencies of vitamin included in formula (some contain multiple vitamins whose content varies among products, others contain only vitamins A, D and C).

## DOSAGE & USAGE INFORMATION

**How to take:**
- Chewable tablets—Chew or crush before swallowing.
- Oral liquid—Take by mouth measured with specially marked dropper. May mix with food, fruit juice, cereal.

**When to take:**
- Bedtime or with or just after meals.
- If at bedtime, brush teeth first.

**If you forget a dose:**
Take as soon as you remember up to 2 hours late. If more than 2 hours, wait for next scheduled dose (don't double this dose).

*Continued next column*

## OVERDOSE

**SYMPTOMS:**
**Minor overdose—Black, brown or white spots on teeth.**
**Massive overdose—Shallow breathing, black or tarry stools, bloody vomit.**
**WHAT TO DO:**
- **Dial 0 (operator) or 911 (emergency) for an ambulance or medical help. Then give first aid immediately.**
- **See emergency information on inside covers.**

**What drug does:**
Provides supplemental fluoride to combat tooth decay.

**Time lapse before drug works:**
8 weeks to provide maximum benefit.

**Don't take with:**
- Other medicine simultaneously.
- See Interaction column and consult doctor.

## POSSIBLE ADVERSE REACTIONS OR SIDE EFFECTS

| SYMPTOMS | WHAT TO DO |
|---|---|
| **Life-threatening:** | |
| Fainting, bloody vomit, bloody or black stool. | Discontinue. Seek emergency treatment. |
| **Common:** | |
| White, black or brown spots on teeth; nausea; vomiting. | Discontinue. Call doctor right away. |
| **Infrequent:** | |
| • Drowsiness; abdominal pain; increased salivation; watery eyes; weight loss; sore throat, fever, mouth sores; constipation; bone pain; rash; muscle stiffness; weakness; tremor; agitation. | Discontinue. Call doctor right away. |
| • Diarrhea. | Continue. Call doctor when convenient. |
| **Rare:** | |
| None expected. | |

## WARNINGS & PRECAUTIONS

**Don't take if:**
- Your water supply contains 0.7 parts fluoride per million. Too much fluoride stains teeth permanently.
- You are allergic to any fluoride-containing product.
- You have underactive thyroid.

**Before you start, consult your doctor or dentist:**
For proper dosage.

**Over age 60:**
No problems expected.

**Pregnancy:**
No problems expected.

**Breast-feeding:**
No problems expected.

**Infants & children:**
No problems expected in children over 3 years of age except accidental overdose. Keep vitamin-mineral supplements out of children's reach.

**Prolonged use:**
Excess may cause discolored teeth and decreased calcium in blood.

**Skin & sunlight:**
No problems expected.

**Driving, piloting or hazardous work:**
No problems expected.

**Discontinuing:**
No problems expected.

**Others:**
- Store in original plastic container. Fluoride decomposes glass.
- Check with dentist once or twice a year to keep cavities at a minimum. Topical applications of fluoride may also be helpful.
- Fluoride probably not necessary if water contains about 1 part per million of fluoride or more. Check with health department.
- Don't freeze.
- Don't keep outdated medicine.

## POSSIBLE INTERACTION WITH OTHER DRUGS

| GENERIC NAME OR DRUG CLASS | COMBINED EFFECT |
|---|---|
| Anticoagulants | Decreased anticoagulant effect. |
| Iron supplements | Decreased effect of any vitamin E if present in multivitamin product. |
| Vitamin D | May lead to vitamin D toxicity if vitamin D is in combination. |

## POSSIBLE INTERACTION WITH OTHER SUBSTANCES

| INTERACTS WITH | COMBINED EFFECT |
|---|---|
| Alcohol: | None expected. |
| Beverages: Milk. | Prevents absorption of fluoride. Space dose 2 hours before or after milk. |
| Cocaine: | None expected. |
| Foods: | None expected. |
| Marijuana: | None expected. |
| Tobacco: | None expected. |

# XANTHINE BRONCHODILATORS

## BRAND NAMES

See complete list of brand names in the *Brand Name Directory,* page 959.

## BASIC INFORMATION

**Habit forming? No**
**Prescription needed?**
  **Canada—No**
  **U.S.: High strength—Yes**
      **Low strength—No**
**Available as generic? Yes**
**Drug class: Bronchodilator (xanthine)**

## USES

Treatment for bronchial asthma symptoms.

## DOSAGE & USAGE INFORMATION

**How to take:**
- Tablet or capsule—Swallow with liquid.
- Extended-release tablets or capsules—Swallow each dose whole. If you take regular tablets, you may chew or crush them.
- Suppositories—Remove wrapper and moisten suppository with water. Gently insert larger end into rectum. Push well into rectum with finger.
- Syrup—Take as directed on bottle.
- Enema—Use as directed on label.

**When to take:**
Most effective taken on empty stomach 1 hour before or 2 hours after eating. However, may take with food to lessen stomach upset.

**If you forget a dose:**
Take as soon as you remember up to 2 hours late. If more than 2 hours, wait for next scheduled dose (don't double this dose).

**What drug does:**
Relaxes and expands bronchial tubes.

*Continued next column*

## OVERDOSE

**SYMPTOMS:**
**Restlessness, irritability, confusion, delirium, convulsions, rapid pulse, coma.**
**WHAT TO DO:**
- **Dial 0 (operator) or 911 (emergency) for an ambulance or medical help. Then give first aid immediately.**
- **See emergency information on inside covers.**

**Time lapse before drug works:**
15 to 30 minutes.

**Don't take with:**
See Interaction column and consult doctor.

## POSSIBLE ADVERSE REACTIONS OR SIDE EFFECTS

| SYMPTOMS | WHAT TO DO |
|---|---|
| **Life-threatening:** None expected. | |
| **Common:** Headache, irritability, nervousness, restlessness, insomnia, nausea, vomiting, stomach pain. | Continue. Call doctor when convenient. |
| **Infrequent:** • Rash or hives, flushed face, diarrhea, appetite loss, rapid breathing, irregular heartbeat. | Discontinue. Call doctor right away. |
| • Dizziness or lightheadedness. | Continue. Call doctor when convenient. |
| **Rare:** None expected. | |

## WARNINGS & PRECAUTIONS

**Don't take if:**
- You are allergic to any bronchodilator.
- You have an active peptic ulcer.

**Before you start, consult your doctor:**
- If you have had impaired kidney or liver function.
- If you have gastritis.
- If you have a peptic ulcer.
- If you have high blood pressure or heart disease.
- If you take medication for gout.

**Over age 60:**
Adverse reactions and side effects may be more frequent and severe than in younger persons.

**Pregnancy:**
Risk to unborn child outweighs drug benefits. Don't use.

**Breast-feeding:**
Drug passes into milk. Avoid drug or discontinue nursing until you finish medicine. Consult doctor for advice on maintaining milk supply.

**Infants & children:**
Use only under medical supervision.

**Prolonged use:**
Stomach irritation.

**Skin & sunlight:**
No problems expected.

**Driving, piloting or hazardous work:**
Avoid if lightheaded or dizzy. Otherwise, no problems expected.

**Discontinuing:**
May be unnecessary to finish medicine. Follow doctor's instructions.

**Others:**
No problems expected.

## POSSIBLE INTERACTION WITH OTHER DRUGS

| GENERIC NAME OR DRUG CLASS | COMBINED EFFECT |
|---|---|
| Allopurinol | Decreased allopurinol effect. |
| Ephedrine | Increased effect of both drugs. |
| Epinephrine | Increased effect of both drugs. |
| Erythromycin | Increased bronchodilator effect. |
| Furosemide | Increased furosemide effect. |
| Lincomycins | Increased bronchodilator effect. |
| Lithiuim | Decreased lithiuim effect. |
| Probenecid | Decreased effect of both drugs. |
| Propranolol | Decreased bronchodilator effect. |
| Rauwolfia alkaloids | Rapid heartbeat. |
| Sulfinpyrazone | Decreased sulfinpyrazone effect. |
| Troleandomycin | Increased bronchodilator effect. |

## POSSIBLE INTERACTION WITH OTHER SUBSTANCES

| INTERACTS WITH | COMBINED EFFECT |
|---|---|
| **Alcohol:** | None expected. |
| **Beverages:** Caffeine drinks. | Nervousness and insomnia. |
| **Cocaine:** | Excess stimulation. Avoid. |
| **Foods:** | None expected. |
| **Marijuana:** | Slightly increased antiasthmatic effect of bronchodilator. |
| **Tobacco:** | Decreased bronchodilator effect. |

# Brand Name Directory

The following drugs are alphabetized by generic name or drug class, shown in large capital letters. The brand and gneeric names that follow each title in this list are the complete list referred to on the drug charts. Generic names are in all capital letters on the lists.

## ACETAMINOPHEN

A'Cenol
Acephen
Aceta
Ace-Tabs
Aceta w/Codeine
Acetaco
Acetaminophen w/Codeine
Actamin
Algisin
Amacodone
Amaphen
Amphenol
Anacin-3
Anapap
Anaphen
Anoquan
Anuphen
Apamide Tablets
APAP
Apo-Acetaminophen
Arthralgen
Aspirin-Free Excedrin
Atasol
Axotal
Bancap w/Codeine
Banesin
Banesin Forte
Bayapap,
Bromo-Seltzer
C2A
Campain
Capital
Capital w/Codeine
Chlorzone Forte
Co-Gesic
Co-Tylenol
Coastaldyne
Coastalgesic
Codalan
Codap
Colrex
Compal
Comtrex
Conacetol
Congespirin
Covangesic
D-Sinus
Dapa
Dapase
Darvocet-N
Datril
Dia-Gesic
Dialog
Dolacet
Dolanex
Dolene AP-65
Dolor
Dolprin
Dorcol
Dorcol Children's Fever and Pain
  Reducer
Dristan
Duadacin

Dularin
Duradyne DHC
Dynosal
Empracet w/Codeine
Endecon
Esgic
Excedrin
Exdol
Febrigesic
Febrinol
Febrogesic
Fendol
G-1
G-2
G-3
Gaysal
Genapap
Genebs
Genetabs
Guaiamine
Halenol
Hasacode
Hi-Temp
Hyco-Pap
Hycomine Compound
Korigesic
Liquiprin
Liquix-C
Lorcet
Lyteca
Meda Cap
Meda Tab
Mejoral without aspirin
Mejoralito
Metrogesic
Midol PMS
Midrin
Migralam
Minotal
Naldegesic
NAPAP
Nebs
Neopap
Oraphen-PD
Ornex
Ossonate-Plus
Pacaps
Pain Relief without aspirin
Panadol
Panasorb
Panex
Paracetamol
Parafon Forte
Paraphen
Pavadon
Pedric
Peedee Dose Aspirin
Percocet-5
Percogesic
Phenaphen
Phenaphen w/Codeine
Phendex
Phrenilin
Presalin

Prodolor
Protid
Proval
Repan
Rhinocaps
Robigesic
Ronuvex
Rounox
S-A-C
SK-65 APAP
SK-APAP
SK-Oxycodone w/Acetaminophen
Salatin
Saleto
Salimeph Forte
Salphenyl
Sedapap
Sinarest
Sine-Aid
Sine-Off
Singlet
Sinubid
Sinulin
Sinutab
St. Joseph Aspirin Free
Stopayne
Strascogesic
Sudoprin
Summit
Supac
Suppap
Sylapar
T.P.I.
Talacen
Tapanol
Tapar
Temlo
Tempra
Tenlap
Tenol
Triaminicin
Trigesic
Trind Sryup
Two-Dyne
Ty-tabs
Tylenol
Tylenol w/Codeine
Tylox
Valadol
Valorin
Vanquish
Vicodin
Wygesic

## ACETAMINOPHEN & SALICYLATES

445 Anti-Pain Compound
Accurate Forte
ACETAMINOPHEN & ASPIRIN
ACETAMINOPHEN, ASPIRIN &
  SALICYLAMIDE
ACETAMINOPHEN &
  SALICYLAMIDE

## ACETAMINOPHEN & SODIUM SALICYLATE
APAP Fortified
Arthralgen
Banesin
Buffets II
Dinol
Double-A
Duoprin
Duoprin-S
Duradyne
Dynosal
Excedrin
Gaysal-S
Gemnisyn
Goody's Extra Strength Tablets
Goody's Headache Powders
Presalin
Rid-A-Pain Compound
S-A-C
Salatin
Saleto
Salimeph Forte
Salocol
Supac
Tisma
Trigesic
Vanquish

## ADRENOCORTICOIDS (TOPICAL)
Acticort
Adcortyl
Aeroseb-Dex
Aeroseb-HC
Alphatrex
Aristocort
Aristocort A
Aristocort C
Aristocort D
Aristocort R
Bactine Hydrocortisone
Barriere-HC
Beben
Benisone
Beta-Val
Betacort
Betacort Scalp Lotion
Betaderm
Betaderm Scalp Lotion
Betatrex
Betnovate
CaldeCORT
Caldecort Anti-Itch
Carmol-HC
Celestoderm-V
Celestone
Cetacort
Clinicort
Cloderm
Cordran
Cordran SP
Cort-Dome
Cortaid
Cortate
Cortef
Corticosporin
Corticreme
Cortifoam
Cortiment
Cortisol

Cortizone
Cortril
Cremocort
Cyclocort
Decaderm
Decadron
Decaspray
Delacort
Dermacort
DermiCort
Dermolate
Dermophyl
Dermovate
Dermovate Scalp Application
Dermtex HC
DesOwen
Dioderm
Diprolene
Diprosone
Drenison
EF cortelan
Ectosone
Ectosone Scalp Lotion
Eldecort
Emo-Cort
Epifoam
Florone
Fluocet
Fluoderm
Fluolar
Fluolean
Fluonid
Fluonide
Flurosyn
Flutex
Flutone
Gynecort
H2 Cort
HC-Jel
Halciderm
Halog
Halog E
Hexadrol
Hi-Cor
Hi-Cort
Hyderm
Hydro-Corilean
Hydro-Tex
Hydrocortone
Hytone
Kenalog
Kenalog-E
Kenalog-H
Lacticare-HC
Lanacort
Lidemol
Lidex
Lidex-E
Locoid
Locacorten
Lyderm
Maxiflor
Medrol
Metaderm
Meti-Derm
Metosyn
Metosyn FAPG
Neo-Cortef
Neo-Decadron
Novobetamet
Novohydrocort
Nutracort

Oxylone
Penecort
Pharma-Cort
Proctocort
Psorcon
Psorcon-E
Racet-SE
Rhulicort
Spencort
Stie-Cort
Synacort
Synalar
Synamol
Synandone
Synemol
Temovate
Texacort
Topicort
Topsyn
Triacet
Triaderm
Trianide
Tridesilon
Trymex
Unicort
Uticort
Valisone
Valisone Scalp Lotion
Vioform
Westcort
Some of these brands are available as oral medicine. Look under specific generic name for each brand.

## ALUMINUM HYDROXIDE
Alagel
Algenic Alka
Alka-mag
ALternaGEL
Alu-Cap
Alu-Tab
Aludrox
Alumid
Aluscop
Amphojel
Basaljel
Bisodol
Camalox
Chemgel
Creamalin
De Witts
Delcid
Di-Gel
Dialume
Dioval Ex
Ducon
Estomul-m
Gaviscon
Gelusil
Kolantyl
Kolantyl Wafers
Kudrox
Lowsium
Maalox
Magmalin
Magnagel
Magnatril
Maox
Marblen
Max-Ox 40

Maxamag
M.O.M.
Mucotin
Mygel
Mylanta
Neosorb Plus
Nephrox
Neutracomp
Neutralca-S
Par-mag
Pepsogel
Phillips Milk of Magnesia
Ratic
Riopan
Robalate
Rolaids
Rulox
Spastoced
Sterazolidin
Tralmag
Univol
Uro-Mag
Vanquish
Win Gel

## ALUMINUM & MAGNESIUM ANTACIDS

Algenic Alka
Alka-Med
Alma-Mag
Aludrox
Alumid
ALUMINA & MAGNESIA
ALUMINA & MAGENSIUM
   CARBONATE
ALUMINA, MAGNESIUM
   CARBONATE & MAGNESIUM
   OXIDE
ALUMINA & MAGNESIUM
   TRISILICATE
Aluscop
Creamalin
Delcid
DIHYDROXYALUMINUM
   AMINOACETATE & MAGNESIA
DIHYDROXYALUMINUM
   AMINOACETATE, MAGNESIA &
   ALUMINA
Diovol Ex
Estomul-M
Gaviscon
Kolantyl
Kudrox
Lowsium
Maalox
Maalox TC
Magmalin
Magnagel
Magnatril
MAGNESIUM TRISILICATE,
   ALUMINA & MAGNESIA
Neosorb Plus
Neutracomp
Neutralca-S
Riopan
Rolox
Rulox
Tralmag
Univol
WinGel

## ALUMINUM, MAGNESIUM, MAGALDRATE & SIME-THICONE ANTACIDS

Alma-Mag  4 Improved
Almacone
Alumid Plus
ALUMINA, MAGNESIA &
   SIMETHICONE
Amphojel Plus
Di-Gel
Diovol
Gelusil
Maalox Plus
MAGALDRATE & SIMETHICONE
Mygel
Mylanta
Mylanta-2
Mylanta-2 Extra Strength
Riopan Plus
Silain-Gel
Simaal Gel
Simeco
SIMETHICONE, ALUMINA,
   MAGNESIUM CARBONATE
   & MAGNESIA

## ANDROGENS

Anabolin
Anabolin LA 100
Anadrol-50
Anapolon 50
Anavar
Andro
Andro-Cyp
Andro-LA
Android
Android-F
Android-T
Androlone
Andron
Andronaq
Andronaq-LA
Andronate
Androyd
Andryl
Bay-Testone
Danabol
Deca-Durabolin
Delatestryl
Dep Andro
Depo-Testosterone
Depotest
Dianabol
Durabolin
Duratest
Durathate
ETHYLESTRENOL
Everone
FLUOXYMESTERONE
Halotestin
Histerone
Malogen
Malogex
Maxibolin
Metandren
Metandren Linguets
METHANDROSTENOLONE
METHYLTESTOSTERONE
NANDROLONE
Ora-Testryl

Oratestin
Oreton Methyl
OXANDROLONE
OXYMETHOLONE
STANOZOLOL
T-Cypionate
Tesionate
Testa-C
Testaqua
Testex
Testoject
Testoject-LA
Testolin
Testone L.A.
TESTOSTERONE
Testostroval P.A.
Testred
Testrin P.A.
T-Iontae
Virilon
Winstrol

## ANESTHETICS (TOPICAL)

Aero Caine
Aero Caine Aerosol
Aerotherm
Americaine
Americaine Aerosol
Americaine Ointment
Anbesol
Anestacon
Bactine
Benzocaine
Benzocaine Topical
Benzocal
BiCozene
Burntame
BUTACAINE
BUTAMBEN
Butesin Picrate
Butyl aminobenzoate
Butyn Sulfate
Caine Spray
Cal-Vi-Nol
Cetacaine
Cetacine
Chiggerex
Chiggertox
Clinicaine
Cyclaine
Cyclaine Solution
CYCLOMETHYCAINE
Derma-Medicone
Dermacoat
Dermo-Gen
Dermoplast
Dibucaine
Diothane
DIPERODON
Dyclone
DYCLONINE
Ethyl Aminobenzoate
Foille
Hexathricin Aerospra
HEXYLCAINE
Hurricaine
Isotraine
Ivy-Dry Cream
Lanacane
Lida-Mantle
Lidocaine

Lidocaine Ointment
Lignocaine
Medicone
Medicone Dressing
Mercurochrome II
Morusan
Nupercainal
Nupercainal Cream
Nupercainal Ointment
Nupercainal Spray
Panthocal A & D
Perifoam
Pontocaine
Pontocaine Cream
Pontocaine Ointment
PRAMOXINE
Prax
Proctodon
Proctofoam
Proxine
Quotane
Rectal Medicone
Soft-N-Soothe
Solarcaine
Surfacaine
Tega-Caine
Tega-Dyne
TETRACAINE
Tronolane
Tronothane
Unguentine
Unguentine Plus
Unguentine Spray
Urolocaine
Velvacaine
Xylocaine
Xylocaine Ointment

# APPETITE
## SUPPRESSANTS

Adipex-D
Adipex-P
Adipost
Adphen
Anorex
Bacarate
BENZPHETAMINE
B.O.F.
Bontril PDM
Bontril Slow Release
Chlor-Tripolon
Chlorophen
CHLORPHENTERMINE
CLORTERMINE
Dapex
Dapex-37.5
Delcozine
D.E.P.—75
Depletite
Dexatrim
Di-Ap-Trol
Didrex
Dietec
DIETHYLPROPION
Dyrexan-OD
Elephemet
Ex-Obese
Fastin
FENFLURAMINE
Hyrex

Hyrex-105
Inifast Unicelles
Ionamin
Limit
Limitite
MASINDOL
Mazanor
Melfiat
Menrium
Metra
Minus
Nobesine
Nobesine-75
Nu-Dispoz
Obalan
Obe-Nil TR
Obe-Nix
Obephen
Obermine
Obestin
Obestin-30
Obestrol
Obeval
Obezine
Oby-Trim
Parmine
Penderal Pacaps
Phendiet
PHENDIMETRAZINE
PHENMETRAZINE
Phentamine
PHENTERMINE
Phentrol
Phenzine
Plegine
Ponderal
Pondimin
Pre-Sate
Prelu-2
Preludin
Propion
P.S.P.R.X. 1,2 &3
Reducto
Regibon
Ro-Diet
Sanorex
Slim-Tabs
Slynn-LL
Span-RD
Sprx-1
Sprx-105
Sprx-3
Statobex
Statobex-G
Symetra
Tenuate
Tenuate Dospan
Tepanil
Tepanil Ten-Tab
Teramine
Tora
Trimcaps
Trimstat
Trimtabs
Unicelles
Unifast
Voranil
Wehless
Weightrol
Wilpowr
X-Trozine
X-Trozine LA

# ASPIRIN

4-Way Cold Tablets
8-Hour Bayer Timed Release
Acetophen
Acetylsalicylic Acid
Alka Seltzer
Alka-Seltzer
Alka-Seltzer Effervescent Pain
    Reliever & Antacid
Aluminum ASA
Amytal and Aspirin
Anacin
Anaphen
Ancasal
Anexsia w/Codeine
A.P.C.
A.P.C w/Codeine
Apo-Asen
Arthritis Bayer Timed-Release
Arthritis Pain Formula
A.S.A.
A.S.A. & Codeine Compound
A.S.A. Compound
A.S.A. Enseals
Ascodeen-30
Ascriptin
Ascriptin A/D
Ascriptin w/Codeine
Asperbuf
Aspergum
Aspir-10
Aspirin Compound w/Codeine
Aspirjen Jr.
Astrin
Axotal
Bancap w/Codeine
Bayer
Bayer Timed-Release Arthritic Pain
    Formula
Bexophene
Buff-A
Buff-A-Comp
Buffaprin
Buffered ASA
Bufferin
Buffex
Buffinol
Buf-Tabs
Calciphen
Cama Arthritis Pain Reliever
Cama Inlay
Causalin
Cefinal
Cirin
Codalan
Codasa
Congespirin
Coralsone
Coricidin D
Coryphen
Cosprin
Darvon Compound
Dasicon
Decagesic
Dia-Gesic
Dihydrocodein Compound
Dolene Compound-65
Dolor
Dolprn #3
Dynosal
Easprin

Ecotrin
Elder 65 Compound
Emagrin
Empirin
Empirin Compound
Empirin Compound w/Codeine
Emprazil
Encaprin
Entrophen
Equagesic
Excedrin
Fiorinal
Fiorinal w/Codeine
Hiprin
Histadyl and ASA Compound
Hyco-Pap
ICN 65 Compound
Kengesin
Lanorinal
Lemidyne w/Codeine
Magnaprin
Maprin
Maprin I-B
Measurin
Mepro Compound
Metrogesic
Mobidin
Norgesic
Norwich Aspirin
Nova-Phase
Novasen
Pabirin Buffered
P-A-C Compound
P-A-C Compound w/Codeine
Pargesic Compound 65
Percodan
Persistin
Phenodyne w/Codeine
Poxy Compound-65
Presalin
Progesic Compound-65
Propoxychel Compound
Propoxyphene HCl Compound
Repro Compound 65
Rhinocaps
Riphen-10
Safety Coated APF Arthritis Pain
   Formula
St. Joseph
St. Joseph Aspirin for Children
Sal-Adult
Salatin
Salatin w/Codeine
Saleto
Salimeph Forte
Sal-Infant
Salocol
Salsprin
SK-65 Compound
Soma Compound
Soma Compound w/Codeine
Stero-Darvon
Supac
Supasa
Synalgos
Talwin Compound
Triaminic
Triaphen-10
Trigesic
Vanquish
Verin
Wesprin Buffered

Zorprin

## ATROPINE

Almezyme
Amocine
Antrocol
Arco-Lase
Atrobarbital
Atromal
Atropine Bufopto
Atropisol
Atrosed
Barbella
Barbeloid
Barbidonna
Barbidonna-CR
Bar-Cy-Amine
Bar-Cy-A-Tab
Bar-Don
Bar-Tropin
Belbutal
Belkaloids
Belladenal
Bellergal-S
Bioxatphen
Briabell
Briaspaz
Brobella
Buren
Butibel
Cerebel
Chardonna
Comhist
Contac
Copin
Dallergy
Ditropan
Donnacin
Donnagel
Donnamine
Donnatal
Donnazyme
Drinus
Eldonal
G.B.S.
HASP
Haponal
Harvitrate
Hyatal
Hybephen
Hycodan
Hyonal
Hyonatol
Hytrona
Isopto Atropine
Kalmedic
Kinesed
Koryza
Levamine
Lyopine Vari-Dose
Magnased
Magnox
Maso-Donna
Neogel w/Sulfa
Nilspasm
Oxybutynin
P & A
Palbar No. 2
PAMA
Peece
Prydon
Renalgin

Ro Trim
Ru-Tuss
Sedamine
Sedapar
Sedatabs
Sedralex
Seds
SK-Diphenoxylate
SMP Atropine
Spabelin
Spasaid
Spasdel
Spasidon
Spasloids
Spasmate
Spasmolin
Spasquid
Spastolate
Spastosed
Stannitol
Thitrate
Trac
Unitral
Urised
Uriseptin
Urogesic
Zemarine

## BELLADONNA

Amobel
Atrocap
Atrosed
Barbidonna
Bebetab
Belap
Belatol
Belbarb
Bellachar
Belladenal
Bellafedrol
Bellergal
Bellkatal
Bello-phen
Belphen
B & O Supprettes
B-Sed
Butabar
Butabar Elixir
Butibel
Butibel Elixir
Butibel-Zyme
Chardonna
Comhist
Coryztime
Decobel
Donabarb
Donnafed Jr.
Donnatal
Donnazyme
Fitacol
Gastrolic
Gelcomul
Hycoff Cold Caps
Hynaldyne
Kamabel
Kinesed
Lanothal
Mallenzyme
Medi-Spas
Nilspasm
Phebe
Phen-o-bel

944

Rectacort
Sedapar
Sedatromine
Spabelin
Spasnil
Trac 2X
Ultabs
Urilief
Urised
U-Tract
Wigraine
Woltac
Wyanoids

## BELLADONNA ALKALOIDS & BARBITURATES

Amobell
Anaspaz PB
Antrocol
ATROPINE, HYOSCYAMINE, SCOPOLAMINE & BUTABARBITAL
ATROPINE, HYOSCYAMINE, SCOPOLAMINE & PHENOBARBITAL
ATROPINE & PHENOBARBITAL
Barbidonna
Barophen
Bay-Ase
Belap
BELLADONNA & AMOBARBITAL
BELLADONNA & BUTABARBITAL
Bellalphen
Bellastal
Bellkatal
Chardonna-2
Donna-Sed
Donnapine
Donnatal
Donnatal Extentabs
Donphen
Hybephen
HYOSCYAMINE & PHENOBARBITAL
Hyosophen
Kinesed
Levsin-PB
Levsin with Phenobarbital
Levsinex with Phenobarbital Timecaps
Malatal
Palbar
Palbar No. 2
Pheno-Bella
Relaxadon
Seds
Spaslin
Spasmolin
Spasmophen
Spasquid
Susano
Vanatal
Vanodonnal

## BENZOYL PEROXIDE

Acetoxyl
Acne-Aid
Allercreme Clear-Up
Alquam-X
Ben-Aqua

Benoxyl
Benzac
Benzac W
Benzagel
Buf-Oxal
Clear By Design
Clearasil
Clearasil BP(M)
Cuticura Acne
Dermodex
Dermoxyl
Desquam-X
Dry and Clean
Dry and Clear
Eloxyl
Epi-Clear
Fostex
Fostex BPO
$H_2Oxyl$
Intraderm-19
Loroxide
Neutrogena Acne Mask
Oxyderm
Oxy-5
Oxy-10
PanOxyl
PanOxyl AQ
Persadox
Persadox HP
Persa-Gel
Persa-Gel W
PHisoAc BP
Porox 7
Propa P.H.
Propa P.H. Porox
Teen
Topex
Vanoxide
Vanoxide-HC
Xerac BP
Zeroxin

## BETAMETHASONE

17-Valerate Celestone
17-Valerate Diprosone
Alphatrex
Beben
Benzoate
Beta-Val
Betacort
Betnelan
Betnesol
Betratrex
B-S-P
Celestoderm
Celestoject
Celestone
Cel-U-Sec
Dipropinate Metaderm
Diprosone
Disodium Phosphate Betnovate
Lotrisone
Uticort
Valerate Betaderm
Valerate Novobetamet
Valisone
Vancerace

## BROMPHENIRAMINE

Brocon
Bromamine

Brombay
Bromepath
Bromfed
Bromphen
Dehist
Dimetane
Dimetane Extentabs
Dimetane-Ten
Dimetapp
Disophrol Chronotabs
Drixoral
Dura Tap-PD
Eldatapp
E.N.T. Syrup
Histaject modified
Histatapp
Nasahist B
ND-Stat Revised
Oraminic II
Poly-Histine
Ralabromophen
Rynatapp
S-T Decongestant
Symptom 3
Taltapp
Tamine S.R.
Tapp
Tolabromophen
Veltane
Veltap

## BUTABARBITAL

Broncholate
Brondilate
Butabell HMB
Butalan
Butaserpazide
Butatran
Butibel
Buticaps
Butisol
Butizide
Cyclo-Bell
Cytospaz-SR
Day-Barb
Levamine
Neo-Barb
Numa-Dura-Tablets
Pyridium Plus
Quibron Plus
Sarisol No. 2
Scolate
Sidonna
Sinate-M
Tedral

## CAFFEINE

Amaphen
Amaphen w/Codeine #3
Anacin
Anaphen
Anexsia w/Codeine
Anoquan
A.P.C.
A.S.A. Compound
Asphac-G
Aspirin Compound w/Codeine
Ban-Drow 2
Bexophene
Buff-A-Comp
Buffadyne

945

Butigetic
Cafacetin
Cafecon
Cafergot
Cafermine
Cafetrate
Cefinal
Cenagesic
Citrated Caffeine
Coastalgesic
Codalan #3
Colrex
Compal
Coryban D
Coryzaid
Darvon Compound
Dasicon
Dexatrim
Dexitac
Dia-Gesic
Dihydrocodeine Compound
Dolor
Duadacin
Dularin
Dynosal
Elder 65 Compound
Emagrin
Empirin Compound
Emprazil
Esgic
Excedrin Extra Strength
Fendol
Fiorinal
G-1 Capsules
Hista-Derfule
Histadyl Compound
ICN 65 Compound
Kengesin
Kirkaffeine
Korigesic
Lanorinal
Lemidyne w/Codeine
Midol
Migralam
Nodaca
Nodoz
Pacaps
P-A-C Compound w/Codeine
Pargesic Compound 65
Percodan
Phenodyne
Phenodyne w/Codeine
Phensal
Phrenilin
Poxy Compound-65
Prodolor
Progesic Compound-65
Propoxychel Compound-65
Propoxyphene Compound
Pyrroxate
Quick Pep
Repro Compound 65
S-A-C
Salatin
Salatin w/Codeine
Saleto
Salocol
Sinarest
SK-65 Compound
Supac
Synalgos
Synalgos-DC

Tirend
Triaminic
Triaminicin
Trigesic
Two-Dyne
Vanquish
Vivarin
Wigraine

## CALCIUM CARBONATE

Alka-mints
Alka-2
Alkets
Amitone
Bio Cal
Calcet
Calcilac
Calcitrate 600
Calglycine
Cal-Sup
Caltrate
Camalox
Chooz
Dicarbosil
Ducon
El-Da-Mint
Equilet
Fosfree
Gustalac
Iromin-G
Mallamint
Mission
Natacomp-FA
Natalins
Nu-Iron-V
Os-Cal
Os-Cal 500
Pama No. 1
Pramet FA
Pramilet FA
Prenate 90
Ratio
Suplical
Theracal
Titracid
Titralac
Trialka
Tums
Tums E-X
Zenate

## CALCIUM SUPPLEMENTS

BioCal
CALCIUM CARBONATE (also used
   as an antacid)
CALCIUM CITRATE
CALCIUM GLUBIONATE
CALCIUM GLUCONATE
CALCIUM GLYCEROPHOSPHATE
   & CALCIUM LACTATE
CALCIUM LACTATE
Calphosan
Cal-Sup
Caltrate
Citracal
DIBASIC CALCIUM PHOSPHATE
Neo-Calglucon
Os-Cal 500
Posture
Suplical
Theracal

TRIBASIC CALCIUM PHOSPHATE
Tums
Tums E-X

## CHLORDIAZEPOXIDE & CLIDINIUM

Apo-Chlorax
Clindex
Clinoxide
Clipoxide
Corium
Librax
Lidox

## CHLORPHENIRAMINE

4-Way Cold Tablets
Acutuss
Acutuss Expectorant w/Codeine
Alermine
Alka-Seltzer Plus
Aller-chlor
Allerbid Tymcaps
Allerest
Allerform
Allergesic
Allerid - O.D.
AL-R
Alumadrine
Anafed
Anamine
Anatuss
Antagonate
Brexin
Bronkotuss
Cerose Compound
Children's Allerest
Chlo-Amine
Chlorafed
Chloramate Unicelles
Chlor-Histine
Chlor-MAL
Chlormine
Chlor-Niramine
Chlor-100
Chlorphen
Chlor-PRO
Chlor-Span
Chlortab
Chlor-Trimeton
Chlor-Trimeton w/Codeine
Chlor-Trimeton Repetabs
Chlor-Tripolon
Ciramine
Ciriforte
Citra Forte
Codimal
Coldene
Colrex
Comhist
Comtrex
Conex w/Codeine
Conex-DA
Cophene-X
Co-Pyronil 2
Coricidin
Coricidin "D"
Corilin
Coryban-D
Coryzaid

Cosea
Co-Tylenol
Covanamine
Covangesic
Dallergy
Deconamine
Dehist
Demazin
Dextromal
Dextro-Tussin
DM Plus
Donatussin
Dorcol
Drinus
Dristan
Drize M
Duadacin
Duphrene
Dura-Vent/A
E.N.T.
Expectrosed
Extendryl
Fedahist
Fernhist
Ginsopan
Guaiahist TT
Guaiamine
Guistrey Fortis
Hal-Chlor
Histalet
Histalon
Histamic
Histaspan
Hista-Vadrin
Histex
Histor-D Timecelles
Historal
Histrey
Hycoff
Hycomine Compound
Iophen-C
Isoclor
Korigesic
Koryza
Kronofed-A
Kronohist Kronocaps
Lanatuss
Marhist
Naldecon
Naldetuss
Napril Plateau
Narine Gyrocaps
Narspan
Nasahist
Neo-Codenyl-M
Neotep Granucaps
Nilcol
Nolamine
Novafed A
Novahistine
Novopheniram
Omni-Tuss
Ornade Spansule
P.R. Syrup
P-V-Tussin
Palohist
Partuss T.D.
Pediacof
Phenacol-DM
Phenate
Phenetron
Phenetron Lanacaps

Polaramine
Probahist
Protid Improved Formula
Pseudo-Hist
Pyma
Pyrroxate
Pyrroxate w/Codeine
Quadrahist
Quelidrine
Queltuss
Resaid T.D.
Rhinex
Rhinolar
Rhinolar-EX
Ru-Tuss
Rynatan
Rynatuss
Salphenyl
Scot-Tussin
Sinarest
Singlet
Sinovan
Sinulin
T.D. Alermine
Tedral Anti-H
Teldrin
Teldrin Spansules
T.P.I.
Triaminicin
Trymegen
Tusquelin
Tuss-Ornade
Tussar
Tussi-Organidin
U.R.I.
Wesmatic Forte

## CONTRACEPTIVES (ORAL)

Anoryol
Brevicon
Demulen
Enovid
Loestrin
Lo-Ovral
Micronor
Min-Ovral
Modacon
Modicon
Nordette
Norlestrin
Norlinyl
Nor-Q.D.
Ortho-Novum
Ovcon
Ovral
Ovrette
Ovulen
Tri-Norinyl
Triphasil

## DEXAMETHASONE

Aeroseb-Dex
Ak-Dex
Congespirin
Cremacoat 1
Dalalone
Dalalon L.A.
Decaderm
Decadrol
Decadron
Decadron L.A.

Decadron Respihaler
Decadron Turbinaire
Decadron with Xylocaine
Decajet
Decameth
Decaspray
Delsym
Demo-Cineol
Deronil
Dexacen
Dexasone
Dexon
Dexone
DM Cough
Extend-12
Hexadrol
Hexandrol
Hold
Maxidex
Mediquell
Oradexon
Pedia Care 1
Pertussin 8 Hour Cough Formula
SK-Dexamethasone
Solurex
Sucrets

## DEXTROMETHORPHAN

2/C-DM
216 DM
Anti-Tuss DM
Balminil DM
Benylin DM
Broncho-Grippol-DM
Cheracol
Congespirin
Contratuss
Cosanyl DM
Cremacoat 1
Delsym
Delsym Polistirex
Demo-Cineol
Dextro-Tussin GG
DM Cough
DM Syrup
Dormethan
Dristan
Dristan Cough Formula
Duad Koff Balls
Endotussin-NN
Extend-12
Formula 44-D
Glycotuss-dM
Guiatuss D-M
Hold
Hold Cough Suppressant
Koffex
Lixaminol AT
Mediquell
Neo-DM
Novahistine DMX
Nyquil
Ornacol
Pedia Care 1
Pertussin 8 Hour Cough Formula
Queltuss
Robidex
Robitussin
Robitussin-DM
Romilar
Romilar CF

947

Romilar Children's Cough
Sedatuss
Silence is Golden
Silexin
Sorbase
Sorbutuss
St. Joseph
St. Joseph Cough Syrup
St. Joseph for Children
Sucrets
Trind DM
Trocal
Tussagesic
Tussaminic
Unproco
Vicks
Vicks Cough Syrup

## DICYCLOMINE

Antispas
A-Spas
Baycyclomine
Bentyl
Bentylol
Byclomine
Cyclobec
Cyclocen
Dibent
Dicen
Dilomine
Di-Spaz
Dyspas
Formulex
Lomine
Menospasm
Neoquess
Nospaz
Or-Tyl
Protylol
Spasmoban
Spasmoject
Triactin
Viscerol

## DIMENHYDRINATE

Apo-Dimenhydrinate
Calm X
Dimentabs
Dinate
Dommanate
Dramaban
Dramamine
Dramilin
Dramocen
Dramoject
Dymenate
Eldodram
Gravol
Hydrate
Marine
Marmine
Motion-Aid
Nauseatol
Novodimenate
PMS-Dimenhydrinate
Reidamine
Travamine
Trav-Arex
Vertiban
Wehamine

## DIPHENHYDRAMINE

Allerdryl
Ambenyl Expectorant
Bena-D
Benadryl
Benadryl Children's Allergy
Benadryl Complete Allergy
Benahist
Bendylate
Benoject-10
Benylin Cough Syrup
Caladryl
Compoz
Diahist
Dihydrex
Diphen
Diphenacen
Diphenadril
Eldadryl
Fenylhist
Fynex
Hydramine
Hydril
Hyrexin-50
Insomnal
Nervine Nighttime Sleep-Aid
Noradryl
Nordryl
Nytol
Nytol with DPH
Phen-Amin
Robalyn
SK-Diphenhydramine
Sleep-Eze
Sleep-Eze 3
Sominex
Sominex Formula 2
SominiFere
Tusstat
Twilite
Valdrene
Wehydryl

## DOCUSATE SODIUM

Afko-Lube
Bilax
Bu-Lax
Colace
Colax
Coloctyl
Dialose
Dilax
Diocto
Dioctyl Sodium Sulfosuccinate
Dioeze
DioMedicone
Diosuccin
Dio-Sul
Disonate
Di-Sosul
Doctate
Doss
Doxidan
Doxinate
D-S-S
Duosol
Ferro-sequels
Geriplex-FS
Laxagel
Laxinate
Liqui-Doss

Modane Plus
Modane Soft
Molatoc
Neolax
Peri-Colase
Peritinic
Prenate 90
Pro-Sof 100
Regulex
Regutol
Senokot-S
Stulex
Trilax

## EPHEDRINE

Acet-Am
Aladrine
Amesec
Amodrine
Asminyl
Benadryl w/Ephedrine
Broncholate
Brondilate
Bronkaid
Bronkolixir
Bronkotabs
Bronkotuss
Calcidrine
Coryza Brengle
Co-Xan Elixir
Dainite
Derma Medicone-HC
Duovent
Ectasule III
Ectasule Minus
Ephed-Organidin
Ephedrine and Amytal
Ephedrine and Nembutal-25
Ephedrine and Seconal
Ephedrol
Ephedrol w/Codeine
Epragen
Iso-Asminyl
Isuprel
Luasmin
Lufyllin-EPG
Marax
Mudrane
Numa-Dura-Tablets
Nyquil
Phyldrox
Primatene
Pyribenazmine w/Ephedrine
Quadrinal
Quelidrine
Quibron Plus
Slo-Fedrin A-60
Tedfern
Tedral
T.E.H.
T-E-P
Thalfed
Theofedral
Theotabs
Theozine
Wesmatic
Wyanoids

## EPINEPHRINE

Adrenalin
Asmolin
Asthma Haler

Asthma Nefrin
Ayerst Epitrate
Bronitin
Bronkaid
Bronkaid Mist
Dysne-Inhal
Epifrin
EpiPen-Epinephrine Auto-Injector
Epi-Pen Jr.
Epitrate
Eppy
Glaucon
Marcaine Hydrochloride
  w/Epinephrine
Medihaler-Epi
microNEFRIN
Murocoll
Mytrate
Primatene
Primatene Mist
Simplene
Sus-phrine
Vaponefrin

## ERYTHROMYCINS

Apo-Erythro-S
A/T/S
Bristamycin
Dowmycin
E-Biotic
E.E.S.
E-Mycin
E-Mycin E
Eryc
Ery-derm
EryPed
Erymax
Erypar
Ery-Tab
Erythrocin
Erythrocin Ethyl Succinate
Erythromid
ERYTHROMYCIN
ERYTHROMYCIN ESTOLATE
ERYTHROMYCIN
  ETHYLSUCCINATE
ERYTHROMYCIN GLUCEPTATE
ERYTHROMYCIN LACTOBIONATE
ERYTHROMYCIN STEARATE
Ethril
Ilosone
Ilosone Estolate
Ilotycin
Ilotycin Gluceptate
Kesso-mycin
Novorythro
Pediazole
Pediamycin
Pendiamycin
Pfizer-E
Robimycin
RP-Mycin
SK-Erythromycin
Staticin
T-Star
Wyamycin
Wyamycin E
Wyamycin S

## ESTROGEN

Amnestrogen
Clinestrone

Delestrogen
DES
DIENESTROL (vaginal)
DV (vaginal)
Estinyl
Estomed
Estrace
Estrace (vaginal)
ESTRADIOL (vaginal)
Estraguard (vaginal)
Estratab
Estrocon
ESTROGENS, CONJUGATED
  (vaginal)
ESTRONE (vaginal)
ESTROPIPATE (vaginal)
Estrovis
Evex
Feminone
Femogen
Formatrix
Hormonin
Menest
Menotrol
Menrium
Milprem
Oagen
Oestrilin
Oestrilin (vaginal)
Ogen
Ogen (vaginal)
Ortho Dienestrol (vaginal)
Piperazine Estrone Sulfate (vaginal)
PMB-200
PMB-400
Premarin
Premarin (vaginal)
Progens
Stilphostrol
Theogen

## FERROUS FUMARATE

Cevi-Fer
Chromagen
Feco-T
Femiron
Feostat
Ferancee
Ferrofume
Ferro-sequels
Fersamal
Fetrin
Fumasorb
Fumerin
Hemocyte
Hemo-Vite
Ircon
Ircon-FA
Laud-Iron
Maniron
Natalins
Neo-Fer
Neo-Fer-50
Novofumar
Palafer
Palmiron
Poly-Vi-Flor
Pramilet FA
Prenate 90
Stuartinic
Toleron
Tolfrinic

Tolifer
Trinsicon
Vitron C
Zenate

## FERROUS SULFATE

Apo-Ferrous Sulfate
Feosol
Fer-In-Sol
Fer-Iron
Fero-folic-500
Fero-Grad
Fero-Grad-500
Fero-Gradumet
Ferospace
Ferralyn
Fesofor
Geritol Tablets
Hematinic
Iberet
Iberet-500
Iberet-Folic-500
Iromal
Mol-Iron
Novoferrosulfa
PMS Ferrous Sulfate
Slow-Fe

## GUAIFENESIN

2/G
2/G-DM
Actol
Ambenyl
Anti-Tuss
Asbron
Asma
Balminil
Baytussin
Breonesin
Brexin
Bromphen
Broncholate
Brondecon
Bronkolizir
Bronkotabs
Bronkotuss
Caldrex Expectorant
Cetro Cirose
Cheracol
Cheracol Cough
Chlor-Trimeton
Codimal
Coditrate
Colrex Expectorant
Conar
Conex
Conex w/Codeine
Congess Jr. & Sr.
Corutol
Coryban-D
Co-Xan
Cremacoat
Cremacoat 2
Deproist w/Codeine
Detussin
Dilaudid
Dilor-G
Dimetane
Donatussin
Dorcol
Dristan
Dristan Cough

Duovent
Dura-Vent
Elixophyllin-GG
Emfaseen
Entex
Entuss-D
Expectorant
Fedahist
Formula
Formula 44-D
Gee-Gee
GG-CEN
Glyceryl Guaiacolate
Glycotuss
Glytuss
Guaiahist
Guaifed
Guiamid
Guiatuss
Gylate
Halotussin
Histalet X
Hycotuss
Hytuss
Hytuss-2X
Luftodil
Lufyllin
Malotuss
Mudrane GG
Naldecon
Neo-Spec
Neospect
Neothyllin-G
Nortussin
Novahistine
Nucofed
Pee Dee Dose Expectorant
Poly-Histine
P-V-Tussin
Queltuss
Quibron
Respaire-SR
Resyl
Robafen
Robitussin
Scot-Tussin Sugar-Free
Silexin
Sinufed Timecelles
Slo-Phyllin GG
Sorbase
Sorbutuss
S-T Expectorant
S-T Forte
Synophylate-GG
Syrup
Tedral
Theo-Guaia
Theolair-Plus
Triafed-C
Triaminic
Triaminic w/Codeine
Trind
Tussar
Tussend
Uproco
Vicks
Vicks Cough
Zephrex

## HYDROCHLOROTHIAZIDE

Aldactazide
Aldoril

Apo-Hydro
Butaserpazide
Butizide
Diuchlor H
Diupres
Dyazide
Esidrix
Esimil
H-H-R
Hydrid
Hydro-Aquil
HydroDIURIL
Hydropres
Hydroserp
Hydroserpine
Hydrotensin
Hydrozide-Z-50
Hyperetic
Inderide
Mallopress
Maxzide
Moduretic
Naquival
Natrimax
Nefrol
Neo-Codema
Novohydrazide
Oretic
Oreticyl
Reserpazide
Ser-Ap-Es
Serpasil-Esidrix
Singoserp-Esidrix
SK-Hydrochlorothiazide
Spironazide
Thiuretic
Timolide
Timolol and Hydrochlorothiazide
Tri-Hydroserpine
Unipres
Urozide
Zide

## HYDROCORTISONE (CORTISOL)

Aeroseb-HC
A-hydroCort
Barseb
Biosone
Cortaid
Cortamed
Cortate
Cort-Dome
Cortef
Cortef Fluid
Cortenema
Corticreme
Cortifoam
Cortiment
Cortisol
Cortoderm
Cortril
Dermacort
Emo-Cort
Fernisone
Hyderm
Hydro-Cortilean
Hydrocortone
Hytone
Microcort
Novohydrocort

Orabase HCA
Proctocort
Rectoid
Restocort
Solu-Cortef
Texacort
Unicort
Westcort

## HYDROXYZINE

Anxanil
Atarax
Ataraxoid
Atozine
Cartrax
Durrax
Enarax
E-Vista
Hydroxacen
Hy-Pam
Hyzine
Marax
Multipax
Neucalm 50
Orgatrax
Quiess
T.E.H. Tablets
Theozine
Vamate
Vistacon
Vistaject
Vistaquel
Vistaril
Vistazine
Vistrax

## HYOSCYAMINE

Almezyme
Anaspa 3
Anaspaz
Anaspaz PB
Arco-Lase Plus
Barbella
Barbeloid
Barbidonna-CR
Bar-Cy-Amine
Bar-Cy-A-Tab
Bar-Don
Belbutal
Belkaloids
Bellafoline
Bellaspaz
Brobella-PB
Buren
Cytospa
De Tal
Donnacin
Donnagel
Donnamine
Donnatal
Donnazyme
Eldonal
Elixiril
Ergobel
Floramine
Gylanphen
Haponal
Hyatal
Hybephen
Hyonal
Hyonatol

Hytrona
Kinesed
Koryza
Kutrase
Levamine
Levsin
Levsinex
Levsinex Timecaps
Maso-Donna
Neoquess
Nevrotase
Nilspasm
Omnibel
Peece
Pyridium Plus
Renalgin
Restophen
Ru-Tuss
Sedajen
Sedamine
Sedapar
Sedatromine
Sedralex
Seds
Spabelin
Spasaid
Spasdel
Spasloids
Spasmolin
Spasquid
Spastolate
Trac 2X
Ultabs
Urised
Uriseptin
Urogesic
Zemarine

## INSULIN
Actrapid
Globin Insulin
Humulin
Humulin BR
Humulin L
Humulin N
Humulin R
Insulatard
Insultard NPH
Lentard
Lente
Lente Iletin I
Lente Iletin II
Lente Insulin
Mixtard
Monotard
NPH
NPH Iletin I
NPH Iletin II
Novolin
Novolin L
Novolin N
Novolin R
Novolin 70/30
PZI
Protamine Zinc & Iletin
Protamine Zinc & Iletin I
Protamine Zinc & Iletin II
Protophane NPH
Regular
Regular (Concentrated) Iletin
Regular (Concentrated) Iletin II,
  U-500

Regular Iletin I
Regular Iletin II
Regular Insulin
Semilente
Semilente Iletin
Semilente Iletin I
Semitard
Ultralente
Ultratard
Utralente Iletin I
Velosulin
Velosulin Human

## MAGNESIUM HYDROXIDE
Aludrox
Arthritis Pain Formula
Camalox
Creamalin
Delcid
Di-Gel
Dolprn 3
Ducon
Gelusil
Kolantyl
Maalox
Magnatril
Maxamag
Milk of Magnesia
M.O.M.
Mucotin
Mygel
Mylanta
Phillips' Milk of Magnesia
Silain-Gel
Simeco
Univol
Vanquish
Win-Gel

## MEPROBAMATE
Apo-Meprobamate
Arcoban
Bamate
Bamo 400
Coprobate
Deprol
Equagesic
Equanil
Equanil Wyseals
Evenol
Kalmn
Lan-Dol
Medi-Tran
Mep-E
Mepriam
Mepro Compound
Meprocon
Meprospan
Meprotabs
Meribam
Miltown
Neo-Tran
Neuramate
Neurate
Novo-Mepro
Novomepro
Pathibamate
Pax 400
PMB
Protran
Quietal

Robam
Robamate
Sedabamate
SK-Bamate
Tranmep

## METHYLPREDNISOLONE
A-methaPred
dep Medalone
Depoject
Depo-Medrol
Depo-medrone
Depopred
Depo-Pred-40
Depo-Pred-80
Duralone
Duralone-40
Duralone-80
Durameth
Medralone
Medralone-40
Medralone-80
Medrol
Medrol Enpak
Medrone
Medrone-80
Mepred-40
Methylone
m-Prednisol
Pre-Dep
Pro-Dep-40
Pro-Dep-80
Rep-Pred
Solu-Medrol
Solu-medrone

## NARCOTIC & ACETAMINOPHEN
ACETAMINOPHEN & CODEINE
Aceta with Codeine
Amacodone
Atasol with Codeine
Bancap-HC
Bayapap with Codeine
Capital with Codeine
Codap
Co-gesic
Cotabs
Darvocet-N
Demerol-APAP
Dolacet
Dolene-AP
Dolo-Pap
Duradyne DHC
Empracet with Codeine
Exdol with Codeine
Hycodaphen
HYDROCODONE & ACETAMINOPHEN
Hydrogesic
Lortab 5
Lortab 7
MEPERIDINE & ACETAMINOPHEN
Norcet
Oxycocet
OXYCODONE & ACETAMINOPHEN
PENTAZOCINE & ACETAMINOPHEN
Percocet
Percocet-Demi
Phenaphen with Codeine

PROPOXYPHENE &
   ACETAMINOPHEN
Proval
SK-APAP with Codeine
SK-Oxycodone and Acetaminophen
SK-65 APAP
Talacen
T-Gesic Forte
Tylenol with Codeine
Tylox
Ty-Tabs
Vicodin
Wygesic

# NARCOTIC ANALGESICS
642
Aceta w/Codeine
Acetaco
Acetaminophen w/Codeine
Actifed-C
Actifed-C Expectorant
Adatuss
Algodex
Ambenyl
Anaphen
A.P.C. w/Codeine Phosphate
   Tablets
A.P.C. w/Codeine Phosphate
Arthralgen
Ascriptin w/Codeine
Aspirin Compound w/Codeine
Axotal
Bancap w/Codeine
Banesin Forte
BUTORPHANOL
Calcidrine
Calcidrine Syrup
Capital w/Codeine
Cetro Cirose
Cheracol
Coastaldyne
Coastalgesic
Codalan
Codalex
Codap
CODEINE
Codeine Sulfate
Codimal PH
Coditrate
Codone
Colrex Compound
Copavin
Corutol DH
Cotussis
Co-Xan
Dapase
Darvocet-N 100
Darvon
Demer-Idine
Demerol
Depronal-SA
Dialog
Dicodid
Dihydromorphinone
Dilaudid
Dilaudid-HP
Dimetane-DC
Dimetane Expectorant-DC
Dolene
Dolophine
Dolor

Doxaphene
Dromoran
Dularin
Duramorph PF
Dynosal
Empirin w/Codeine
Empracet w/Codeine
Emprazil-C
Ephedrol w/Codeine
Epimorph
Esgic
FL-Tussex
Fiorinal w/Codeine
Fortral
Gaysal
G-2
G-3
Hasacode
Hycodan
Hycotuss
HYDROCODONE
HYDROMORPHONE
Isoclor
Levo-Dromoran
Levorphan
LEVORPHANOL
Liquix-C
Lo-Tussin
Maxigesic
Mepergan Fortis
MEPERIDINE
METHADONE
Methadose
Metrogesic
Minotal
MORPHINE
Morphitec
M.O.S. Syrup
MS Contin
MSIR
MST Continus
NALBUPHINE
Novahistine DH
Novahistine Expectorant
Novopropoxyn
Nubain
Numorphan
OPIUM
Ossonate-Plus
OXYCODONE
OXYMORPHONE
Pantapon
PAREGORIC
Pargesic
Pavadon
Paveral
Pediacof
PENTAZOCINE
Percodan
Pethadol
Pethidine
Phenaphen w/Codeine
Phenergan
Phrenilin
Physeptone
Poly-Histine w/Codeine
Presalin
Prodolor
Profene
Promethazine HCl w/Codeine
PROPOXYPHENE
Pro-65

Proxagesic
Proxene
Prunicodeine
RMS Uninserts
Robidone
Robitussin A-C
Roxanol
Roxanol SR
S-A-C
Salatin
Saleto
Salimeph Forte
Sedapap
SK-65
SK-APAP w/Codeine
Soma Compound w/Codeine
Sorbase II
Stadol
Statex
Strascogesic
Supac
Supeudol
Sylapar
Synalgos-DC
Talwin
Talwin-NX
Terpin Hydrate w/Codeine
Triaminic w/Codeine
Trigesic
Tussar
Tussend
Tussi-Organidin
Tylenol w/Codeine
Tylox
Vicodin
Wygesic

# NARCOTIC & ASPIRIN
222
282
292
A&C with Codeine
A.C.&C.
Ancasal
Anexsia with Codeine
Anexsia-D
A.S.A. and Codeine Compound
Ascriptin with Codeine
ASPIRIN & CODEINE
ASPIRIN, CODEINE & CAFFEINE
Bexophene
BUFFERED ASPIRIN & CODEINE
Codoxy
Coryphen with Codeine
C2 with Codeine
Damason-P
Darvon Compound
Darvon with A.S.A.
Darvon-N with A.S.A.
Dolene Compound
Doxaphene Compound
DROCODE, ASPIRIN & CAFFEINE
Emcodeine
Empirin with Codeine
HYDROCODONE, ASPIRIN &
   CAFFEINE
Instantine Plus
Novo AC&C
Oxycodan
OXYCODONE & ASPIRIN
PENTAZOCINE & ASPIRIN
Percodan

Percodan-Demi
PROPOXYPHENE & ASPIRIN
PROPOXYPHENE ASPIRIN &
  CAFFEINE
SK-65 Compound
SK-Oxycodone with Aspirin
Synalgos-DC
Talwin Compound

## NIACIN (NICOTINIC ACID)

Diacin
N-Caps
Niac
Niacin
Nicalex
Nico-400
Nico-Span
Nicobid
Nicocap
Nicolar
Nicotinex
Nicotinyl alcohol
Nicotym
Novoniacin
SK-Niacin
Span-Niacin
Tega-Span
Vasotherm
Numerous other multiple
  vitamin-mineral supplements.

## NITRATES

Ang-O-Span
Cardilate
Coronex
Dilatrate-SR
Duotrate
ERYTHRITYL TETRANITRATE
Glyceryl Trinitrate
Iso-Bid
Isochron
Isogard
Isonate
Isonate TR
Isordil
ISOSORBIDE DINITRATE
Isotrate
Kaytrate
Klavikordal
Naptrate
N-G-C
Niong
Nitro-Bid
Nitrobon
Nitrocap
Nitrocap T.D.
Nitrocardin
Nitrodisc
Nitro-Dur
Nitrogard-SR
NITROGLYCERIN (GLYCERYL
  TRINITRATE)
Nitroglyn
Nitrol
Nitrolin
Nitro-Long
Nitronet
Nitrong
Nitrospan
Nitrostablin
Nitrostat

Nitro-Time
Novosorbide
Onset
PENTAERYTHRITOL
  TETRANITRATE
Pentestan
Pentol
Pentol S.A.
Pentraspan
Pentraspan SR
Pentritol
Pentylan
Peritrate
Peritrate SA
P.E.T.N.
Sorate
Sorbide
Sorbide T.D.
Sorbitrate
Sorbitrate SA
Susadrin
Tranderm-Nitro
Trates
Tridil
Vaso-80
Vasoglyn

## OXYMETAZOLINE

4-Way Long-Acting Nasal
Afrin
Bayfrin
Dristan Long Lasting
Duramist Plus
Duration
Nafrine
Neo-Synephrine 12 Hour
Nostrilla
NTZ Long Lasting Nasal
Ocuclear
Otrivin
Oxymeta-12 Nasal Spray
Sinex Long-Lasting
St. Joseph Decongestant for
  Children

## PAPAVERINE

Cerebid
Cerespan
Copavin
Dipav
Durapav
Dylate
Hyobid
Kavrin
Lapav
Myobid
Octapav
Orapav
P-200
P-A-V
Pavabid
Pavabid HP
Pavacap
Pavadon
Pavadur
Pavagen
Pavakey
Pavased
Pavasule
Pavatest
Pavatran

Pavatym
Paverolan
Payadur
Ro-Papan
Sustaverine
Therapav
Vasal
Vasospan

## PHENOBARBITAL

Aminophylline-Phenobarbital
Anaspaz-PB
Antrocol
Asminyl
Banthine w/Phenobarbital
Barbidonna
Barbita
Bardase Filmseal
Bar-Tropin
Belap
Belbarb
Belladenal
Bellergal
Bellkatal
Bentyl Phenobarbital
Bronkolixir
Bronkotabs
Cantil w/Phenobarbital
Chardonna
Cyclo-Bell
Dactil Phenobarbital
Dainite-KI
Daricon PB
Donna-Lix
Donnatal
Duovent
Eskabarb
Gardenal
Gastrolic
HASP
Hybephen
Hytrona
Iso-Asminyl
Isuprel Compound
Kinesed
Levsin PB
Levsin w/Phenobarbital
Luasmin
Luftodil
Lufyllin-EPG
Luminal
Matropinal
Mesopin PB
Mudrane
Neospect
Nova-Pheno
Oxoids
Pamine PB
Pathilon w/Phenobarbital
PBR/12
Phyldrox
Primatene, P Formula
Pro-Banthine w/Phenobarbital
Probital
Pyrdonnal Spansules
Quadrinal
Robinul-PH
Sedadrops
SK-Phenobarbital
Solfoton
Spasdel
Spasticol

Tedral
T-E-P
Thalfed
Theofedral
Theotabs
Tral w/Phenobarbital
Valpin-PB

## PHENYLEPHRINE
4-Way Nasal Spray
4-Way Tablets
Albatussin
Alconefrin
Alka-Seltzer Plus
Anamine T.D.
Bromepaph
Bromphen Compound
Callergy
Cenagesic
Children's Allerest
Chlor-Histine
Chlor-Trimeton
Citra
Clistin D
Codalex
Codimal
Colrex
Comhist
Conar
Congespirin
Contac
Coricidin
Coricidin Mist
Coryban-D
Coryban-D Cough Syrup
Coryzaid
Cosea-D
Co-Tylenol
Covanamine
Covangesic
Dallergy
Dehist
Demazin
Dimetapp
doKtors Nose Drops
Donatussin DC
Dri-Hist No. Meta-Caps
Drinus Graduals
Dristan Advanced Formula
Dristan Nasal Spray
Drize M
Duadacin
Duo-Medihaler
Duphrene
Dura Tap-PD
Duration Mild
Dura-Vent/DA
Emagrin Forte
E.N.T.
Entex
Extendryl
Fendol
Fernhist
Ginospan
Guaiahist
Hista-Vadrin
Histabid Duracaps
Histalet
Histaspan
Histatapp
Histor-D Timecelles
Historal No. 2

Hycomine Compound
Isophrin
Korigesic
Koryza
Marhist
Mydrin
Naldecon
Napril Plateau
Narine Cyrocaps
Narspan
Nasahist
Neo-Mist
Neo-Synephrine
NeoSynephrin Compound
Neotep Granucaps
Nostril
Novahistine
Palohist
Pediacof
Phenate
Phenergan VC
Phenergan VC w/Codeine
Prefrin
Protid Improved Formula
P-V-Tussin
Pyma Timed
Pyracort-D
Quelidrine
Rhinall
Rhinex
Rolabromophen
Rolahist
Ru-Tuss
Rynatan
Rynatapp
Salphenyl
Sinarest Nasal
Sinex
Singlet
Sinophen Intransal
Sinoran
S-T Forte
Super Anahist
Synasal
Taltapp
Tamine S.R.
Tapp
T.P.I.
Tussar DM
Tussirex
Tympagesic
U.R.I.
Vacon
Veltar

## PHENYLPROPANOLAMINE
4-Way Cold Tablets
4-Way Nasal Spray
Acutrim Maximum Strength
Alka-Seltzer Plus
Allerest
Alumadrine
Asbron
Axon
Bayer Cold Tablets
Bayer Cough Syrup
Blu-Hist
Bromphen Compound
Caldecon
Children's Allerest
Cinsospan
Citra

Codimal
Coffee-Break
Colrex
Comtrex
Conex-DA
Congespirin
Conhist
Contac
Control
Coricidin "D" Decongestant
Cornex Plus
Coryban-D
Coryztime
CoTylenol Children's Liquid Cold
    Formula
Covanamine
Cremacoat
Dal-Sinus
Decongestant-P
Dehist
Dex-A-Diet
Dexatrim
Diadox
Dietac
Dieutrim
Dimetane
Dimetapp
Dri-Hist Meta-Kaps
Drinus Syrup
D-Sinus
Dura Tap-PD
Dura-Vent, /A
Efed II
Eldatapp
Endecon
E.N.T
Entex
Fiogesic
Formula 44-D
Help
Histalet Forte
Histapp
Histatapp
Hycomine
Korigesic
Koryza
Kronohist Kronocaps
MSC Triaminic
Naldecon
Napril Plateau
Nasahist
Nolamine
Novahistine
Obestat
Ornacol
Ornade
Ornex
Partuss T.D.
Phenate
Phenylin
Poly-Histine-D
PPA
Prolamine
Prolamine, Maximum Strength
Propadrine
Propagest
Quadrahist
Resaid T.D.
Rescaps-D T.D.
Resolution I Maximum Strength
Resolution II Half-Stregth
Rhindecon

Rhinex Ty-Med
Rhinidrin
Rhinocaps
Rhinolar
Robitussin-CF
Rolabromophen
Ru-Tuss
Rynatapp
Saleto-D
Sinarest
Sine-Off
Sinubid
Sinulin
Sinutab
S-T Decongestant
S-T Forte
Symtrol
Taltapp
Tapp
Tavist-D
T.P.I.
Triaminic
Triaminicin
Triaminicol
Tuss-Ade
Tussagesic
Tussaminic
Tuss-Ornade
Unitrol
U.R.I.
Ursinus
Veltap
Vernata Granucaps
Westrim
Westrim LA

## PHENYLTOLOXAMINE

Amaril D
Amaril D Spantab
Comhist
Condecal
Decongestabs
Kutrase
Magsal
Naldecol
Naldecon
Naldelate
Percogesic
Poly-Histine-D
Quadra Hist
Sinocon
Sinubid
Sinutab
Trihista-Phen-25
Tri-Phen-Chlor
Tudecon
Tussionex

## POTASSIUM SUPPLEMENTS

Apo-K
Bayon
Bi-K
Cena-K
CHLORIDE
EM-K-10%
Infacyte
K-10
Kalium Durules
Kaochlor
Kaochlor S-F

Kaochlor-Eff
Kaon
Kaon-Cl
Kaon-Cl 10
Kaon-Cl 20
Kao-Nor
Kato
Kay Ciel
Kaylixir
KCL
K-Dur
KEFF
K-G Elixir
K-Long
K-Lor
Klor-10%
Klor-Con
Klor-Con/EF
Klor Con/25
Klorvess
Klotrix
K-Lyte
K-Lyte DS
K-Lyte/Cl
K-Lyte/Cl 50
Kolyum
K-Tab
Micro-K
Micro-K 10
Neo-K
Novo-Lente-K
Pfiklor
Potachlor
Potage
Potasalan
Potassine
POTASSIUM ACETATE
POTASSIUM BICARBONATE
POTASSIUM BICARBONATE &
    POTASSIUM CHLORIDE
POTASSIUM BICARBONATE &
    POTASSIUM CITRATE
POTASSIUM CHLORIDE
POTASSIUM CHLORIDE,
    POTASSIUM BICARBONATE &
    POTASSIUM CITRATE
POTASSIUM GLUCONATE
POTASSIUM GLUCONATE &
    POTASSIUM CHLORIDE
POTASSIUM GLUCONATE &
    POTASSIUM CITRATE
POTASSIUM GLUCONATE,
    POTASSIUM CITRATE &
    AMMONIUM
Potassium Triplex
Potassium-Rougier
Potassium-Sandoz
Roychlor
Royonate
Rum-K
SK-Potassium Chloride
Slo-Pot
Slow-K
Tri-K
TRIKATES
Twin-K
Twin-K-Cl

## PREDNISOLONE

Ak-Pred
Ak-Tate
Articulose

Codesol
Cortalone
Delta-Cortef
Deltastab
Econopred
Fernisolone-P
Hydeltrasol
Hydeltra-TBA
Inflamase
Key-Pred
Metalone-TBA
Meticortelone
Meti-Derm
Metimyd
Metreton
Nor-Pred-TBA
Nova-Pred
Novaprednisolone
Predaject
Predate
Predcor
Pred Cor-TBA
Pred Forte
Pred Mild
Prednisol TBA
Predulose
Prelone
PSP-IV
Savacort 50 & 100
Sterane

## PROMETHAZINE

Anergan
Baymethazine
Dihydrocodeine Compound
Fellozine
Ganphen
Histantil
Historest
K-Phen
Mallergan
Mepergan Fortis
Phenazine
Phenccn-50
Phenoject-50
Pentazine
Phenameth
Phenergan
Phenerhist
PMS Promethazine
Promet 50
Prometh
Prorex
Prosedin
Prothazine
Provigan
Remsed
V-Gan
ZiPan

## PSEUDOEPHEDRINE

Actifed
Afrinol
Afrinol Repetabs
Ambenyl-D
Anafed
Anamine
Brexin
Bromfed
Bronchobid
Cardec DM

955

Cenafed
Children's Sudafed Liquid
Chlorafed
Chlor-Trimeton
Codimal
Co-Pyronil 2
Cosanyl
Co-Tylenol
Cotrol-D
Decofed
Deconamine
D-Feda
Deproist w/Codeine
Detussin
Dimacol
Disobrom
Disophrol
Dorcol
Dorcol Pediatric Formula
Drixoral
Eltor
Emprazil
Entuss-D
Fedahist
Fedrazil
Guaifed
Halofed
Hista-Clopane
Histalet DM
Histamic
Historal
Isoclor
Kronofed-A Kronocaps
Naldegesic
Neo-Synephrinol Day Relief
Neobid
Neofed
Novafed A
Novahistine DMX
Nucofed
PediaCare
Peedee Dose Decongestant
Phenergan
Phenergan-D
Poly-Histine-DX
Probahist
Pseudo-Hist
Pseudofrin
Redahist Gyrocaps
Respaire-SR
Ro-Fedrin
Robidrine
Robitussin-DAC
Rondec
Sherafed
Sine-Aid Sinus Headache Tablets
Sinufed
Sinufed Timecelles
Sudafed
Sudafed S.A.
Sudagest
Sudahist
Suda-Prol
Sudolin
Sudrin
Triafed
Trifed
Trinalin Repetabs
Triphed
Tripodrine
Tussend

Tylenol Maximum Strength Sinus
    Medicine
Zephrex

## PSYLLIUM

Cillium
Effersyllium
Fiberall
Hydrocil
Konsyl
Konsyl-D
L.A. Formula
Metamucil
Modane Bulk
Mucillium
Mucilose
Naturacil
Perdiem Plain
Plova
Pro-Lax
Prompt
Regacilium
Reguloid
Saraka
Senokot with Psyllium
Serutan
Siblin
Sof-Cil
Syllact
V-Lax

## PYRILAMINE

4-Way Nasal Spray
Albatussin
Allerstat
Allertoc
Citra Forte
Codimal DH, DM, PH
Covanamine
Dormarex
Duphrene
Excedrin P.M.
Fiogesic
Histalet Forte
Kronohist Kronocaps
Midol PMS
Napril Plateau
Nervine Nighttime Sleep-Aid
Panadyl
Poly-Histine D
Primatene, M Formula
P-V-Tussin
Relemine
Ru-Tuss
Rynatan
Sominex
Somnicaps
Triaminic
Trihista-Phen-25
Tussanil

## RADIO-
    PHARMACEUTICALS

Cyanocobalamin Co 57
Cyanocobalamin Co 60
Ferrous Citrate Fe 59
Gallium Citrate Ga 67
Indium In 111 Pentetate
Iodinated I 131 Albumin
Iodohippurate Sodium I 123
Iodohippurate Sodium I 131

Iothalamate Sodium I 125
Krypton Kr 81m
Selenomethionine Se 75
Sodium Chromate Cr 51
Sodium Iodide I 123
Sodium Iodide I 131
Sodium Pertechnetate Tc 99m
Sodium Phosphate P 32
Technetium Tc 99m Albumin
    Aggregated
Technetium Tc 99m Disofenin
Technetium Tc 99m Gluceptate
Technetium Tc 99m Human Serum
    Albumin
Technetium Tc 99m Medronate
Technetium Tc 99m Oxidronate
Technetium Tc 99m Pentetate
Technetium Tc 99m Pyrophosphate
Technetium Tc 99m Succimer
Technetium Tc 99m Sulfur Colloid
Thallous Chloride Tl 201
Xenon Xe 127
Xenon Xe 133

## RAUWOLFIA ALKALOIDS

Alkarau
ALSEROXYLON
Bonapene
Broserpine
Butiserpazide-50 Prestabs
Buytizide-25 Prestabs
Chloroserpine
Demi-Regroton
DESERPIDINE
Diupres
Diutensin-R
Dralserp
Enduronyl
Harmonyl
Harmonyl-D
H-H-R
Hydro-Fluserpine
Hydromox R
Hydropres
Hydroserp
Hydroserpine
Hydrotensin-50
Mallopress
Metatensin
Naquival
Novoreserpine
Oreticyl
Raudixin
Raulfia
Raunormine
Raupoid
Rauraine
Rau-Sed
Rauserpa
Rautrax
Rauverid
Rauwiloid
Rauzide
RAUWOLFIA SERPENTINA
Regroton
Releserp-5
Renese-R
Reserfia
Reserpazide
RESERPINE
Reserpoid

Salutensin
Sandril
Ser-Ap-Es
Serpalan
Serpanray
Serpasil
Serpasil-Apresoline
Serpasil-Esidrix
SK-Reserpine
Serpate
Singoserp-Eisdrix
T-Serp
Unipres
Wolfina

## RAUWOLFIA & THIAZIDE DIURETICS

Demi-Regroton
DESERPIDINE & HYDROCHLOROTHIAZIDE
DESERPIDINE & METHYCLOTHIAZIDE
Diupres
Diutensen-R
Enduronyl
Hydromox-R
Hydropres
Metatensin
Naquival
Oreticyl
Oreticyl Forte
RAUWOLFIA SERPENTINA & BENDROFLUMETHIAZIDE
Rauzide
Regroton
Renese-R
RESERPINE & CHLOROTHIAZIDE
RESERPINE & CHLORTHALIDONE
RESERPINE & HYDROCHLOROTHIAZIDE
RESERPINE & HYDROFLUMETHIAZIDE
RESERPINE & METHYCLOTHIAZIDE
RESERPINE & POLYTHIAZIDE
RESERPINE & QUINETHAZONE
RESERPINE & TRICHLORMETHIAZIDE
Salutensin
Salutensin-Demi
Serpasil-Esidrix

## SALICYLATES

Arcylate
Artha-G
Arthropan
CHOLINE MAGNESIUM SALICYLATES
Choline Magnesium Trisalicylate
CHOLINE SALICYLATE
DIFLUNISAL
Disalcid
Doan's Pills
Durasil
Magan
MAGNESIUM SALICYLATE
Mobidin
SALICYLAMIDE
SALSALATE
SODIUM SALICYLATE
S-60

Uracel
Uromide

## SCOPOLAMINE (HYOSCINE)

Allerspan
Almezyme
Aluscop
Bar-Cy-Amine
Bar-Cy-A-Tab
Barbella
Barbeloid
Barbidonna
Barbidonna-CR
Bar-Don
Belbutal
Belkaloids
Bobid
Brobella-PB
Buren
Cenahist
Chlorpel
Conalsyn
Dallergy
Donnacin
Donnagel
Donnamine
Donnatal
Donnazyme
Drinus
Drize
Eldonal
Eulcin
Extendryl
Haponal
Histaspan-D
Historal
Hyatal
Hybephen
Hydrochol-Plus
Hyonal
Hyonatol
Hytrona
Kinesed
Kleer
Kleer-Tuss
Koryza
Levamine
Maso-Donna
Methnite
MSC Triaminic
Narine
Narspan
Nilspasm
Omnibel
Pamine
Pamine PB
Paraspan
Renalgin
Ru-Tuss
Sanhist
Scoline
Scoline-Amobarbital
Scopolamine Trans-Derm
Scotnord
Sedamine
Sedapar
Sedralex
Seds
Sinaprel
Sinodec

Sinoran
Sinunll
Spabelin
Spasdel
Spasloids
Spasmid
Spasmolin
Spasquid
Spastolate
Symptrol
Transderm
Transderm-Scop
Transderm-V
Triptone
Trisohist
Uriseptin
Urogesic
Vanodonnal
Zemarine

## SULFISOXAZOLE

Apo-Sulfisoxazole
Azo-Gantrisin
Azo-Soxazole
Barazole
Chemovag
Gantrisin
G-Sox
Lipo Gantrisin
Koro-Sulf
Novosoxazole
Pediazole
Rosoxol
SK-Soxazole
Sosol
Soxa
Sulfafurazole
Sulfagen
Sulfizin
Sulfizole
Urisoxin

## TESTOSTERONE & ESTRADIOL

Andrest
Andro-Estro
Andro/Fem
Androgyn L.A.
De-Comberol
Deladumone
Deladumone OB
depAndrogyn
Depo-Testadiol
Depotestogen
Ditate
Ditate DS
Duo-Cyp
Duo-Gen L.A.
Duoval PA
Duratestrin
Estra-Testrin
Menoject-L.A.
Span-Est-Test
Teev
T.E.-Ionate P.A.
Testadiate-Depo
Test-Estra-C
Test-Estro Cypionates
TESTOSTERONE CYPIONATE & ESTRADIOL CYPIONATE

957

## TESTOSTERONE ENANTHATE & ESTRADIOL VALERATE
Testradiol
Valertest

## TETRACYCLINES
Achromycin
Achromycin V
Achrostatin V
Apo-Tetra
Bicycline
Bio-Tetra
Bristacycline
Cefracycline
Centet
Comycin
Cyclopar
Declomycin
DEMECLOCYCLINE
Desamycin
Doxy
Doxy-Caps
Doxychel
DOXYCYCLINE
Doxy-Lemmon
Doxy-Tabs
Fed-Mycin
G-Mycin
Kesso-Tetra
Lemtrex
Maytrex-BID
Medicycline
METHACYCLINE
Minocin
MINOCYCLINE
Muracine
Mysteclin F
Neo-Tetrine
Nor-Tet
Novotetra
Oxlopar
Oxy-Kesso-Tetra
OXYTETRACYCLINE
Paltet
Panmycin
Piracaps
PMS Tetracycline
Q'Dtet
Retet
Retet-S
Robitet
Ro-Cycline
Rondomycin
Sarocyclin
Scotrex
SK-Tetracycline
Sumycin
T-Caps
TETRACYCLINE
Terramycin
Tet-Cy
Tetet
Tetrachel
Tetra-Co
Tetracrine
Tetracyn
Tetracyrine
Tetralean
Tetram
Tetramax
Tetramine
Tetrastatin (M)

Tetrex
Tetrex-S
Topicycline
Trexin
Ultramycin
Urobiotic
Vibramycin
Vibratabs

## TRIAMCINOLONE
Acetospan
Amcort
Aristocort
Aristospan
Articulose-L.A.
Azmacort
Cenocort
Cenocort Forte
Cinalone 40
Cino-40
Cinonide 40
Cremocort
Kenacort
Kenaject
Kenalog
Kenalog in Orabase
Kenalog-E
Kenalone
Ledercort
Lederspan
Mycolog
Myco-Triacet
Mytrex
Nust-Olone
Spencort
Tramacort
Triacet
Triacort
Triaderm
Trialean Acetonide
Triam
Triamcinair
Triamonide
Tri-Kort
Trilog
Trilone
Trimalone
Tristoject
Trymex
Some of these brands are available as topical medicines (ointments, creams or lotions).
See ADRENOCORTICOIDS (TOPICAL), page 16.

## TRICYCLIC ANTIDEPRESSANTS
Adapin
Amitid
Amitril
AMITRYPTILINE
AMOXAPINE
Anafranil
Anemtyl
Apo-Amitriptyline
Apo-Imipramine
Ascendin
Aventyl
CLOMIPRAMINE
DESIPRAMINE
Elavil
Emitrip

Endep
Enovil
Etrafon
IMIPRAMINE
Impril
Janimine
Levate
Meravil
Norpramin
NORTRIPTYLINE
Novopramine
Novotriptyn
Pamelor
Pertofrane
Presamine
PROTRIPTYLINE
Sinequan
SK-Amitriptyline
SK-Pramine
Surmontil
Tipramine
Tofranil
Tofranil-PM
Triadapin
Triavil
TRIMIPRAMINE
Triptil
Vivactil

## VITAMIN B-12 (CYANOCOBALAMIN)
Alphamin
Alpha Redisol
Anocobin
Bedoz
Berubigen
Betalin 12
Betalin 12 Crystalline
Cyanabin
Kaybovite
Kaybovite-1000
Neo-Betalin
Neo-Rubex
Redisol
Rubion
Rubramin
Rubramin-PC
Sytobex
Numerous other multiple vitamin-mineral supplements.

## VITAMIN C (ASCORBIC ACID)
Adenex
Apo-C
Arco-Cee
Ascorbajen
Ascorbicap
Ascoril
Calscorbate
Cecon
Cemill
Cenolate
Ceri-Bid
Cetane
Cevalin
Cevi-Bid
Ce-Vi-Sol
Cevita
C-Ject
Flavorcee

Liqui-Cee
Megascorb
Redoxon
Numerous other multiple
    vitamin-mineral supplements.

## XANTHINE
##   BRONCHODILATORS

Accurbron
Aerolate
Aerophylline
Airet
Amesec
Aminodur
Aminodur Dura-tabs
Aminophyl
Aminophyllin
AMINOPHYLLINE
Aminophylline and Amytal
Aminophylline-Phenobarbital
Amodrine
Amoline
Amophylline
Apo-Oxtriphylline
Aquaphyllin
Asbron
Asma
Asmalix
Asminyl
Asthmophylline
Bronohobid Duracaps
Broncholate
Brondecon
Brondilate
Bronkodyl
Bronkodyl S-R
Bronkolixir
Bronkotabs
Brosema
Choledyl
Choledyl SA
Chophylline
Constant-T
Corophyllin
Corophylline
Co-Xan
Dilin
Dilor
Dilor-G
Droxine
Droxine L.A.
Droxine S.F.
Duovent
Duraphyl
Dyflex
Dylline
DYPHILLINE
Dy-Phyl-Lin
Elixicon
Elixomin
Elixophyllin
Elixophyllin SR
Emfaseem
G-Bron
Iso-Asminyl
Isuprel Compound
Klophyllin
LABID
Lanophyllin
Liquophylline
Lixaminol
Lixaminol AT

Llxolin
Lodrane
Luasmin
Luftodil
Lufyllin
Marax
Marax DF
Mersalyl-Theophylline
Mini-Lix
Mudrane
Neospect
Neothylline
Neothylline-G
Novotriphyl
Numa-Dura-Tabs
Orthoxine & Aminophylline
OXTRIPHYLLINE
Oxystat
Palaron
Phenylin
Phyldrox
Phyllocontin
Physpan
PMS Theophylline
Primatene, M Formula
Primatene, P Formula
Protophylline
Pulmophylline
Quadrinal
Quibron
Quibron Plus
Quibron-T
Quibron-T/SR Dividose
Respbid
Slo-Phyllin GG
Slo-bid Gyrocaps
Slophyllin
Somophyllin
Somophyllin-12
Somophyllin-CRT
Somophyllin-DF
Somophyllin-T
Sudolin
Sustaire
Synophylate-GG
Tedfern
Tedral
T.E.H.
Thalfed
Theobid
Theobid Duracaps
Theobid Jr. Duracaps
Theochron
Theoclear
Theoclear L.A. Cenules
Theo-Dur
Theo-Dur Sprinkle
Theofedral
Theo-Guaia
Theolair
Theolair-Plus
Theolair-SR
Theolixir
Theon
Theo-Nar 100
Theo-Organidin
Theophyl
Theophyl-SR
THEOPHYLLINE
Theophylline Choline
Theospan
Theospan SR

Theostat
Theostate 80
Theotabs
Theo-Time
Theo-24
Theovent Long-acting
Theozine
Truphylline
Uniphyl

# Additional Drug Interactions

The following lists of drugs and their interactions with other drugs are continuations of lists found in the alphabetized drug charts beginning on page 2. These lists are alphabetized by generic name or drug class name, shown in large capital letters. Only those lists too long for the drug charts are included in this section. For complete information about any generic drug, see the alphabetized charts.

| GENERIC NAME OR DRUG CLASS | COMBINED EFFECT | GENERIC NAME OR DRUG CLASS | COMBINED EFFECT |
|---|---|---|---|

## ACETAMINOPHEN & SALICYLATES

| GENERIC NAME OR DRUG CLASS | COMBINED EFFECT | GENERIC NAME OR DRUG CLASS | COMBINED EFFECT |
|---|---|---|---|
| Phenytoin | Increased phenytoin effect. | Sulfinpyrazone | Decreased sulfinpyrazone effect. |
| Probenecid | Decreased probenecid effect. | Tetracyclines (effervescent granules or tablets) | May slow tetracycline absorption. Space doses 2 hours apart. |
| Propranolol | Decreased aspirin effect. | Vancomycin | Hearing loss. |
| Rauwolfia alkaloids | Decreased aspirin effect. | Verapamil | Increased risk of toxicity. |
| Spironolactone | Decreased spironolactone effect. | Vitamin C (large doses) | Possible aspirin toxicity. |

## ASPIRIN

| GENERIC NAME OR DRUG CLASS | COMBINED EFFECT | GENERIC NAME OR DRUG CLASS | COMBINED EFFECT |
|---|---|---|---|
| Spironolactone | Decreased spironolactone effect. | Terfenadine | May conceal symptoms of aspirin overdose, such as ringing in ears. |
| Sulfinpyrazone | Decreased sulfinpyrazone effect. | Vitamin C (large doses) | Possible aspirin toxicity. |
| Suprofen | Increased risk of stomach ulcer. | | |

## ATROPINE, HYOSCYAMINE, METHENAMINE, METHYLENE BLUE, PHENYLSALICYLATE & BENZOIC ACID

| GENERIC NAME OR DRUG CLASS | COMBINED EFFECT | GENERIC NAME OR DRUG CLASS | COMBINED EFFECT |
|---|---|---|---|
| Meperidine | Increased atropine and hyoscyamine effect. | Phenothiazines | Increased atropine and hyoscyamine effect. |
| Methylphenidate | Increased atropine and hyoscyamine effect. | Phenytoin | Increased phenytoin effect. |
| Minoxidil | Decreased minoxidil effect. | Pilocarpine | Loss of pilocarpine effect in glaucoma treatment. |
| Orphenadrine | Increased atropine and hyoscyamine effect. | Potassium supplements | Possible intestinal ulcers with oral potassium tablets. |
| Oxprenolol | Decreased antihypertensive effect of oxprenolol. | Probenecid | Decreased probenecid effect. |
| Para-aminosalicylic acid (PAS) | Possible salicylate toxicity. | Propranolol | Decreased salicylate effect. |
| Penicillins | Increased effect of both drugs. | Rauwolfia alkaloids | Decreased salicylate effect. |
| Phenobarbital | Decreased salicylate effect. | Salicylates (other) | Likely salicylate toxicity. |

| GENERIC NAME OR DRUG CLASS | COMBINED EFFECT | GENERIC NAME OR DRUG CLASS | COMBINED EFFECT |
|---|---|---|---|

## ATROPINE, HYOSCYAMINE, METHENAMINE, METHYLENE BLUE, PHENYLSALICYLATE & BENZOIC ACID continued

| GENERIC NAME OR DRUG CLASS | COMBINED EFFECT | GENERIC NAME OR DRUG CLASS | COMBINED EFFECT |
|---|---|---|---|
| Sodium bicarbonate | Decreased methenamine effect. | Terfenadine | May conceal symptoms of salicylate overdose, such as ringing in ears. |
| Spironolactone | Decreased spironolactone effect. | Vitamin C (1 to 4 grams per day) | Increased effect of methenamine, contributing to urine acidity; decreased atropine effect; possible salicylate toxicity. |
| Sulfa drugs | Possible kidney damage. | | |
| Sulfinpyrazone | Decreased sulfinpyrazone effect. | | |

# BELLADONNA ALKALOIDS & BARBITURATES

| GENERIC NAME OR DRUG CLASS | COMBINED EFFECT | GENERIC NAME OR DRUG CLASS | COMBINED EFFECT |
|---|---|---|---|
| Meperidine | Increased belladonna effect. | Pilocarpine | Loss of pilocarpine effect in glaucoma treatment. |
| Methylphenidate | Increased belladonna effect. | Potassium supplements | Possible intestinal ulcers with oral potassium tablets. |
| Mind-altering drugs | Dangerous sedation. Avoid. | Sedatives | Dangerous sedation. Avoid. |
| Narcotics | Dangerous sedation. Avoid. | Sleep inducers | Dangerous sedation. Avoid. |
| Nitrates | Increased internal-eye pressure. | Tranquilizers | Dangerous sedation. Avoid. |
| Orphenadrine | Increased belladonna effect. | Valproic acid | Increased barbiturate effect. |
| Pain relievers | Dangerous sedation. Avoid. | Vitamin C | Decreased belladonna effect. Avoid large doses of vitamin C. |
| Phenothiazines | Increased belladonna effect. Danger of oversedation. | | |

# BETA-ADRENERGIC BLOCKING AGENTS & THIAZIDE DIURETICS

| GENERIC NAME OR DRUG CLASS | COMBINED EFFECT | GENERIC NAME OR DRUG CLASS | COMBINED EFFECT |
|---|---|---|---|
| Antidiabetics | Increased antidiabetic effect. | Digitalis preparations | Excessive potassium loss that causes dangerous heart rhythms. Can either increase or decrease heart rate. Improves irregular heartbeat. |
| Antihistamines | Decreased antihistamine effect. | Diuretics (thiazide) | Increased effect of other thiazide diuretics. |
| Antihypertensives | Increased antihypertensive effect. | Indapamide | Increased diuretic effect. |
| Anti-inflammatory drugs | Decreased anti-inflammatory effect. | MAO inhibitors | Increased hydrochlorothiazide effect. |
| Barbiturates | Increased barbiturate effect. Dangerous sedation. | Narcotics | Increased narcotic effect. Dangerous sedation. |
| Cholestyramine | Decreased hydrochlorothiazide effect. | | |
| Cortisone drugs | Excessive potassium loss that causes dangerous heart rhythms. | | |

| GENERIC NAME OR DRUG CLASS | COMBINED EFFECT | GENERIC NAME OR DRUG CLASS | COMBINED EFFECT |
|---|---|---|---|

## BETA-ADRENERGIC BLOCKING AGENTS & THIAZIDE DIURETICS continued

| | | | |
|---|---|---|---|
| Nitrates | Excessive blood-pressure drop. | Probenecid | Decreased probenecid effect. |
| Oxprenolol | Increased antihypertensive effect. Dosages of both drugs may require adjustment. | Quinidine | Slows heart excessively. |
| | | Reserpine | Increased reserpine effect. Excessive sedation and depression. |
| Phenytoin | Increased beta-adrenergic effect. | | |
| Potassium supplements | Decreased potassium effect. | Tocainide | May worsen congestive heart failure. |

# BUTALBITAL & ASPIRIN (Also contains caffeine)

| | | | |
|---|---|---|---|
| Anti-inflammatory drugs (non-steroid) | Risk of stomach bleeding and ulcers. | Mind-altering drugs | Dangerous sedation. Avoid. |
| Aspirin (other) | Likely aspirin toxicity. | Minoxidil | Decreased minoxidil effect. |
| Beta-adrenergic blockers | Decreased effect of beta-adrenergic blocker. | Narcotics | Dangerous sedation. Avoid. |
| Contraceptives (oral) | Decreased contraceptive effect. | Pain relievers | Dangerous sedation. Avoid. |
| Cortisone drugs | Increased cortisone effect. Risk of ulcer and stomach bleeding. | Salicylates (others) | Likely aspirin toxicity. |
| | | Sedatives | Dangerous sedation. Avoid. |
| Digitoxin | Decreased digitoxin effect. | Sleep inducers | Dangerous sedation. Avoid. |
| Doxycycline | Decreased doxycycline effect. | Spironolactone | Decreased spironolactone effect. |
| Dronabinol | Increased effect of both drugs. | Sulfinpyrazone | Decreased sulfinpyrazone effect. |
| Furosemide | Possible aspirin toxicity. | | |
| Gold compounds | Increased likelihood of kidney damage. | Terfenadine | May conceal symptoms of aspirin overdose, such as ringing in ears. |
| Griseofulvin | Decreased griseofulvin effect. | | |
| Indapamide | Increased indapamide effect. | Tranquilizers | Dangerous sedation. Avoid. |
| Indomethacin | Risk of stomach bleeding and ulcers. | Valproic acid | Increased butalbital effect. |
| MAO inhibitors | Increased butalbital effect. | Vitamin C (large doses) | Possible aspirin toxicity. |
| Methotrexate | Increased methotrexate effect. | | |

# BUTALBITAL, ASPIRIN & CODEINE (Also contains caffeine)

| | | | |
|---|---|---|---|
| Antidepressants | Decreased antidepressant effect. Possible dangerous oversedation. | Antidiabetics (oral) | Increased butalbital effect. Low blood sugar. |
| | | Antihistamines | Dangerous sedation. Avoid. |

| GENERIC NAME OR DRUG CLASS | COMBINED EFFECT | GENERIC NAME OR DRUG CLASS | COMBINED EFFECT |
|---|---|---|---|

## BUTALBITAL & ASPIRIN (Also contains caffeine) continued

| GENERIC NAME OR DRUG CLASS | COMBINED EFFECT | GENERIC NAME OR DRUG CLASS | COMBINED EFFECT |
|---|---|---|---|
| Anti-inflammatory drugs (non-steroid) | Risk of stomach bleeding and ulcers. | Pain relievers | Dangerous sedation. Avoid. |
| Aspirin (other) | Likely aspirin toxicity. | Para-aminosalicylic acid (PAS) | Possible aspirin toxicity. |
| Beta-adrenergic blockers | Decreased effect of beta-adrenergic blocker. | Penicillins | Increased effect of drugs. |
| Contraceptives (oral) | Decreased contraceptive effect. | Phenobarbital | Decreased aspirin effect. |
| Cortisone drugs | Increased cortisone effect. Risk of ulcer and stomach bleeding. | Phenothiazines | Increased phenothiazine effect. |
| Digitoxin | Decreased digitoxin effect. | Phenytoin | Increased phenytoin effect. |
| Doxycycline | Decreased doxycycline effect. | Probenecid | Decreased probenecid effect. |
| Dronabinol | Increased effect of drugs. | Propranolol | Decreased aspirin effect. |
| Furosemide | Possible aspirin toxicity. | Rauwolfia alkaloids | Decreased aspirin effect. |
| Gold compounds | Increased likelihood of kidney damage. | Salicylates (others) | Likely aspirin toxicity. |
| Griseofulvin | Decreased griseofulvin effect. | Sedatives | Dangerous sedation. Avoid. |
| Indapamide | Increased indapamide effect. | Sleep inducers | Dangerous sedation. Avoid. |
| Indomethacin | Risk of stomach bleeding and ulcers. | Spironolactone | Decreased spironolactone effect. |
| MAO inhibitors | Increased butalbital effect. | Sulfinpyrazone | Decreased sulfinpyrazone effect. |
| Methotrexate | Increased methotrexate effect. | Terfenadine | May conceal symptoms of aspirin overdose, such as ringing in ears. |
| Mind-altering drugs | Dangerous sedation. Avoid. | Tranquilizers | Dangerous sedation. Avoid. |
| Minoxidil | Decreased minoxidil effect. | Valproic acid | Increased phenobarbital effect. |
| Narcotics | Dangerous sedation. Avoid. | Vitamin C (large doses) | Possible aspirin toxicity. |
| Nitrates | Excessive blood-pressure drop. | | |

# CAPTOPRIL & HYDROCHLOROTHIAZIDE

| GENERIC NAME OR DRUG CLASS | COMBINED EFFECT | GENERIC NAME OR DRUG CLASS | COMBINED EFFECT |
|---|---|---|---|
| Nitrates | Excessive blood-pressure drop. | Potassium supplements | Excessive potassium in blood. |
| Oxprenolol | Increased antihypertensive effect. Dosages of both drugs may require adjustments. | Probenecid | Decreased probenecid effect. |
| | | Spironolactone | Possible excessive potassium in blood. |
| | | Triamterene | Possible excessive potassium in blood. |

## CHLORDIAZEPOXIDE & AMITRIPTYLINE

| | | | |
| --- | --- | --- | --- |
| **Thyroid hormones** | Irregular heartbeat. | **Tranquilizers** | Increased sedative effect of both drugs. |

## CHLORDIAZEPOXIDE & CLIDINIUM

| | | | |
| --- | --- | --- | --- |
| **Pilocarpine** | Loss of pilocarpine effect in glaucoma treatment. | **Sleep inducers** | Increased sedative effect of both drugs. |
| **Potassium supplements** | Possible intestinal ulcers with oral potassium tablets. | **Tranquilizers** | Increased sedative effect of both drugs. |
| **Sedatives** | Increased sedative effect of both drugs. | **Vitamin C** | Decreased clidinium effect. Avoid large doses of vitamin C. |

## CLONIDINE & CHLORTHALIDONE

| | | | |
| --- | --- | --- | --- |
| **Digitalis preparations** | Excessive potassium loss that causes dangerous heart rhythms. | **MAO inhibitors** | Increased chlorthalidone effect. |
| **Diuretics** | Excessive blood-pressure drop. | **Nitrates** | Possible excessive blood-pressure drop. |
| **Fenfluramine** | Possible increased clonidine effect. | **Oxprenolol** | Increased antihypertensive effect. Dosages of both drugs may require adjustments. |
| **Indapamide** | Increased diuretic effect. | **Potassium supplements** | Decreased potassium effect. |
| **Lithium** | Increased effect of lithium. | **Probenecid** | Decreased probenecid effect. |

## CORTISONE

| | | | |
| --- | --- | --- | --- |
| **Suprofen** | Increased risk of stomach ulcer and bleeding. | **Sympathomimetics** | Possible glaucoma. |

## DEXAMETHASONE

| | | | |
| --- | --- | --- | --- |
| **Rifampin** | Decreased dexamethasone effect. | **Sympathomimetics** | Possible glaucoma. |

## ENALAPRIL & HYDROCHLOROTHIAZIDE

| | | | |
| --- | --- | --- | --- |
| **Potassium supplements** | Excessive potassium in blood. | **Spironolactone** | Possible excessive potassium in blood. |
| **Probenecid** | Decreased probenecid effect. | **Triamterene** | Possible excessive potassium in blood. |

## ERGOTAMINE, BELLADONNA & PHENOBARBITAL

| | | | |
| --- | --- | --- | --- |
| **Contraceptives (oral)** | Decreased contraceptive effect. | **Cortisone drugs** | Decreased cortisone effect. Increased internal-eye pressure. |

ADDITIONAL DRUG INTERACTIONS

| GENERIC NAME OR DRUG CLASS | COMBINED EFFECT | GENERIC NAME OR DRUG CLASS | COMBINED EFFECT |
|---|---|---|---|

## ERGOTAMINE, BELLADONNA & PHENOBARBITAL continued

| GENERIC NAME OR DRUG CLASS | COMBINED EFFECT | GENERIC NAME OR DRUG CLASS | COMBINED EFFECT |
|---|---|---|---|
| Digitoxin | Decreased digitoxin effect. | Nitrates | Increased internal-eye pressure. |
| Doxycycline | Decreased doxycycline effect. | Orphenadrine | Increased belladonna effect. |
| Dronabinol | Increased effect of drugs. | Pain relievers | Dangerous sedation. Avoid. |
| Ephedrine | Dangerous blood-pressure rise. | Phenothiazines | Increased belladonna effect. |
| Epinephrine | Dangerous blood-pressure rise. | Pilocarpine | Loss of pilocarpine effect in glaucoma treatment. |
| Griseofulvin | Decreased griseofulvin effect. | Potassium supplements | Possible intestinal ulcers with oral potassium tablets. |
| Haloperidol | Increased internal-eye pressure. | | |
| Indapamide | Increased indapamide effect. | Sedatives | Dangerous sedation. Avoid. |
| MAO inhibitors | Increased belladonna and phenobarbital effect. | Sleep inducers | Dangerous sedation. Avoid. |
| | | Tranquilizers | Dangerous sedation. Avoid. |
| Meperidine | Increased belladonna effect. | Troleandomycin | Increased adverse reactions of ergotamine. |
| Methylphenidate | Increased belladonna effect. | Valproic acid | Increased phenobarbital effect. |
| Mind-altering drugs | Dangerous sedation. Avoid. | Vitamin C | Decreased belladonna effect. Avoid large doses of vitamin C. |
| Narcotics | Dangerous sedation. Avoid. | | |

# ERGOTAMINE, CAFFEINE, BELLADONNA & PENTOBARBITAL

| GENERIC NAME OR DRUG CLASS | COMBINED EFFECT | GENERIC NAME OR DRUG CLASS | COMBINED EFFECT |
|---|---|---|---|
| Anticoagulants (oral) | Decreased anticoagulant effect. | Beta-adrenergic blockers | Decreased effect of beta-adrenergic blocker. |
| Anticonvulsants | Changed seizure patterns. | Contraceptives (oral) | Decreased contraceptive effect. |
| Antidepressants (tricyclics) | Decreased antidepressant effect. Possible dangerous oversedation. | Cortisone drugs | Decreased cortisone effect. Increased internal-eye pressure. |
| Antidiabetics (oral) | Increased pentobarbital effect. | Digitoxin | Decreased digitoxin effect. |
| Antihistamines | Dangerous sedation. Avoid. | Doxycycline | Decreased doxycycline effect. |
| Anti-inflammatory drugs (non-steroidal) | Decreased anti-inflammatory effect. | Dronabinol | Increased effect of drugs. |
| | | Ephedrine | Dangerous blood-pressure rise. |
| Aspirin | Decreased aspirin effect. | Epinephrine | Dangerous blood-pressure rise. |

## ERGOTAMINE, CAFFEINE, BELLADONNA & PENTOBARBITAL continued

| GENERIC NAME OR DRUG CLASS | COMBINED EFFECT | GENERIC NAME OR DRUG CLASS | COMBINED EFFECT |
|---|---|---|---|
| Griseofulvin | Decreased griseofulvin effect. | Phenothiazines | Increased belladonna effect. |
| Haloperidol | Increased internal-eye pressure. | Pilocarpine | Loss of pilocarpine effect in glaucoma treatment. |
| Indapamide | Increased indapamide effect. | Potassium supplements | Possible intestinal ulcers with oral potassium tablets. |
| Isoniazid | Increased caffeine effect. | | |
| MAO inhibitors | Increased belladonna effect, dangerous blood-pressure rise. | Sedatives | Dangerous sedation. Avoid. |
| | | Sleep inducers | Dangerous sedation. Avoid. |
| Meperidine | Increased belladonna effect. | Sympathomimetics | Overstimulation, blood-pressure rise. |
| Methylphenidate | Increased belladonna effect. | Thyroid hormones | Increased thyroid effect. |
| Mind-altering drugs | Dangerous sedation. Avoid. | Tranquilizers | Dangerous sedation. Avoid. |
| Narcotics | Dangerous sedation. Avoid. | Troleandomycin | Increased adverse reactions of ergotamine. |
| Nitrates | Increased internal-eye pressure. | Valproic acid | Increased pentobarbital effect. |
| Orphenadrine | Increased belladonna effect. | Vitamin C | Decreased belladonna effect. Avoid large doses of vitamin C. |
| Pain relievers | Dangerous sedation. Avoid. | | |

# GUANETHIDINE & HYDROCHLOROTHIAZIDE

| GENERIC NAME OR DRUG CLASS | COMBINED EFFECT | GENERIC NAME OR DRUG CLASS | COMBINED EFFECT |
|---|---|---|---|
| Indapamide | Possible increased effects of both drugs. When monitored carefully, combination may be beneficial in controlling hypertension. | Nitrates | Excessive blood-pressure drop. |
| | | Oxprenolol | Increased antihypertensive effect. Dosages of both drugs may require adjustments. |
| Lithium | Increased lithium effect. | Potassium supplements | Decreased potassium effect. |
| MAO inhibitors | Increased hydrochlorothiazide effect. | Probenecid | Decreased probenecid effect. |
| Minoxidil | Dosage adjustments may be necessary to keep blood pressure at proper level. | | |

# HYDRALAZINE & HYDROCHLOROTHIAZIDE

| GENERIC NAME OR DRUG CLASS | COMBINED EFFECT | GENERIC NAME OR DRUG CLASS | COMBINED EFFECT |
|---|---|---|---|
| Lithium | Increased effect of lithium. | Oxprenolol | Increased antihypertensive effect. Dosages of both drugs may require adjustments. |
| MAO inhibitors | Increased effect of drugs. | | |
| Nitrates | Excessive blood-pressure drop. | | |

ADDITIONAL DRUG INTERACTIONS

967

| GENERIC NAME OR DRUG CLASS | COMBINED EFFECT | GENERIC NAME OR DRUG CLASS | COMBINED EFFECT |
|---|---|---|---|

## HYDRALAZINE & HYDROCHLOROTHIAZIDE continued

| | | | |
|---|---|---|---|
| Potassium supplements | Decreased potassium effect. | Probenecid | Decreased probenecid effect. |

# KAOLIN, PECTIN, BELLADONNA & OPIUM

| | | | |
|---|---|---|---|
| Mind-altering drugs | Increased sedative effect. | Potassium supplements | Possible intestinal ulcers with oral potassium tablets. |
| Narcotics (other) | Increased narcotic effect. | Sedatives | Excessive sedation. |
| Nitrates | Increased internal-eye pressure. | Sleep inducers | Increased effect of sleep inducers. |
| Orphenadrine | Increased belladonna effect. | Tranquilizers | Increased tranquilizer effect. |
| Phenothiazines | Increased sedative effect of paregoric. | Vitamin C | Decreased belladonna effect. Avoid large doses of vitamin C. |
| Pilocarpine | Loss of pilocarpine effect in glaucoma treatment. | All other oral medicines | Decreases absorption of other medicines. Separate doses by at least 2 hours. |

# MEPROBAMATE & ASPIRIN

| | | | |
|---|---|---|---|
| Para-aminosalicylic acid (PAS) | Possible aspirin toxicity. | Sleep inducers | Increased effect of sleep inducer. |
| Penicillins | Increased effect of both drugs. | Spironolactone | Decreased spironolactone effect. |
| Phenobarbital | Decreased aspirin effect. | Sulfinpyrazone | Decreased sulfinpyrazone effect. |
| Phenytoin | Increased phenytoin effect. | Terfenadine | Possible excessive sedation. May conceal symptoms of aspirin overdose, such as ringing in ears. |
| Probenecid | Decreased probenecid effect. | | |
| Propranolol | Decreased aspirin effect. | Tranquilizers | Increased tranquilizer effect. |
| Rauwolfia alkaloids | Decreased aspirin effect. | Vitamin C (large doses) | Possible aspirin toxicity. |
| Salicylates (other) | Likely aspirin toxicity. | | |
| Sedatives | Increased sedative effect. | | |

# METHYLDOPA & THIAZIDE DIURETICS

| | | | |
|---|---|---|---|
| MAO inhibitors | Dangerous blood-pressure changes. | Oxprenolol | Increased antihypertensive effect. Dosages of both drugs may require adjustments. |
| Nitrates | Excessive blood-pressure drop. | | |
| | | Potassium supplements | Decreased potassium effect. |

# METHYLPREDNISOLONE

| GENERIC NAME OR DRUG CLASS | COMBINED EFFECT | GENERIC NAME OR DRUG CLASS | COMBINED EFFECT |
| --- | --- | --- | --- |
| Potassium supplements | Decreased potassium effect. | Rifampin | Decreased methylprednisolone effect. |
| | | Sympathomimetics | Possible glaucoma. |

# NARCOTIC & ASPIRIN

| GENERIC NAME OR DRUG CLASS | COMBINED EFFECT | GENERIC NAME OR DRUG CLASS | COMBINED EFFECT |
| --- | --- | --- | --- |
| Phenobarbital | Decreased aspirin effect. | Spironolactone | Decreased spironolactone effect. |
| Phenytoin | Increased phenytoin effect. | Sulfinpyrazone | Decreased sulfinpyrazone effect. |
| Probenecid | Decreased probenecid effect. | Terfenadine | Possible excessive sedation. May conceal symptoms of aspirin overdose, such as ringing in ears. |
| Propranolol | Decreased aspirin effect. | | |
| Rauwolfia alkaloids | Decreased aspirin effect. | Tranquilizers | Increased sedative effect. |
| Salicylates (other) | Likely aspirin toxicity. | Vitamin C (large doses) | Possible aspirin toxicity. |
| Sedatives | Increased sedative effect. | | |
| Sleep inducers | Increased sedative effect. sleep inducer. | | |

# ORPHENADRINE, ASPIRIN & CAFFEINE

| GENERIC NAME OR DRUG CLASS | COMBINED EFFECT | GENERIC NAME OR DRUG CLASS | COMBINED EFFECT |
| --- | --- | --- | --- |
| Antidepressants (tricyclic) | Increased sedation. | Levodopa | Increased effect of levodopa. (Improves effectiveness in treating Parkinson's disease.) |
| Antidiabetics (oral) | Low blood sugar. | | |
| Anti-inflammatory drugs (non-steroid) | Risk of stomach bleeding and ulcers. | MAO inhibitors | Dangerous blood-pressure rise. |
| Aspirin (other) | Likely aspirin toxicity. | Methotrexate | Increased methotrexate effect. |
| Chlorpromazine | Hypoglycemia (low blood sugar). | Minoxidil | Decreased minoxidil effect. |
| Contraceptives (oral) | Increased caffeine effect. | Nitrates | Increased internal-eye pressure. |
| Cortisone drugs | Increased cortisone effect. Risk of ulcers and stomach bleeding. | Oxprenolol | Decreased antihypertensive effect of oxprenolol. |
| Furosemide | Possible aspirin toxicity. | Para-aminosalicylic acid (PAS) | Possible aspirin toxicity. |
| Gold compounds | Increased likelihood of kidney damage. | Penicillins | Increased effect of drugs. |
| Griseofulvin | Decreased griseofulvin effect. | Phenobarbital | Decreased aspirin effect. |
| Indomethacin | Risk of stomach bleeding and ulcers. | Potassium supplements | Increased possibility of intestinal ulcers with oral potassium tablets. |
| Isoniazid | Increased caffeine effect. | | |

| GENERIC NAME OR DRUG CLASS | COMBINED EFFECT | GENERIC NAME OR DRUG CLASS | COMBINED EFFECT |
|---|---|---|---|

## ORPHENADRINE, ASPIRIN & CAFFEINE continued

| GENERIC NAME OR DRUG CLASS | COMBINED EFFECT | GENERIC NAME OR DRUG CLASS | COMBINED EFFECT |
|---|---|---|---|
| Probenecid | Decreased probenecid effect. | Sulfinpyrazone | Decreased sulfinpyrazone effect. |
| Propoxyphene | Possible confusion, nervousness, tremors. | Sympathomimetics | Overstimulation. |
| Propranolol | Decreased aspirin effect. | Terfenadine | May conceal symptoms of aspirin overdose, such as ringing in ears. Possible increased orphenadrine effect. |
| Rauwolfia alkaloids | Decreased aspirin effect. | | |
| Salicylates (other) | Likely aspirin toxicity. | Thyroid hormones | Increased thyroid effect. |
| Sedatives | Decreased sedative effect. | Tranquilizers | Decreased tranquilizer effect. |
| Sleep inducers | Decreased sedative effect. | Vitamin C (large doses) | Possible aspirin toxicity. |
| Spironolactone | Decreased spironolactone effect. | | |

## PANCREATIN, PEPSIN, BILE SALTS, HYOSCYAMINE, ATROPINE, SCOPOLAMINE & PHENOBARBITAL

| GENERIC NAME OR DRUG CLASS | COMBINED EFFECT | GENERIC NAME OR DRUG CLASS | COMBINED EFFECT |
|---|---|---|---|
| Indapamide | Increased indapamide effect. | Pilocarpine | Loss of pilocarpine effect in glaucoma treatment. |
| MAO inhibitors | Increased atropine effect. | Potassium supplements | Possible intestinal ulcers with oral potassium tablets. |
| Meperidine | Increased atropine effect. | | |
| Methylphenidate | Increased atropine effect. | Sedatives | Dangerous sedation. Avoid. |
| Mind-altering drugs | Dangerous sedation. Avoid. | Sleep inducers | Dangerous sedation. Avoid. |
| Narcotics | Dangerous sedation. Avoid. | Tranquilizers | Dangerous sedation. Avoid. |
| Nitrates | Increased internal-eye pressure. | Valproic acid | Increased phenobarbital effect. |
| Orphenadrine | Increased atropine effect. | Vitamin C | Decreased atropine effect. Avoid large doses of vitamin C. |
| Phenothiazines | Increased atropine effect. | | |

## PARGYLINE & METHYCLOTHIAZIDE

| GENERIC NAME OR DRUG CLASS | COMBINED EFFECT | GENERIC NAME OR DRUG CLASS | COMBINED EFFECT |
|---|---|---|---|
| Antihypertensives | Excessively low blood pressure. | Cortisone drugs | Excessive potassium loss that causes dangerous heart rhythms. |
| Barbiturates | Increased methyclothiazide effect. | | |
| Caffeine | Irregular heartbeat or high blood pressure. | Cyclobenzaprine | Fever, seizures. Avoid. |
| Carbamazepine | Fever, seizures. Avoid. | Digitalis preparations | Excessive potassium loss that causes dangerous heart rhythms. |
| Cholestyramine | Decreased methyclothiazide effect. | | |

## PARGYLINE & METHYCLOTHIAZIDE continued

| GENERIC NAME OR DRUG CLASS | COMBINED EFFECT | GENERIC NAME OR DRUG CLASS | COMBINED EFFECT |
|---|---|---|---|
| Diuretics (other) | Excessively low blood pressure. | Nitrates | Excessive blood-pressure drop. |
| Guanethidine | Blood-pressure rise to life-threatening level. | Oxprenolol | Possible blood-pressure rise if MAO inhibitor is discontinued after simultaneous use with oxprenolol. |
| Indapamide | Increased indapamide and diuretic effect. | | |
| Levodopa | Sudden, severe blood-pressure rise. | Potassium supplements | Decreased potassium effect. |
| Lithium | Increased effect of lithium. | Probenecid | Decreased probenecid effect. |
| MAO inhibitors (other, when taken together) | High fever, convulsions, death. Increased methyclothiazide effect. | Terfenadine | Increased side effects of MAO inhibitors. |

# PERPHENAZINE & AMITRIPTYLINE

| GENERIC NAME OR DRUG CLASS | COMBINED EFFECT | GENERIC NAME OR DRUG CLASS | COMBINED EFFECT |
|---|---|---|---|
| Guanethidine | Decreased guanethidine effect. | Quinidine | Impaired heart function. Dangerous mixture. |
| Levodopa | Decreased levodopa effect. | Sedatives | Dangerous oversedation. |
| MAO inhibitors | Fever, delirium, convulsions. | Sympathomimetics | Increased sympathomimetics effect. |
| Methyldopa | Decreased methyldopa effect. | Thyroid hormones | Irregular heartbeat. |
| Mind-altering drugs | Increased effect of mind-altering drugs. | Tranquilizers (other) | Increased tranquilizer effect. |
| Narcotics | Increased narcotic effect and dangerous sedation. | | |

# PHENPROCOUMON

| GENERIC NAME OR DRUG CLASS | COMBINED EFFECT | GENERIC NAME OR DRUG CLASS | COMBINED EFFECT |
|---|---|---|---|
| Chloramphenicol | Increased phenprocoumon effect. | Digitalis preparations | Decreased phenprocoumon effect. |
| Chlorpromazine | Decreased phenprocoumon effect. | Disulfiram | Increased phenprocoumon effect. |
| Cholestyramine | Unpredictable increased or decreased phenprocoumon effect. | Estrogens | Decreased phenprocoumon effect. |
| | | Ethacrynic acid | Increased phenprocoumon effect. |
| Cimetidine | Increased phenprocoumon effect. | Ethchlorvynol | Decreased phenprocoumon effect. |
| Clofibrate | Unpredictable increased or decreased phenprocoumon effect. | Furosemide | Decreased phenprocoumon effect. |
| Contraceptives (oral) | Unpredictable increased or decreased phenprocoumon effect. | Glucagon | Increased phenprocoumon effect. |
| | | Glutethimide | Decreased phenprocoumon effect. |
| Cortisone drugs | Unpredictable increased or decreased phenprocoumon effect. | Griseofulvin | Decreased phenprocoumon effect. |

ADDITIONAL DRUG INTERACTIONS

| GENERIC NAME OR DRUG CLASS | COMBINED EFFECT | GENERIC NAME OR DRUG CLASS | COMBINED EFFECT |
|---|---|---|---|

## PHENPROCOUMON continued

| GENERIC NAME OR DRUG CLASS | COMBINED EFFECT | GENERIC NAME OR DRUG CLASS | COMBINED EFFECT |
|---|---|---|---|
| Guanethidine | Increased phenprocoumon effect. | Phenylbutazone | Unpredictable increased or decreased phenprocoumon effect. |
| Haloperidol | Decreased phenprocoumon effect. | Phenylpropanolamine | Decreased anticoagulant effect. |
| Hydroxyzine | Increased phenprocoumon effect. | Phenyramidol | Increased phenprocoumon effect. |
| Indomethacin | Increased phenprocoumon effect. | Probenecid | Increased phenprocoumon effect. |
| Insulin | Increased insulin effect. | Propoxyphene | Increased phenprocoumon effect. |
| Isocarboxazid | Increased phenprocoumon effect. | Propylthiouracil | Increased phenprocoumon effect. |
| Isoniazid | Increased phenprocoumon effect. | Quinidine | Increased phenprocoumon effect. |
| Mefenamic acid | Increased phenprocoumon effect. | Rauwolfia alkaloids | Unpredictable increased or decreased phenprocoumon effect. |
| Meprobamate | Decreased phenprocoumon effect. | Salicylates (including aspirin) | Increased phenprocoumon effect. |
| Mercaptopurine | Increased phenprocoumon effect. | Sulfa drugs | Increased phenprocoumon effect. |
| Methyldopa | Increased phenprocoumon effect. | Sulfinpyrazone | Increased phenprocoumon effect. |
| Methylphenidate | Increased phenprocoumon effect. | Tetracyclines | Increased phenprocoumon effect. |
| Metronidazole | Increased phenprocoumon effect. | Thyroid hormones | Increased phenprocoumon effect. |
| Nalidixic acid | Increased phenprocoumon effect. | Trimethoprim | Increased phenprocoumon effect. |
| Nortriptyline | Increased phenprocoumon effect. | Vitamin C (large doses) | Decreased phenprocoumon effect. |
| Oxyphenbutazone | Increased phenprocoumon effect. | Vitamin E (large doses) | Increased phenprocoumon effect. |
| Para-aminosalicylic acid (PAS) | Increased phenprocoumon effect. | | |
| Phenelzine | Increased phenprocoumon effect. | | |

# PHENYTOIN

| GENERIC NAME OR DRUG CLASS | COMBINED EFFECT | GENERIC NAME OR DRUG CLASS | COMBINED EFFECT |
|---|---|---|---|
| Gold compounds | Increased phenytoin blood levels. Phenytoin dose may require adjustment. | Methotrexate | Increased methotrexate effect. |
| Griseofulvin | Increased griseofulvin effect. | Methylphenidate | Increased phenytoin effect. |
| Isoniazid | Increased phenytoin effect. | Molindone | Increased phenytoin effect. |
| MAO inhibitors | Increased polythiazide effect. | Nitrates | Excessive blood-pressure drop. |
| Methadone | Decreased methadone effect. | Oxyphenbutazone | Increased phenytoin effect. |

| GENERIC NAME OR DRUG CLASS | COMBINED EFFECT | GENERIC NAME OR DRUG CLASS | COMBINED EFFECT |
|---|---|---|---|

## PHENYTOIN continued

| GENERIC NAME OR DRUG CLASS | COMBINED EFFECT | GENERIC NAME OR DRUG CLASS | COMBINED EFFECT |
|---|---|---|---|
| Oxprenolol | Increased antihypertensive effect. Dosages of both drugs may require adjustments. | Probenecid | Decreased probenecid effect. |
| | | Propranolol | Increased propranolol effect. |
| Para-aminosalicylic acid (PAS) | Increased phenytoin effect. | Quinidine | Increased quinidine effect. |
| Phenothiazines | Increased phenytoin effect. | Sedatives | Increased sedative effect. |
| Phenylbutazone | Increased phenytoin effect. | Sulfa drugs | Increased phenytoin effect. |
| Potassium supplements | Decreased potassium effect. | Theophylline | Reduced anticonvulsant effect. |

## PRAZOSIN & POLYTHIAZIDE

| GENERIC NAME OR DRUG CLASS | COMBINED EFFECT | GENERIC NAME OR DRUG CLASS | COMBINED EFFECT |
|---|---|---|---|
| Cholestyramine | Decreased polythiazide effect. | Lithium | Increased effect of lithium. |
| Chlorpromazine | Acute agitation. | MAO inhibitors | Blood-pressure drop. Increased polythiazide effect. |
| Cortisone drugs | Excessive potassium loss that causes dangerous heart rhythms. | Nitrates | Possible excessive blood-pressure drop. |
| Digitalis preparations | Excessive potassium loss that causes dangerous heart rhythms. | Oxprenolol | Increased antihypertensive effect. Dosages may require adjustments. |
| Diuretics (other) | Increased effect of other thiazide diuretics. | Potassium | Decreased potassium effect. |
| Indapamide | Increased diuretic effect. | Probenecid | Decreased probenecid effect. |

## PREDNISONE

| GENERIC NAME OR DRUG CLASS | COMBINED EFFECT | GENERIC NAME OR DRUG CLASS | COMBINED EFFECT |
|---|---|---|---|
| Ethacrynic acid | Potassium depletion. | Isoniazid | Decreased isoniazid effect. |
| Furosemide | Potassium depletion. | | |
| Glutethimide | Decreased prednisone effect. | Oxyphenbutazone | Possible ulcers. |
| | | Phenylbutazone | Possible ulcers. |
| Indapamide | Possible excessive potassium loss, causing dangerous heartbeat irregularity. | Potassium supplements | Decreased potassium effect. |
| | | Rifampin | Decreased prednisone effect. |
| Indomethacin | Increased prednisone effect. | Sympathomimetics | Possible glaucoma. |
| Insulin | Decreased insulin effect. | | |

| GENERIC NAME OR DRUG CLASS | COMBINED EFFECT | GENERIC NAME OR DRUG CLASS | COMBINED EFFECT |
|---|---|---|---|

# PROBENECID & COLCHICINE

| GENERIC NAME OR DRUG CLASS | COMBINED EFFECT | GENERIC NAME OR DRUG CLASS | COMBINED EFFECT |
|---|---|---|---|
| Pyrazinamide | Decreased probenecid effect. | Sleep inducers | Oversedation. |
| Salicylates | Decreased probenecid effect. | Sulfa drugs | Slows elimination. May cause harmful accumulation of sulfa. |
| Sedatives | Oversedation. | Tranquilizers | Oversedation. |

# PROCHLORPERAZINE & ISOPROPAMIDE

| GENERIC NAME OR DRUG CLASS | COMBINED EFFECT | GENERIC NAME OR DRUG CLASS | COMBINED EFFECT |
|---|---|---|---|
| Nitrates | Increased internal-eye pressure. | supplements | ulcers with oral potassium tablets. |
| Orphenadrine | Increased isopropamide effect. | Quinidine | Impaired heart function. Dangerous mixture. |
| Phenothiazines | Increased isopropamide effect. | Sedatives | Increased sedative effect. |
| Phenytoin | Increased phenytoin effect. | Tranquilizers (other) | Increased tranquilizer effect. |
| Pilocarpine | Loss of pilocarpine effect in glaucoma treatment. | Vitamin C | Decreased isopropamide effect. Avoid large doses of vitamin C. |

# PYRILAMINE & PENTOBARBITAL

| GENERIC NAME OR DRUG CLASS | COMBINED EFFECT | GENERIC NAME OR DRUG CLASS | COMBINED EFFECT |
|---|---|---|---|
| Griseofulvin | Decreased griseofulvin effect. | Pain relievers | Dangerous sedation. Avoid. |
| Hypnotics | Excess sedation. Avoid. | Sedatives | Dangerous sedation. Avoid. |
| Indapamide | Increased indapamide effect. | Sleep inducers | Dangerous sedation. Avoid. |
| MAO inhibitors | Increased pentobarbital effect. Avoid mixture. May be toxic. | Tranquilizers | Dangerous sedation. Avoid. |
| Mind-altering drugs | Dangerous sedation. Avoid. | Valproic acid | Dangerous sedation. Avoid. |
| Narcotics | Dangerous sedation. Avoid. | | |

# RAUWOLFIA & THIAZIDE DIURETICS

| GENERIC NAME OR DRUG CLASS | COMBINED EFFECT | GENERIC NAME OR DRUG CLASS | COMBINED EFFECT |
|---|---|---|---|
| Beta-adrenergic blockers | Increased effect of rauwolfia alkaloids. Excessive sedation. | Digitalis preparations | Excessive potassium loss that causes dangerous heart rhythms. |
| Cholestyramine | Decreased hydrocholorthiazide effect. | Diuretics (thiazide) | Increased effect of other thiazide diuretics. |
| Cortisone drugs | Excessive potassium loss that causes dangerous heart rhythms. | Dronabinol | Increased effect of both drugs. Avoid. |
| | | Indapamide | Increased diuretic effect. |
| | | Levodopa | Decreased levodopa effect. |

| GENERIC NAME OR DRUG CLASS | COMBINED EFFECT | GENERIC NAME OR DRUG CLASS | COMBINED EFFECT |
|---|---|---|---|

## RAUWOLFIA & THIAZIDE DIURETICS continued

| GENERIC NAME OR DRUG CLASS | COMBINED EFFECT | GENERIC NAME OR DRUG CLASS | COMBINED EFFECT |
|---|---|---|---|
| Lithium | Increased effect of lithium. | Oxprenolol | Increased antihypertensive effect. Dosages of both drugs may require adjustments. |
| MAO inhibitors | Increased hydrochlorothiazide effect. Severe depression. | | |
| | | Potassium supplements | Decreased potassium effect. |
| Mind-altering drugs | Excessive sedation. | Probenecid | Decreased probenecid effect. |
| Nitrates | Excessive blood-pressure drop. | | |

# RESERPINE & HYDRALAZINE

| GENERIC NAME OR DRUG CLASS | COMBINED EFFECT | GENERIC NAME OR DRUG CLASS | COMBINED EFFECT |
|---|---|---|---|
| Aspirin | Decreased aspirin effect. | Dronabinol | Increased effect of both drugs. Avoid. |
| Beta-adrenergic blockers | Increased effect of rauwolfia alkaloids. Excessive sedation. | Levodopa | Decreased levodopa effect. |
| | | MAO inhibitors | Severe depression. |
| Digitalis preparations | Irregular heartbeat. | Mind-altering drugs | Excessive sedation. |
| Diuretics (oral) | Increased effect of both drugs. When monitored carefully, combination may be beneficial in controlling hypertension. | | |

# RESERPINE, HYDRALAZINE & HYDROCHLOROTHIAZIDE

| GENERIC NAME OR DRUG CLASS | COMBINED EFFECT | GENERIC NAME OR DRUG CLASS | COMBINED EFFECT |
|---|---|---|---|
| Allopurinol | Decreased allopurinol effect. | Beta-adrenergic blockers | Increased effect of rauwolfia alkaloids. Excessive sedation. |
| Amphetamines | Decreased hydralazine effect. | Cholestyramine | Decreased hydrochlorothiazide effect. |
| Anticoagulants (oral) | Unpredictable increased or decreased effect of anticoagulant. | Cortisone drugs | Excessive potassium loss that causes dangerous heart rhythms. |
| Anticonvulsants | Serious change in seizure pattern. | | |
| Antidepressants (tricyclic) | Dangerous drop in blood pressure. Avoid combination unless under medical supervision. | Digitalis preparations | Excessive potassium loss that causes dangerous heart rhythms. |
| Antihistamines | Increased antihistamine effect. | Diuretics (oral) | Increased effects of drugs. When monitored carefully, combination may be beneficial in controlling hypertension. |
| Antihypertensives (other) | Increased antihypertensive effect. | | |
| Aspirin | Decreased aspirin effect. | Dronabinol | Increased effects of drugs. |
| Barbiturates | Increased hydrochlorothiazide effect. | Indapamide | Increased diuretic effect. |

ADDITIONAL DRUG INTERACTIONS

975

| GENERIC NAME OR DRUG CLASS | COMBINED EFFECT | GENERIC NAME OR DRUG CLASS | COMBINED EFFECT |
|---|---|---|---|

## RESERPINE, HYDRALAZINE & HYDROCHLOROTHIAZIDE continued

| GENERIC NAME OR DRUG CLASS | COMBINED EFFECT | GENERIC NAME OR DRUG CLASS | COMBINED EFFECT |
|---|---|---|---|
| Levodopa | Decreased levodopa effect. | Oxprenolol | Increased antihypertensive effect. Dosages of drug may require adjustments. |
| Lithium | Increased lithium effect. | | |
| MAO inhibitors | Increased effects of drugs. Severe depression. | Potassium supplements | Decreased potassium effect. |
| Mind-altering drugs | Excessive sedation. | Probenecid | Decreased probenecid effect. |
| Nitrates | Excessive blood-pressure drop. | | |

# SALICYLATES

| GENERIC NAME OR DRUG CLASS | COMBINED EFFECT | GENERIC NAME OR DRUG CLASS | COMBINED EFFECT |
|---|---|---|---|
| Propranolol | Decreased salicylate effect. | Spironolactone | Decreased spironolactone effect. |
| Rauwolfia alkaloids | Decreased salicylate effect. | Sulfinpyrazone | Decreased sulfinpyrazone effect. |
| Salicylates (other) | Likely salicylate toxicity. | Vitamin C (large doses) | Possible salicylate toxicity. |

# SPIRONOLACTONE & HYDROCHLOROTHIAZIDE

| GENERIC NAME OR DRUG CLASS | COMBINED EFFECT | GENERIC NAME OR DRUG CLASS | COMBINED EFFECT |
|---|---|---|---|
| Antihypertensives (other) | Increased antihypertensive effect. | Lithium | Increased effect of lithium. Likely lithium toxicity. |
| Aspirin | Decreased spironolactone effect. | MAO inhibitors | Increased hydrochlorothiazide effect. |
| Barbiturates | Increased hydrochlorothiazide effect. | Nitrates | Excessive blood-pressure drop. |
| Cholestyramine | Decreased hydrochlorothiazide effect. | Oxprenolol | Increased antihypertensive effect. Dosages of both drugs may require adjustment. |
| Cortisone drugs | Excessive potassium loss that causes dangerous heart rhythms. | Potassium supplements | Decreased potassium effect. Dangerous potassium retention, causing possible heartbeat irregularity. |
| Diuretics (other) | Increased effect of both drugs. Beneficial if needed and dose is correct. | | |
| Indapamide | Increased diuretic effect. | Probenecid | Decreased probenecid effect. |
| Laxatives | Reduced potassium levels. | Sodium bicarbonate | Reduces high potassium levels. |
| | | Triamterene | Dangerous potassium retention. |

# THEOPHYLLINE, EPHEDRINE, & BARBITURATES

| GENERIC NAME OR DRUG CLASS | COMBINED EFFECT | GENERIC NAME OR DRUG CLASS | COMBINED EFFECT |
|---|---|---|---|
| Antihypertensives | Decreased antihypertensive effect. | Anti-inflammatory drugs (non-steroidal) | Decreased anti-inflammatory effect. |

| GENERIC NAME OR DRUG CLASS | COMBINED EFFECT | GENERIC NAME OR DRUG CLASS | COMBINED EFFECT |
|---|---|---|---|

## THEOPHYLLINE, EPHEDRINE, & BARBITURATES continued

| GENERIC NAME OR DRUG CLASS | COMBINED EFFECT | GENERIC NAME OR DRUG CLASS | COMBINED EFFECT |
|---|---|---|---|
| Aspirin | Decreased aspirin effect. | Indapamide | Increased indapamide effect. |
| Beta-adrenergic blockers | Decreased effect of drugs. | Lincomycins | Increased bronchodilator effect. |
| Contraceptives (oral) | Decreased contraceptive effect. | Lithium | Decreased lithium effect. |
| Cortisone drugs | Decreased cortisone effect. | MAO inhibitors | Increased ephedrine effect. Dangerous blood-pressure rise. |
| Digitalis preparations | Serious heart-rhythm disturbances. | Mind-altering drugs | Dangerous sedation. Avoid. |
| Doxycycline | Decreased doxycycline effect. | Narcotics | Dangerous sedation. Avoid. |
| Dronabinol | Increased effect of drugs. Avoid. | Nitrates | Possible decreased effect of drugs. |
| Ephedrine | Increased effect of drugs. | Probenecid | Decreased effect of drugs. |
| Epinephrine | Increased effect of drugs. | Propranolol | Decreased bronchodilator effect. |
| Ergot preparations | Serious blood-pressure rise. | Pseudoephedrine | Increased pseudoephedrine effect. |
| Erythromycin | Increased bronchodilator effect. | Rauwolfia alkaloids | Rapid heartbeat. |
| Furosemide | Increased furosemide effect. | Sulfinpyrazone | Decreased sulfinpyrazone effect. |
| Griseofulvin | Decreased griseofulvin effect. | Troleandomycin | Increased bronchodilator effect. |
| Guanethidine | Decreased effect of drugs. | Valproic acid | Increased barbiturate effect. |

## THEOPHYLLINE, EPHEDRINE, GUAIFENESIN & BARBITURATES

| GENERIC NAME OR DRUG CLASS | COMBINED EFFECT | GENERIC NAME OR DRUG CLASS | COMBINED EFFECT |
|---|---|---|---|
| Antidepressants (tricyclics) | Decreased antidepressant effect. | Digitalis preparations | Serious heart-rhythm disturbances. |
| Antidiabetics (oral) | Increased phenobarbital effect. | Digitoxin | Decreased digitoxin effect. |
| Antihistamines | Dangerous sedation. Avoid. | Doxycycline | Decreased doxycycline effect. |
| Anti-inflammatory drugs (non-steroid) | Decreased anti-inflammatory effect. | Dronabinol | Increased effect of drugs. |
| Aspirin (other) | Decreased aspirin effect. | Ephedrine | Increased effect of drugs. |
| Beta-adrenergic blockers | Decreased effect of drugs. | Ergot preparations | Serious blood-pressure rise. |
| Contraceptives (oral) | Decreased contraceptive effect. | Erythromycin | Increased bronchodilator effect. |
| Cortisone drugs | Increased cortisone effect. | Furosemide | Increased furosemide effect. |

ADDITIONAL DRUG INTERACTIONS

977

| GENERIC NAME OR DRUG CLASS | COMBINED EFFECT | GENERIC NAME OR DRUG CLASS | COMBINED EFFECT |
|---|---|---|---|

## THEOPHYLLINE, EPHEDRINE, GUAIFENESIN & BARBITURATES continued

| GENERIC NAME OR DRUG CLASS | COMBINED EFFECT | GENERIC NAME OR DRUG CLASS | COMBINED EFFECT |
|---|---|---|---|
| Griseofulvin | Decreased griseofulvin effect. | Probenecid | Decreased effect of drugs. |
| Guanethidine | Decreased effect of drugs. | Propranolol | Decreased bronchodilator effect. |
| Indapamide | Increased indapamide effect. | Pseudoephedrine | Increased pseudoephedrine effect. |
| Lincomycins | Increased bronchodilator effect. | Rauwolfia alkaloids | Rapid heartbeat. |
| Lithium | Decreased lithium effect. | Sedatives | Dangerous sedation. Avoid. |
| MAO inhibitors | Increased phenobarbital effect. | Sleep inducers | Dangerous sedation. Avoid. |
| Mind-altering drugs | Dangerous sedation. Avoid. | Sulfinpyrazone | Decreased sulfinpyrazone effect. |
| Narcotics | Dangerous sedation. Avoid. | Tranquilizers | Dangerous sedation. Avoid. |
| Nitrates | Possible decreased effect of drugs. | Troleandomycin | Increased bronchodilator effect. |
| Pain relievers | Dangerous sedation. Avoid. | Valproic acid | Increased phenobarbital effect. |

# THEOPHYLLINE, EPHEDRINE & HYDROXYZINE

| GENERIC NAME OR DRUG CLASS | COMBINED EFFECT | GENERIC NAME OR DRUG CLASS | COMBINED EFFECT |
|---|---|---|---|
| Beta-adrenergic blockers | Decreased effect of drugs. | MAO inhibitors | Increased ephedrine effect. Dangerous blood-pressure rise. |
| Digitalis preparations | Serious heart-rhythm disturbances. | Nitrates | Possible decreased effect of drugs. |
| Dronabinol | Increased effect of drugs. | Pain relievers | Increased effect of drugs. |
| Ephedrine | Increased effect of drugs. | Probenecid | Decreased effect of drugs. |
| Epinephrine | Increased effect of drugs. | Propranolol | Decreased bronchodilator effect. |
| Ergot preparations | Serious blood-pressure rise. | Pseudoephedrine | Increased pseudoephedrine effect. |
| Erythromycin | Increased bronchodilator effect. | Rauwolfia alkaloids | Rapid heartbeat. |
| Furosemide | Increased furosemide effect. | Sulfinpyrazone | Decreased sulfinpyrazone effect. |
| Guanethidine | Decreased effect of drugs. | Tranquilizers | Increased effect of drugs. |
| Lincomycins | Increased bronchodilator effect. | Troleandomycin | Increased bronchodilator effect. |
| Lithium | Decreased lithium effect. | | |

# TRIAMETERINE & HYDROCHOLOROTHIAZIDE

| GENERIC NAME OR DRUG CLASS | COMBINED EFFECT | GENERIC NAME OR DRUG CLASS | COMBINED EFFECT |
| --- | --- | --- | --- |
| **Oxprenolol** | Increased antihypertensive effect. Dosages may require adjustments. | **Probenecid** | Decreased probenecid effect. |
| **Potassium supplements** | Possible excessive potassium retention. Decreased potassium effect. | **Spironolactone** | Dangerous retention of potassium. |

# Glossary The following medical terms are found in the drug charts.

## A

**A.C.E. inhibitor**—Angiotensin-converting enzyme (A.C.E.) inhibitor reduces aldosterone secretion and reduces blood pressure. The inhibitors decrease the rate of conversion of Angiotensin I into Angiotensin II, which is the normal process for the angiotensin-converting enzyme.

**Acute**—Having a short and relatively severe course.

**Addiction**—Psychological or physiological dependence upon a drug.

**Addison's Disease**—Changes in the body caused by a deficiency of hormones manufactured by the adrenal gland. Usually fatal if untreated.

**Adrenal Cortex**—Center of the adrenal gland.

**Adrenal Gland**—Gland next to the kidney that produces cortisone and epinephrine (adrenalin).

**Alkylating Agent**—Chemical used to treat malignant diseases.

**Allergy**—Excessive sensitivity to a substance.

**Amebiasis**—Infection with amoeba, one-celled organisms. Causes diarrhea, fever and abdominal cramps.

**Amphetamine**—Drug that stimulates the brain and central nervous system, increases blood pressure, reduces nasal congestion and is habit-forming.

**Analgesic**—Agent that reduces pain without reducing consciousness.

**Anaphylaxis**—Severe allergic response to a substance. Symptoms are wheezing, itching, hives, nasal congestion, intense burning of hands and feet, collapse, loss of consciousness and cardiac arrest. Symptoms appear within a few seconds or minutes after exposure. Anaphylaxis is a severe medical emergency. Without appropriate treatment, it can cause death. Instructions for home treatment for anaphylaxis are on the front inside cover.

**Anemia**—Not enough healthy red-blood cells in the bloodstream or too little hemoglobin in the red-blood cells. Anemia is caused by imbalance of blood loss and blood production.

**Anemia, Hemolytic**—Anemia caused by a shortened life span of red-blood cells. The body can't manufacture new cells fast enough to replace old cells.

**Anemia, Iron-Deficiency**—Anemia caused when iron necessary to manufacture red-blood cells is not available.

**Anemia, Pernicious**—Anemia caused by a vitamin B-12 deficiency. Symptoms include weakness, fatigue, numbness and tingling of the hands or feet, and degeneration of the central nervous system.

**Anemia, Sickle-Cell**—Anemia caused by defective hemoglobin that deprives red-blood cells of oxygen, making them sickle-shaped.

**Anesthetic**—Drug that eliminates the sensation of pain.

**Angina (Angina Pectoris)**—Chest pain with a sensation of suffocation and impending death. Caused by a temporary reduction in the amount of oxygen to the heart muscle through diseased coronary arteries.

**Antacid**—Chemical that neutralizes acid, usually in the stomach.

**Antibiotic**—Chemical that inhibits the growth of or kills germs.

**Anticholinergic**—Drug that chemically inhibits nerve impulses through the parasympathetic nervous system.

**Anticoagulant**—Drug that inhibits blood clotting.

**Antiemetic**—Drug that prevents or stops nausea and vomiting.

**Antihypertensive**—Medication to reduce blood pressure.

**Appendicitis**—Inflammation or infection of the appendix. Symptoms include loss of appetite, nausea, low-grade fever and tenderness in the lower right of the abdomen.

**Artery**—Blood vessel carrying blood away from the heart.

**Asthma**—Recurrent attacks of breathing difficulty due to spasms and contractions of the bronchial tubes.

# B

**Bacteria**—Microscopic organism. Some bacteria contribute to health; others (germs) cause disease.

**Basal Area of Brain**—Part of the brain that regulates muscle control and tone.

**Blood Count**—Laboratory studies to count white-blood cells, red-blood cells, platelets and other elements of the blood.

**Blood Pressure, Diastolic**—Pressure (usually recorded in millimeters of mercury) in the large arteries of the body when the heart muscle is relaxed and filling for the next contraction.

**Blood Pressure, Systolic**—Pressure (usually recorded in millimeters of mercury) in the large arteries of the body at the instant the heart muscle contracts.

**Blood Sugar (Blood Glucose)**—Necessary element in the blood to sustain life.

# C

**Cataract**—Loss of transparency in the lens of the eye.

**Cell**—Unit of protoplasm, the essential living matter of all plants and animals.

**Cephalosporin**—Antibiotic that kills many bacterial germs that penicillin and sulfa drugs can't destroy.

**Cholinergic (also Parasympathomimetic)**—Chemical that facilitates passage of nerve impulses through the parasympathetic nervous system.

**Cirrhosis**—Disease that scars and destroys liver tissue.

**Cold Urticaria**—Hives that appear in areas of the body exposed to the cold.

**Colitis, Ulcerative**—Chronic, recurring ulcers of the colon for unknown reasons.

**Collagen**—Support tissue of skin, tendon, bone, cartilage and connective tissue.

**Colostomy**—Surgical opening from the colon, the large intestine, to the outside of the body.

**Congestive**—Excess accumulation of blood. In congestive heart failure, congestion occurs in the lungs, liver, kidney and other parts to cause shortness of breath, swelling of the ankles and feet, rapid heartbeat and other symptoms.

**Constriction**—Tightness or pressure.

**Contraceptive**—Something that prevents pregnancy.

**Convulsions**—Violent, uncontrollable contractions of the voluntary muscles.

**Corticosteroid (Adrenocorticosteroid)**—Steroid hormones produced by the body's adrenal cortex or their synthetic equivalents.

**Cystitis**—Inflammation of the urinary bladder.

# D

**Delirium**—Temporary mental disturbance characterized by hallucinations, agitation and incoherence.

**Diabetes**—Metabolic disorder in which the body can't use carbohydrates efficiently. This leads to a dangerously high level of glucose (a carbohydrate) in the blood.

**Dialysis**—Procedure to filter waste products from the bloodstream of patients with kidney failure.

**Dilation**—Enlargement.

**Disulfiram Reaction**—Disulfiram (Antabuse) is a drug to treat alcoholism. When alcohol in the bloodstream interacts with disulfiram, it causes a flushed face, severe headache, chest pains, shortness of breath, nausea, vomiting, sweating and weakness. Severe reactions may cause death.

A disulfiram reaction is the interaction of any drug with alcohol or another drug to produce these symptoms.

**Duodenum**—The first 12 inches of the small intestine.

# E

**Eczema**—Disorder of the skin with redness, itching, blisters, weeping and abnormal pigmentation.

**Electrolyte**—Substance that can transmit electrical impulses when dissolved in body fluids.

**Embolism**—Sudden blockage of an artery by a clot or foreign material in the blood.

**Emphysema**—Disease in which the lung's air sacs lose elasticity, and air accumulates in the lungs.

**Endometriosis**—Condition in which uterus tissue is found outside the uterus. Can cause pain, abnormal menstruation and infertility.

**Enzyme**—Protein chemical that can accelerate a chemical reaction in the body.

**Epilepsy**—Episodes of brain disturbance that cause convulsions and loss of consciousness.

**Esophagitis**—Inflammation of the lower part of the esophagus, the tube connecting the throat and the stomach.

**Estrogens**—Female sex hormones that stimulate female characteristics and prepare the uterus for fertilization.

**Eustachian Tube**—Small passage from the middle ear to the sinuses and nasal passages.

**Extremity**—Arm, leg, hand or foot.

# F

**Fecal Impaction**—Condition in which feces become firmly wedged in the rectum.

**Fibrocystic Breast Disease**—Overgrowth of fibrous tissue in the breast, producing non-malignant cysts.

**Fibroid Tumors**—Non-malignant tumors of the muscular layer of the uterus.

**Flu (Influenza)**—A virus infection of the respiratory tract that lasts three to ten days. Symptoms include headache, fever, runny nose, cough, tiredness and muscle aches.

**Folliculitis**—Inflammation of a follicle.

# G

**G6PD**—Deficiency of glucose 6-phosphate, necessary for glucose metabolism.

**Gastritis**—Inflammation of the stomach.

**Gastrointestinal**—Stomach and intestinal tract.

**Gland**—Cells that manufacture and excrete materials not required for their own metabolic needs.

**Glaucoma**—Eye disease in which increased pressure inside the eye damages the optic nerve, causes pain and changes vision.

**Glucagon**—Injectable drug that immediately elevates blood sugar by mobilizing glycogen from the liver.

# H

**Hangover Effect**—The same feelings as a "hangover" after too much alcohol consumption. Symptoms include headache, irritability and nausea.

**Hemochromatosis**—Disorder of iron metabolism in which excessive iron is deposited in and damages body tissues, particularly liver and pancreas.

**Hemoglobin**—Pigment that carries oxygen in red-blood cells.

**Hemorrhage**—Heavy bleeding.

**Hemosiderosis**—Increase of iron deposits in body tissues without tissue damage.

**Hepatitis**—Inflammation of liver cells, usually accompanied by jaundice.

**Hiatal Hernia**—Section of stomach that protrudes into the chest cavity.

**Histamine**—Chemical in body tissues that dilates the smallest blood vessels, constricts the smooth muscle surrounding the bronchial tubes and stimulates stomach secretions.

**History**—Past medical events in a patient's life.

**Hives**—Elevated patches on the skin that are redder or paler than surrounding skin and often itch severely.

**Hormone**—Chemical substance produced in the body to regulate other body functions.

**Hypertension**—High blood pressure.

**Hypocalcemia**—Abnormally low level of calcium in the blood.

**Hypoglycemia**—Low blood sugar (blood glucose). A critically low blood-sugar level will interfere with normal brain function and can damage the brain permanently.

# I

**Ichthyosis**—Skin disorder with dryness, scaling and roughness.

**Ileitis**—Inflammation of the ileum, the last section of the small intestine.

**Ileostomy**—Surgical opening from the ileum, the end of the small intestine, to the outside of the body.

**Impotence**—Male's inability to achieve or sustain erection of the penis for sexual intercourse.

**Insomnia**—Sleeplessness.

**Interaction**—Change in the body's response to one drug when another is taken. Interaction may increase the effect of one or both drugs, decrease the effect of one or both drugs, or cause toxicity.

**J**

**Jaundice**—Symptoms of liver damage, bile obstruction or red-blood-cell destruction. Includes yellowed whites of the eyes, yellow skin, dark urine and light stool.

**K**

**Keratosis**—Growth that is an accumulation of cells from the outer skin layers.
**Kidney Stones**—Small, solid stones made from calcium, cholesterol, cysteine and other body chemicals.

**L**

**Lupus**—Serious disorder of connective tissue that primarily affects women. Varies in severity with skin eruptions, joint inflammation, low white-blood cell count and damage to internal organs, especially the kidney.
**Lymph Glands**—Glands in the lymph vessels throughout the body that trap foreign and infectious matter and protect the bloodstream from infection.

**M**

**Manic-Depressive Illness**—Psychosis with alternating cycles of excessive enthusiasm and depression.
**Mast Cell**—Connective-tissue cell.
**Menopause**—The end of menstruation in the female, often accompanied by irritability, hot flushes, changes in the skin and bones and vaginal dryness.
**Metabolism**—Process of using nutrients and energy to build and break down wastes.
**Migraine**—Periodic headaches caused by constriction of arteries to the skull. Symptoms include severe pain, vision disturbances, nausea, vomiting and light sensitivity.
**Mind-Altering Drugs**—Any drug that decreases alertness, perception, concentration, contact with reality or muscular coordination.
**Myasthenia Gravis**—Disease of the muscles characterized by fatigue and progressive paralysis. It is usually confined to muscles of the face, lips, tongue and neck.

**N**

**Narcotic**—Drug, usually addictive, that produces stupor.

**O**

**Osteoporosis**—Softening of bones caused by a loss of chemicals usually found in bone.
**Ovary**—Female sexual gland where eggs mature and ripen for fertilization.

**P**

**Palpitations**—Rapid heartbeat noticeable to the patient.
**Pancreatitis**—Serious inflammation or infection of the pancreas that causes upper abdominal pain.
**Parkinson's Disease**—Disease of the central nervous system. Characteristics are a fixed, emotionless expression of the face, tremor, slower muscle movements, weakness, changed gait and a peculiar posture.
**Pellagra**—Disease caused by a deficiency of the water-soluble vitamin, thiamine (vitamin B-1). Symptoms include brain disturbance, diarrhea and skin inflammation.
**Penicillin**—Chemical substance (antibiotic) originally discovered as a product of mold, which can kill some bacterial germs.
**Phlegm**—Thick mucus secreted by glands in the respiratory tract.
**Pinworms**—Common intestinal parasite that causes rectal itching and irritation.
**Pituitary Gland**—Gland at the base of the brain that secretes hormones to stimulate growth and other glands to produce hormones.
**Platelet**—Disc-shaped element of the blood, smaller than red- or white-blood cells, necessary for blood clotting.
**Polyp**—Growth on a mucous membrane.
**Porphyria**—Inherited metabolic disorder characterized by changes in the nervous system and kidney.
**Post-partum**—Following delivery of a baby.
**Potassium**—Important chemical found in body cells.
**Potassium Foods**—Foods high in potassium content, including dried apricots and peaches, lentils, raisins, citrus and whole-grain cereals.
**Prostate**—Gland in the male that surrounds the neck of the bladder and the urethra.
**Prothrombin**—Blood substance essential in clotting.

**Prothrombin Time**—Laboratory study used to follow prothrombin activity and keep coagulation safe.

**Psoriasis**—Chronic, inherited skin disease. Symptoms are lesions with silvery scales on the edges.

**Psychosis**—Mental disorder characterized by deranged personality, loss of contact with reality and possible delusions, hallucinations or illusions.

**Purine Foods**—Foods that are metabolized into uric acid. Foods high in purines include anchovies, liver, brains, sweetbreads, sardines, kidney, oysters, gravy and meat extracts.

# R

**RDA**—Recommended daily allowance of a vitamin or mineral.

**Rebound Effect**—Return of a condition, often with increased severity, once the prescribed drug is withdrawn.

**Renal**—Pertaining to the kidney.

**Retina**—Innermost covering of the eyeball on which the image is formed.

**Reye's Syndrome**—Rare, sometimes fatal, disease of children that causes brain and liver damage.

**Rickets**—Bone disease caused by vitamin-D deficiency. Bones become bent and distorted during infancy or childhood.

# S

**Sedative**—Drug that reduces excitement or anxiety.

**Seizure**—Brain disorder causing changes of consciousness or convulsions.

**Sinusitis**—Inflammation or infection of the sinus cavities in the skull.

**Streptococcus**—Bacteria that causes infections in the throat, respiratory system and skin. Improperly treated, can lead to disease in the heart, joints and kidneys.

**Stroke**—Sudden, severe attack. Usually sudden paralysis from injury to the brain or spinal cord caused by a blood clot or hemorrhage in the brain.

**Stupor**—Near unconsciousness.

**Sublingual**—Under the tongue. Some drugs are absorbed almost as quickly this way as by injection.

# T

**Tardive Dyskinesia**—Involuntary movements of the jaw, lips and tongue caused by an unpredictable drug reaction.

**Thrombophlebitis**—Inflammation of a vein caused by a blood clot in the vein.

**Thyroid**—Gland in the neck that manufactures and secretes several hormones.

**Tic-douloureaux**—Painful condition caused by inflammation of a nerve in the face.

**Toxicity**—Poisonous reaction to a drug that impairs body functions or damages cells.

**Tranquilizer**—Drug that calms a person without clouding consciousness.

**Tremor**—Involuntary trembling.

**Trichomoniasis**—Infestation of the vagina by *trichomonas,* an infectious organism. The infection causes itching, vaginal discharge and irritation.

**Triglyceride**—Fatty chemical manufactured from carbohydrates for storage in fat cells.

**Tyramine**—Normal chemical component of the body that helps sustain blood pressure. Can rise to fatal levels in combination with some drugs.

Tyramine is found in many foods:

Beverages—Alcoholic beverages, especially Chianti or robust red wines, vermouth, ale, beer.

Breads—Homemade bread with a lot of yeast and breads or crackers containing cheese.

Fats—Sour cream.

Fruits—Bananas, red plums, avocados, figs, raisins.

Meats and meat substitutes—Aged game, liver, canned meats, salami, sausage, cheese, salted dried fish, pickled herring.

Vegetables—Italian broad beans, green-bean pods, eggplant.

Miscellaneous—Yeast concentrates or extracts, marmite, soup cubes, commercial gravy, soy sauce, any protein food that has been stored improperly or is spoiled.

# U

**Ulcer, Peptic**—Open sore on the mucous membrane of the esophagus, stomach or duodenum caused by stomach acid.

**Urethra**—Hollow tube through which urine (and semen in men) is discharged.

**Urethritis**—Inflammation or infection of the urethra.

**Uterus**—Also called *womb*. A hollow muscular organ in the female in which the embryo develops into a fetus.

## V
**Vascular**—Pertaining to blood vessels.
**Virus**—Infectious organism that reproduces in the cells of the infected host.

## Y
**Yeast**—A single-cell organism that can cause infections of the mouth, vagina, skin and parts of the gastrointestinal system.

# GUIDE TO INDEX

Alphabetical entries in the index include three categories—generic names, brand names and drug-class names.

1. Generic names appear in capital letter, followed by their chart page number:

   ASPIRIN, 66

2. Brand names appear in *italic*, followed by their generic ingredient and chart page number.

   *Bayer*—See ASPIRIN, 66

   Some brands contain two or more generic ingredients. These generic ingredients are listed in capital letters following the brand name:

   *Cefinal*—See
   ASPIRIN, 66
   CAFFEINE, 128

   Some brands contain generic ingredients that are not included in this book because of space limitations. These generics are designated by (NL), which means "not listed."

   *Fedrazil*—See
   CHLORCYCLIZINE (NL)
   PSEUDOEPHEDRINE, 752

3. Drug-class names appear in regular type, capital and lower-case letters. All generic drug names in this book that fall into a drug class are listed after the class name.

   Analgesics
   ACETAMINOPHEN, 4
   ASPIRIN, 66
   CARBAMAZEPINE, 140
   PHENACETIN, 672
   SALICYLATES, 796

---

Amaril D—See
    PHENYLTOLOXAMINE 692
AMBENONIUM 36
Ambenyl—See
    GUAIFENESIN 404
    NARCOTIC ANALGESICS 594
Ambenyl-D—See
    PSEUDOEPHEDRINE 752
Ambenyl Expectorant—See
    BROMODIPHENHYDRAMINE 108
    DIPHENHYDRAMINE 296
Ambodryl—See
    BROMODIPHENHYDRAMINE 108
Amcill—See AMPICILLIN 52
Amcort—See TRIAMCINOLONE 890
Amen—See
    MEDROXYPROGESTERONE 512
Americaine Aerosol—See
    ANESTHETICS (TOPICAL) 56
Americaine Ointment—See
    ANESTHETICS (TOPICAL) 56
Americaine—See
    ANESTHETICS (TOPICAL) 56
Amersol—See IBUPROFEN 438
Amesec—See
    EPHEDRINE 326
    XANTHINE BRONCHODILATORS 938
A-methaPred—See
    METHYLPREDNISOLONE 562
AMILORIDE 38
AMILORIDE &
    HYDROCHLOROTHIAZIDE 40
AMINOBENZOATE POTASSIUM 42
Aminodur—See XANTHINE
    BRONCHODILATORS 938
Aminodur Dura-tabs—See XANTHINE
    BRONCHODILATORS 938
Aminophyl—See XANTHINE
    BRONCHODILATORS 938
Aminophyllin—See XANTHINE
    BRONCHODILATORS 938
AMINOPHYLLINE—See XANTHINE
    BRONCHODILATORS 938
Aminophylline and Amytal—See
    XANTHINE BRONCHODILATORS 938
Aminophylline-Phenobarbital—See
    PHENOBARBITAL 678
    XANTHINE BRONCHODILATORS 938
AMIODARONE 44
Amitid—See TRICYCLIC
    ANTIDEPRESSANTS 900
Amitone—See CALCIUM
    CARBONATE 130
Amitril—See TRICYCLIC
    ANTIDEPRESSANTS 900
AMITRYPTILINE—See TRICYCLIC
    ANTIDEPRESSANTS 900
AMITRIPTYLINE &
    CHLORDIAZEPOXIDE 178
AMITRIPTYLINE & PERPHENAZINE 670
Amnestrogen—See
    ESTERIFIED ESTROGENS 346
Amnestrogen—See ESTROGEN 350
AMOBARBITAL 46
Amobel—See BELLADONNA 84
Amobell—See BELLADONNA
    ALKALOIDS & BARBITURATES 86
Amocine—See ATROPINE 70
Amodrine—See
    EPHEDRINE 326
    XANTHINE BRONCHODILATORS 938
Amoline—See XANTHINE
    BRONCHODILATORS 938
Amophylline—See XANTHINE
    BRONCHODILATORS 938
AMOXAPINE—See TRICYCLIC
    ANTIDEPRESSANTS 900
AMOXICILLIN 48
Amoxil—See AMOXICILLIN 48
Amphaplex—See
    DEXTROAMPHETAMINE 272
Amphaplex 10 & 20—See
    AMPHETAMINE 50
Amphenol—See ACETAMINOPHEN 4
AMPHETAMINE 50

Amphicol—See
    CHLORAMPHENICOL 174
Amphojel Plus—See ALUMINUM,
    MAGNESIUM, MAGALDRATE &
    SIMETHICONE AMPICILLIN 52
Amphojel—See
    ALUMINUM HYDROXIDE 26
Ampicin—See AMPICILLIN 52
Ampilean—See AMPICILLIN 52
A-M-T—See
    MAGNESIUM TRISILICATE 502
Amytal—See AMOBARBITAL 46
Amytal and Aspirin—See ASPIRIN 66
Anabolin—See ANDROGENS 54
Anabolin LA 100—See ANDROGENS 54
Anacin—See
    ASPIRIN 66
    CAFFEINE 128
Anacin-3—See ACETAMINOPHEN 4
Anadrol-50—See ANDROGENS 54
Anafed—See
    CHLORPHENIRAMINE 190
    PSEUDOEPHEDRINE 752
Anafranil—See TRICYCLIC
    ANTIDEPRESSANTS 900
Analgesic
    ACETAMINOPHEN 4
    ACETAMINOPHEN & SALICYLATES 6
    ASPIRIN 66
    BUTALBITAL & ASPIRIN
        (Also contains caffeine) 122
    BUTALBITAL, ASPIRIN & CODEINE
        (Also contains caffeine) 124
    CARBAMAZEPINE 140
    CHLORZOXAZONE &
        ACETAMINOPHEN 202
    ERGOTAMINE, BELLADONNA &
        PHENOBARBITAL 336
    ERGOTAMINE & CAFFEINE 338
    ISOMETHAPRINE,
        DICHLORALPHENAZONE &
        ACETAMINOPHEN 452
    MEPROBAMATE & ASPIRIN 524
    NARCOTIC & ACETAMINOPHEN 592
    NARCOTIC & ASPIRIN 596
    ORPHENADRINE, ASPIRIN &
        CAFFEINE 626
    PHENACETIN 672
    SALICYLATES 796
    SUPROFEN 836
Analgesic (non-steroidal anti-inflammatory
    analgesic)—See KETOPROFEN 474
Analgesic (urinary) sulfonamide—See
    PHENAZOPYRIDINE 674
    SULFONAMIDES &
        PHENAZOPYRIDINE 832
Anamine—See
    CHLORPHENIRAMINE 190
    PSEUDOEPHEDRINE 752
Anamine T.D.—See
    PHENYLEPHRINE 688
Anapap—See ACETAMINOPHEN 4
Anaphen—See
    ACETAMINOPHEN 4
    ASPIRIN 66
    CAFFEINE 128
    NARCOTIC ANALGESICS 594
Anapolon 50—See ANDROGENS 54
Anaprox—See NAPROXEN 590
Anaspa 3—See HYOSCYAMINE 436
Anaspaz PB—See
    BELLADONNA ALKALOIDS &
        BARBITURATES 86
    HYOSCYAMINE 436
    PHENOBARBITAL 678
Anatuss—See CHLORPHENIRAMINE 190
Anavar—See ANDROGENS 54
Anbesol—See
    ANESTHETICS (TOPICAL) 56
Ancasal—See
    ASPIRIN 66
    NARCOTIC & ASPIRIN 596
Andrest—See TESTOSTERONE &
    ESTRADIOL 848
Andro—See ANDROGENS 54

Andro-Cyp—See ANDROGENS 54
Andro-Estro—See
    TESTOSTERONE & ESTRADIOL 848
Andro/Fem—See
    TESTOSTERONE & ESTRADIOL 848
Andro-LA—See ANDROGENS 54
ANDROGENS 54
Androgens-estrogens—See
    TESTOSTERONE & ESTRADIOL 848
Androgyn L.A.—See
    TESTOSTERONE & ESTRADIOL 848
Android—See ANDROGENS 54
Android-F—See ANDROGENS 54
Android-T—See ANDROGENS 54
Androlone—See ANDROGENS 54
Andron—See ANDROGENS 54
Andronaq—See ANDROGENS 54
Andronaq-LA—See ANDROGENS 54
Andronate—See ANDROGENS 54
Androyd—See ANDROGENS 54
Andryl—See ANDROGENS 54
Anemtyl—See TRICYCLIC
    ANTIDEPRESSANTS 900
Anergan—See PROMETHAZINE 746
Anestacon—See
    ANESTHETICS (TOPICAL) 56
ANESTHETICS (TOPICAL) 56
Anexsia w/Codeine—See
    ASPIRIN 66
    CAFFEINE 128
    NARCOTIC & ASPIRIN 596
Anexsia-D—See NARCOTIC &
    ASPIRIN 596
Ang-O-Span—See NITRATES 608
Anhydron—See CYCLOTHIAZIDE 252
ANISINDIONE—See
    ANTICOAGULANTS (ORAL) 58
Anocobin—See VITAMIN B-12
    (CYANOCOBALAMIN) 926
Anoquan—See
    ACETAMINOPHEN 4
    CAFFEINE 128
Anorex—See
    APPETITE SUPPRESSANTS 64
Anorex-CCK—See
    METHYLCELLULOSE 552
Anoryol—See
    CONTRACEPTIVES (ORAL) 236
Anspor—See CEPHRADINE 164
Antabuse—See DISULFIRAM 308
Antacid—See
    ALUMINUM HYDROXIDE 26
    ALUMINUM, MAGNESIUM,
        MAGALDRATE & SIMETHICONE
        ANTACIDS 30
    ALUMINUM, MAGNESIUM & SODIUM
        BICARBONATE ANTACIDS 32
    CALCIUM CARBONATE 130
    CALCIUM & MAGNESIUM
        ANTACIDS 132
    MAGNESIUM CARBONATE 494
    MAGNESIUM HYDROXIDE 498
    MAGNESIUM TRISILICATE 502
    SODIUM BICARBONATE 808
    SODIUM CARBONATE 810
ANTACIDS 30—See
    ALUMINUM, CALCIUM & MAGNESIUM
        ANTACIDS 24
    ALUMINUM & MAGNESIUM
        ANTACIDS 28
Antagonate—See
    CHLORPHENIRAMINE 190
Antazone—See SULFINPYRAZONE 828
Anthrombin-K—See
    ANTICOAGULANTS (ORAL) 58
Antiacne—See ISOTRETINOIN 462
Antiacne (topical)—See
    BENZOYL PEROXIDE 90
    TRETINOIN 888
Antianginal (nitrate)—See NITRATES 608
Antianginal—See
    DILTIAZEM 290
    NIFEDIPINE 606
    VERAPAMIL 922
Antianxiety (tranquilizer)—See

INDEX

INDEX

991

INDEX

Chromagen—See
FERROUS FUMARATE 370
Chronulac—See LACTULOSE 478
Cibalith-S—See LITHIUM 488
Cillium—See PSYLLIUM 756
CIMETIDINE 206
Cinalone 40—See TRIAMCINOLONE 890
Cino-40—See TRIAMCINOLONE 890
Cinobac—See CINOXACIN 208
Cinobactin—See CINOXACIN 208
Cinonide 40—See TRIAMCINOLONE 890
CINOXACIN 208
Cin-Quin—See QUINIDINE 772
Cinsospan—See
PHENYLPROPANOLAMINE 690
Ciramine—See
CHLORPHENIRAMINE 190
Circanol—See
ERGOLOID MESYLATES 330
Circlidrin—See NYLIDRIN 620
Ciriforte—See CHLORPHENIRAMINE 190
Cirin—See ASPIRIN 66
Citra Capsules—See PHENIRAMINE 676
Citra—See
PHENYLEPHRINE 688
PHENYLPROPANOLAMINE 690
Citra Forte—See
CHLORPHENIRAMINE 190
PHENIRAMINE 676
PYRILAMINE 762
Citracal—See CALCIUM
SUPPLEMENTS 134
Citrate of Magnesia—See
MAGNESIUM CITRATE 496
Citrated Caffeine—See
CAFFEINE 128
CITRATES 210
Citrocarbonate—See
SODIUM BICARBONATE 808
Citrolith—See CITRATES 210
Citroma—See MAGNESIUM
CITRATE 496
Citro-Mag—See MAGNESIUM
CITRATE 496
Citro-Nesia—See MAGNESIUM
CITRATE 496
Citrucel—See METHYLCELLULOSE 552
C-Ject—See ASCORBIC ACID
(VITAMIN C) 928
Claripex—See CLOFIBRATE 218
Clear By Design—See
BENZOYL PEROXIDE 90
Clearasil—See BENZOYL PEROXIDE 90
Clearasil BP(M)—See
BENZOYL PEROXIDE 90
CLEMASTINE 212
Cleocin—See
CLINDAMYCIN 216
LINCOMYCIN 482
Cleocin-T—See CLINDAMYCIN 216
CLIDINIUM 214
CLIDINIUM & CHLORDIAZEPOXIDE 180
Climestrone—See
ESTERIFIED ESTROGENS 346
Clinazine—See TRIFLUOPERAZINE 904
CLINDAMYCIN 216
CLINDAYCIN—See LINCOMYCIN 482
Clindex—See CHLORDIAZEPOXIDE &
CLIDINIUM 180
Clinestrone—See ESTROGEN 350
Clinicaine—See ANESTHETICS
(TOPICAL) 56
Clinicort—See
ADRENOCORTICOIDS (TOPICAL) 16
Clinoril—See SULINDAC 834
Clinoxide—See CHLORDIAZEPOXIDE &
CLIDINIUM 180
Clipoxide—See CHLORDIAZEPOXIDE &
CLIDINIUM 180
CLIDINIUM 214
Clistin—See CARBINOXAMINE 146
Clistin D—See PHENYLEPHRINE 688
Clistin R-A—See CARBINOXAMINE 146
Cloderm—See
ADRENOCORTICOIDS (TOPICAL) 16

CLOFIBRATE 218
Clomid—See CLOMIPHENE 220
CLOMIPHENE 220
CLOMIPRAMINE—See TRICYCLIC
ANTIDEPRESSANTS 900
CLONIDINE 222
CLONIDINE & CHLORTHALIDONE 224
CLORAZEPATE 226
Clorazine—See CHLORPROMAZINE 192
CLORTERMINE—See
APPETITE SUPPRESSANTS 64
CLOXACILLIN 228
Cloxapen—See CLOXACILLIN 228
Cloxilean—See CLOXACILLIN 228
Clysodrast—See BISACODYL 104
CM with Paregoric—See
PAREGORIC 652
CoTylenol Children's Liquid Cold
Formula—See
PHENYLPROPANOLAMINE 690
Coastaldyne—See
ACETAMINOPHEN 4
NARCOTIC ANALGESICS 594
ACETAMINOPHEN 4
CAFFEINE 128
NARCOTIC ANALGESICS 594
Coco-Quinine—See QUININE 774
Codalan—See
ACETAMINOPHEN 4
ASPIRIN 66
NARCOTIC ANALGESICS 594
Codalan  3—See CAFFEINE 128
Codalex—See
NARCOTIC ANALGESICS 594
PHENYLEPHRINE 688
Codap—See
ACETAMINOPHEN 4
NARCOTIC & ACETAMINOPHEN 592
NARCOTIC ANALGESICS 594
Codasa—See ASPIRIN 66
CODEINE—See NARCOTIC
ANALGESICS 594
CODEINE, BUTALBITAL & ASPIRIN
(Also contains caffeine) 124
Codeine Sulfate—See NARCOTIC
ANALGESICS 594
Codelsol—See PREDNISOLONE 722
Codimal—See
CHLORPHENIRAMINE 190
GUAIFENESIN 404
PHENYLEPHRINE 688
PHENYLPROPANOLAMINE 690
PSEUDOEPHEDRINE 752
Codimal DH, DM, PH—See
PYRILAMINE 762
Codimal PH—See NARCOTIC
ANALGESICS 594
Coditrate—See
GUAIFENESIN 404
NARCOTIC ANALGESICS 594
Codone—See NARCOTIC
ANALGESICS 594
Codoxy—See NARCOTIC & ASPIRIN 596
Codylax—See BISACODYL 104
Coffee-Break—See
PHENYLPROPANOLAMINE 690
Cogentin—See BENZTROPINE 94
Co-Gesic—See ACETAMINOPHEN 4
NARCOTIC &
ACETAMINOPHEN 592
ColBENEMID—See PROBENECID 728
PROBENECID & COLCHICINE 730
ColBenemid—See COLCHICINE 230
Colabid—See PROBENECID &
COLCHICINE 730
Colace—See DOCUSATE SODIUM 316
Colax—See DOCUSATE SODIUM 316
COLCHICINE 230
COLCHICINE & PROBENECID 730
Coldene—See CHLORPHENIRAMINE 190
Colestid—See COLESTIPOL 232
COLESTIPOL 232
Colidrate—See CHLORAL HYDRATE 170
Colisone—See PREDNISONE 724
Coloctyl—See DOCUSATE SODIUM 316

Cologel—See METHYLCELLULOSE 552
Colonil—See DIPHENOXYLATE &
ATROPINE 300
Col-Probenecid—See
COLCHICINE 230
PROBENECID 728
Colrex—See
ACETAMINOPHEN 4
CAFFEINE 128
CHLORPHENIRAMINE 190
PHENYLEPHRINE 688
PHENYLPROPANOLAMINE 690
Colrex Compound—See NARCOTIC
ANALGESICS 594
Colrex Expectorant—See
GUAIFENESIN 404
Combid—See
ISOPROPAMIDE 456
PROCHLORPERAZINE 738
Combid Spansules—See
PROCHLORPERAZINE &
ISOPROPAMIDE 740
Combipres—See
CHLORTHALIDONE 198
CLONIDINE 222
CLONIDINE & CHLORTHALIDONE 224
Comhist—See
ATROPINE 70
BELLADONNA 84
CHLORPHENIRAMINE 190
PHENYLEPHRINE 688
PHENYLTOLOXAMINE 692
Compal—See
ACETAMINOPHEN 4
CAFFEINE 128
Compazine—See
PROCHLORPERAZINE 738
Compocillin VK—See PENICILLIN V 662
Compoz—See DIPHENHYDRAMINE 296
Comtrex—See
ACETAMINOPHEN 4
CHLORPHENIRAMINE 190
PHENYLPROPANOLAMINE 690
Comycin—See TETRACYCLINES 850
Conacetol—See ACETAMINOPHEN 4
Conalsyn—See
SCOPOLAMINE (HYOSCINE) 798
Conar—See
GUAIFENESIN 404
PHENYLEPHRINE 688
Condecal—See
PHENYLTOLOXAMINE 692
Conex—See GUAIFENESIN 404
Conex-DA—See
CHLORPHENIRAMINE 190
PHENYLPROPANOLAMINE 690
Conex w/Codeine—See
CHLORPHENIRAMINE 190
GUAIFENESIN 404
Congespirin—See
ACETAMINOPHEN 4
ASPIRIN 66
DEXAMETHASONE 268
DEXTROMETHORPHAN 274
PHENYLEPHRINE 688
PHENYLPROPANOLAMINE 690
Congess Jr. & Sr.—See
GUAIFENESIN 404
Conhist—See
PHENYLPROPANOLAMINE 690
CONJUGATED ESTROGENS 234
Constant-T—See XANTHINE
BRONCHODILATORS 938
Contac—See
ATROPINE 70
PHENYLEPHRINE 688
PHENYLPROPANOLAMINE 690
Contraceptive—See
CONTRACEPTIVES (ORAL) 236
CONTRACEPTIVES (ORAL) 236
Contratuss—See
DEXTROMETHORPHAN 274
Control—See
PHENYLPROPANOLAMINE 690
Copavin—See

# D

998

INDEX

Foille—See ANESTHETICS (TOPICAL) 56
Foldan—See THIABENDAZOLE 860
Folex—See METHOTREXATE 546
Folex PFS—See METHOTREXATE 546
FOLIC ACID (VITAMIN B-9) 386
Folvite—See
    FOLIC ACID (VITAMIN B-9) 386
Forbaxin—See METHOCARBAMOL 544
Forhistal—See DIMENTHINDENE 294
Formatrix—See ESTROGEN 350
Formula—See GUANEFESIN 404
Formula 44-D—See
    DEXTROMETHORPHAN 274
    GUAIFENESIN 404
    PHENYLPROPANOLAMINE 690
Formulex—See DICYCLOMINE 280
Fortral—See NARCOTIC
    ANALGESICS 594
Fosfree—See
    CALCIUM CARBONATE 130
    FERROUS GLUCONATE 372
Fostex—See BENZOYL PEROXIDE 90
Fostex BPO—See
    BENZOYL PEROXIDE 90
Foygen Aqueous—See ESTRONE 352
Fructines-Vichy—See
    PHENOLPHTHALEIN 680
Fulvicin P/G—See GRISEOFULVIN 402
Fulvicin U/F—See GRISEOFULVIN 402
Fumasorb—See
    FERROUS FUMARATE 370
Fumerin—See
    FERROUS FUMARATE 370
Furadantin—See NITROFURANTOIN 610
Furalan—See NITROFURANTOIN 610
Furaloid—See NITROFURANTOIN 610
Furantoin—See NITROFURANTOIN 610
Furatine—See NITROFURANTOIN 610
FUROSEMIDE 388
Furoside—See FUROSEMIDE 388
Fynex—See DIPHENHYDRAMINE 296

## G

G-1—See ACETAMINOPHEN 4
G-1 Capsules—See CAFFEINE 128
G-2—See ACETAMINOPHEN 4
G-2—See NARCOTIC ANALGESICS 594
G-3—See ACETAMINOPHEN 4
G-3—See NARCOTIC ANALGESICS 594
G-Bron—See XANTHINE
    BRONCHODILATORS 938
GALLBLADDER X-RAY
    TEST DRUGS 390
Gallium Citrate Ga 67—See
    RADIO-PHARMACEUTICALS 776
Ganphen—See PROMETHAZINE 746
Gantanol—See
    SULFAMETHOXAZOLE 824
Gantrisin—See
    SULFAMETHOXAZOLE 824
    SULFISOXAZOLE 830
Gardenal—See PHENOBARBITAL 678
Gas-Is-Gon—See ALUMINUM,
    MAGNESIUM, MAGALDRATE &
        SODIUM BICARBONATE ANTACIDS
        32
Gastrolic—See BELLADONNA 84
Gastrolic—See PHENOBARBITAL 678
Gas-X—See SIMETHICONE 806
Gaviscon—See
    ALUMINUM HYDROXIDE 26
    ALUMINUM & MAGNESIUM
        ANTACIDS 28
    MAGNESIUM CARBONATE 494
    MAGNESIUM TRISILICATE 502
Gaysal—See
    ACETAMINOPHEN 4
    NARCOTIC ANALGESICS 594
Gaysal-S—See ACETAMINOPHEN &
    SALICYLATES 6
G.B.S.—See
    ATROPINE 70
    DEHYDROCHOLIC ACID 266
Gelcomul—See BELLADONNA 84

Gelusil—See
    ALUMINUM HYDROXIDE 26
    ALUMINUM, MAGNESIUM,
        MAGALDRATE & SIMETHICONE
        ANTACIDS 30
    MAGNESIUM HYDROXIDE 498
    MAGNESIUM TRISILICATE 502
    SIMETHICONE 806
Gelusil-M—See
    MAGNESIUM TRISILICATE 502
GEMFIBROZIL 392
Gemnisyn—See ACETAMINOPHEN &
    SALICYLATES 6
Gemonil—See METHARBITAL 538
Genapap—See ACETAMINOPHEN 4
Genebs—See ACETAMINOPHEN 4
Genetabs—See ACETAMINOPHEN 4
Geocillin—See CARBENICILLIN 143
Geopen—See CARBENICILLIN 143
Geriplex-FS—See
    DOCUSATE SODIUM 316
Geritol Tablets—See
    FERROUS SULFATE 374
GG-CEN—See GUAIFENESIN 404
Ginospan—See
    PHENYLEPHRINE 688
    CHLORPHENIRAMINE 190
Gitaligen—See DIGITALIS
    PREPARATIONS 288
GITALIN—See
    DIGITALIS PREPARATIONS 288
Glaucon—See EPINEPHRINE 328
Glibenclamide—See GLYBURIDE 396
GLIPIZIDE 394
Globin Insulin—See INSULIN 444
Glucamide—See
    CHLORPROPAMIDE 194
Glucotrol—See GLIPIZIDE 394
Glutofac—See
    MAGNESIUM SULFATE 500
    PYRIDOXINE (VITAMIN B-6) 760
GLYBURIDE 396
Glyceryl Gualacolate—See
    GUAIFENESIN 404
Glyceryl Trinitrate—See NITRATES 608
Glycery T—See
    THEOPHYLLINE & GUAIFENESIN 858
GLYCOPYRROLATE 398
Glycotuss—See GUAIFENESIN 404
Glycotuss-dM—See
    DEXTROMETHORPHAN 274
Glysennid—See SENNOSIDES A & B 804
Glytinic—See
    FERROUS GLUCONATE 372
Glytuss—See GUAIFENESIN 404
G-Mycin—See TETRACYCLINES 850
GOLD COMPOUNDS 400
Gold compounds—See
    GOLD COMPOUNDS 400
Gold Sodium Thiomalate—See GOLD
    COMPOUNDS 400
Gonad stimulant—See CLOMIPHENE 220
Gonadotropin inhibitor—See
    DANAZOL 258
Gonio-Gel—See
    METHYLCELLULOSE 552
Goody's Extra Strength Tablets—See
    ACETAMINOPHEN & SALICYLATES 6
Goody's Headache Powders—See
    ACETAMINOPHEN & SALICYLATES 6
Granulex—See CASTOR OIL 156
Gravol—See DIMENHYDRINATE 292
Grifulvin V—See GRISEOFULVIN 402
Grisactin Ultra—See GRISEOFULVIN 402
Grisactin—See GRISEOFULVIN 402
GRISEOFULVIN 402
Grisovin-FP—See GRISEOFULVIN 402
grisOwen—See GRISEOFULVIN 402
Gris-PEG—See GRISEOFULVIN 402
G-Sox—See SULFISOXAZOLE 830
Guaiaphed—See THEOPHYLLINE,
    EPHEDRINE, GUAIFENESIN &
        BARBITURATES 854
Guaifed—See PSEUDOEPHEDRINE 752
GUAIFENESIN 404

GUAIFENESIN, BARBITURATES,
    THEOPHYLLINE & EPHEDRINE 854
GUAIFENESIN & OXTRIPHYLLINE 634
GUAIFENESIN & THEOPHYLLINE 858
Gualahist—See
    GUAIFENESIN 404
    PHENYLEPHRINE 688
Gualahist TT—See
    CHLORPHENIRAMINE 190
Gualamine—See
    ACETAMINOPHEN 4
    CHLORPHENIRAMINE 190
Gualfed—See GUAIFENESIN 404
GUANABENZ 406
GUANADREL 408
GUANETHIDINE 410
GUANETHIDINE &
    HYDROCHLOROTHIAZIDE 412
Guiatuss D-M—See
    DEXTROMETHORPHAN 274
Guistrey Fortis—See
    CHLORPHENIRAMINE 190
Gulamid—See GUAIFENESIN 404
Gulatuss—See GUAIFENESIN 404
Gustalac—See CALCIUM
    CARBONATE 130
Gylanphen—See HYOSCYAMINE 436
Gylate—See GUAIFENESIN 404
Gynecort—See
    ADRENOCORTICOIDS (TOPICAL) 16
Gynergen—See ERGOTAMINE 334
Gynogen—See ESTRONE 352

## H

H2Oxyl—See BENZOYL PEROXIDE 90
H2 Cort—See
    ADRENOCORTICOIDS (TOPICAL) 16
H-H-R—See HYDRALAZINE 422
H-H-R—See
    HYDROCHLOROTHIAZIDE 426
H-H-R—See
    RAUWOLFIA ALKALOIDS 780
HALAZEPAM 414
Hal-Chlor—See
    CHLORPHENIRAMINE 190
Halciderm—See
    ADRENOCORTICOIDS (TOPICAL) 16
Halcion—See TRIAZOLAM 896
Haldol—See HALOPERIDOL 416
Haldol Decanoate—See
    HALOPERIDOL 416
Haldol LA—See HALOPERIDOL 416
Haldrone—See PARAMETHASONE 650
Halenol—See ACETAMINOPHEN 4
Halofed—See PSEUDOEPHEDRINE 752
Halog—See
    ADRENOCORTICOIDS (TOPICAL) 16
Halog E—See
    ADRENOCORTICOIDS (TOPICAL) 16
HALOPERIDOL 416
Halotestin—See ANDROGENS 54
Halotussin—See GUAIFENESIN 404
Haltran—See IBUPROFEN 438
Haponal—See
    ATROPINE 70
    HYOSCYAMINE 436
    SCOPOLAMINE (HYOSCINE) 798
Harmonyl—See
    RAUWOLFIA ALKALOIDS 780
Harmonyl-D—See
    RAUWOLFIA ALKALOIDS 780
Harvitrate—See ATROPINE 70
Hasacode—See
    ACETAMINOPHEN 4
    NARCOTIC ANALGESICS 594
HASP—See
    ATROPINE 70
    PHENOBARBITAL 678
HC-JEL—See
    ADRENOCORTICOIDS (TOPICAL) 16
Hedulin—See
    ANTICOAGULANTS (ORAL) 58
Help—See
    PHENYLPROPANOLAMINE 690

MAGNESIUM CITRATE 496
MAGNESIUM SULFATE 500
SODIUM PHOSPHATE 814
Laxative (stimulant)—See
  BISACODYL 104
  CASCARA 154
  CASTOR OIL 156
  DANTHRON 260
  DEHYDROCHOLIC ACID 266
  PHENOLPHTHALEIN 680
  SENNA 802
  SENNOSIDES A & B 804
Laxinate—See DOCUSATE SODIUM 316
Ledercillin VK—See PENICILLIN V 662
Ledercort—See TRIAMCINOLONE 890
Lederspan—See TRIAMCINOLONE 890
Lemidyne w/Codeine—See
  ASPIRIN 66
  CAFFEINE 128
Lemtrex—See TETRACYCLINES 850
Lentard—See INSULIN 444
Lente—See INSULIN 444
Lente Iletin I—See INSULIN 444
Lente Iletin II—See INSULIN 444
Lente Insulin—See INSULIN 444
Letter—See THYROXINE
  (T-4, LEVOTHYROXINE) 872
Leukeran—See CHLORAMBUCIL 172
Levamine—See
  ATROPINE 70
  BUTABARBITAL 120
  HYOSCYAMINE 436
  SCOPOLAMINE (HYOSCINE) 798
Levate—See TRICYCLIC
  ANTIDEPRESSANTS 900
LEVODOPA 480
LEVODOPA & CARBIDOPA 144
Levo-Dromoran—See NARCOTIC
  ANALGESICS 594
Levoid—See THYROXINE
  (T-4, LEVOTHYROXINE) 872
Levopa—See LEVODOPA 480
Levorphan—See NARCOTIC
  ANALGESICS 594
LEVORPHANOL—See NARCOTIC
  ANALGESICS 594
Levothroid—See
  THYROID 870
  THYROXINE
  (T-4, LEVOTHYROXINE) 872
LEVOTHYROXINE T-4, (THYROXINE) 872
Levsin—See HYOSCYAMINE 436
Levsin-PB—See BELLADONNA
  ALKALOIDS & BARBITURATES 86
Levsin PB—See PHENOBARBITAL 678
Levsin w/Phenobarbital—See
  BELLADONNA ALKALOIDS &
  BARBITURATES 86
  PHENOBARBITAL 678
Levsinex—See HYOSCYAMINE 436
Levsinex with Phenobarbital
  Timecaps—See BELLADONNA
  ALKALOIDS & BARBITURATES 86
Librax—See
  CHLORDIAZEPOXIDE &
  CLIDINIUM 180
  CLIDINIUM 214
Libritabs—See
  CHLORDIAZEPOXIDE 176
  CHLORDIAZEPOXIDE &
  CLIDINIUM 180
Librium—See CHLORDIAZEPOXIDE 176
Lida-Mantle—See
  ANESTHETICS (TOPICAL) 56
Lidemol—See
  ADRENOCORTICOIDS (TOPICAL) 16
Lidex—See
  ADRENOCORTICOIDS (TOPICAL) 16
Lidex-E—See
  ADRENOCORTICOIDS (TOPICAL) 16
Lidocaine—See
  ANESTHETICS (TOPICAL) 56
Lidocaine Ointment—See
  ANESTHETICS (TOPICAL) 56

Lidox—See CHLORDIAZEPOXIDE &
  CLIDINIUM 180
Lignocaine—See
  ANESTHETICS (TOPICAL) 56
Limbitrol—See CHLORDIAZEPOXIDE &
  AMITRIPTYLINE 178
Limbitrol DS—See CHLORDIAZEPOXIDE
  & AMITRIPTYLINE 178
Limit—See
  APPETITE SUPPRESSANTS 64
Limitite—See
  APPETITE SUPPRESSANTS 64
Lincocin—See LINCOMYCIN 482
LINCOMYCIN 482
Lioresal—See BACLOFEN 80
LIOTHYRONINE 484
LIOTRIX 486
Lipancreatin—See PANCRELIPASE 642
Lipo Gantrisin—See
  SULFISOXAZOLE 830
Lipoxide—See
  CHLORDIAZEPOXIDE 176
  CHLORDIAZEPOXIDE &
  CLIDINIUM 180
Liprinal—See CLOFIBRATE 218
Liquamar—See
  ANTICOAGULANTS (ORAL) 58
  PHENPROCOUMON 682
Liqui-Cee—See
  ASCORBIC ACID (VITAMIN C) 928
Liqui-Doss—See
  DOCUSATE SODIUM 316
Liquid-Pred—See PREDNISONE 724
Liquiprin—See ACETAMINOPHEN 4
Liquix-C—See
  ACETAMINOPHEN 4
  NARCOTIC ANALGESICS 594
Liquophylline—See XANTHINE
  BRONCHODILATORS 938
Lithane—See LITHIUM 488
LITHIUM 488
Lithizine—See LITHIUM 488
Lithobid—See LITHIUM 488
Lithonate—See LITHIUM 488
Lithostat—See
  ACETOHYDROXAMIC ACID (AHA) 10
Lithotabs—See LITHIUM 488
Lixaminol—See XANTHINE
  BRONCHODILATORS 938
Lixaminol AT—See
  DEXTROMETHORPHAN 274
  XANTHINE BRONCHODILATORS 938
Lixolin—See XANTHINE
  BRONCHODILATORS 938
Lobac—See CHLORZOXAZONE &
  ACETAMINOPHEN 202
Locacorten—See
  ADRENOCORTICOIDS (TOPICAL) 16
Locoid—See
  ADRENOCORTICOIDS (TOPICAL) 16
Lodrane—See XANTHINE
  BRONCHODILATORS 938
Loestrin—See
  CONTRACEPTIVES (ORAL) 236
  ETHINYL ESTRADIOL 360
Lofene—See
  DIPHENOXYLATE & ATROPINE 300
Lomanate—See
  DIPHENOXYLATE & ATROPINE 300
Lomine—See DICYCLOMINE 280
Lomotil—See DIPHENOXYLATE &
  ATROPINE 300
Loniten—See MINOXIDIL 576
Lonox—See
  DIPHENOXYLATE & ATROPINE 300
Lo-Ovral—See
  ETHINYL ESTRADIOL 360
  CONTRACEPTIVES (ORAL) 236
  NORGESTREL 618
LOPERAMIDE 490
Lopid—See GEMFIBROZIL 392
Lopressor—See METOPROLOL 570
Lopressor HCT—See
  BETA-ADRENERGIC BLOCKING
  AGENTS & THIAZIDE DIURETICS 96

Lopressor SR—See METOPROLOL 570
Lopurin—See ALLOPURINOL 20
Loraz—See LORAZEPAM 492
LORAZEPAM 492
Lorcet—See ACETAMINOPHEN 4
Lorelco—See PROBUCOL 732
Loroxide—See BENZOYL PEROXIDE 90
Lortab 5—See NARCOTIC &
  ACETAMINOPHEN 592
Lortab 7—See NARCOTIC &
  ACETAMINOPHEN 592
Lotrisone—See BETAMETHASONE 98
Lo-Trol—See DIPHENOXYLATE &
  ATROPINE 300
Lotusate—See
  TALBUTAL (BUTALBITAL) 838
Lo-Tussin—See NARCOTIC
  ANALGESICS 594
Low-Quel—See
  DIPHENOXYLATE & ATROPINE 300
Lowsium—See ALUMINUM &
  MAGNESIUM ANTACIDS 28
Lowsium—See
  ALUMINUM HYDROXIDE 26
Lozide—See INDAPAMIDE 440
Lozol—See INDAPAMIDE 440
L-PAM—See MELPHALAN 516
L-Thyroxine—See THYROXINE
  (T-4, LEVOTHYROXINE) 872
L-T-S—See THYROXINE
  (T-4, LEVOTHYROXINE) 872
Luasmin—See
  EPHEDRINE 326
  PHENOBARBITAL 678
  XANTHINE BRONCHODILATORS 938
Ludiomil—See MAPROTILINE 506
Luftodil—See
  GUAIFENESIN 404
  PHENOBARBITAL 678
  XANTHINE BRONCHODILATORS 938
Lufyllin—See
  GUAIFENESIN 404
  XANTHINE BRONCHODILATORS 938
Lufyllin-EPG—See
  EPHEDRINE 326
  PHENOBARBITAL 678
Luminal—See PHENOBARBITAL 678
Luride—See SODIUM FLUORIDE 812
Luride-SF—See SODIUM FLUORIDE 812
Lyderm—See
  ADRENOCORTICOIDS (TOPICAL) 16
Lyopine Vari-Dose—See ATROPINE 70
Lysodren—See MITOTANE 578
Lyteca—See ACETAMINOPHEN 4

M

Maalox—See
  ALUMINUM & MAGNESIUM
  ANTACIDS 28
  ALUMINUM HYDROXIDE 26
  MAGNESIUM HYDROXIDE 498
Maalox Plus—See ALUMINUM,
  MAGNESIUM, MAGALDRATE &
  SIMETHICONE ANTACIDS 30
Maalox TC—See ALUMINUM &
  MAGNESIUM ANTACIDS 28
Macrodantin—See
  NITROFURANTOIN 610
MAGALDRATE & SIMETHICONE—See
  ALUMINUM, MAGNESIUM,
  MAGALDRATE & SIMETHICONE
  ANTACIDS 30
MAGALDRATE, SIMETHICONE
  ANTACIDS, ALUMINUM &
  MAGNESIUM 30
Magan—See SALICYLATES 796
Magmalin—See
  ALUMINUM & MAGNESIUM
  ANTACIDS 28
  ALUMINUM HYDROXIDE 26
Magnagel—See
  ALUMINUM & MAGNESIUM
  ANTACIDS 28
  ALUMINUM HYDROXIDE 26

HYOSCYAMINE 436
SCOPOLAMINE (HYOSCINE) 798
*Spasticol*—See PHENOBARBITAL 678
*Spastoced*—See ALUMINUM
HYDROXIDE 26
*Spastolate*—See
ATROPINE 70
HYOSCYAMINE 436
SCOPOLAMINE (HYOSCINE) 798
*Spastosed*—See
ATROPINE 70
CALCIUM & MAGNESIUM
ANTACIDS 132
*Spectrobid*—See BACAMPICILLIN 78
*Spencort*—See
ADRENOCORTICOIDS (TOPICAL) 16
TRIAMCINOLONE 890
*Spinaxin*—See METHOCARBAMOL 544
SPIRONOLACTONE 816
SPIRONOLACTONE &
HYDROCHLOROTHIAZIDE 818
*Spironazide*—See
HYDROCHLOROTHIAZIDE 426
SPIRONOLACTONE 816
*Sprx-1*—See APPETITE
SUPPRESSANTS 64
*Sprx-3*—See APPETITE
SUPPRESSANTS 64
*Sprx-105*—See APPETITE
SUPPRESSANTS 64
*S-P-T*—See THYROID 870
*S-T Decongestant*—See
BROMPHENIRAMINE 110
PHENYLPROPANOLAMINE 690
*S-T Expectorant*—See GUAIFENESIN 404
*S-T Forte*—See
GUAIFENESIN 404
PHENIRAMINE 676
PHENYLEPHRINE 688
PHENYLPROPANOLAMINE 690
*St. Joseph*—See
ASPIRIN 66
DEXTROMETHORPHAN 274
*St. Joseph Aspirin Free*—See
ACETAMINOPHEN 4
*St. Joseph Aspirin for Children*—See
ASPIRIN 66
*St. Joseph Cough Syrup*—See
DEXTROMETHORPHAN 274
*St. Joseph Decongestant For
Children*—See OXYMETAZOLINE 636
*St. Joseph for Children*—See
DEXTROMETHORPHAN 274
*Stabinol*—See CHLORPROPAMIDE 194
*Stadol*—See NARCOTIC
ANALGESICS 594
*Stannitol*—See ATROPINE 70
*STANOZOLOL*—See ANDROGENS 54
*Staphcillin*—See METHICILLIN 542
*Statex*—See NARCOTIC
ANALGESICS 594
*Staticin*—See ERYTHROMYCINS 342
*Statobex*—See APPETITE
SUPPRESSANTS 64
*Statobex-G*—See APPETITE
SUPPRESSANTS 64
*Stay-Flo*—See SODIUM FLUORIDE 812
*Stelazine*—See TRIFLUOPERAZINE 904
*Stemetic*—See
TRIMETHOBENZAMIDE 912
*Stemetil*—See
PROCHLORPERAZINE 738
*Sterane*—See PREDNISOLONE 722
*Sterapred*—See PREDNISONE 724
*Sterazolidin*—See
ALUMINUM HYDROXIDE 26
MAGNESIUM TRISILICATE 502
PHENYLBUTAZONE 686
PREDNISONE 724
*Sterine*—See METHENAMINE 540
*Stero-Darvon*—See ASPIRIN 66
*Stie-Cort*—See ADRENOCORTICOIDS
(TOPICAL) 16
*StieVAA*—See TRETINOIN 888
*Stilbestrol*—See
DIETHYLSTILBESTROL 282

*Stilbilium*—See
DIETHYLSTILBESTROL 282
*Stilphostrol*—See
DIETHYLSTILBESTROL 282
ESTROGEN 350
Stimulant (xanthine)—See
CAFFEINE 128
ERGOTAMINE & CAFFEINE 338
ERGOTAMINE, CAFFEINE,
BELLADONNA &
PENTOBARBITAL 340
Stimulant—See ORPHENADRINE,
ASPIRIN & CAFFEINE 626
*Stimuzyme Plus*—See CASTOR OIL 156
*Stopayne*—See ACETAMINOPHEN 4
*Strascogesic*—See
ACETAMINOPHEN 4
NARCOTIC ANALGESICS 594
*Strema*—See QUININE 774
*Stress-Pam*—See DIAZEPAM 276
*Stuartinic*—See FERROUS
FUMARATE 370
*Studaflor*—See SODIUM FLUORIDE 812
*Stulex*—See DOCUSATE SODIUM 316
*Sub-Quin*—See PROCAINAMIDE 734
SUCRALFATE 820
*Sucrets*—See
DEXAMETHASONE 268
DEXTROMETHORPHAN 274
*Sudafed*—See PSEUDOEPHEDRINE 752
*Sudafed S.A.*—See
PSEUDOEPHEDRINE 752
*Sudagest*—See
PSEUDOEPHEDRINE 752
*Sudahist*—See PSEUDOEPHEDRINE 752
*Suda-Prol*—See
PSEUDOEPHEDRINE 752
*Sudolin*—See
PSEUDOEPHEDRINE 752
XANTHINE BRONCHODILATORS 938
*Sudoprin*—See ACETAMINOPHEN 4
*Sudrin*—See PSEUDOEPHEDRINE 752
*Sulcrato*—See SUCRALFATE 820
*Suldiazo*—See SULFONAMIDES &
PHENAZOPYRIDINE 832
Sulfa (sulfonamide)—See
ERYTHROMYCIN &
SULFISOXAZOLE 344
SULFACYTINE 822
SULFAMETHOXAZOLE 824
SULFASALAZINE 826
SULFISOXAZOLE 830
SULFACYTINE 822
*Sulfafurazole*—See SULFISOXAZOLE 830
*Sulfafurazole & Phenazopyridine*—See
SULFONAMIDES &
PHENAZOPYRIDINE 832
*Sulfagen*—See SULFISOXAZOLE 830
*Sulfamethoprim*—See
SULFAMETHOXAZOLE 824
SULFAMETHOXAZOLE 824
*SULFAMETHOXAZOLE &
PHENAZOPYRIDINE*—See
SULFONAMIDES &
PHENAZOPYRIDINE 832
SULFASALAZINE 826
SULFINPYRAZONE 828
SULFISOXAZOLE 830
SULFISOXAZOLE &
ERYTHROMYCIN 344
*SULFISOXAZOLE &
PHENAZOPYRIDINE*—See
SULFONAMIDES &
PHENAZOPYRIDINE 832
*Sulfizin*—See SULFISOXAZOLE 830
*Sulfizole*—See SULFISOXAZOLE 830
SULFONAMIDES &
PHENAZOPYRIDINE 832
Sulfone—See DAPSONE 264
Sulfonurea—See
ACETOHEXAMIDE 8
CHLORPROPAMIDE 194
GLIPIZIDE 394
GLYBURIDE 396

TOLAZAMIDE 880
TOLBUTAMIDE 882
SULINDAC 834
*Summit*—See ACETAMINOPHEN 4
*Sumox*—See AMOXICILLIN 48
*Sumycin*—See TETRACYCLINES 850
*Supac*—See
ACETAMINOPHEN 4
ACETAMINOPHEN & SALICYLATES 6
ASPIRIN 66
CAFFEINE 128
NARCOTIC ANALGESICS 594
*Supasa*—See ASPIRIN 66
*Supen*—See AMPICILLIN 52
*Super Anahist*—See
PHENYLEPHRINE 688
*Supeudol*—See NARCOTIC
ANALGESICS 594
*Suplical*—See
CALCIUM CARBONATE 130
CALCIUM SUPPLEMENTS 134
*Suppap*—See ACETAMINOPHEN 4
SUPPRESSANTS, APPETITE 64
*Suprazine*—See TRIFLUOPERAZINE 904
SUPROFEN 836
*Suprol*—See SUPROFEN 836
*Surfac*—See DOCUSATE
POTASSIUM 314
*Surfacaine*—See ANESTHETICS
(TOPICAL) 56
*Surfak*—See DOCUSATE CALCIUM 312
*Surmontil*—See TRICYCLIC
ANTIDEPRESSANTS 900
*Susadrin*—See NITRATES 608
*Susano*—See BELLADONNA ALKALOIDS
& BARBITURATES 86
*Sus-phrine*—See EPINEPHRINE 328
*Sust-A*—See VITAMIN A 924
*Sustaire*—See XANTHINE
BRONCHODILATORS 938
*Sustaverine*—See PAPAVERINE 646
*Swiss Kriss*—See SENNA 802
*Sylapar*—See
ACETAMINOPHEN 4
NARCOTIC ANALGESICS 594
*Syllact*—See PSYLLIUM 756
*Symetra*—See APPETITE
SUPPRESSANTS 64
*Symmetrel*—See AMANTADINE 34
Sympathomimetic—See
ALBUTEROL 18
EPHEDRINE 326
EPINEPHRINE 328
ISOPROTERENOL 458
ISOPROTERENOL &
PHENYLEPHRINE 460
METAPROTERENOL 530
METHYLPHENIDATE 560
OXYMETAZOLINE 636
PHENYLEPHRINE 688
PHENYLPROPANOLAMINE 690
PSEUDOEPHEDRINE 752
TERBUTALINE 842
THEOPHYLLINE, EPHEDRINE &
BARBITURATES 852
THEOPHYLLINE, EPHEDRINE,
GUAIFENESIN &
BARBITURATES 854
THEOPHYLLINE, EPHEDRINE &
HYDROXYZINE 856
Sympathomimetic (bronchodilator)—See
ISOETHARINE 450
*Symptom 3*—See
BROMPHENIRAMINE 110
*Symptrol*—See
PHENIRAMINE 676
SCOPOLAMINE (HYOSCINE) 798
*Symtrol*—See
PHENYLPROPANOLAMINE 690
*Synacort*—See ADRENOCORTICOIDS
(TOPICAL) 16
*Synalar*—See ADRENOCORTICOIDS
(TOPICAL) 16
*Synalgos*—See
ASPIRIN 66

**INDEX**

PHENIRAMINE 676
PHENYLPROPANOLAMINE 690
*Tussaminic*—See
DEXTROMETHORPHAN 274
PHENIRAMINE 676
PHENYLPROPANOLAMINE 690
*Tussanil*—See PYRILAMINE 762
*Tussar*—See
CHLORPHENIRAMINE 190
GUAIFENESIN 404
NARCOTIC ANALGESICS 594
*Tussar DM*—See PHENYLEPHRINE 688
*Tussend*—See
GUAIFENESIN 404
NARCOTIC ANALGESICS 594
PSEUDOEPHEDRINE 752
*Tussionex*—See
PHENYLTOLOXAMINE 692
*Tussi-Organidin*—See
CHLORPHENIRAMINE 190
NARCOTIC ANALGESICS 594
*Tussirex*—See PHENYLEPHRINE 688
*Tussirex Sugar-Free*—See
PHENIRAMINE 676
*Tuss-Ornade*—See
CHLORPHENIRAMINE 190
PHENYLPROPANOLAMINE 690
*Tusstat*—See DIPHENHYDRAMINE 296
*Twilite*—See DIPHENHYDRAMINE 296
*Twin-K*—See POTASSIUM
SUPPLEMENTS 714
*Twin K-Cl*—See POTASSIUM
SUPPLEMENTS 714
*Two-Dyne*—See
ACETAMINOPHEN 4
CAFFEINE 128
*Tylenol*—See ACETAMINOPHEN 4
*Tylenol Maximum Strength Sinus
Medicine*—See
PSEUDOEPHEDRINE 752
*Tylenol w/Codeine*—See
ACETAMINOPHEN 4
NARCOTIC ANALGESICS 594
NARCOTIC & ACETAMINOPHEN 592
*Tylox*—See
ACETAMINOPHEN 4
NARCOTIC & ACETAMINOPHEN 592
NARCOTIC ANALGESICS 594
*Tympagesic*—See PHENYLEPHRINE 688
*TYROPANOATE*—See GALLBLADDER
X-RAY TEST DRUGS 390
*Ty-Tabs*—See NARCOTIC &
ACETAMINOPHEN 592
*Ty-tabs*—See ACETAMINOPHEN 4

# U

*UAA*—See ATROPINE, HYOSCYAMINE,
METHENAMINE, METHYLENE BLUE,
PHENYLSALICYLATE & BENZOIC
ACID 72
*Ultabs*—See
BELLADONNA 84
HYOSCYAMINE 436
*Ultracef*—See CEFADROXIL 160
*Ultralente*—See INSULIN 444
*Ultralente Iletin I*—See INSULIN 444
*Ultramycin*—See TETRACYCLINES 850
*Ultratard*—See INSULIN 444
*Unguentine*—See ANESTHETICS
(TOPICAL) 56
*Unguentine Plus*—See ANESTHETICS
(TOPICAL) 56
*Unguentine Spray*—See ANESTHETICS
(TOPICAL) 56
*Unicelles*—See APPETITE
SUPPRESSANTS 64
*Unicort*—See
ADRENOCORTICOIDS (TOPICAL) 16
HYDROCORTISONE (CORTISOL) 428
*Unifast*—See APPETITE
SUPPRESSANTS 64
*Unigen*—See ESTRONE 352
*Unipen*—See NAFCILLIN 586
*Unipes*—See HYDRALAZINE 422

*Uniphyl*—See XANTHINE
BRONCHODILATORS 938
*Unipres*—See
HYDROCHLOROTHIAZIDE 426
RAUWOLFIA ALKALOIDS 780
RESERPINE, HYDRALAZINE &
HYDROCHLOROTHIAZIDE 786
*Uniserp*—See HYDRALAZINE 422
*Unisoil*—See CASTOR OIL 156
*Unisom Nighttime Sleep Aid*—See
DOXYLAMINE 318
*Unitral*—See ATROPINE 70
*Unitrol*—See
PHENYLPROPANOLAMINE 690
*Univol*—See
ALUMINUM & MAGNESIUM
ANTACIDS 28
MAGNESIUM HYDROXIDE 498
*Unproco*—See
DEXTROMETHORPHAN 274
*Uproco*—See GUAIFENESIN 404
*Uracel*—See SALICYLATES 796
*Uramine*—See ATROPINE,
HYOSCYAMINE, METHENAMINE,
METHYLENE BLUE,
PHENYLSALICYLATE & BENZOIC
ACID 72
*Urecholine*—See BETHANECHOL 100
*Urex*—See METHENAMINE 540
*U.R.I.*—See
CHLORPHENIRAMINE 190
PHENYLEPHRINE 688
PHENYLPROPANOLAMINE 690
*Uridon Modified*—See ATROPINE,
HYOSCYAMINE, METHENAMINE,
METHYLENE BLUE,
PHENYLSALICYLATE & BENZOIC
ACID 72
*Uridon*—See CHLORTHALIDONE 198
*Urilief*—See BELLADONNA 84
*Urimed*—See ATROPINE,
HYOSCYAMINE, METHENAMINE,
METHYLENE BLUE,
PHENYLSALICYLATE & BENZOIC
ACID 72
Urinary acidifier—See
POTASSIUM PHOSPHATES 710
POTASSIUM & SODIUM
PHOSPHATES 712
Urinary alkalizer—See CITRATES 210
Urinary anti-infective—See
CINOXACIN 208
METHENAMINE 540
*Urinary Antiseptic No. 2*—See ATROPINE,
HYOSCYAMINE, METHENAMINE,
METHYLENE BLUE,
PHENYLSALICYLATE & BENZOIC
ACID 72
Urinary tract analgesic—See ATROPINE,
HYOSCYAMINE, METHENAMINE,
METHYLENE BLUE,
PHENYLSALICYLATE & BENZOIC
ACID 72
*Urised*—See
ATROPINE 70
ATROPINE, HYOSCYAMINE,
METHENAMINE, METHYLENE BLUE,
PHENYLSALICYLATE & BENZOIC
ACID 72
BELLADONNA 84
HYOSCYAMINE 436
METHENAMINE 540
*Urisep*—See ATROPINE,
HYOSCYAMINE, METHENAMINE,
METHYLENE BLUE,
PHENYLSALICYLATE & BENZOIC
ACID 72
*Uriseptin*—See
ATROPINE 70
HYOSCYAMINE 436
SCOPOLAMINE (HYOSCINE) 798
*Urisoxin*—See SULFISOXAZOLE 830
*Urispas*—See FLAVOXATE 376
*Uritab*—See ATROPINE, HYOSCYAMINE,
METHENAMINE, METHYLENE BLUE,

PHENYLSALICYLATE & BENZOIC
ACID 72
*Urithol*—See ATROPINE,
HYOSCYAMINE, METHENAMINE,
METHYLENE BLUE,
PHENYLSALICYLATE & BENZOIC
ACID 72
*Uritin*—See ATROPINE, HYOSCYAMINE,
METHENAMINE, METHYLENE BLUE,
PHENYLSALICYLATE & BENZOIC
ACID 72
*Uritol*—See FUROSEMIDE 388
*Urobiotic*—See
PHENAZOPYRIDINE 674
TETRACYCLINES 850
*Uroblue*—See
ATROPINE, HYOSCYAMINE,
METHENAMINE, METHYLENE BLUE,
PHENYLSALICYLATE & BENZOIC
ACID 72
METHENAMINE 540
*Urocit-K*—See CITRATES 210
*Urogesic*—See
ATROPINE 70
HYOSCYAMINE 436
SCOPOLAMINE (HYOSCINE) 798
*Uro-KP-Neutral*—See POTASSIUM &
SODIUM PHOSPHATES 712
*Urolocaine*—See ANESTHETICS
(TOPICAL) 56
*Uro-Mag*—See ALUMINUM
HYDROXIDE 26
*Uromide*—See SALICYLATES 796
*Uro-phosphate*—See METHENAMINE 540
*Uroquid-Acid*—See METHENAMINE 540
*Urotoin*—See NITROFURANTOIN 610
*Uro-Ves*—See ATROPINE,
HYOSCYAMINE, METHENAMINE,
METHYLENE BLUE,
PHENYLSALICYLATE & BENZOIC
ACID 72
*Urozide*—See
HYDROCHLOROTHIAZIDE 426
*Ursinus*—See
PHENIRAMINE 676
PHENYLPROPANOLAMINE 690
*Uticillin VK*—See PENICILLIN V 662
*Uticort*—See
ADRENOCORTICOIDS (TOPICAL) 16
BETAMETHASONE 98
*Utimox*—See AMOXICILLIN 48
*U-Tract*—See
ATROPINE, HYOSCYAMINE,
METHENAMINE, METHYLENE BLUE,
PHENYLSALICYLATE & BENZOIC
ACID 72
BELLADONNA 84

# V

*Vacon*—See PHENYLEPHRINE 688
*Valadol*—See ACETAMINOPHEN 4
*Valdrene*—See DIPHENHYDRAMINE 296
*Valerate Betaderm*—See
BETAMETHASONE 98
*Valerate Novobetamet*—See
BETAMETHASONE 98
*Valertest*—See TESTOSTERONE &
ESTRADIOL 848
*Valisone*—See
ADRENOCORTICOIDS (TOPICAL) 16
BETAMETHASONE 98
*Valisone Scalp Lotion*—See
ADRENOCORTICOIDS (TOPICAL) 16
*Valium*—See DIAZEPAM 276
*Valorin*—See ACETAMINOPHEN 4
*Valpin-PB*—See PHENOBARBITAL 678
VALPROIC ACID (DIPROPYLACETIC
ACID) 920
*Valrelease*—See DIAZEPAM 276
*Vamate*—See HYDROXYZINE 434
*Vanatal*—See BELLADONNA ALKALOIDS
& BARBITURATES 86
*Vancenase Inhaler*—See
BECLOMETHASONE 82

INDEX

1025

# Z

Zantac—See RANITIDINE 778
Zapex—See OXAZEPAM 630
Zarontin—See ETHOSUXIMIDE 364
Zaroxolyn—See METOLAZONE 568
Zemarine—See
  ATROPINE 70
  HYOSCYAMINE 436
  SCOPOLAMINE (HYOSCINE) 798
Zenate—See
  CALCIUM CARBONATE 130
  FERROUS FUMARATE 370
Zendole—See INDOMETHACIN 442
Zephrex—See
  GUAIFENESIN 404
  PSEUDOEPHEDRINE 752
Zeroxin—See BENZOYL PEROXIDE 90
Zetran—See
  CHLORDIAZEPOXIDE 176
  CHLORDIAZEPOXIDE &
    CLIDINIUM 180
ZiPan—See PROMETHAZINE 746
Zide—See
  HYDROCHLOROTHIAZIDE 426
ZIDOVUDINE, Also Called AZT
  (AZIDOTHYMIDINE) 76
Zorprin—See ASPIRIN 66
Zovirax—See ACYCLOVIR (ORAL &
  TOPICAL) 14
Zovirax Ointment—See ACYCLOVIR
  (ORAL & TOPICAL) 14
Zoxaphen—See CHLORZOXAZONE &
  ACETAMINOPHEN 202
Zurinol—See ALLOPURINOL 20
Zyloprim—See ALLOPURINOL 20
Zyloric—See ALLOPURINOL 20
Zynol—See SULFINPYRAZONE 828

# NOTES

# EMERGENCY GUIDE FOR OVERDOSE VICTIMS

This section lists *basic* steps in recognizing and treating immediate effects of drug overdose.

Study the information before you need it. If possible, take a course in first aid and learn external cardiac massage and mouth-to-mouth breathing techniques, called *cardiopulmonary resuscitation* (CPR).

For quick reference, list emergency telephone numbers in the spaces provided on the inside front cover for fire department paramedics, ambulance, poison-control center and your doctor. These numbers, except for doctor, are usually listed on the inside cover of your telephone directory.

## *IF VICTIM IS UNCONSCIOUS, NOT BREATHING:*

1. Yell for help. Don't leave victim.

2. Begin mouth-to-mouth breathing immediately.

3. If there is no heartbeat, give external cardiac massage.

4. Have someone call 0 (operator) or 911 (emergency) for an ambulance or medical help.

5. Don't stop CPR until help arrives.

6. Don't try to make victim vomit.

7. If vomiting occurs, save vomit to take to emergency room for analysis.

8. Take medicine or empty bottles with you to emergency room.

## *IF VICTIM IS UNCONSCIOUS AND BREATHING:*

1. Dial 0 (operator) or 911 (emergency) for an ambulance or medical help.

2. If you can't get help immediately, take victim to the nearest emergency room.

3. Don't try to make victim vomit.

4. If vomiting occurs, save vomit to take to emergency room for analysis.

5. Watch victim carefully on the way to the emergency room. If heart or breathing stops, use cardiac massage and mouth-to-mouth breathing (CPR).

6. Take medicine or empty bottles with you to emergency room.